C0-AZW-441

The Growing Spine

Behrooz A. Akbarnia
Muharrem Yazici
George H. Thompson (Eds.)

The Growing Spine

Management of Spinal Disorders in Young Children

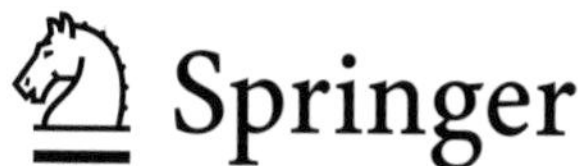

Behrooz A. Akbarnia, MD
Clinical Professor, Orthopaedic Surgery,
University of California, San Diego
Medical Director, San Diego Center for
Spinal Disorders
4130 La Jolla, Village Drive
La Jolla, CA 92037
USA
akbarnia@ucsd.edu

George H. Thompson, MD
Professor, Orthopaedic Surgery and Pediatrics
Director, Pediatric Orthopaedics
Rainbow Babies & Children's Hospital,
Case Western Reserve University
11000 Euclid Avenue
Cleveland, OH 44106-6003
USA
ght@po.cwru.edu

Muharrem Yazici, MD
Professor, Orthopaedic Surgery
Department of Orthopaedics &
Traumatology, Hacettepe University
06100 Sihhiye, Ankara
Turkey
yazioglu@hacettepe.edu.tr

With Editorial Assistance of:
Pooria Salari, MD
Sarah Canale, BS

ISBN: 978-3-540-85206-3 e-ISBN: 978-3-540-85207-0

DOI: 10.1007/978-3-540-85207-0

Springer Heidelberg Dordrecht London New York

Library of Congress Control Number: 2009933271

Cover design: eStudioCalamar, Figueres/Berlin

Printed on acid-free paper

Springer is part of Springer Science+Business Media (www.springer.com)

Dedication

The diverse nature of this textbook, the reasons for its existence, and the important people who made its completion possible warranted this dedication to be rendered in three parts. *First*, we dedicate this book to children with early onset spine deformity (EOS). This constitutes a group of challenging patients with varying natural histories. The text provides the first attempt to define these natural histories as well as patient treatment options and results in a unified approach; such efforts will hopefully lead to the development of more accurate and effective treatment protocols. It is well known that children with EOS have cardiopulmonary and gastrointestinal problems and also suffer from short stature and possibly from pain. One of our main goals in presenting current treatment methods is to enable decisions that will make these patients functional and productive adults with minimal residual deformities. This book will undoubtedly require numerous revisions as our knowledge advances and newer treatment concepts and techniques become available.

Secondly, we dedicate this book to the members of the Growing Spine Study Group (GSSG) and the faculty and participants of the International Congress on Early Onset Scoliosis and Growing Spine (ICEOS). These individuals have devoted a significant portion of their careers to the study of EOS. They have demonstrated a willingness to work cooperatively in furthering our understanding of the various disorders associated with EOS and to share this information with others. Their contributions and generosity of spirit are leading to the development of newer and better techniques for the correction of spinal deformity while simultaneously maintaining maximum growth and development of the spine and chest. Certainly, newer non-fusion approaches must be developed in the future, such as spinal tethers, self-expanding implants, and minimally invasive techniques, all of which aim to decrease the number of surgical procedures that these children must currently endure. This should result in better spinal alignment, fewer surgeries, fewer complications, and more normal growth.

Finally, we dedicate this work to our families. The creation of this textbook has taken a considerable amount of time away from our homes and loved ones. Nevertheless, our families have always recognized our dedication to others and our major goal of improving their lives. Our endeavor would not have been possible without their understanding and support. In particular, *Behrooz Akbarnia* would like to thank his wife, Nasrin Owsia, for her unyielding love and encouragement, his children (Halleh, Ladan, and Ramin), their spouses (Stu and Gil), and his grandchildren (Simia and Kian); as well as his associates Ramin Bagheri and Greg Mundis and support team at San Diego Center for Spinal Disorders, in particular Pat Kostial and Jeff Pawelek for allowing him to take as much time as needed to work on this book. *Muharrem Yazici* would like to thank his parents, Ayyildiz and Zekeriya, for having taught him that the greatest virtue in life lies in earning by producing; and Ruya, Yildiz Naz, and Mehmed Emir, for silently condoning his borrowing from their time, and for never depriving him of their support. Finally, *George Thompson* would especially like to thank his wife, Janice Thompson, for her support for the past 3–4 years, both during his Presidency of the Scoliosis Research Society and in the preparation of this textbook. There has been little time for family activities.

We hope that this book will be a foundation for future work in this exciting and developing field.

La Jolla, USA Behrooz A. Akbarnia, MD
Ankara, Turkey Muharrem Yazici, MD
Cleveland, USA George H. Thompson, MD

Foreword I

Spinal disorders, commonly encountered in the growing spine, are particularly prevalent among adolescents, who continue to receive the lion's share of attention and study. However, the spinal disorders present at birth or beginning in the first decade of life are the ones that most threaten a patient's quality and extent of life, and they are the focus of this timely and much-needed book.

While there are many diseases resulting in spinal disorders, the individual incidence of most is small; many have become known as orphan diseases. But, for most of the affected patients, the resulting spinal disorder is a lifetime condition, thus making the cumulative prevalence substantial. These factors conspire to limit the experience of even the largest centers. This and the fact that many of these young children often have comorbidities foster the need for collaboration among subspecialists.

A common denominator for almost all young children with spinal disorders is diminished spine growth. It is now realized that for many of them there is also diminished thoracic growth. The problem is compounded as the diminished growth is usually asymmetrical, resulting in not only a shortened spine and diminished thorax but also angular deformity. To quantify the abnormal, one must know what is normal; this topic is thoroughly documented in *Growing Spine*.

Management of spinal disorders in young children may be as simple as periodic observation or as complex as the outer limits of surgical art and science. The choice hinges on the natural history of the disorder. Long-term observational studies, including critical imaging interpretation, have added greatly to natural history knowledge. Advances in imaging techniques have made it possible to more clearly define the anatomical abnormalities and plan the appropriate corrective surgery.

Management of spinal disorders in young children often requires surgery. Traction, bracing, and/or casting are sometimes utilized to help decrease or at least control spinal deformity until as much spine growth as is reasonably possible has been achieved, thus delaying surgical treatment. As is described in this book, bracing and/or casting are occasionally the successful, definitive treatment for disorders with relatively favorable natural histories.

Surgical goals are to correct as much as possible the existing deformity, optimize normal growth, prevent abnormal growth, maintain maximum mobility, and protect neurological function. The essential tools of surgery are instrumentation and arthrodesis, and generally two approaches have been taken.

In one, posterior distraction instrumentation without arthrodesis was used with the hope that as the straighter spine grew; it would continue to grow straighter. When this did not occur, the process was modified to include planned, periodic re-operation to reapply distraction load. As the distraction rod-spine construct was not intrinsically stable, supplemental external immobilization with a brace or cast became necessary. Because the distraction hooks often became dislodged, arthrodesis of the upper and lower end two vertebrae was added. After as much lengthening as could be achieved was obtained, the posterior spinal arthrodesis of the spanned vertebrae was performed.

In the other approach, arthrodesis of the convex side of the scoliosis curve was performed, thereby encouraging concave side growth to catch up. The result was not satisfactory. Eventually, concave distraction instrumentation was added to the convex apex convex arthrodesis with somewhat better results.

The next step in the development of the posterior instrumentation approach was propelled by the desire to avoid supplemental brace or cast immobilization and periodic lengthening. Segmental posterior instrumentation utilizing multiple level sublaminar wire anchors and two parallel rods was introduced. This proved unsatisfactory because of auto-arthrodesis and instrumentation breakage.

This was followed by a return to the limited vertebrae anchor approach. Initially, stable end instrumented vertebrae anchor foundations (initially four hooks, transversely connected dual rods, and expandable connectors at the thoracolumbar junction) were used. Periodic lengthening at approximately 6-month intervals is done until further lengthening is no longer possible, at which point definitive arthrodesis is done. Currently, with some modifications, this is probably the most widely used approach. Two related developments are now occurring. The first is experimentation with periodic lengthening utilizing external magnetic power. The second development shifts focus from the end vertebrae to the apex vertebrae. Bilateral apex and end vertebrae pedicle screw anchorage is utilized to provide three-dimensional apex correction, and apex arthrodesis is performed. Spine growth on either side of the apex is then guided by end vertebrae pedicle screw anchors whose connections are free to slide along the rods.

The last several years have brought a number of innovations. The most thoroughly researched and widely used are the techniques and instrumentation utilized with thoracic expansion. Growth modulation through fixation of the convex apex vertebrae continues to be researched as does the possibility of stopping growth of the concave neurocentral synchondrosis.

An important part of the development of this field has been the improved surgical capability of mobilizing the spine. This includes kyphectomy, hemivertebrectomy, vertebral osteotomy, and vertebral resection. The possibility of safely performing these important but invasive procedures has been aided by continued improvement in anesthesia, neurological monitoring, and postoperative care.

Finally, molecular biology has not as yet impacted this field. However, it is not unreasonable to think that the underlying diseases' abnormal metabolic pathways will gradually begin to be understood, raising the possibility of preventative medical therapies.

The compilation of the rapid advances in knowledge about the management of spinal disorders in young children during the past several years has been badly needed. Without it progress is difficult to achieve. The editors and authors of *Growing Spine: Management of Spinal Disorders in Young Children* are at the forefront of this field and are to be congratulated for consolidating the diffuse knowledge base into one easily accessible tome.

Marc A. Asher, MD
Professor Emeritus
Kansas University Medical Center
Kansas City, KS, USA

Foreword II

Behrooz Akbarnia, MD, Muharrem Yazici, MD, and George Thompson, MD have all put together a wonderful book regarding aspects of management of the pediatric spine. There are 50 chapters in this textbook. There is a very substantial international flavor as well. To my count, portions of 18 chapters were written by deformity experts outside North America.

The textbook is very complete as it covers aspects of infantile, juvenile, and adolescent deformity and also covers operative and nonoperative management and not only deformity, but also issues of infection, tumor, trauma, and back pain.

Several chapters in this book should be considered classic and probably represent the definitive work by the definitive expert in a particular topic.

Chapter 2, regarding normal growth of the spine and thorax, by Dr. Alan Dimeglio from Montpellier, France, is the most concise and up-to-date manuscript covering this topic, which is perhaps the most important topic to understand if one is to treat complex pediatric spine problems.

Chapter 15, regarding spinal manifestations of the skeletal dysplasias, by Dr. Michael Ain, is certainly the most definitive source of recommendations and suggestions for treatment of complex skeletal dysplasia problems in the pediatric population.

Likewise, Chap. 16, regarding Marfan, Ehlers-Danlos, and other rare syndromes, by Dr. Paul Sponseller, is a very definitive work that is not available in other sources.

Chapter 23, regarding neurofibromatosis, by Dr. Alvin Crawford, is the most complete work regarding treatment of this disorder in the pediatric population that I have seen. Dr. Crawford and Dr. Akbarnia are considered the international experts on neurofibromatosis.

Dr. Johnston and his institution, The Texas Scottish Rite Hospital in Dallas, have the world's experience with utilizing traction for spinal deformities and there is a wealth of extraordinarily useful information included. Also, Dr. Suzuki's career of experience on fusion in the growing child is extremely valuable and apparent in Chap. 29.

The works by Dr. George Thompson and Dr. Behrooz Akbarnia, Chaps. 35 and 36, regarding single growing rod and dual growing rod fusionless techniques, are likewise extremely up-to-date and definitive. Drs. Thompson and Akbarnia, of course, are the international experts on utilizing techniques of "growing rods." There is an extensive amount of useful information and data in those chapters.

Chapter 37, regarding thoracic expansion, by Dr. Robert Campbell, Jr., should be read carefully as well. Dr. Campbell is the world expert on this topic and the information contained in this chapter is unparalleled.

All chapters in this textbook are written by experts in the field, are very informative, and are well referenced. The chapters represent a nice blend of basic factual data, the author's extensive experience, and a bit of innovation. All chapters are excellent. The chapters I mentioned are those that stand above the rest and are, to my mind, the go-to source for any student of complex pediatric spine disease. I look forward to seeing this textbook in print.

The three editors have done a wonderful job. Thank you for allowing me to write this foreword. It is an honor and a pleasure.

Keith Bridwell, MD
Washington University in St. Louis
One Barnes Jewish Hospital Plaza
Suite 11300, West Pavilion
Campus Box 8233
St. Louis, MO 63110
USA

Foreword III

A foreword in a textbook is customarily written as an explanation of why the authors are adding yet another text to the already crowded world of medical publishing. Although the pediatric spine is well represented in both spine and pediatric Orthopaedics textbooks, neither of these can provide the in-depth presentation of a text solely devoted to the subject. It has been 25 years since *The Pediatric Spine* by Bradford and Hensinger, and 15 years since *Disorders of the Pediatric Spine* by Pang. Much has been learned during those many years.

As I looked at the Contents of this book, two things struck me: the thorough and excellent coverage of the topic, and the truly unique and international scope of those chosen to lend their expertise. In all, ten different countries are represented with 47 total authors.

Basic science is well represented, along with the latest proven and as yet unproven techniques of treatment. Since we have to wait until the end of growth to really know whether our efforts are truly effective, we must be patient and willing to monitor various landmarks of progress over time. These landmarks are coronal curve control, sagittal curve control, torso length, and vital capacity.

Those who read this book will know that they possess the latest knowledge in this unique field.

Robert B. Winter, MD
Research Consultant
Twin Cities Spine Center
Clinical Professor
Department of Orthopaedic Surgery
University of Minnesota

Preface

Early onset scoliosis (EOS) is a major topic in pediatric spine deformity today. These challenging deformities occur in almost all differential diagnostic categories. Unfortunately, each diagnosis has a different natural history, making it even more demanding. This is the first textbook on this topic. It is a compilation of the current concepts of evaluation and treatment of the various deformities of the growing spine. We have tried to explore the normal growth of the spine and other associated organs as well as natural history of the various differential diagnostic categories and possible treatment options. It is anticipated that this textbook will need to be updated every two to three years in the future as concepts and treatment guidelines change. Treating the spinal deformity is not the major issue, but controlling the deformity to allow for growth of the spine and the associated organ systems, such as pulmonary, cardiac, and gastrointestinal, is the major goal. Controlling deformity allows for improved spinal growth of the involved child and the controlling associated development of these organ systems. A short trunk has an adverse effect on these organ systems. As a consequence, EOS requires a multidisciplinary care. It involves genetics, pediatrics, pulmonology, cardiology, neurology, neurosurgery, as well as orthopaedic surgery.

Treatment options for very young children are controversial. Bracing, serial Risser casts, and surgery (growth modulation and the use of distraction based or growth-guided techniques such as growing rods) are explored in this textbook.

Preliminary treatment results have demonstrated that growth friendly surgical techniques are effective in controlling or modulating curve progression and allowing for spinal growth. Spinal growth allows for improved capacity of the thoracic and abdominal cavities. Cosmesis is less than ideal as crankshaft remains a significant problem even in the growing rod systems. Surgical treatment complications are high, particularly, infection and implant failure, especially rod breakage. Management of complications is an important aspect of the treatment of EOS. Because of the high complication rate, it is important to make the right decision regarding patient and family selection. They must be cooperative and understanding and be willing to be cooperative during the postoperative period.

Future research is important. The Growing Spine Study Group (GSSG) and other databases will hopefully guide future investigations. Only by defining the results of treatment in a relatively large volume of children over a long period of time can the true effectiveness of each of these techniques be determined. Predicting who will worsen, improving spinal tethers to control progressive deformities and the development of self-expanding or remotely controlled devices that would obviate the need for repeated surgical procedures.

We thank our contributors who are all specialists and experts in a variety of areas involved with early onset scoliosis. We also acknowledge the contribution of the members of Growing Spine Study Group who have continuously provided the information that is the basis for a significant portion of the data presented in this book. Special thanks for assistance in preparing and organizing this textbook are to Sarah Canale and Pooia Salari, without their assistance, the completion of this project would have been very difficult.

La Jolla, USA
Ankara, Turkey
Cleveland, USA

Behrooz A. Akbarnia, MD
Muharrem Yazici, MD
George H. Thompson, MD

Contents

Contributors

R. Emre Acaroglu Ankara Spine Center, Iran Caddesi 45/2, Kavaklidere, Ankara 06700, Turkey
acaroglue@gmail.com

Jaimo Ahn Department of Orthopaedic Surgery, University of Pennsylvania, 2 Silverstein, 3400 Spruce Street, Philadelphia, PA 19104, USA
jaimo.ahn@uphs.upenn.edu

Michael C. Ain Department of Orthopaedic Surgery, Johns Hopkins Bayview Medical Center, The Johns Hopkins University, 4940 Eastern Avenue, A665, Baltimore, MD 21224-2780, USA
ehenze1@jhmi.edu

Nejat Akalan Department of Neurosurgery, Institute of Neurological Sciences, Hacettepe University, 06100 Ankara, Turkey
nakalan@hacettepe.edu.tr

Behrooz A. Akbarnia Department of Orthopaedics, University of California, San Diego and San Diego Center for Spinal Disorders 4130 La Jolla Village Drive, Suite 300, La Jolla, CA 92037, USA
akbarnia@ucsd.edu

İbrahim Akel Kent Hospital, Cigli 35580 Izmir, Turkey
akel02@yahoo.com

Ahmet Alanay Istanbul Spine Center, Florence Nightingale Hospital, Sisli, Istanbul, 34403 Turkey
aalanay@gmail.com

Phyllis D'Ambra Children's Hospital Los Angeles, 4650 Sunset Blvd, Mailstop 69, Los Angeles, CA 90027, USA
pdambra@chla.usc.edu

Kerry Armet Shriners Hospitals for Children, 1645 West 8th Street, Erie, PA 16505, USA
karmet@shrinenet.org

Jahangir Asghar Shriners Hospitals for Children, 3551 North Broad Street, Philadelphia, PA 19140, USA
jasghar@shrinenet.org

Ramin Bagheri San Diego Center for Spinal Disorders, 4130 La Jolla Village Drive, Suite 300, La Jolla, CA 92037, USA
rbagherimd@yahoo.com

Shay Bess Rocky Mountain Hospital for Children, 1721 East 19th Avenue, Denver, CO 80218, USA
shay_bess@hotmail.com

Randal R. Betz Shriners Hospitals for Children, 3551 North Broad Street, Philadelphia, PA 19140, USA
rbetz@shrinenet.org

Oheneba Boachie-Adjei The Scoliosis Service, Hospital for Special Surgery, New York, NY 10021, USA
boachie@hss.edu

Gérard Bollini Hôpital Timone Enfants, 264 Rue Saint Pierre, 13385 Marseille Cedex 5, France
gerard.bollini@ap-hm.fr

François Bonnel 2 rue de la Faculté de Médecine, 34 000 Montpellier, France
profbonnel@Free.Fr

Susan Bukata Shriners Hospitals for Children, 1645 West 8th Street, Erie, PA 16505, USA
susan_bukata@urmc.rochester.edu

Danielle B. Cameron The Children's Hospital of Philadelphia, Division of Orthopaedic Surgery, 2nd Floor, Wood Center, 34th Street and Civic Center Blvd., Philadelphia, PA 19104, USA
cameron.danielle@gmail.com

Robert M. Campbell The Children's Hospital of Philadelphia, Division of Orthopaedic Surgery, 2nd Floor, Wood Center, 34th Street and Civic Center Blvd., PA 19104, USA
campbellrm@email.chop.edu

Federico Canavese Chu Lapeyronie, 371 Avenue Doyen Gaston Giraud, 34264 Montpellier Cedex 5, France
canavese_federico@yahoo.fr

Kenneth M.C. Cheung Department of Orthopaedics and Traumatology, 5F Professorial Block, Queen Mary Hospital, 102 Pokfulam Road, Hong Kong, SAR, China
ken-cheung@hku.hk

Alvin H. Crawford Cincinnati Children's Hospital, 3333 Burnet Avenue, MLC 2017, Cincinnati, OH 45229, USA
alvin.crawford@cchmc.org

Matthew E. Cunningham Hospital for Special Surgery, New York, NY 10510, USA
cunninghamM@hss.edu

Ozgur Dede Department of Orthopaedics and Traumatology, Hacettepe University, 06100 Sihhiye, Ankara, Turkey
ozgrdd@hacettepe.edu.tr

Gokhan Demirkiran Ankara Spine Center, Iran Caddesi 45/2, Kavaklidere, 06700 Ankara, Turkey
gokhan@ankaraomurga.com

Alain Dimeglio Service de Chirurgie Orthopédique Pédiatrique, Chu Lapeyronie, 371 Avenue Doyen Gaston Giraud, 34264 Montpellier, Cedex 5, France
a-dimeglio@chu-montpellier.fr

Pierre-Louis Docquier Department of Orthopaedic Surgery, Saint-Luc Hospital, Catholic University of Louvain, Avenue Hippocrate 10, 1200 Brussels, Belgium
pierre-louis.docquier@clin.ucl.ac.be

John P. Dormans Department of Orthopaedic Surgery, Children's Hospital of Philadelphia, University of Pennsylvania, Philadelphia, PA 19104–4399, USA
dormans@email.chop.edu

Jean Dubousset Saint Vincent de Paul Hospital, 26 rue des Cordelières, Paris 75013, France
jean.dubousset@wanadoo.fr

Hazem B. Elsebaie Department of Orthopaedics, Cairo University, 22 Degla Street, Mohandessin Giza, PO. Box 12411, Egypt
hazembelsebaie@yahoo.com

John B. Emans Department of Orthopaedic Surgery, Children's Hospital, Boston, MA 02115, USA
john.emans@childrens.harvard.edu

John M. Flynn The Children's Hospital of Philadelphia, Division of Orthopaedic Surgery, 2nd Floor, Wood Center, 34th Street and Civic Center Blvd., Philadelphia, PA 19104, USA
flynnj@email.chop.edu

Ivan Florentino-Pineda Department of Anesthesiology, Children's Medical Center, 1446 Harper Street, BT-2651, Augusta, GA 30912-2700, USA
iflorentino@mail.mcg.edu

Tamás Fülöp Fekete Spine Unit, Schulthess Clinic, Lengghalde 2, 8008 Zürich, Switzerland
amas.fekete@kws.ch

Yann Glard Hôpital Timone Enfants, 264 Rue Saint Pierre, 13385 Marseille Cedex 5, France
yann.glard@ap-hm.fr

Daniel W.H. Ho Department of Biochemistry, L6-01, Laboratory Block, The University of Hong Kong, 21 Sassoon Road, Pokfulam, Hong Kong, SAR, China
dwhho@hku.hk

Neel Jain Children's Memorial Hospital, 2300 Children's Plaza, Chicago, IL 60614, USA
neel-jain@md.northwestern.edu

Viral V. Jain Cincinnati Children's Hospital, 3333 Burnet Avenue, MLC 2017, Cincinnati, OH 45069, USA
viral.jain@cchmc.org

Dezsö Jeszenszky Spine Unit, Schulthess Clinic, Lengghalde 2, 8008 Zürich, Switzerland
dezsoe.jeszenszky@kws.ch

Charles E. Johnston II Texas Scottish Rite Hospital, 2222 Welborn Street, Dallas, TX 75219–3924, USA
charles.johnston@tsrh.org

Jean-Luc Jouve Hôpital Timone Enfants, 264 Rue Saint Pierre, 13385 Marseille Cedex 5, France
jean-luc.jouve@ap-hm.fr

Lawrence I. Karlin Department of Orthopaedic Surgery, Children's Hospital Medical Center, 300 Longwood Avenue, Boston, MA 02115, USA
lawrence.karlin@childrens.harvard.edu

Patricia N. Kostial San Diego Center for Spinal Disorders, 4130 La Jolla Village Drive, Suite 300, La Jolla, CA 92037, USA
pkostial@sandiego-spine.com

Franck Launay Hôpital Timone Enfants, 264 Rue Saint Pierre, 13385 Marseille Cedex, France
franck.launay@ap-hm.fr

Lawrence G. Lenke Washington University School of Medicine, 660 South Euclid Avenue, Campus Box 8233, St. Louis, MO 63110, USA
lenkel@wudosis.wustl.edu

Andrew T. Mahar Department of Orthopaedic Surgery, University of California San Diego, San Diego, CA 92103, USA
andrew.mahar@gmail.com

Richard E. McCarthy University of Arkansas for Medical Sciences, Arkansas Children's Hospital, 800 Marshal, Little Rock, AR 72202, USA
rmccarthy@uams.com

Lotfi Miladi Saint Vincent de Paul Hospital, 82 Avenue Denfert Rochereau, 75014 Paris, France
l.miladi@svp.aphp.fr

Gregory M. Mundis San Diego Center for Spinal Disorders, 4130 La Jolla Village Drive, Suite 300, La Jolla, CA 92037, USA
gmundis1@gmail.com

Peter O. Newton University of California San Diego,
Rady Children's Hospital and Health Center, 3030 Children's Way,
Suite 410, San Diego, CA 92123, USA
pnewton@rchsd.org

James W. Ogilvie Shriners Hospital for Children, 3182 Silver Fork Brighton,
Salt Lake City, Utah 84121, USA
jwogilvie@msn.com

Acke Ohlin Department of Orthopaedic Surgery, Malmö University Hospital,
Lund University, 205 02 Malmö, Sweden
acke.ohlin@med.lu.se

Jeff Pawelek San Diego Center for Spinal Disorders, 4130 La Jolla Village Drive,
Suite 300, La Jolla, CA 92037, USA
jpawelek@sandiego-spine.com

Francisco S. Pérez-Grueso Hospital La Paz, Pedro Rico, 31 8 G 28029,
Madrid, Spain
pérezgrueso@terro.es

Connie Poe-Kochert Division of Pediatric Orthopaedic Surgery,
Rainbow Babies and Children's Hospital, 11100 Euclid Avenue,
Cleveland, OH 44106, USA
connie.poe-kochert@uhhospitals.org

Mikko Poussa ORTON Orthopaedic Hospital,
Tenholantie 10, 00280 Helsinki, Finland
mikko.poussa@pp.inet.fi

Gregory J. Redding Pulmonary Division, Seattle Children's Hospital, University
of Washington, Seattle, WA, USA
gredding@u.washington.edu

Pooria Salari San Diego Center for Spinal Disorders, 4130 La Jolla
Village Drive, Suite 300, La Jolla, CA 92037, USA
psalari@sandiego-spine.com

Amer F. Samdani Shriners Hospitals for Children, 3551 North Broad Street,
Philadelphia, PA 19140, USA
asamdani@shrinenet.org

James O. Sanders Department of Orthopaedics and Rehabilitation,
University of Rochester, 601 Elmwood Avenue, Rochester, NY 14642, USA
james_sanders@urmc.rochester.edu

John F. Sarwark Department of Orthopaedic Surgery,
The Children's Memorial Hospital, 2300 Children's Plaza,
Chicago, IL 60614, USA
jsarwark@childrensmemorial.org

Dietrich K.A. Schlenzka ORTON Orthopaedic Hospital, Invalid Foundation,
Tenholantie 10, 00280 Helsinki, Finland
dschlenzka@aospine.org

Daniel M. Schwartz Surgical Monitoring Associates, 900 Old Marple Road, Springfield, PA, 19064, USA
dan@surgmon.com

Anthony K. Sestokas Surgical Monitoring Associates, 900 Old Marple Road, Springfield, PA 19064, USA
tonys@surgmon.com

Ritesh R. Shah Children's Memorial Hospital, 2300 Children's Plaza, Chicago, IL 60614, USA
ritesh-shah@md.northwestern.edu

Suken A. Shah Department of Orthopaedics, Alfred I. duPont Hospital for Children, 1600 Rockland Road, PO Box 269, Wilmington, DE 19899, USA
sshah@nemours.org

Eric D. Shirley Naval Medical Center Portsmouth, 620 John Paul Jones Circle, Portsmouth, VA 23708, USA
eric.shirley@med.navy.mil

David L. Skaggs Childrens Hospital Los Angeles, University of Southern California School of Medicine, 4650 Sunset Boulevard, #69 Los Angeles, CA 90027, USA
dskaggs@chla.usc.edu

John T. Smith University of Utah, Department of Orthopaedics, Primary Childrens Medical Center, 100 North Mario Capecchi Drive, Suite 4550, Salt Lake City, UT 84113, USA
john.smith@hsc.utah.edu

You-Qiang Song The University of Hong Kong, Room L3-75, Biochemistry, Li Ka Shing Faculty of Medicine, Hong Kong, SAR, China
songy@hku.hk

Jochen P. Son-Hing Rainbow Babies and Children's Hospital, University Hospitals Case Medical Center, 11100 Euclid Avenue, Cleveland, OH 44106-5043, USA
jochen.son-hing@uhhospitals.org

Paul D. Sponseller Johns Hopkins Medical Institution, 601 N. Caroline Street, Baltimore, MD 21287-0882, USA
psponse@jhmi.edu

Nobumasa Suzuki Saiseikai Central Hospital, Scoliosis Center, 1-4-17 Mita, Minato-ku, Tokyo,108-0073, Japan
nobumasa@po.jah.ne.jp

George H. Thompson Division of Pediatric Orthopaedic Surgery, Rainbow Babies and Children's Hospital, University Hospitals Case Medical Center, 11100 Euclid Avenue, Cleveland, Ohio 44106, USA
ght@po.cwru.edu

Ejovi Ughwanogho Department of Orthopaedic Surgery, University of Pennsylvania, 2 Silverstein, 3400 Spruce Street, Philadelphia, PA 19104, USA
ejovi.ughwanogho@uphs.upenn.edu

Vidyadhar V. Upasani Rady Children's Hospital and Health Center, 3020 Children's Way, MC5054, San Diego, CA 92123, USA
vupasani@rchsd.org

Koki Uno National Hospital Organization, Kobe Medical Center, 3-1-1 Nishiochiai Sumaku, Kobe, Japan 654-0155
uno@kobemc.go.jp

Vikas V. Varma Manhattan Orthopaedic and Sports Medicine Group, 1065 Park Avenue, New York, NY 10128, USA
vvarm001@umaryland.edu

Elke Viehweger Hôpital Timone Enfants, 264 Rue Saint Pierre, 13385 Marseille Cedex 5, France
elke.viehweger@efort.org

Michael G. Vitale MS Children's Hospital of New York, 3959 Broadway, 8 North, New York, NY 10032, USA
mgv1@columbia.edu

Kota Watanabe Department of Orthopaedic Surgery, School of Medicine, Keio University, 35 Shinanomati, Shinjuku-ku, Tokyo 160-8582, Japan
kw197251@sc.itc.keio.ac.jp

James Wright Hospital for Sick Children, 555 University Avenue, Room 1254, Toronto, ON M5G 1X8, Canada
jgwright@sickkids.on.ca

Justin Yang Johns Hopkins Medical Institution, 601 North Caroline Street, Baltimore, MD 21287-0882, USA
justiny@jhmi.edu

Burt Yaszay Pediatric Orthopaedics and Scoliosis Center, Rady Children's Hospital, San Diego, 3030 Children's Way, Suite 410, San Diego, CA 92131, USA
byaszay@rchsd.org

Muharrem Yazici Department of Orthopaedics and Traumatology, Hacettepe University, Faculty of Medicine, 06100 Sihhiye, Ankara, Turkey
yazioglu@hacettepe.edu.tr

Guney Yilmaz Department of Orthopaedics, Alfred I. duPont Hospital for Children, 1600 Rockland Road, PO Box 269, Wilmington, DE 19899, USA
aflguney@gmail.com

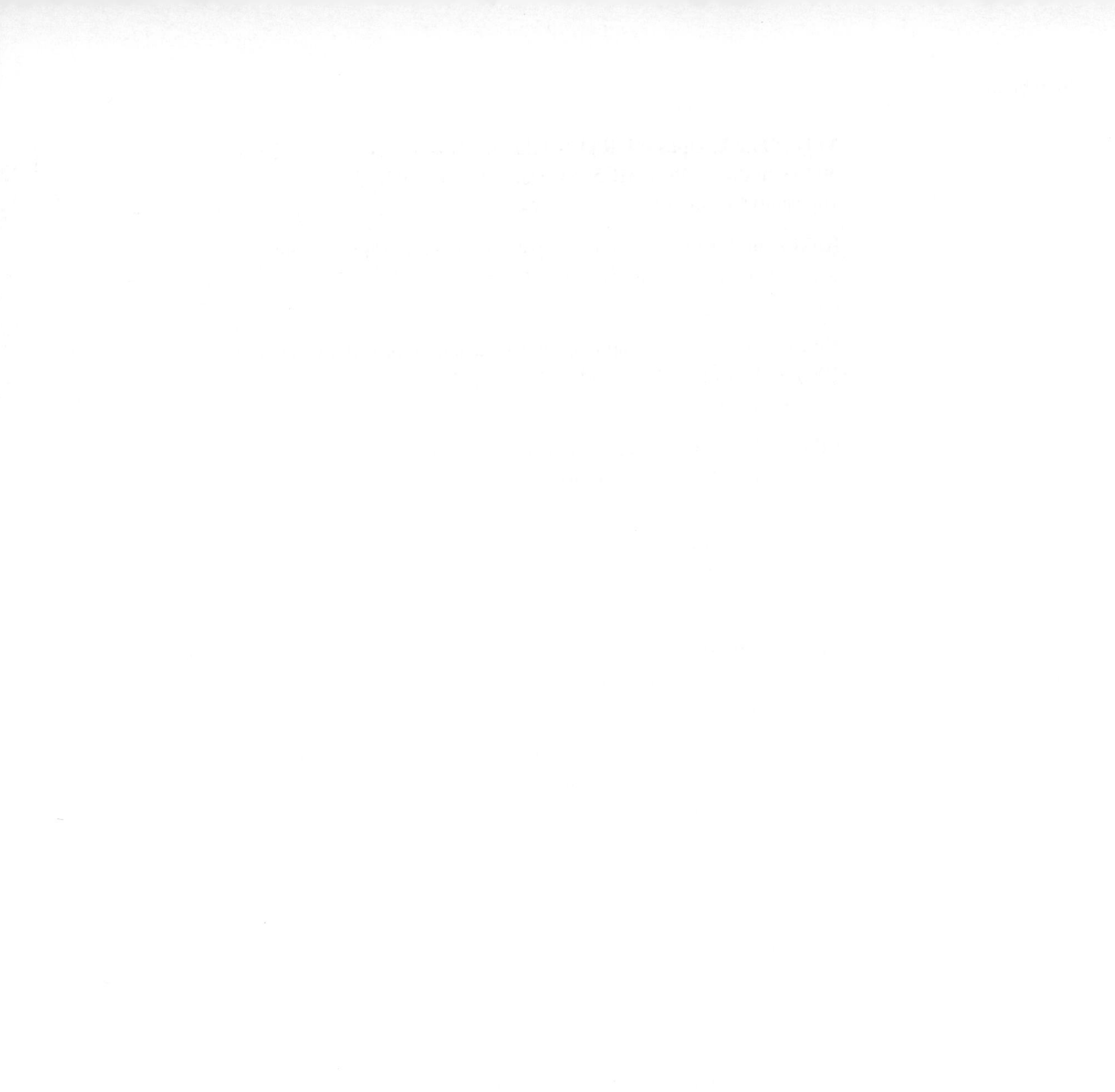

Section I

General

1 Embryology and Anatomy: Spine/Spinal Cord

Shay Bess and Vikas Varma

Key Points

- Development of the spine and spinal cord begins during the third week of gestation.
- Early development includes formation of primitive neural tissue, notochord development, and of the axes of the embryo. The axial skeleton eventually arises from the somites.
- Normal vertebral and neural formation is dependent upon development of these early structures to induce the adjacent cell lines to form the neural arch and distinct vertebral bodies.
- Errors in the formation of these structures lead to induction failure and subsequent spinal dysraphism and congenital scoliosis. Mesodermal vertebrae eventually give way to a cartilaginous anlage, which then ossifies forming the mature vertebral column.
- Neurocentral synchondroses allow continued growth of the spinal canal, and secondary vertebral ossification centers persist until the third decade of life.

1.1 Introduction

Development of the spine and spinal cord begins during the third week of gestation. Early development includes formation of primitive neural tissue, notochord development, and of the axes of the embryo. The axial skeleton eventually arises from the somites, while the central nervous system (CNS) arises from primordial mesoderm. Neurons within the CNS sprout axons form mixed spinal nerves that extend to the appropriate end organs creating the peripheral nervous system (PNS). Mesodermal vertebrae eventually give way to a cartilaginous anlage, which is then progressively ossified, forming the mature vertebrae. Secondary vertebral ossification centers and the neurocentral synchondroses persist until the third decade of life and allow growth of the spinal canal during development. This chapter discusses these key elements of spine and spinal cord development and highlight critical moments during development that can lead to bony and neural malformation.

1.2 Early Development

Initial spine development begins during the third week of gestation. At this stage of development, the embryo exists as a two cell layered structure called the bilaminar germ disc. Approximately on day 15, a groove forms in the midline of the germ disc and progressively elongates. The groove itself is termed the primitive groove. The embryonic cranial and caudal axis is formed as the primitive groove deepens at the cranial end of the embryo, and extends caudally. This central depression is termed the primitive pit, and the mound of cells surrounding the primitive pit is called the

S. Bess (✉)
Rocky Mountain Hospital for Children, 1721 East 19th Avenue, Denver, CO 80218, USA
e-mail: shay_bess@hotmail.com

B. A. Akbarnia et al. (eds.), *The Growing Spine*,
DOI: 10.1007/978-3-540-85207-0_1, © Springer-Verlag Berlin Heidelberg 2011

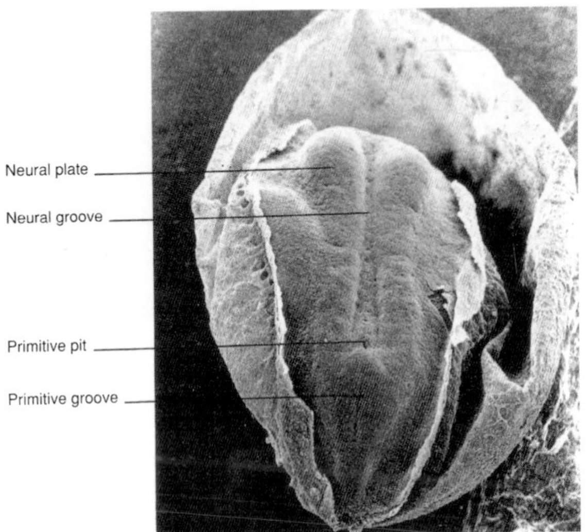

Fig. 1.1 Photomicrograph of primitive streak in the bilaminar germ disc. The primitive pit, primitive groove, and primitive node form the primitive streak. The head of the embryo will eventually form at the primitive pit and primitive node, and the entire structure (the primitive streak) establishes the embryonic longitudinal axis. (Adapted with permission from ref. [10])

primitive node (Fig. 1.1). The head of the embryo will eventually form at the primitive pit and primitive node. The entire structure (primitive pit, node and groove) is called the primitive streak. The primitive streak establishes the embryonic longitudinal axis, giving rise to left and right sides of the embryo. The cranial/caudal, left/right and ventral/dorsal axes are thus formed in the third week of gestation.

A three layered embryo is subsequently formed by proliferation and migration of epiblast cells through the primitive streak (Fig. 1.2a–c). Epiblast cells invade and replace the hypoblast cell layer, forming the definitive endoderm. Migration of epiblast cells between the epiblast and endoderm layers continues, forming a third cell layer, the mesoderm. Upon establishment of the mesodermal layer, the epiblast is renamed and is now termed the ectoderm or ectodermal layer.

Two midline structures develop in the mesoderm: the prechordal plate and the notochordal process. The notochordal process begins as a hollow mesodermal tube and goes on to become a solid rod structure, called the notochord. The notochord induces formation of the vertebral bodies, and as the early vertebral bodies coalesce around the notochord, the notochord becomes the nucleus pulposus (Fig. 1.3a, b).

Following development of notochord, three distinct structures form in the mesoderm: the paraxial mesoderm, intermediate mesoderm, and lateral plate mesoderm. The paraxial mesoderm lies adjacent to the notochord and gives rise to cell lines that differentiate into the axial skeleton, voluntary musculature and skin

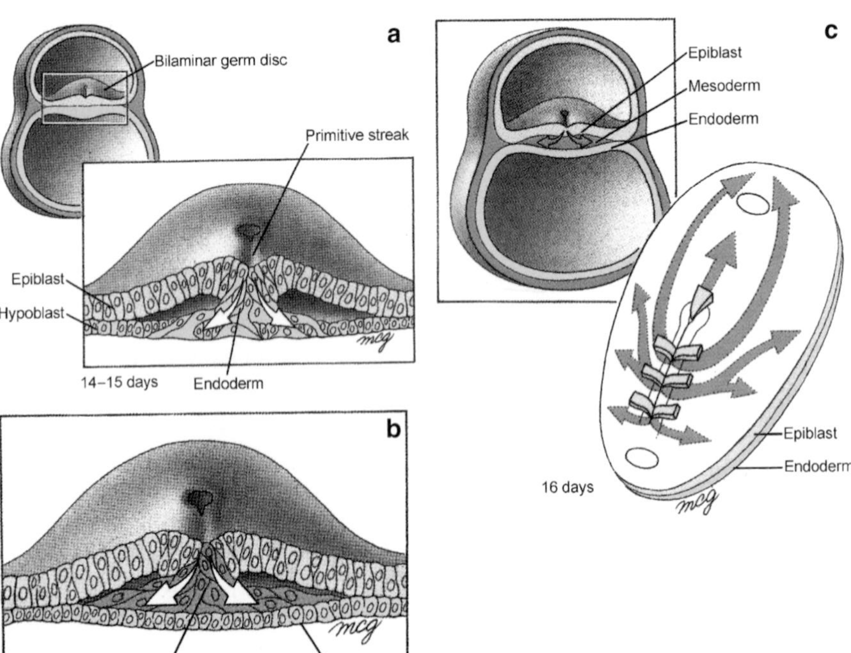

Fig. 1.2 (**a–c**) Proliferation and migration of epiblast cells. Epiblast cells proliferate and migrate through the primitive streak eventually forming the endoderm, mesoderm and ectoderm; the definitive three cell layered embryo. (Adapted with permission from ref. [6])

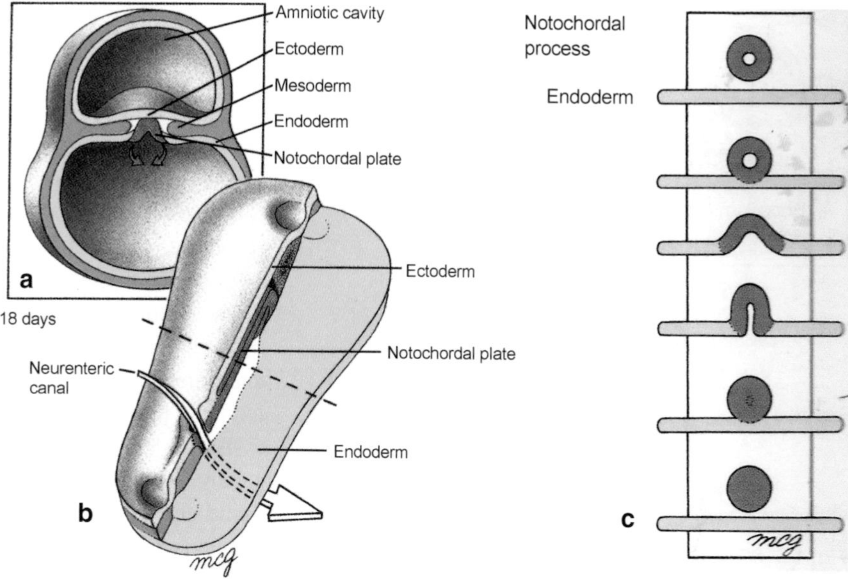

Fig. 1.3 (**a, b**) Formation of Notochordal Process and Notochord. The hollow notochordal process forms within the mesoderm, and goes on to form the solid notochord. The notochord induces vertebral body formation and eventually becomes the nucleus pulposus. (Adapted with permission from ref. [6])

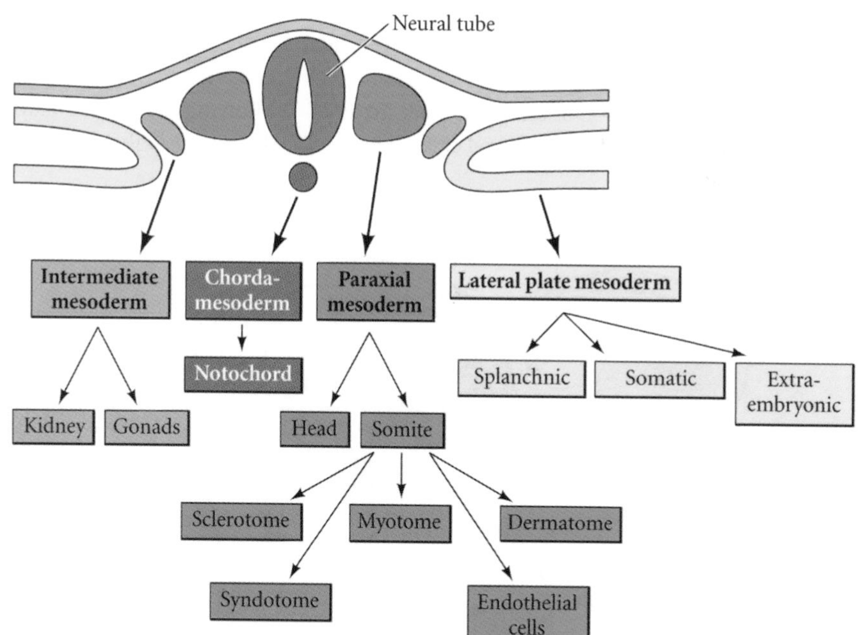

Fig. 1.4 Paraxial mesoderm, intermediate mesoderm, and lateral plate mesoderm formation, location and eventual structures. (Adapted with permission from ref. [4], Figure 16.1 (Section II))

dermis, via formation of somites. The intermediate mesoderm gives rise to the urinary and genital system. The lateral plate mesoderm splits into a ventral and a dorsal layer. The ventral layer forms the mesothelial covering of the visceral organs, and the dorsal layer gives rise to the skin dermis and the parietal lining of the body wall (Fig. 1.4).

1.3 Somite Formation and Differentiation

As indicated above, the axial skeleton, voluntary muscle, and the dermis of the neck and trunk are derived from the somites. The paired somites appear approximately on gestational day 20. The somites arise from the

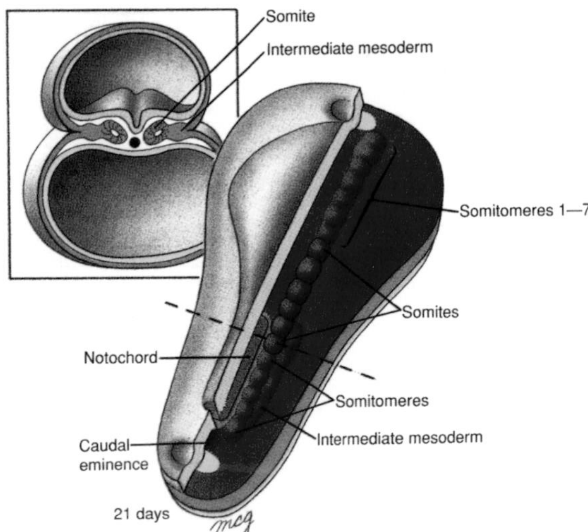

Fig. 1.5 Somite formation. The paired somites arise from the paraxial mesoderm and form the axial skeleton, voluntary muscle, and the dermis of the neck and trunk. (Adapted with permission from ref. [6])

paraxial mesoderm, and develop in a cranial to caudal fashion at a rate of approximately 3–4 somites per day (Fig. 1.5). Initially, 42–44 somite pairs flank the notochord forming the base of the skull and extending to the embryonic tail. The terminal 5–7 somites eventually regress, forming a final total of 37 somite pairs. Somite pairs 1–4 form the occiput, and bones of the face and inner ear. Somites 5–12 form the cervical spine (there are 8 cervical somites, but only 7 cervical vertebrae, because the first cervical somite participates in occiput formation). Somites 13–24 form the thoracic vertebrae, somites 25–29 form the lumbar vertebrae, and somites 30–34 form the sacral vertebrae. The three caudal, terminal somite pairs persist after regression of the terminal embryonic tail, forming the coccyx. The somite pairs and somite positioning on the embryo form an anatomic template that organizes the spinal column and PNS.

As the embryo develops, the somites separate into subdivisions. Each subdivision gives rise to the ultimate tissue structure that develops from each somite. The first somite subdivisions to appear are the sclerotomes. The sclerotomes ultimately form the bony spinal column. Sclerotomes are formed when a hollow central cavity forms within the somite. This cavity develops in the medial region of the somite, adjacent to the midline notochord and neural tube. The central cavity fills with cells, termed loose core cells, and eventually ruptures, allowing the core cells to migrate towards the midline and envelop the notochord and neural tube (Fig. 1.6).

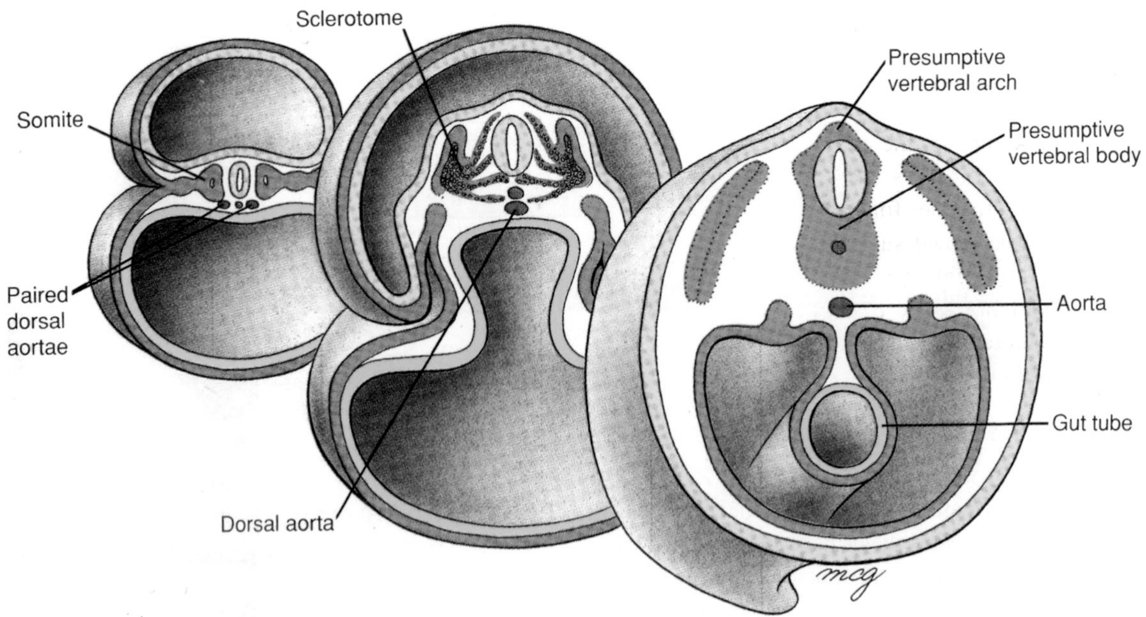

Fig. 1.6 Sclerotome formation. The central cavity within the somite fills with loose core cells, and eventually ruptures. Core cells migrate toward the midline and envelop the notochord and neural tube forming a sclerotome. The ventral sclerotome forms the vertebral body, and the dorsal sclerotome becomes the vertebral arch. (Adapted with permission from ref. [6])

The cellular structure that eventually surrounds the notochord and neural tube is termed sclerotome. The ventral sclerotome that surrounds the notochord forms the vertebral body, and the dorsal sclerotome that envelops the neural tube eventually becomes the vertebral arch.

Normal vertebral body and vertebral arch development is dependent upon normal sclerotome induction by the underlying notochord and neural tube. Spinal dysraphism, is a spectrum of birth defects originating from failure of neural tube closure (see Chap. 21). This leads to abnormal cell signaling and induction of the overlying sclerotome. Spina bifida is defined as incomplete closure of the neural arch. In the setting of spina bifida, the underlying neural elements are uncovered. Spina bifida occulta indicates that only the neural arch failed to close completely. However, in more severe conditions of spina bifida, the contents of the neural canal can bulge out and become continuous with the overlying skin. The contents of the spina bifida defect are contained by a membranous tissue, a cele. The cele is on the skin surface overlying the spina bifida defect. The contents of the cele may include only the neural meninges (dura and arachnoid) and is termed as meningocele. If the cele contains neural tissue and meninges, it is termed as meningomyelocele.

Once the sclerotomes form and become positioned adjacent to the notochord and neural tube, each sclerotome divides, allowing the spinal nerves to emerge from the neural tube, and exit at their respective level (Fig. 1.7a–d). When the sclerotome division is complete, the caudal half of the suprajacent sclerotome merges with the cranial half of the subjacent sclerotome, forming the vertebra precursor. The division and subsequent refusion explains why there are eight cervical nerves, but only seven cervical vertebrae. The cranial division of the first cervical somite contributes to form the base of the occiput, while the caudal division of the first cervical somite and the cranial division of the second cervical somite form the first cervical vertebra. The first cervical nerve exits above the C1 vertebra, the second cervical nerve exits between C1 and C2, this pattern persists to C7-T1 foramen where the C8 nerve root exits. The sclerotomal cells that remain in the original region of the sclerotome division surround the notochord, and form the fibrous portion of the intervertebral disc, the annulus fibrosis. The enveloped notochord goes on to form the infantile and childhood nucleus pulposis. As the child ages, the original notochord cells of the nucleus pulposis are replaced by fibrocartilageous cells.

1.4 Central Nervous System Development

During early development, two key structures originate in the mesoderm; the notochordal process and the prechordal plate. The prechordal plate induces the overlying epiblast cell layer to form the neural plate. In response to inductive factors produced by the prechordal plate, the neural plate cells differentiate into neurectoderm and proliferate in a cranial to caudal fashion. The cranial portion of the neural plate is broad and gives rise to the brain, while the tapered caudal region of the neural plate forms the spinal cord. The caudal portion of the neural plate overlies the notochord and is bordered by the somite pairs. This positioning allows the caudal neural plate, which will become the spinal cord, to become enveloped by the sclerotomes, forming the spinal canal (Fig. 1.8). The neural plate becomes the neural tube by a process called neurulation, in which the neural plate involutes, until the lateral edges of the folded neural plate and overlying ectoderm meet and fuse in the midline (Fig. 1.9).

Once the neural tube fuses in the midline, it separates from the overlying ectoderm, and differentiates into three distinct layers (Fig. 1.10). The innermost cell layer of the neural tube, the ventricular layer, lays adjacent to the lumen of the neural tube (the neural canal). The ventricular layer contains neuroepithelial cells, which are the precursors to the cells that eventually comprise the CNS. The first generation of cells produced by the neuroepithelial cells is neuroblasts. Neuroblasts eventually become neurons in the CNS. Once formed, neuroblasts migrate away from the ventricular layer to form the mantle layer. The mantle layer eventually becomes the grey matter of the CNS. The neuroblasts in the mantle layer organize into four columns during the fourth week of gestation, forming paired dorsal and ventral columns. The cells of the dorsal column form association neurons that serve to interconnect the motor neurons of the ventral columns with the sensory neurons in the dorsal root

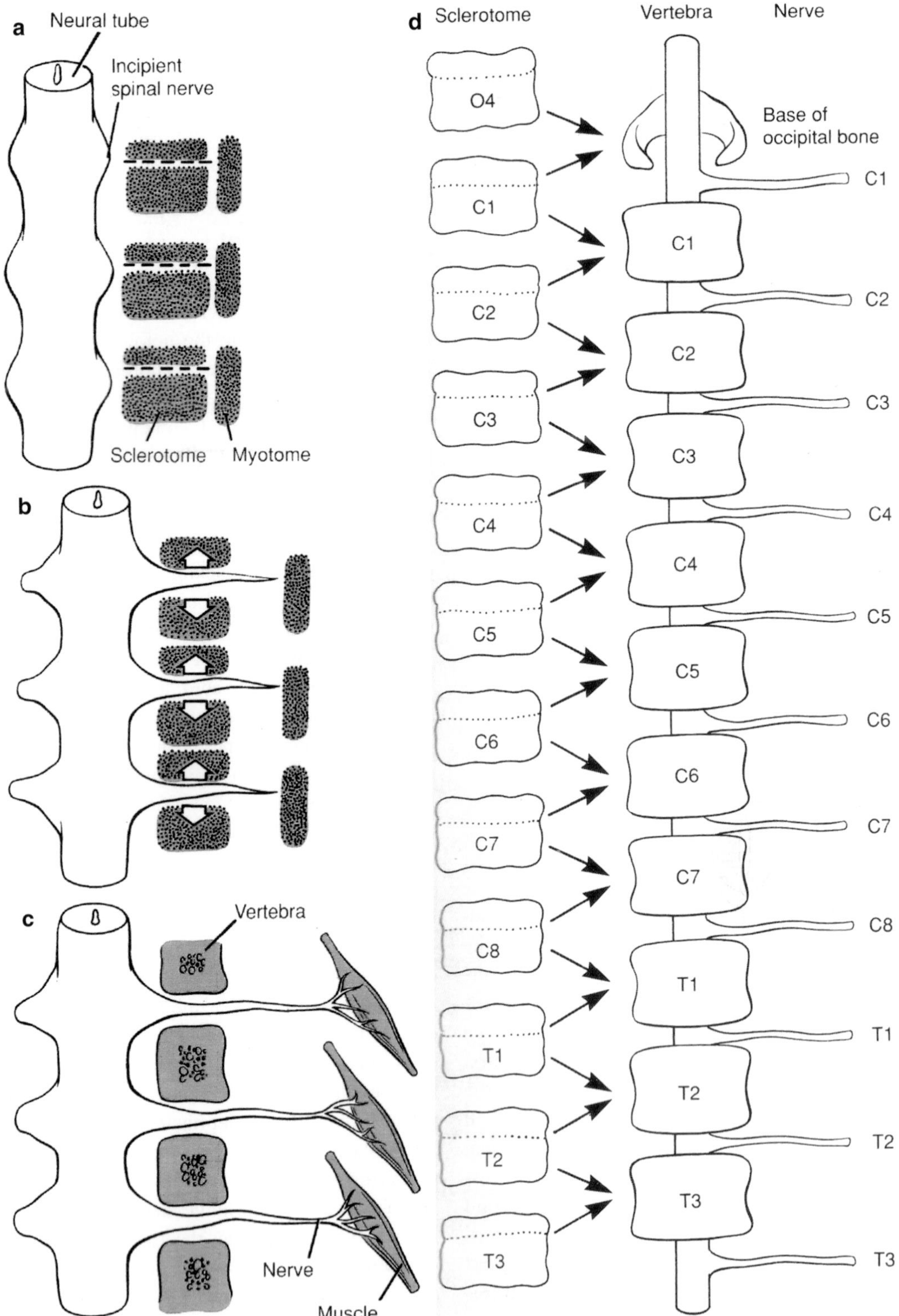

Fig. 1.7 (**a–d**) Sclerotome division and reconvergence. Sclerotome division allows the spinal nerves to emerge from the neural tube, and extend to the periphery. The sclerotomes then reconverge to form the final vertebrae. (Adapted with permission from ref. [6])

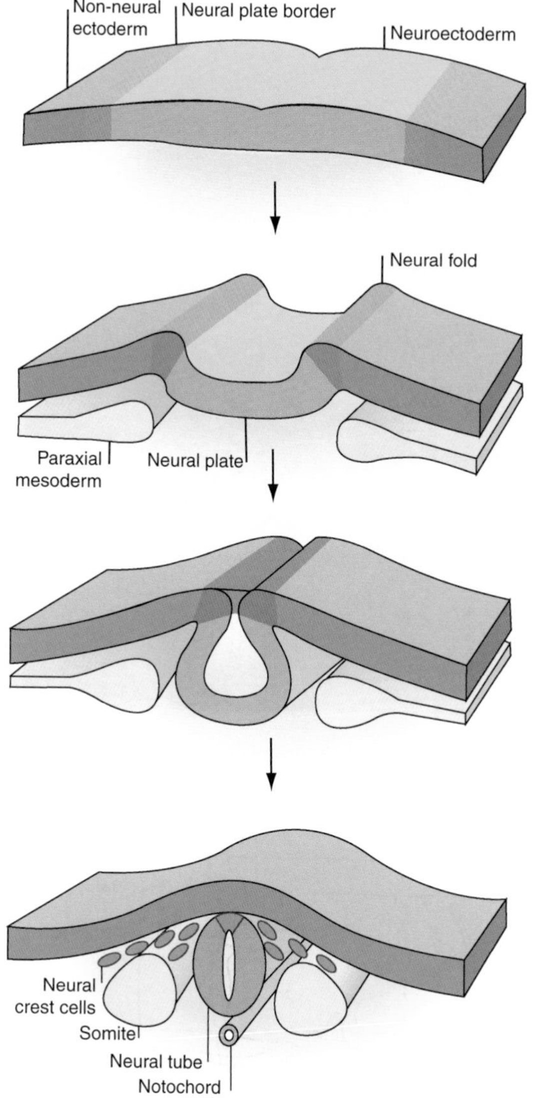

Fig. 1.8 Neural Plate and CNS Formation. The neural plate differentiates from the epiblast, neurectoderm cells and migrate in a cranial and caudal fashion, giving rise to the cranial (brain) and caudal (spinal cord) neural plate. The caudal neural plate is eventually enveloped by the sclerotomes, forming the spinal cord and bony spinal canal, respectively. (Adapted with permission from ref. [3])

ganglia (DRG). Neuronal processes that germinate from the neuroblasts extend peripherally to form the third layer of the neural tube, the marginal layer. The marginal layer becomes the axonal white matter of the CNS.

1.5 Peripheral Extension of the CNS; Formation of the Peripheral Nervous System

Formation of the PNS begins approximately on gestational day 30. Somatic motor neurons in the ventral gray columns extend axon sprouts towards the adjacent sclerotome tissue (Fig. 1.11). The axon sprouts begin at the cervical region, and progressive axonal sprouting extends in a cranial to caudal manner. The ventral axons coalesce as they reach the adjacent sclerotomes, forming distinct segmental nerves and the ventral roots. The somatic system is formed as ventral roots extend past the DRG, inducing the neurons in the DRG to sprout axons. Unlike the somatic neurons in the ventral column, the neurons in the DRG are derived from neural crest cells. The neural crest cells arise from the lateral margins of the neural folds during neurulation. These cells detach from the neural plate, and migrate to different regions of the developing embryo, forming melanocytes, sympathetic and parasympathetic ganglia, and the sensory neurons that reside in the DRG. The axons that extend ventrolaterally from the DRG join the axons in the ventral roots to form mixed spinal nerves. The mixed spinal nerves extend to and penetrate the adjacent sclerotomes and eventually function to innervate the end organs. Other DRG axons grow medially, extending into the dorsal column to synapse with the newly formed association neurons.

1.6 Vertebral Ossification

At approximately the sixth week of gestation, the mesodermal spine precursor transforms into a cartilage model forming the chondrification centers within each vertebra. Two chondrification centers develop in the vertebral body, called the centrum, that go on to fuse in the midline forming a single vertebral body cartilage precursor. If one of the centrum chondrification centers fails to form, a hemivertebra is formed, leading to congenital scoliosis (Figs. 1.12 and 1.13; see Chap. 18). The vertebral arches derive from chondrification centers adjacent to the vertebral body. One chondrification center exists for each neural arch. Chondrification centers for the transverse processes and spinal process

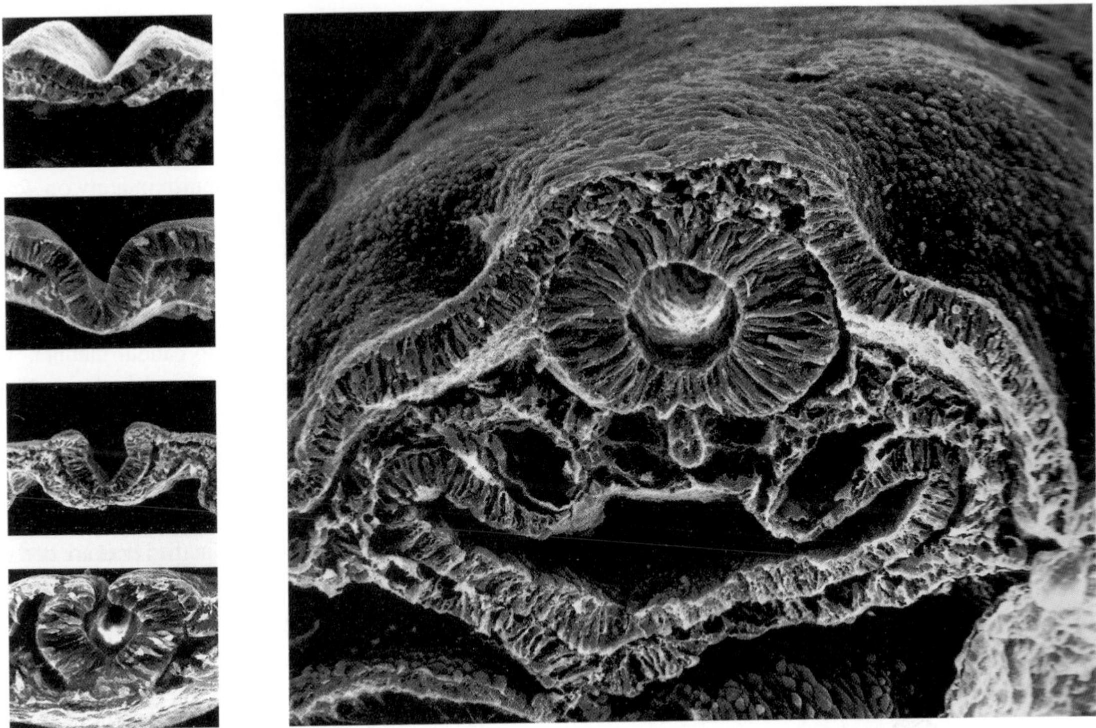

Fig. 1.9 Neurulation. The neural plate becomes the neural tube during neurulation, in which the neural plate involutes and the lateral edges of the folded neural plate fuse in the midline. (Adapted with permission from ref. [6])

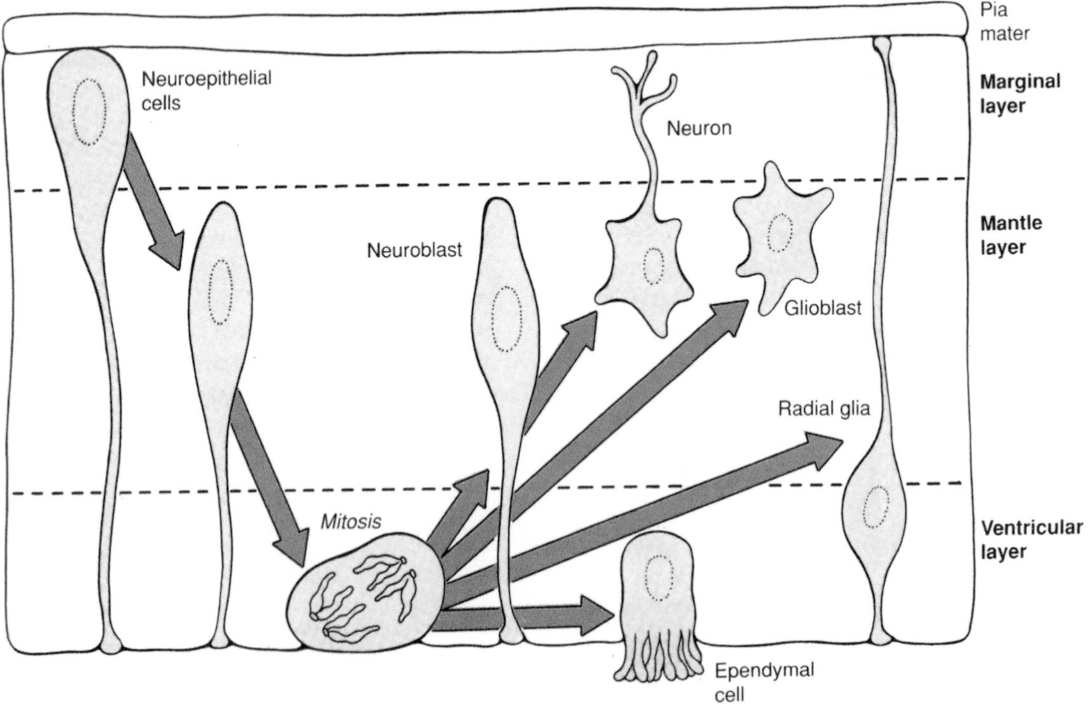

Fig. 1.10 Neural tube differentiation. The neural tube differentiates into three distinct layers. The ventricular layer forms the precursor cells that eventually populate the mantle and marginal layers, and comprise the CNS. The mantle layer forms the grey matter of the CNS. The marginal layer becomes the axonal white matter of the CNS. (Adapted with permission from ref. [6])

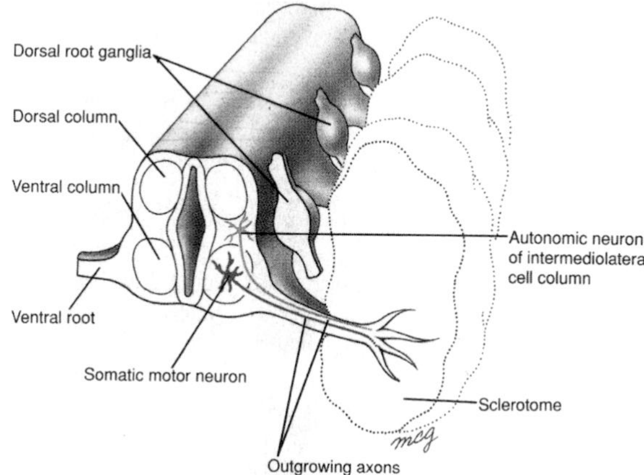

Fig. 1.11 PNS formation. Axon sprouts emerge from the primordial spinal cord and coalesce as they reach the adjacent sclerotomes, forming segmental nerves and providing end organ innervation. (Adapted with permission from ref. [6])

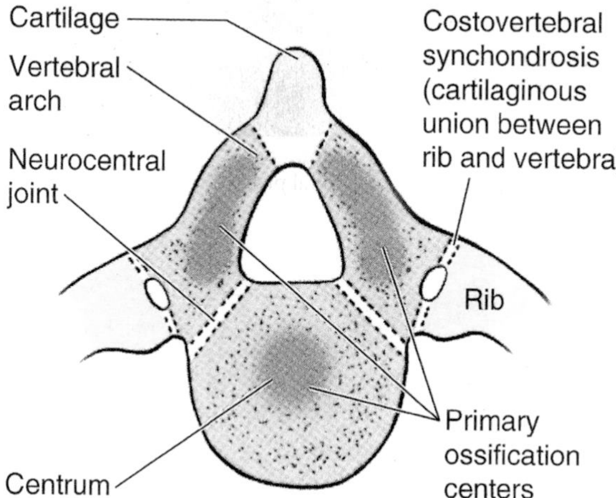

Fig. 1.12 Vertebral chondrification centers. The mesodermal spine precursor transforms into a cartilage model via the chondrification centers. The chondrification centers are eventually ossified forming the mature vertebrae. (Adapted with permission from ref. [7])

subsequently form, completing the cartilage anlage for the vertebra.

Each vertebra derives from three primary ossification centers; one for the body (centrum) and two adjacent centers for the vertebral arches (Fig. 1.14). The centra are first ossified in the lower thoracic and upper lumbar regions. Centra ossification progresses more rapidly in the caudal vertebrae, while the vertebral arches are more rapidly ossified in the cervical spine. The cervical lamina are ossified as early as the eighth week, well before the cervical centra ossify. Dorsal, midline fusion of the lamina initially occurs in the lumbar spine, then progresses cranially. Once ossified, the lamina do not fuse to the centrum. Instead, an embryologic joint, the neurocentral synchondroses, persists between the centrum and each lamina. The neurocentral

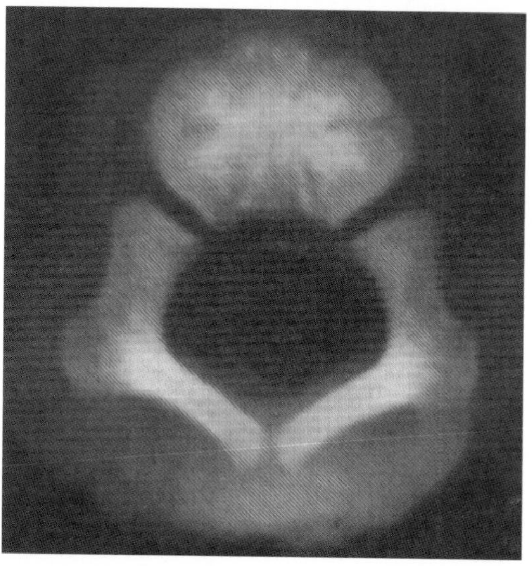

Fig. 1.14 Vertebral ossification centers. The three primary ossification centers of the vertebrae. (Adapted with permission from ref. [5])

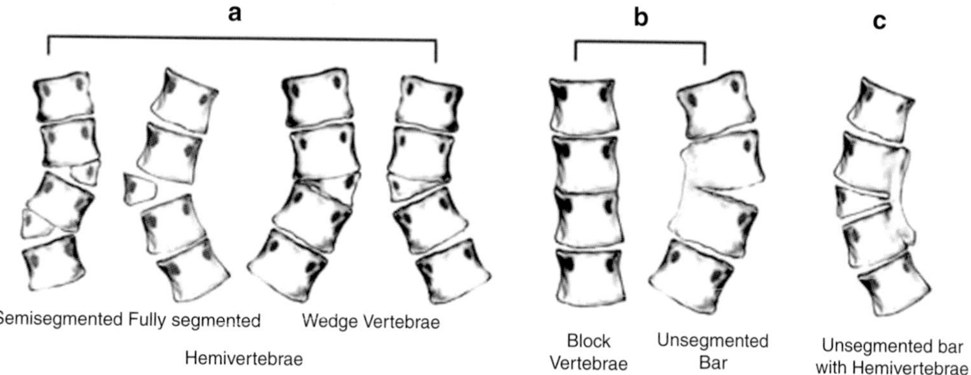

Fig. 1.13 Congenital scoliosis. (Adapted with permission from ref. [2])

synchondroses allow expansion of the spinal canal during growth of the centrum and lamina, and eventually disappear by 6 years of age. Secondary ossification centers at the tips of the transverse processes, spinous process, and ring apophysis develop after birth, and eventually fuse during the third decade (Fig. 1.12).

1.7 Conclusion

Embryological formation of the spine and spinal cord progresses in an organized manner, beginning with formation of the primitive streak, notochord, somites, and sclerotomes. Normal vertebral and neural formation is dependent upon development of these early structures to induce the adjacent cell lines to form the neural arch and distinct vertebral bodies. Errors in formation of these structures lead to induction failure and subsequent spinal dysraphism and congenital scoliosis. These embryological events have been previously described [8–10].

References

1. Bono CM, Parke WW, Garfin SR (2006) Development of the spine. In: Herkovitz GS, Garfin SR, Eismont FJ, Bell GR, Balderston RA (eds) Rothman-Simeone: the spine. Saunders, Philadelphia
2. Erol B, Kusumi K, Lou J et al (2002) Etiology of congenital scoliosis. UPOJ 15:37–42
3. Gammill LS, Bronner-Fraser M (2003) Neural crest specification: migrating into genomics. Nat Rev Neurosci 4, 795–805
4. Gilbert SF (2006) Developmental biology, 8th edn. Sinauer, Sunderland
5. Herkowitz HH, Garfin SR, Balderston RA et al (1999) Rothman-Simeone: the spine, 4th edn. Saunders, Philadelphia
6. Larsen W (1993) Human embryology. Churchill Livingstone, New York
7. Moore KL, Dalley AF (1999) Clinically oriented anatomy, 4th edn. Lippincott, Williams & Wilkins, Philadelphia, PA
8. Moore KL, Persaud TVN (2003) The developing human; clinically oriented embryology, 7th edn. Saunders, Philadelphia
9. Noback CR, Demarest RJ, Ruggiero DA et al (2005) The human nervous system; structure and function, 6th edn. Humana, Totowa
10. Tamarin A (1983) Stage 9 macaque embryo studied by electron microscopy. J Anat 137:765

Normal Growth of the Spine and Thorax

2

Alain Dimeglio, François Bonnel, and Federico Canavese

Key Points

- The growing spine is a mosaic of physes.
- Growth is characterized by changes in rhythm.
- The thorax is part of the spine, it is the "fourth dimension of the spine".
- Lung growth is essentially completed by the age of 8 years with a golden period of maximum growth occurring before 5 years of age.
- Anticipation is the best strategy when dealing with complex spinal deformities.
- The goal of management is to control spinal deformity without impending spinal growth.
- The best strategy is to open the thorax before 5 years of age and keep the spine supple before puberty.
- The immature spine is dominated by the crankshaft phenomenon.
- Early arthrodesis before 10 years of age has a negative effect on the development of the thorax.
- Puberty is a turning point for scoliosis, and skeletal maturation is a precious parameter for follow-up.

2.1 Growth Holds the Basics

It is growth that distinguishes pediatric from adult orthopaedics. It is this ongoing 17-year adventure, punctuated by upheavals that gives this discipline its originality and makes it so interesting. Growth analysis is the evaluation of the effects of time on the growing child. Growth is a complex and well-synchronized phenomenon with a hierarchical pattern that organizes the different types and rates of growth in various tissues, organs, and individuals through time [6, 20, 26].

Growth can be considered as "microgrowth", which is mainly the growth at the cellular level (e.g., in the physes). Although the histologic structure is the same, each physes has its own characteristics and dynamics [20]. The study of height, weight, and body proportions may be considered as the study of "macrogrowth". This study is the culmination of all the effects of microgrowth on the individual: the combined effect of growth of the lower limbs, the trunk, and the upper limbs, increase in weight, and so on [20, 26].

The scope of this process called *growth,* and the changes it brings about, can be better perceived by considering these facts: from birth onward, height will increase by 350% and weight will increase 20 fold, and the spine will double in length [24, 26].

Growth is an essential element in the natural history of any orthopaedic disorder in the growing child [24, 26]. It would be a mistake to assume that only growth in terms of increase in height is important. It is equally important to consider the manner in which the skeletal system develops, that is, the timing of growth in various parts of the body and the changing proportions o f various body segments.

The spine surgeon needs to know the normal values for many parameters and how to measure them. He or she needs to know the significance of these values, for

A. Dimeglio (✉)
Service de Chirurgie Orthopédique Pédiatrique,
Chu Lapeyronie, 371 Avenue Doyen Gaston Giraud,
34264 Montpellier, Cedex 5, France
e-mail: a-dimeglio@chu-montpellier.fr

B. A. Akbarnia et al. (eds.), *The Growing Spine*,
DOI: 10.1007/978-3-540-85207-0_2, © Springer-Verlag Berlin Heidelberg 2011

example, the effect of a ten-level spinal fusion in a boy who has a bone age of 10 years. Bone age, Tanner classification, stages of puberty, and measurement of the upper and lower portions of the body are all parameters that may need to be considered in the analysis of any particular case [20, 24, 26].

Knowledge of the synchronization of the various events in growth will also allow the orthopaedist to anticipate certain events, for example, the onset of puberty characterized by an increase in growth velocity in a girl with early breast development. However, these values vary with the individual, and average values may not apply to a particular individual. What is most important is the pattern and rate of growth for a particular individual. It is the rate of growth that will influence orthopedic decisions, more than the final height. A sequence of measurements of the important parameters is far superior to a single measurement [20, 24, 26].

The criticism often directed at growth data is that such data are ethnically specific, and it is difficult to transfer parameters from one population to another. For example, bone age atlases are not transferable between populations nor are growth curves, from one country to another. A comparison of data relating to children in England, Switzerland, France, and the United States reveals no significant differences in final heights, bone ages, or other parameters of growth [33, 50, 55, 56, 58]. Looking beyond racial diversity, there are growth constants (i.e., stages through which every child must pass regardless of chronologic age) that are the same in ethnic groups.

A few simple tools are required at the time of consultation: a height gauge, scales, a metric tape, and a bone age atlas. With these tools, the specialist will be able to form a rapid mental arithmetic and reach a reasonable decision. A few simple questions will provide the orthopedic surgeon the information that is required [20, 24, 26] (Table 2.1).

Table 2.1 Clinical examination must answer to these basic questions

How tall is the child?
What is the child's sitting height?
How long is the subischial leg length?
How much has the child grown in a single year?
What is the child's chronologic age?
What is the bone age?
How much growth does the child have left in the trunk and in the lower limbs?
Exactly what point has the child reached on his or her developmental peak?
Where is the child in relation to puberty and the pubertal peak?
What about the Tanner signs?
Are the child's proportions within normal limits?
How much does the child weigh?

2.2 Biometric Measurements

There is not much useful data that can be obtained from a single measurement. A single measurement can be an error and two measurements constitute an indication, while three measurements define a tendency.

Measurements of growth should be taken at regular intervals. Checking the child every 6 months, one of the two checkups being preferably around his or her birthday, allows an easy assessment of the growth velocity of the child and the different body segments [20, 24, 26]. These measurements provide a real-time image of growth and, when carefully recorded in a continually updated "growth notebook," they provide charts that make decisions easier. Growth velocity is an excellent example, because it provides the best indicator of the beginning of puberty, on which so many decisions rest. The first sign of puberty is the increase in growth rate of the standing height to more 0.5 cm/month or more than 6 cm/year.

The spine surgeon should be familiar with the measurements of these parameters. Regarding standards of growth, several good references are available [3, 20, 24, 26, 35, 37, 50].

2.2.1 Standing Height

Measuring the height is to the orthopaedic specialist as listening to the heart is to the cardiologist. In children younger than 5 years, standing height is measured with the child lying down because in this age group, this position is both easier and more reliable [20, 24, 26].

Between birth and maturity, the body will grow by approximately 1.20 m, or even 1.30 m. Growth is brisk up to 5 years of age. After that, it slows considerably until the onset of puberty, which occurs at approximately 11 years in girls and 13 years in boys. At 2 years of age, the standing height is approximately 50% of the adult height, at 5 years of age it is approximately 60%, by the age of 9 years approximately 80%, and at puberty approximately 86%. In this latter period, standing height increases more rapidly.

Standing height is a global marker and is composed of two specific measurements known as subischial height (i.e., the growth of the lower limbs) and sitting height (i.e., the growth of the trunk). These two different regions often grow at different rates at different times, which is valuable information for decisions in orthopaedics. Values for the standing heights of girls and boys at various age were given in previous publications [59–61].

2.2.2 Sitting Height

In children 2 years of age or younger, the sitting height is measured with the child lying down for the same reasons that the standing height is also measured supine in this age group. After 2 years of age, the child to be measured should be placed on a stool or table at a convenient height. The most important consideration is that the child should always be measured under the same conditions using the same measuring instruments. The sitting height averages 34 cm at birth and averages 88 cm for girls for a standing height of 165 cm at skeletal maturity, and, 92 cm (sitting height) for boys at the end of growth for a standing height of 175 cm [20, 22, 24, 26, 52] (Figs. 2.1–2.3).

In patients with scoliosis, it can be instructive to follow the changes in the sitting height rather than in the standing height. If a 6-year-old girl with juvenile scoliosis is being treated, her sitting height will be approximately 64 cm and will increase to about 88 cm. Therefore, the spine surgeon will have to control the spinal curve while her trunk grows 24 cm. The measurement of sitting height can also be useful in anticipating the onset of puberty. In an average population, puberty starts at approximately 75 cm sitting height in girls and 78 cm in boys. When the sitting height is approximately 84 cm, 80% of girls have menarche (Figs. 2.4–2.6).

2.2.3 Subischial Limb Length

The segment of the body consisting of the lower extremities is measured to determine the subischial limb length. As implied by the name, subischial limb length is measured by subtracting the sitting height from the standing height.

At birth, the subischial limb length averages 18 cm. At the completion of growth, it will average 81 cm in boys and 74.5 cm in girls. These 63 cm of growth in boys and 56.5 cm of growth in girls contribute to a far greater percentage of growth in height than does trunk growth. This accounts for the changing proportions of the body during growth (See Figs. 2.4–2.6).

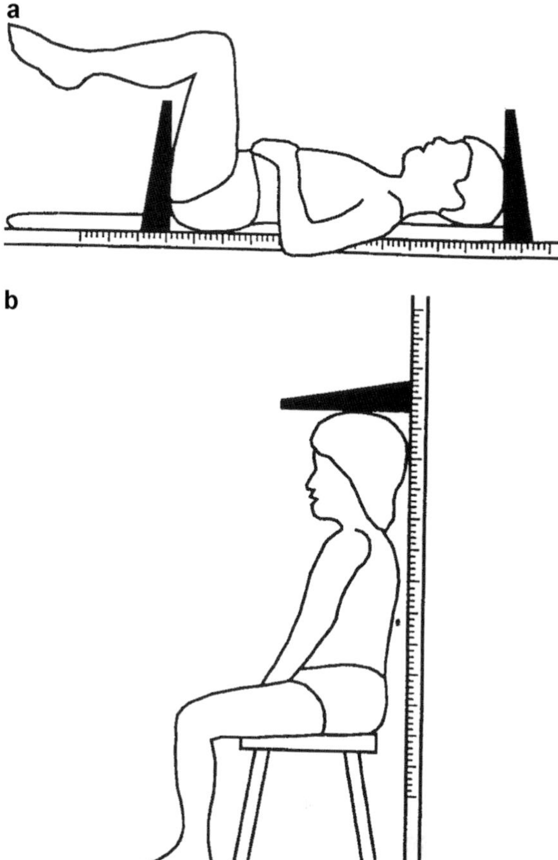

Fig. 2.1 Sitting height measurement: in children younger than 2 years (**a**) and in children older than 2 years (**b**)

2.2.4 Arm Span

The measurement of arm span provides an indirect control parameter for the measurement of standing height. Combining these two measurements avoids virtually all errors. To measure arm span, the patient simply raises the arms to a horizontal position, and the distance between the tips of the middle fingers is measured with a tape measure. There is an excellent correlation between arm span and standing height, as standing height is about 97% of arm span. If the trunk

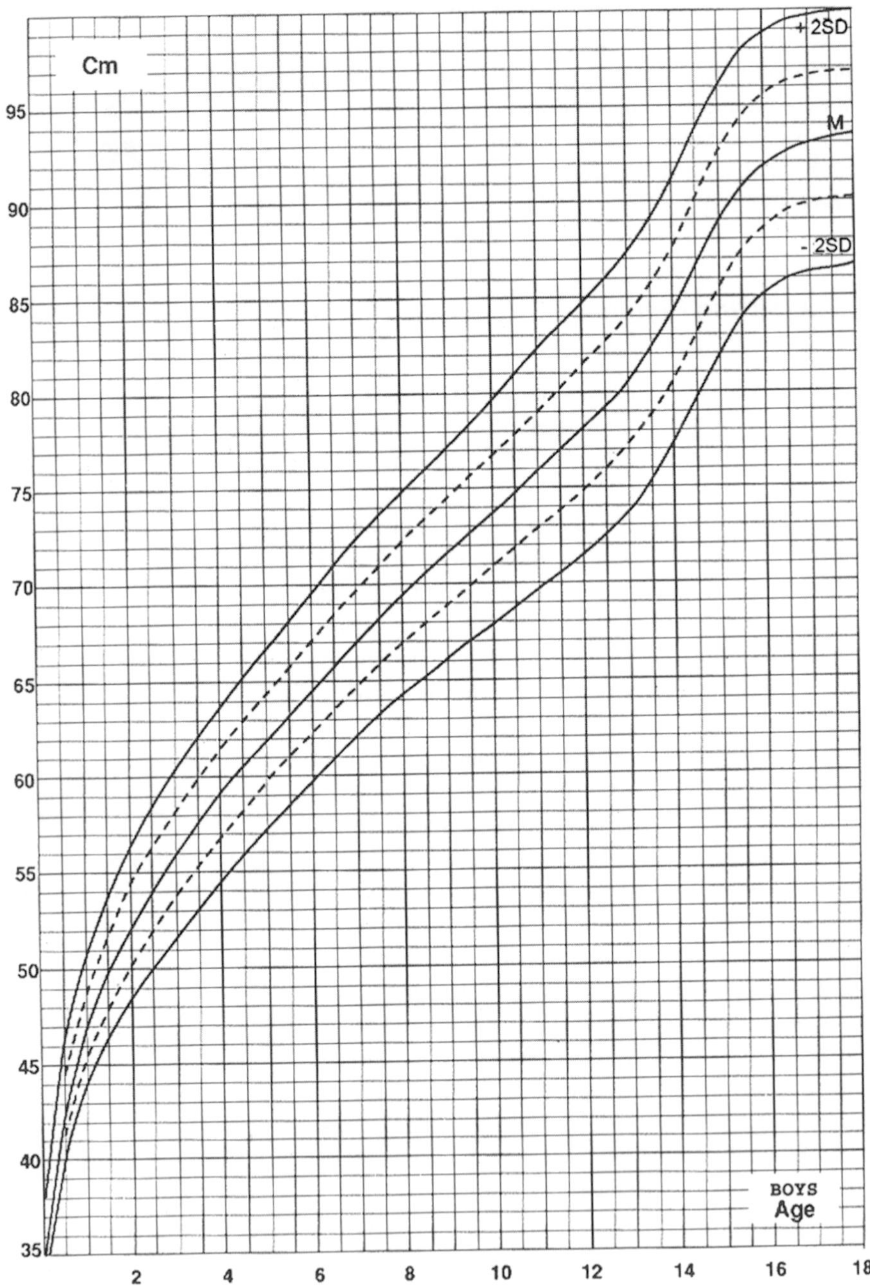

Fig. 2.2 Sitting height-for-age (birth to 18 years: boys)

is normal (i.e., without deformity), its length will equal approximately 52% of arm span, and the lower limbs will be equal to approximately 48%, or will be the same as their proportions in the standing height.

The relation of arm span to normal height is useful in determining the normal height of a child who is wheelchair bound; this allows the calculation of the child's height [39]. It is a routine used for any child who has a spine deformity (e.g., scoliosis) for calculating the normal values for pulmonary function. With spinal deformity, arm is a good estimate of what the standing height would be if there was no scoliosis.

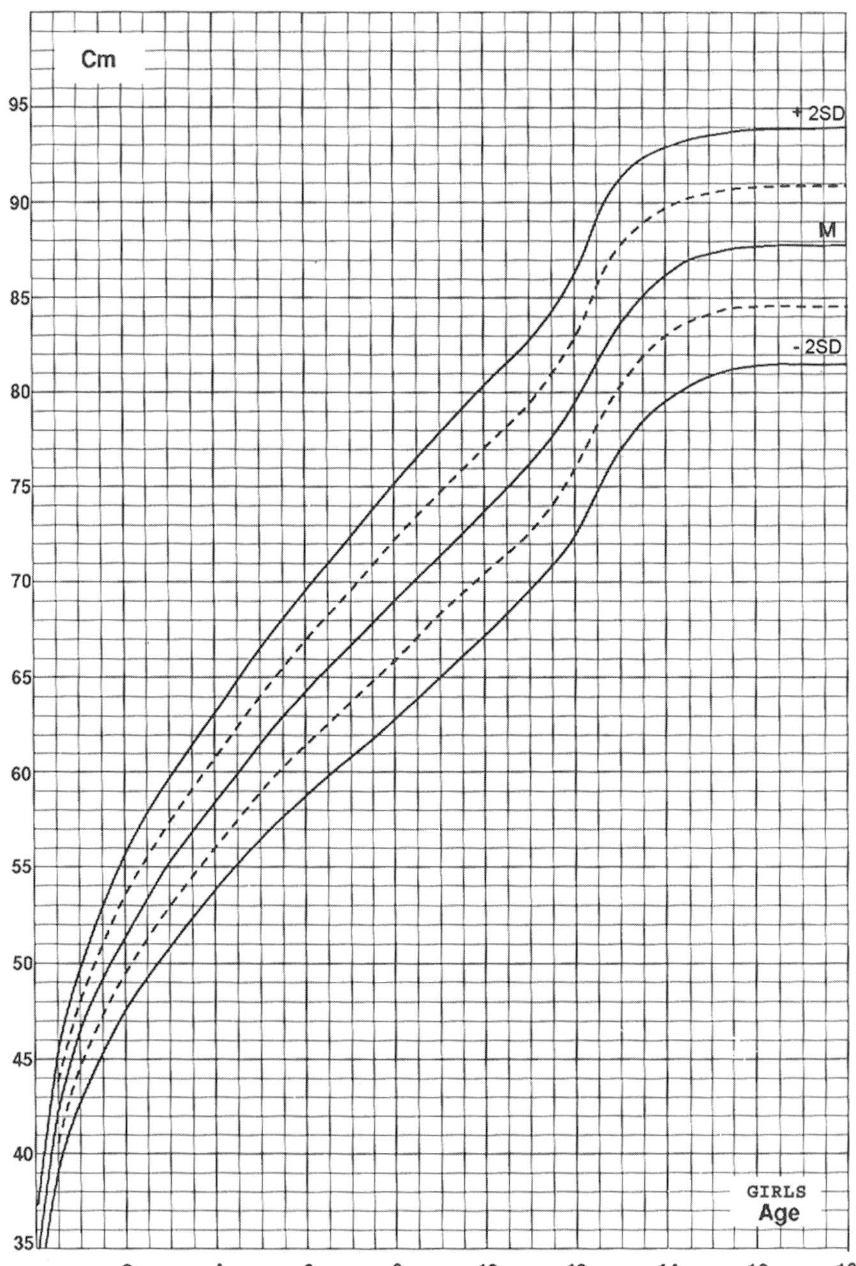

Fig. 2.3 Sitting height-for-age (birth to 18 years: girls)

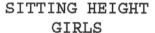

2.2.5 Weight

Weight should always be brought into the equation when making a surgical decision, whether the orthopaedic is dealing with a case of idiopathic scoliosis or paralytic scoliosis. Children should always be weighed at consultations. There may be striking morphologic changes from 1 year to the next. If weight evaluation becomes an integral part of each consultation, changes will become obvious and can be incorporated into the orthopedic specialist's deliberations. A simple trend in the increase in a boy's weight is 18–20 kg at 5 years

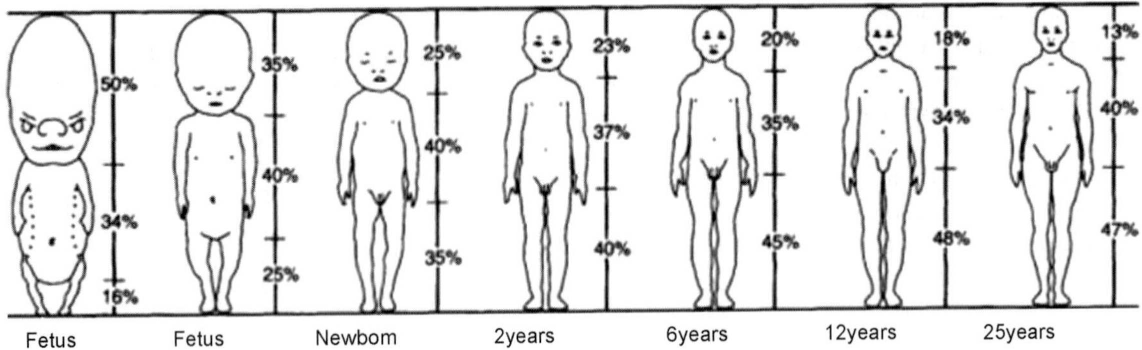

Fig. 2.4 Sitting height and lower limb length proportion. Sitting height is 65% of standing height at birth and 52%, at 12 years

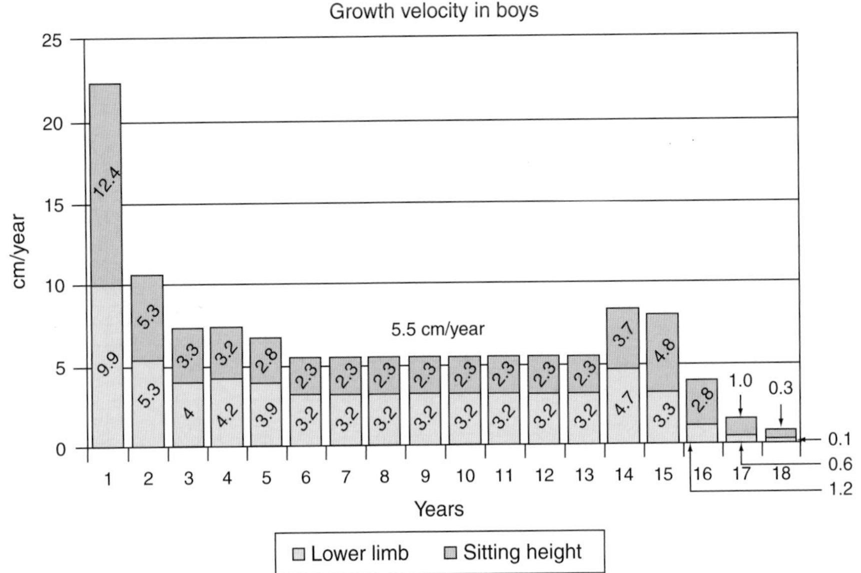

Fig. 2.5 Growth velocity of sitting height and lower limb (1–18 years: boys)

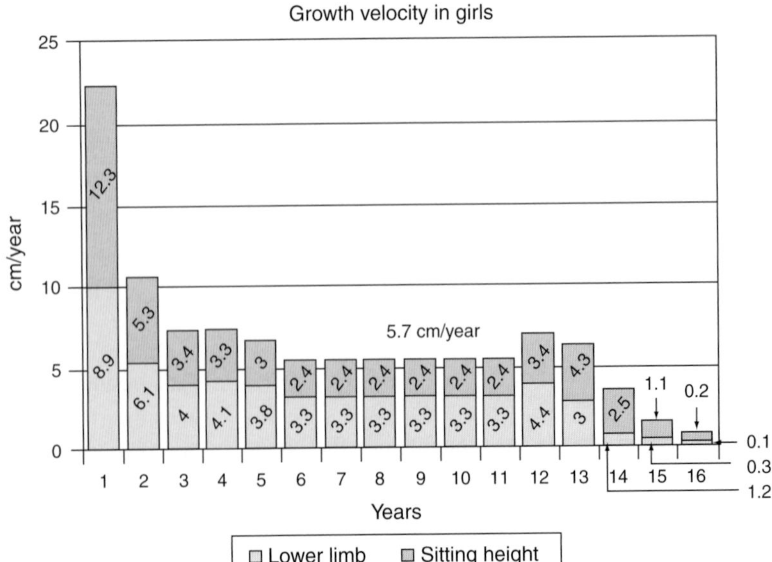

Fig. 2.6 Growth velocity of sitting height and lower limb (1–16 years: girls)

of age; 30 kg at 10 years of age; and 60 kg at 17 years of age [26]. Note that weight doubles between 10 and 17 years of age. At 5 years of age, the child's weight reaches 32% of the final normal weight yet only 48% of the final normal weight is achieved at 10 years of age. In a patient whose weight is 10% or more above normal, a scoliosis brace may no longer correct the spinal curve as it did before. A low weight, on the other hand, can explain the delay in the onset of menarche because girls generally need to attain a weight of 40 kg for menarche to occur. Hypotrophy is frequent in severe infantile scoliosis. A generally accepted estimate of body fat is expressed in Quetelet body mass index: weight (kg)/height (m^2). Using this index, 20–25 kg/m^2 is normal, 25–30 kg/m^2 is moderate obesity, 30–40 kg/m^2 is major obesity, and more than 40 kg/m^2 is morbid obesity. Obesity is a major problem in Willi–Prader syndrome with scoliosis [20, 24, 26].

2.2.6 The Multiplying Coefficient

Lefort [42] outlined the concept of "multiplying coefficient," which can be applied to growth measurements in children at any age. This has also been extensively described by Paley [49]. It is easy to calculate this coefficient, which is obtained by considering the percentage of growth that has been attained. For example, once a child has reached 40% of his or her expected adult standing height, the multiplying coefficient can be calculated as 100/40 = 2.5. The multiplying coefficient can be applied to all biometric data- standing height, sitting height, subischial limb length, and length of the femur, tibia, humerus, radius, and ulna.

At birth, the sitting height of boys reaches 37% of its final value. The multiplying factor is 2.85. At 10 years, sitting height of boys reaches 77% of its final value; the multiplying factor is 1.28.

2.3 Chronology

2.3.1 Intrauterine Development

Growth starts before birth. During the first trimester of gestation, the systems are busy organizing themselves and develop at a brisk pace [34, 46]. During this period, the fetus makes daily progress, so that when the infant is born, it reaches a weight six million times that of the original egg. By the second month of life, the sitting height increases at a rate of 1 mm daily, which subsequently increases to 1.5 mm/day. Were this rate of growth to continue until the age of 10 years, the child would ultimately stand 6 m tall [6, 20, 24, 26, 34, 62].

From the third month onward, the embryo becomes a fetus and turns into a miniature adult. At the end of the second trimester of gestation, the fetus reaches 70% of its expected length at birth (it measures 30 cm at this stage) but achieves no more than 20% of the expected birth weight (it weighs approximately 800 g). During the third trimester, the fetus gains weight at the highest rate (700 g/month). This means that various stages of growth do not occur simultaneously during intrauterine life. Length increases steadily and rapidly during the first 6 months in *utero,* whereas weight gain is most rapid during the final 3 months of gestation.

With high-resolution ultrasonography, it is possible to follow the growth of the fetus and to detect even the slightest abnormality. It can be anticipated that many orthopedic spine conditions characterized by abnormal growth will be diagnosed prenatally.

2.3.2 From Birth to 5 Years

Birth marks a very obvious transition in the growth of the child. After birth, not only does the overall rate of growth vary at different ages, but the rates at which various segments of the body grow also differ. For example, during the first 5 years of life, sitting height and subischial leg length increase at about the same rate; from 5 years of age to puberty, the sitting height accounts for one-third of the gain and the subischial limb length accounts for two-thirds; from puberty to maturity, the ratio is reversed, with the sitting height accounting for two-thirds of the gain in height and the subischial limb length accounting for one-third. The extent of increase in sitting height and subischial leg length for boys and girls of various ages are shown [20, 22–24, 26].

At birth, the standing height of the neonate (50–54 cm) is 30% of the final height. By 5 years of age, the standing height increases to 108 cm, which is double the birth height and 62% of the final height. The first year of life sees particularly vigorous growth rates, with the infant's height increasing by 22cm. This means that the height gain during a single year is as great as it is during the entire surge of puberty. After the age of 1 year, the growth rate starts to slow down but remains strong, with the infant growing another 11cm between 1 and 2 years of age, and 7cm between 3 and 4 years of age.

At birth, the sitting height of the neonate is approximately 34cm, which is roughly two-thirds of the standing height and 37% of the final sitting height. The sitting height gains about 12cm from birth to age 1; 5.3cm from 1 to 2; 3.3cm from 2 to 3; and 3.2cm from 3 to 4; 2.8cm from 4 to 5 (average). In 5 years, the trunk gains about 28cm for girls, 29 for boys, much more than during the puberty spurt (11.5cm for girls, 13cm for boys!).

During the first 5 years of growth after birth, the proportions change. The cephalic end of the body becomes relatively smaller, whereas the subischial leg length increases

During this period, growth is not only a vertical phenomenon but also a volumetric one. At birth, weight is between 3,000 and 3,500g, which is 5% of the final figure.

At 5 years of age, the weight averages 18–20kg, which is 32% of *the* final adult weight. In 5 years, the weight gain is 15–17kg. Birth weight triples in a single year and quadruples by the age of 3 years.

The circumference of the chest is 32cm at birth but increases by 25cm to reach 57cm by the age of 5 years [2, 3, 8, 45]. Chest morphology has undergone dramatic changes (Figs. 2.5, 2.6).

2.3.3 From 5 Years to Beginning of Puberty

Between 5 years of age and the onset of puberty, 11 years of bone age in girls and 13 years of bone age in boys, there is a marked deceleration in growth, with standing height increasing at approximately 5.5cm/year. About two-thirds of this growth (3.2cm) occurs in the lower limb and about one-third (2.3cm) occurs in the sitting height. The trunk is now growing at a slower rate, whereas the lower limbs are growing faster than the trunk, thereby altering the proportions of the body. During this period, in boys, standing height will increase by 27% (approximately 44cm), sitting height by 20% (approximately 18cm), and subischial limb length by 32% (approximately 26cm); in girls, standing height will increase by 22% (approximately 34cm), sitting height by 17% (approximately 14cm), and subischial limb length by 28% (approximately 20cm) [20, 22–24, 26].

From 5 years of age to the beginning of puberty, the average weight gain is about 2.5kg/year [26]. At 10 years of age, the weight represents about 50% of the final weight. In contrast, the standing height at this age is 78% of the final standing height in the case of boys and 83% in the case of girls [26].

By 5 years of age, the sitting height increases to 60cm, approximately 66% of the final sitting height, with only another 26–30cm to grow. This information is useful in anticipating the effects of deformity and the consequences of arthrodesis in spinal deformity in young patients.

2.3.4 Puberty: A Turning Point

At the beginning of puberty, approximately 22.5cm of growth remains to be attained in standing height (12.5cm in sitting height and 10cm in lower limb) in the case of boys and 20.5cm (11.5cm in sitting height and 9cm in lower limb) in the case of girls (Figs. 2.7–2.10).

Chronologic age is a poor indicator of puberty. We may start anticipating puberty at 10 years of age in girls and 12 years in boys. The acceleration in growth velocity best characterizes the beginning of puberty. From a clinical viewpoint, puberty will be recognized by a combination of factors other than growth: sexual development, chronologic age, and bone age. After 11 years of age, the growth patterns of boys and girls proceed differently. On an average, girls will experience the onset of puberty at 11 years (bone age), and boys at 13 years (bone age). Puberty and its accompanying rapid growth is a period of great importance to the orthopedic surgeon. It is therefore crucial to recognize the period just before puberty.

There are four main characteristics that dominate the phase of growth called puberty:

1. Dramatic increase in stature
2. Change in the proportions of the upper and lower body segments
3. Change in overall morphology: biachromial diameter, pelvic diameter, fat distribution, and so on [32]
4. Development of secondary sexual characteristics

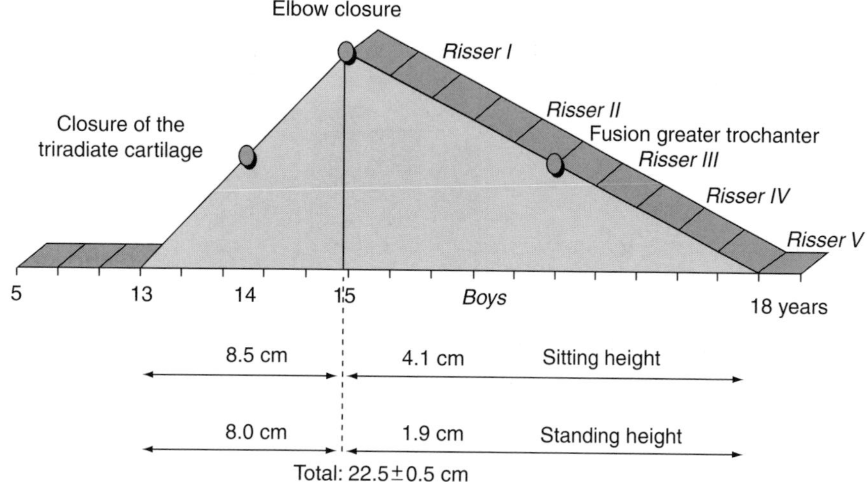

Fig. 2.7 Pubertal diagram in boys

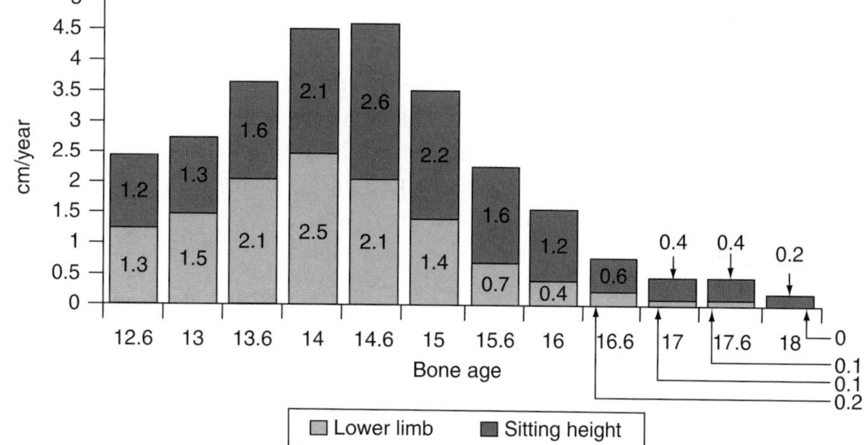

Fig. 2.8 Growth velocity for bone age (boys). The peak velocity of growth during puberty occurs between 13 and 15 years of bone age in boys

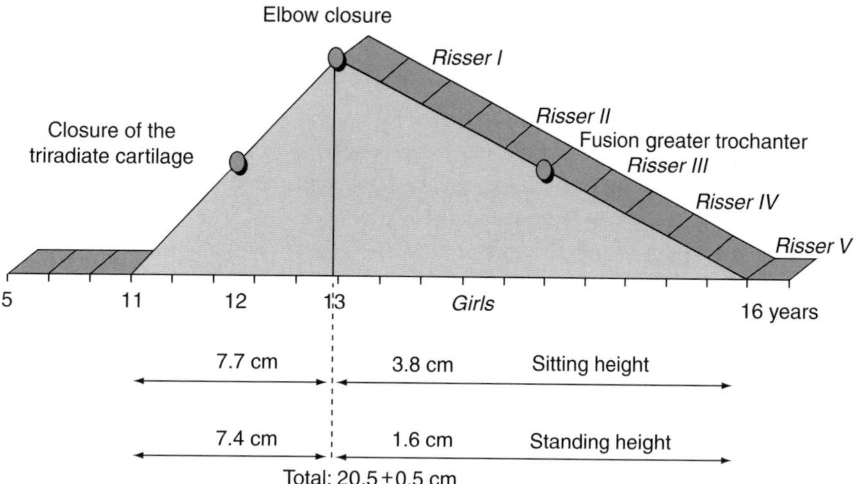

Fig. 2.9 Pubertal diagram for girls

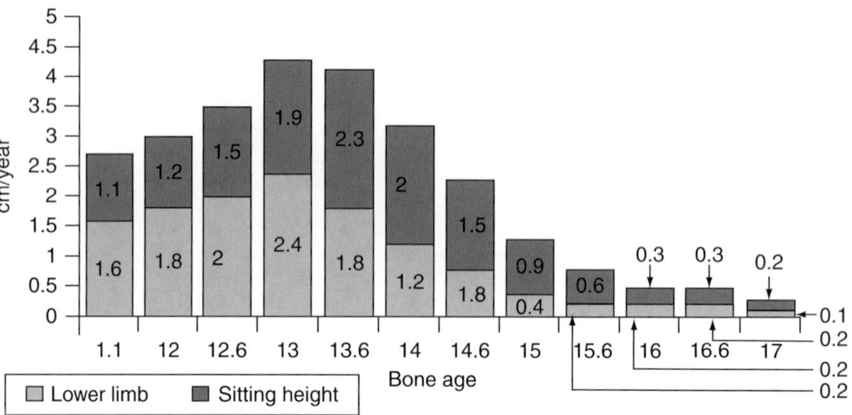

Fig. 2.10 Growth velocity for bone age (girls). Menarche usually occurs on the descending side, after elbow closure at 13 years 6 months bone age, around Risser I

During puberty from 11 to 15 years of age in girls and from 13 to 17 years in boys there is a dramatic increase in the growth rate. However, during this period, the growth is far more noticeable in the trunk than in the lower limbs: two-thirds of the growth goes toward increasing sitting height and only one-third is toward increasing subischial limb length. It is during this period that boys overtake girls in height. On an average, boys are between 12 and 15 cm taller than girls. This is accounted for by two factors. First, boys have approximately 2 years of growth more than girls. Second, boys have a slightly greater increase in the rate of growth during puberty than do girls, accounting for approximately 2 cm of additional height [20, 24, 26].

During puberty, the standing height increases by approximately 1 cm/month. At the onset of puberty, boys have 14% (±1%) of their remaining standing height to grow; this is approximately 22.5 cm (±1 cm), made up of 12.5 cm in sitting height and 10 cm in subischial limb length. Girls have 13% (±1%) of their standing height to grow. This is approximately 20.5 cm (±1 cm), made up of 11.5 cm in sitting height and 9 cm in subischial leg length.

The peak velocity of growth during puberty occurs between 13 and 15 years of bone age in boys and between 11 and 13 years of bone age in girls. After bone age of 13 years in girls and 15 years in boys, there is a considerable decrease in the annual velocity of height gain. The lower limbs stop growing rapidly; the total remaining growth is 5.5 cm, about 4 cm in the sitting height and about 1.5 cm in the lower limb. This variation in growth velocity is an extremely important factor to consider in the treatment of many disorders, especially scoliosis and limb-length discrepancy.

These figures, ratios, and rates provide only a partial view of the growth phenomenon. Precise evaluation of the characteristics of puberty, using the bone age assessment, the Tanner classification, the onset of menstruation, the Risser sign, and the annual height velocity, is something that needs to be undertaken with a great deal of care and consideration. One of the major problems with using only the onset of menarche and the Risser sign is that, they occur after the growth associated with puberty has begun to slow.

2.3.5 Secondary Sexual Characteristics

Secondary sexual characteristics develop throughout the course of puberty; the first appearance of pubic hair, the budding of the nipples, and the swelling of the testes are the first physical signs to signal the onset of puberty. The first physical sign of puberty in boys, testicular growth in 77%, occurs, on average, 1.7 years before the peak height velocity and 3.5 years before attaining adult height [53].

The bone age will be approximately 13 years at the onset of puberty; the Risser sign is 0 and the triradiate cartilage is open.

The first physical sign of puberty in girls, breast budding in 93%, occurs about 1 year before peak height velocity [26]. This averages 11 years in bone age. The Risser sign is still 0, and the triradiate cartilage is still open at the onset of puberty. Menarche occurs about 2 years after breast budding, and final height is usually achieved 2.5–3 years after menarche. After menarche, girls will gain the final 5% of their standing height, about 3–5 cm [26]. The appearance of axillary hair, although variable, occurs after the peak of the pubertal growth diagram.

The secondary sexual characteristics generally develop in harmony with bone age, but there are discrepancies in 10% of cases. Puberty may be accelerated and growth can end more quickly than usual, catching the unwary physician off guard. In fact, it has been demonstrated that it is not uncommon to see an acceleration of the bone age during puberty.

2.3.6 Pubertal Diagram and Peak Height Velocity *(Figs. 2.7–2.10)*

Using all of these landmarks, it is possible to draw a diagram relating the events occurring during puberty. Even if one indicator is missing or does not match the other, it is still possible to have a good idea of where the child is, on his or her own path through puberty. By plotting the gains in standing height and sitting height every 6 months, a picture of the period of puberty is developed. It is also easy to divide this into two parts. The first phase (i.e., the ascending phase of the growth velocity curve) is characterized by an increase in the velocity of growth and is the major portion of the pubertal growth spurt. The second phase (i.e., the descending phase of the growth velocity curve) is characterized by a slowing of the rate of growth [57].

The first phase of the pubertal growth spurt is the ascending phase, which corresponds to the acceleration in the velocity of growth. This phase lasts 2 years, from approximately 11–13 years of bone age in girls and from 13 to 15 years of bone age in boys. The gain in standing height in girls during this phase is about 15.1 cm, made up of 7.7 cm in sitting height and 7.4 cm in subischial limb length. The gain in standing height in boys during this phase is about 16.5 cm, made up of 8.5 cm in sitting height and 8 cm in subischial limb length. During this first phase of pubertal growth spurt, the increase in sitting height contributes 53% and the increase in subischial length contributes 47%. Therefore, more growth comes from the trunk than from the legs during this phase growth.

The peak height velocity occurs on the ascending side of the growth velocity curve. It does not occur at just one point on the curve but takes place during a period of 2 years [26, 54]. It can be roughly identified by accurate assessment of standing height and sitting height at 6-month interval.

Triradiate cartilage closure occurs about halfway up the ascending phase of the pubertal growth velocity diagram. This closure corresponds to an approximate bone age of 12 years in girls and 14 years in boys. After closure of the triradiate cartilage, there is still a considerable amount of growth remaining: greater than 12 cm of standing height in girls and more than 14 cm in boys. Sanders et al. [54] has shown that the crankshaft phenomenon decreases substantially after closure of the tri-radiate cartilage.

The second phase of the pubertal growth spurt is the descending side, which corresponds to the deceleration of the velocity of growth. The closure of the elbow (discussed in subsequent text) divides the ascending and descending phases of puberty. The descending phase lasts 3 years from 13 to 16 years of bone age in girls and from 15 to 18 years of bone age in boys. During this phase, both boys and girls will gain about 6 cm in standing height, with 4.5 cm attained from an increase in sitting height and 1.5 cm attained from an increase in subischial limb length. During this phase, the increase in sitting height contributes 80% of the gain in the standing height [20, 22, 24, 26].

Menarche usually occurs after closure of the olecranon apophysis, on the descending phase of the growth curve when the rate of growth is slowing. This decrease in rate of growth is usually between bone ages of 13, and 13 years 6 months and corresponds to Risser sign I on the iliac apophysis. After this stage, the average girl will gain an additional 4 cm of sitting height and 0.6 cm of subischial limb length. Menarche is not as precise as many other indicators during puberty. Forty-two percent of girls experience menarche before Risser I, 31% at Risser II, 8% at Risser III, and 5% at Risser IV [20, 22, 24, 26]; after 2 years of menarche, there is no more growth.

The descending phase of puberty is characterized by a significant growth of the thorax (Fig. 2.11).

During puberty, the peak growth is a combination of three micropeaks: the first peak involves the lower limb at the very beginning of this period, and the second peak involves the trunk (these two peaks are on the ascending phase of the growth velocity curve); the third peak involves growth of the thorax and occurs during the descending phase of the curve.

At skeletal maturity, the final standing height is about 175 cm (±6.6 cm) for boys and about 166 cm (±6 cm) for girls.

Puberty is characterized by a great increase in weight. At the beginning of puberty, the average weight

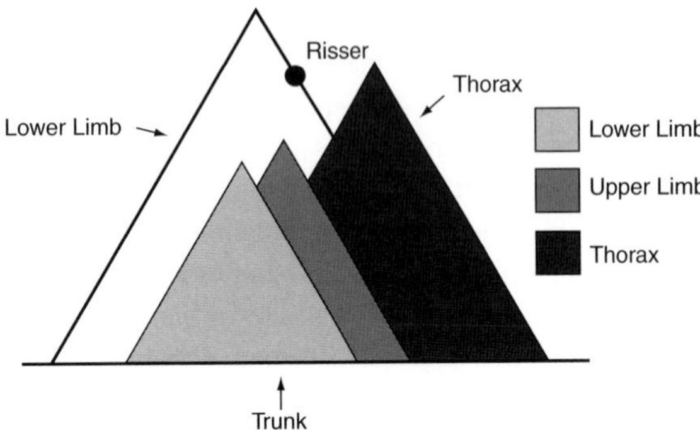

Fig. 2.11 During puberty, the peak growth is a combination of three micropeaks: 1, lower limb growth peak; 2, trunk growth peak; and 3, thorax growth peak

is 40 kg for boys and 33 kg for girls. At skeletal maturity, the average weight of boys is 65 kg (a gain of 25 kg) and the average weight of girls is 56 kg (a gain of 23 kg). During the growth spurt of puberty, the average gain in weight each year is 5 kg [20, 24, 26].

2.4 Estimation of Skeletal Maturity

In pediatric orthopaedics, chronologic age is of no significance. Everything depends on bone age. Personal data indicate that about 50% of children have a bone age that is significantly different from their chronologic age. Delayed bone age is characteristic of severe cerebral palsy (total body) involvement. All, reasoning, analyses, forecasting, and decision making, should be based on bone age [2, 14, 19, 20, 22, 24, 25, 55, 56, 58].

Accurate assessment of bone age is not easy. The younger the child, especially before puberty, the more difficult it is to determine future growth, and the more likely it is for errors to be made. In addition, children are often bone age mosaics. Bone age determinations carried out in the hands, elbows, pelvis, and knees will not always agree with one another.

Often, the bone age determination is made too quickly and with too little information. The standard deviations for determining bone age must be understood, as well as the nuances of what to look for in the interpretation of the radiograph. When using a particular method (e.g., the Greulich and Pyle Atlas), [33] it is important to read the entire book to understand what to look for and to know the standard error, rather than simply comparing radiographs. If there is a major decision to be made, it is better to have two interpretations of the child's bone age and to enlist the support of pediatric radiologists with experience in bone age determination.

Cundy et al. [19] demonstrated that four radiologists' interpretations of skeletal age differed by more than 2 years in 10% of patients.

Carpenter and Lester [14] evaluated bone age in children younger than 10 years. They showed that taking separate readings of the distal radius and ulna, the carpal bones, the metacarpals, and the phalanges could magnify these errors, and that the ages of the carpal bones and the distal radius and ulna often lag behind the ages of the metacarpals and phalanges. This means that excessive haste in reading the bone age can result in fatal strategic errors.

There are three basic approaches to the radiographic assessment of skeletal maturity: atlas, sum of scores, and statistical combination of scores. Knowledge of these methods and their limitations is important for the orthopedist, especially in difficult cases. The Greulich and Pyle Atlas [33] is the most familiar and commonly applied approach and involves qualitatively matching the subject's hand and wrist radiographs against a series of gender-specific standards. This atlas is based on a collection of radiographs of children born between 1917 and 1942. In comparing this atlas with its French counterpart, Sempé and Pavia Atlas [56], we learned that there is no major difference between these two atlases. One of the shortcomings in using the Greulich and Pyle Atlas is that there are few changes in the hand during the critical time of puberty (ascending side of pubertal growth velocity diagram) [20, 26, 28].

For this reason, the author has found the method by Sauvegrain et al. [25, 55] to be of enormous value in assessing children during puberty. This method is the scoring system that evaluates anteroposterior and lateral views of the elbow and assigns a value to the epiphyses. This value is then plotted on a chart to give the bone age. Four ossification centers are taken into consideration: condyle and epicondyle, trochlea, olecranon, and radial epiphysis. This method is reliable and is based on the skeletal maturation of the elbow, which occurs during a 2-year period corresponding to the ascending phase of the growth velocity curve. Therefore, it is extremely helpful in boys aged 13–15 years and in girls aged 11–13 years, a period in which many of the clinical decisions involving future growth are made (spinal arthrodesis). In addition, it shows good correlation with the Greulich and Pyle Atlas but is much easier to use.

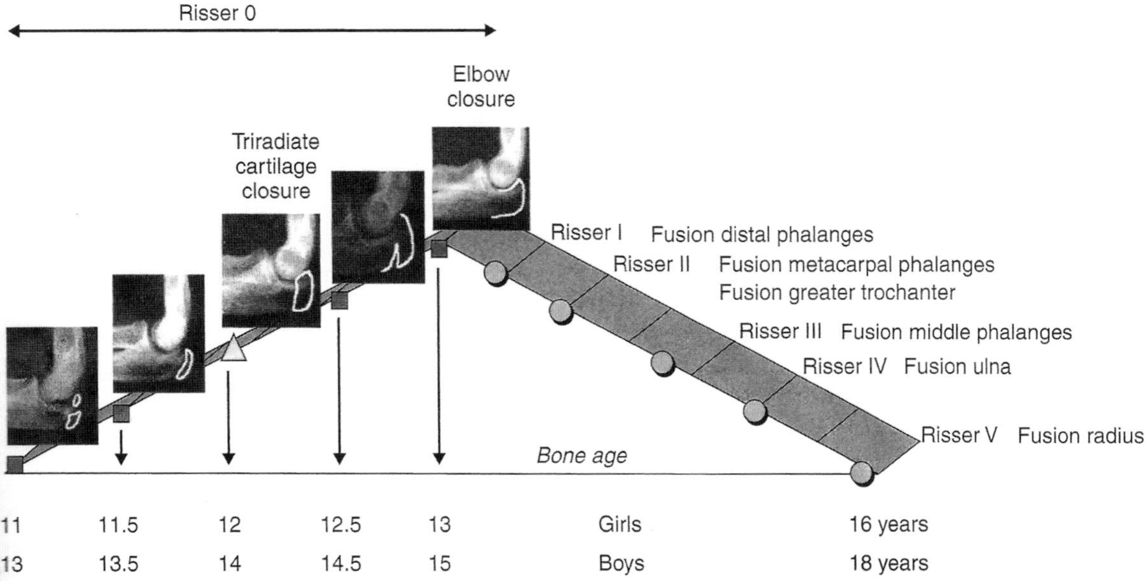

Fig. 2.12 Examination of skeletal maturity (bone age) by Olecranon method (described by Dimeglio)

At the beginning of puberty, growth centers of the elbow are wide open, but 2 years later, when the peak velocity of the pubertal growth spurt is reached and growth begins to slowdown, they are all completely closed. This complete closure occurs 6 months before Risser I. In the method by Sauvegrain et al., the olecranon is the bone that shows the most characteristic and clear-cut sequences during the first 2 years of puberty [17, 25]. For this reason, the author has described the olecranon method, at the beginning of puberty (at bone age of 11 years in girls and 13 years in boys), two ossification centers appear (Fig. 2.12). Six months later (at bone age of 11.5 years in girls and 13.5 years in boys), they merge to form a half-moon shape. At bone age of 12 years in girls and 14 years in boys, the olecranon apophysis has a rectangular appearance. Six months later (at bone age of 12.5 years in girls and 14.5 years in boys), the olecranon apophysis begins to fuse with the ulna, a process that takes another 6 months, being completed by the bone age of 13 years in girls and 15 years in boys. In our clinical practice experience, the olecranon alone can give rapid and valuable information about bone age. The olecranon method is more accurate in itself because it allows differentiation of bone age in semesters, which is not true for the Greulich and Pyle Atlas for the considered time of puberty [33].

Other methods are described: the Tanner et al. [58] system scores 20 indicators on hand and wrist radiograph, yielding total scores ranging from 0 to 100. The Fels method is a sophisticated approach, scoring hand and wrist radiographs and using a computer program. Both of these methods are time consuming and not useful in daily practice.

The Oxford scoring method for assessing skeletal maturity from pelvic radiographs is based on nine indicators, three of which are useful during puberty: the triradiate cartilage, the greater trochanter, and the Risser sign [2]. The triradiate cartilage dosure occurs on the ascending side of the pubertal growth diagram at bone age of 12 years in girls and 14 years in boys. After its dosure, a significant amount of growth in standing height still remains: 13 cm in girls and 14 cm in boys. The greater trochanter dosure occurs on the descending phase of the pubertal growth diagram, at bone age of 14 years in girls and 16 years in boys (i.e., between Risser II and Risser III).

2.5 The Concept of Risser sign is Misleading (Figs. 2.13, 2.14)

The Risser sign is one of the most commonly used markers of skeletal maturation, especially in the treatment of scoliosis. The sign appears on the radiograph of the pelvis, which is often studied during the assessment of

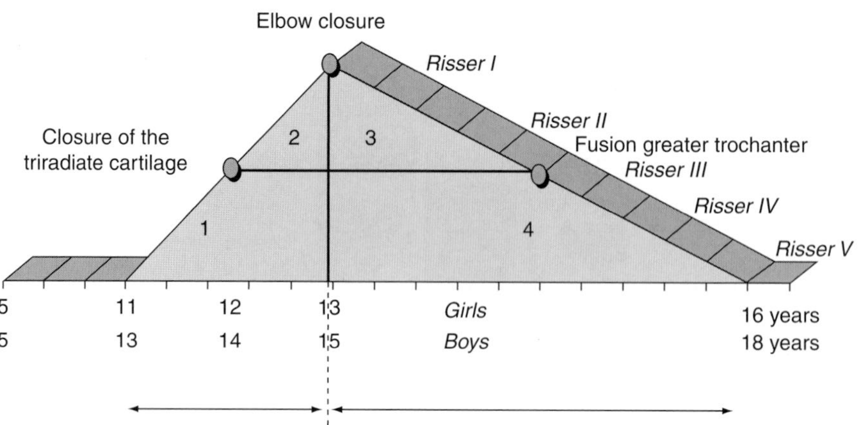

Fig. 2.13 Pubertal diagram and Risser stages

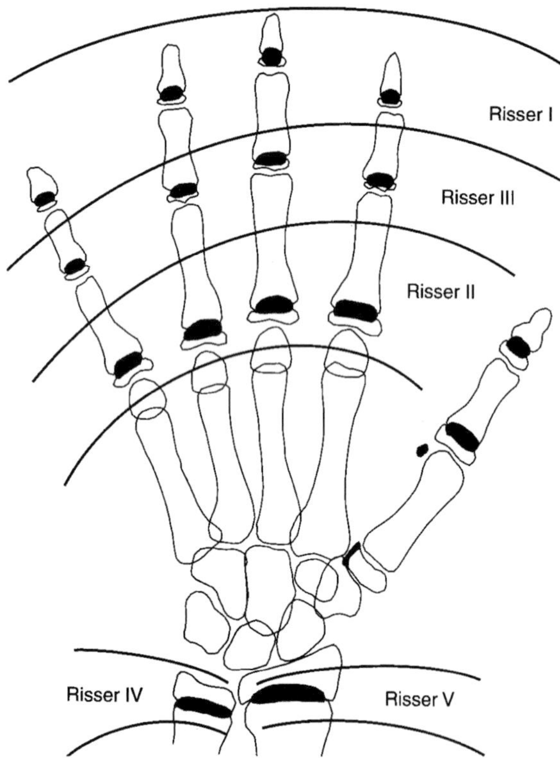

Fig. 2.14 Epiphyseal closure and Risser stages in hand

this disorder, thereby obviating the need for an additional radiograph. The duration of excursion of the Risser sign is also variable, and may range from 1 to 3 years [4]. However, the value of this sign in accurate decision making has been questioned. Little and Sussman [43] concluded that, all things considered, it is better to rely on chronologic age. Although the author does not agree with their conclusions, when important decisions are made, the Risser sign should be supplemented with the bone age, as determined by the method of Greulich and Pyle [33].

Risser 0 covers the first two-thirds of the pubertal growth, which corresponds to the ascending limb of the pubertal growth diagram. However, this period of Risser 0 is important in decision making in many conditions; therefore, it is important to have more precise markers of stage of puberty (growth) during this period, such annual growth velocity, elbow maturation (olecranon), and changes in morphology of the triradiate cartilage [16]. Risser 0 gives little information, other than indicating that the peak of the growth velocity curve has not been reached [16]. The author has recommended dividing this period of the ascending phase of the pubertal growth diagram, characterized by Risser 0, into three periods, based on the triradiate cartilage and the closure of the olecranon apophysis: triradiate cartilage open, triradiate cartilage closed but olecranon open, and olecranon closed [17, 20, 22, 24, 26].

Risser I heralds the beginning of the descending slope of the pubertal growth velocity diagram. It generally appears after the elbow closure, when the epiphyses of the distal phalanges (II, III, IV, and V) of the hand fuse. The rate of growth in sitting height and standing height decreases abruptly. Axillary hair generally appears during this period [17, 20, 22, 24, 26].

Risser II corresponds to a bone age of 14 years in girls and 16 years in boys. It generally appears when the greater trochanteric apophysis unites with the femur. When the proximal phalangeal epiphyses fuse in the hand, there is approximately 3 cm left to grow in sitting height and no more growth of the lower limb.

Risser III corresponds to bone ages of 14.5 years in girls and 16.5 years in boys. The phalangeal epiphyses of P1 and P2 fuse during this period; the greater trochanter is closed; and 1 year of growth and an increase of 2 cm in sitting height still remain.

Risser IV corresponds to a bone age of 15 years in girls and 17 years in boys. The distal epiphysis of the ulna is united to the shaft. At this stage, the remaining growth in sitting height is 1 cm.

Risser V is very much like Risser 0: it is a long period that does not provide much information to the dinician. The distal radial epiphysis generally fuses around Risser V. The iliac apophysis may fuse at age 22 or 23 years, but in some cases it never fuses [7].

Regardless of the method of its determination, bone age is meaningless as an isolated parameter. It should be constantly measured against chronologic age, the rate of annual growth in standing height, and secondary sexual characteristics [53].

Before 10 years of age, evaluation of bone age is difficult: the appearance of the ossification center on the hand or on the elbow can give useful informations but the most important is to look at the growth curves of the standing and sitting height, and mainly the weight, to evaluate the biologic age.

On the ascending side of puberty, olecranon evaluation is more precise than the hand; on the descending side of puberty, ossification centers of the hand must be balanced with the Risser sign [25].

2.6 Growth of the Trunk

2.6.1 Growth in the Spinal Column

Measurement of sitting height provides an indirect indication of spinal growth. The spine makes up 60% of the sitting height, whereas the head represents 20%, and the pelvis represents 20% [22]. If we accept the fact that there are at least three growth zones per vertebra (sometimes four), the resulting morphology of the spinal column is the product of 130 physes. The pattern of growth in the posterior arch, where closure is linked, in particular, to the presence of the neural stem, differs from that seen in the body of the vertebra, which behaves like a long bone [21, 22].

If one were to compare any of the vertebrae of a newborn, one would find very little morphologic variation between them. The process by which cervical, thoracic, and lumbar vertebrae acquire their individual identities is gradual. In the vertebral body, ossification first appears in the dorsal region; from this hub, the process of ossification radiates to the cranial and caudal parts of the spine. The process of ossification is extremely slow, and does not finish until the 25th year of life.

At birth, the lumbosacral vertebrae are relative smaller than the thoracic and cervical vertebrae. However during the first years of growth, they grow more rapidly. Between 3 and 15 years of age, the lumbar vertebrae and their discs increase in size by about 2 mm/year, whereas the thoracic vertebrae and their discs increase by 1 mm.

The discs account for approximately 30% of the height of the spinal segment at birth. At maturity, this proportion decreases to 25%, with the discs constituting 22% of the cervical spine, 18% of the thoracic spine, and 35% of the lumbar spine.

The anterior and posterior portions of the vertebrae do not grow at the same rate. In the thoracic region, the posterior components grow at a faster pace than their anterior counterparts. The reverse occurs in the lumbar region. Growth potential therefore varies from one level to the next, differing from anterior to posterior. In addition, as the vertebrae develop, there is a constant remodeling of the anatomic organization of the spine; for example, the articular apophyses change in both morphology and direction.

The neurocentral synchondroses is at the junction between the vertebral body and the posterior arch. There are two physes developing in two directions, the neurocentral physes contribute to 30% of the ossification of the vertebral body and participate mostly in the posterior arch ossification.

Zhang et al. [64] have studied in normal children, the evolution of the neurocentral synchondroses by MRI axial images. The neurocentral growth plate is opened in all patients less than 3 years. It closes from the lumbar and proximal thoracic spine to the middle and distal thoracic spine. At 4 years, the neurocentral synchondroses had 50–74% closure in the lumbar region. At 5 years, the proximal thoracic (T1–T6) had 25% less closure with the middle T7–T9 and distal (T10–T12) thoracic demonstrated no closure. At 9 years, the neurocentral synchondroses of the spine are closed. This excellent study provided significant information for growing modulation treatment of early onset deformities.

The length of the spine will nearly triple between birth and adulthood. At birth, the vertebral column is approximately 24cm long. In the newborn, only 30% of the spine is ossified. There is little substantial difference in morphology between one vertebra and another. The length of a thoracic vertebra is about 7.6mm and that of a lumbar vertebra is about 8 mm [22]. The average adult spine is approximately 70cm long in men, with the cervical spine measuring 12cm, the thoracic spine 28cm, the lumbar spine 18cm, and the sacrum 12cm. The average female spine is approximately 63cm long at maturity [21, 22].

2.6.2 Cervical Spine

At birth, the cervical spine measures 3.7cm; it will grow about 9cm, to reach the adult length of 12–13cm. The length of the cervical spine will nearly double by 6 years of age. It will gain an additional 3.5cm during the pubertal growth spurt. The cervical spine represents 22% of the C1 S1 segment and 15–16% of sitting height.

The diameter of the cervical spinal canal varies with location, typically decreasing in width from Cl to C7 or from C1 to C3, and then widening slightly. These differences are important in the clinical setting because the room available for the spinal cord can be very consequential. It should be remembered that, regardless of the size of the child (e.g., in dwarfing conditions), the spinal cord will attain the usual adult diameter. The average width of the cervical cord is 13.2mm, and the average anteroposterior depth is 7.7mm [22]. Therefore, the transverse and sagittal diameters of the cervical canal are important. In the adult, at C3, the norrmal transverse diameter is 27mm and the average sagittal diameter is approximately 19mm. The cervical canal is wide enough to permit the entry of the thumb of an adult finger.

2.6.3 T1–S1 Segment *(Figs. 2.15, 2.16)*

The Tl–S1 segment is very important because the most frequent disorders of the spine during growth originate in this segment. The Tl-S1 segment measures about 19cm at birth, and 45cm at the end of growth in the average man, and 42–43cm in the average woman. This segment makes up 49% of the sitting height at maturity. Knowledge of the effects of arthrodesis on this segment of the spine requires precise knowledge of the growth remaining at various ages (Figs. 2.17, 2.18).

2.6.4 Thoracic Spine T1–T12 *(Figs. 2.19, 2.20)*

The thoracic spine is about 11cm long at birth and reaches a length of about 28cm in boys and 26cm in girls at the end of growth. Its length more than doubles between birth and the end of the growth period. The growth of the thoracic segment has a rapid phase from birth to 5 years of age (7cm), a slower phase from 5 to 10 years of age (4cm), and rapid growth through puberty (7cm) [22–24, 26]. The T1–T12 segment represents 30% of the sitting height, so a single thoracic vertebra and its disc represents 2.5% of the sitting height. By knowing the amount of growth that each vertebra contributes to the final height, the effect of a circumferential arthrodesis, which stops all growth in the vertebrae and discs, can be calculated [21, 22, 24, 26].

Posterior arthrodesis results in only one-third of this deficit (2.5% of sitting height for each thoracic vertebra), which is about 0.8% of the remaining sitting height.

The thoracic spinal canal is narrower than either the lumbar or the cervical canals. At the age of 5 years, this canal attains its maximum volume, and is wide enough to permit the entry of the little finger of an adult hand. The average of the transverse and anteroposterior diameters at T7 is approximately 15mm.

2.6.5 Lumbar Spine *(L1–L5)*

The L1–L5 lumbar spine is approximately 7cm in length at birth, and it grows to approximately 16cm in men and 15.5cm in women. As in the thoracic spine, growth is not linear: there is rapid growth from 0 to 5 years of age (gain of about 3cm); slow growth from 5 to 10 years (gain of about 2cm); and rapid growth again from 10 to 18 years of age (gain of about 3cm). The height of the lumbar spine doubles between birth and maturity (Figs. 2.21, 2.22).

The lumbar spine represents 18% of the sitting height and a single lumbar vertebra and its disc account for 3.5 of the sitting height. Values for the remaining growth of the lumbar segment at various ages are given

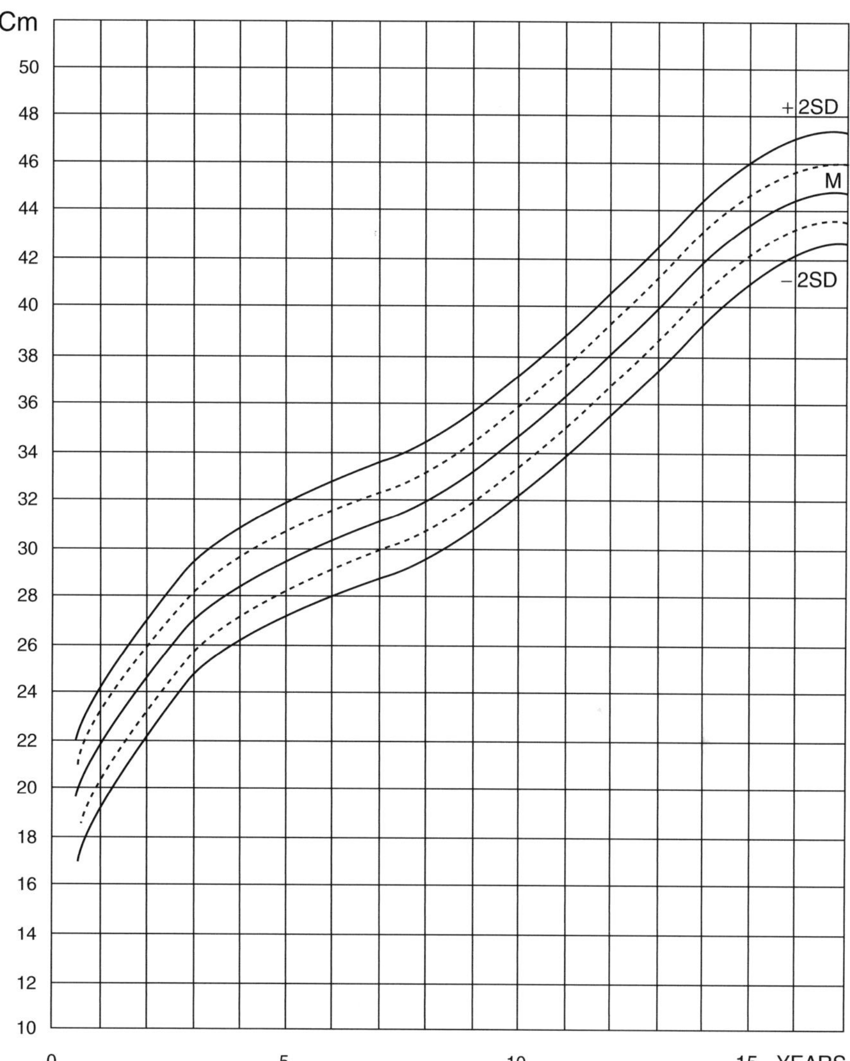

Fig. 2.15 T1–S1segment length-for-age (birth to skeletal maturity: boys)

in figures. A posterior vertebral arthrodesis results in a deficit of only one-third of this value, that is, slightly more than 1% of the remaining sitting height.

At the skeletal age of 10 years, the lumber spine reaches 90% of its final height but only 60% of its final volume. The medullar canal in the lumbar spine is wider than that in the thoracic spine. At skeletal maturity, the dimensions of the canals are such that the adult thumb can be introduced into the cervical canal, the forefinger into the thoracic canal, and the thumb into the lumbar canal. At birth, the spinal cord ends at L3, and at maturity, it ends between L1 and L2.

2.6.6 The Thoracic Growth is the Fourth Dimension of the Spine [20]

The thoracic circumference is a rough but valuable indicator of this fourth dimension of spinal growth. The thorax has a circumference of 32 cm at birth, and it will grow to 56 cm in boys and 53 cm in girls, that is, to almost three times of its birth size.

In boys, the thoracic circumference is 36% of its final size at birth, 63% at 5 years of age 73% at 10 years, 91% at 15 years, and 100% at 18 years. From birth to

Fig. 2.16 T1–S1segment length-for-age (birth to skeletal maturity: girls)

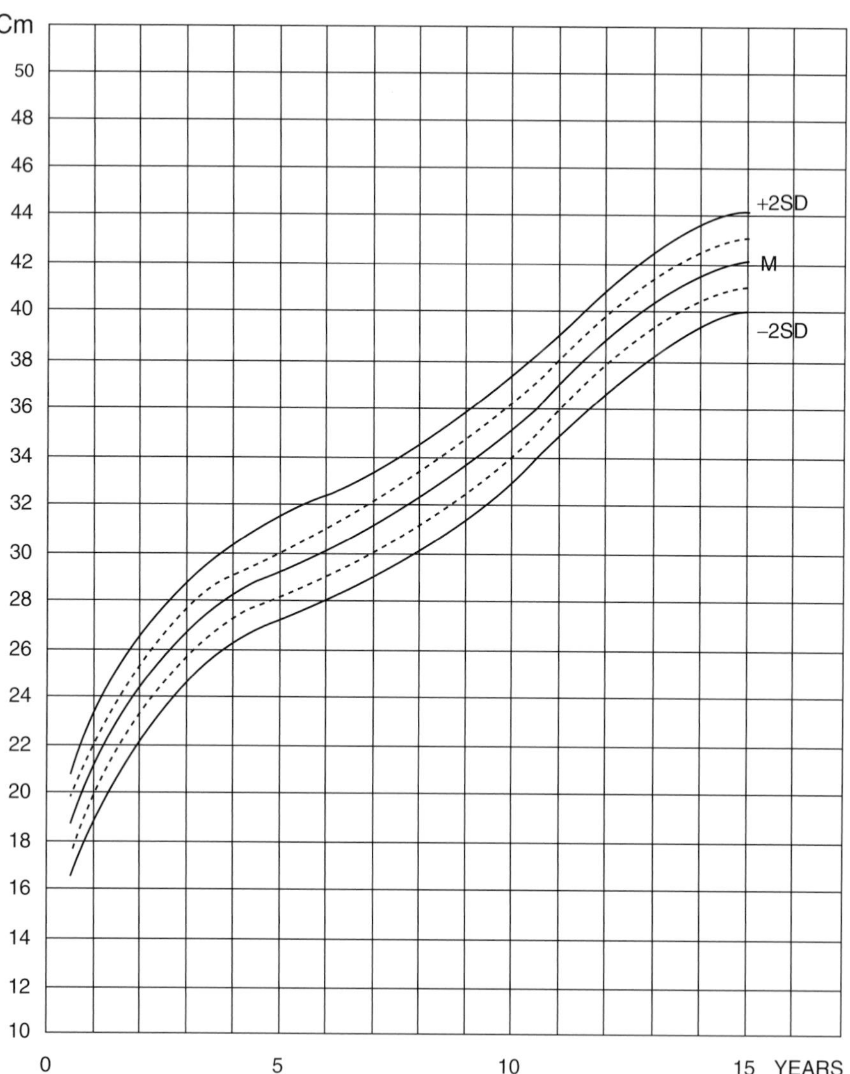

5 years of age, the thoracic circumference grows exponentially and increases by 24 cm. From the ages of 5–10 years, the increase is slower; the thoracic circumference is 66 cm at 10 years of age, which means that its growth is only 10 cm in 5 years. At that stage, it is at 73% of its final dimension. Another spurt occurs between the ages of 10 and 18 years, particularly during puberty. The thoracic circumference then increases by 23 cm, that is, as much as between birth and 5 years.

The thoracic circumference measures approximately 96% of the sitting height [22, 26]. These two meausures do not grow simultaneously, especially during puberty. At 10 years of age the thoracic circumference is at 74% of its final size, whereas the sitting height is almost at 80% of the expected measurement at the end of growth. The transverse and anteroposterior diameters, which can be measured with obstetrical calipers, are two more parameters to assess the growth of the thorax. At the end of growth, the thorax has an anteroposterior diameter of about 21 cm in boys and 17 cm in girls; that is, it has increased by 9 cm since birth. The transverse diameter is 28 cm in boys and 24 cm in girls at the end of growth; that is, it has increased by 14 cm since birth. The transversal

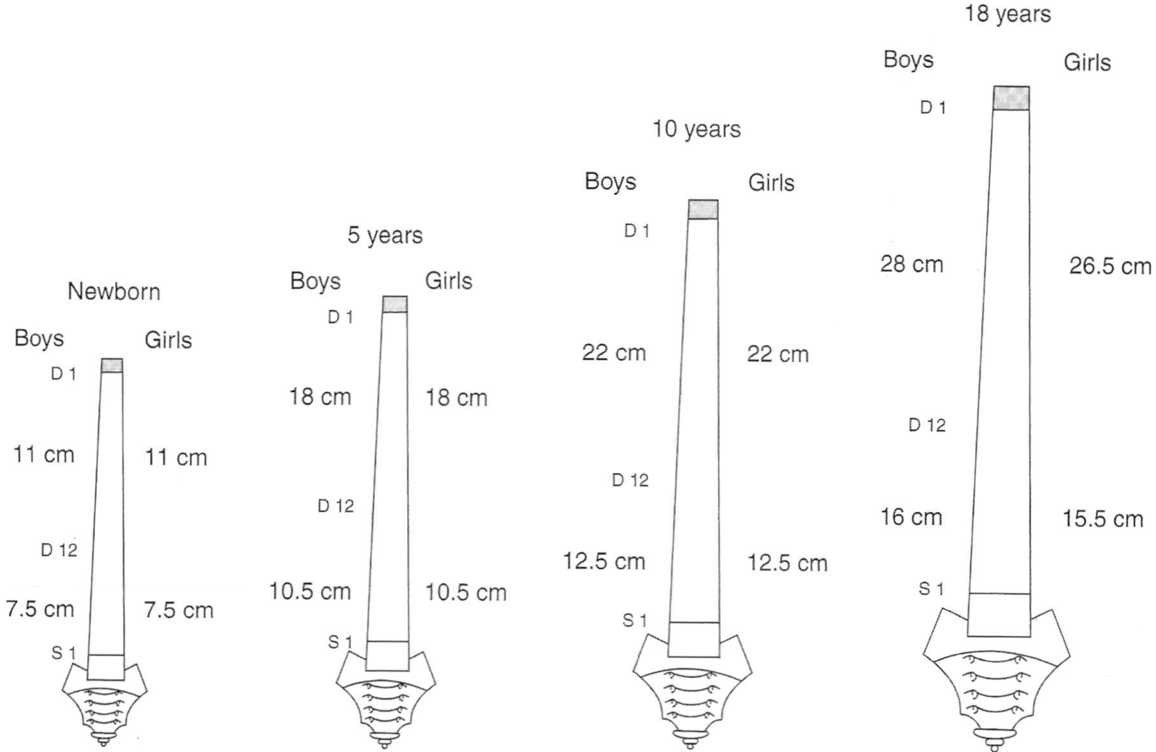

Fig. 2.17 Evaluation of T1–S1; thoracic segment T1–T12, and lumbar segment L1–L5 at birth, 5, 10 and 18 years (the figures are average values)

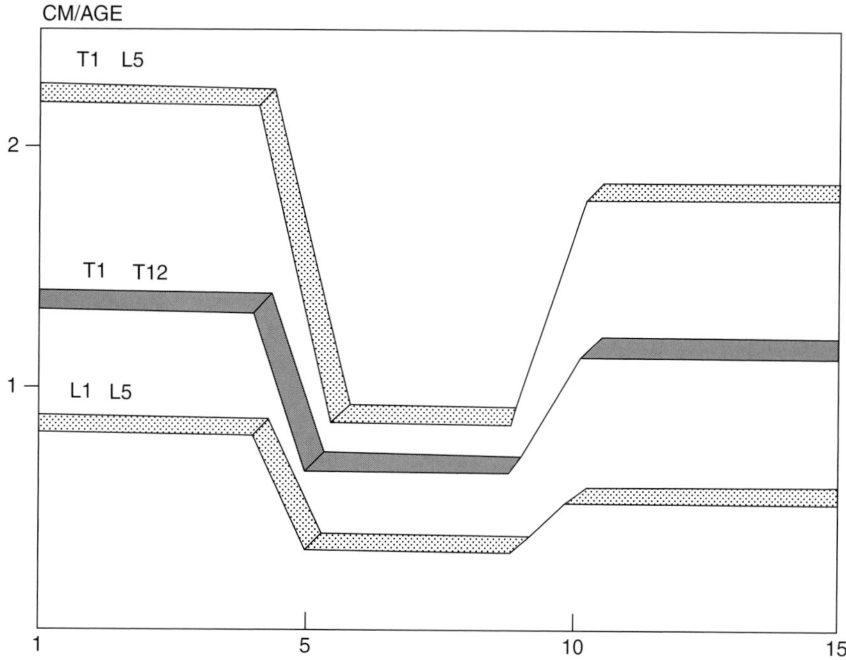

Fig. 2.18 Growth velocity of T1–L5, thoracic segment T1–T12, and lumbar segment L1–L5

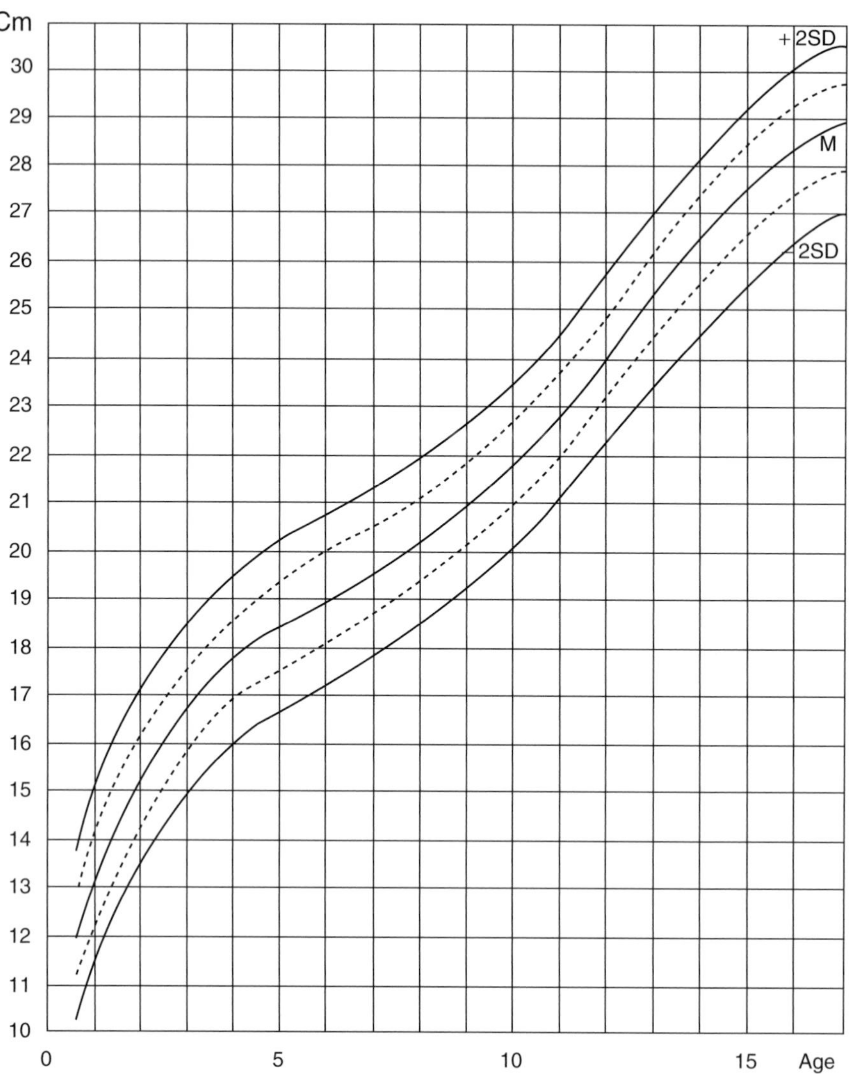

Fig. 2.19 T1–T12 segment length-for-age (birth to skeletal maturity: boys)

diameter makes up 30% of the sitting height and the anteroposterior diameter constitutes 20%. The sum of the measurements of the transverse and anteroposterior diameters of the thorax should equal 50% or more of the sitting height.

All parameters do not progress at the same speed, at the same pace. At 5 years of age, the increased weight and thoracic volume remain offset relative to the other parameters: sitting height and standing height. At birth the thoracic volume is about 6% [23].

At 5 years it is 30%. From birth to the age of 5, thoracic circumference grows exponentially and thoracic volume increases fivefold. During this period, the thorax experiences its most rapid growth. At 10 years it is 50%. The thoracic volume doubles between 10 years and skeletal maturity. At 5 years, the remaining growth of the thorax is about 70% and the remaining sitting height is about 35%. In treating scoliosis, the morphology of the thorax must be taken into consideration [22]. As the curve progresses, not only the growth of the spine is affected but the size of the chest cavity is diminished. This will affect the development of the lungs which can create significant respiratory problems [8–11, 28].

Campbell et al. [8–11] has described the thoracic insufficiency syndrome, defined as the inability of the thorax to support usual respiration and lung growth. The opening wedge thoracostomy increases the volumetric thoracic growth (parasol effect); Dubousset et al. [28] has shown that severe scoliosis leads to

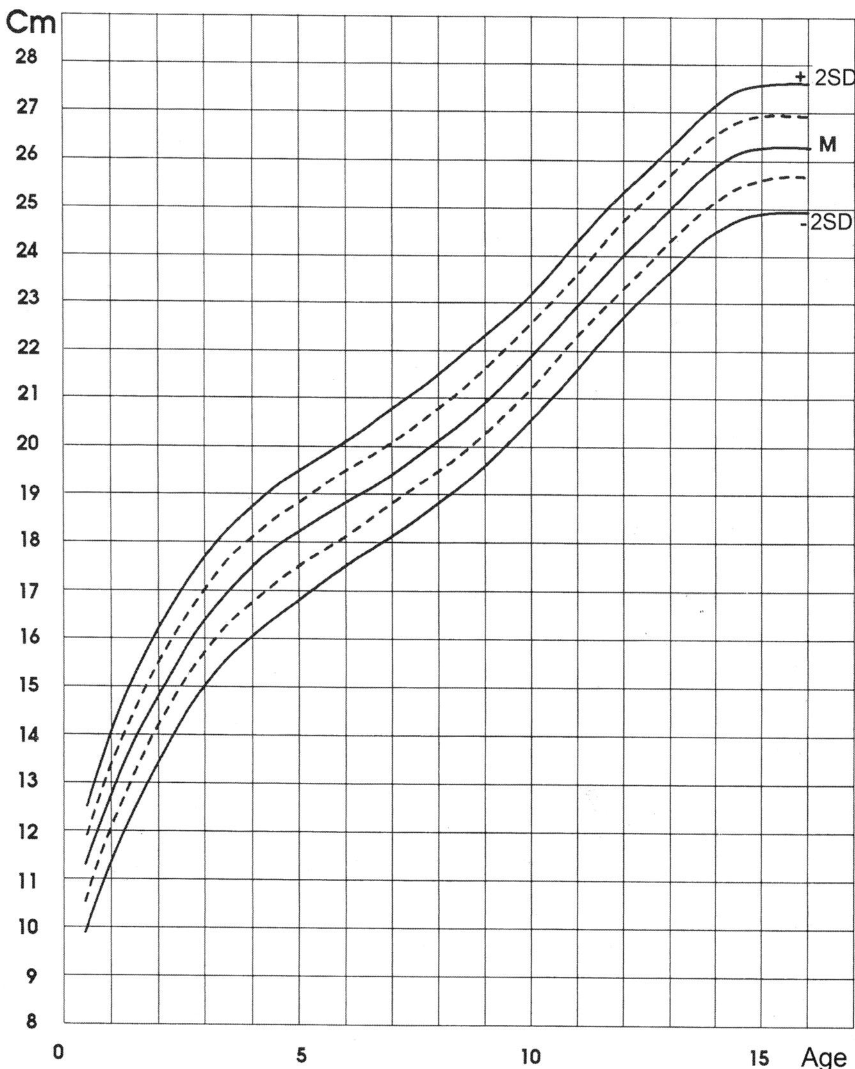

Fig. 2.20 T1–T12 segment length-for-age (birth to skeletal maturity: girls)

penetration of the vertebra inside the thorax, and has described the spinal penetration index. Severe scoliosis has a negative effect on the sitting height and the morphology of the thorax.

2.6.7 Scoliosis and Puberty

The sitting height plays an essential part in the treatment of scoliosis; unfortunately, it is not recorded often enough. Gain in sitting height always needs to be compared with angular development of the spine. This relation is ail that is needed for the proper assessment of treatment efficacy. If there is an increase of the sitting height without worsening of the curve angulation, the treatment is definitely working well. If, on the other hand, it is accompanied by deterioration of angulation, the treatment needs to be reconsidered.

When we treat scoliosis, we must also think of growth. In congenital scoliosis, the intrauterine growth and that occurring in the first few years of life can reveal a great deal about the future behavior of the spinal curvature. In idiopathic infantile and juvenile scoliosis, the growth during the first 10 years of life can be very important and may give dues to the behavior of the spinal curvature during the pubertal growth spurt [22–24, 26, 30].

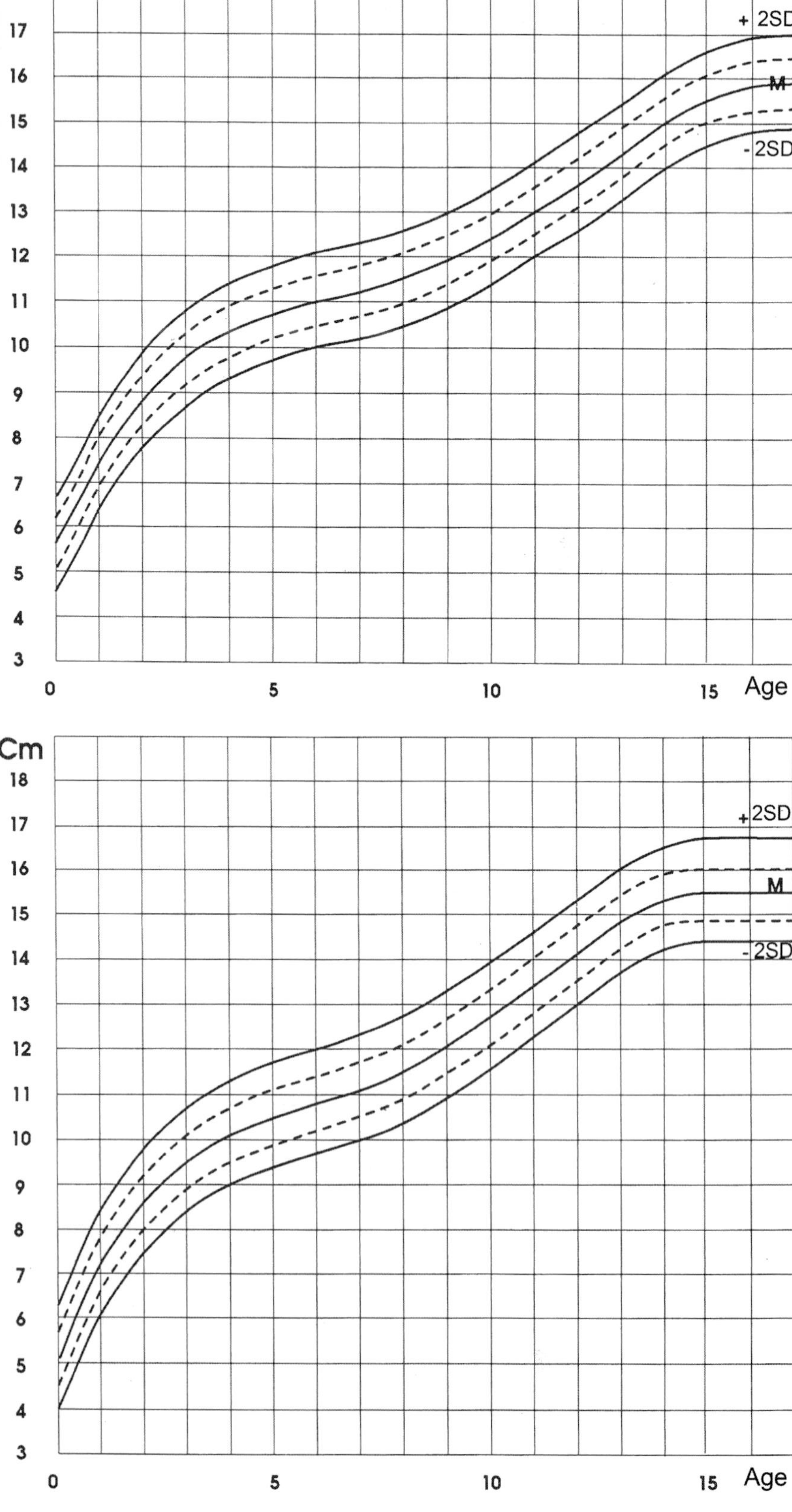

Fig. 2.21 L1–L5 segment length-for-age (birth to skeletal maturity: boys)

Fig. 2.22 L1–L5 segment length-for-age (birth to skeletal maturity: girls)

However, in adolescent idiopathic scoliosis, the most common form of scoliosis, there is no such information available before the spine begins to curve in puberty. The ultimate outcome of the curve will be determined during the pubertal growth spurt. Therefore, monitoring the behavior of the spinal curve during this short and decisive period gives the only dues to its natural history. To detect these dues, it is necessary to know the onset of puberty.

The natural history of the curve of the spine can be judged on the ascending side of the pubertal growth velocity diagram corresponding to the first 2 years of puberty (from 11 to 13 years of bone age in girls and from 13 to 15 years of bone age in boys). Any spinal curve increasing by 1° each month (12°/year) during the ascending phase of the pubertal growth diagram is likely to be a progressive curve that will require treatment. Any curve that increases by 0.5° each month during this phase must be monitored closely, whereas a curve that increases by less than 0.5° each month during this phase can be considered mild [16, 26]. This observation of the natural history of the spinal curve during the early part of puberty gives information about the behavior of the curve during the last phase of puberty, as growth is slowing, and thereby gives guidance about the frequency of follow-up visits and the duration of bracing.

2.6.8 The Scoliotic Risk

It is therefore clear that scoliotic risk evaluation plays an essential role in the treatment of the disease. During the ascending phase of the pubertal growth diagram a 5° curve is associated with a 10% risk of progression, a 10° curve represents a 20% risk, a 20° curve carries a 30% risk, and a 30° curve raises the risk to virtually 100% [15, 16, 44].

The risk of scoliosis decreases on the descending phase of the puberty growth diagram. At Risser I (13.6 years of bone age in girls and 15.6 years of bone age in boys), there is a 10% risk of progression for an angulation of 20° and a 60% risk for a 30° curve [20, 24, 26, 45] (Fig. 2.23).

At Risser II (14 years of bone age in girls and 16 years of bone age in boys), there is still a 30% risk of progression (5° or more) for a 30° curve and a 2% risk for a 20° curve [57].

At Risser III (14.6 years of bone age in girls and 16.6 years of bone age in boys), there is a 12% risk of a curve of 20° or greater progressing by 5° or more [11]. At Risser IV (15 years of bone age in girls and 17 years of bone age in boys), the risk of the progression of scoliosis is markedly decreased, although, for boys, a slight risk remains. At Risser V (16 years of bone age in girls and 18 years of bone age in boys), it would be futile, if

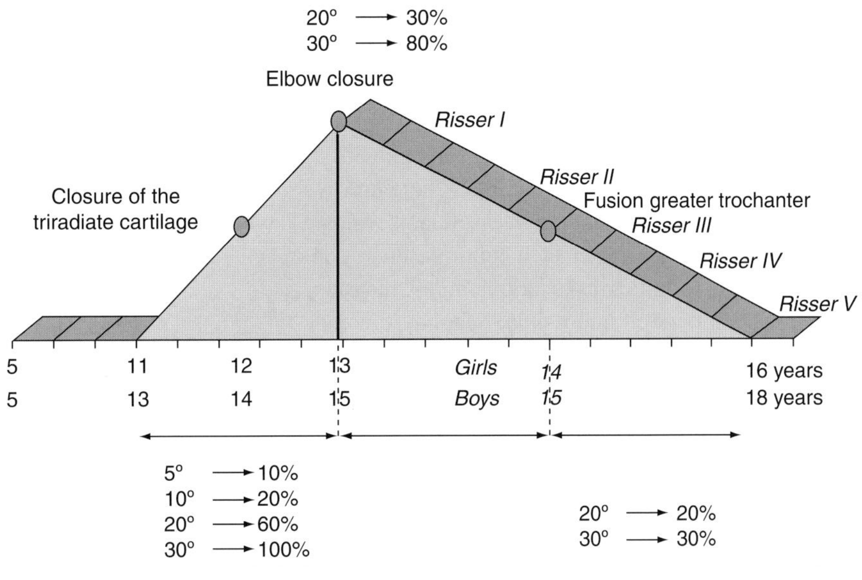

Fig. 2.23 Evaluation of scoliosis progression risk in pubertal growth diagram

not naive, to wait until the iliac crest is completely ossified, before discontinuing the treatment of scoliosis, but there is still a risk of worsening in boys who has idiopathic scoliosis between Risser IV and Risser V [40].

However imprecise and approximate the Risser sign may be, it is widely used as a deciding factor in many reports of brace treatment or surgery. Nevertheless, its limitations must be understood. The data of the studies by Lonstein and Carlson [45] relating Risser sign and the curve magnitude have been discussed. As was discussed previously, because two-thirds of the pubertal growth spurt occurs before the appearance of Risser I, and often ambiguous relation exists between Risser stage and bone age, its value in both dinical decision making and research should be questioned [22–24, 43]. Bone age, abnormal growth velocity, and secondary sexual characteristics are the most reliable parameters. Risser stages must not be regarded as a first-choice indicator; they must always be compared with bone age [53] especially when making decisions that will have major consequences, such as ordering or removing a brace or scheduling vertebral fusion. Does growth stop at Risser V? What is the best parameter? Growth stops when standing height does not progress (the best parameter …) When the distal epiphysis of the ulna and the radius are closed; at the same period, the proximal epiphysis of the humerus closes [38].

2.6.9 Growth in the Paralytic Child

The growth pattern is abnormal in many children with paralytic disorders (e.g., cerebral palsy, spina bifida, and poliomyelitis). In these children, therefore, it is essential to record and follow the parameters of growth closely to establish an indication for surgery with as much accuracy and safety as possible. There are two problems that make it difficult to measure and evaluate the parameters of growth in such children. First, contractures and deformities make morphometric measurements difficult or even impossible. Second, reference values of children with normal growth and development are not applicable to these children [26, 48].

Nevertheless, it is still possible to gain valuable information about growth, first by measuring arm span when the child is in a wheelchair and, second, by scrutinizing the child carefully from head to foot. The length of even one bone that has been more or less spared by the deficit could be sufficient to determine the standing height of the child. For example, after 8 years of age, the proportions of the body segments remain the same; therefore, the length of the femur represents 28% of standing height, and the length of the tibia and fibula represents 24% of standing height. For the upper extremities, the humerus represents 19% of standing height and 36.5% of sitting height, the radius represents 14.5% of standing height and 27.8% of sitting height, respectively, and the ulna represents 15.5% and 29.5%, respectively [18, 39].

Weight is an important parameter to take into consideration. Many children, especially those with cerebral palsy and total body involvement, have a deficit of 20–30 kg. Surgical procedures are not the same for children who weigh 20, 40, and 60 kg. Being underweight as a result of malnutrition creates a risk of infection after surgery. There are many parameters that are used to assess nutritional status, such as measurements of the triceps and the subscapular skinfold, or determination of the total lymphocyte count. Whichever tests the surgeon relies on, should be carried out on underweight children before surgery, especially on those children with chronic conditions.

On the other hand, obesity can also be a problem in surgery. The obesity of children with muscular dystrophy or spina bifida may restrict the choice of surgical approaches and instrumentation. The gain in weight during puberty is the main enemy of children with diplegia or ambulatory quadriplegia.

The assessment of bone age is more difficult in paralyzed children. Bone age retardation is frequent in severe cerebral palsy. These patients sometimes display a wide range of bone ages, with the bone age of the hand not matching that of the elbow or the pelvis (this observation is made from the author's personal experience). The real bone age, therefore, must be approximately assessed, and this information must be correlated with the results of anthropometric measurements.

2.7 Lessons Learned from Growth

Charts and diagrams are only models or templates. They do not by themselves define a true age. They define trends and outline the evolution of growth. They should be taken as just what they are: a convenient means to map the route through puberty. They record ephemeral points in the processes of growth and anticipate the events that lie in the future.

Their use helps the surgeon in avoiding uncertain or unnecessary treatments and aids in developing successful strategies. Nothing can produce worse results than decisions leading into uncharted territory.

Annual growth velocity is an essential parameter, mainly to detect the pubertal peak velocity. Birthdays are a convenient reminder for annual evaluations such as measurements of growth. Percentages provide an extremely valuable and objective tool for evaluating residual growth, particularly with respect to the proportions between the lengths of various segments of the limbs, and between the limbs and the trunk. The multiplying coefficient can be applied to all biometric data. However diverse their ethnic origins, and although stature has been increasing in succeeding generations over the centuries, boys of all generations and ethnic backgrounds will always have approximately 14% of outstanding growth in standing height (13% for girls). Neither the percentage nor the proportions change, and even the ratios are stable. The humerus is equivalent to, and will always be equivalent to, approximately 19% of standing height and 36.5% of sitting height [20]. Whatever be the population profile, *the chronology of growth and stages of puberty remain the same*.

A figure in isolation is meaningless; a ratio is more reliable. For instance, the length of the thoracic segment in relation to sitting height, provides more objective values. To gain this information, the examiner should try to obtain a general overview of the child's growth and plot the child's anthropometric chart. The ratios of the various body segments are important in many conditions, especially the various types of dwarfism. The ratio of sitting height to subischial leg length is essential when analyzing chondrodystrophy. Special curves can be used to follow such patients. Dwarfism can be divided into two families: short-trunk dwarfism, the prime example of which is represented by Morquio syndrome; and normal-trunk dwarfism, which is characterized by the limbs being shorter than normal. The prime example here is achondroplasia.

The various processes that make up growth are well synchronized, organized, and interdependent, but they vary widely in the time of occurrence during growth. For instance, the growth of the trunk accounts for most of the increase in standing height during the last part of puberty. Also, weight gain lags behind growth in length until puberty, after which the percentage gain in weight far exceeds the percentage gain in height. All changes are gradual. Growth itself is a succession of phases, periods of deceleration or acceleration, spurts, and alternating processes.

The pubertal growth velocity diagram is very useful in decision making. The peak height growth velocity takes place during the first 2 years of puberty. By measuring the standing height, the sitting height, and the subischial leg length every 6 months, it becomes much easier to understand the puberty growth spurt. Bone age must be analyzed with a critical mind and constantly compared to the rate of annual growth in standing height and secondary sexual characteristics [20, 24, 26].

Treatment of children often requires a consideration of remaining growth. Puberty is the time when most of these decisions will be made. In children in whom growth disturbance is anticipated, it is best to record several parameters over time in order to have an accurate picture of growth.

Treatment is easiest when it is done in anticipation of future growth. The milestones that mark the growth path during puberty must be noted and understood by the orthopedic surgeon [20, 24, 26].

2.8 The Growing Spine: from the Normal to Abnormal

2.8.1 *The Pathologic Spine is Dominated by the Crankshaft Phenomenon*

Theoretically, when dealing with a severe scoliosis, the best arthrodesis is the peri-veretebral arthrodesis. posterior arthrodesis in the immature spine induces the cranckshaft phenomenon. For severe cases, and, particularly in congenital scoliosis, early hemiarthrodesis before 5 years of age has been proposed, but experience has shown that early arthrodesis has negative effect [27, 51].

2.8.2 *Growth Disturbances After Spinal Arthrodesis*

Mehta et al. [47] has shown that in a growing rabbit model, there is an interaction between growth of the spine and thorax: a unilateral deformity of the spine or

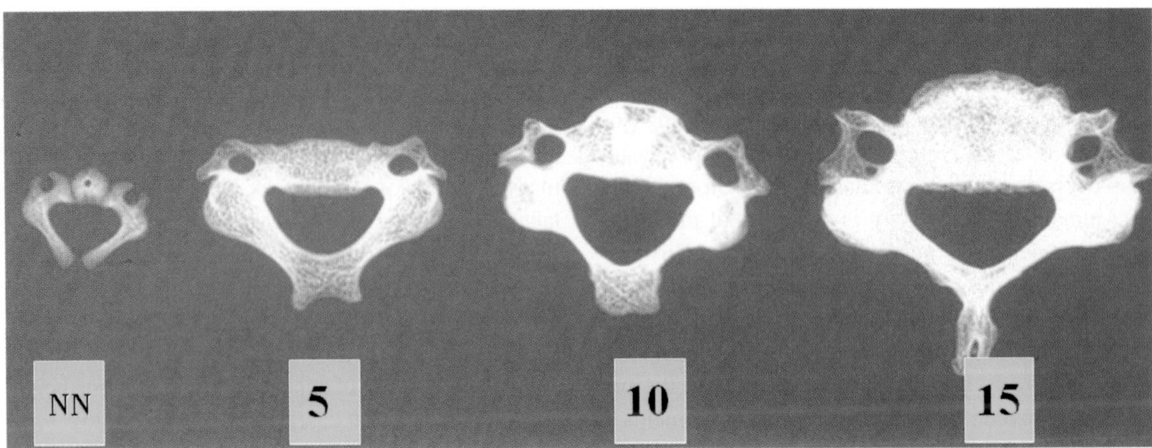

Fig. 2.24 Vertebral body ossification and spinal canal size from birth to skeletal maturity; by the age of 5 years ossification raises up to 65% and the spinal canal has grown to 95% of its definitive size

the thorax induces both scoliosis and thoracic cage deformity with asymmetric lung volumes.

Karol et al. [41] has shown that early arthrodesis reduces the AP diameter and shortens the T1–T12 index. Fusion is a cause of respiratory insufficiency and adds to the spinal deformity, the loss of pulmonary function. The forced vital capacity may decrease to less than 50% of predicted volume if more than 60% of the thoracic spine (i.e., eight thoracic volume) is fused before the age of 8 years. Emans et al. [31] has confirmed this negative effect of early arthrodesis.

Canavese et al [12, 13] has shown that dorsal arthrodesis in prepubertal rabbits changes thoracic growth patterns in operated rabbits. The dorsoventral diameter grows more slowly than latero-lateral diameter. The sternum, as well as the lengths of the thoracic vertebral bodies in the spinal segment, where the dorsal arthrodesis were performed grew less. The cranckshaft phenomenon is evident at the fused vertebral levels where there is a reduction of thoracic kyphosis [12].

The weight of the lung will increase by 10-fold, from 60 g at birth to 750 g. Up to 85% of alveoli develop after birth. Alveoli are added by multiplication after birth until the age of 8 years.

The golden period of the thoracic spine and rib cage coincides with lung development. The source of the respiratory failure is twofold: intrinsic alveolar hypoplasia and extrinsic disturbances of the chest wall function. The chest deformity prevents hyperplasia of the lung tissues (Campbell (2000) personnal communication) [8, 10, 11].

At birth the spine is mainly cartilaginous. Only 30% of the spine is ossified; by 5 years of age ossification raises up to 65%. At this age the spinal canal has grown to 95% of its definitive size [21–23] (Fig. 2.24).

From birth to 5 years, the morphology of the thorax changes: it is cylindrical at birth and becomes ovoid at 5; the frontal diameter grows more than the anteroposterior diameter [22] (Fig. 2.25)

2.9 From Birth to 5 Years of Age, the Spine-Rib-Lung Complex

Growth requires an enormous amount of energy. The nutritional requirements in the first 3 years of life are much greater than those of adulthood: calories, 110 vs. 40 calories/kg/day; protein, 2 vs. 1 gm/kg/day; and water, 150 vs. 5 mL/kg/day. Skeletal mineralization alone requires storage of 1 kg of calcium between birth and adulthood.

2.9.1 A Thorough Pediatric Evaluation is a Priority

Because of the great diversity of diseases involved in early spine deformities, a complete pediatric investigation is strongly recommended:

- severe scoliosis has negative effect on the standing height, sitting height, thoracic perimeter, T1 S1 length, weight, vital capacity [22–24].

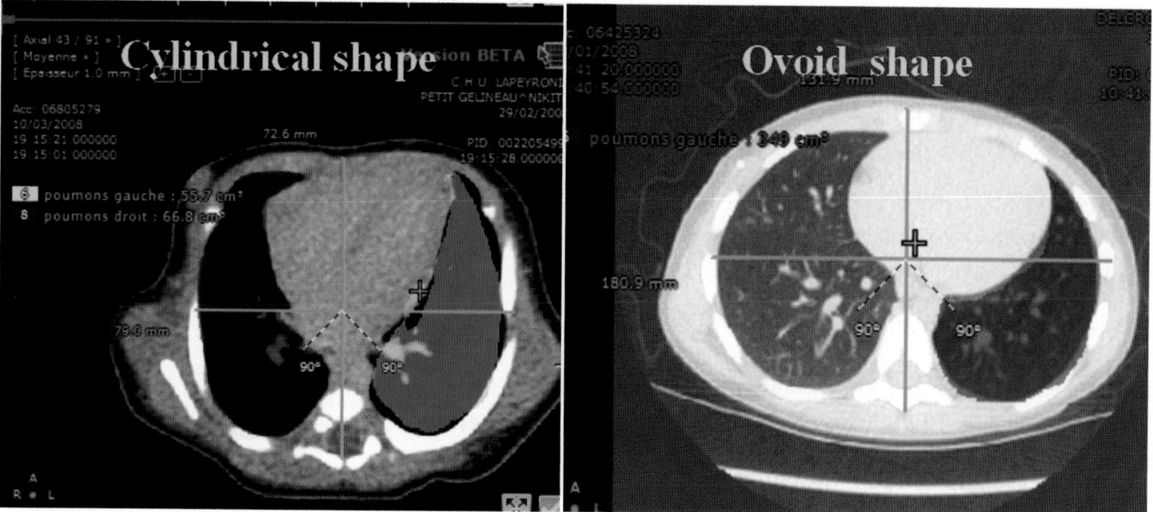

Fig. 2.25 Morphology of the thorax; It is cylindrical at birth and becomes ovoid at 5 years

- the weight is an important reference; most of these children have a severe deficit in weight.
- measurement of the standing and sitting height in supine position avoids many mistakes in the evaluation of the child and allows a standardized report, confortation of different growth curves gives a better strategic visibility [22–24].

The priority is to preserve the growth of the thorax and increased lung volume throughout this critical period of life. T1–S1 will increase 10 cm. The thoracic spine grows.

2.9.2 From Five to Puberty, a Quiescent Period

The growth velocity of the sitting height and T1–S1 slows down. T1–S1 will increase from 5 to 10, 6 cm. The annual growth velocity on the standing height is 5.7 cm: 2.4 cm on the trunk, 3.3 cm on the lower limbs [21–23].

At 5 years of age, the remaining growth on T1–S1 is about 15 cm. 2/3 on the thoracic spine, 10 cm, 1/3 on the lumbar spine (5 cm). Remaining standing growth is about 65 cm at 5 years. Remaining sitting growth is about 32 cm [21–23].

At 10 years of age, the thoracic volume will increase from 30 to 50% [17, 21–23]. When curves are severe, dual distraction rods are indicated to control the crankshaft phenomenon [1]. A distraction of 1 cm/ year is recommended.

Effect on the impact of the distraction can be appreciated by measuring the sitting height [21–24, 26].

Other surgical alternatives are possible, like staples or distraction rods and fixation of the thorax.

At 10 years of age, the remaining growth of T1–S1 is about 11 cm for boys, 7 cm for girls. Remaining standing height is 38 cm for boys and 26 cm for girls. Remaining sitting height is 20 cm for boys and 15 cm for girls. The remaining growth on the thoracic perimeter is about 33 cm for boys and 31 cm for girls.

- A curve of 20° at the onset of puberty has a surgical risk of 16%.
- A curve of 20–30° at the onset of puberty has a surgical risk of 75%.
- A curve of 30° at the onset of puberty has a surgical risk of 100% [16].

Puberty, a period characterized by progression of the curve [22–24, 29, 30].

T1–S1 will increase from ten to skeletal maturity, about 9.5 cm for boys, 6.5 cm for girls [22–24, 26].

Aggressive scoliosis in the first year of puberty should be detected soon and offensive strategy be chosen.

Severe scoliosis should be treated early, and if necessary, on the ascending side of puberty.

If the annual curve progression is less than 6°/year on the ascending side of puberty, 33% of cases are high candidates for surgery. If the progression is between 6–10°/year, the rate becomes 71%. If the progression is more than 10°/year, the surgical risk is 100%.

When treating scoliosis on the ascending side of puberty, during the Risser 0 period, two important parameters should be carefully observed:

- the olecranon morphologic changes [21–24, 26]
- the annual curve progression velocity

The risk of crankshaft phenomenon is low if the spine curvature is reduced to 0° or when the triradiate cartilage is closed [54]. It is 75% when the triradiate cartilage is open. It drops to 40% after the closure of the triradiate cartilage.

When planning a perivertebral arthrodesis, we should know what the deficit of the trunk will be [63]. The remaining sitting height and the figure 2.5% of sitting height for thoracic vertebra, and 3.5% for lumbar vertebra are the elements to take into consideration.

For girls, a perivertebral arthrodesis at the beginning of puberty will cause a deficit of 3.6cm on the thoracic segment and 2.1 on the lumbar segment.

For boys, a perivertebral arthrodesis at the beginning of puberty will cause a deficit of 3.9cm on the thoracic segment and 2.3 on the lumbar segment.

The deficit on the trunk will be outbalanced by the correction of the deformity.

2.9.3 What we Know, Where we are, and Which Way to Follow?

There is a normal interaction between the organic components of the spine, the thoracic cage and the lungs.

Deformities of the spine adversely affect the development of the thorax by changing its shape and reducing its normal mobility [32]. The rib vertebral complex which fits the thoracic cavity three dimensionally tends to constitute an elastic structural model similar to a cube in shape, but in the presence of scoliosis it becomes flat, rigid and turns elliptical, thus preventing the lungs from expanding [13].

Early posterior arthrodesis in the central portion of the spine (T1–T6) disturbs significantly, the morphology of the thorax and blocks the thoracic volume [5].

Before the age of 5 years, the retractions of the thorax should be treated to preserve the pulmonary growth [8].

Innovative techniques such as expansion thoracoplasty [8] and dual rod distraction [1], stapling, screwing of the neurocentral growth plate, offer the possibility of preventing thoracic insufficiency and spinal deformity.

Challenging the growing spine means how to maintain the spinal growth, the thoracic growth, the lung growth and to keep the spine supple [22].

The principle that a short spine produced by early fusion is better than a long curved spine is no longer generally accepted [36].

References

1. Acheson RM (1957) The Oxford method of assessing skeletal maturity. Clin Orthop 10:19
2. Akbarnia BA, Marks DS, Boachie-Adjei O, Thompson A, Asher MA (2005) Dual growing rod technique for the treatment of progressive early-onset scoliosis: a multicenter study. Spine 30(17S):S46–S57
3. Bailey DK, Pinneau S (1952) Tables for predicting adult height from skeletal age. J Pediatr 40:421
4. Biondi J, Weiner DS, Bethem D et al (1985) Correlation of Risser's sign and bone age determination in adolescent idiopathic scoliosis. J Pediatr Orthop 5:697
5. Bowen R, Scaduto A, Banuelos S (2008) Does early thoracic fusion exacerbate preexisting restrictive lung disease in congenital scoliosis patients? J Pediatr Orthop 28:506–511
6. Buckwalter JA, Ehrlich MG Sandell LI et al (eds) (1997) Skeletal growth and development: clinical issues and basic science advances, vol 3. American Academy of Orthopaedic Surgeons, Rosemont, p 577
7. Bunch W, Dvonch V (1983) Pitfalls in the assessment of skeletal immaturity: an anthropologic case study. J Pediatr Orthop 3:220
8. Campbell RM, Smith MD, Mayes TC et al (2003) The characteristic of thoracic insufficiency syndrome associated with fused ribs and congenital scoliosis. J Bone Joint Surg Am 85:399–408
9. Campbell RM, Hell-Voecke AK (2003) Growth of the thoracic spine in congenital scoliosis after expansion thoracoplasty. J Bone Joint Surg Am 85:409–420
10. Campbell RM, Smith MD, Hell-Voecke AK (2004) Expansion thoracoplasty: the surgical technique of opening-wedge thoracostomy. J Bone Joint Surg Am 86(Suppl I): 51–64
11. Campbell RM Jr, Smith MD, Mayes TC et al (2004) The effect of opening wedge thoracostomy on thoracic insufficiency syndrome associated with fused ribs and congenital scoliosis. J Bone Joint Surg Am 86A(8):1659–1674
12. Canavese F, Dimeglio A, Volpatti D, Stebel M (2007) Dorsal arthrodesis of thoracic spine and effects on thorax growth in prepubertal New Zealand white rabbits. Spine 32(16): E443–E450
13. Canavese F, Dimeglio A, Cavalli F (2007) Arthrodesis of the first six dorsal vertebrae in prepubertal New Zealand white rabbits and thoracic growth to skeletal maturity: the role of

the rib-vertebral-sternal complex. Minerva Orthop Traumatol 58:369–77
14. Carpenter CT, Lester EL (1993) Skeletal age determination in young children: analysis of three regions of the hand/wrist film. Pediatr Orthop 13:76
15. Charles YP, Dimeglio A (2006) Progression risk of idiopathic juvenile scoliosis during pubertal growth. Spine 31:7
16. Charles YP, Dimeglio A, Canavese F et al (2007) Skeletal age assessment from the olecranon for idiopathic scoliosis at Risser grade 0. J Bone Joint Surg Am 89(12):2737–2744
17. Charles YP, Dimeglio A, Marcoul, Bourgin JF, Marcoul A, Bozonnat MC (2008) Influence of idiopathic scoliosis on three-dimensional thoracic growth. Spine 33(11): 1209–1218
18. Cheng JCY, Leung SSF, Chin BSK et al (1998) Can we predict body height from segmental bone length measurements? A study of 3,647 children. J Pediatr Orthop 18:387
19. Cundy P, Paterson D, Morris L et al (1988) Skeletal age estimation in leg length discrepancy. J Pediatr Orthop 8:513
20. Diméglio A (1987) La croissance en orthopedie. Sauramps Medical, Montpellier
21. Dimeglio A, Bonnel F (1989) Growth of the spine. In: Raimondi AJ, Choux M, Di Rocco C (eds) Principales of pediatric neuro-surgery: the pediatric spine, development and the dysraphic stage, vol 9. Springer-Verlag, New York, p 39
22. Dimeglio A, Bonnel F (1990) Le rachis en croissance. Springer-Verlag, Paris
23. Dimeglio A (1993) Growth of the spine before age 5 years. J Pediatr Orthop B 1:102
24. Dimeglio A (2001) Growth in pediatric orthopaedics. J Pediatr Orthop 21:549–555
25. Dimeglio A, Charles YP, Daures JP Accuracy of the Sauvegrain method in determining skeletal age during puberty. J Bone Joint Surg Am 87(8):1689–1696
26. Dimeglio A (2005) Growth in pediatric orthopedics. In: Morrissy T, Weinstein SL (eds) Lovell and Winter's pediatric orthopedics, 6th edn. Lippincott William & Wilkins, Philadelphia, pp 35–65
27. Dubousset J, Herring JA, Shufflebarger HL (1989) The crankshaft phenomenon. J Pediatr Orthop 9:541
28. Dubousset J, Wicart P. Pomero V (2002) Scolioses thoraciques: les gibbosités exo et endo-thoraciques et l'index de pénétration rachidienne. Rev Chir Orthop 88:9–18
29. Duval-Beaupère G (1970) Les repères de maturation dans la surveillance des scolioses. Rev Chir Orthop 56:59
30. Duval-Beaupère G (1976) Croissance residuelle de la taille et des segments apres la premiere menstruation chez la fille. Rev Chir Orthop 62:501
31. Emans JB, Caubet JF, Ordonez CL et al (2005) The treatment and chest wall deformities with fused ribs by expansion thoracostomy and insertion of vertical expandable prothetic titanium rib: growth of thoracic spine and improvement of long volumes. Spine 30:558
32. Grassi V, Tantucci C (1993) Respiratory prognosis in chest wall diseases. Arch Chest Dis 48(2):183–7
33. Greulich WW, Pyle SI (1959) Radiographic atlas of skeletal development of the hand and wrist, 2nd edn. Stanford University Press, Stanford, p 50
34. Gruenwald P (1966) Growth of the human fetus. Am J Obstet Gynecol 94:1112
35. Hamill PVV, Drizd TA, Johnson CL et al (1979) National center for health statistics percentiles. Am J Clin Nutr 32:607
36. Herring JA (ed) (2008) Scoliosis. In: Tachdjian's pediatric orthopaedics, 4th edn, vol 1. Saunders–Elsevier, pp 358–376
37. Hensinger RN (1986) Standards in pediatric orthopaedic: charts, tables and graphs illustrating growth. Raven Press, New York
38. Hoppenfeld S, Lonner B, Murthy V et al (2003) The rib epiphysis and other growth centers as indicators of the end of spinal growth. Spine 29:47–50
39. Jarzem PF, Gledhill RB (1993) Predicting height from arm measurement. J Pediatr Orthop 13:761
40. Karol LA, Johnston CE, Browne RH et al (1993) Progression of the curve in boys who have idiopathic scoliosis. J Bone Joint Surg Am 75:1804
41. Karol LA, Johnston CE, Mladenov K, Schochet P, Walters P (2008) Pulmonary function following early thoracic fusion in non-neuromuscular scoliosis. J Bone Joint Surg Am 90: 1272–1281
42. Lefort J (1981) Utilisation du coefficient de croissance résiduelle dans le calcul prévisionnel des inégalités de longueur des membres inférieurs. Rev Chir Pediatr Orthop 67:753
43. Little DG, Sussman MD (1994) The Risser sign: a critical analysis. J Pediatr Orthop 14:569
44. Little DG, Song KM, Katz D et al (2000) Relationship of peak height velocity to other maturity indicators in idiopathic scoliosis in girls. J Bone Joint Surg Am 82:685–693
45. Lonstein JE, Carlson JM (1984) The prediction of curve progression in untreated idiopathic scoliosis during growth. J Bone Joint Surg Am 66:1061–1071
46. Lonstein JE (1995) Embryology and spine growth. In: Lonstein JL, Bradford DS, Winter RB et al (eds) Moes' textbook of scoliosis and other spinal deformities, 3rd edn. WB Saunders, Philadelphia, p 23
47. Mehta HP, Snyder BD, Callender NN, Bellardine CL, Jackson AC (2006) The reciprocal relationship between thoracic and spinal deformity and its effect on pulmonary function in a rabbit model. A pilot study. Spine 31(23): 2654–2664
48. Miller F, Koreska J (1992) Height measurement of patients with neuromuscular disease and contractures. Dev Med Child Neurol 35:55
49. Paley D, Bhave A, Herznberg JE et al (2000) Multiplier method for predicting limb-length discrepancy. J Bone Surg Am 82:1432–1446
50. Prader A, Lango RH, Molinari L et al (1989) Physical growth of Swiss children from birth to 20 years of age: first longitudinal study of growth and development. Helv Paediatr Acta 52:(Suppl): 1–25
51. Richards BS (1997) The effects of growth on the scoliotic spine following posterior spinal fusion. In: Buckwalter JA, Ehrlich MG, Sandell LJ et al (eds) Skeletal growth and development: clinical issues and basic science advances, vol 3. American Academy of Orthopaedic Surgeons, Rosemont, p 577
52. Risser J, Agostini S, Sampaio J et al (1973) The sitting-standing height ratio as a method of evaluating early spine fusion in the growing child. Clin Orthop 24:7
53. Roberto RF, Lonstein JE, Winter RB et al (1997) Curve progression in Risser stage 0 on patients after posterior spinal fusion for idiopathic scoliosis. J Pediatr Orthop 17: 718

54. Sanders JO, Herring JA, Browne RH (1995) Posterior arthrodesis a instrumentation in the immature (Bisser-grade-0) spine in pathic scoliosis. J Bone Joint Surg Am 77:39
55. Sauvegrain J, Nahm H, Bronstein N (1962) Etude de la maturation osseuse du coude. Ann Radiol 5:542
56. Sempé M, Pavia C (1979) Atlas de la maturation sequelettique. SIMEP, Paris
57. Tanner JM, Whitehouse RH, Takaishi M (1966) Standards from birth to maturity for height, weight height velocity and weight velocity. British children 1965, parts I and II. Arch Dis Child 41:454
58. Tanner JM, Whiteouse RH, Marshall WA et al (1975) Assessment of skeletal maturity and prédiction of aduit height (TW2 method). Academic Press, London
59. Tanner JM, Whitehouse RH (1976) Clinical longitudinal standards for height, weight, height velocity and the stages of puberty. Arch Dis Child 51:170
60. Tanner JM (1978) Physical growth and development. In: Forfar JO, Arneil GC (eds) Textbook of paediatrics, vol 7, 2nd edn. Churchill Livingstone, New York, p 249
61. Tanner JM, Davies PSW (1985) Clinical longitudinal standards for height and height velocity for North America children. J Pediatr 107:317
62. Uhthoff HK (1990) The embryology of the human locomotor system. Springer-Verlag, New York
63. Winter RW (1977) Scoliosis and spinal growth. Orthop Rev 6:17
64. Zhang H, Sucato D, Nuremberg P et al (2008) Characterize neuro-central synchondrosis developmental stages in normal pediatric patients using magnetic resonance imaging. In: Scoliosis Research Society 43rd Annual Meeting Poster, Salt Lake City

3 Biomechanics in the Growing Spine

Andrew T. Mahar

Key Points

- Early onset scoliosis is a biomechanical challenge to the treating orthopaedic surgeon as typical treatment methods such as bracing or arthrodesis may be ineffective or contraindicated.
- The biomechanical requirements of instrumentation must be to provide some initial deformity correction, stabilize the growing spine, allow for growth of the spine, and they ideally would not adversely affect the spinal anatomy.
- The dual growing rod instrumentation has demonstrated improved clinical outcomes compared with single rod systems, due to theoretically greater biomechanical stability.
- The most biomechanically stable construct within which to attach the dual growing rods is a bilateral pedicle screw system in the cephalad and caudal constructs.
- The distraction forces are distributed along the length of spine and thus should not adversely affect the spinal anatomy of singular areas within the spine.
- The immature porcine spine has been utilized for both in vivo and in vitro biomechanical studies and may be the most appropriate based on growth rates and anatomical dimensions.
- Intraoperative distraction in patients exhibit high variability most likely related to the inherent differences in spine stiffness associated with different disease processes.
- In future, research should be carried out in human subjects to evaluate deformity correction as well as spinal growth as it relates to the type of instrumentation system used and the distraction force applied at each surgery.

3.1 Background

Early onset scoliosis (EOS) presents an extremely challenging clinical scenario. While bracing/casting may be utilized, these techniques may often fail or be contraindicated [20, 22]. Spinal fusion and instrumentation may be the gold standard for adolescent or adult deformity correction, but is contraindicated in EOS since spinal arthrodesis may limit truncal growth and adversely affect pulmonary development/function [8, 16, 22]. Surgical treatment that allows both deformity correction and spinal growth has existed since Harrington's initial study in 1962 [17]. He advocated instrumentation without fusion in patients 10 years of age or less. Moe et al. [29] used a "subcutaneous rod technique" specifically for children with remaining growth potential. However, this "growing rod" did not provide stable fixation, and the use of Luque rods followed to achieve better results [24]. This technique was also associated with poor outcomes related to autofusions that were thought to occur due to the requisite subperiosteal exposure [14, 27, 33].

Modifications to both the instrumentation and surgical method have developed into the current dual

A. T. Mahar
Department of Orthopaedic Surgery, University of California San Diego, San Diego, CA 92103, USA
e-mail: andrew.mahar@gmail.com

B. A. Akbarnia et al. (eds.), *The Growing Spine*,
DOI: 10.1007/978-3-540-85207-0_3,

growing rod technique [2–5]. Currently, the dual rod growing technique appears to provide better initial correction and maintenance of correction, as well as greater overall spinal growth compared with the previously used single rods [36]. The construction of the dual rod technique can typically employ either laminar hooks or pedicle screws to create "foundations" to which the system is anchored. While the growth of the immature spine has been well documented [11, 12], little is known regarding the biomechanics of spinal deformity in this age group. In addition, there is sparse literature regarding what instrumentation should be used or what models may be used for scientific investigations. The goal of this chapter is to review the literature that exists on the topic and provide direction to those who choose to study the biomechanics of the growing spine.

3.2 Biomechanical Considerations for Instrumenting the Growing Spine

The surgeon has several options with which to obtain fixation at the foundations of the construct. Laminar hooks or pedicle screws may be used at either foundation and can potentially be supplemented with cross-links. (Fig. 3.1a, b) There have been multiple reports of implant failures at the bone-implant interface with use of the instrumentation without fusion technique [1, 7, 21, 28], but to the authors' knowledge, few biomechanical studies exist comparing different configurations. Although many previous studies have explored the failure of individual anterior vertebral screws or posterior pedicle screws [13, 18, 19, 23, 25, 30–32, 34, 37], only one previous biomechanics study attempted to address this issue for the specific patient population with EOS. Using an immature porcine spine, the study compared laminar hooks with a cross-link, a hybrid hook and screw construct with a cross-link, pedicle screws with a cross-link and pedicle screws without a cross-link in a pulloff or "failure" test. These data found that the pedicle screw constructs were significantly more stable than any construct containing a laminar hook ($p < 0.002$) (Fig. 3.2).

Although pedicle screws may have increased biomechanical stability and greater three column control, there have been general concerns with their use [35], and this may be especially true in the EOS population [38]. In this population, the pedicle dimensions are smaller than in the adult, and typical thoracolumbar screws may not be appropriate. In the aforementioned study, Yazici et al. [38] used immature porcine vertebrae to determine if sequential dilation of the pedicle would adversely affect the biomechanical stability of the screw. The study did find that pedicle expansion was possible but significantly reduced the pullout force of control pedicles (408 N ± 102) compared to dilated pedicles (320 N ± 84). While in vivo forces on the spine are not well understood, it may be assumed that the pedicles would remodel following dilation and that the potential pullout force would increase in this group. It should also be noted that a survival study in a similar immature porcine model found that unilateral pedicle screws significantly altered pedicle/hemi-canal growth compared to contralateral controls with no instrumentation [10]. How stable constructs are and their effect on anatomical growth requires further studies.

Another particular consideration is the ability to distract the spine and lengthen it which should in turn provide some deformity correction. The ability to distract is based in part on the viscoelastic behavior of the spine and the stability of the implants between which distraction is placed. In a dual growing rod system, distraction is applied between the rods joined by a connector. Expandable or growing rods are placed within the pediatric spine, which act as an "internal brace", allowing continued growth of the unfused portion of the spine while maintaining correction and control of the scoliotic curve. Serial lengthening procedures are performed until the child reaches skeletal maturity with a reported average growth rate of 0.87 cm/year [36]. Owing to the increased stability when pedicle screws are used, it may theoretically be possible to deliver greater distraction forces to the spine during the initial lengthening and during subsequent lengthenings. However, differences in distraction forces related to the type of foundation are currently unclear. In addition, it is currently unclear whether posterior distraction maneuvers affect the anterior column by altering intradiscal biomechanics [26]. It is theoretically possible that a single distraction maneuver may primarily affect the disc space adjacent to the foundation rather than have a "global" spinal affect. It is also possible that the posterior distraction maneuver may in fact create a focal kyphotic deformity as the motion segment used for the foundation rotates on the inferior disc creating a compressive load. A previous study has examined this specifically by varying

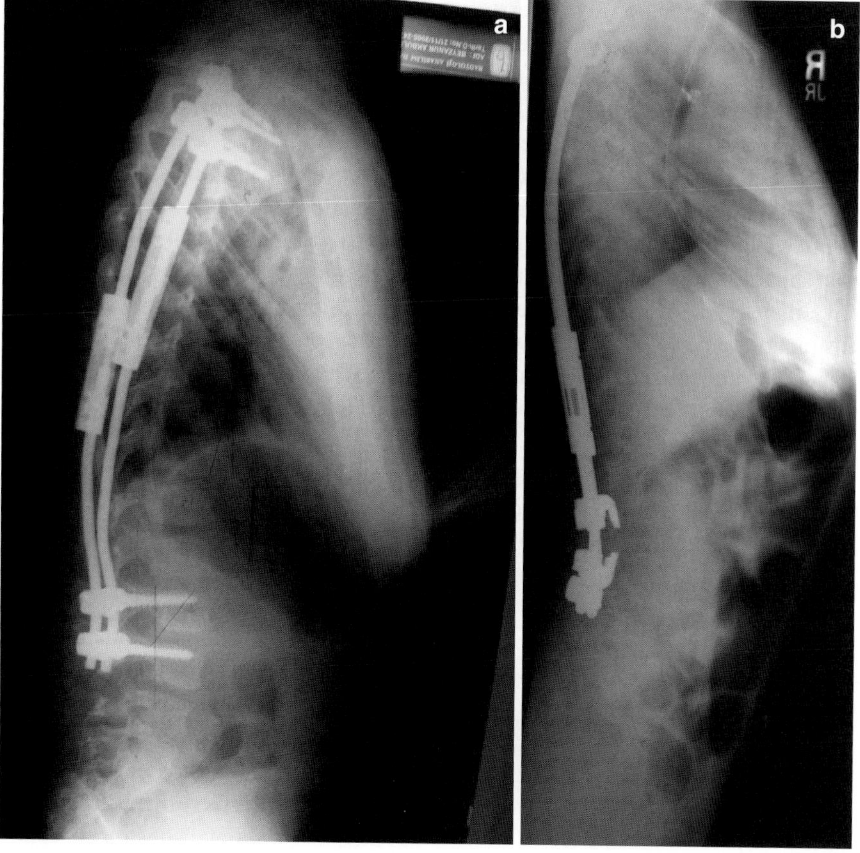

Fig. 3.1 (**a**) Sagittal views for potential foundations for use in the dual growing rod system with segmental pedicle screws in the cephalad and caudal foundations. (**b**) Fluoroscopy imaging employing segmental laminar hooks and a cross-link at each foundation

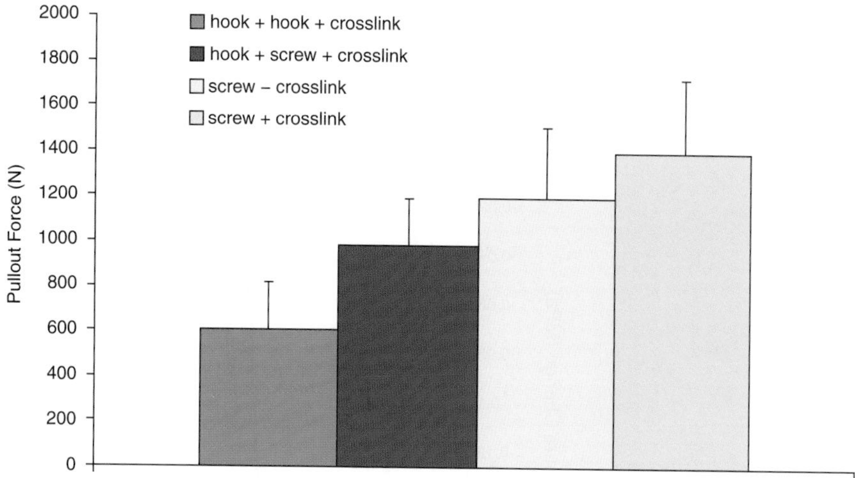

Fig. 3.2 Biomechanical comparison of different foundations demonstrating significantly increased pullout force (N) strength when using pedicle screws compared to laminar hooks

the foundations at the cephalad construct and inserting needle-type pressure transducers at the level immediately below the upper construct and another transducer in the central disc within the construct [26]. The ability to generate distraction forces was calculated by placing a bonded strain gage at the tip of the distractor tool and by running the signal through custom amplification. The use of pedicle screws in the upper construct allowed for significantly greater distraction force application (416 ± 101 N) than upper level hooks (349 ± 100 N)

($p < 0.04$). The intradiscal pressures were seen to decrease during distraction, representing separation of the endplates, although these data were not different between constructs (Table 3.1). The loading and pressure data also confirmed the time-dependent viscoelastic nature of spinal loading (Fig. 3.3). However, translation of in vitro information to the in situ situation is often quite difficult, and it is unclear what happens to the spine in situ during distraction. For this reason, investigations are currently underway to explore how distraction force application may be different between patients with curves of varying stiffness and how the distraction forces may correlate with clinical outcomes.

An alternative to the growing rod technique that has been utilized effectively to treat chest wall deformities and scoliosis is the vertical expandable prosthetic expandable rib (VEPTR). A variety of diseases such as Jeune's syndrome or Jarcho–Levin syndrome may result in severe pulmonary compromise and other organ system issues, resulting in shortened life expectancy [6]. However, expansion thoracostomy and serial lengthenings of the VEPTR have proven to improve and maintain lung function [9, 15]. Benchtop investigations to analyze this procedure are difficult as the hypoplastic chest wall and spinal deformity have not yet been simulated in an animal survival model and animal/human cadaveric tissue would be unsuitable due to the complexity of the deformities of the chest. The biomechanical effectiveness of the VEPTR technique cannot be disputed though as the patient's show marked improvement in vital lung capacity with deformity correction.

Table 3.1 Intradiscal pressure (MPa) changes at each level for both Types of instrumentation

	Adjacent pressure		Middle pressure	
	Hooks	Screws	Hooks	Screws
Mean	0.183	0.194	0.161	0.173
SD	0.098	0.062	0.065	0.083

3.3 Conclusions

The biomechanics of deformity correction in the growing spine is clinically and technically challenging. The biomechanical concerns for instrumentation often mirror the clinical concerns wherein patient age/size, dimensions of the spinal anatomy, bone quality, and curve stiffness influence the implant selection. Pedicle screw constructs appear to provide the greatest

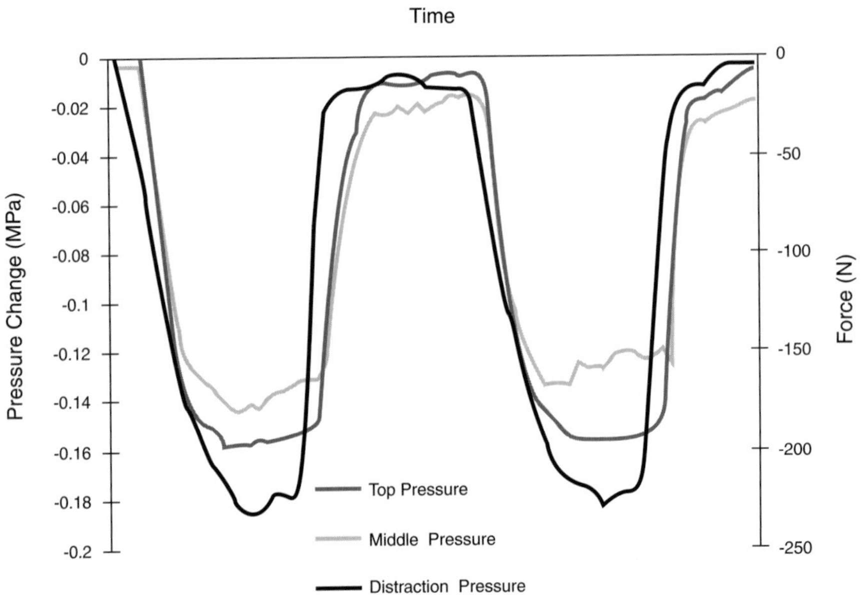

Fig. 3.3 A typical data collection during distraction loading while measuring intradiscal pressure changes

stability and the greatest ability to distract the spine. However, smaller patients may not tolerate pedicle screws placed following pedicular dilation. Thus, laminar hooks may prove a suitable initial construct until spinal growth will accommodate pedicle screw placement at a revision surgery. The immature porcine spine appears to provide a similar growth rate and have similar anatomical dimensions making it appropriate as a model for this patient population. Distraction appears to uniformly "stretch" the spine, and maximizing this effort intraoperatively is cautiously recommended. The use of the VEPTR technique to expand the chest and partially correct the spinal deformity has been used with significant improvements for treating thoracic insufficiency syndrome. Although biomechanical data may not be available for this technique, the clinical data supports the use of this system. Subsequent in vivo and in situ information is needed to further elucidate biomechanical needs and considerations for this complex patient population with growing *spines*.

References

1. Acaroglu E, Yazici M, Alanay A, Surat A (2002) Three-dimensional evolution of scoliotic curve during instrumentation without fusion in young children. J Pediatr Orthop 22:492–496
2. Akbarnia BA, McCarthy R (1998) Pediatric Isola instrumentation without fusion for the treatment of progressive early onset scoliosis. In: McCarthy R (ed) Spinal instrumentation techniques. Scoliosis Research Society, Chicago
3. Akbarnia BA, Marks D (2000) Instrumentation with limited arthrodesis for the treatment of progressive early-onset scoliosis. Spine: state of the art reviews, vol 14, pp 181–189
4. Akbarnia BA, Marks DS, Boachie-Adjei O et al (2005) Dual growing rod technique for the treatment of progressive early-onset scoliosis: a multicenter study. Spine 30:S46–S57
5. Asher M (1997) Isola spinal instrumentation system for scoliosis. In: Bridwell K (ed) Textbook of spinal surgery. Lippincott-Raven, Philadelphia, pp 569–609
6. Betz RR, Mulcahey MJ, Ramirez N et al (2008) Mortality and life-threatening events after vertical expandable prosthetic titanium rib surgery in children with hypoplastic chest wall deformity. J Pediatr Orthop 28(8):850–853
7. Blakemore LC, Scoles PV, Poe-Kochert C, Thompson GH (2001) Submuscular Isola rod with or without limited apical fusion in the management of severe spinal deformities in young children: preliminary report. Spine 26:2044–2048
8. Campbell RM Jr, Smith MD, Mayes TC et al (2003) The characteristics of thoracic insufficiency syndrome associated with fused ribs and congenital scoliosis. J Bone Joint Surg Am 85-A:399–408
9. Campbell RM Jr, Smith MD, Mayes TC et al (2004) The effect of opening wedge thoracostomy on thoracic insufficiency syndrome associated with fused ribs and congenital scoliosis. J Bone Joint Surg Am 86-A(8):1659–1674
10. Cil A, Yazici M, Daglioglu K et al (2005) The effect of pedicle screw placement with or without application of compression across the neurocentral cartilage on the morphology of the spinal canal and pedicle in immature pigs. Spine 30(11):1287–1293
11. Dimeglio A, Bonnel F (1989) Growth of the spine. In: Raimondi AJ, Choux M, Di Rocco C (eds) Principles of pediatric neurosurgery. The pediatric spine, development and dysraphic state. Springer, New York, pp 39–83
12. Dimeglio A (2001) Growth in pediatric orthopaedics. J Pediatr Orthop 21(4):549–555
13. Dvorak M, MacDonald S, Gurr R et al (1993) An anatomic, radiographic, and biomechanical assessment of extrapedicular screw fixation in the thoracic spine. Spine 12:1689–1694
14. Eberle CF (1988) Failure of fixation after segmental spinal instrumentation without arthrodesis in the management of paralytic scoliosis. J Bone Joint Surg Am 70:696–703
15. Emans JB, Caubet JF, Ordonez CL et al (2005) The treatment of spine and chest wall deformities with fused ribs by expansion thoracostomy and insertion of vertical expandable prosthetic titanium rib: growth of thoracic spine and improvement of lung volumes. Spine 30(17 Suppl):S58–S68
16. Emery JL, Mithal A (1960) The number of alveoli in the terminal respiratory unit of man during late intrauterine life and childhood. Arch Dis Child 35:544–547
17. Harrington PR (1962) Treatment of scoliosis. Correction and internal fixation. Bone Joint Surg Am 44-A:591–610
18. Heller JG, Shuster JK, Hutton WC (1999) Pedicle and transverse process screws of the upper thoracic spine. Biomechanical comparison of loads to failure. Spine 24:654–658
19. Inceoglu S, Ferrara L, McLain RF (2004) Pedicle screw fixation strength: pullout versus insertional torque. Spine J 4:513–518
20. Kennedy JD, Robertson CF, Olinsky A et al (1987) Pulmonary restrictive effect of bracing in mild idiopathic scoliosis. Thorax 42:959–961
21. Klemme WR, Denis F, Winter RB, Lonstein JW, Koop SE (1997) Spinal instrumentation without fusion for progressive scoliosis in young children. J Pediatr Orthop 17:734–742
22. Kose N, Campbell RM (2004) Congenital scoliosis. Med Sci Monit 10:RA104–RA110
23. Lowe T, O'Brien M, Smith D et al (2002) Central and juxta-endplate vertebral body screw placement. A biomechanical analysis in a human cadaveric model. Spine 27:369–373
24. Luque ER (1982) Paralytic scoliosis in growing children. Clin Orthop Relat Res 163:202–209
25. Mahar AT, Brown DS, Oka RS, Newton PO (2006) Biomechanics of cantilever "plow" during anterior thoracic scoliosis correction. Spine J 6:572–576
26. Mahar A, Flippin M, Oka R et al (2007) Biomechanical differences in distraction forces and anterior column intradiscal pressures when using different constructs for the dual growing rod technique. 53rd Annual Meeting of the Orthopaedic Research Society, San Diego, CA, Poster 1003
27. Mardjetko SM, Hammerberg KW, Lubicky JP et al (1992) The Luque trolley revisited. Review of nine cases requiring revision. Spine 17:582–589

28. Mineiro J, Weinstein SL (2002) Subcutaneous rodding for progressive spinal curvatures: early results. J Pediatr Orthop 22:290–295
29. Moe JH, Kharrat K, Winter RB, Cummine JL (1984) Harrington instrumentation without fusion plus external orthotic support for the treatment of difficult curvature problems in young children. Clin Orthop Relat Res 185:35–45
30. Mohamad F, Oka R, Mahar A, Wedemeyer M, Newton P (2006) Biomechanical comparison of the screw-bone interface: optimization of 1 and 2 screw constructs by varying screw diameter. Spine 31:E535–E539
31. Morgenstern W, Ferguson SJ, Berey S et al (2003) Posterior thoracic extrapedicular fixation: a biomechanical study. Spine 28:1829–1835
32. Ogon M, Haid C, Krismer M et al (1996) Comparison between single-screw and triangulated, double-screw fixation in anterior spine surgery. A biomechanical test. Spine 21:2728–2734
33. Sengupta D, Freeman B, Grevitt M et al (2002) Long term follow-up of the Luque trolly growing-rod construct in the surgical treatment of early onset idiopathic scoliosis. Scoliosis Research Society 37th Annual Meeting. Seattle, Washington
34. Snyder BD, Snaltz I, Hall JE et al (1995) Predicting the integrity of vertebral bone screw fixation in anterior spinal instrumentation. Spine 20:1568–1574
35. Suk SI, Kim WJ, Lee SM et al (2001) Thoracic pedicle screw fixation in spinal deformities: are they really safe? Spine 26(18):2049–2057
36. Thompson GH, Akbarnia BA, Kostial P et al (2005) Comparison of single and dual growing rod techniques followed through definitive surgery: a preliminary study. Spine 30:2039–2044
37. White KK, Oka R, Mahar AT, Lowry A, Garfin SR (2006) Pullout strength of thoracic pedicle screw instrumentation: comparison of the transpedicular and extrapedicular techniques. Spine 31:E355–E358
38. Yazici M, Pekmezci M, Cil A et al (2006) The effect of pedicle expansion on pedicle morphology and biomechanical stability in the immature porcine spine. Spine 31(22):E826–E829

Genetics

4

Kenneth M. C. Cheung, Daniel W. H. Ho, and You-Qiang Song

Key Points

- DNA is the blueprint of our human body. Variations in DNA are the source for the phenotypes of different individuals.
- The two most common types of variations, also called polymorphisms, are microsatellites and single nucleotide polymorphisms (SNPs) in our DNA.
- Mendelian disease refers to a simple form of disease in which alternation or mutation in a single gene is enough for its manifestation. Linkage analysis has been proven to be a useful method for studying this type of disease.
- Complex genetic disorders are caused by multiple genes with small effects combined with environmental factors. Candidate gene and genome-wide association studies using case–control design are best used to analyze these disorders.
- Idiopathic scoliosis is likely a complex genetic disorder. With the recent new developments in human genetics, the cause of idiopathic and congenital scoliosis will most likely be elucidated in the not-too-distant future.

4.1 Basic Genetics

Today's human genetics and genetic epidemiology are based on the Mendelian laws of inheritance, which explains the pattern of segregation of genes through generations. With the help of modern technology, we are able to determine the status of potential or causative genetic variants that might lead to the development of disease. This chapter aims to provide the reader with a basic concept of the terminology and principles involved in disease gene hunting, so that the readers will have a better understanding of the advances in genetics and scoliosis that will undoubtedly appear in the literature in future.

4.2 The Chromosome and DNA

To understand the principle of genetics and disease gene mapping, concepts concerning the chromosome and its structure, DNA, genetic polymorphisms, and different types of diseases need to be clarified.

The human genome consists of 23 pairs of homologous chromosomes. This complete set of chromosomes is called diploid, while the halved set of a gamete is called haploid. For each pair of these homologous chromosomes, one is derived from the father (paternal), while the other is from the mother (maternal). The chromosomes are made up of deoxyribonucleic acid (DNA), which is a long stretch of nucleotide sequence of 4 bases – adenine (A), cytosine (C), guanine (G), and thymine (T). Each single strand of DNA has two ends, namely, 5′ and 3′. Hydrogen bonds make the pairing of A with T, and C with G. With the existence of base complementarity between bases of two DNA strands running in opposite directions (5′–3′ and 3′–5′),

K. M. C. Cheung (✉)
Department of Orthopaedics and Traumatology,
5F Professorial Block, Queen Mary Hospital, 102 Pokfulam Road, Hong Kong, SAR, China
e-mail: ken-cheung@hku.hk

B. A. Akbarnia et al. (eds.), *The Growing Spine*,
DOI: 10.1007/978-3-540-85207-0_4, © Springer-Verlag Berlin Heidelberg 2011

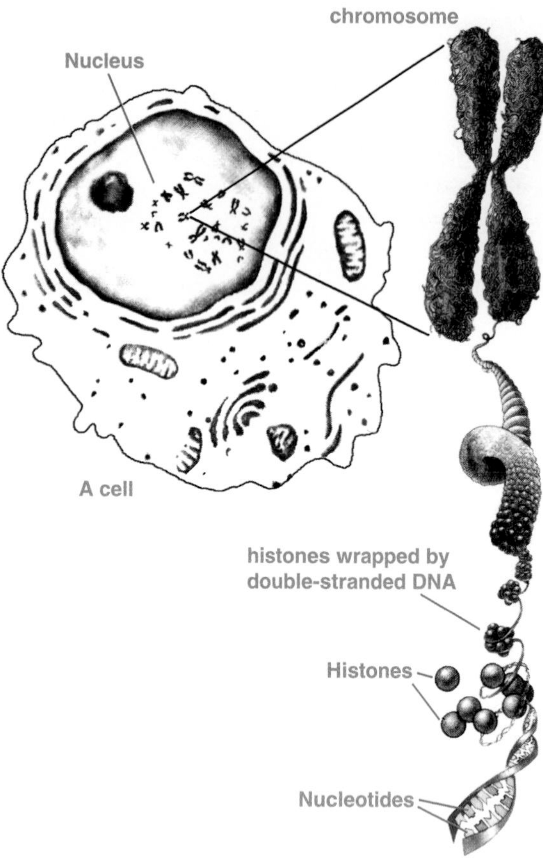

Fig. 4.1 Chromosomal organisation

a double-stranded DNA is formed. This is the primary structure of DNA. Upon further interaction with histone and scaffold protein, which are the major proteins to package DNA into a smaller volume to fit in the cell, the DNA is tightly wound together into chromosomes (Fig. 4.1).

The DNA contained in the chromosomes provides the blueprint for making all the structures inside the human body, as well as all the "software" needed to regulate its processes at the molecular level. All the necessary information is stored in the DNA sequence as a series of codes. A sequence of DNA that contains coding information is called "exons", while the noncoding sequences are called "introns". A series of steps occurs inside each cell to decode the information and translate them into protein products that are essential for metabolism as well as other normal functions of the human body. Through the process of *transcription*, a single DNA strand is used as a template for constructing a complementary RNA strand. Apart from the intrinsic chemical difference between DNA and RNA, the most important difference is that uracil (U) replaces T in RNA. In a certain region of the genome, which we call a gene, the transcribed RNA sequence encodes for information (codons – every three bases of RNA determine an amino acid) on how to make a certain protein (depending on the gene) with a specific amino acid sequence. Any genes will contain regulatory sequences and variable numbers of intervening exons and introns. The transcription of genes forms messenger RNA (mRNA), and would include all the intron and exon regions. Although the introns are noncoding region and are removed eventually, they may have regulatory functions during the processes of transcription. Eventually, with posttranscriptional modification called splicing, these intron regions are removed, and the coding exons are linked together to form mature mRNA. The mRNA then undergoes *translation*. This is the process in which the specific amino acid sequence coded for by the mRNA is translated by ribosomes into amino acids. The amino acid sequences assemble into peptides and proteins (Fig. 4.2). Upon further posttranslational folding, twisting and interaction with other proteins, the secondary, tertiary, as well as quaternary structure of proteins are formed. These are important for the proper functioning of the active protein.

These proteins may form part of the structural elements of the tissue, such as collagen types 1 and 2; they may contribute to the extracellular matrix to form proteoglycans; or they may form regulatory enzymes, such as metalloproteinases, that help to regulate the metabolic processes inside the tissue.

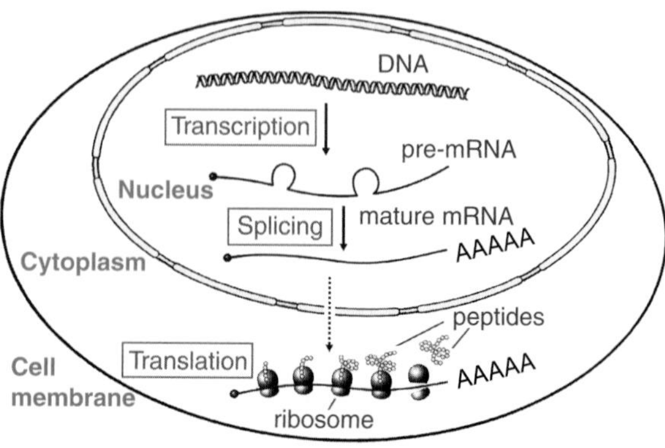

Fig. 4.2 Central dogma from DNA through RNA to protein

4.3 Genetic Polymorphisms and Their Relation to Diseases

The haploid genome is comprised of about 3 billion base pairs (bp). There are about 30,000 genes located in the genome [22, 46]. Majority of the genome is shared in common among the population, with only a small part of it having variation. Such small proportion of difference may cause great influence on the phenotype of different individuals. The two most common types of variation, also called polymorphisms, are microsatellites and single nucleotide polymorphisms (SNPs). At the locus where the polymorphism is located, variants are called alleles. These alleles of the polymorphism are inherited through generations with each individual having two alleles at each locus and are determined by both the paternal and maternal lineages. Microsatellites are tandem repeats of short sequence of 2–8 bp, and the number of tandem repeats differentiates alleles (Fig. 4.3). It is highly polymorphic. SNPs are polymorphisms that differ at a single nucleotide (Fig. 4.4), and the number of known SNPs exceeded 10 million in the human genome [12, 44]. Although an individual SNP is not as polymorphic as a microsatellite due to the limited number of alleles. They are compensated by the large numbers of SNPs scattered throughout the gene and the genome; thus, with high-throughput genotyping technology, SNP markers are more commonly used for genetic analysis nowadays. There are various types of SNP, such as nonsynonymous coding SNPs that change the amino acid sequence encoded, synonymous coding SNPs that do not modify the encoded amino acid, intronic SNPs located in the introns that might affect proper splicing, SNPs located in the 5′ and 3′ untranslated regions (UTRs), and intergenic SNPs that are not located within a gene.

Changes in gene sequences that result in disease are generally called mutations, while changes in the gene sequence without significant external effects are termed polymorphisms, of which the allele frequency should be over 1% in a population. Nonsense mutations result in an amino acid change to a stop codon. Deletion mutations delete one or more nucleotides from a sequence, and insertion mutations insert one or more nucleotides into a sequence. The most recorded pathogenic mutations are

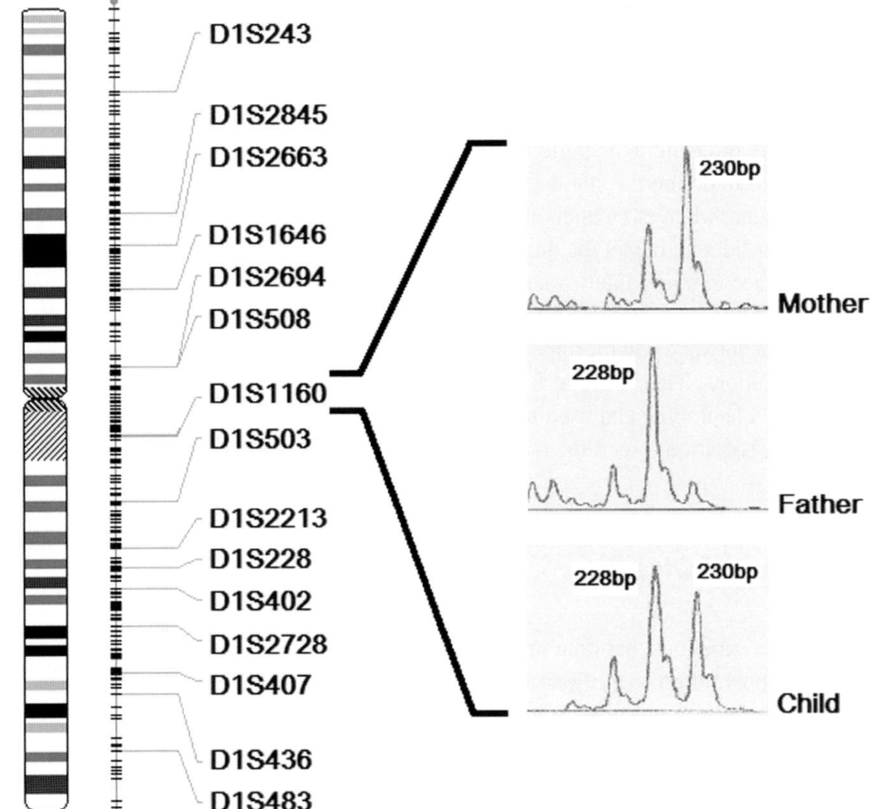

Fig. 4.3 Microsatellite markers and their inheritance. The mother is homozygous for 230 bp allele at marker D1S1160, while the father is homozygous for 228 bp allele. As a result, their child inherited one copy of both the alleles simultaneously from the parents and hence heterozygous at the marker

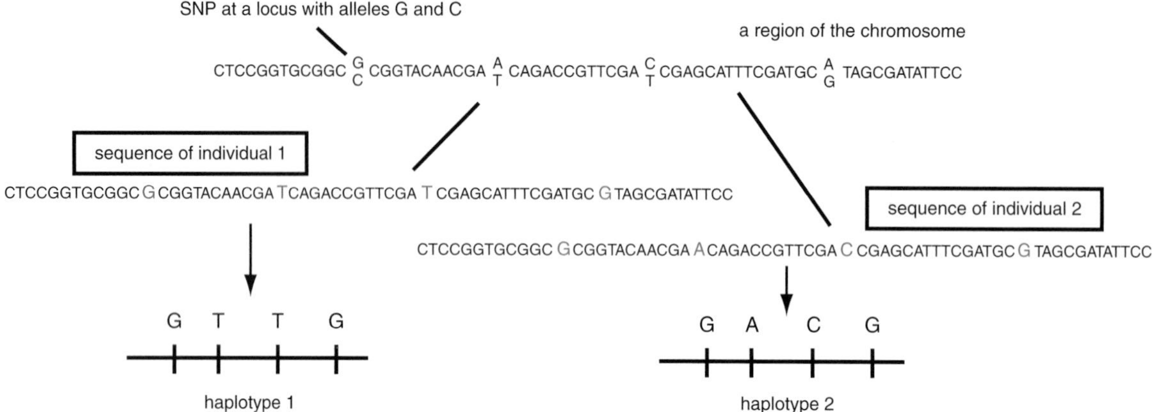

Fig. 4.4 SNP and haplotype. On the sequence of a chromosome region, there are 4 SNP loci. When considering the haplotype of these 4 loci, individual 1 is having GTTG, while individual 2 is having GACG

detected in the coding sequence, such as nonsynonymous mutations and frameshift mutations. Promoter is the regulatory region that is located upstream of a gene and it provides regulation to transcription so that gene expression is controlled. Mutations in promoter that control gene transcription would prevent the promoter from working, resulting in a change in the level of gene expression. These products of mutations may have reduced or no function called loss-of-function mutation [7], while gain-of-function mutation takes place when the gene product has a positive abnormal effect [15, 40].

If we are referring to a single locus, the term genotype is used to define the status of the two alleles. On the other hand, when more than one locus on a chromosome is considered, haplotype denotes their allele configuration according to their order in physical position (see Fig. 4.4). As a single SNP locus has only two alleles, it is not very polymorphic, with a limited number of variations. Thus, several SNP loci can be combined into a haplotype and used to increase the ability to detect associations (see Fig. 4.4).

4.4 Types of Disease

Phenotypic variations between individuals are determined by polymorphisms of particular genes resulting in differences in genotypes. These phenotypic outcomes may be expressed subtly at the molecular level (e.g., expressional level difference of a protein) or more obviously resulting in notable body changes (e.g., height) or even symptoms of diseases. However, risk-conferring genotype in one individual may not necessarily result in disease or symptoms of disease in another. This is due to a phenomenon known as penetrance. Incomplete penetrance refers to the case in which the risk-conferring genotype is not fully expressed, and therefore does not actually cause disease. This maybe due to the risk-conferring genotypes that may require additional exposure to environmental factors, as well as interaction with other susceptibility genes in order to develop disease. Such conditions requiring an interaction of multiple genes with the environment are known as complex genetic disorders. Osteoarthritis, degenerative disc disease, hypertension, and diabetes are examples. Mendelian disease refers to a simpler form of disease in which alternation or mutation at a single gene is enough for its manifestation [32, 35]. These tend to be rarer diseases with more severe phenotype, such as osteogenesis imperfect or Duchenne muscular dystrophy. Furthermore, phenotypic outcomes may be qualitative (i.e., with or without the disease) or quantitative, presenting with a spectrum of severity from mild to severe, which can be measured by number of units (e.g., blood pressure and scores of intervertebral disc degeneration) [42].

4.5 Disease Gene Mapping

Before claiming a disease has a genetic component and trying to find the gene, commonly called mapping, it is important to estimate the relative importance of the genetic risk factor on the disease. One way to do so is to assess familial aggregation; if the disease occurs in multiple members of the same family, this is an indication. However, one needs to remember that members of the same family are likely to be exposed to similar environmental factors, such that the appearance pattern of a disease may not be ultimately due to genes but merely to nongenetic factors. An even better method is to examine disease occurrence between twins, especially as monozygotic (identical) twins share the same genes; on the other hand, dizygotic (nonidentical) twins only share 50% of similar genes. Therefore, for a purely genetic disease, both the monozygotic twins should have the disease (high concordance rate). However, if both the mono and dizygotic twin have similar concordance rates, it would be a stronger evidence for shared environmental factors being a major factor. While if low concordance rates are found among twins, the disease could be affected by some unshared environmental factors. In summary, for a disease predisposition to be genetic, high and low concordance rates must be obtained from monozygotic and dizygotic twin pairs, respectively [8]. These classical twin studies are a common feature of many diseases that are suspected to have a genetic component.

Once a disease has been confirmed to have a substantial genetic component, one can attempt to map the disease gene to a particular location in the genome by using a number of strategies, including linkage analysis on familial subjects, case–control association studies using population-based subjects on either biologically relevant candidate genes, or case–control association studies on a genome-wide scale using gene-chip arrays.

4.6 Linkage Analysis on Familial Subjects

Linkage analysis is a classical method for mapping disease genes, and it has been successfully used to identify numerous disease genes in the past decades. Families, preferably large and having multiple affected members are recruited and genotyped for hundreds of microsatellite markers. If a disease gene is located in the proximity of one of these markers, so that recombination is unlikely to occur at a position in between the marker and the disease gene, that region of the chromosome is likely to be transmitted to the affected members within the family together with the marker. Hence, the marker is said to be in linkage with the disease gene, and it produces a characteristic pattern of transmission (Fig. 4.5). With the usage of microsatellite markers covering the whole genome, genome-wide linkage analysis can locate the rough chromosomal localization of an unknown disease gene without any prior knowledge. It is a powerful strategy that can maximize the chance of finding a disease gene.

If the marker is on the same chromosome as the disease gene, recombination will be responsible for breaking them up so that their alleles will not be transmitted together on the same chromosome. The further apart they are, the higher the chance that they will be affected by recombination. Hence, from the rate of recombination, we can estimate the distance between the marker and the unknown disease gene. Generally speaking, a 1% recombination rate (θ) is referred to as 1 centimorgan (cM) apart, and it is roughly equivalent to 1 million bp distance on the chromosome [31, 41].

In parametric linkage analysis, one tests either the test hypothesis (that the marker linked to the disease gene is true) or the null hypothesis (that the marker is not linked to the disease gene). After making the assumption of disease model (e.g., mode of inheritance, penetrance, and disease allele frequency), one performs sequential test at various θ to compare the likelihoods of the test and null hypotheses. The likelihood of the test hypothesis to the likelihood of the null hypothesis is called the likelihood ratio or odds. Taking the logarithm to base 10 of this likelihood ratio will give us the logarithm of odds (LOD) score. The point with the highest LOD score indicates the most likely distance between the marker and the disease gene locus [28]. To achieve a genome-wide significant level equivalent to $P = 0.05$, a LOD score of 3.3 is required [21].

The advantage of the LOD score method is that one can combine the results from different studies to strengthen the significance (considering they are studying the same disease with the same disease model assumption) [28]. For instance, one may have relatively small sample sizes across studies and find suggestive linkage evidence with LOD score <3.3. Although the LOD score does not reach the threshold of 3.3 in an individual study, their LOD scores can be added up so that the combined LOD score may reach statistical significance.

An alternative to parametric linkage is nonparametric linkage analysis. Without making an assumption on the disease model, which is usually unknown, this still allows the usage of the power of linkage analysis. The

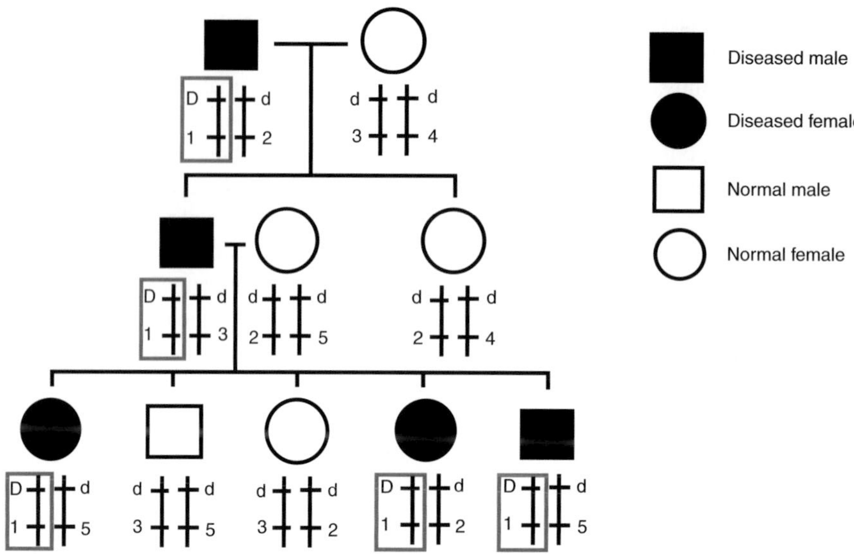

Fig. 4.5 Typical inheritance pattern of linkage. In the figure, 2 loci are considered. The upper locus is the disease gene locus with disease allele D and normal allele d, while the lower one is a nearby microsatellite marker locus with many alleles (1–5). If the 2 loci are in linkage, they will be transmitted together to the offsprings without being disrupted by recombination during meiosis. In this example, the 2 loci are in linkage and allele D is linked with allele 1. The resulting haplotype D-1 is transmitted to every diseased family member. Since the disease gene locus is unknown, linkage analysis relies on correlating the marker locus inheritance (genotype) with disease status (phenotype) to detect linkage. As the marker locus is in linkage with the phenotype, it is an evidence that the unknown disease gene locus is somewhere nearby and thus its rough chromosomal localization can be determined. By using large amount of markers covering the whole genome, genome-wide linkage analysis can be performed. As the markers are not the actual disease-causing mutation and they only denote a certain status of the chromosome, each family may have a different allele in linkage with the disease-causing allele

affected sib pair (ASP) method [19, 33] and the affected pedigree member (APM) method [47, 48] were developed. The latter case uses all the affected members instead of using only the affected siblings for analysis. The idea of nonparametric linkage analysis is that if there is a disease-causing mutation at a locus near a marker, they are in linkage and their alleles on the same chromosome are likely to be transmitted among the APMs unless recombination disrupts them. As a result, the affected members within the same family are expected to share marker alleles in common more often than by chance alone (50% for siblings) if there is a disease-causing mutation at a gene nearby.

A number of computer programs Allegro [14], Genehunter [20], and Merlin [1] have been developed for performing linkage analysis.

The merit of linkage analysis is that we need not have any prior knowledge on where the disease gene is, and we can determine its location based on the evidence of linkage with markers; thus it is a method used to discover new and unexpected predisposing genes. However, it works best in diseases where relatively few genes are involved, and that these genes exert relatively major effects (i.e., disease causing). It lacks the power to detect the effect of common alleles with modest effects on disease, and these maybe important as our understanding of genetic predisposition increases. It is likely that common diseases such as hypertension, diabetes, osteoarthritis, and intervertebral disc degeneration are the result of multiple genes with modest effects interacting with the environment to produce a phenotype. For these, a population-based, genome-wide case–control association study maybe the better approach.

4.7 Case–Control Association Studies on Population-Based Subjects

Instead of testing for allele sharing within families in linkage described earlier, population-based association looks for an allele to be associated with a trait (symptom or characteristic of a disease) across the population. The principles are similar to linkage but it searches for an allele for a disease-causing gene mutation in an extended family (i.e., individuals of a population believed to share a common ancestry). In this special kind of linkage study, the "family" considered is the whole population, and the linkage is so tight (distance between the disease-gene locus and the marker locus is extremely close) that it will not be disrupted by recombination even after thousands of generations. To test for association, we test whether a particular allele of a locus (i.e., a marker) is overrepresented in cases and at the same time under-represented in controls. If so, we can claim that such locus is associated with the studied disease.

In general, there are two types of association – direct and indirect [11]. Direct association targets polymorphisms that have functional consequences and predisposes to disease. This kind of association is the most powerful, but the chance of selecting a marker that is also a disease predisposing allele is not high. On the other hand, in indirect association, the association is between the marker and the nearby disease predisposing allele. It relies on the principle of linkage disequilibrium (LD), whereby due to the proximity of the marker to the predisposing allele, the marker will be associated with the predisposing allele, and therefore results in a disease in a higher frequency than would be expected. Thus, identification of such a marker would provide clues that a disease-causing polymorphism is nearby, and narrows the search for this polymorphism.

There are two methodologies for association studies. The first is by using a candidate gene approach, in which one guesses the likely genes that are involved in the disease and directly screens them for disease association by using a set of markers as described earlier. The identification of such genes is usually based on previous studies that suggest the candidate genes are biologically involved in the disease or that they reside within the functional pathway of the disease process. One such example would be for the testing of the Asporin (*ASPN*) gene in degenerative disc disease [42], when this gene has already been shown to be involved in osteoarthritis [18].

Once the candidate genes are selected, the next step would be the selection of markers within the gene or region of interest. The most commonly used markers are called SNPs. These are single nucleotide changes within the human genome that do not have a functional consequence. These have been identified and are provided within the HapMap database [44]. This type of association study is also often the final part of a linkage analysis study. Although linkage analysis described earlier can identify a region within a particular chromosome, it is unable to identify a particular gene. Thus, the best candidate genes can be selected within the confined interval and tested using a case-association approach. Such a two-stage approach would minimize the candidates to be tested as well as maximize the chance of disease gene hunting.

The second type of case-association study is the so-called genome-wide association study. The principle is the same as that described earlier, except that due to advancements in technology, rather than to test single candidate genes, a high-density SNP map of the whole genome is generated, and all these SNPs are tested for association with disease by comparing their frequencies between the diseased and control cohorts. This type of study is only made possible recently by the availability of high-throughput genotyping platforms such as DNA genechips [34]. It is now feasible to genotype hundreds of thousands of SNPs at a reasonable cost and time. By using large amounts of SNP markers that cover the whole genome, genome-wide association studies need not select candidates and thus does not rely on "best guess" selection of candidate genes. With the availability of initial results highlighting a particular chromosomal region, the indicated genes can be studied in detail by a direct association approach, in which polymorphisms that result in a change in the coding sequence of the gene (often referred to as nonsynonymous SNPs) are examined.

4.8 Genetic Mutations to Spinal Abnormalities

Nonsynonymous coding mutations, SNPs in the introns of splicing sites, and SNPs in the 5′ and 3′ UTR may affect gene function. As genes encode peptides and proteins that may form structural elements of the spine (e.g., collagens), extracellular matrix components (e.g., proteoglycans), or enzymes in regulating metabolic processes (e.g., metalloproteinases), alterations in their gene function may result in altered levels of expression or altered structure of the involved protein, leading to disease.

For example, radiological studies of spondyloepiphyseal dysplasia (SED) Omani type showed minor metaphyseal changes but major manifestations in the spine and the epiphyses. With age, the vertebral endplates became increasingly irregular, the intervertebral space diminished further, and individual vertebrae started to fuse resulting in a severe short-trunk dwarfism with kyphoscoliosis [37]. A mutation (R304Q) in the *CHST3* gene was identified in these patients [45]. *CHST3* encodes chondroitin 6-*O*-sulfotransferase 1 (C6ST-1), which catalyzes the modifying step of chondroitin sulfate (CS) synthesis by transferring sulfate to the C-6 position of the *N*-acetylgalactosamine of chondroitin. The mutation is essential for the structure of the cosubstrate binding site that leads to defective sulfation of CS chain and chondrodysplasia, with major involvement of the spine [45].

CHD7 gene is widely expressed in undifferentiated neuroepithelium and in mesenchyme of neural crest origin. Toward the end of the first trimester, it is expressed in dorsal root ganglia, cranial nerves and ganglia, and auditory, pituitary, and nasal tissues as well as in the neural retina [39]. Gao et al. [10], in 2007, identified an SNP, an A-to-G change in intron 2 of the *CHD7* gene that was predicted to disrupt a caudal-type (cdx) transcription factor binding site, which affects the *CHD7* gene expression leading to association with late-onset idiopathic scoliosis (IS) [13].

Osteogenesis imperfecta type IIB is an autosomal recessive form of perinatal lethal osteogenesis imperfecta with excess posttranslational modification of type I collagen, indicative of delayed folding of the collagen helix [6]. CRTAP protein interacts with the enzyme responsible for posttranslational prolyl 3-hydroxylation of collagen. Without CRTAP protein, collagen structure was abnormal. A homozygous single-base pair (T) deletion in exon 4 (879delT) caused a frameshift and was expected to cause a null allele due to nonsense-mediated decay [6]. Other homozygous or compound heterozygous mutations in the *CRTAP* gene also have been identified to cause low levels of *CRTAP* mRNA and a lack of CRTAP protein [27].

4.9 Genetics of Idiopathic Scoliosis

IS is the most common spinal deformity in children and its etiology is unknown. Inherence models of IS are complex. Twin studies gave evidence for a genetic etiology in adolescent IS (AIS) [3, 51]. The severity of the disease within families can change and sometimes miss or skip generations. It is also possible that more than one gene is involved in the disease.

Ogilvie et al. [30] in 2006 investigated a cohort of 145 AIS probands, to ascertain whether they have a family history of AIS, and found that nearly all (97%) AIS patients have familial origins. The authors suggested at least one major gene with different penetrance and expressivity. They also detected a major gene effect by segregation analysis using a model with age and gender effects in 101 pedigrees ascertained through a proband. Their model indicates that only 30% of the male and 50% of the female carriers of the predisposing allele develop pronounced forms of the disease [5].

Family linkage analysis and case–control association have been used to detect disease susceptibility genes. Miller et al. [25] and Cheung et al. [10] in 2007 gave good reviews on the genetics of familial IS in four published data sets. Significant linkage regions were identified through a genome-wide analysis of a large family on chromosome 6, 10, and 18, with the highest LOD score on chromosome 18 [49].

Genome scans of seven multiplex families of southern Chinese descent with AIS were carried out. A two-point linkage gave an LOD score of 3.63 with a flanked region (5.2 cM) between D19S894 and D19S1034 on chromosome 19p13.3 [9]. This region was later confirmed to be significantly linked to a subset of families with probands having a curve ≥30° [2]. The X chromosome was reported to link to a subset families with a maximum LOD score of 1.69 (θ = 0.2) at marker GATA172D05 [17], and chromosomes 5 and 13 were found to link to a subset of families with kyphoscoliosis [24]. A positive LOD score of 3.20 at θ = 0.00 was detected with marker D17S799 in a three-generation IS Italian family. Then, six additional flanking microsatellites confirmed the linkage between D17S947 and D17S798 [38]. More recently, significant linkage was detected to the telomeric regions of chromosomes 9q at marker D9S2157, with a maximum LOD score of 3.64 and 17q at marker AAT095 with a maximum LOD score of 4.08 in AIS pedigrees of the British population. The 9q region was further narrowed down to approximately 21 Mb at 9q31.2-q34.2 between markers D9S930 and D9S1818, and the 17q candidate region was 3.2 Mb between the distal to marker D17S1806 on chromosome 17q25.3-qtel [29].

In addition, evidence of linkage and association with (multipoint LOD 2.77; P = 0.0028) was detected in a cohort of 52 families of AIS on 8q12 loci of genome-wide scans. Haplotypes of the *CHD7* gene were detected to be associated with the CHARGE syndrome after fine mapping in the region. The resequencing of *CHD7* gene revealed at least one potentially functional polymorphism that is overtransmitted ($P = 0.005$) to the affected offspring and predicts disruption of a caudal-type (cdx) transcription factor binding site. These results suggest etiological overlap between the rare, early onset CHARGE syndrome and the common, late-onset IS [13].

Several genes have been studied by using case–control design. *MATN1* gene was analyzed in a population of 81 trios, each consisting of a daughter or son affected by IS and both parents. An allele of a microsatellite marker in *MATN1* was found to have been significantly overtransmitted from parents to the affected probands. The results suggest that familial IS is associated with the *MATN1* gene [26]. Melatonin receptor 1B (*MTNR1B*) is one of the candidate genes. A chicken pinealectomy model suggested that melatonin deficiency could play a significant role in AIS. The authors initially screened 472 cases and 304 controls with five tag SNPs and replicated the study with 342 cases and 347 controls. A promoter SNP (rs4753426) was significant with the CC genotype, which had an odds ratio of 1.29 for AIS. However, they could not rule out the possibility that some other unrecognized variants might be present and may contribute to the observed association [36]. The XbaI polymorphism site of the estrogen receptor gene was studied in 304 girls with IS using Cobb's method. The authors detected that this polymorphism was associated with curve severity [16]. This association was confirmed by a Chinese data set consisting of 202 patients with AIS and 174 healthy controls [50]. However, the association with curve severity could not be replicated in 364 Chinese AIS patients and 260 controls [43]. Although other candidate genes such as *IGF-I* [52], growth hormone receptor [23], and aggrecan [37] did not appear to be significantly associated with AIS in a particular study data set, further studies are still required.

In summary, several loci have been detected by linkage analysis as listed in Table 4.1. Although the linkage analysis to map AIS was proven to be successful, nonetheless, the progress of detecting disease genes remains slow and so far only *CHD7* gene has been discovered by linkage approach.

This maybe because in complex diseases, multiple genes with only moderate effects are involved, and as previously mentioned, linkage analysis may not have the ability to detect all of them in an individual, leading to inconsistent results. Case–control studies also identified genes associated with sporadic (nonfamilial) AIS; however, there is a need to carefully interpret these results as case-association studies can give rise to false-positive information. It is important to remember that for genetic association studies to be successful, one needs large sample sizes, small *P* values, reported associations that make biological sense, and alleles that affect the gene product in a physiologically meaningful way [4]. Therefore, many such studies and identified genetic risk factors need further confirmation with larger samples and different populations.

Table 4.1 Linkage Loci and genetic risk factors have been reported

Linkage regions	Reference
6p, 10q, and 18q	Wise et al. [49]
19p13.3	Chan et al. [9]
Xq23–26	Justice et al. [17]
5p13, 13q13, and 13q32	Miller et al. [24]
17p11	Salehi et al. [38]
9q31.2-q34.2, 17q25.3-qtel	Ocaka et al. [29]
8q12 (*CHD7*)	Gao et al. [13]
Case–control studies	
MATN1	Montanaro et al. [26]
MTNR1B	Qiu et al. [36]
ER	Inoue et al. [16], Wu et al. [50], Tang et al. [43]
IGF-I	Yeung et al. [52]
GHR	Marosy et al. [23]

With the completion of the human HapMap project and with new technologies, one can foresee that case–control studies using a set of high-density SNP marker to cover the whole genome will become an increasingly popular approach. With international collaboration with well-defined phenotypes and large sample sizes, study of gene interaction and gene–environment interaction will be performed to speed the discovery of genetic risk factors for scoliosis.

The study of genetic factors that predispose to scoliosis has come a long way in the past 10 years. Our understanding of the human genome and the development of new high-throughput techniques and computational methods have provided us with the tools to really embark on large-scale studies on scoliosis. The cause of IS and congenital scoliosis, factors that may influence their progression, will likely be elucidated in the not-too-distant future.

References

1. Abecasis GR, Cherny SS, Cookson WO et al (2002) Merlin – rapid analysis of dense genetic maps using sparse gene flow trees. Nat Genet 30:97–101
2. Alden KJ, Marosy B, Nzegwu N, Justice CM, Wilson AF, Miller NH (2006) Idiopathic scoliosis: identification of candidate regions on chromosome 19p13. Spine 31:1815–1819
3. Andersen MO, Thomsen K, and Kyvik KO (2007) Adolescent idiopathic scoliosis in twins-a population-based survey. Spine 32:927–930
4. Anonymous (1999) Freely associating (editorial). Nat Genet 22:1–2
5. Axenovich TI, Zaidman AM, Zorkoltseva IV, Tregubova IL, Borodin PM (1999) Segregation analysis of idiopathic scoliosis: demonstration of a major gene effect. Am J Med Genet 86:389–394
6. Barnes AM, Chang W, Morello R, Cabral WA, Weis M, Eyre DR, Leikin S, Makareeva E, Kuznetsova N, Uveges TE, Ashok A, Flor AW, Mulvihill JJ, Wilson PL, Sundaram UT, Lee B, Marini JC (2006) Deficiency of cartilage-associated protein in recessive lethal osteogenesis imperfecta. New Engl J Med 355:2757–2764
7. Bateman JF, Wilson R, Freddi S, Lamande SR, Savarirayan R (2005) Mutations of COL10A1 in Schmid metaphyseal chondrodysplasia. Hum Mutat 25:525–534
8. Burmeister M (1999) Basic concepts in the study of diseases with complex genetics. Biol Psychiatry 45:522–532
9. Chan V, Fong GC, Luk KD, Yip B, Lee MK, Wong MS, Lu DD, Chan TK (2002) A genetic locus for adolescent idiopathic scoliosis linked to chromosome 19p13.3. Am J Hum Gene 71:401–406
10. Cheung KM, Wang T, Qiu GX, Luk KD (2007) Recent advances in the aetiology of adolescent idiopathic scoliosis. Int Orthop 15:2:16
11. Cordell HJ, Clayton DG (2005) Genetic association studies. Lancet 366:1121–1131
12. Crawford DC, Nickerson DA (2005) Definition and clinical importance of haplotypes. Annu Rev Med 56:303–320
13. Gao X, Gordon D, Zhang D, Browne R, Helms C, Gillum J, Weber S, Devroy S, Swaney S, Dobbs M, Morcuende J, Sheffield V, Lovett M, Bowcock A, Herring J, Wise C (2007) CHD7 gene polymorphisms are associated with susceptibility to idiopathic scoliosis. Am J Hum Genet 80:957–965
14. Gudbjartsson DF, Jonasson K, Frigge ML et al (2000) Allegro, a new computer program for multipoint linkage analysis. Nat Genet 25:12–13
15. Humphries SE, Luong LA, Talmud PJ et al (1998) The 5A/6A polymorphism in the promoter of the stromelysin-1 (MMP-3) gene predicts progression of angiographically determined coronary artery disease in men in the LOCAT gemfibrozil study. Lopid Coronary Angiography Trial. Atherosclerosis 139:49–56
16. Inoue M, Minami S, Nakata Y, Kitahara H, Otsuka Y, Isobe K, Takaso M, Tokunaga M, Nishikawa S, Maruta T, Moriya H (2002) Association between estrogen receptor gene polymorphisms and curve severity of idiopathic scoliosis. Spine 27:2357–2362
17. Justice CM, Miller NH, Marosy B, Zhang J, Wilson AF (2003) Familial idiopathic scoliosis: evidence of an X-linked susceptibility locus. Spine 28:589–594
18. Kizawa H, Kou I, Iida A, Sudo A, Miyamoto Y, Fukuda A, Mabuchi A, Kotani A, Kawakami A, Yamamoto S, Uchida A, Nakamura K, Notoya K, Nakamura Y, Ikegawa S (2005) An aspartic acid repeat polymorphism in asporin inhibits chondrogenesis and increases susceptibility to osteoarthritis. Nat Genet 37(2):138–144
19. Kruglyak L, Lander ES (1995) Complete multipoint sib-pair analysis of qualitative and quantitative traits. Am J Hum Genet 57:439–454
20. Kruglyak L, Daly MJ, Reeve-Daly MP et al (1996) Parametric and nonparametric linkage analysis: a unified multipoint approach. Am J Hum Genet 58:1347–1363
21. Lander E, Kruglyak L (1995) Genetic dissection of complex traits: guidelines for interpreting and reporting linkage results. Nat Genet 11:241–247
22. Lander ES, Linton LM, Birren B et al (2001) Initial sequencing and analysis of the human genome. Nature 409:860–921
23. Marosy B, Justice CM, Nzegwu N, Kumar G, Wilson AF, Miller NH (2006) Lack of association between the aggrecan gene and familial idiopathic scoliosis. Spine 31:1420–1425
24. Miller NH (2007) Genetics of familial idiopathic scoliosis. Clin Orthop Rel Res 462:6–10
25. Miller NH, Marosy B, Justice CM, Novak SM, Tang EY, Boyce P, Pettengil J, Doheny KF, Pugh EW, Wilson AF (2006) Linkage analysis of genetic loci for kyphoscoliosis on chromosomes 5p13, 13q13.3, and 13q32. Am J Med Genet A 140:1059–1068
26. Montanaro L, Parisini P, Greggi T, Di Silvestre M, Campoccia D, Rizzi S, Arciola CR (2006) Evidence of a linkage between matrilin-1 gene (MATN1) and idiopathic scoliosis. Scoliosis 1:21
27. Morello R, Bertin TK, Chen Y, Hicks J, Tonachini L, Monticone M, Castagnola P, Rauch F, Glorieux FH, Vranka J, Bachinger HP, Pace JM, Schwarze U, Byers PH, Weis M, Fernandes RJ, Eyre DR, Yao Z, Boyce BF, Lee B (2006) CRTAP is required for prolyl 3-hydroxylation and mutations cause recessive osteogenesis imperfecta. Cell 127:291–304
28. Morton NE (1955) Sequential tests for the detection of linkage. Am J Hum Genet 7:277–318
29. Ocaka L, Zhao C, Reed JA, Ebenezer ND, Brice G, Morley T, Mehta M, O'dowd J, Weber JL, Hardcastle AJ, Child AHJ (2007) Med Genet. Assignment of two loci for autosomal dominant adolescent idiopathic scoliosis (AIS) to chromosomes 9q31.2-q34.2 and 17q25.3-qtel. J Med Genet 45(2):87–92
30. Ogilvie JW, Braun J, Argyle V, Nelson L, Meade M, Ward K (2006) The search for idiopathic scoliosis genes. Spine 31:679–681
31. Ott J (1999) Analysis of human genetic linkage. Johns Hopkins University Press, Baltimore
32. Pagon RA (2002) Genetic testing for disease susceptibilities: consequences for genetic counseling. Trends Mol Med 8:306–307
33. Penrose LS (1953) The general purpose sibpair linkage test. Ann Eugen 18:120–4
34. Peters T, Sedlmeier R (2006) Current methods for high-throughput detection of novel DNA polymorphisms. Drug Discov Today 3:123–29
35. Pritchard JK, Cox NJ (2002) The allelic architecture of human disease genes: common disease-common variant…or not? Hum Mol Genet 11:2417–2423
36. Qiu XS, Tang NL, Yeung HY, Lee KM, Hung VW, Ng BK, Ma SL, Kwok RH, Qin L, Qiu Y, Cheng JC (2007) Melatonin

receptor 1B (MTNR1B) gene polymorphism is associated with the occurrence of adolescent idiopathic scoliosis. Spine 32:1748–753

37. Rajab A, Kunze J, Mundlos S (2004) Spondyloepiphyseal dysplasia Omani type: a new recessive type of SED with progressive spinal involvement. Am J Med Genet 126A:413–419
38. Salehi LB, Mangino M, De Serio S, De Cicco D, Capon F, Semprini S, Pizzuti A, Novelli G, Dallapiccola B (2002) Assignment of a locus for autosomal dominant idiopathic scoliosis (IS) to human chromosome 17p11. Hum Genet 111:401–404
39. Sanlaville D, Etchevers HC, Gonzales M, Martinovic J, Clement-Ziza M, Delezoide A-L, Aubry M-C, Pelet A, Chemouny S, Cruaud C, Audollent S, Esculpavit C et al (2006) Phenotypic spectrum of CHARGE syndrome in fetuses with CHD7 truncating mutations correlates with expression during human development. J Med Genet 43:211–217
40. Seki S, Kawaguchi Y, Chiba K et al (2005) A functional SNP in CILP, encoding cartilage intermediate layer protein, is associated with susceptibility to lumbar disc disease. Nat Genet 37:607–612
41. Sham P (1998) Statistics in human genetics. Arnold, London
42. Song YQ, Cheung KMC, Ho DWH, Poon SCS, Chiba K, Kawaguchi Y, Hirose Y, Alini M, Yee AFY, Leong JCY, Luk KDK, Yip SP, Cheah KSE, Sham P, Ikegawa S, Chan D (2008) Asporin D14 allele increases the risk of lumbar disc degeneration in Chinese and Japanese populations. Am J Hum Genet 82(3):744–747
43. Tang NL, Yeung HY, Lee KM, Hung VW, Cheung CS, Ng BK, Kwok R, Guo X, Qin L, Cheng JC (2006) A relook into the association of the estrogen receptor [alpha] gene (PvuII, XbaI) and adolescent idiopathic scoliosis: a study of 540 Chinese cases. Spine 31:2463–2468
44. The International HapMap Consortium (2003) The International HapMap Project. Nature 426:789–796
45. Thiele H, Sakano M, Kitagawa H, Sugahara K, Rajab A, Hohne W, Ritter H, Leschik G, Nurnberg P, Mundlos S (2004) Loss of chondroitin 6-O-sulfotransferase-1 function results in severe human chondrodysplasia with progressive spinal involvement. Proc Natl Acad Sci USA 101: 10155–10160
46. Venter JC, Adams MD, Myers EW et al (2001) The sequence of the human genome. Science 291:1304–1351
47. Weeks DE, Lange K (1988) The affected-pedigree-member method of linkage analysis. Am J Hum Genet 42:315–326
48. Whittemore AS, Halpern J (1994) A class of tests for linkage using affected pedigree members. Biometrics 50:118–127
49. Wise CA, Barnes R, Gillum J, Herring JA, Bowcock AM, Lovett M (2000) Localization of susceptibility to familial idiopathic scoliosis. Spine 15:25:2372–2380
50. Wu J, Qiu Y, Zhang L, Sun Q, Qiu X, He Y (2006) Association of estrogen receptor gene polymorphisms with susceptibility to adolescent idiopathic scoliosis. Spine 31:1131–1136
51. Wynne-Davies R (1969) Familial idiopathic scoliosis: a family survey. J Bone Joint Surg 50B:24–30
52. Yeung HY, Tang NL, Lee KM, Ng BK, Hung VW, Kwok R, Guo X, Qin L, Cheng JC (2006) Genetic association study of insulin-like growth factor-I (IGF-I) gene with curve severity and osteopenia in adolescent idiopathic scoliosis. Stud Health Technol Inform 123:18–24

Section II

Evaluation of the Growing Child

5 Clinical Examination

Jeff Pawelek, Vikas V. Varma, and Ramin Bagheri

Key Points

- Carefully evaluate the spinal deformity but look beyond the curve for associated and underlying medical conditions.
- Secondary diagnoses that introduce additional comorbidities can significantly affect the prognosis and treatment plan.
- Understanding pulmonary health is paramount to preserving and improving the overall health of the child.

5.1 Introduction

The physical examination of a young child with a spinal deformity begins with a thorough medical history documenting the onset of the spinal deformity and its changes over time as well as associated medical conditions such as skin, pulmonary, and syndromic abnormalities. The overall health of the child can be assessed with a routine patient evaluation with a special consideration of the child's neurologic status and musculoskeletal features. The information obtained from the patient's history is paramount in conducting an appropriate physical examination and formulating an effective treatment plan.

J. Pawelek (✉)
San Diego Center for Spinal Disorders, 4130 La Jolla Village Drive, Suite 300, La Jolla, CA 92037, USA
e-mail: jpawelek@sandiego-spine.com

5.2 Medical History

5.2.1 Birth History

The child's complete medical history should be well understood before initiating a treatment plan for his or her spinal disorder. Significant facts relating to the birth of the child should be noted, with particular attention to neurologic and skeletal abnormalities. The Apgar score (activity, pulse, grimace, appearance, and respiration) may reveal important information related to the child's primary diagnosis and secondary musculoskeletal abnormalities (e.g., clubfoot and loss of limb) by noting muscle tone, heart rate, reflex irritability, skin coloration, and breathing immediately after childbirth [1]. Additional notes from previous physical examinations as an infant may be of special interest in identifying possible neurologic causes of the spinal deformity.

5.2.2 Family History

Spinal deformities that exist within the child's family may predict the potential for progression of the deformity during growth and should be considered when developing a treatment plan [4]. Syndromes, neuropathies, and myopathies that are present in immediate family members may also provide clues to the child's diagnosis and potential comorbidities.

5.2.3 Spinal Deformity History

Previous spinal deformity treatments, including Risser casting, bracing, and surgery, should be well understood

B. A. Akbarnia et al. (eds.), *The Growing Spine*,
DOI: 10.1007/978-3-540-85207-0_5, © Springer-Verlag Berlin Heidelberg 2011

before planning new treatment. If the child's spinal deformity is due to a congenital or neuromuscular condition, historical details of the primary diagnosis should be noted, including prior hospitalizations, surgeries, and medical complications. A thorough review of existing comorbidities and previous medical complications will help maximize treatment outcomes and limit future complications. The age of onset of the child's spinal deformity is important for an accurate assessment of the rate of growth and progression of the deformity [3].

5.3 Physical Examination

5.3.1 Overall Health and Review of Systems

The child's overall health, with particular attention to nutrition and pulmonary status, is an critical factor in the decision to proceed with surgery. Current medications should be noted and appropriate medications should be discontinued prior to surgery. Any known allergies should be carefully documented in the medical record and accommodated. A review of respiratory, cardiovascular, gastrointestinal, urinary, hematologic, and endocrine systems should be performed subsequent to a routine physical examination. Knowledge of any history of pneumonia or dysphagia, as well as pulmonary, cardiac, or renal abnormalities must be considered prior to surgical intervention and monitored postoperatively.

5.3.2 Neurological Status

A neurologic evaluation will help identify any neurologic causes of the spinal deformity (i.e., intraspinal neoplasm). The examination should include a complete motor, reflex, and sensory evaluation. Abnormal abdominal reflexes may suggest the presence of an intraspinal disorder [5]. The child's pre- and post-treatment ambulatory status should also be monitored for significant changes.

5.3.3 Mental Status

Developmental delays may suggest that the etiology of the spinal deformity is related to an underlying syndrome with more global involvement, so the child's mental status should be noted, especially if the child has limited communication abilities or evidence of a developmental delay. Changes in verbal communication should also be monitored before and after treatment.

5.3.4 Pain Status

If the child is experiencing pain, note the region, severity, and frequency (see Chap. 9).

5.3.5 Musculoskeletal Status and Examination of the Thorax

A detailed musculoskeletal examination include basic clinical measurements such as height and weight, a thorough evaluation of spinal balance, and any abnormalities of the thorax. The height and weight of the patient is recorded at every visit to monitor growth and nutrition. Standing height is measured to quantify linear extremity growth and total height over time. Because some patients may be unable to stand comfortably, sitting height may be measured while the patient is supine to assess linear truncal growth and its relationship to total height over time (Fig. 5.1a, b).

Clinical photographs are an useful tool for documenting a child's growth over time as well as the correction, or progression, of spinal deformity. Routine photographs include posteroanterior, anteroposterior, lateral (left- and right-sided) views, and views of the thoracic and lumbar prominences present during an Adams forward bend test.

Coronal balance and trunk shift are used to measure the translation of the head and thorax relative to the center of the pelvis, respectively (Fig. 5.2). Preoperative and annual postoperative clinical photographs of coronal balance are helpful in monitoring the child's spinal balance.

Thoracic kyphosis and lumbar lordosis are the major factors contributing to a patient's overall sagittal balance. The thoracolumbar junction links the kyphotic and lordotic regions of the spine and is neutral in normal patients. Sagittal balance, also known as sagittal alignment or sagittal profile, is most often evaluated using a standing lateral radiograph as well as clinically. Pre- and post-operative clinical photographs can also provide valuable information to assess sagittal balance.

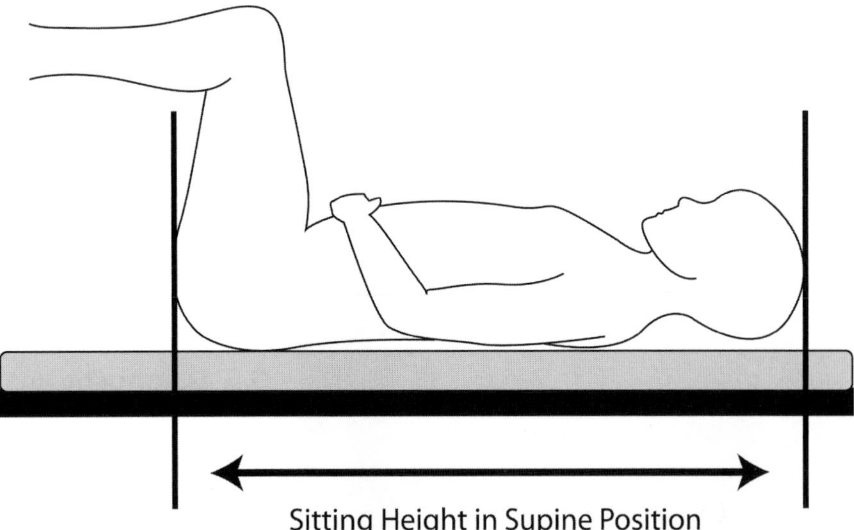

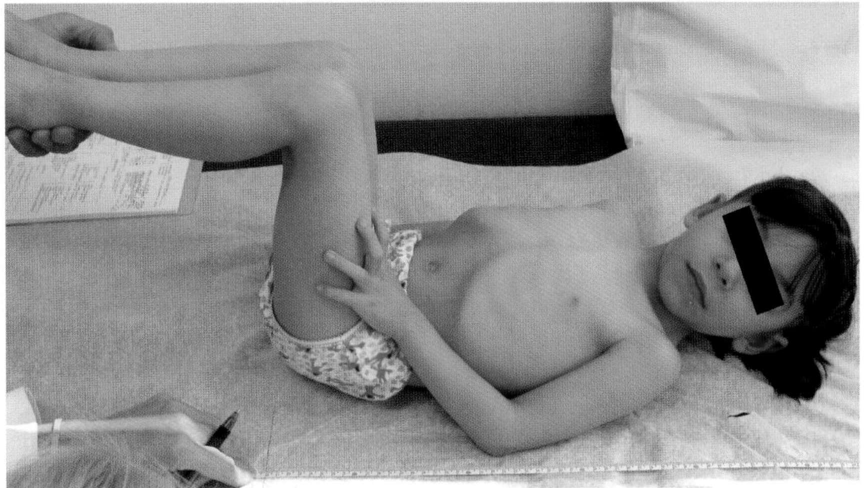

Fig. 5.1 Measurement of sitting height in supine position; (**a**) drawing, (**b**) clinical photo

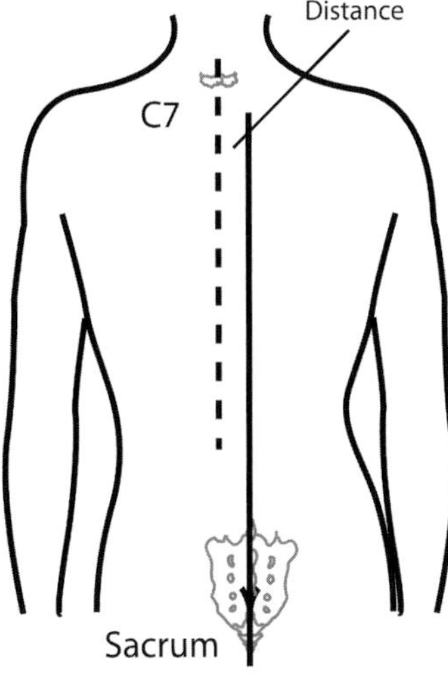

Fig. 5.2 Measurement of coronal balance

Rotational deformity of the trunk is often the most obvious spinal abnormality. The magnitude of trunk rotation can be visualized with an Adams forward bend test and measured using a scoliometer. Rib prominence of the thoracic spine and lumbar prominence of the lumbar spine can also be recorded photographically to document progression.

Chest and rib deformities are evaluated by observation of a child's breathing, recording respiratory rate, and measuring the circumference of the chest throughout treatment (Fig. 5.3). The expansion of the thorax over time may be useful in gauging the growth of the child as well as correlating growth with pulmonary function. The thorax should be evaluated for symmetrical or asymmetrical expansion during inhalation.

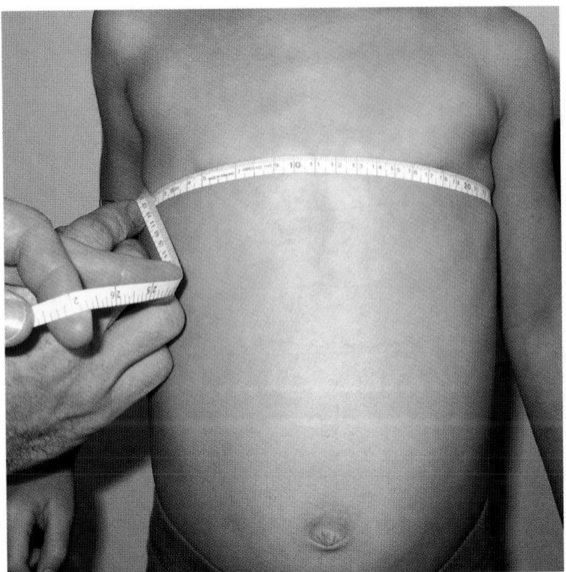

Fig. 5.3 Measurement of chest-wall circumference

A unique method in determining chest-wall motion in a flail chest with absent ribs is known as the "Thumb Excursion Test" and was described by Campbell [2]. To perform this test, the base of the chest is encircled from the back by the examiner's hands, with the examiner's fingers just anterior to the anterior axillary line of the patient (Fig. 5.4). The tips of the examiner's thumbs are positioned equidistant from the spine. The distance between each thumb tip is graded during inhalation as the thumbs move laterally away from the spine.

5.4 Diagnostic Laboratory Testing

A child who is to undergo surgical intervention requires a preoperative complete blood count and a metabolic panel to identify disorders such as anemia, infection, and other diseases. If the patient is cooperative, a pulmonary function test should be performed to assess lung capacity and expiratory volume.

5.5 Diagnostic Imaging

5.5.1 Radiographs

Routine primary evaluation radiographs should include a standing posteroanterior and a standing lateral; both of which should span the lower cervical spine to the femoral heads. If planning surgical treatment, preoperative films should also include coronal supine left- and right-bending films. Traction or bolster films are also useful to determine the degree of curve flexibility, appropriate levels of instrumentation, and expected degree of correction (see Chap 8).

5.5.2 Magnetic Resonance Imaging (MRI)

MRI studies are not routinely used in the evaluations of patients with early onset scoliosis. However, if there is

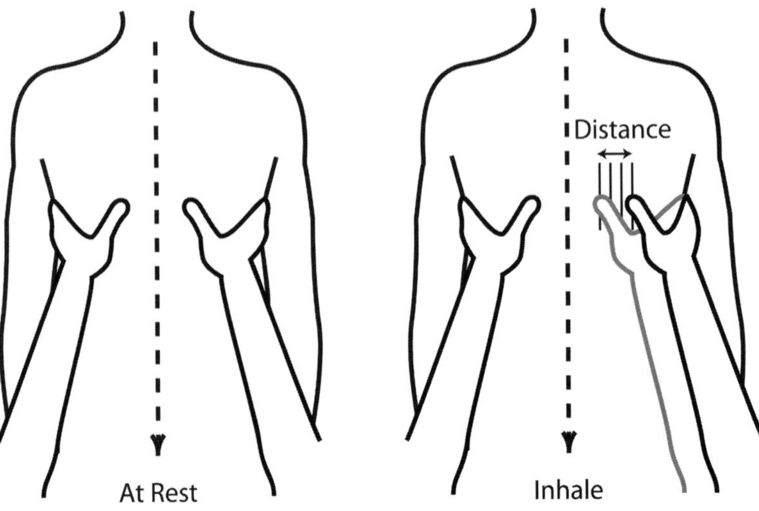

Fig. 5.4 Thumb excursion (modified from ref. [1])

concern for an intraspinal anomaly (e.g., a syrinx, tethered cord, tumor, and diastemetomyelia), then an MRI should be performed to identify abnormal neural elements.

5.5.3 Computed Tomography (CT)

If the child's radiographs demonstrate congenital abnormalities, a CT scan (preferably with 3-dimensional reconstruction) is obtained to further investigate bony abnormalities, such as failure of vertebral segmentation or formation. Accurate detection and classification of abnormalities may alter management and treatment decisions. Intravenous contrast is not routinely needed. However, intrathecal contrast may be warranted if an MRI is contraindicated for medical reasons and further evaluation for intraspinal anomalies (e.g., cord tethering or diastematomyelia) is required.

5.6 Developing a Comprehensive Treatment Plan

Managing early onset spinal deformities requires the commitment and flexibility of both the surgeon and the family. A carefully developed treatment plan is likely to span over several years as the child grows. Short-term and long-term goals of the treatment plan should be identified and clearly discussed with the patient's family. Input from the family, clinical evaluation, consultations, and the results of the imaging studies form the basis of decision making for the treatment plan.

5.6.1 Postoperative Examination

If the child undergoes surgery, a postoperative evaluation should include an examination of the skin incision, assessment of neurologic status, and evaluation for prominent implants. Spinal alignment should be assessed by clinical examination with photographic documentation and standing radiographs.

Acknowledgement The authors would like to acknowledge J.D. Bomar for his assistance with the illustrations in this chapter.

References

1. Apgar V (1953) A proposal for a new method of evaluation of the newborn infant. Curr Res Anesth Analg 32:(4): 260–267
2. Campbell RM Jr, Smith MD, Mayes TC, Mangos JA, Willey-Courand DB, Kose N, Pinero RF, Alder ME, Duong HL, Surber JL (2003) The characteristics of thoracic insufficiency syndrome associated with fused ribs and congenital scoliosis. Bone Joint Surg Am 85:399–408
3. Charles YP, Daures JP, de Rosa V, Diméglio A (2006) Progression risk of idiopathic juvenile scoliosis during pubertal growth. Spine 31(17):1933–42
4. Ogilvie JW, Braun J, Argyle V, Nelson L, Meade M, Ward K (2006) The search for idiopathic scoliosis genes. Spine 31(6): 679–81
5. Zadeh HG, Sakka SA, Powell MP, Mehta MH (1995) Absent superficial abdominal reflexes in children with scoliosis. An early indicator of syringomyelia. J Bone Joint Surg Br 77(5):762–7

6 Comorbidities Associated with Early Onset Scoliosis

Hazem B. Elsebaie

Key Points

- Spinal deformities in the growing spine can be associated with other organ system abnormalities.
- Different nonvertebral abnormalities occur with variable frequencies in different types of spinal deformities.
- Comorbidities can be easily diagnosed by clinical examination or may need to be searched for by specific investigations.
- It is important to identify these comorbidities to avoid the potential problems that might affect and jeopardize the results of management.

6.1 Introduction

Spinal deformities in the growing spine can be associated with other organ system abnormalities; such association, which implies a greater-than-random tendency for abnormalities to occur together, can be attributable to many causes. Both spinal deformity and the other abnormalities can have the same origin, they can have a cause effect relationship in a reciprocal way and sometimes no clear reason for this association could be identified. The time of presentation may not be synchronous and, in many times, depends on the causal relationship.

H. B. Elsebaie
Department of Orthopaedics, Cairo University
22 Degla Street, Mohandessin Giza, PO. Box 12411, Egypt
e-mail: hazembelsebaie@yahoo.com

This chapter is concerned with the most common and clinically relevant comorbidities associated with different types of spinal deformities in order to develop clinical guidelines for investigation and management; one of the main purposes is to discuss nonvertebral abnormalities and the potential problems that might affect and jeopardize the results of treatment or expose these patients to uncalculated risks during their management. No attempt will be made to categorize the spinal deformities and their associated abnormalities by syndrome.

Associated comorbidities will be discussed separately with possible reference to their occurrence in different types of scoliosis; they will be discussed under the following headings:

1. Neural axis
2. Cardiac
3. Urogenital
4. Musculoskeletal
5. Gasterointestinal
6. Cutaneous
7. Pain and disability

6.2 Organ System Comorbidities

6.2.1 *Neural Axis*

When evaluating spinal deformity in a growing child, the physician who treats must be aware that scoliosis in children can be the presenting sign of an asymptomatic neural axis abnormality. These abnormalities include Arnold–Chiari malformation, syringomyelia, hydromyelia, low-lying conus, tethered cord, and tumors. If these neural axis abnormalities remain undetected, there is a risk of neurological sequelae resulting from

B. A. Akbarnia et al. (eds.), *The Growing Spine*,
DOI: 10.1007/978-3-540-85207-0_6, © Springer-Verlag Berlin Heidelberg 2011

the use of instrumentation for correction of the scoliosis [25, 26]. Detailed neurological examination of scoliosis should consist of an evaluation of the motor, sensory, and reflex function of the upper and lower extremities as well as an evaluation of abnormal neurologic signs such as sustained hyperactive reflex, unilateral superficial abdominal reflex, muscle atrophy, motor weakness, sensory loss, and sometimes eliciting gag reflex. History of complaint of severe headache, backache, and the presence of neurologic symptoms should be noted.

6.2.1.1 Idiopathic Scoliosis

For infantile and juvenile idiopathic scoliosis with curves more than 20°, the reports in the literature have demonstrated an approximately 20% (range, 17.6–26%) prevalence of neural axis abnormalities [14, 15, 19]; of additional concern is the reported need for neurosurgical intervention between the time of birth and 10 years of age in more than 50% of patients with idiopathic scoliosis who have neural axis abnormalities on magnetic resonance imaging (MRI). Screening by total spine MRI examination in these young children is recommended at the time of presentation in early onset scoliosis with curves more than 20° even if the findings of neurological examination are normal, and despite the fact that many children at that age may need intravenous sedation or general anesthesia [14]. Once neural axis abnormality is detected, neurosurgical consultation is mandatory for evaluation, treatment, follow-up or possible intervention usually in the form of decompression of the posterior fossa, surgical decompression and/or shunting of a syrinx, and cord untethering.

The association between "idiopathic" scoliosis in all age groups and craniovertebral abnormalities has been well established. It has been reported that the mean position of the cerebellar tonsils in patients with "idiopathic" scoliosis was 4 mm below the foramen magnum and that 50% of patients with "idiopathic" scoliosis had cerebellar tonsils below the foramen magnum [27]. With the development of MRI, neural axis abnormalities such as syringomyelia or Chiari malformations, tonsillar ectopia, and low conus medullaris are increasingly being found in patients with asymptomatic "idiopathic" scoliosis [20].

At 10 years of age and older, the routine use of MRI in patients with idiopathic scoliosis before surgery remains controversial, the classical guidelines for MRI screening in scoliosis are valuable, and the proposed indications for ordering MRI in the literature include neurologic deficits, infantile and juvenile onset, male gender, abnormal sagittal profile of the spine, atypical curve pattern (left-sided curve), rapid curve progression, and the presence of pain [20]. Advocates of a safer routine MRI point out that a higher risk of neurologic complications has been reported during surgery of scoliosis associated with syringomyelia; in addition, to prevent potential neurologic complications [13], neural axis malformations need to be addressed before the treatment of scoliosis; therefore, every attempt should be made to identify these patients clinically or by MRI [25, 32]. However, selective approach is advised by some investigators suggesting that MRI study is not necessary for a neurologically intact patient with adolescent idiopathic scoliosis as patients with "idiopathic" scoliosis, whose neurologic status is normal, might entail little risk of neurologic complications as a result of scoliosis surgery even if these patients have a neural axis malformation on MRI [12, 33, 41].

6.2.1.2 Congenital Scoliosis

Congenital scoliosis is often associated with intraspinal abnormalities. The embryonic development of vertebrae is closely related with that of the spinal cord and the organs of the mesoderm [22]. An incidence of intra spinal anomalies between 30 and 38% is reported in association with congenital spinal deformities when using total spine MRI for assessment of these patients [3, 5, 28]. The intraspinal anomalies can cause progressive neural loss with growth and curve progression. In addition, they greatly increase the risk of neurologic injury during surgical correction of the deformity.

Neurocutaneous stigmas and neurological findings of intraspinal lesions can appear from history or examination; these include hairy patches (Fig 6.1) and pigmentation overlying the spine, bladder symptoms, paraesthesia in one leg, foot deformity, obvious wasting of one leg, asymmetrical abdominal reflexes, and abnormality of posterior column sensation. However, the presence of neurocutaneous stigmas is not a reliable indicator of intraspinal abnormality [5, 20, 23, 24].

Tethered spinal cord (Fig. 6.2a) is the most common MRI-identified intraspinal anomaly in congenital spinal deformity in many reports; syrinx (Fig. 6.2b) is

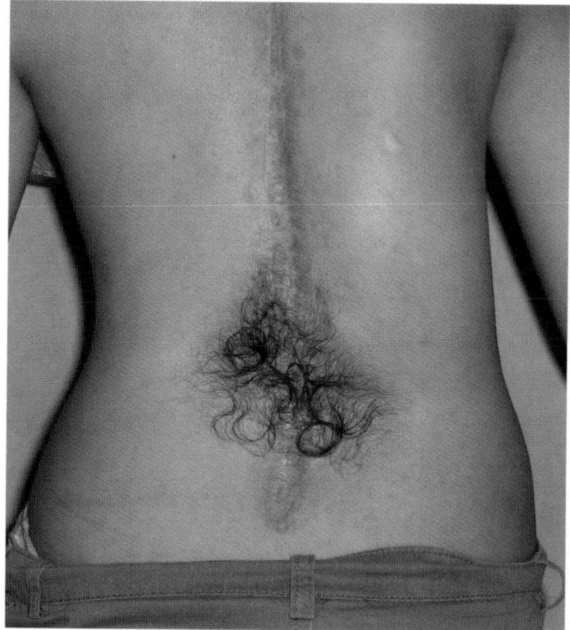

Fig. 6.1 A hairy patch found in the back of a child with congenital spinal deformity; it can be associated with occult spinal dysraphism. The presence of neurocutaneous stigmas is an unreliable indicator of intraspinal abnormality

the second, then thickened and fatty filum, low conus, diastematomyelia (Fig 6.2c) intradural mass/ lipoma, extradural mass, Chiari malformation arachnoid cyst, and Dandy–Walker malformation [3, 5, 36].

Neurologic deficit caused by tethered spinal cord in congenital spinal deformity may not be manifested in very young children, and in older ages, there is lack of clear association between intraspinal anomalies and detectable clinical manifestations; therefore, MRI is generally recommended in evaluation of patients with congenital spinal deformity even in the absence of clinical findings [36]. The performance of MRI in young children, especially 5 years of age or less, involves administration of sedation or general anesthesia, with the attendant risks of respiratory complications in these children who already may suffer from pulmonary compromise; as a result, a selective approach probably is wise; an MRI scan must be obtained in older age groups before surgical correction of the spinal deformity in cases with established or developing neurologic signs, and probably also in cases with progressive deformity, in which surgery is to be considered sooner, but for younger children, MRI with the patient under general anesthesia is to be considered only if surgery is imminent or neurologic signs develop [3].

6.2.1.3 Marfan Syndrome

Dural ectasia is ballooning or widening of the dural sac, fibrillin deficiency resulting in connective tissue abnormality, and weakness in the dural sac has been suggested as the cause for dural ectasia in Marfan syndrome; it usually occurs in the most caudal portion of the lumbosacral spinal column, at the point of greatest cerebrospinal fluid pressure in the upright patient. The neural symptoms are thought to be related to stretching and traction mechanisms, which may be clinically manifested with back pain and headaches. The consequences of dural ectasia include bony erosion or anterior meningoceles. Widened interpediculate distance, increased vertebral scalloping, and increased sagittal diameter can detect dural ectasia in patients with Marfan syndrome. Dural ectasia is a major diagnostic criterion used in Marfan syndrome especially in patients who previously have not had sufficient major and minor diagnostic criteria [17, 35].

An incidence of dural ectasia of 63% was reported in Marfan syndrome [29], this incidence was noted to be 76% in patients with Marfan syndrome and back pain and 41% in patients with Marfan syndrome without back pain [1]. Because the calculation of dural volume requires sophisticated software programs that are not widely available, and because dural ectasia is important as a major diagnostic criterion for Marfan syndrome many guidelines were developed to detect the presence of dural ectasia on Computed Tomography or MRI scan with trials to establish normative values for lumbosacral dural sac dimensions [2]. An abnormal dural sac ratio (the dural sac diameter corrected for vertebral size) has also been used to identify dural ectasia in patients with Marfan syndrome. In symptomatic dural ectasia, posterior laminectomy has been sometimes implemented as a means of relieving back pain.

6.2.1.4 Neurofibromatosis

Dystrophic neurofibromatosis scoliosis is characterized by early onset, rapidly progressive curves that are difficult to treat and has a tendency to progress to a severe deformity. Dystrophic curves may be associated with kyphosis and have a higher incidence of neurologic injury. Most of these patients present with skin lesions (Fig 6.3) as well as associated neurofibromas that envelope the bone or come from the canal (dumbbell lesion) [34].

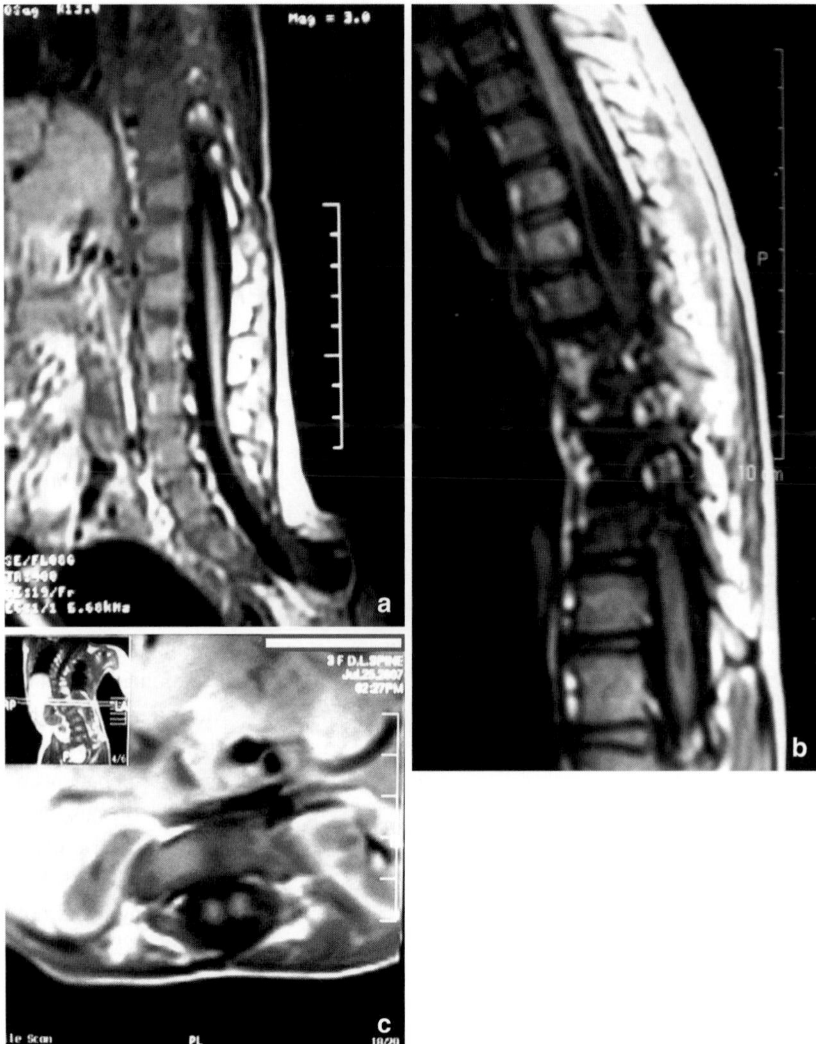

Fig. 6.2 Intraspinal anomalies associated with spinal deformities requiring neurosurgical consultation. (**a**) A sagittal T1-weighted MRI showing a tethered spinal cord, the most common MRI-identified intraspinal anomaly in congenital spinal deformity. Syrinx and tethered cord can also be found in case diagnosed as idiopathic scoliosis. (**b**) A sagittal T1-weighted MRI showing multiple variable sized dorsal syrinx associated with congenital scoliosis. (**c**) An axial T1-weighted magnetic resonance image (MRI) showing diastematomyelia with complete split of the cord at the dorsal region in a child with congenital scoliosis

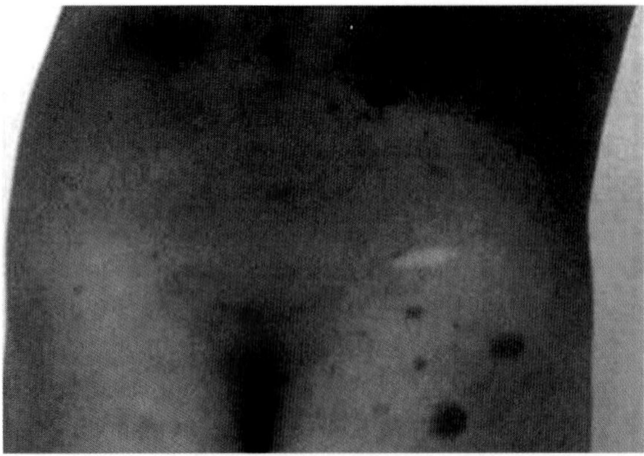

Fig. 6.3 Café au lait spots, cutaneous markers of systemic disorders observed in children with neurofibromatosis scoliosis

Enlargement of the spinal canal caused by intraspinal tumors or dural ectasia is common, it erodes the bony and ligamentous structures causing vertebral scalloping and meningocele formation. Meningoceles, pseudomeningoceles, dural ectasia, and dumbbell lesions are related to the presence of neurofibroma or abnormal pressure phenomena in and around the spinal canal neuraxis. Paraplegia is an uncommon finding in patients who have dystrophic curves; it is more prevalent in patients who have severe vertebral angulation (kyphosis), vertebral subluxation, and soft tissue tumors in the spinal canal [10]. Occasionally, these intraspinal elements may compromise the cord directly when instrumentation and stabilization are attempted, or they may cause erosive changes in the bone, preventing primary fusion. A rare, but important, cause of paraparesis in scoliotic patients is spinal cord compression due to rib penetration [11, 36]. A CT scan is the most sensitive tool to diagnose intraspinal rib dislocation. A resection of the rib will prevent or improve paraparesis in most patients who have dislocation.

It is the surgeon's responsibility to correct and stabilize the spine with the most expedient, safe, and permanent method without causing neurologic injury. Therefore, it is imperative to evaluate such a condition in the preoperative period. MRI should be used in the investigation of all dystrophic curves before surgical treatment [8, 9].

6.2.1.5 Neuromuscular and Myelomeningocele Scoliosis

By definition, neuromuscular disorders are a group of diseases that affect any part of the nerve and muscle. These nerve tissue disorders include motor neuron diseases such as amyotrophic lateral sclerosis and spinal muscular atrophy, which may involve motor neurons in the brain, spinal cord, and periphery, and ultimately weaken the muscle. Many of these diseases can cause early onset scoliosis due to a primary affection in the neural axis.

Spinal deformity also may be caused by paralysis secondary to the spinal cord injury, the scoliosis is secondary to spinal cord affection in the very young age; traumatic paralysis of the spinal cord may also lead to syringomyelia or traumatic tethering in 20% of patients and should be looked for when patients with spinal cord injury have worsening symptoms. Another type of scoliosis is defined by the presence of a clear anomaly in the spinal cord "myelomeningocele scoliosis". Both the types of scoliosis, neuromuscular and myelomeningocele, have their own characteristics, complications, and way of management meriting a separate detailed discussion.

6.3 Cardiac

The relationship between cardiac abnormalities and scoliosis is a complex one, both can orginate from the same tissue defect: in Marfan syndrome, due to connective tissue disorder or in neuromuscular scoliosis, due to different types of myopathy; scoliosis and congental heart disease can occur as a part of multiorgan congenital anomalies; in addition, there is an unexplained higher incidence of minor cardiac anomalies with idiopathic scoliosis. Conversely, scoliosis has a higher tendency to be present in children with congenital heart disease (CHD) with or without previous thoracotomy.

6.3.1 *Idiopathic Scoliosis*

Mitral valve prolapse (MVP) is known to be associated with thoracic skeletal anomalies and MVP is four times more common in patients with severe idiopathic scoliosis than in the normal adolescent population. MVP and other valvular anomalies have been detected by echocardiogram and or ultrasound Doppler in 13.6–24.4% of patients with idiopathic scoliosis as compared to 3.2% in age- and weight-matched controls [12].

Patients with MVP are mostly asymptomatic and only a systolic click or murmur can be detected on examination. The electrocardiogram (ECG) is abnormal in 21% of patients with MVP as compared to only 1.6% of patients with idiopathic scoliosis but no MVP. The persistent nature of MVP, even after corrective spinal surgery, may be related to factors other than geometric changes of the heart caused by abnormal thoracic curvature [13]. Looking at other comorbidities associated with idiopathic soliosis, a significant relationship was found between valvular anomalies and other comorbidities, valvular anomalies were detected in (17.2%) with no comorbidity and in (50%) with a comorbid condition. In this latter group of patients, routine echocardiographic study seems advisable in the preoperative evaluation. [7]

6.3.2 *Congenital Scoliosis*

CHD was found to be associated with congenital spinal deformity in 7–26% of the patients; these include ventricular septal defects, atrial septal defects, patent ductus arteriosus, Fallot transposition of great arteries, pulmonary stenosis, sick sinus syndrome, and dextrocardia. Almost half of these children need medical therapy, some would require surgery for the cardiac condition in the future, and others will need to be kept under observation. This underscores the importance of a systematic clinical cardiac assessment and using echocardiography for these patients. All patients in whom surgery is planned for correction of congenital spinal deformity should have echocardiography as part of preoperative workup. In addition, it has been suggested that patients with congenital scoliosis resulting from mixed bony defects and those with congenital kyphosis should have a routine echocardiogram because of the higher risk for CHD. These patients should be referred subsequently to a cardiologist for further management [3, 4].

6.3.3 Neuromuscular Scoliosis

Cardiac involvement may occur in most of the primary myopathies, including Duchenne muscular dystrophy (DMD), Becker muscular dystrophy (BMD), myotonic muscular dystrophy (MMD), and some cases of limb girdle muscular dystrophy. Dystrophin has been localized to the membrane surface of cardiac Purkinje fibers; this localization probably contributes to the cardiac conduction disturbances seen in DMD and BMD.

A high (60–80%) occurrence of cardiac involvement is present in patients of all ages with DMD and BMD; this can be detected via ECG and echocardiogram; however, only about 30% of patients with DMD have clinically significant cardiac complications. Pulmonary hypertension also has been implicated in the cardiorespiratory insufficiency associated with DMD and some investigators blame congestive heart failure as the cause of death in as many as 40% of patients with DMD. The cardiac compromise may be disproportionately severe relative to respiratory compromise in some patients with BMD. Thus, ECG and echocardiography screening are indicated at regular intervals for all patients with BMD because severe cardiac involvement in BMD may occasionally precede the clinical presentation of skeletal myopathy. Patients with myocardial involvement need close follow-up and treatment by a cardiologist with expertise in this area. Some patients with BMD may be suitable candidates for cardiac transplantation [6].

A high prevalence of abnormalities found via ECG exists in MMD. Studies have shown that about one-third of patients with MMD have first-degree atrioventricular block, while about one-fifth have left axis deviation, only 5% have left bundle branch block. Complete heart blockage, requiring pacemaker placement, is rare but can occur. Patients with MMD should receive routine cardiac evaluations [6, 38].

6.3.4 Marfan Syndrome

Marfan syndrome is characterized by connective tissue disorder with classic triad affection ocular, skeletal, and cardiac. Cardiovascular system anomalies account for a significant proportion of the shortened life span with Marfan syndrome.

The most prominent cardiovascular manifestations of Marfan syndrome are known to be caused by defects in fibrillin 1. MVP occurs in (35–100%), aortic dilatation in (75%), mitral regurge in (44–58%), and aortic regurge in (15–44%). Many patients present with silent MVP, diagnosis by echocardiography (78–100%) largely exceed the auscultatory diagnosis (45–70%); therefore, it is recommended that all patients suspected for Marfan syndrome be evaluated echocardiographically [40]. As the progressive aortic root dilatation, aortic regurgitation, dissection, or rupture is the most common life-threatening feature. Aortic regurge is an indicator of high risk for subsequent complications such as dissection; in general, morbidity and mortality are associated with aortic abnormalities rather than with mitral valve dysfunction. Investigators reported that sporadic cases of Marfan syndrome have more severe cardiovascular involvement compared to familial cases [40].

Due to early diagnosis, the awareness for milder forms of the disease, advances in aortic surgery and medical treatment, the life expectancy of Marfan patients has increased from 37 years in the seventies to more than 60 years in the nineties [40].

6.3.5 Congenital Heart Disease

It has been well established that the incidence of scoliosis is higher in patients with CHD than in normal subjects. The incidence of scoliosis in patients with CHD has been reported in the literature to be from 2 to 19%. The relative wide range in the incidence of scoliosis associated with CHD is, though to be, due to differences in types of CHD, criteria of patient's selection, the effect of cardiac surgery, and the definition of scoliosis. In other words, the etiology of scoliosis associated with CHD is still unknown, and many factors such as CHD itself, cardiac surgery, thoracotomy, cyanosis, and other abnormalities may affect the onset of scoliosis. Some reports found strong correlation between thoracotomy done for cardiac surgery and the development of scoliosis in up to 22% of their patients [31], whereas others found no correlation [39]. A number of theories have been proposed to explain the etiology of scoliosis associated with CHD, impaired oxygenation, and deficient or asymmetrical blood supply to the vertebral bodies or supporting tissues may be causative factors [21].

6.4 Urogenital

6.4.1 Congenital Scoliosis

The genitourinary and musculoskeletal systems are both of mesodermal origin and develop at the same time in the embryo. As a result, any genetic defect or other insult acting at a crucial stage of organogenesis, which results in a congenital vertebral abnormality, may also lead to a congenital genitourinary malformation. There is also the possibility that other developing organ systems will be affected. Thus, a cluster of disparate congenital abnormalities may occur. Renal anomalies are mostly nonhereditary, which supports the suggested etiology of an insult to the embryo between the fifth and seventh week. This period corresponds to the stage of organogenesis when the stem cell population is being established for the primordial organs. These interactions are sensitive to insult from genetic and environmental influences. In a 4-week-old embryo, the mesonephros is located from the sixth cervical vertebra to the lumbar spine. A stimulus in the lower cervical or upper thoracic area between the fourth and seventh week of gestation could simultaneously affect the developing mesodermal structures [30].

The frequent occurrence of congenital genitourinary abnormalities in patients with congenital scoliosis was reported in the 1980s [37]. The incidence of genitourinary abnormalities between 20 and 34% has been found to occur in patients with congenital vertebral anomalies in different series using intravenous pyelography (IVP) and ultrasound. The most common urogenital anomalies associated with congenital spinal deformities are renal hypoplasia, horseshoe kidney, single kidney, congenital Megaureter, ectopic kidney (pelvic), hypospadius, pelviureteric junctional obstruction, posterior urethral valve, cloacal anomaly, epispadius, exstrophy of the bladder, hydronephrosis, and undescended testis [4]. It has been observed that the association of some malformation of the urinary system seems to be directly related to the occurrence of hemivertebrae; the location of the hemivertebra also seems important in relation to the side of agenesis of the kidney [37].

While these anomalies may remain asymptomatic, some can be associated with significant morbidity. Infection, obstruction, and the formation of calculus are the main reported problems; these patients are also at increased risk of proteinuria, hypertension, and renal insufficiency, and it is essential to have prolonged and careful follow-up. Some patients with urogenital anomalies (up to25% in some series) required surgery, others had abnormal renal function requiring medical therapy including dialysis, and the rest had abnormalities that do not affect renal function or do not require treatment [3].

Historically, IVP has been the investigation of choice in the evaluation of the morphology of the urinary tract, but diagnostic ultrasonography has been shown to be an acceptable alternative method of screening. Some centers reserve IVP for confirmation in those patients in whom an abnormality has been identified ultrasonographically, or when the study is inconclusive. Ultrasonography is noninvasive, less expensive, and has a reduced exposure to radiation. This is relevant in patients in whom multiple anomalies have been identified and repeated imaging is required. Recently, the trend has been for an initial ultrasonographic evaluation; this can be difficult in the overweight patient and in those with severe spinal deformity in whom the chest is abutting against the pelvis; in these circumstances, IVP is recommended [30].

6.4.2 Neuromuscular Scoliosis

Urinary tract infections are frequently seen with paralytic spinal deformities as a consequence of paralysis of the muscles that control the bowel and bladder. Patients with paralytic spinal deformity classically have a higher postoperative infection rate, and the chronic urinary tract infections in these patients are often thought to be a potential cause. Patients with urinary tract infections should be treated preoperatively in an effort to eradicate the infection and eliminate the urinary tract as a potential source of bacteremia. It can be helpful to consult with a urologist who can evaluate the renal function of the child with regard to the child's ability to withstand major spinal surgery and can also be instrumental in optimizing the renal function of the child [16].

6.5 Musculoskeletal

6.5.1 Idiopathic Scoliosis

Early onset scoliosis has been noted to be associated with ipsilateral plagiocephaly (Fig. 6.4) (an asymmetric and twisted head in reference to the spine), which is very common in children with pelvic flattening and obliquity and hip adduction. Subsequently, a correlation between infant positioning and early onset scoliotic deformities has been proposed, which was later questioned warranting further research [18]. Developmental dysplasia of the hip is also found at a higher frequency in patients with early onset idiopathic scoliosis than in children without scoliosis. Other comorbidities associated with idiopathic soliosis include isthmic spondylolisthesis, hereditary exostosis, and slipped capital femoral epiphysis [7].

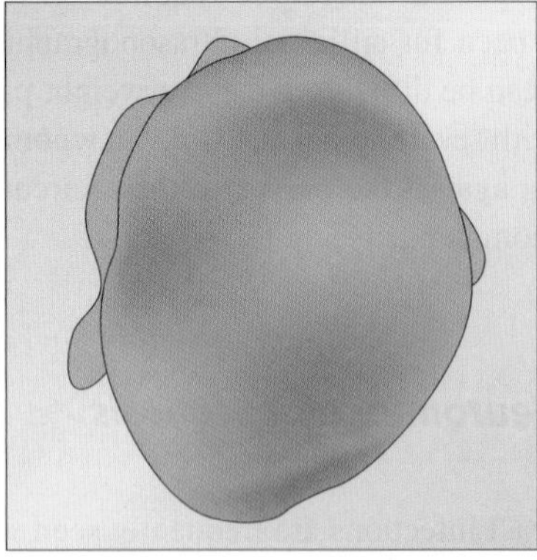

Fig. 6.4 Plagiocephaly, an asymmetric flattening and twisting of the head in reference to the spine, is common in children with early onset scoliosis; it may be related to the long-standing tilted position of the soft head of the infant when lying supine

6.5.2 Congenital Scoliosis

Hypoplasia of upper extremity and lower extremity, wasting of one leg, club foot, and other foot deformities, Sprengel's deformity, dislocated hip, and polydactyly can be associated with congenital spinal deformities [3].

6.5.3 Neuromuscular Scoliosis

In neuromuscular scoliosis there is an affection of different groups of muscles caused by the disease itself causing weakness, deformities and difficult ambulation, or the affection can occur secondary to the spinal deformity resulting in pelvic obliquity, hip subluxation and dislocation, equines foot, and apparent leg length discrepancy.

6.5.4 Marfan Syndrome

The association of protrusio acetabuli and Marfan syndrome has been confirmed in many studies with an incidence reaching around 30% of the cases. Planovalgus foot deformity is sometimes observed in patients with Marfan syndrome with a reported incidence reaching 25% and it has been postulated to be caused by increased ligamentous laxity resulting from underlying connective pathology. Several investigators also reported decreased bone mineral density (BMD) in patients with Marfan syndrome, the significance of this finding in relation to fracture risk remains uncertain [17].

6.5.5 Neurofibromatosis

Patients with neurofibromatosis scoliosis may present with some type of bony dysplasia. The orthopaedic complications with neurofibromatosis usually appear early, they include congenital tibial dysplasia with bowing and pseudarthrosis of the tibia, forearm, other bones, as well as overgrowth phenomenon of an extremity, and soft tissue tumors (Fig. 6.3) [8].

6.6 Gastrointestinal

Inguinal hernia is found at a higher frequency in patients with early onset idiopathic scoliosis than in children without scoliosis; celiac disease, cystic fibrosis, and lactose intolerance were also found to be associated more with idiopathic scoliosis [7].

Imperforate anus, hernia, esophageal atresia, and situs inversus were found to occur with congenital spinal deformities [3].

6.7 Cutaneous

A thorough physical examination in early onset scoliosis should be performed, beginning with a search for cutaneous markers of systemic disorders, such as the café au lait spots and axillary or inguinal freckling observed in neurofibromatosis (see Fig. 6.3) and the hairy patch (see Fig. 6.1) associated with occult spinal dysraphism. Additionally, pigmented nevus, hemangioma, and dimples can be associated with congenital spinal deformities sometimes denoting an underlying neurological abnormality. Skin scarring and defects can also be associated with myelomeningocele scoliosis, clearly affecting the outcome of these patients and warranting detailed assessment.

6.8 Pain and Disability

Idiopathic pediatric scoliosis patients have more pain than asymptomatic pediatric age group without scoliosis and those with Schmorl's nodes often had greater pain than those without, however the overall degree of disability is clinically mild. This is different than neuromuscular scoliosis, which usually results in a considerable degree of both pain and disability.

The etiology for painful idiopathic scoliosis is thought to include muscular pain due to eccentric loading about the apex of a curvature, asymmetric facet joint loading resulting in facet arthritis or synovitis, discogenic pain, or a combination. Human studies have shown disc degeneration at the concave aspect of scoliotic discs. However, the progression from disc degeneration to discogenic pain is not fully understood. The location of the pain is mainly over the apex of the primary curvature; to a lesser extent, at the midline at levels corresponding to patients' Schmorl's nodes, and finally in the interscapular and low back regions.

Overall, disc degeneration was similar in scoliosis and asymptomatic control groups; however, specific aspects of degeneration, such as Schmorl's nodes and inflammatory end plate changes, were more common suggesting that symptoms in the scoliosis patients may, in part, have a discogenic etiology and that pain in scoliosis may occur in an abnormal loading environment combined with abnormal endplates [6].

Mental disabilities can be associated with some types of neuromuscular scoliosis due to brain affection. The presence of cognitive delay has been shown to correlate with curve progression in early onset scoliosis and particular attention should be paid to whether the child has appropriately reached developmental milestones [18].

References

1. Ahn NU, Sponseller PD, Ahn UM et al (2000) Dural ectasia is associated with back pain in Marfan syndrome. Spine 25:1562–1568
2. Ahn NU, Sponseller PD, Ahn UM et al (2000) Dural ectasia in the Marfan syndrome: MR and CT findings and criteria. Genet Med 2:173–179
3. Basu PS, Elsebaie H, Noordeen MHH (2002) Congenital spinal deformity a comprehensive assessment at presentation. Spine 27:2255–2259
4. Beals RK, Robbins JR, Rolfe B (1993) Anomalies associated with vertebral malformations. Spine 18:1329–1332
5 Bradford DS, Heithoff KB, Cohen M (1991) Intraspinal abnormalities and congenital spine deformities: A radiographic and MRI study. J Paediatr Orthop 11:36–41
6. Buttermann GR, Mullin WJ (2008) Pain and disability correlated with disc degeneration via magnetic resonance imaging in scoliosis patients. Eur Spine J 17:240–249
7. Colomina MJ, Puig L, Godet C et al (2002) Prevalence of asymptomatic cardiac valve anomalies in idiopathic scoliosis. Pediatr Cardiol 23(4):426–429
8. Crawford AH, Herrera-Soto J (2007) Scoliosis associated with neurofibromatosis. Orthop Clin N Am 38:553–562
9. Crawford AH, Parikh S, Schorry EK et al (2007) The immature spine in type-1 neurofibromatosis. J Bone Joint Surg Am 89:123–142
10. Curtis BH, Fisher RL, Butterfield WL et al (1969) Neurofibromatosis with paraplegia. Report of eight cases. J Bone Joint Surg Am 51(5):843–861
11. Deguchi M, Kawakami N, Saito H et al (1995) Paraparesis after rib penetration of the spinal canal in neurofibromatous scoliosis. J Spinal Disord 8(5):363–367

12. Dhuper S, Ehlers KH, Fatica NS et al (1997) Incidence and risk factors for mitral valve prolapse in severe adolescent idiopathic scoliosis. Pediatr Cardiol 18(6):425–428
13. Do T, Fras C, Burke S et al (2001) Clinical value of routine preoperative magnetic resonance imaging in adolescent idiopathic scoliosis. J Bone Joint Surg Am 83:577–579
14. Dobbs MB, G Lenke LG, Bridwell KH et al (2002) Prevalence of neural axis abnormalities in patients with infantile idiopathic scoliosis. J Bone Joint Surg Am 84:2230–2234
15. Evans SC, Edgar MA, Hall-Graggs MA et al (1996) MRI of 'idiopathic' juvenile scoliosis: a prospective study. J Bone Joint Surg Br 78:314–317
16. Ferguson RL (2007) Medical and congenital comorbidities associated with spinal deformities in the immature spine. J Bone Joint Surg Am 89:34–41
17. Giampietro PF, Raggio C, Davis JG (2002) Marfan syndrome: orthopaedic and genetic review. Curr Opin Pediatr 14:35–41
18. Gillingham BL, Fan RA, Akbarnia BA (2006) Early onset idiopathic scoliosis. J Am Acad Orthop Surg 14: 101–112
19. Gupta P, Lenke LG, Bridwell KH (1998) Incidence of neural axis abnormalities in infantile and juvenile patients with spinal deformity. Is a magnetic resonance image screening necessary. Spine 23:206–210
20. Inoue M, Minami S, Nakata Y et al (2004) Preoperative MRI analysis of patients with idiopathic scoliosis. Spine 30: 108–114
21. Kawakami N, Mimatsu K, Deguchi M et al (1995) Scoliosis and congenital heart disease. Spine 20:1252–1256
22. McMaster MJ Ohtsuka K (1982) The natural history of congenital scoliosis: A study of two hundred and fifty-one patients. J Bone Joint Surg Am 64:1128–1147
23. McMaster MJ (1984) Occult intraspinal anomalies and congenital scoliosis. J Bone Joint Surg Am 66:588–601
24. McMaster MJ (1998) Congenital scoliosis caused by a unilateral failure of vertebral segmentation with a contralateral hemivertebra. Spine 23:998–1005
25 Noordeen MHH, Taylor BA, Edgar MA (1994) Syringomyelia: a potential risk factor in scoliosis surgery. Spine 12:1406–1409
26. Peer S, Krismer M, Judmaier W, Kerber W (1994) The value of MRI in the preoperative assessment of scoliosis. Orthopäde 23:318–322
27. Porter RW, Hall-Craggs M, Walker AE et al (2000) The position of the cerebellar tonsils and the conus in patients with scoliosis. J Bone Joint Surg Br 82(Suppl III):286
28. Prahinski JR, Polly DW, McHale KA et al (2000) Occult intraspinal anomalies in congenital scoliosis. J Paediatr Orthop 20:59–63
29. Pyeritz RE, Fishman EK, Bernhardt BA et al (1988) Dural ectasia is a common feature of the Marfan syndrome. Am J Hum Genet 43:726–732
30. Rai AS, Taylor TKF, Smith GHH et al (2002) Congenital abnormalities of the urogenital tract in association with congenital vertebral malformations. J Bone Joint Surg Br 84-B: 891–895
31. Reckles LN, Peterson HA, Bianco AJ Jr et al (1975) The association of scoliosis and congenital heart defects. J Bone joint Surg Am 57:449–455
32. Samuelsson L, Lindell D, Kogler H (1991) Spinal cord and brain stem anomalies in scoliosis: MR screening of 26 cases. Acta Orthop Scand 62:403–406
33. Shen WJ, McDowell GS, Burke SW et al (1996) Routine preoperative MRI and SEP studies in adolescent patients with idiopathic scoliosis before spinal instrumentation and fusion. J Pediatr Orthop 16:350–353
34. Sirois JL III, Drennan JC (1990) Dystrophic spinal deformity in neurofibromatosis. J Pediatr Orthop 10(4):522–526
35. Sponseller PD, Sethi N, Cameron DE et al (1997) Infantile scoliosis in Marfan syndrome. Spine 22:509–516:33
36. Suh SW, Sarwark JF, Vora A et al (2001) Evaluating congenital spine deformities for intraspinal anomalies with magnetic resonance imaging. J Pediatr Orthop 21:525–531
37 Tori JA, Dickson JH (1980) Association of congenital anomalies of the spine and kidneys. Clin Orthop Rel Res 148: 259–262
38. Tysnes OB, Vollset SE, Larsen JP et al (1994) Prognostic factors and survival in amyotrophic lateral sclerosis. Neuroepidemiology 13(5):226–235
39. Van Biezen FC, Bakx PAGM, De Villeneuve VH et al (1993) Scoliosis in children after thoracotomy for aortic coarctation. J Bone Joint Surg Am 75:514–518
40. Van Karnebeek, Naeff MSJ, Mulder BJM et al (2001) Natural history of cardiovascular manifestations in Marfan syndrome. Arch Dis Child 84:129–137
41. Winter RB, Lonstein JE, Heithoff KB et al (1997) Magnetic resonance imaging evaluation of the adolescent patient with idiopathic scoliosis before spinal instrumentation and fusion: a prospective, double-blinded study of 140 patients. Spine 22:855–858

Thoracic Insufficiency Syndrome (TIS)

7

Gregory J. Redding

Key Points

- Thoracic insufficiency syndrome includes spine and chest wall disorders that produces progressive restrictive respiratory disease.
- Respiratory features of TIS include reduced chest wall excursion and distensibility, distortion of the lung, respiratory muscles, and increased respiratory work.
- Functional assessments of breathing complement structural assessments of the spine and chest wall as indicators of surgical intervention and effectiveness of different operative strategies.

7.1 Introduction

Thoracic insufficiency syndrome (TIS) is defined as the inability of the thorax to support normal respiratory function and postnatal lung growth in children with skeletal immaturity [6]. It is a purposefully vague term that includes several disorders of the spine, ribs, sternum, and surrounding muscles that restrict lung expansion and normal chest wall excursion. Primary TIS refers to disorders of thoracic and spine structures that directly impair lung function. Secondary TIS includes abnormalities of spine and thoracic structures produced as a result of underlying neuromuscular weakness syndromes. Children with either primary or secondary TIS may have additional pulmonary disease, such as aspiration pneumonias or primary pulmonary hypoplasia, but the functional assessment of breathing in children with TIS presumes that these other pulmonary issues have been optimally treated and that they contribute minimally to the restrictive respiratory disease.

The major spine deformities that produce TIS are congenital and infantile idiopathic scoliosis involving the thoracic vertebrae with or without kyphosis. These deformities can be severe initially on presentation or mild but progressive over time. The deformities are complex with different sites of spine curvature, numbers of vertebrae involved, and the types of vertebral anomalies, e.g., block vertebrae, unsegmented vertebrae, and hemivertebrae, all with or without rib fusion [28]. These lead to variable degrees of scoliosis, kyphosis, lordosis, and rotation of thoracic vertebrae and their associated ribs. They also produce abnormal rib alignment, reduction in costovertebral joint motion, and localized chest wall deformities, such as a rib hump. The impact of each structural feature on lung function is difficult to assess. Several studies have shown that different lung functions have little relation to the Cobb angle alone in children with TIS [15, 24]. Given the combinations of structural abnormalities of the vertebrae and ribs producing TIS, and the variations in severity of each structural deformity, it is not surprising that combinations of thoracic and spine structural features, in general, do not correlate well with respiratory functional abnormalities.

An alternative approach is to use both the structural and functional measures in conjunction with one another to determine severity and, when used serially, to assess the rate of progression of TIS in young children. This chapter describes the respiratory functional abnormalities that result from TIS because of the early onset of

G. J. Redding
Pulmonary Division, Seattle Children's Hospital, University of Washington, Seattle, WA, USA
e-mail: gredding@u.washington.edu

B. A. Akbarnia et al. (eds.), *The Growing Spine*,
DOI: 10.1007/978-3-540-85207-0_7, © Springer-Verlag Berlin Heidelberg 2011

Table 7.1 Pulmonary function domains

Pulmonary function domains
Lung and chest wall mechanics
Lung and chest wall compliance
Chest wall excursion
Lung volumes
Gas exchange
Oxygenation efficiency
Carbon dioxide removal
Regional lung function
Ventilation and perfusion distribution
Respiratory muscles
Inspiratory and expiratory force generation
Thresholds for respiratory muscle fatigue
Pulmonary hemodynamics
Pulmonary hypertension and cor pulmonale
Pulmonary host defenses
Cough effectiveness

scoliosis and the tests available to quantify these abnormalities. Respiratory function is not limited to the function of the lung and can be categorized in several domains (Table 7.1). The most commonly used tests measure respiratory mechanics (and hence the work of breathing) and gas exchange. It is reasonable to presume that as the spine and thoracic deformities progress, respiratory function deteriorates. Although this is likely globally, different aspects of lung function may be preserved until severe deformity develops, e.g., pulmonary hypertension. Not every test mentioned later has been uniformly used to assess children with early onset scoliosis. However, several pilot studies have been completed and the prevalence of respiratory abnormalities in this high-risk group of children in (Fig. 7.1) has been traced.

7.2 Lung and Chest Wall Mechanics

The shape and compliance of a child's thorax change with increasing age. The depth and width of an infant's chest are equal at birth and achieve the adult's AP/lateral dimension ratio of 0.7 by 2–3 years of age [5]. Ribs project at right angles from vertebrae at birth and

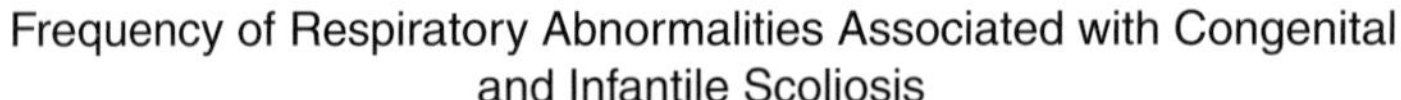

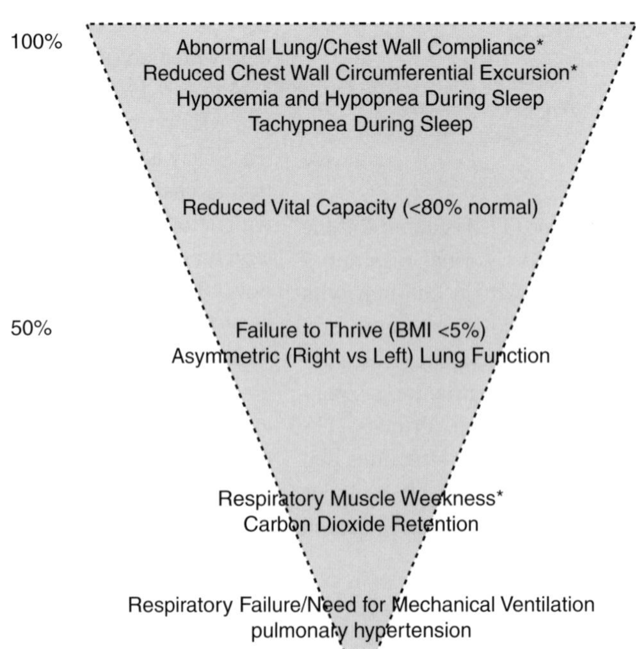

Fig. 7.1 Frequency of respiratory abnormalities associated with congenital and infantile idiopathic scoliosis and other children with thoracic insufficiency syndrome

achieve degrees of angulation seen in adulthood by the third year of life. Chest wall compliance is greatest in infancy and becomes stiffer with increasing thoracic muscle development and ossification of bony structures. "Normal" stiffness of the chest wall is therefore age dependent. In newborns, the chest wall is seven times more compliant than the lung and active chest wall and diaphragmatic muscle tone is required to maintain resting lung volumes [26]. In children up to 5 years of age, the chest wall is almost twice as compliant as the lung during quiet breathing [23]. In adults, the ratio of chest wall to lung compliance is close to 1.0 [29]. In children with scoliosis, chest wall compliance is reduced as is rib cage excursion. In response to increasingly stiff chest wall, children choose to breathe shallowly to reduce the work needed to stretch the lungs and chest wall with each breath and breathe rapidly to maintain normal minute ventilation. Respiratory rate during wakefulness is higher due to activity, excitement, and speech, and is more reflective of respiratory mechanics when measured during sleep. The normal respiratory rates of children, which are age dependent, are portrayed in Fig. 7.2 [8, 27]. Tachypnea due to scoliosis is common but the exact prevalence of tachypnea during wakefulness and sleep have not been reported.

Lung volumes increase as the thorax increases in size, with vertebral and rib lengthening. Thoracic volume (at maximum inspiration) at birth increases by 33-fold to reach the adult size [33]. Processes that slow thoracic growth therefore reduce lung volume. Lung compliance, apart from chest wall compliance, is volume dependent. At very low lung volumes, the lung resists expansion more when intrathoracic pressure changes. At normal lung volumes during tidal breathing, the lung is maximally distensible. It is possible that surgical procedures that increase thoracic volume may increase lung volumes and thus render the lungs more compliant independent of changes in chest wall compliance. Lung volumes and lung compliance have been measured in one series of young children with early onset scoliosis under anesthesia and found to be low, but these results were complicated by concurrent atelectasis [18]. With prolonged constraint of the lungs by a small thorax, alveolar development may be hampered postnatally [4]. Lung growth after birth primarily occurs in the distal or acinar regions of the lung, and include increased alveolar number, size, and alveolar-capillary surface area. These attributes of alveolar growth change at different times, so that alveolar number and complexity increase early in life, while increased alveoli enlarge later in proportion to height [1].

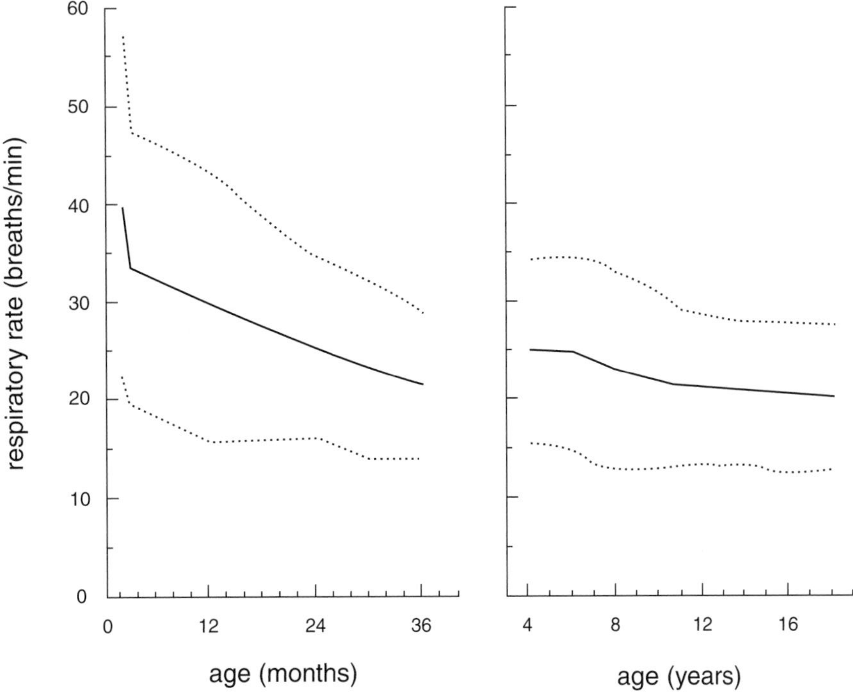

Fig. 7.2 Normal respiratory rates in awake children (*panel a*) [27] and (*panel b*) [8]

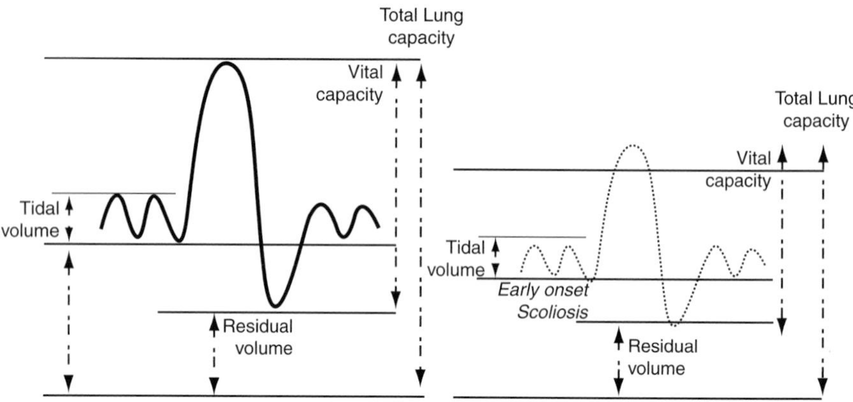

Fig. 7.3 Lung volumes and capacities in normal children and children with early onset scoliosis

Scoliosis impacts respiratory mechanics in several ways and does so more when it begins in early life than with onset during adolescence [21]. Abnormal lung volumes have been measured using infant lung function techniques as early as 6 months of age in infants with chest wall disorders [25]. Lung volumes are subdivided as illustrated in (Fig. 7.3); combinations of lung volumes are described as lung "capacities". The *vital capacity* is that portion of total lung capacity that can be voluntarily inhaled or exhaled with maximal efforts and reflects ventilatory reserve that could be used if needed. In contrast, the residual volume is that volume of gas in the chest that cannot be altered with breathing efforts but assists with transfer of oxygen and carbon dioxide.

In children and adults with scoliosis, the vital capacity is preferentially reduced as a result of reduced lung volumes and reduced lung and chest wall compliance (see Fig. 7.3). Residual volume is reduced less than vital capacity as it depends on thoracic cage volume but not on chest wall stiffness or reduced excursions. *Total lung capacity*, the combination of vital capacity and *residual volume*, is reduced less than the vital capacity because residual volume is least compromised [14]. Studies of these measurements in children with TIS suggest that there is greater reduction in vital capacity per degree Cobb angle if scoliosis begins earlier in life than when it begins in adolescence [21].

Vital capacity is measured by spirometry in children old enough to understand and perform maximal inspiratory and expiratory efforts. Reproducible artifact-free efforts that reflect lung function rather than how a child performs the test occur between 4 and 6 years of age. All spirometric indices, including vital capacity, are compared to published norms that are created using height to normalize across different ages. In children with scoliosis, heights are dependent on spine curvature and arm span is used instead to estimate height and vital capacity as a percent of predicted normal value [9]. In contrast to spirometry, measures of total lung capacity and all of its volume components requires either gas dilution techniques or measurements with a body plethysmograph. These two techniques are available for children in tertiary care centers with a pediatric focus but are much less available than routine spirometry. Vital capacity is therefore the most clinically available spirometric test for clinicians managing children with TIS.

Spirometry also measures inspiratory and expiratory airflow. Diseases that reduce flow as a result of narrowed conducting airways produce obstructive lung disease. The degree of airway obstruction is most commonly quantified using the forced expiratory volume at 0.5 and 1 s (FEV 0.5 or FEV 1) after the onset of a forced expiratory effort and the forced expiratory flow in the mid-half of the exhaled vital capacity. (FEF 25–75% VC) FEV 1 is usually normalized for vital capacity and the normal ratio of FEV1/FVC is 80–85% and independent of age. The thoracic disorders that produce TIS, including early onset scoliosis, do not often produce obstructive lung disease [2, 15]. If these indices are abnormal during evaluation with spirometry, other conditions, such as asthma, should also be considered and treated.

Pulmonary function tests in children can be subdivided by those that do and do not require cooperation and those that are invasive in nature. Spirometric measures are noninvasive but require cooperation. Lung and chest wall compliance measurements do not require cooperation but do require placement of a pressure transducer within the esophagus to estimate

Table 7.2 Invasive and pulmonary function tests

	Pulmonary function testing in infants and children	
	Invasive	*Noninvasive*
Effort–dependent[a]	Transdiaphragm pressures	Spirometry Respiratory muscle strength and endurance Exercise tests
Effort –independent[a]	Chest wall and lung compliance	Respiratory rate Oximetry Lung volumes Blood gas tensions Lung ventilation/ perfusion scans Sleep study Echocardiogram

[a]Voluntary effort at 5–6 years of age

pleural pressure. The invasive nature of esophageal balloons has led to measurements of lung compliance in the operating room under anesthesia but not during outpatient visits with children awake [18]. The issue of cooperation is particularly important as it limits the use of many tests in very young children with TIS who are being considered for surgical therapies. Table 7.2 lists commonly used tests of respiratory function based on need for cooperation and for invasive procedures.

7.2.1 Gas Exchange

Respiratory gas exchange is measured by efficiency of oxygenation and sufficiency of ventilation. Oxygenation is most often measured as percent of hemoglobin saturated by oxygen using noninvasive pulse oximeters. These devices have replaced direct measures of partial pressure of oxygen in arterial blood except in intensive care units. Oxygenation varies with wakefulness and sleep and oxyhemoglobin saturation (SaO_2 or SpO_2) may fall by 2% in normal children and adults during sleep [17]. In children with TIS, SaO2 is normal (>96%) in most children when awake. In the initial study of 218 children with TIS who underwent expansion thoracoplasty, only 22% received supplemental oxygen therapy [30]. However, a recent abstract studying children with TIS during sleep reported that brief hypoxemic episodes occurred in 11 of 12, regardless of age [31]. Hypoxmeic events during sleep were associated with periods of shallow breathing, hypopneas, and were more common during REM stage sleep. An alternative setting to measure efficiency of oxygenation is during exercise. However, many children with TIS are too young to perform formal exercise testing.

Ventilation is assessed using arterial or arterialized measurement of carbon dioxide partial pressures in blood. Capillary sampling of arterialized blood is commonly used to measure PCO_2 in the outpatient setting. Retention of carbon dioxide above normal levels, i.e., PCO_2>50 mmHg, is uncommon and a late finding in children with TIS, reflecting acute and/or chronic respiratory failure. An alternative way to measure CO_2 status is with a capnograph, which measures CO_2 concentration in exhaled gas. The end-tidal PCO_2 can be used as a noninvasive surrogate measure of arterial pCO_2 in children who have no underlying lung disease and only spine and chest wall disease. End-tidal PCO_2 has been used during sleep studies to identify frequency, duration, and severity of hypercapnia. Gas exchange measures are not dependent on voluntary efforts and noninvasive techniques are available and commonly used in clinical practice.

7.2.2 Lung Function Asymmetry

One consequence of progressive chest wall deformity due to early onset scoliosis is an asymmetric chest wall shape and increasingly different volumes in the right and left hemithoraces. Different capabilities to move the right and left chest walls due to differences in rib alignment, diaphragm configuration, and regional chest wall compliances, may accompany the asymmetric lung volumes, leading to a change in the distribution of ventilation and perfusion between the right and left lungs. Relative regional ventilation and perfusion are measured with lung scans. Ventilation is measured using inhalation of a radiotracer gas; regional lung perfusion is measured using intravenous radiolabeled agents. Both lung ventilation and perfusion scans require minimal cooperation and can be used in children of all ages. In infants, the normal distribution of ventilation and perfusion to the right and left lungs is 50%:50%. As the chest wall becomes more oblong transversely, there is a shift to the adult distribution of 55% right lung: 45% left lung function for both ventilation and perfusion [11]. Perfusion is normally well matched to ventilation, but when a primary maldistribution of ventilation occurs, perfusion asymmetry will be similar but less in magnitude.

Among children with congenital or infantile scoliosis, lung function asymmetry can be severe with less than 10% of function residing in the right or left lung [24]. In 39 children with these forms of scoliosis, half had >5% deviation from the normal right and left lung distribution of ventilation. Although reduced function occurred more often in the lung in the concave chest, this was not invariable. The degree of lung function asymmetry did not correlate with Cobb angle [24]. The child with TIS due to scoliosis can thus be described as someone with increased work of breathing, minimal chest wall excursion, who relies increasingly on one lung as the spine and chest wall deformity progresses.

7.2.3 Respiratory Muscle Function

The more rigid the chest wall, the less effective are chest wall and accessory muscles for breathing. With minimal rib motion, the child with TIS becomes particularly dependent on function of the diaphragm. Force is generated in the costal region of the diaphragm that lies parallel to the chest and abdominal walls. The diaphragm attaches at the base of the sternum anteriorly and descends to attach at the level of T8–T12 in the lateral and posterior aspects of the thoracoabdominal wall [20]. Contractile fibers are normally aligned in the cuadad to cephalad direction and shortening moves the diaphragm downward during inspiration. In normal individuals, diaphragmatic motion also raises the lower ribs, prompting the "bucket handle" motion that increases the thorax in the anterior–posterior and lateral dimensions. This action is lost when the chest wall becomes rigid. The diaphragm is the principal muscle of inspiration accounting for 65% of inspiratory muscle force generation in upright individuals and more in the supine position [16].

Inspiratory muscle force can be measured noninvasively with inspiratory efforts against a closed system that measures pressure. This measure is lung volume dependent; the greatest inspiratory force is generated when the effort originates at the end of exhalation. This test is termed the maximum inspiratory muscle pressure (MIP) and is dependent on voluntary effort. The invasive way to assess diaphragmatic force more specifically is the transdiaphragmatic pressure measuring the pressure differential above and below the diaphragm during maximum effort. Data in adults with severe scoliosis have shown that as transdiaphragmatic pressure falls, vital capacity diminishes and carbon dioxide is retained [13]. Normal MIP values are age and gender dependent with preadolescents and girls having lower values (−83 ±27 cm H_2O for boys; −66 ± −20 cm H_2O for girls, ages 7–14 years) [34]. Causes of reduced respiratory muscle force generation in children without underlying neuromuscular conditions likely relate to the orientation of the diaphragm fibers and the insertion of the diaphragm into the abdominal wall at the normal position. Abnormal diaphragm insertion has been described in up to 5% of children with TIS (R. Campbell personal communication). Rotation of the diaphragm in each hemithorax with rotation of the vertebrae in early onset scoliosis may effect the orientation of diaphragmatic muscle fibers and hence inspiratory movement and force generation [12].

Maximum expiratory muscle pressure (MEP) that develops after a full inspiration is reduced in some adults and adolescents with late-onset scoliosis [10]. This measure does not depend on the diaphragm but does depend on force generated by abdominal muscles. One explanation for reduced MEP is that maximal pressure during expiration is volume dependent and at lower values of total lung capacity, less force can be generated compared to normal people. Patients with progressively reduced lung volumes due to TIS would be expected to be at a mechanical disadvantage when exhaling forcefully [10]. The apparatus to measure MIPs is the same used to measure MEPs. Reduction in MEPs will reduce the effectiveness of the cough reflex and predispose children to retained airway secretions and atelectasis during respiratory infections and postoperatively. The prevalence of impaired respiratory muscle force has not been described among young children with early onset scoliosis, in part, because it requires strenuous sustained voluntary efforts. Among adolescents with idiopathic scoliosis, this finding occurs primarily in those with moderate or severe spinal deformities [32].

In contrast to respiratory muscle strength and force generation, respiratory muscles can fatigue when respiratory mechanics worsen. Although there are techniques to assess respiratory muscle fatiguability [19], these have not been broadly utilized in clinical medicine.

7.3 Pulmonary Hypertension

Respiratory disease that is severe enough to produce respiratory failure often leads to pulmonary hypertension and cor pulmonale. These conditions are markers of severe and prolonged hypoxemia but they can also directly predispose a patient to right heart failure and death. Previous reports of lung pathology in adults with advanced scoliosis have noted the remodeling of pulmonary vessels characteristic of pulmonary hypertension [7]. However, in recent decades, the advent of long-term use of oxygen therapy at home in both children and adults has made pulmonary hypertension a rare pulmonary complication. Echocardiograms are currently used to assess both right heart morphology (right ventricular hypertrophy) and abnormal septal motion as evidence of chronic pulmonary hypertension and cor pulmonale. Additionally, the velocity of the regurgitant jet from the tricuspid valve provides estimates of current pulmonary artery pressures. More importantly, the echocardiogram can identify unsuspected congenital heart disease that may complicate surgical and medical management of children with TIS. In one report, 26% of 126 children with congenital spine deformities had associated congenital heart disease [3]. The noninnvasive nature of the test and the need for minimal patient cooperation make the echocardiogram easy to use for screening of pulmonary vascular disease and associated cardiac conditions.

7.4 Nutritional Status as a Pulmonary Assessment

Abnormal respiratory mechanics lead to increased respiratory work to breathe and increased oxygen consumption. Restrictive chest wall disease in particular leads to dependence of the diaphragm to perform this work within a rigid thorax. Gastrointestinal processes that distend the abdomen, e.g., constipation, produce an additional restrictive element from below that affects diaphragmatic motion. Children with TIS avoid large meals and tend to graze in order to minimize gastric distension. Their eating patterns, their choice of foods, and their increased work of breathing likely contribute to inadequate caloric intake and excessive caloric use over time. In a study of 80 children with TIS from three referral centers, 55% of children had body mass indicesof <5% predicted when arm span rather than height was used in the calculation [25]. The relationship of lung function to nutritional status has been described for other chronic pediatric lung diseases, but correlates of abnormal lung function and nutritional status in children with TIS have not been made [22]. Poor subcutaneous tissues predisposes to poor wound healing and wound infections when prostheses are implanted in the chest wall to correct scoliosis. For these reasons, the nutritional assessment of children with TIS is an important adjunct to the pulmonary assessment in children with TIS.

References

1. Ad hoc Statement Committee ATS (2004) Mechanisms and limits of induced postnatal lung growth. Am J Respir Crit Care Med 170:319–343
2. Al-Kattan K, Simonds A, Chung KF et al (1997) Kyphoscoliosis and bronchial torsion. Chest 111:1134–1137
3. Basu PS, Elsebaie H, Noordeen MH (2002) Congenital spinal deformity: a comprehensive assessment at presentation. Spine 15:2255–2259
4. Berend N, Marlin GE (1970) Arrest of alveolar multiplication in kyphoscoliosis. Pathology 11:485–491
5. Bryan AC, Gaultier C (1985) Chest wall mechanics in the newborn. In: Roussos C, Macklem PT (eds) The Thorax. Marcel Dekker, New York
6. Campbell RM, Smith MD, Mayes TC et al (2003) The characteristics of thoracic insufficiency syndrome associated with fused ribs and congenital scoliosis. J Bone and Joint Surgery Am 85:399–408
7. Davies G, Reid L (1971) Effect of scoliosis on growth of alveoli and pulmonary arteries and on right ventricle. Arch Dis Child 46:623–32
8. Hooker EA, Danzl DF, Brueggmeyer M et al (1992) Respiratory rates in pediatric emergency patients. J Emerg Med 10:407–410
9. Jarzem PF, Gledhill RB (1993) Predicting height from arm measurements. J Pediatr Orthop 13:761–765
10. Jones RS, Kennedy JD, Hashham F et al (1981) Mechanical inefficiency of the thoracic cage in scoliosis. Thorax 36:456–61
11. Kao CH, Liao SQ, Wang SJ et al (1992) Pulmonary scintigraphic findings in children with pectus excavatum by the comparison of chest radiograph indices. Clin Nucl Med 17:874–876
12. Kotani T, Minami S, Takahashi K et al (2004) An analysis of chest wall and diaphragm motions in patients with idiopathic scoliosis using dynamic breathing MRI. Spine 29:298–302
13. Lisboa C, Moreno R, Fava M et al (1985) Inspiratory muscle function in patients with severe kyphoscoliosis. Am Rev Respir Dis 132:48–52

14. Mayer O, Redding G (2008) Infant lung functions in children with thoracic insufficiency syndrome (TIS). American Thoracic Society, NewYork, Abstract 516
15. Mayer OH, Redding G (2007) Change in Cobb angle and lung function after VEPTR insertion in children with thoracic insufficiency syndrome. Am J Respir Crit Care Med 175:A721
16. Mead J, Smith JC, Loring SH (1985) Volume displacements of the chest wall and their mechanical significance. In: Roussos C, Macklem PT (eds) The Thorax. Marcel Dekker, New York
17. Montgomery-Downs HE, O'Brien LM, Gulliver TE et al (2006) Polysomnographic characteristics in normal preschool and early school-aged children. Pediatrics 117: 741–753
18. Motoyama EK, Deeney VF, Fine GF et al (2006) Effects of lung function of multiple expansion thoracoplasty in children with thoracic insufficiency syndrome: a longitudinal study. Spine 31:284–290
19. Nickerson BG, Keens TG (1982) Measuring ventilatory muscle endurance in humans as sustainable inspiratory pressure. J Appl Physiol 52:768–772
20. Osmond DG (1985) Functional anatomy of the chest wall. In: Roussos C, Macklem PT (eds) The Thorax. Marcel Dekker, New York
21. Owange-Iraka JW, Harrison A, Warner JO (1984) Lung function in congenital and idiopathic scoliosis. Eur J Pediatr 142:198–200
22. Padman R, McColley SA, Miller DP et al (2207) Infant care patterns at epidemiologic study of cystic fibrosis sites that achieve superior childhood lung function. Pediatrics 119:e531–537
23. Papastamelos C, Panitch HB, England SE et al (1995) Developmental changes in chest wall compliance in infancy and early childhood. J Appl Physiol 78:179–184
24. Redding G, Song K, Inscore S et al (2007) Lung function asymmetry in children with congenital and infantile scoliosis. Spine 8(4):639–644
25. Redding G, Mayer O, Flynn J et al (2007) Infant lung functions in children with thoracic insufficiency syndrome (TIS). Presented at 14th International Meeting of Advanced Spine Techniques (IMAST), July 11–14, Paradise Island, Bahamas
26. Reynolds RN, Etsen BE (1966) Mechanics of respiration in apneic anesthetized infants. Anesthesiology 27:13–19
27. Rusconi F, Castagneto M, Gagliard L et al (1994) Reference values for respiratory rate in the first 3 years of life. Pediatrics 94:350–355
28. Shahcheraghi GH, Hobbi MH (1999) Patterns and progression in congenital scoliosis. J Pediatr Orthop 19:766–775
29. Sharp M, Druz W, Balgot R et al (1970) Changes in ventilation and chest wall mechanics in infants and children. J Appl Physiol 2:775–779
30. Song KM, Redding G (2005) Changes in respiratory failure of children with thoracic insufficiency syndrome (TIS) following expansion thoracoplasty: effect of age and diagnosis. Presented at the Annual Meeting of the Pediatric Orthopaedic Society of North America, May 13–15, Ottawa, Ontario, Canada
31. Striegl AM, Chen ML, Kifle Y et al (2008) Sleep disordered breathing in children with thoracic insufficiency syndrome. American Thoracic Society, NewYork, Am J Resp. Crit Care Med 177:A706
32. Szeinberg A, Canny GJ, Rashed N et al (1988) Forced vital capacity and maximal respiratory pressures in patients with mild and moderate scoliosis. Pediatr Pulmonol 4:8–12
33. Thorsteinsson A, Larsson A, Jonmarker C et al (1994) Pressure-volume relations of the respiratory system in healthy children. Am J Respir Crit Care Med 150: 421–430
34. Tomalak W, Pogorzelski A, Prusak J (2002) Normal values for maximal static inspiratory and expiratory pressures in healthy children. Pediatr Pulmonol 34:42–46

8 Imaging of the Growing Spine

John T. Smith and Jean Dubousset

Key Points

- New technology for three-dimensional (3D) imaging is significantly reducing radiation exposure in children.
- 3D imaging technology allows for the development of new classification systems for spinal deformity.
- Functional imaging such as dynamic MRI shows promise for a novel method for assessment of outcomes in the management of pediatric deformity.

8.1 Introduction

Since the introduction of X-rays by Wilhelm Roentgen in 1895, there has been a steady increase in the ability to use imaging modalities to assess disease and deformity. Management of deformity in the growing spine presents unique challenges to the treating physician. The cause of the deformity, future growth, spinal balance, and the three-dimensional (3D) nature of the deformity must all be considered. It demands selectivity in deciding the appropriate imaging studies to make efficient decisions for future management, while not overlooking significant comorbidities that can contribute to the overall natural history of a given deformity. In addition, one must consider the amount of radiation that a child will receive through the course of management during growth.

In recent years, there has been increasing interest and ability to assess spinal deformity in three dimensions. The ability to use 3D reconstruction has revolutionized preoperative planning of surgical strategy to correct the most challenging complex spinal deformities. It has also facilitated a better understanding of the effect of spinal deformity on the chest wall and shows promise in predicting the effect of chest and spine deformity on pulmonary function in young children. There is also increasing interest in using magnetic resonance imaging (MRI) to perform dynamic assessment of pulmonary function avoiding the considerable radiation associated with traditional computed tomography (CT) scanning.

The evolution of imaging techniques is a continuously evolving field. The purpose of this chapter is to provide an overview of current imaging techniques and considerations for this unique population of children with deformity in the growing spine.

8.2 Plain Radiography

The initial evaluation of suspected spinal deformity in a child begins with a thorough history and physical examination. If there is a strong suspicion of spinal deformity, then plain radiographs should be obtained. Plain radiographs allow for the initial assessment of the potential etiology of the deformity (idiopathic, congenital, neuromuscular, etc.), the severity of the curve, and should direct the next steps in imaging and management. There is often a general lack of understanding or technical

J. T. Smith (✉)
University of Utah, Department of Orthopaedics,
Primary Childrens Medical Center, 100 North Mario
Capecchi Drive, Suite 4550, Salt Lake City, UT 84113, USA
e-mail: john.smith@hsc.utah.edu

B. A. Akbarnia et al. (eds.), *The Growing Spine*,
DOI: 10.1007/978-3-540-85207-0_8, © Springer-Verlag Berlin Heidelberg 2011

ability in some instances in the primary care community and among radiologists regarding the optimal technique to obtain these initial radiographs in an efficient manner while minimizing radiation.

The general principles for obtaining initial spine radiographs in children are well known to spine surgeons. All initial spine radiographs should be taken in the upright position when possible (sitting or standing), and taken in the posterior–anterior (PA) and lateral planes. The use of PA exposure lessens the amount of radiation to breast tissue and reproductive organs, particularly in teenage females. Levy et al. [19] showed that taking radiographs in the PA view, compared with the AP view, results in a sevenfold reduction in cumulative radiation dose to the thyroid and breast, resulting in a threefold to fourfold reduction in the risk of developing breast cancer and halving the risk of thyroid cancer. Radiographs should be taken on long cassettes (36 in.) allowing for single exposures rather than multiple views that increase radiation and do not allow assessment of spinal balance in the coronal and saggital plane. The use of grids reduces the amount of radiation scatter, allowing restriction of the size of the radiation beam to the area of interest. Shielding of radiation sensitive structures (ovaries, testicles, and thyroid) should be routine when possible, as long as they do not block visualization of essential structures including the ribs and iliac crest for assessment of skeletal maturity (Fig. 8.1).

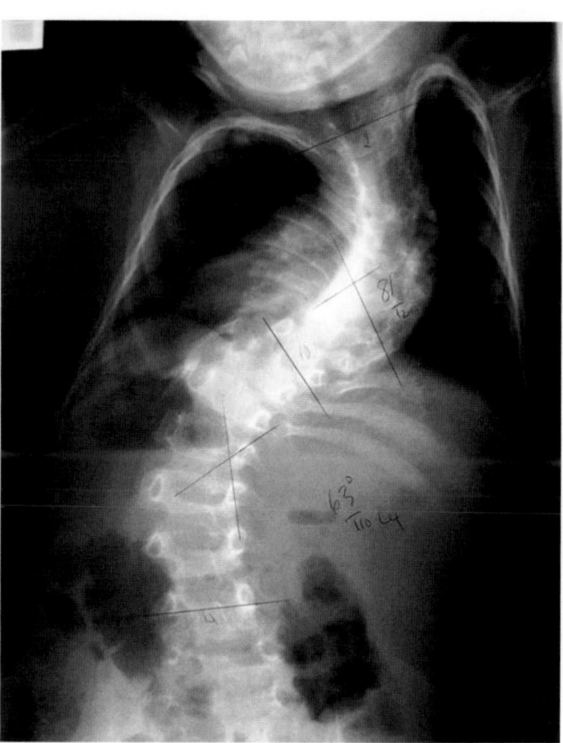

Fig. 8.1 Upright (*standing*) PA view of the spine obtained on a long 36 in. cassette. This view not only shows the entire spine on a single exposure but allows for assessment of coronal balance, measurement of the effect of the curve on the chest, and estimation of skeletal maturity

There are several unique considerations when obtaining plain radiographs in children with complex spinal deformity. The treating surgeon must specify these inclusions unless the medical imaging facility obtains these films routinely. It is important in children with thoracic deformity to include the entire chest wall in the initial image. Many children will have a significant chest wall deformity in addition to spinal curvature, which may be an important consideration in future management. It is essential to include a measurement standard (ruler) on the films for evaluation of growth of the spine over time. This marker will take into account radiographic magnification which can vary with the technique used for film acquisition. Standard measurements of spinal deformity are made from these initial films using the Cobb Angle. Measurements of thoracic deformity in the coronal and saggital plane including thoracic height, sitting height, thoracic depth, and the *Space Available for the Lung* described by Campbell et al. [5] may have indirect implications regarding pulmonary function and growth (Fig. 8.2). Inclusion of

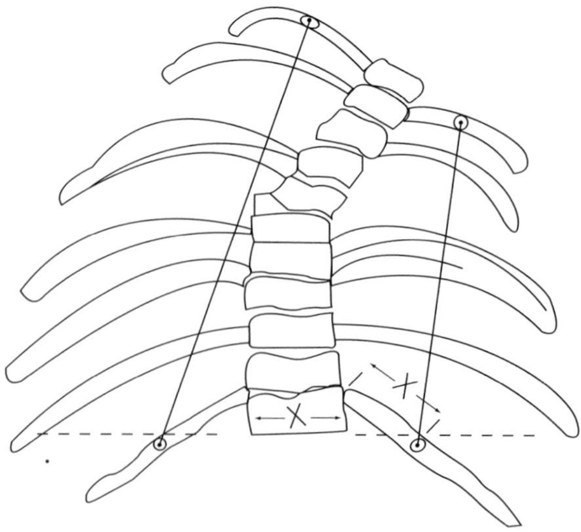

Fig. 8.2 Space available for the lung (SAL). The SAL is a ratio expressed as a percentage of the distance from the diaphragm to the apex of the lung measured on an upright radiograph of the chest when comparing one side to the other. In this example, the SAL is 70% when comparing the right to the left

the iliac crest and hip joints allows the estimation of skeletal maturity and growth potential, especially in the preadolescent age group. The Risser sign is useful in predicting if peak growth velocity has occurred. An open triradiate cartilage at the acetabulum would predict that there is significant growth remaining.

Films to assess flexibility are useful for preoperative planning for surgical constructs and instrumentation levels. There are a variety of techniques for this, including supine right and left bending films, supine traction views, and films taken over bolsters. These films are valuable only in anticipation of treatment and not as an initial screening technique.

An additional consideration is the timing and frequency of obtaining radiographs to follow children for progression of deformity. As a general rule, a rapidly progressing curve during active growth changes as much as 1–2° per month. The average intra-observer measurement error for measuring the Cobb angle in scoliosis or kyphosis is about 3°. Therefore, to see a significant difference in curve progression greater than measure error, it is logical to wait at least 6 months between obtaining new radiographs in a child who is actively growing. In younger children compared to teenagers, the rate of growth is slow and steady and it is reasonable to wait as long as one year between radiographs unless otherwise indicated. The risks associated with repeated radiation exposure of breast tissue in females are not insignificant. Doody et al. [7] reported that females with multiple scoliosis radiographs had a two-fold increase in mortality from breast cancer when compared to age-matched controls. This risk correlated with increasing numbers of radiographs and cumulative radiation dose.

8.3 The EOS System

Dubousset et al. [9] have recently described the new method for acquisition of images in two dimensions and reconstruction in three dimensions using the EOS system (Biospace Med, Atlanta, GA, USA). This system uses microstrip gas detectors able to change radiographic photons into electrons, allowing to get a digital radiographic image with a very low dose of radiation (8–10 times less than conventional radiographs). This led to the design of a machine built with two radiographic sources and their detector located at 90° from one another and linked by a rigid frame. This makes it possible to scan a patient from head to toe in 15–20 s with the beam continuously orthogonal to the target, avoiding any distortion. In addition, there is a modeling technique capable of making an accurate 3D reconstruction of the external envelop of the osteoarticular structures, as complex as those existing in the spine. All the data obtained can be accurately validated and is comparable to the 3D reconstruction coming from CT scans with considerably less radiation. An additional advantage is that images can be obtained in a standing posture where the resultant gravity factor plays an important role that cannot be achieved in conventional supine CT scans (Fig. 8.3a–j). The dose of radiation using the EOS is estimated at 800–1000 times less when compared to 3D reconstruction with CT scan. Some limitations of the technique include the requirement for subjects to stand still for at least 10 seconds, making it difficult to use in small children. In addition, images cannot be acquired in the supine position at this point.

This new technique opens a number of potential opportunities for the analysis of spinal deformity in three dimensions. These 3D images provide comprehensive assessment of the horizontal or axial plane when seen from the top "view from the airplane" showing the helicoïdal pile of the vertebrae with their volumetric value. This allows for the development of new methods more comprehensive than the Cobb angle to quantify scoliosis measurements such as the assessment of pre- and post-operative correction of the deformity on volumetric and real balance criteria instead of angle. Another application is to measure the volume and deformity of the thoracic cage, the amount of penetration of the spinal structures inside the thorax in surface or volume. Using simulation software, surgical scoliosis correction can be simulated preoperatively using various positioning of the implants.

8.4 Computed Tomography (CT Scans)

The clinical use of CT is attributed to Hounsfield [15] in 1973. The basic principle of CT scans is that the internal structure of an object can be reconstructed using multiple images in the form of sections obtained sequentially. The radiographic beam is highly collimated and moves around the patient at 360° to obtain a single slice. This information is processed by computer to display

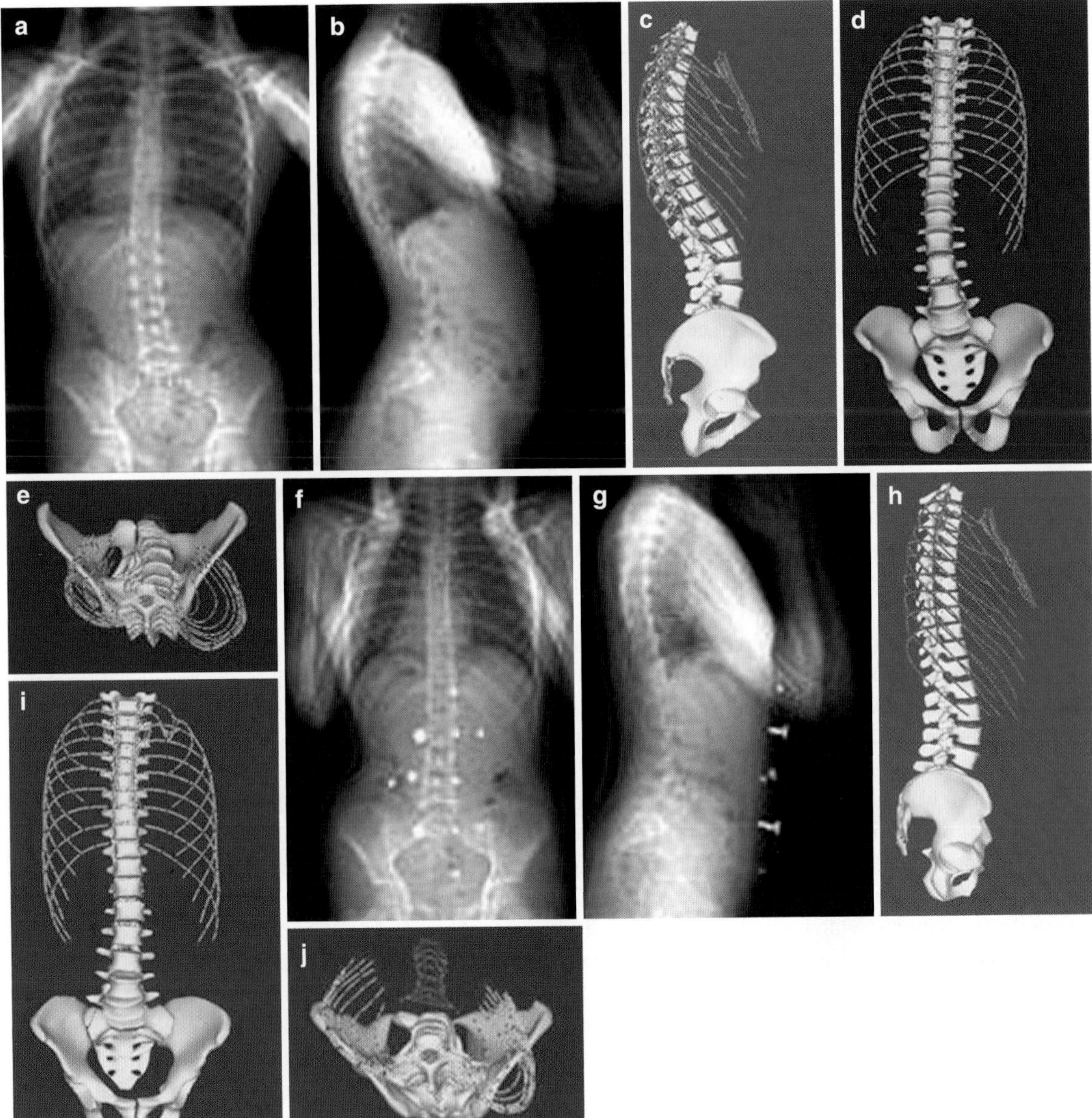

Fig. 8.3 (**a–e**) Images using the EOS system. (Courtesy of Biospace Med, USA). (**a, b**) Plain radiographs of a lumbar scoliosis obtained with the EOS System. (**c, d**) 3D reconstruction of the curve before the use of a brace. (**e**) "Top down" reconstruction of the curve. (**f, g**) Plain radiographs of the scoliosis after initiation of brace treatment. (**h, i**) 3D reconstruction of the spine after brace treatment. (**j**) "Top down" view of the spine after initiation of brace treatment

the images on a 512×512 grid of small squares termed pixels. Pixels are given a mathematical number by the computers that are displayed as shades of gray based on the density of the imaged object. This allows for manipulation of the images to emphasize bone vs. soft tissue detail. Recent ongoing advances in both CT technology and imaging software have allowed for the ability to produce 3D reconstruction of the images which is essential to the current understanding of the 3D nature of spinal deformity and preoperative planning.

CT scans are an invaluable tool for diagnosis and treatment planning related to complex deformity of the spine in growing children. However, there is a significant cost in terms of radiation exposure that must be considered when requesting these images. Depending on the technique of image acquisition, quality of the specific scanner, and the extent of the spine imaged, radiation exposure is estimated to be the equivalent of 115–600 chest radiographs [11]. If the average radiation from a single chest radiograph is 0.02 mSV, a thoracic spine film is 0.07 mSV, a CT scan of the chest is 8.0 mSV, the equivalent of 400 chest radiographs. Some of this radiation exposure can be reduced by requesting a specific imaging sequence that uses wider spacing of image acquisition and is non-enhanced. In our institution, we request a CT scan protocol that uses 5-mm cuts and a non-enhanced technique that in part reduces radiation when compared with a standard high-resolution protocol.

8.5 Unique Applications of Using CT Scans in the Growing Spine

Despite the radiation cost, CT scans allow for accurate measurement of spinal deformity including spinal length, rotation, and the amount of distortion of the chest invoked by the spinal deformity. Dubousset et al. [8] described the spine penetration index as a way to measure the space occupied by the spine inside the thorax, which correlates with increased thoracic lordosis. Gollogly et al. [12] described the thoracic distortion index, which measures the cross-sectional area of the thorax in patients with chest wall and spine deformity and compares this to age-matched normal children. In this study, the extent of thoracic distortion correlated closely with impairment of thoracic function as measured by pulmonary function studies (Fig. 8.4a, b).

Understanding the 3D nature of spinal deformity in the growing child and understanding its effect on the thorax is essential to plan a future management strategy. One of the challenges in small children is estimating the effect of large spinal curves on distortion of the thorax and pulmonary function. Campbell et al. [5] described the CT finding of the "windswept thorax" associated with thoracic insufficiency syndrome (TIS). TIS is defined as the inability of the thorax to support normal respiration and lung growth. The effect of a large thoracic deformity on the shape and volume of the thorax is obvious by CT scan. Evaluation of the thorax allows the ability to quantify the degree of rotation of the spine and loss of space for lung development and function. (Fig. 8.5) In addition, it provides

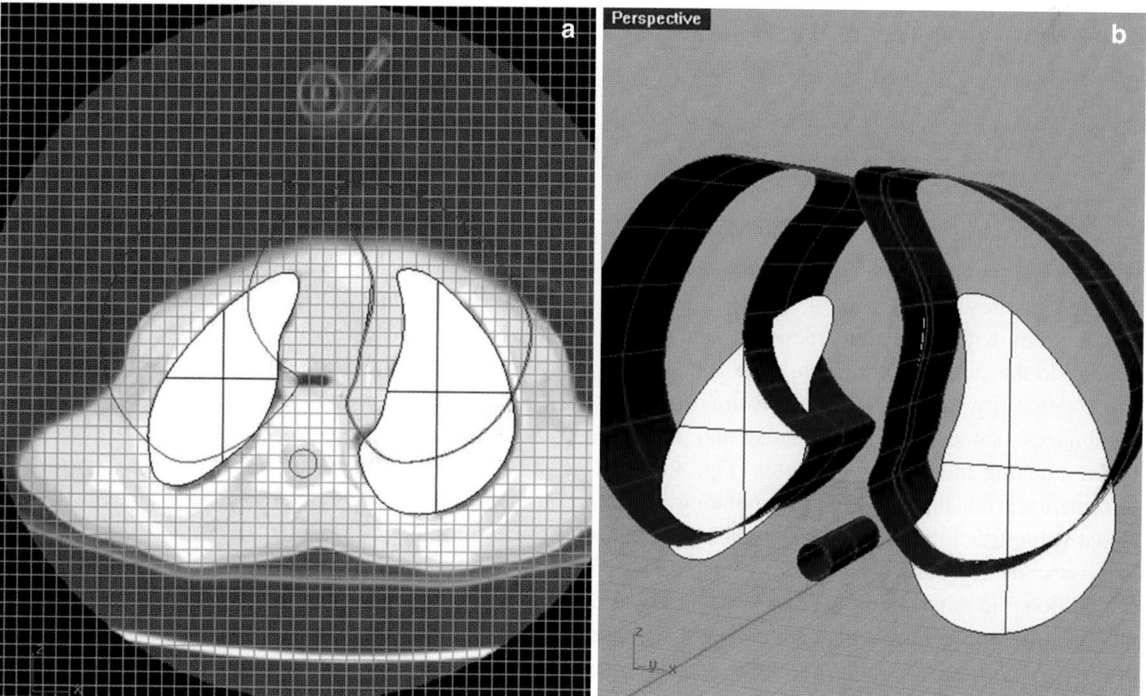

Fig. 8.4 (a) An axial CT cut and a perspective view graphically demonstrates the thoracic deformity index as a percentage of overlap of the distorted lung fields with normal lung fields. (b) The extent of thoracic distortion is calculated as a percentage of normal

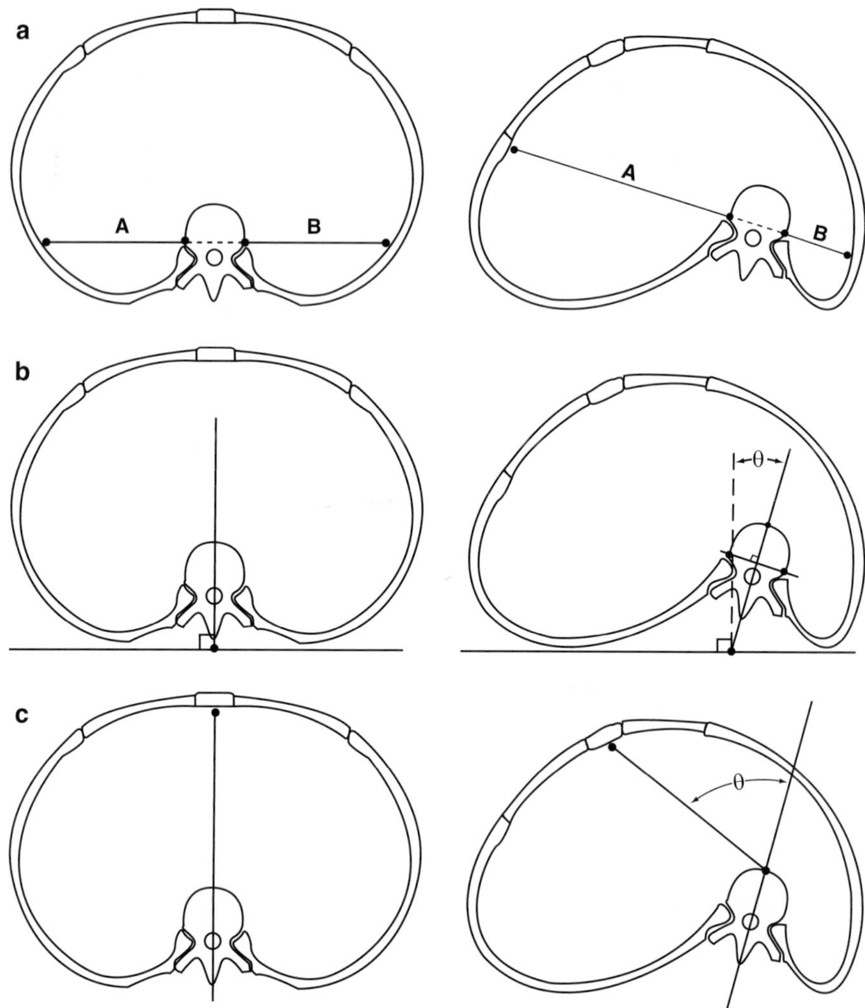

Fig. 8.5 Measurement of thoracic rotation and deformity. (**a**) Posterior hemithorax ratio, (**b**) spine rotation, and (**c**) thoracic rotation

the opportunity to estimate lung volume in children who are too young to participate in standard pulmonary function testing.

CT scans with 3D reconstruction is an essential adjunct to the surgical care of children with complex spinal deformity. Reconstruction software can provide 3D images that can be manipulated and measured before entering the operating theater (Fig. 8.6). This information is invaluable when contemplating complex spinal reconstruction procedures such as osteotomies, hemivertebrae resection of vertebral column resection. In addition, 3D data can be used to create a physical model of the spine allowing simulation of a complex procedure before the actual procedure (Fig. 8.7) [4].

Gollogly et al. [13] first reported using CT scans to measure lung volumes in children with congenital scoliosis and fused ribs (Fig. 8.8). The volume of the lung parenchyma can be measured by CT scan using a software package designed for volumetric analysis (e.g., VoxTool Version 3.0.26e, GE Advantage Workstation 4.0, General Electric, Milwaukee, WI). A 3D image of the lungs, consisting of multiple voxels, can be generated for the entire pulmonary system. A "voxel" is a combination of the words "volume" and "pixel", the two-dimensional picture element generated by the CT scan. Multiple voxels are combined to generate the 3D image from the CT scan data. Each voxel has a defined volume and density, and therefore by setting tissue imaging thresholds the lung tissue can be isolated from other tissues of differing density such as bone or cartilage. The computer can then generate a 3D reconstruction of the lungs and measure volume of that structure.

The technique of measuring lung volume using CT scans is a useful tool when attempting to quantify

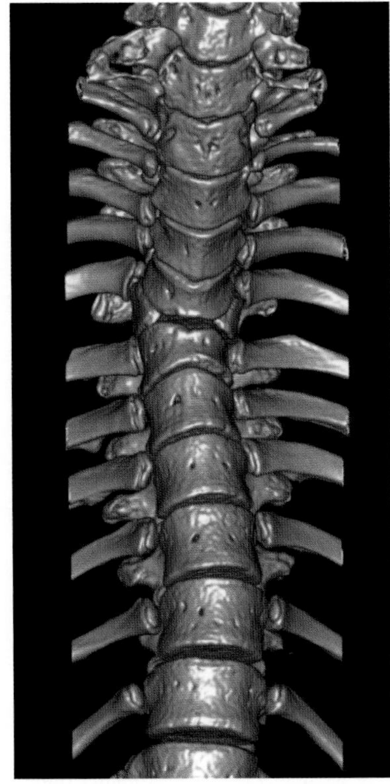

Fig. 8.6 3D reconstruction of the lumbar spine showing a hemivertebrae at L5

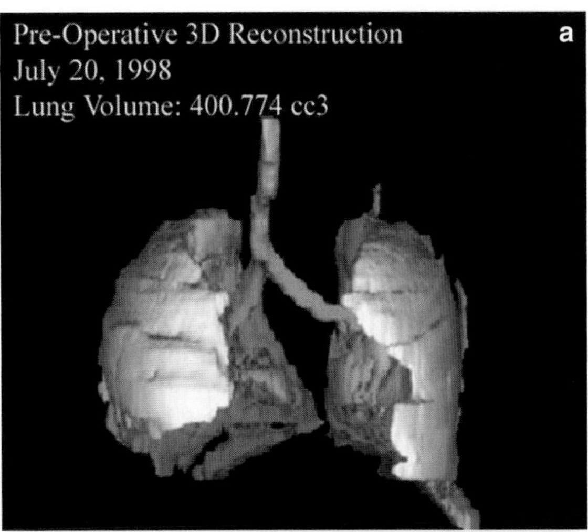

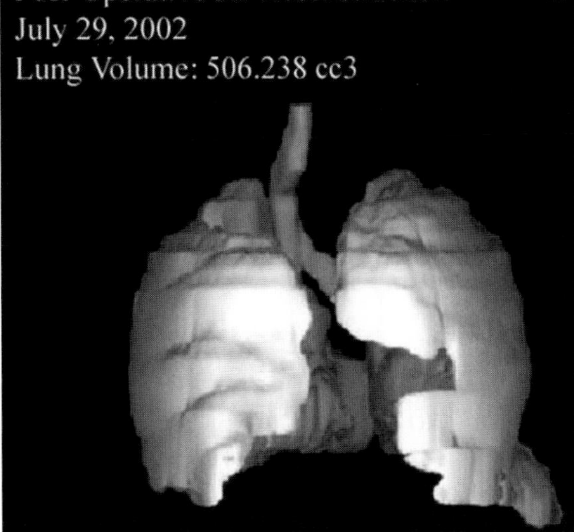

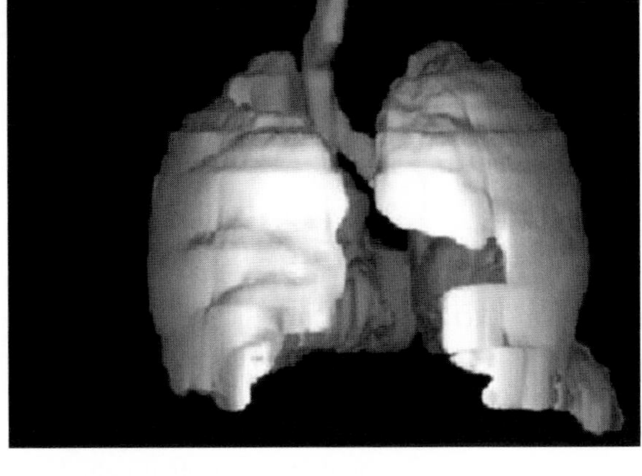

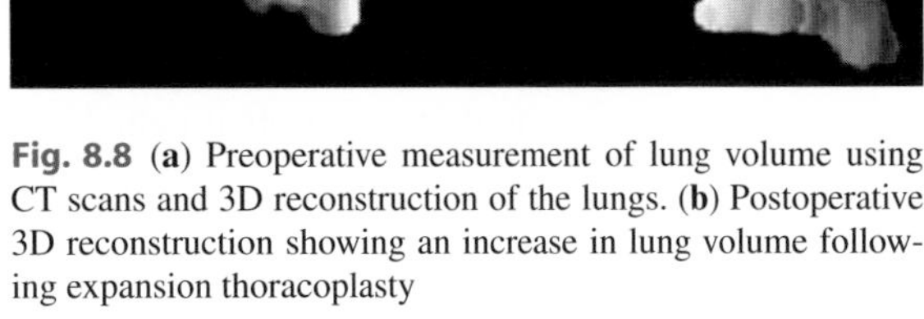

Fig. 8.8 (**a**) Preoperative measurement of lung volume using CT scans and 3D reconstruction of the lungs. (**b**) Postoperative 3D reconstruction showing an increase in lung volume following expansion thoracoplasty

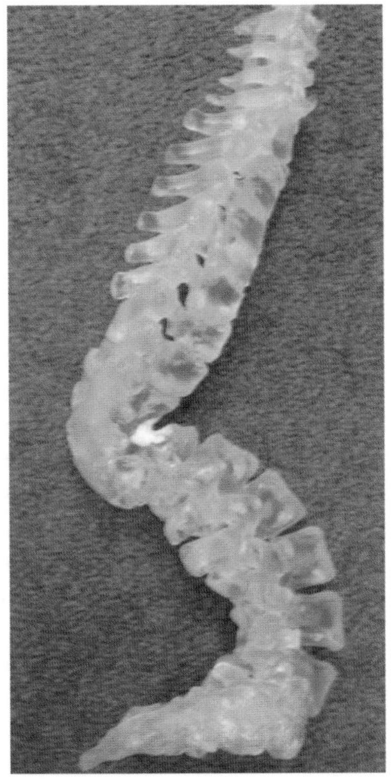

Fig. 8.7 3D plastic model of the spine made using CT data and rapid prototyping technology. This is a valuable tool when considering complex spinal reconstruction

response to treatment of thoracic deformity. Age-related normative data for CT lung volumes were established by Gollogy et al. [14] for normal children in a study of 1,050 CT scans of the chest in children without spinal deformity [14]. In a pilot study evaluating the effect of expansion thoracoplasty on lung volume in children with congenital scoliosis with fused ribs, Smith et al. showed an average increase in lung volume of 257 cc at an average follow-up of 12 months [22]. Another study showed that expansion thoracoplasty increased the lung volume on the convex non-instrumented side of the chest [23].

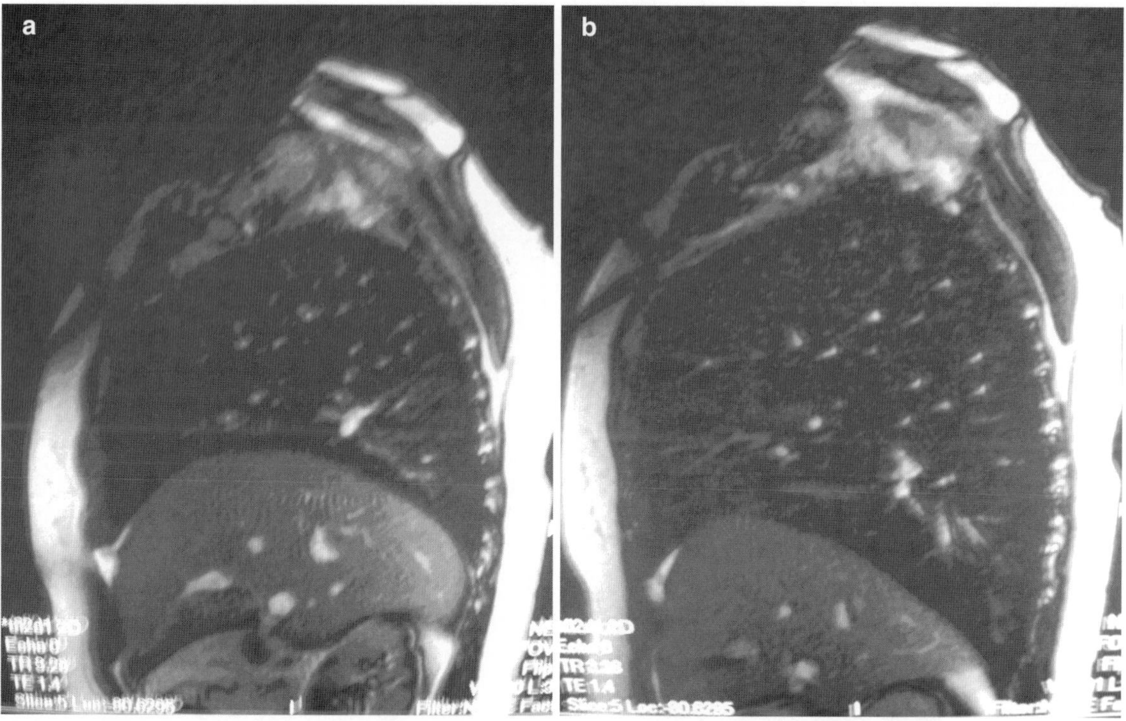

Fig. 8.9 (**a**) Dynamic MRI imaging used to measure the movement of the diaphragm in maximum expiration. (**b**) Dynamic MRI showing diaphragm excursion in maximum inspiration

8.6 Magnetic Resonance Imaging (MRI)

The use of MRI has become a standard of care in the evaluation of significant spinal deformity in growing children. It has replaced more invasive and less specific imaging modalities such as myelograms and CT myelograms as a screening tool for intraspinal pathology. The incidence of intraspinal pathology varies depending on the etiology of the spinal deformity. In congenital scoliosis, the incidence of intraspinal pathology associated with vertebral malformations varies from 3 to 52% [1–3, 20, 21, 24]. This is dependent in part on the type of malformation, with multiple hemivertebrae with contralateral failure of segmentation (bar) having the highest incidence of intraspinal pathology. Congenital kyphosis also has a high association with intraspinal anomalies.

Dynamic MRI: as image acquisition technology has improved, there is new interest in the use of dynamic MRI for understanding the intricacies of lung and chest wall function. Dynamic MRI can be performed in children at rest or under sedation during tidal breathing. The excursion of the diaphragm can be measured during inspiration and expiration (Fig. 8.9). This type of measurement can then be used to quantify the impact of spinal deformity on pulmonary function and its' response to treatment. Dynamic MRI offers the promise of further understanding the effect of intervention in the growing spine of pulmonary development and diaphragmatic function.

Functional MRI: recent improvements in MRI technology have resulted in the emerging use of functional MRI scanning to analyze the effect of varying pulmonary diseases on lung function. These techniques may be more specific and provide unique information replacing standard radiographic measurements and scintigraphy. The use of hyperpolarized gases such as helium-3 or xenon 129 as inhaled aerosols allows for measurement of regional lung ventilation, perfusion, and V/Q ratios. Reported advantages are lack of radiation, high spatial and temporal resolution, and a broad range of functional information such as air space size, regional oxygen partial pressure, etc. [16, 18]. Although currently a research tool is not clinically available, early clinical trials show significant promise [6, 10, 17, 18, 25].

References

1. Basu PS, Elsebaie H, Noordeen MH (2002) Congenital spinal deformity: a comprehensive assessment at presentation. Spine 27:2255–2259
2. Belmont PJ, Kuklo TR,Taylor, KF et al (2004) Intraspinal anomalies associated with isolated congenital hemivertebra: the role of routine magnetic resonance imaging. J Bone Joint Surg Am 86-A:1704–1710
3. Bradford DS, Heithoff KB, Cohen M (1991) Intraspinal abnormalities and congenital spine deformities: a radiographic and MRI study. J Pediatr Orthop 11:36–41
4. Brown GA, Firoozbakhsh K, DeCoster TA et al (2003) Rapid prototyping: the future of trauma surgery? J Bone Joint Surg Am 85:49–55
5. Campbell RM, Smith M, Mayes TC et al (2003) The characteristics of thoracic insufficiency syndrome associated with fused ribs and congenital scoliosis. J Bone Joint Surg 85-A:399–408
6. Deninger AJ, Mansson S, Peterson JS et al (2002) Quantitative measurement of regional lung ventilation using 3He MRI. Magn Reson Med 48:223–232
7. Doody MM, Lonstein JE, Stovall M et al (2000) Breast cancer mortality after diagnostic radiography. Spine 25: 2052–2063
8. Dubousset J, Wicart P, Pomero V et al (2003) Spinal penetration index: new threedimensional quantified reference for lordoscoliosis and other spinal deformities. J Orthop Sci 8:41–49
9. Dubousset J, Charpak G, Skalli W et al (2008) Skeletal and spinal imaging with EOS system. Arch Pediatr Adolesc Med 15:665–666
10. Eberle B, Markstaller K, Schreiber WG et al (2001) Hyperpolarised gases in magnetic resonance: a new tool for functional imaging of the lung. Swiss Med Wkly 131:503–509
11. Behealthy.com, Information for healthy life style (2008) Get wise about radiation exposure from CT scans.
12. Gollogly S, Smart MP, Smith JT (2004) The thoracic distortion index: a new technique for quantifying the effects of spinal deformities on pulmonary impairment. In: Scoliosis Research Society 39th Annual Meeting and Course, Buenos Aires, Argentina
13. Gollogly S, Smith JT, Campbell RM (2004) Determining lung volume with three-dimensional reconstructions of CT scan data: a pilot study to evaluate the effects of expansion thoracoplasty on children with severe spinal deformities. J Pediatr Orthop 24:323–328
14. Gollogly S, Smith J, White SK et al (2004) The volume of lung parenchyma as a function of age: a review of 1050 normal CT scans of the chest with three-dimensional volumetric reconstruction of the pulmonary system. Spine 29: 2061–2066
15. Hounsfield GN (1973) Computerized transverse axial scanning (tomography): part 1. Description of system. Br J Radiol 46:1016–1022
16. Kauczor HU (2003) Hyperpolarized helium-3 gas magnetic resonance imaging of the lung. Top Magn Reson Imag 14: 223–230
17. Kauczor HU, Chen XJ, van Beek EJR et al (2001) Pulmonary ventilation imaged by magnetic resonance: at the doorstep of clinical application. Eur Resp J 17:1008–1023
18. Kauczor HU, Hanke A, Van Beek EJ (2002) Assessment of lung ventilation by MR imaging: current status and future perspectives. Eur J Radiol 12:1962–1970
19. Levy AR, Goldberg MS, Mayo NE et al (1996) Reducing the lifetime risk of cancer from spinal radiographs among people with adolescent idiopathic scoliosis. Spine21:1540–1547
20. McMaster MJ (1984) Occult intraspinal anomalies and congenital scoliosis. J Bone Joint Surg Am 66:588–601
21. Prahinski JR, Polly DW, McHale KA et al (2000) Occult intraspinal anomalies in congenital scoliosis. J Ped Orthop 20:59–63
22. Smith JT, Gollogly S, White SK et al (2004) The effect of expansion thoracoplasty on lung volume in congenital scoliosis with fused ribs. A pilot study of 10 patients using CT scan reconstruction of the lung. In: Pediatric Orthopaedic Society of North America Annual Meeting, St. Louis, Missouri
23. Smith JT, Jerman J, Stringham J et al (2005) Does expansion thoracoplasty improve volume of the convex lung in a windswept thorax? In: Scoliosis Research Society 40th Annual Meeting and Course, Miami, Florida
24. Suh SW, Sarwark JF, Vora A et al (2001) Evaluating congenital spine deformities for intraspinal anomalies with magnetic resonance imaging. J Ped Orthop 21:525–531
25. Zapke M, Topf HG, Zenker M et al (2006) Magnetic resonance lung function – a breakthrough for lung imaging and functional assessment? A phantom study and clinical trial. Resp Res 7:106

9 Back Pain in Children

Mikko Poussa

Key Points

- Despite previous beliefs, new data has revealed that there is a high prevalence of back pain among adolescents.
- Girls tend to have more back pain than boys, though contradictory evidence does exist.
- There does not seem to exist a high correlation between adolescent back pain and tallness.
- There exists no correlation between good posture (good sagittal balance), lumbar spinal mobility and strong back and abdominal muscles.
- Though it still remains controversial, sporting activities during adolescence seem to reduce LBP in adulthood.
- Disc pathology as a causative factor is still unclear.

Low back pain in the adult population of the Western world is a major problem and includes personal, healthcare and socioeconomic factors [7]. On the other hand, backache in children and adolescent was considered to be a rare and serious condition in the past and in the majority of cases because of tumour infection or systemic disease.

In recent years, however, several epidemiological studies have revealed a high prevalence of back pain among children. These findings have stimulated several epidemiological studies with the aim of detecting possible risk factors, in which young people could also predict back pain in adulthood. Currently, one study claims that the roots of adult back problems lie in the youth [16].

At present, data showing that a high frequency of co-morbidity exists in those suffering from low back pain, both adolescents and adults are also available. This makes it difficult to determine from the majority of studies whether low back pain is the cause or the effect of the associated problem.

9.1 Epidemiology of Back Pain in Children

Some parameters concerning the occurrence of low back pain are firstly defined here and used throughout the text. Annual incidence means new cases during a single year. Lifetime prevalence is the proportion that have experienced symptoms by the age concerned. There is an unambiguous consensus that increasing age brings more low back pain in children. The majority of the studies are cross-sectional and give frequencies from 23 to 33% in children aged between 6–13 and 14–18 years, respectively. [30] Poussa et al. [37] in their longitudinal prospective study reported lifetime prevalence at 14 years to be 17.6% rising to 78.6% at the age of 22 years. In another longitudinal study by Burton et al. [9], the children were monitored annually from the ages of 11–15, and there was a rise in the annual incidence from 11.8% at 12 years to 21.5% at 15 years and in the lifetime prevalence from 11.6% at 11 years to 50.4% at 15 years.

In the majority of studies concerning low back pain in children, girls tend to have more pain, but the Burton et al. study [9] study was an exception, boys having more

M. Poussa
ORTON Orthopaedic Hospital, Tenholantie 10,
00280 Helsinki, Finland
e-mail: mikko.poussa@pp.inet.fi

B. A. Akbarnia et al. (eds.), *The Growing Spine*,
DOI: 10.1007/978-3-540-85207-0_9, © Springer-Verlag Berlin Heidelberg 2011

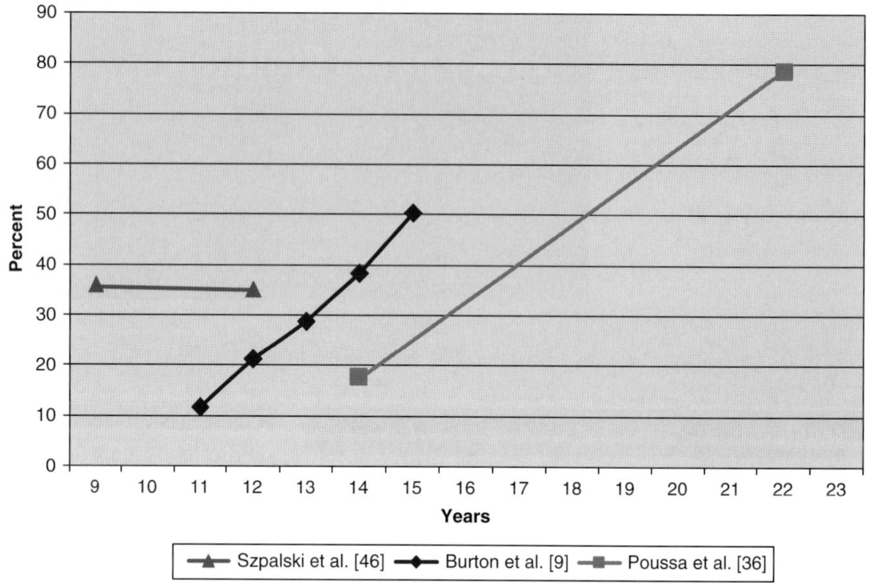

Fig. 9.1 Frequency of low back pain in three longitudinal studies. The *horizontal line* in the study by Szpalski et al. [46] can mean that before the age of 12 there is no tendency for increase of pain

pain, especially by the age of 15 years, which was thought to be due to the sporting activities of the boys at that age.

Because the increasing frequency of low back pain with increasing age has been displayed, factors related to growth and lifestyle are scrutinized in more detail.

9.2 Age

The significance of age was clearly demonstrated in previous studies when the lifetime prevalence of low back pain increased from 17.6% at the age of 14 to 78.6% at the age of 22 [33, 36]. The participants were personally interviewed at the ages of 11, 12, 13, 14 and 22. A questionnaire about low back pain was sent to them beforehand and checked in the study. In addition to an increase in the number of participants with low back pain the duration of the pain in pain sufferers was also longer.

In the Burton et al. [9] longitudinal study, both the annual incidence and point and lifetime prevalence increased between the ages of 11 and 15. Szpalski et al. [46] performed longitudinal study on the back pain of school children aged 9–12. At the end of the study, 17.8% of the children reported as having a back pain episode during the follow up period. The figure is quite close to other similar studies [33, 35]. In the Olsen et al. study [35], a 4-year follow-up was performed and at the age of 15 years the lifetime prevalence had doubled to 36%. In the cross-sectional study of 11,276 participants aged 12–18 years, Vikat et al. [47] found that neck and shoulder pain were more prevalent than low back pain, but both increased with age.

It seems that puberty leads to an exaggeration of low back symptoms [47]. Furthermore, in the majority of studies, girls tend to have higher levels of back pain when compared with boys. An exception is the study by Burton et al. [9], where one explanation for the higher frequency of low back pain in boys was their sporting activity at the age of 15 years. Maybe also that the different growth pattern between boys and girls give rise to different amount of pain between them during the growth period.

In Fig. 9.1 there are three longitudinal surveys on lifetime prevalence of low back pain during growth.

9.3 Gender

The majority of studies on non-specific back pain in children and adolescents reveal that girls have more pain than boys. In Finland, Salminen et al. [38, 39] described the prevalence for girls as being 24.2% and 15.2% for boys. The study was a cross-sectional survey and the participants were personally studied by the author. The age range of the participants was between 11 and 17 years. In another study by Salminen et al. [40] on 1,503 adolescents aged 15 years, the prevalence of back pain was 33.9% among girls and 27% among boys. There was also a subgroup comprising

8% of the whole sample with permanent or recurrent low back pain, and girls reported more disability than boys.

In the longitudinal studies by Nissinen et al. [33] and Poussa et al. [36], the lifetime prevalence of low back pain at 14 years of age was 18.4% for girls and 16.9% for boys, increasing to 78.9% and 78:4 at the age of 22 years.

Similar results reporting girls to have more back pain are given by Balague et al. [3], Vikat et al. [47], Hakala et al. [14], Brattberg and Wickman [8] and Fairbank et al. [13].

Szpalski et al. [44] found no risk factors including gender in schoolchildren aged 9–12 years. Also Widhe [48] in 2001 in his longitudinal study found no difference in low back pain between boys and girls.

In contrast to earlier studies, Burton et al. [9] in their longitudinal 5-year study reported the prevalence of back pain as being 52.6% among boys and 34.3% among girls. A possible explanation of this result was that many of the boys in this study were involved in sporting activities at the age of 15 years at the end of the study.

The reasons for the difference in pain between genders remain speculative, but there are differences in growth patterns, development of posture and also mobility of the spine during growth.

9.4 Anthropometric Factors

In the literature there are controversial studies concerning the association between anthropometric parameters (height, weight, body mass index (BMI) and growth) and low back pain. A common opinion is that increased body height is a risk factor for low back pain in adulthood, but its importance is obscure during childhood and adolescence [3, 13, 18]. In a study by Fairbank et al. [13], body height was increased in low back pain sufferers and they also had decreased lower limb mobility. The explanation for this was that because the LBP sufferers avoided sports the effect was decreased mobility of the lower limb joints.

In Salminen et al. [42] 3-year follow-up study, the height of the boys suffering from LBP was greater at the baseline, and both boys and girls with disc protrusions were also taller. The registration of growth in this study was not possible because girls usually stop growing at the age of 15 years, which was the starting point of this study.

In the studies by Nissinen et al. [33] and Poussa et al. [36], an attempt was made to clarify the role of anthropometric factors, especially the significance of growth, in the development of low back pain during growth. The longitudinal study design made it possible to find out predictive factors for low back pain at a certain phase of a child's growth period. The participants in the study were assessed annually at the ages of 11, 12, 13, 14 and 22. The history of LBP was obtained by a structured questionnaire at the ages of 14 and 22. To obtain the history of LBP the lower back region was pictured in a questionnaire and also shown to the respondent by the examiner. One-year incidence of LBP was obtained (from 13 to 14 years). A 1-year change of anthropometric factors (from 12 to 13 years) and cross-sectional anthropometric measurements at 13 years were made. Thus, predictors for 1-year incidence of LBP were registered, as were inquiries concerning possible visits to a physician and whether standing, sitting, walking, running, leisure time sports or physical education at school had provoked LBP. The following anthropometric measurements were made annually by the examining doctor: rib or lumbar hump and leg length inequality. In addition, nurses measured height and weight on every visit. This follow-up study was finished when the participants were approximately 22 years old and the same protocol including the questionnaire and measurements was repeated. At both the measurement points (14 and 22 years), growth-related issues, i.e. sitting height and the size of the thoracic or lumbar hump at 14 years and the growth from 11 to 14 years at 22 years, predicted LBP. The reasons for these results remain speculative. Excessive BMI, limb-length inequality or other anthropometric measurements had no predictive value for LBP either at 14 or 22 years of age. It is known that majority of children and adolescents develop a hump of a size of 4–6 mm and the appearance of the hump occurs at the ascending phase of the peak height velocity. Maybe this rapid growth can, at least theoretically, give rise to temporary dysfunction in the back. The role of the anthropometric characteristics, however, seems only modest.

9.5 Spinal Posture

Good posture was considered of utmost importance in the past [26]. Good posture, however, is an undefined issue.

There are not many longitudinal studies, in which the development of spinal sagittal curves are clarified. In the Poussa et al. [37] study the participants were measured by spinal pantograph and followed from the ages of 11–22 years. In this survey, there was an increase in the kyphosis in boys and girls during the follow-up and a tendency for a decrease for lordosis in girls. Boys were always more kyphotic and girls more lordotic. However, no correlation with the changes in sagittal profiles and LBP was observed.

In Widhe's survey [48] 90 children were studied first at the ages of 5–6 years and re-examined at 15–16 years. Measurements were made using De-brunner's kyphometer. Both kyphosis and lordosis increased during the 10 year follow-up. Here, too, here boys were more kyphotic than girls and girls had a tendency to be more lordotic. No correlation with the sagittal profiles and LBP was observed. There are two more comprehensive cross-sectional studies on the development of sagittal curves during growth; Willner and Johnson [49] used a pantograph on 1,101 children between the ages of 8 and 16 years and they also found that kyphosis increases with age. A similar trend was not observed in lordosis. Cil et al. [10] radiologically studied 151 children in their cross-sectional survey. During growth, both thoracic kyphosis and lumbar lordosis increased. In the two latter investigations, back pain was not taken into consideration.

In all the four studies mentioned above, a wide variation in the sagittal curves was observed, and, therefore, it is difficult to give boundaries between normal and possible abnormal posture.

Based on the current studies, it seems that faults in spinal posture as such cannot be regarded as risk factors for non-specific low back pain.

9.6 Spinal Mobility

Difficulties are encountered in assessing the relationship between spinal mobility, muscle flexibility and adolescent low back pain. This is due to the variation of methods for measuring mobility or flexibility and also due to the fact that there are slight changes in the mobility of the spine during growth and also gender differences.

Mellin et al. [28] studied the spinal mobility of 13–14 year old boys and girls. The measurements were made by goniometric methods. The main differences were in the thoracic spine, where the girls were stiffer than the boys. In the lumbar spine no differences between the genders were found. Mellin and Poussa [27] carried out a cross-sectional study on 294 children aged 8–16-years. The girls in this study were also stiffer in the thoracic spine and at 14 years of age there seemed to be a decrease in thoracic mobility, perhaps corresponding to pubertal events. The results in the lumbar spine were more difficult to interpret and no clear deviations were observed. In both of these studies low back pain was not included in the scheme.

Widhe [48] performed a longitudinal study of 90 children who were analyzed twice; at 5–6 and 15–16 years of age. The mobility in the sagittal plane was performed using Debrunner's kyphometer. The total sagittal mobility of the spine decreased significantly during the 10-year study period; in the thoracic spine 27° and in the lumbar spine 4°. About one-third of the children stated that they had occasional low back pain at the age of 16. This pain had no correlation to spinal posture, spinal mobility or physical activity.

In the Salminen et al. [40] study from a group of 1,503 schoolchildren aged 15 years, 38 children with back pain and 38 asymptomatic controls were selected for testing spinal mobility and trunk muscle strength. The measurements were made using flexicurve technique. Lumbar extension, straight leg raising, endurance of the back and abdominal muscles were decreased in the pain group. If the pupil had sciatica flexion of the lumbar spine was also diminished. It is probable that the restrictions are due to spinal pain and disc degeneration.

In the Burton et al. [9] follow-up study, 216 children were monitored for 5 years. The severity of pain and flexibility were not related. The mean lumbar spine mobility increased during the follow-up. This increase could be accounted for by a significant increase in extension. Mean flexion was reduced, significantly so for girls.

According to Kujala et al. [23] study, decreased lower lumbar segment extension mobility may cause overloading of the low back among athletes and that it predicts future low back pain in the future. In another study Kujala et al. [24] stated that training does not increase maximal lumbar extension in healthy adolescents. This knowledge according to the authors should be considered when the rules of sports and choreography of dance performances are considered.

Ohlen et al. [34] studied spinal sagittal configuration and mobility among 12 year-old gymnasts. Measurements by Debrunner's kyphometer and Myrin's inclinometer were highly correlated. On average, 1° of the total sagittal lumbar mobility was lost for every 1° of increased lordosis. Low back pain was reported by 20% of the girls, and these girls had significantly larger lordosis (41°) than girls with no history of LBP (35°).

Thus the causative relationship between lumbar spinal mobility and low back pain remains obscure. Around the growth spurt there can be restrictions on the mobility in certain segments of the lumbar spine and these restrictions must be respected to avoid unnecessary spine injuries.

9.7 Muscle Strength

Adult LBP sufferers have been advised to strengthen their abdominal and back muscles. Although it could be tempting to assume that, nowadays, young people have weaker muscles and that they are also heavier than they were in the past, no correlation between weak muscles, increased BMI (body mass index) and low back pain has been proven.

Kujala et al. [22] performed a longitudinal 5-year follow-up study with the aim investigating predictive factors on healthy adult people at the baseline. Height and heavy physical loading predicted low back pain but not aerobic power or muscle strength characteristics.

Balaque et al. [4] in their cross-sectional survey on children 10–16 years of age could not show that low back pain and trunk muscle strength were correlated. In Salminen et al.'s studies [40, 41] from a group of 1,503 children aged 15 years, 38 with recurrent LBP and 38 with no LBP were compared. The endurance strength of the abdominal and back muscles was decreased in the LBP group. It is probable that the results reflect secondary events to LBP. Contradictory results about the role of abdominal muscles in the etiopathogenesis of LBP were presented by Newcomer and Sinaki [32]. They found in their longitudinal study that those who were suffering from LBP had stronger back flexors at the baseline and follow-up compared with the pain-free counterparts. They believed that the majority of low back pain in children is due to musculotendinous strains and ligamentous sprains.

9.8 Leisure Time and Sporting Activities

Analyzing the epidemiological data from various studies shows that the prevalence of pain seems to be quite constant below the age of 15 years: in the Burton et al. [9] study 12% at the age of 12 years, in Nissinen et al. [33] study 18% at 14 years of age. There is also a clear annual rise in pain in both longitudinal and cross-sectional studies. Also, the explanation for this tend to be uniform: sitting at school or watching television, competitive or leisure time sports, sometimes back injury in competitive sports. All these factors mentioned earlier increase the load on intervertebral disks, vertebral endplates and posterior elements.

There are some studies which demonstrate that sporting activities during adolescence reduce LBP in adult age. Harreby et al. [17] studied a cohort of 38-year-old men and women, who at the age of 14 years had been interviewed by their school doctors. Physical activity for at least 3 h/week reduced the lifetime risk for LBP. In the study by Mikkelsson et al. [31], primary measurements were made when the participants were 9–21 year old and the follow-up was 25 years. The result was that physical activity during adolescence reduced LBP in adulthood in men and. physical activity in adulthood may reduce LBP in women. In addition, the higher the BMI, the greater the risk of LBP in both the genders.

Sports and physical activities, especially at the competitive level, may provoke low back symptoms and even back injuries. In the Burton et al. study [9], boys aged 15 years had more pain, which is contrary to other studies. The explanation was that out of the participants there were lot of boys who were active in sports and, therefore, had more pain. Auvinen et al.'s study [2] on 5,999 boys and girls born in 1986 also revealed that very active participation in physical activities is related to self-reported LBP. In contrast to this, Salminen et al. [41] in his study assembled two groups of 38 participants aged 15 years, one with recurrent or continuous LBP and the other being totally asymptomatic. Low physical activity and restrictions in lumbar spine mobility were characteristic of the former group. However, it is not possible to draw conclusions from this study as to what is the cause and effect.

Kujala et al. [23] carried out a 3-year follow-up study among athletes and non-athletes both being free of pain upon entry to the study. During the follow-up time, there were five times as many people with LBP among athletes. Low lumbar extension mobility among the athletes was thought to be predictive of future low back pain. Magnetic Resonance Imaging (MRI) examinations were also carried out on 43 girls participating in a baseline and follow-up study; new abnormalities were detected in 6 of 8 reporting acute back injury. The significance of an MRI and bone scan in detecting sports-related back injuries was emphasized by Kujala et al. [25]. Their series comprised 19 athletes aged 12–18, who had low-back pain that had interfered with their training for at least 4 weeks. Twelve had changes in the disc-vertebral end plate complex and eight had positive bone scan indicative posterior vertebral arch stress reaction. Restricting painful activities usually led to a good recovery.

Micheli and Wood [29] compared the findings between adults and young athletes suffering from LBP. They found significant differences between the two groups; the majority of young people had derangements of their posterior elements while the majority of adults were interpreted as having symptomatic disc abnormalities or muscle-tendon strain as a cause of their LBP.

To give accurate counsel and management in spine problems of active athletes, understanding the possible pain source is crucial. A restriction on activities for 3 months led to a recovery in the majority of cases. Also, in the study by El Rassi et al. [12] those who stopped playing soccer for 3 months had better results than those who did not comply with this restriction.

9.9 Back Pain and Co-Morbidity

It is a known fact that adult low-back patients have a lot of neck problems. It is also known that headache and gastrointestinal complaints are common in young schoolchildren. Brattberg and Wickman [8] made a cross-sectional survey asking 8–17-year-old children about headaches and low back pain. The prevalence of both increased with age, and more children complained about headache than LBP. Girls had more trouble in both. Similar results were obtained by Hakala et al. [14] from Finland when they made a nationwide postal survey on close to 190,000 young people aged between 12 and 18. Girls had more pain in the neck, shoulders and low back. And both had more pain in the neck-shoulder region than in the low back. In the study by El-Metwally et al. [11] 11-year-old children, free of pain at baseline were followed for 1 year. They separated two types of pain: traumatic and non-traumatic. The independent risk factors for non-traumatic musculoskeletal pain were headache and daytime tiredness. The risk factors for traumatic musculoskeletal pain were vigorous exercise and day-time tiredness. The authors suggest that school healthcare professional should pay attention to children reporting headache and practicing vigorous exercise.

Hakala et al. [15] carried out a survey that was mailed to 6,003 participants who were 14–18-year-old. Neck-shoulder pain was more frequent than low back pain. Daily use of computers exceeding 2–3 h seemed to be the threshold for neck-shoulder pain and exceeding 5 h for low back pain.

There are studies from Denmark based on their twin register and where co-morbidity around low back pain was studied. The first study by Hestbaek et al. [19] was cross-sectional and revealed that if young people have LBP they also have an increased risk of suffering from asthma and headache. The second survey [20] was longitudinal with an 8-year follow-up and the result was the same; there is a clustering of LBP, headache and asthma in adolescence.

On the other hand, in the group of adolescent pain sufferers there may be individuals who have widespread pain symptoms and who have low pain threshold, depressive symptoms and sleep problems.

9.10 Disc Pathologies as Causative Factors for Low Back Pain in Adolescents

On the basis of twin studies, it seems that disc degeneration is mostly hereditary and physical loading such as sporting activities and occupation-related factors play a minor role in disc degeneration [5, 6].

In children and adolescents, there are few studies that can elucidate this issue. Kujala et al. [25] investigated the prognosis of low back pain and the association of clinical symptoms and MRI/bone scan findings in 12–18-year-old athletes. A total of 19 athletes were included and in 15 of them anatomic abnormalities that corresponded to the location and type of clinical symptoms were found. One subject had typical disc extrusion and nine had disc protrusion either with or without vertebral end plate changes. In addition, two had vertebral end plate irregularities without disc degeneration. Eight had changes in the posterior arch complex, which was detected by bone scan. Because of the nature of the study, no etiopathogenetic conclusions on the possible causes of the disc degeneration can be drawn. However, it seems reasonable to assume that the changes in the posterior vertebral arch are traumatic and the disc changes degenerative.

Swärd et al. [45] reported vertebral ring apophysis injuries in young (14–25 years) wrestlers and female gymnasts. The changes were found at the thoracic and thoracolumbar junction and led to excavation in the anterior part of the vertebral ring apophysis. The same authors [44] found that in elite male gymnasts disc degeneration was significantly more common than in non-athletes.

An example of posterior annular tear and posterior disc protrusion is given in (Fig. 9.2).

Salminen et al. [43] made a comprehensive follow-up study on 1,503 schoolchildren aged 15 year at the baseline from whom 38 with recurrent LBP cases and 38 totally free of pain were compared. Three interviews at 15, 18 and 23 years of age were made and an MRI at 15 and 18 years was taken. Eleven participants (35% from the original 38) persistently reported recurrent low back pain. Disc degeneration at 15 years gave a risk of 16 as having recurrent low Back pain at 23 years when compared with those having no disc degeneration. In addition to disc protrusion, Scheuermann-type changes at 15 years made an extra impact on the risk of persistently recurrent low back pain. It should be noticed that MRI changes at 18 years had much less predictive value for future low back pain. This may be interpreted as there being perhaps 2–3% of the population at risk for chronic low back pain and those by whom genetic risk factors can be associated with the disc degeneration.

Kjaer et al. [21] examined 439 children aged 13 years with MRI and interviewed them about LBP. One third of the children had disc degeneration. They separated the upper and lower lumbar spine in the sense that degeneration in the lower lumbar spine and especially disc protrusions were associated with contacts to medical professionals. Alyas et al. [1] studied 33 asymptomatic elite tennis players who were 17–19-year-old. The Survey revealed that only 15% of the participants had normal and 85% had abnormal MRI; 9/33 had posterior arch lesions and 13/33 had disc desiccation, facet joint arthrosis was also relatively common.

It seems feasible to say that the role of disc degeneration in children and adolescents is still controversial like it is in adults. Prospective longitudinal studies are required to envisage the natural history of adolescent disc degeneration and its role in low back pain.

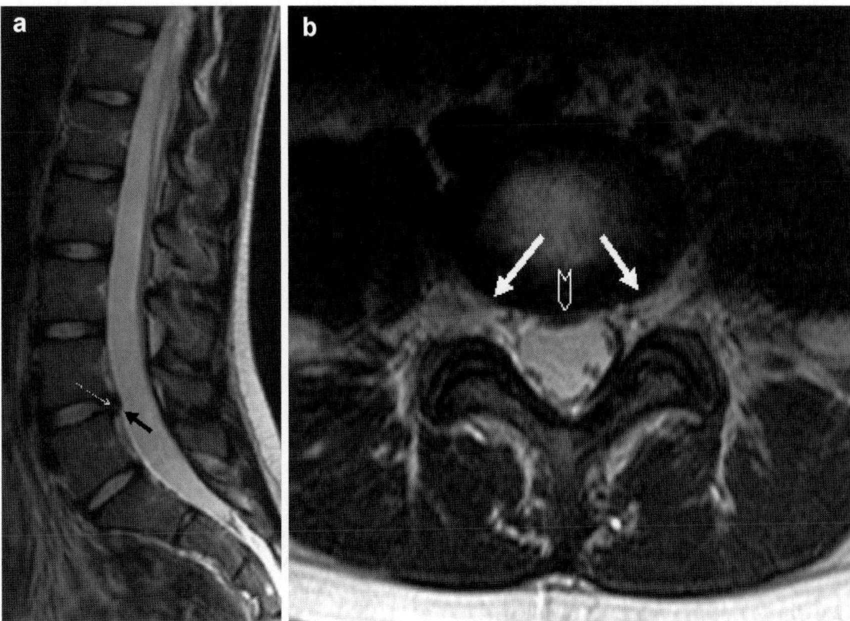

Fig. 9.2 A 13-year-old female with a history of prolonged low back pain. Sagittal (**a**) and axial (**b**) T2-weighted MR images show disc protrusion (*arrows* (**a, b**)) with annular tear (*arrow with dotted line* (**a**), *arrowhead*, (**b**)). Also, there is a history of intense weight lifting exercise. (Courtesy of Dr Seppo Koskinen)

9.11 Summary

The etiopathogenesis of LBP in children and adolescents is multifactorial. In a small segment, 2–3% of the cause may be discogenic due to degeneration. Active sports can cause both disc and posterior element injuries. Growth brings an annually increasing amount of pain, the mechanism is unclear. Possibly stiffening of the spine and soft tissue adaptation difficulties give their contribution to back pain especially around puberty.

The significance of increased BMI, leg-length-inequality and increased lumbar lordosis remains unproven. To recognise those children and adolescents who are at risk to become chonically disabled because of low back pain is currently the big challenge for national sociomedical organisations.

References

1. Alyas F, Turner M, Connel D (2007) MRI findings in the lumbar spine of asymptomatic adolescent elite tennis players. Br J Sports Med 41:836–841
2. Auvinen J, Tammelin T, Taimela S et al (2007) Association of physical activity with low back pain in adolescents. Scand J Med Sci Sports 18:188–194
3. Balague F, Dutoit G, Waldburger M (1988) Low back pain in schoolchildren – an epidemiological study. Scand J Rehabil Med 20:175–179
4. Balague F, Damidot P, Nordin M et al (1993) Cross-sectional study of the isokinetic muscle strength among school children. Spine 18:1199–1205
5. Battie MC, Videman T (2006) Lumbar disc degeneration: epidemiology and genetics. Bone Joint Surg Am 88(Suppl 2):3–9
6. Battie MC, Videman T, Levalahti E et al (2007) Heritability of low back pain and the role of disc degeneration. Pain 131:272–280
7. Biering-Sorensen F (1984) Physical measurements as risk indicators for low trouble over one year period. Spine 9:106–119
8. Brattberg G, Wickman V (1992) Prevalence of back pain and headache in Swedish school children: A questionnaire survey. Pain Clin 4:211–220
9. Burton AK, Clarke RD, McClune TD et al (1996) The natural history of low-back pain in adolescents. Spine 20:2323–2328
10. Cil A, Yazici M, Uzumcugil A et al (2005) The evolution of sagittal segmental alignment of the spine during childhood. Spine 30:93–100
11. El-Metwally A, Salminen JJ, Auvinen A et al (2007) Risk factors for development of non-specific musculoskeletal pain in preteens and early adolescents: a prospective 1-year follow-up study. BMC Musculoskelet Disord 23:46
12. El Rassi G, Takemitsu M, Woratanarat P et al (2005) Lumbar spondylolysis in pediatric and adolescent soccer players. Am J Sports Med 33:1688–1693
13. Fairbank J, Pynsent P, van Poortvliet J et al (1984) Influence of anthropometric factors and joint laxity in the incidence of adolescent back pain. Spine 5:461–464
14. Hakala P, Rimpelä A, Salminen JJ et al (2002) Back neck and shoulder pain in Finnish adolescents: national cross sectional surveys. BMJ 325:743
15. Hakala PT, Rimpelä AH, Saarni LA et al (2006) Frequent computer-raalated activities increase the risk of neck-shoulder and low back pain in adolescents. Eur J Public Health 16: 536–541
16. Harreby M, Kjer J, Hesselsoe G et al (1996) Epidemiological aspects and risk factors for low back pain in 38-year-old men and women: a 25-year prospective cohort study of 640 school children. Eur Spine J 5:312–318
17. Harreby M, Hesselsoe G, Kjer J et al (1997) Low back pain and physical exercise in leisure time in 38 year old men and women: a 25-year prospective cohort study of 640 school children. Eur Spine J 6:181–186
18. Heliövaara M, Mäkelä M, Knekt P et al (1991) Determinants of sciatica and low back pain. Spine 6:608–614
19. Hestbaek L, Leboeuf-Yde C, Kyvik KO et al (2004) Comorbidity with low back pain: a cross-sectional population-based survey of 12- to 22-year-olds. Spine 29:1483–1491
20. Hestbaek L, Lebooeuf-Yde C, Kyvik KO (2006) Is comorbidity in adolescence a predictor for adult low back pain? A prospective study of a young population. BMC Musculoskeletal Disord 16:29
21. Kjaer P, Leboeuf-Yde C, Sorensen JS et al (2005) An epidemiologic study of MRI and low back pain in 13-year-old children. Spine 30:798–806
22. Kujala UM, Taimela S, Viljanen T et al (1996) Physical loading and performance as predictors of back pain in healthy adults. Eur J Appl Physiol 73:452–458
23. Kujala UM, Taimela S, Oksanen A et al (1997) Lumbar mobility and low back pain during adolescence. A longitudinal three-year follow-up study in athletes and controls. Am J Sports Med 25:363–368
24. Kujala UM, Oksanen A, Taimela S (1997) Training does not increase maximal lumbar extension in healthy adolescents. Clin Biomech 12:181–184
25. Kujala UM, Kinnunen J, Helenius P et al (1999) Prolonged low-back pain in young athletes: a prospecrive case series study of findings and prognosis. Eur Spine J 8:480–484
26. Lindqvist C, Signell H, Wasz-Höckert C (1962) Synpunkter på hållningsfel hos barn (in Swedish) Finska Läkarsällskapets Handlingar 106:146–157
27. Mellin G, Poussa M (1992) Spinal mobility and posture in 8- to 16-year-old children. J Orthop Res 10:211–216
28. Mellin G, Härkönen H, Poussa M (1988) Spinal mobility and posture and their correlations with growth velocity in structurally normal boys and girls aged 13 to 14. Spine 13:152–154
29. Micheli LJ, Wood R (1995) Back pain in young athletes. Significant differences from adults in causes and patterns. Arch Pediatr Adolesc Med 149:15–18
30. Mierau D, Cassidy JD, Yong-Hing K (1989) Low-back pain and straight leg raising in children and adolescents. Spine 14:526–528

31. Mikkelsson LO, Nupponen H, Kaprio J et al (2006) Adolescent flexibility, endurance strength, and physical activity as predictor of adult tension neck, low back pain and knee injury: a 25 year follow up study. Br J Sports Med 40:107–113
32. Newcomer K, Sinaki M (1996) Low-back pain in children and its relationship to back strength and level of physical activity. Acta Paedriatr 85:433–439
33. Nissinen M, Heliövaara M, Seitsamo J et al (1994) Anthropometric measurements and the incidence of low back pain in a cohort of pubertal children. Spine 12:1367–1370
34. Ohlen G, Wredmark T, Spangfort E (1989) Spinalsa gittal configuration and mobility related to low-back pain in the female gymnast. Spine 14:847–850
35. Olsen TL, Anderson RL, Dearwater SR et al (1992) The epidemiology of low-back pain in an adolescent population. Am J Public Health 82:606–608
36. Poussa M, Heliövaara M, Seitsamo J et al (2005) Anthropometric measurements and growth as predictors of low back pain:a cohort study of children followed up from the age of 11 to 22 years. Eur Spine J 14:595–598
37. Poussa M, Heliövaara M, Seitsamo J et al (2005) Development of spinal posture in a cohort of children from the age of 11 to 22 years. Eur Spine J 14:738–742
38. Salminen JJ (1984) The adolescent back. A field survey of 370 Finnish schoolchildren. Acta Paediatr Scand Suppl 315: 8–122
39. Salminen JJ, Pentti J, Terho P (1992) Low back pain and disability in 14-year-old schoolchildren. Acta Paediatr 81: 1035–1039
40. Salminen J, Mäki P, Oksanen A et al (1992) Spinal mobility and trunk muscle strength in 15-year-old school children with and without low-back pain. Spine 17:405–411
41. Salminen J, Tertti M, Paajanen H (1993) Magnetic resonance imaging findings of lumbar spine in the young: correlation with leisure time physical activity, spinal mobility, and trunk muscle strength in 15-year old pupils with and without low-back pain. J Spinal Disord 5:386–391
42. Salminen JJ, Erkintalo M, Laine M et al (1995) Low-back pain in the young. A prospective three-year follow-up study of subjects with and without low back pain. Spine 20: 2101–2108
43. Salminen JJ, Erkintalo MO Pentti J et al (1999) Recurrent low back pain and early disc degeneration in the young. Spine 24:1316–1321
44. Swärd L, Hellström M, Jacobsson B et al (1991) Disc degeneration and associated abnormalities of the spine in elite gymnasts. A magnetic resonance imaging study. Spine 16: 437–443
45. Swärd L, Hellström M, Jacobsson B et al (1993) Vertebral ring apophysis injury in athletes. Is the etiology different in the thoracic and lumbar spine. Am J Sports Med 21: 841–845
46. Szpalski M, Gunzburg R, Balaque F et al (2002) A 2-year prospective longitudinal study on low back pain in primary school children. Eur Spine J 11:459–464
47. Vikat A, Rimpelä M, Salminen JJ et al (2000) Neck or shoulder pain and low back pain in Finnish adolescents. Scand J Public Health 28:164–173
48. Widhe T (2001) Spine: posture mobility and pain. A Longitudinal study from childhood to adolescence. Eur Spine J 2:118–123
49. Willner S, Johnson B (1983) Thoracic kyphosis and lumbar lordosis during growth period in children. Acta Paediatr Scand 72:873–878

10 Pediatric Spinal Infections

Ahmet Alanay and İbrahim Akel

Key Points

- Clinical workup for pediatric spinal infections begins with a high level of suspicion.
- Discitis can usually be managed by medical treatment, while surgical irrigation and debridement may be necessary for patients with vertebral osteomyelitis.
- Tuberculosis is a slowly progressing infection, thus the clinical picture is completely different than the nonspecific infections of the spine.
- Early diagnosis and effective chemotherapy in spinal tuberculosis make the process a well-controlled medical disease. Surgical treatment should be considered as an adjuvant to effective drug therapy.
- Early and late spinal infections following spinal surgery mostly require surgical intervention.

10.1 Pediatric Spinal Infections

Spinal infections are uncommon in childhood; therefore, the clinical workup begins with a high level of suspicion. Spinal infections can be classified as either disc or vertebral body infections (i.e., discitis or vertebral osteomyelitis, respectively). Indeed, both diseases have distinct epidemiologic, clinical, and radiographic features [78]. In this chapter, pathophysiology, clinical evaluations, and management of discitis, vertebral osteomyelitis, tuberculosis, and postoperative spinal infections observed in childhood will be reviewed.

A. Alanay (✉)
Istanbul Spine Center, Florence Nightingale Hospital
Sisli, Istanbul, 34403 Turkey
e-mail: aalanay@gmail.com

10.1.1 Discitis

Discitis is mostly seen among children around 5 years of age and primarily involves the lumbar region. Consequently, the symptomatic child refuses to walk or has a progressive limp, allowing a Gower's sign to potentially be present at the beginning of the disease. Complaint of back pain is typically expressed by approximately 50% of the patients. Additionally, the families of the patients commonly report an antecedent or concurrent illness, and a confounding history of trauma. Duration of the symptoms may vary from hours to weeks. Incidence of discitis in childhood is estimated to be 1–2 cases per year [18, 91].

10.1.1.1 Pathophysiology

Discitis is mainly hematogenous in origin for pediatric patients; preceding infections may be otitis media, urinary tract infections, or pulmonary infections [30]. Histological examinations revealed that nutrient arteries are the route of infection for the hematogenous spread rather than the paraspinal venous system, which is primarily the course in adult discitis. Furthermore, a similar mechanism is involved as seen in osteomyelitis of the long bone metaphysis in children. The cause of infection may rarely be direct inoculation or a contigious spread from an adjacent infection locus [93].

Intervertebral discs are avascular with hyaline cartilage and end plates lying on both sides of the disc in

B. A. Akbarnia et al. (eds.), *The Growing Spine*,
DOI: 10.1007/978-3-540-85207-0_10, © Springer-Verlag Berlin Heidelberg 2011

children. Those cartilaginous plates, however, contain a vascular supply by means of numerous canals that appear before the 16th gestational week and persist until the third decade at which point the ring apophyses fuse. This rich vascular supply via canal systems to the disc is the unique property of pediatric end plates. Thus, blood-borne bacteria also reach the intervertebral disc via these roots to subsequently spread and contaminate the avascular disc with the hematogenous pathogen. Pediatric vertebral bodies have a higher vascular supply through intraosseos enormous anastamosis compared to the adult vertebral body. High vasculature of the body prevents the risk of pyogenic infection in the vertebrae. The pediatric vertebral body is also less prone to infarction. Additionally, cartilage caps on both sides prevent the spread of the infection to the vertebral body from the disc space [16, 79, 92].

After inoculation of the disc space with the pathogen, the infection is localized to the disc space, and the end plate is not affected. Bacterial enzymes, however, alter the disc biology and annulus fibrosis to cause the typical disc space narrowing as observed in plain radiographic images. If the infection persists, end plate erosion occurs, and a saw-tooth pattern of end plate destruction is seen on the radiograph. Redundant vascular supply at the vertebral body is consequently exposed to the infection at this level. Depending on the proficiency of the host mechanism, the outcome of the infection is determined. The infection may clear up or progress to the classical vertebral osteomyelitis with or without a concomitant soft tissue abscess [70].

10.1.1.2 History and Physical Examination

Children younger than 3 years of age present with an acute onset of limping or refusal to bear weight. Ultimately, symptoms continue to progress and the children become uncomfortable in all positions other than lying supine. Children 3–8 years of age may present with vague abdominal or back pain and have a decline in physical activity. Older children may present with abdominal pain, back pain, or buttock and leg pain due to nerve irritations [17, 91].

Physical examination may reveal no or a low-grade fever, as well as the possibility for the child to not appear as being acutely ill. Refusal to walk and discomfort with hip movements can be observed but not to the degree as seen in patients with septic arthritis. Local spinal tenderness and paraspinal muscle spasms with a decreased spinal range of motion and hamstring tightness is a common finding. Moreover, examination may also yield a positive result for the straight leg raise test. A stiff back may be observed for those children who can walk. Additionally, the child typically shows difficulty in picking up an object from the floor and probably would bend the knees then squat while keeping the back straight [25].

10.1.1.3 Laboratory Workup

Laboratory tests should involve a complete blood count (CBC) with differential white blood cell count, erythrocyte sedimentation rate (ESR), C-reactive protein (CRP) level, and blood cultures in febrile states. Typically, white blood cell count is in the high normal range and a left shift with mild leukocytosis. ESR is elevated in almost all patients. CRP levels are elevated as well and can be used in monitoring the disease's progress. Finally, purified protein derivative (PPD) skin tests should be obtained if tuberculosis is suspected [9, 18, 45, 74].

10.1.1.4 Imaging Studies

Radiographs may demonstrate a loss of lumbar lordosis, observed as a narrowing of the disc space with variable degrees of destruction of adjacent vertebral end plates after 2–3 weeks. Scalloping of the superior and inferior vertebral bodies is seen in long-standing cases. A vertebra magna resulting in a canal narrowing and a block vertebra due to spontaneous disc space fusion may be seen when the infection clears up [33, 50, 83].

Technetium 99m-labeled bone scans may be helpful in suspicious cases without radiological changes especially at the beginning phase of the disease. This technique, although difficult with physical examination in younger children, can help isolate the specific motion segment involved. Scintigraphic changes may appear at the onset of the disease, such as 3–5 days after clinical symptoms appear. Thus, scintigraphy may precede the radiological changes and can aid in an early diagnosis [18, 51].

Additionally, computed tomography (CT) may show bony end plate erosion, which is not overly necessary for the diagnosis. Magnetic resonance imaging (MRI), however, is more helpful for visualization of the soft tissue and more sensitive than bone scans and CT in diagnosis of the discitis. In this way, MRI may help in differentiating discitis from vertebral osteomyelitis. Although MRI is the most sensitive imaging technique, it rarely alters the treatment modality. It is mostly helpful in symptomatic patients with no plain radiographic or nuclear imaging abnormality or who do not improve following intravenous parenteral antibiotic treatment of 2–3 days. Surgical intervention for large soft tissue abscesses, bone destruction, or neural element involvement may be indicated after an MRI examination. It also aids in differential diagnoses for patients with sagittal or coronal deformity as observed on plain radiographs [1, 19, 23, 29, 38, 57, 63, 83, 85].

Differential diagnosis involves both infectious and noninfectious conditions. Scheuermann's kyphosis is a noninfectious condition with back pain that is mostly seen among adolescents. Plain radiography reveals end plate irregularity, wedging of the vertebrae, and the presence of Schmorl's nodules in lumbar spine involvement. Metastatic tumors and leukemia involves vertebral bodies whereby mainly multilevel involvement is seen. Furthermore, eosinophilic granuloma leads to vertebra plana as observed on radiographs. Osteoid osteomas and osteoblastomas commonly involve the posterior elements of the vertebrae [25].

Additionally, differential diagnosis for infectious conditions may be septic arthritis of the hip or sacroiliac joint. Untreated discitis may lead to pyogenic vertebral osteomyelitis, which in turn leads to vertebral body collapse. Acutely ill-looking patients with neurological signs and meningeal irritations may have paraspinal or epidural abscesses [25].

10.1.1.5 Biopsy

Positive cultures in discitis are reported to be as low as 37%, which is probably due to inadequate sampling or culturing techniques such as previous antimicrobial treatments or adequate host responses that neutralize the pathogen. Moreover, biopsy requires anesthesia and may have potential morbidities. Hence, it is not recommended as a routine. *Staphylococcus aureus* is the most commonly isolated pathogen. CT-guided biopsy may yield better results but should be kept for cases unresponsive to empirical intravenous antibiotic treatment. If the specimen is not diagnostic, open biopsy may be necessary to rule out neoplasm, fungal infection, tuberculosis, brucellosis, and nonstaphylococcal pyogenic infections [8, 12, 32, 74].

10.1.1.6 Management

Bed rest or immobilization with orthosis is almost universally recommended. Even though a debate in antibiotic treatment exists, hospitalization duration and recurrence is shown to be lower with antibiotic therapy. Antibiotic treatment also provides a rapid resolution of symptoms. Specifically, oral antibiotic treatment may be successful in treating discitis. Even so, the more favorable results are obtained with a combined 1–2 week parenteral treatment following 4–6 weeks of an oral regime. Concurrent immobilization with antibiotic therapy typically improves the comfort of the patient. An empiric coverage directed to *S aureus* is successful in most of the cases; if not, biopsy is recommended to determine the pathogen and corresponding antibiogram [7, 27, 44, 54, 81].

Systemically, ill patients with documented abscesses or an evolving neurological deficit may need surgical debridement, which is a rarely considered course of action. Patients should be followed up clinically and radiologically for 12–18 months. C-reactive protein and ESR are helpful in monitoring the treatment.

10.1.2 Vertebral Osteomyelitis

Vertebral osteomyelitis in childhood is rare when compared to discitis. Older children are more susceptible to vertebral osteomyelitis than younger children. The mean age of patients with vertebral osteomyelitis is 6–9 years. These patients tend to look more systemically ill compared to discitis patients. Also, management is more in favor of invasive procedures [22, 26].

10.1.2.1 Pathophysiology

Vertebral osteomyelitis is thought to occur when microorganisms lodge in the low-flow, end-organ vasculature adjacent to the subchondral plate region. Recently, some cases of vertebral osteomyelitis in adults have been associated with intravenous drug use. Additionally, the association with urinary tract infections is well known. These associated risk factors, however, have not been noted in pediatric patients [22, 25, 27].

10.1.2.2 History and Physical Examination

Vertebral osteomyelitis is a rare condition and accounts for 1–2% of all children with osteomyelitis. It typically occurs in older children in the lumbar, thoracic, or cervical regions [15]. Children with a history of fever, limping, back pain, or a refusal to walk, in addition to positive laboratory findings should be considered to have the disease even though these symptoms are considered to be nonspecific.

Characteristically, children with discitis have low-grade fever and less severe symptoms. In contrast, children with vertebral osteomyelitis are more likely to be febrile and ill-appearing at the time of presentation of the symptoms than those with discitis. Initial radiographs of the spine, if abnormal, may help distinguish between the two entities, but because these findings often appear late in the course of the disease, additional studies are required to establish a diagnosis. Series describing discitis and vertebral osteomyelitis report a biphasic age distribution. Discitis has a higher incidence early in childhood and a second peak during adolescence. Vertebral osteomyelitis, in contrast, has a peak during adolescence and another peak in patients older than 50 years of age. More specifically, vertebral osteomyelitis is rarely seen among young children (before 3 years of age), while discitis is uncommon in children 8 or more years of age. Children with intermediate ages may have either of these spinal infections, and they should be carefully evaluated [25].

Antecedent trauma has been associated with vertebral osteomyelitis, as well as discitis, but this association was not found among the majority of the patients [25, 27].

10.1.2.3 Laboratory Workup

Laboratory studies, such as CBC, ESR, and CRP provide nonspecific information. Blood cultures and more invasive procedures, including biopsy, should be strongly considered in patients with suspected vertebral osteomyelitis, where the definition of a causal agent is particularly important in selection of the appropriate antimicrobial therapy and in defining the duration of therapy. *S. aureus* is the most common organism isolated both from discitis and osteomyelitis patients. Vertebral osteomyelitis, although infrequently encountered, can be an atypical manifestation of *B henselae* infection. The availability of specific serologic assays allowed the confirmation of this cat scratch disease organism. In patients with cat exposure, this cause should be considered, and serologic testing should be performed [15, 31].

10.1.2.4 Imaging Studies

Radiographs demonstrate localized rarefaction of a vertebral body at the beginning of the disease, and later, destruction of bone (primarily the anterior portion), and lastly the occurrence of osteophytic bridging. Early in the course of the disease, differentiating between discitis and vertebral osteomyelitis is often difficult. Nuclear bone scans, CT scans, and laboratory studies typically provide nonspecific data, and appropriate patient management demands experience by the physician. The widely available MRI technique can both uncover the anatomic spectrum of these spinal infections and also provide sufficient detail to guide the need for invasive diagnostic procedures [19, 27, 65].

Before the advent of more sensitive imaging techniques, the routine radiograph was considered to be the definitive study in establishing a specific diagnosis of discitis. In one series, initial radiographs were abnormal in 76% of children with discitis, but in only 46% of those with vertebral osteomyelitis. Radiographic changes sometimes are evident only late in the disease process making this diagnostic method less reliable early in the illness. Spine radiographs should be obtained in all children with suspected spinal infection; if these demonstrate characteristic findings of discitis or vertebral osteomyelitis, the diagnosis is established. Gallium and technetium 99-m bone scans have been used in the past, but the pattern of uptake is nonspecific and no study can reliably differentiate between discitis and vertebral osteomyelitis. The CT scan also may not be useful in providing a specific diagnosis. MRI has been shown to have a sensitivity of 96% and a specificity of 93% for the diagnosis of vertebral osteomyelitis, making it more sensitive and specific than nuclear bone scans or routine radiographs. MRI is a fast, accurate, and noninvasive method that can distinguish discitis from pyogenic bone involvement (i.e., osteomyleitis), and it also provides information about involvement of surrounding tissue (e.g., abscesses). It has been widely accepted to be the imaging study of choice to evaluate children with possible vertebral osteomyelitis. According to Donovan et al. [21], the optimal MRI technique for evaluation of spinal infection is thin-section surface coil imaging with T1-weighted images in sagittal and axial views, and sagittal T2-weighted images. Edema and pus in the marrow or disc space will appear dark on T1-weighted images and bright on T2-weighted images. A contrast-enhanced MRI should be considered for doubtful results [1, 21, 28, 49, 55, 58, 75, 76].

10.1.2.5 Management

Isolation of the pathogen is vital in planning a management strategy for vertebral osteomyelitis. Hence, percutaneous or open biopsies may be needed. When the organism is determined, an appropriate antibiotic regimen is necessary. Clinical and radiological progression of the disease in spite of antibiotic therapy may necessitate a surgical intervention. Abscess formation is another indication for surgical debridment. Following the debridment, potential instability is assessed and if present, instrumentation and fusion is necessary for stabilization. External stabilization with an orthosis or a cast reduces the pain, and thus may be added to antibiotic therapy [27, 43].

10.1.3 Tuberculosis of the Spine

Tuberculosis is a slowly progressing infection, thus the clinical picture is completely different than the nonspecific infections of the spine. The spine is the most commonly involved osseous site accounting for 5–15% of all patients with tuberculosis. Lower thoracic and lumbar regions are more frequently involved, whereas the cervical region is rarely involved [36, 48]. The causative factor, *Mycobacterium tuberculosis* bacillus is believed to be as old as *Homo sapiens* and the disease has been recognized since 3500 BC. Percivall Pott described tuberculosis spondylitis along with palsy in 1779, which is now known as Pott's disease. This old phenomenon is still challenging to manage for both in terms of surgery and medical treatment. Fortunately, antituberculosis chemotherapy has brought a breakthrough in the management of the disease. Before the antituberculosis chemotherapy era, surgical management of any tuberculosis deformity of the spine had nearly a 50% mortality rate. Drug treatments brought both a safe control of the disease and less need for an operation together with diminished mortality [47, 87].

10.1.3.1 Pathophysiology

Tuberculosis is most commonly identified as being in the form of primary pulmonary. Extrapulmonary spread is primarily seen in childhood tuberculosis with the most common site being the spine in the osseous form of extrapulmonary tuberculosis. If T cell-dependent cellular immunity is not able to overcome the bacilli, hematogenic spread of the bacilli from the primary pulmonary focus to the vertebral body yields the settlement of the disease at the bone. The slowly progressing disease is then transferred to the disc space and subsequently to the subligamentous space of both the anterior and posterior sites. If left untreated, paraspinal abscess formation will occur concurrently with the bony destruction that leads to kyphotic deformity [6, 61].

10.1.3.2 History and Physical Examination

Children with spinal tuberculosis have mild vertebral osteomyelitis symptoms with slow progression. Kyphotic deformity becomes prominent as the collapse of the vertebral body takes place. Additionally, subligamentous spread of the infection yields multilevel involvement and paraspinal abscesses, which may cause adjacent organ symptoms correlated with the size and localization of the abscess(es). Spinal tuberculosis is predominantly seen at lower thoracic and lumbar regions. In 90% of the cases, the anterior region of the vertebral body is involved whereby kyphosis results from the buckling collapse of the vertebral bodies [67, 69].

10.1.3.3 Laboratory Workup

Laboratory workup is the same as done for the specific vertebral osteomyelitis. PPD is also useful. It should be kept in mind that anergic patients may have a false negative response, while immunized patients may have a false positive response to PPD test. Isolation of the bacilli in specific cultures is a long and tedious process and positive cultures can be obtained in 50% of patients. Demonstration of caseification necrosis at the biopsy specimens can help diagnose tuberculosis infection and is a faster diagnostic tool than positive cultures. PCR is another diagnostic tool with a sensitivity of 95% and specificity of 83% [6].

10.1.3.4 Imaging Studies

Vertebral end plate irregularity, sclerosis, and diminished disc space are the common radiological findings associated with spinal tuberculosis. Ongoing bony deterioration eventually causes a kyphotic deformity. Plain radiography is very helpful in evaluating bony changes, but CT and MRI studies provide more valuable information about the disc, longitudinal ligaments, and the presence of an abscess. Andronikou et al. [3] reported 98% paraspinal abscess existence and 68% subligamentous extension along with the spinal tuberculosis. Overall, MRI is the most helpful diagnostic tool in monitoring spinal tuberculosis and the treatment. It may also help in differentiation between tuberculous and pyogenic spondylitis. Rim enhancement of abscess on MRI, a well-defined paraspinal abnormal signal, a thin and smooth abcess wall, subligamentous spread to three or more vertebral levels and multiple vertebral or entire body involvement were shown to be more suggestive of tubercuolus spondylitis than pyogenic spondylitis [42].

10.1.3.5 Management

Antituberculosis drug therapy has been shown to be the mainstay of management by several studies of Medical Research Council. Early diagnosis and effective antituberculosis chemotherapy makes the process a well-controlled medical disease. Surgical treatment should be considered as an adjuvant to effective drug therapy. Surgical management may be necessary for patients with neurological involvement, large abscesses, and with deformity and instability [67].

Anterior debridement and fusion (Hong Kong operation) with a strut graft of rib inserted into the endplates of the vertebra above and below has been the standard surgical approach for tuberculosis. Satisfactory results have been reported for patients with single level disease, minimum destruction of vertebral bodies, limited surgical excision of bone, and for lesions not exceeding more than two disc levels. However, use of rib grafts has resulted with a high rate of failure for patients with a marked intraoperative correction of deformity especially at the lumbar spine [68]. The studies demonstrating that tuberculosis bacilli is less adhesive to stainless steel implants have opened a new era in the surgical treatment of tuberculosis [34, 62]. This study enabled surgeons to stabilize the spine and correct the deformities safely by the aid of metallic instrumentations and satisfactory results have been reported by combined anterior debridement and posterior instrumentation and posterior drainage of abscess in addition to posterior instrumentation [86, 88]. Currently, anterior debridement with anterior strut long bone allografts or titanium mesh grafts and stabilization by anterior instrumentation is the popular procedure with many satisfactory results reported in the literature [4, 59, 66].

Spinal tuberculosis is the most common cause of kyphotic deformity in childhood especially in underdeveloped countries. This is a consequence of children being more prone to deterioration of the deformity compared to adults [68]. Fifteen percent of spinal tuberculosis patients who are treated conservatively develop kyphosis, of which 3–5% have more than 60° of deformity. Untreated spinal tuberculosis may end up with an increasing deformity and neurological deficit [67].

A severe kyphotic deformity leads to secondary cardiopulmonary problems and a late onset of neurological deteriorations as well. Prevention of the deformity is much more important than the surgical treatment. Children 10 years of age or less are more susceptible to experiencing progressive deformity with the disease. The natural history of spinal deformity associated spinal tuberculosis is not clear. Rajasekaran [66] reported 61 spinal tuberculosis pediatric patients that were treated with ambulatory antituberculosis chemotherapy and followed for 15 years. Three types of deformity dynamics (worsening, improvement, and staying constant), a scoring system, and spine at risk signs were all defined. Radiological risk signs were as follows: facet joint separation, posterior retropulsion of the diseased segment, lateral translation of the vertebral column, and indication of toppling. Each of these was scored with a point value of one, if present, which can ultimately reveal a maximum instability score of four. Rajasekaran [67, 68] also defined the biomechanics of the progressive deformity "buckling of the spine." Furthermore, it was reported that patients younger than 7 years of age at the time of disease having thoracolumbar involvement, destruction of more than two vertebral bodies, and an instability score of greater than 2 are indicative of potential buckling and consequently in need of surgical intervention [68].

Management of an established deformity is more complicated than preventive surgery with debridment. More difficult interventions such as posterior osteotomies and staged or simultaneous anterior and posterior procedures may be necessary for correction of late kyphotic deformities (Fig. 10.1)

10.1.4.1 Other Pathogens Involved in Spondylodiscitis

Brucella, *Cryptococcus*, and *Aspergillus* species are rare pathogens reported in pediatric age group spinal infections. Brucella infections have step like vertebral body erosions on the plain radiograph with elevated brucella titers (>1/80). Fungal infections are mostly seen in immune compromised patients [25]. Parasitic infections are reported as cases in the literature and are cyst hydatid manifestations [2, 77].

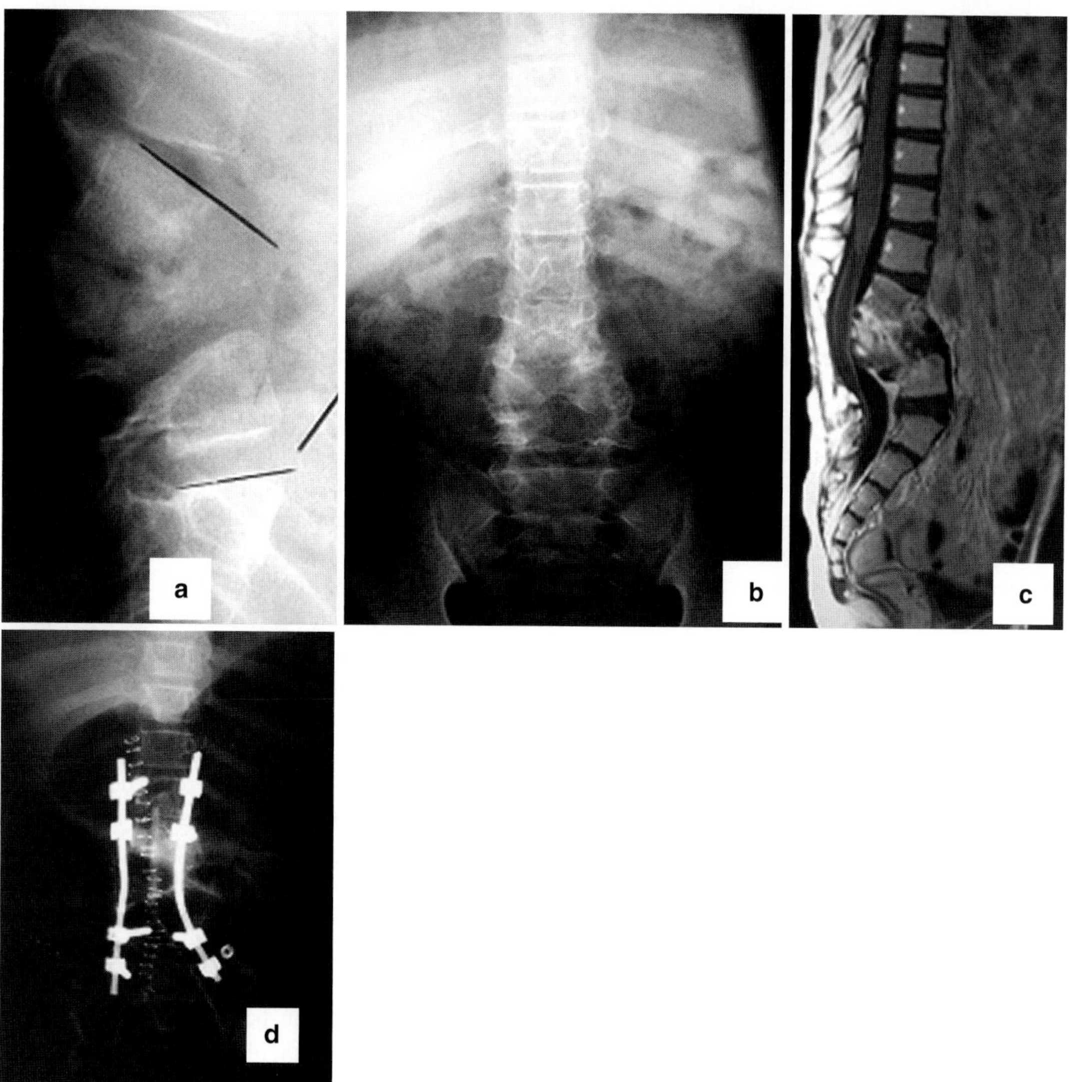

Fig. 10.1 Management of Tuberculosis Spondylitis in a 14 year old male. Preoperative plain radiographs (**a**, **b**) and MRI (**c**) reveal marked spondylodiscitis resulting in kyphotic deformity. Early postoperative (**d**, **e**) and 1 year follow-up (**f**, **g**) radiographs following combined anterior debridement with fibula strut grafting and posterior instrumentation fusion surgery

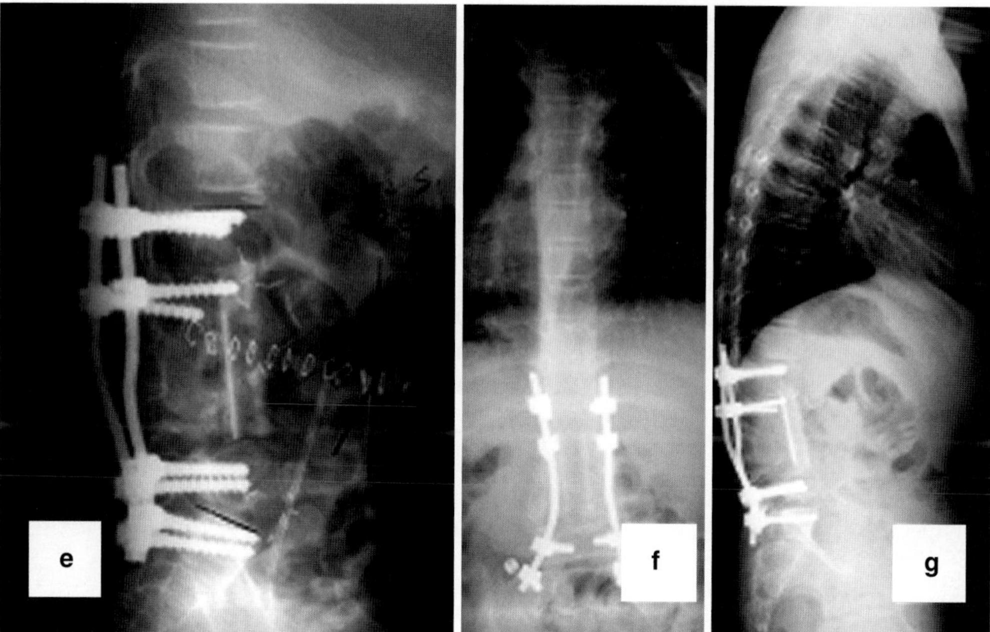

Fig. 10.1 (continued)

10.1.5 Postoperative Infections

Superficial and deep wound infection is not uncommon following pediatric spinal surgery especially when the spinal instrumentation is used. Reported infection rates following pediatric spinal deformity surgery vary between 0.4 and 8.7%. Postoperative infections may cause devastating results causing severe morbidity. Prevention seems to be the most important factor to avoid this unpleasant complication.

10.1.5.1 Pathophysiology

Postoperative wound infections can occur either early or late. Definition of early and late infection is controversial in the literature as there is no consensus on how late an infection should be accepted as early infection. Nevertheless, infections diagnosed from 0 to 12–24 weeks following the index spinal procedure has been widely accepted to be early infections. *S. aureus*, *Staphylococcus epidermidis*, *Propionibacter* sp., and *Enterococcus* sp. are the most commonly isolated microorganisms from infected wounds following spinal surgery. Less virulent microorganisms such as *S. epidermidis* and *Propionibacter* sp. are usually isolated from patients with late infections [13, 72, 73]. The infection rate seems to be higher after posterior surgeries than anterior ones [14].

Immunological problems and poor skin conditions may provoke postoperative infection. Infection following surgery for neuromuscular deformities seems to be more common compared to idiopathic scoliosis, whereas Hahn [35] and Ho et al. [39] found similar infection rates among different etiology of spinal deformities. Ho et al. [40] reported the risk factors for late infections following posterior surgery as, significant medical history, delayed surgical time, distal fusion levels, transfusion need, and wound drainage.

Implants, allogenic grafts, and dead spaces are potential infection sites. Sponseller et al. [82] and McCarthy et al. [52] have suggested that the use of allograft in neuromuscular patients may cause an increased risk of infection, while some have not found use of allograft to carry an increased infection rate in spinal fusion [32]. Moreover, Ho et al. did not find a significant association between use of allograft and eradication of infection [40].

Microorganisms capable of forming biofilm can colonize on the foreign bodies like implants and the allografts. When host immune mechanism is overcome by the pathogen, infection becomes evident [39]. Although there is a belief that titanium implants are less prone for bacteria adhesion, a recent study has shown that *S. epidermidis* can form biofilm on both the titanium and stainless implants. In fact, the number of colonizing units was higher on titanium implants than the stainless steel [34].

10.1.5.2 Clinical Diagnosis and Laboratory Workup

Pain, wound drainage, fever, and fluctuation following a spinal surgery indicate a possible underlying infection. Late onset pain following spinal surgery should be considered as a late infection unless the opposite is proven. High levels of white blood cell count, ESR, and CRP are indicative of infection if the clinical findings are supportive of the diagnosis [39]. Procalcitonin is another laboratory parameter defined as an early phase reactant and is being used in diagnosis and osteomyelitis and septic arthritis [10, 71]. Procalcitonin is elevated early following infection and declined to the normal as soon as the infection settles down. Thus, it is a useful parameter for monitoring the postoperative infections and can be used for spinal infection monitoring as well.

10.1.5.3 Imaging Studies

Conventional radiograms may not be helpful for early postoperative infections. However, radiolucencies around the pedicle screws may indicate an infection at the later stages. Late infections can be concomitant with pseudoarthrosis. Loss of correction or implant failure as observed on plain radiographs and fusion defects shown on CT sections are both indicative of pseudoarthorsis, which may accompany infection. MRI is the most helpful diagnostic tool for infections following a spinal surgery, if implants used are made of titanium. MRI may not be helpful in the case of stainless steel implants, which may cause image distortions. Bone scan, ultrasonography, and fistulograms can be utilized when MRI is not available.

10.1.5.4 Management and Prevention

Both early and late spinal infections following spinal surgery mostly require surgical intervention. It is evident that deep wound infections increase the chance of poor outcome when not treated properly. Therefore, it is of utmost importance to have a very aggressive approach to wound drainage and contaminated hematoma early after the index operation. Irrigation and debridment should not be delayed if infection is highly suspected. An overdiagnosis may even be better than to undertreat early infection that may result with chronic pyogenic spinal infection. Additionally, removal of implants, bone grafts, and substitutes may often be necessary to eradicate the infection. Many authors have found that the retention of implants resulted with recurrent infection up to 50% of patients who had a treatment for postoperative infection and they recommended removal of implants to completely eradicate the infection [39, 82]. However, a shortcoming of early implant removal is the eventual increase in deformity as the fusion has not occurred yet. On the other hand, it is not always possible to tell when a fusion is solid and thick enough, and removal of the implants even years after surgery has been shown to result with progressive spinal deformity [39, 60, 64, 71]. Therefore, the removal of spinal implants to eradicate infection must be weighed against the significant chance of progressive spinal deformity after implant removal. One approach to this difficult situation may be long-term suppression of the infection with antibiotics, followed by removal of spinal implants once the fusion is solid if the infection remains persistent. Several treatment options for the salvage of implants such as multiple I&D and primary closure of the wound [39], leaving the wound open [5, 82, 84], continuous antibiotic solution irrigation [80], and muscle flaps for soft tissue coverage [24, 56] have been reported with successful results. Recently, vacuum-assisted closure (VAC) has been shown to be an effective alternative method, enabling retention of implant and eradication of infection for many orthopaedic procedures. There are few reports with successful results for postoperative infections after spinal surgery in adult patients [41, 53, 90]. van Rhee et al. [89] reported their results utilizing VAC combined with antibiotic therapy in postoperative spinal infections of neuromuscular scoliosis patients. Wound coverage averaged 3 months and implant removal was not needed in any patients.

In summary, high suspicion of infection and early surgical debridement and irrigation of wound in addition to systemic antibiotic treatment sensitive to the isolated micrororganism(s) are the mainstays of treatment for early postoperative infection. Every effort should be given to retain the stable implants to prevent pseudoarthrosis and deterioration of the deformity. VAC treatment seems to be a promising method for effective management with retention of implants after infections which cannot be controlled by multiple I&D's and antibiotic treatment. I&D and antibiotic treatment is also the procedure of choice for late infections. Removal of implants is a controversial issue for late infections as it is not always possible to judge the solidity and thickness of the fusion mass and there are studies reporting high rate of pseudoarthrosis and deterioration of deformities [64, 71]. Therefore, close follow-up of patients and reinstrumentation after eradication of infection is mandatory, if there are any signs of pseudoarthrosis or progression of deformity after implant removal.

Prevention of infection has utmost importance and starts with precise preoperative evaluation including assessment of comorbidities, diagnosis and treatment of urinary infection, and providing nutritional supplementation for malnourished patients [46]. Preoperative antibiotic prophylaxis is an important measure and first generation cephalosporins should be given during the induction of anesthesia and should be continued no more than 48 h. Recently, Ho et al. [39] suggested to use vancomycin and ceftazadine rather than cefazolin, to cover *S. epidermidis* and other organisms. Pulsatile lavage of the wound before closure is thought to be effective in infection prophylaxis. In a prospective, randomized study, Cheng et al. [11] found that irrigation of the spinal wound with dilute betadine solution completely prevented infection in a group of patients. Use of subcutaneous drains should also be considered to prevent hematoma formation, although there is controversy on its efficacy in preventing postoperative infection [20, 37].

References

1. Adatepe MH, Powell OM, Isaacs GH (1986) Hematogenous pyogenic vertebral osteomyelitis: diagnostic value of radionuclide bone imaging. J Nucl Med 27:1680–1685
2. Akhaddar A, Gourinda H, el Alami Z et al (1999) Hydatid cyst of the sacrum. Report of a case. Rev Rhum Engl Ed 66(5):289–291
3. Andronikou S, Jadwat S, Douis H (2002) Patterns of disease on MRI in 53 children with tuberculous spondylitis and the role of gadolinium Pediatr Radiol 32:798–805
4. Bailey HL, Gabriel M, Hodgson AR et al (1972) Tuberculosis of the spine in children: operative findings and results in one hundred consecutive patients treated by removal of the lesion and anterior grafting. J Bone Joint Surg 54A: 1633–1657
5. Banta JV (1990) Combined anterior and posterior fusion for spinal deformity in myelomeningocele. Spine 15:946–952
6. Berk RH, Yazici M, Atabey N et al (1996) Detection of *Mycobacterium tuberculosis* in formaldehyde solution-fixed, paraffin-embedded tissue by polymerase chain reaction in Pott's disease. Spine 21:1991–1995
7. Boston HC Jr, Bianco AJ Jr, Rhodes KH (1975) Disk space infections in children. Orthop Clin North Am 6:953–964
8. Brook I (2001) Two cases of discitis attributable to anaerobic bacteria in children. Pediatrics 107:E26
9. Brown R, Hussain M, McHugh K et al (2001) Discitis in young children. J Bone Joint Surg Br 83:106–111
10. Butbul-Aviel Y, Koren A, Halevy R et al (2005) Procalcitonin as a diagnostic aid in osteomyelitis and septic arthritis. Pediatr Emerg Care 21(12):828–832
11. Cheng MT, Chang MC, Wang ST et al (2005) Efficacy of dilute betadine solution irrigation in the prevention of postoperative infection of spinal surgery. Spine 30:1689–1693
12. Chew FS, Kline MJ (2001) Diagnostic yield of CT-guided percutaneous aspiration procedures in suspected spontaneous infectious discitis. Radiology 218:211–214
13. Clark CE, Shufflebarger HL (1999) Late-developing infection in instrumented idiopathic scoliosis. Spine 24: 1909–1912
14. Collins I, Wilson-MacDonald J, Chami G et al (2008) The diagnosis and management of infection following instrumented spinal fusion. Eur Spine J 17: 445–450. doi:10.1007/s00586-007-0559-8
15. Correa AG, Edwards MS, Baker CJ (1993) Vertebral osteomyelitis in children. Pediatr Infect Dis J 12:228–233
16. Coventry MB, Ghormley RK, Kernohan JW (1945) The intervertebral disc: its microscopic anatomy and pathology: I. Anatomy, development, and physiology. J Bone Joint Surg 27:105–112
17. Crawford AH, Kucharzyk DW, Ruda R, Smitherman HC Jr (1991) Discitis in children. Clin Orthop 266:70–79
18. Cushing AH (1993) Discitis in children. Clin Infect Dis 17:1–6
19. Dagirmanjian A, Schils J, McHenry M (1996) MR imaging of vertebral osteomyelitis revisited. AJR Am J Roentgenol 167:1539–1543
20. Diab MA, Erickson MA, Dormans JP et al (2007) Use and outcome of wound drain in children undergoing operation for idiopathic scoliosis. In: 42nd Annual Meeting of Scoliosis Research Society, Edinburgh, Scotland
21. Donovan Post MJ, Bowen BC, Sze G (1991) Magnetic resonance imaging of spinal infection. Rheum Dis Clin North Am 17:773–794
22. Dormans JP, Moroz L (2007) Infection and tumors of the spine in children. J Bone Joint Surg Am 89:79–97
23. Du Lac P, Panuel M, Devred P et al (1990) MRI of disc space infection in infants and children: report of 12 cases. Pediatr Radiol 20:175–178
24. Dumanian GA, Ondra SL, Liu J et al (2003) Muscle flap salvage of spine wounds with soft tissue defects or infection. Spine 28(11):1203–1211

25. Early SD, Kay RM, Tolo VT (2003) Childhood discitis. J Am Acad Orthop Surg 11:413–420
26. Eismont FJ, Bohlman HH, Soni PL et al (1982) Vertebral osteomyelitis in infants. J Bone Joint Surg Br 64:32–35
27. Fernandez M, Carrol CL, Baker CJ (2000) Discitis and vertebral osteomyelitis in children: an 18-year review. Pediatrics 105:1299–1304
28. Fisher GW, Popich GA, Sullivan DE et al (1978) Discitis: a prospective diagnostic analysis. Pediatrics 62:543–548
29. Gabriel KR, Crawford AH (1988) Magnetic resonance imaging in a child who had clinical signs of discitis: report of a case. J Bone Joint Surg Am 70:938–941
30. Galil A, Gorodischer R, Bar-Ziv J et al (1982) Intervertebral disc infection (discitis) in childhood. Eur J Pediatr 139: 66–70
31. Garron E, Viehweger E, Launay F (2002) Nontuberculous spondylodiscitis in children. J Pediatr Orthop 22:321–328
32. Glazer PA, Hu SS (1996) Pediatric spinal infections. Orthop Clin North Am 27:111–123
33. Grünebaum M, Horodniceanu C, Mukamel M et al (1982) The imaging diagnosis of nonpyogenic discitis in children. Pediatr Radiol 12:133–137
34. Ha KY, Chung YG, Ryoo SJ (2005) Adherence and biofilm formation of *Staphylococcus epidermidis* and *Mycobacterium tuberculosis* on various spinal implants. Spine 30(1):38–43
35. Hahn F, Zbinden R, Min K (2005) Late implant infections caused by *Propionibacterium acnes* in scoliosis surgery. Eur Spine J 14:783–788
36. Harisinghani MG, McLoud TC, Shepard JO et al (2000) Tuberculosis from head to toe. Radiographics 20:449–470
37. Hasley BP, McClung A, Sucato DJ (2007) Closed suction drainage following posterior spinal fusion for adolescent idiopathic scoliosis: is it necessary? In: 42nd Annual Meeting of Scoliosis Research Society, Edinburgh, Scotland
38. Heller RM, Szalay EA, Green NE et al (1988) Disc space infection in children: magnetic resonance imaging. Radiol Clin North Am 26:207–209
39. Ho C, Skaggs DL, Weiss JM et al (2007) Management of infection after instrumented posterior spine fusion in pediatric scoliosis. Spine 32:2739–2744
40. Ho C, Sucato DJ, Richards BS (2007) Risk factors for the development of delayed infections following posterior spinal fusion and instrumentation in adolescent idiopathic scoliosis patients. Spine 32:2272–2277
41. Jones GA, Butler J, Lieberman I et al (2007) Negative-pressure wound therapy in the treatment of complex postoperative spinal wound infections: complications and lessons learned using vacuum-assisted closure. J Neurosurg Spine 6(5):407–411
42. Jung NY, Jee WH, Ha KY et al (2004) Discrimination of tuberculous spondylitis from pyogenic spondylitis on MRI. AJR Am J Roentgenol 182(6):1405–1410
43. Kayser R, Mahlfeld K, Greulich M et al (2005) Spondylodiscitis in childhood: results of a long-term study. Spine 30(3):318–323
44. Kemp HBS, Jackson JW, Jeremiah JD et al (1973) Pyogenic infections occurring primarily in intervertebral discs. J Bone Joint Surg Br 55:698–714
45. King HA (1999) Back pain in children. Orthop Clin North Am 30:467–474
46. Klein JD, Hey LA, Yu CS et al (1996) Perioperative nutrition and postoperative complications in patients undergoing spinal surgery. Spine 21:2676–2682
47. Lichtor J, Lichtor A (1957) Paleopathological evidence suggesting pre-Columbian tuberculosis of spine. J Bone Joint Surg Am 39:1938–1939
48. Loke TK, Ma HT, Chan CS (1997) MRI of tuberculous spinal infection. Australas Radiol 41:7–12
49. Magera BE, Klein SG, Derrick CW Jr et al (1989) Radiological cases of the month. Am J Dis Child 143: 1479–1480
50. Mahboubi S, Morris MC (2001) Imaging of spinal infections in children. Radiol Clin North Am 39:215–222
51. Maliner LI, Johnson DL (1997) Intervertebral disc space inflammation in children. Childs Nerv Syst 13:101–104
52. McCarthy RE, Peek RD, Morrisy RT et al (1986) Allograft bone in spinal fusion for paralytic scoliosis. J Bone Joint Surg Am 68:370–375
53. Mehbod AA, Ogilvie JW, Pinto MR et al (2005) Postoperative deep wound infections in adults after spinal fusion: management with vacuum-assisted wound closure. J Spinal Disord Tech 18(1):14–17
54. Menelaus MB (1964) Discitis: an inflammation affecting the intervertebral discs in children. J Bone Joint Surg Br 46:16–23
55. Miller GM, Forbes GS, Onofrio BM (1989) Magnetic resonance imaging of the spine. Mayo Clin Proc 64:986–1004
56. Mitra A, Mitra A, Harlin S (2004) Treatment of massive thoracolumbar wounds and vertebral osteomyelitis following scoliosis surgery. Plast Reconstr Surg 113:206–213
57. Modic MT, Pavlicek W, Weinstein MA et al (1984) Magnetic resonance imaging of intervertebral disk disease: clinical and pulse sequence considerations. Radiology 152:103–111
58. Modic MT, Feiglin DH, Piraino DW et al (1985) Vertebral osteomyelitis: assessment using MR. Radiology 157:157–166
59. Moon MS, Woo YK, Lee KS et al (1995) Posterior instrumentation and anterior interbody fusion for tuberculous kyphosis of dorsal and lumbar spines. Spine 20:1910–1916
60. Muschik M, Luck W, Schlenzka D (2004) Implant removal for late-developing infection after instrumented posterior spinal fusion for scoliosis: reinstrumentation reduces loss of correction. A retrospective analysis of 45 cases. Eur Spine J 13:645–651
61. Ng Alex WH, Chu Winnie CW, Ng Bobby KW et al (2005) Extensive paraspinal abscess complicating tuberculous spondylitis in an adolescent with Pott kyphosis. J Clin Imaging 29:359–361
62. Oga M, Arizono T, Takasita M et al (1993) Evaluation of the risk of instrumentation as a foreign body in spinal tuberculosis. Spine 18:1890–1894
63. Paushter DM, Modic MT, Masaryk TJ (1985) Magnetic resonance imaging of the spine: applications and limitations. Radiol Clin North Am 23:551–562
64. Potter BK, Kirk KL, Shah SA et al (2006) Loss of coronal correction following instrumentation removal in adolescent idiopathic scoliosis Spine 31(1):67–72
65. Pui MH, Mitha A, Rae WI et al (2005) Diffusion-weighted magnetic resonance imaging of spinal infection and malignancy. J Neuroimaging 15:164–170
66. Rajasekaran S, Soundarapandian S (1989) Progression of kyphosis in tuberculosis of the spine treated by anterior arthrodesis. J Bone Joint Surg 71A:1314–1323

67. Rajasekaran S (2001) The natural history of post-tubercular kyphosis in children radiological signs which predict late ıncrease ın deformity. J Bone Joint Surg Br 83-B:954–962
68. Rajasekaran S (2002). The problem of deformity in spinal tuberculosis. Clin Orthop Relat Res (398):85–92
69. Rajasekaran S (2007) Buckling collapse of the spine in childhood spinal tuberculosis. Clin Ortho Rel Res 460: 86–92
70. Ratcliffe JF (1985) Anatomic basis for the pathogenesis and radiologic features of vertebral osteomyelitis and its differentiation from childhood discitis: a microarteriographic investigation. Acta Radiol Diagn (Stockh) 26:137–143
71. Rathjen K, Wood M, McClung A et al (2007) Clinical and radiographic results after implant removal in idiopathic scoliosis. Spine 32:2184–2188
72. Richards BS (1995) Delayed infections following posterior spinal instrumentation for the treatment of idiopathic scoliosis. J Bone Joint Surg Am 77:524–529
73. Richards BS, Emara KM (2001) Delayed infections after posterior TSRH spinal instrumentation for idiopathic scoliosis: revisited. Spine 26:1990–1996
74. Ring D, Johnston CE II, Wenger DR (1995) Pyogenic infectious spondylitis in children: the convergence of discitis and vertebral osteomyelitis. J Pediatr Orthop 15:652–660
75. Rocco HD, Eyring EJ (1972) Intervertebral disk infections in children. Am J Dis Child 123:448–451
76. Rothman SLG (1996) The diagnosis of infections of the spine by modern imaging techniques. Orthop Clin North Am 27:15–31
77. Rumana M, Mahadevan A, Nayil Khurshid M et al (2006) Cestode parasitic infestation: intracranial and spinal hydatid disease – a clinicopathological study of 29 cases from South India. Clin Neuropathol 25(2):98–104
78. Sapico FL, Montgomerie JZ (1979) Pyogenic vertebral osteomyelitis: report of nine cases and review of the literature. Rev Infect Dis 1:754–776
79. Song KS, Ogden JA, Ganey T et al (1997) Contiguous discitis and osteomyelitis in children. J Pediatr Orthop 17:470–477
80. Soultanis K, Mantelos G, Pagiatakis A et al (2003) Late infection in patients with scoliosis treated with spinal instrumentation. Clin Orthop Relat Res 411:116–123
81. Spiegel PG, Kengla KW, Isaacson AS et al (1972) Intervertebral disc-space inflammation in children. J Bone Joint Surg Am 54:284–296
82. Sponseller PD, LaPorte DM, Hungerford MW et al (2000) Deep wound infections after neuromuscular scoliosis surgery: a multicenter study of risk factors and treatment outcomes. Spine 25:2461–2466
83. Szalay EA, Green NE, Heller RM et al (1987) Magnetic resonance imaging in the diagnosis of childhood discitis. J Pediatr Orthop 7:164–167
84. Szoke G, Lipton G, Miller F et al (1988) Wound infection after spinal fusion in children with cerebral palsy. J Pediatr Orthop 18:727–733
85. Szypryt EP, Hardy JG, Hinton CE et al (1988) A comparison between magnetic resonance imaging and scintigraphic bone imaging in the diagnosis of disc space infection in an animal model. Spine 13:1042–1048
86. Talu U, Gogus A, Ozturk C et al (2006) The role of posterior instrumentation and fusion after anterior radical debridement and fusion in the surgical treatment of spinal tuberculosis: experience of 127 cases. J Spinal Disord Tech 19(8): 554–559
87. Tuli SM (2007). Tuberculosis of the Spine A Historical Review. Clin Ortho and Rel Res 460:29–38
88. Upadhyay SS, Sail MJ, Sell P et al (1994) Spinal deformity after childhood surgery for tuberculosis of the spine a comparison of radical surgery and debridement. J Bone Joint Surg Br 76:91–98
89. van Rhee M, de Klerk L, Verhaar J (2007) Vacuum-assisted wound closure of deep infections after instrumented spinal fusion in six children with neuromuscular scoliosis Spine J 7:596–600
90. Vicario C, de Juan J, Esclarin A, Alcobendas M (2007) Treatment of deep wound infections after spinal fusion with a vacuum-assisted device in patients with spinal cord injury. Acta Orthop Belg 73(1):102–106
91. Wenger DR, Bobechko WP, Gilday DL (1978) The spectrum of intervertebral disc-space infection in children. J Bone Joint Surg 60A:100–108
92. Whalen JL, Parke WW, Mazur JM et al (1985) The intrinsic vasculature of developing vertebral end plates and its nutritive significance to the intervertebral discs. J Pediatr Orthop 5:403–410
93. Wiley AM, Trueta J (1959) The vascular anatomy of the spine and its relationship to pyogenic vertebral osteomyelitis. J Bone Joint Surg Br 41:796–809

Management of Spine Tumors in Young Children

11

R. Emre Acaroglu and H. Gokhan Demirkiran

Key Points

- Tumors are relatively rare in the pediatric spinal column but still constitute a substantial portion of pediatric spinal disorders.
- Presentation may be very unspecific with vague symptoms; a high level of suspicion is required.
- Treatment guidelines are not particularly different compared to primary tumors in appendicular skeleton, or those of adults.
- Surgery is the treatment of choice in most of the pediatric spine tumors, and should not be withheld on the basis of potential complications.

Vertebral neoplasms in the pediatric age group are uncommon and present a significant clinical challenge to the orthopaedic surgeon involved in their diagnosis and management. As most problems in this age group will present with vague symptoms, especially back pain, it should be taken seriously, and the possibility of a tumor should be evaluated in children.

R. E. Acaroglu (✉)
Ankara Spine Center, Iran Caddesi 45/2, Kavaklidere, Ankara 06700, Turkey
e-mail: acaroglue@gmail.com

11.1 Evaluation

11.1.1 Clinical Presentation

The most common symptom is pain, which has been reported to be the presenting problem in 46–83% of patients [2, 17, 32]. Persistent back pain should alert the physician for an underlying pathological process. The characterization of pain in spinal tumors may be progressive pain, predominant night pain, or unrelenting [25, 44]. Severe pain is usually associated with microfractures induced by the rapid growth of neoplasms. In most of the patients, palpation of the affected segments may induce pain.

Another relatively common finding is neurological involvement. Several studies report incidences of 54 and 67% for motor weakness and neurological involvement in pediatric patients with spinal neoplasms [17, 44]. Neurological involvement is most commonly associated with malignant and spinal cord tumors; radicular symptoms and myelopathy may arise from the involvement of neural foramina and spinal canal concordant with the level of involvement. A detailed history and physical examination is essential.

Children with spinal tumors may present with spinal deformity, especially in cases of osteoid osteoma and osteoblastoma [1, 17, 31,32, 45, 52]. It has been reported to be the presenting symptom in 27–63% of these patients [52, 60]. Other tumors such as langerhans cell histiocytosis may also cause subsequent deformity (scoliosis and kyphosis) because of destruction of the vertebral body and collapse.

B. A. Akbarnia et al. (eds.), *The Growing Spine*,
DOI: 10.1007/978-3-540-85207-0_11,

11.1.2 Imaging Studies

The evaluation of a patient with suspected spinal tumor should start with high-quality PA and lateral radiographs. In cases with stigmata that may be associated with tumors such as atypical spinal deformity, masses, bony destruction, vertebral collapse, widened interpedicular distances, erosion of pedicles ("winking owl" sign), sclerosis, enlarged neural foramina, and scalloping of vertebral bodies, advanced imaging studies must be performed. The sensitivity of plain radiographs for detection of spinal tumors varies between 55 and 98% [2, 17]. Computed tomography (CT), magnetic resonance imaging (MRI), and technetium bone scans are the most commonly used advanced imaging studies. CT is well tolerated as it is noninvasive and is usually fast and very efficient in the demonstration of bony lesions such as erosive masses, bone destruction, sclerosis with central radiolucency (nidus), periosteal reaction, and widened spinal canal. On the other hand, CT scan has disadvantages of an increased exposure to radiation as well as of not being very sensitive in the demonstration of soft tissue lesions. MRI appears to be the most sensitive of all imaging studies and should be the first choice, especially in the presence of neurological involvement. It may show the bony and soft tissue masses, bone destruction, lesions extending to or originating from surrounding soft tissues, as well as the spinal canal and neural elements. Furthermore, in patients with malignant neoplasms, MRI may be useful in the monitoring of the response to chemotherapy and/or radiotherapy. Along with gadolinium enhancement, MRI is the most sensitive and specific measure for the detection of metastatic disease. The major disadvantage of MRI happens to be the need for sedation or general anesthesia for younger children. Bone scan is very useful for patients with vague symptoms for whom the presence or location of a problem cannot be ascertained with other studies. Finally, in very rare cases with malignant neoplasms, spinal angiography helps the surgeon in the preoperative surgical planning and may facilitate surgical resection when coupled with embolization.

11.1.3 Staging

11.1.3.1 Oncological Staging

Oncological staging of tumors is aimed to define the biological behavior of primary tumors of musculoskeletal origin. The most commonly used is the Surgical Staging System (SSS) introduced by Enneking, [16] which forms the basis of staging this chapter so forth. In this staging system, benign tumors are evaluated in three stages, latent, active, and aggressive, whereas primary malignant tumors are divided into two stages of localized disease with two sub stages each and a third stage for metastatic disease. This staging was originally described for long bone tumors but proved to be applicable to the primary tumors of the spinal column as well, as demonstrated by several studies [4, 6, 9].

Benign Tumors

Benign tumors are divided into three stages as stage 1 (S1) latent tumors, stage 2 (S2) active tumors, and stage 3 (S3) aggressive tumors. Treatment principles for these tumors located in the pediatric spinal column are similar to those located in the appendicular skeleton and will not be discussed here in detail.

Malignant Tumors

Malignant tumors are studied based on the concept of "grade" and classified into two groups as low grade and high grade. These are further subdivided into two categories of A and B based on the relation of the tumor with the compartment it has originated from. Based on this, a low-grade stage IA tumor is one that remains inside the vertebra itself and by contrast, a stage IB tumor invades paravertebral compartments. High-grade tumors are likewise divided into stages IIA and IIB. Treatment is wide en bloc excision as radical excision in the spinal column is virtually impossible because of the continuous character of various spinal compartments (e.g., epidural space) and the ring shape of the vertebrae [7].

11.1.3.2 Surgical Staging

After the definitive diagnosis and oncological staging has been established, the next step before biopsy should be surgical staging. The most widely used scheme was developed by Weinstein for primary spine tumors and later modified by Boriani et al. to become the Weinstein, Boriani, Biagnini (WBB) system [63] (Fig. 11.1). The major advantage of this system is that it delineates the relation of the lesion with the spinal cord and therefore intrinsically marks out the amenability of the tumor to wide resection [7].

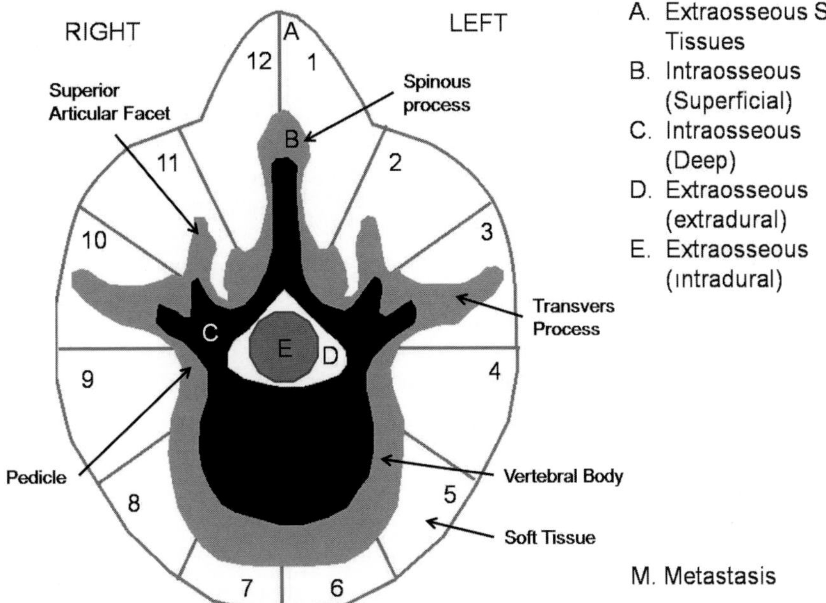

Fig. 11.1 The Weinstein, Boriani, Biagnini classification scheme for vertebral tumors. Adapted and redrawn from ref. [7]

Another classification system is proposed by Tomita et al. [62] This system is composed of a two-part numeric system and incorporates a detonation of tumor location providing a simplified scheme for describing the extent of vertebral involvement [61]. For the sake of simplicity, only the WBB system will be used in this chapter.

11.1.4 Biopsy

Biopsy is usually an essential step before planning the treatment. The most important principle in oncological surgery is to include the biopsy route within the line of incision that will be used at the time of definitive surgery. The most accessible part of the lesion should be biopsied, based on the imaging studies and specifically by the surgeon who will perform the definitive surgery. Selected biopsy tract should be suitable to perform the intervention with minimal morbidity and healthy tissue contamination. Given these principles, biopsy can be performed through percutaneous or open techniques [55]. Percutaneous needle biopsy is a relatively simple procedure and has been proven to be safe and effective when performed under image guidance [62]. On the other hand, open biopsy by definition requires an incision and may result in substantial blood loss and morbidity, but the surgeon can obtain a relatively large amount of tissue for diagnosis, decreasing the likelihood of a sampling error. Selection of the optimal biopsy technique depends on the differential diagnosis, the location and extension of the lesion, and the potential definitive treatment plan. Although there is the theoretical possibility of having intraoperative frozen sections, the authors do not recommend it on a routine basis as, in our hands, it has been associated with a substantial rate of diagnostic errors, totally unacceptable for tumor surgery in spinal column. Therefore, it should be reserved for the confirmation of the adequacy of surgical margins if necessary. Tumors of posterior elements are more easily sampled by open biopsy, whereas anterior elements of spine are more amenable to sampling with image intensifier or CT-guided needle techniques (Fig. 11.3 a–d). Care should be taken not to contaminate the thoracic or abdominal cavities regardless of the technique. It has to be kept in mind that failure of the excision of the biopsy route can increase the risk of recurrence. For this reason, the optimal technique so as to reduce the spread of tumor cells for an anteriorly located lesion appears to be a transpedicular image-guided trocar biopsy and filling the empty pedicle with acrylic cement [7].

11.2 Surgical Treatment of Spinal Tumors

The goals of the surgery for pediatric spinal tumors are as follows:

1. Relief of pain
2. Decompression of neural structures

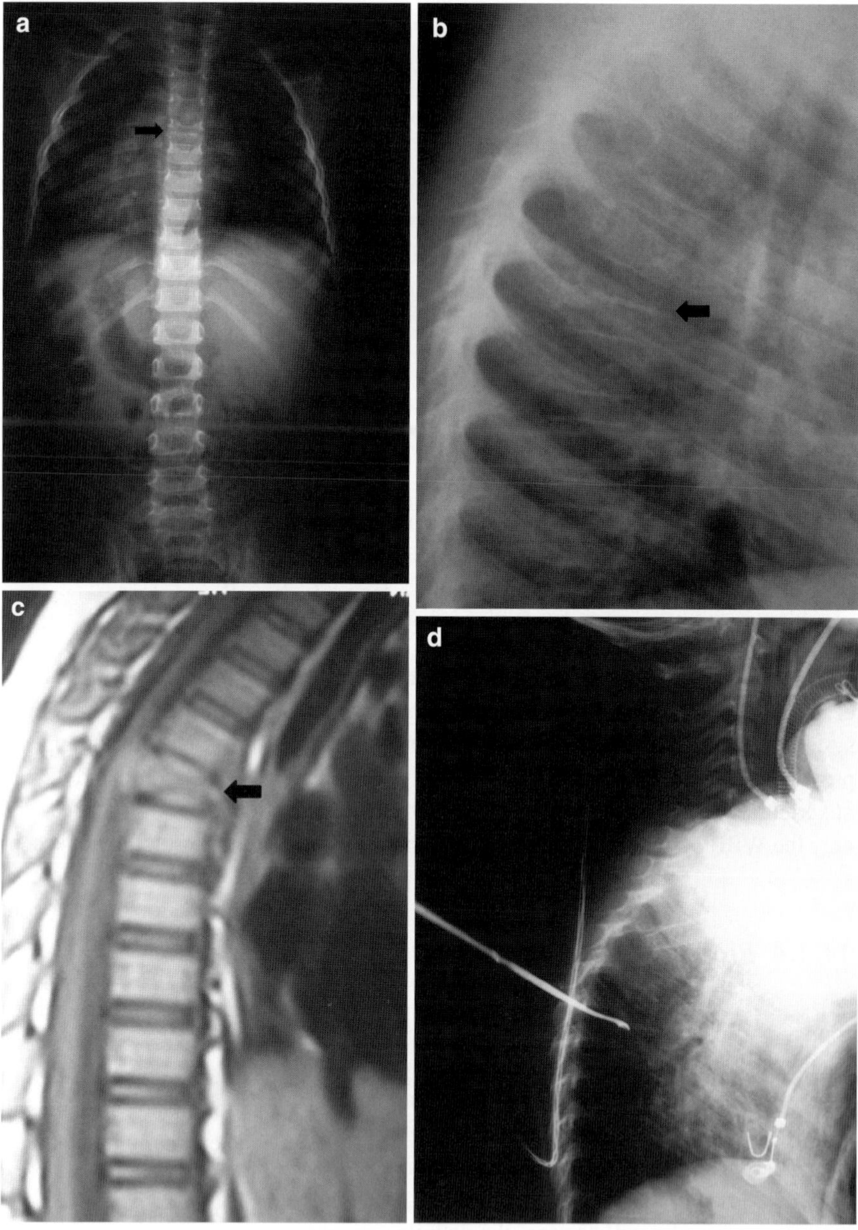

Fig. 11.2 A five year old male presenting with back pain. (**a**, **b**) AP and lateral plain radiographs demonstrating the typical appearance of vertebra plana (*arrows*). (**c**) T1-weighted sagittal MRI demonstrating the totally preserved disc spaces (*arrow*). (**d**) Intraoperative lateral radiograph taken during transpedicular biopsy

3. Possible total resection of tumor and affected osseous structures
4. Reconstruction of spinal alignment and achieve spinal stability [62].

A commonly accepted terminology for surgical procedures and for definition of tumor extent is needed for surgical planning. Lesions in the pediatric spine are often more challenging to treat than lesions of similar behavior elsewhere in the musculoskeletal system. "Curettage" describes the piecemeal removal of the tumor. As such, it is always an intralesional procedure. "En bloc" indicates an attempt to remove the whole tumor in one piece, together with a layer of healthy tissue.

Slow-growing but locally aggressive tumors that may be easily treated elsewhere in the skeleton may be unresectable and potentially lethal in certain locations in the spine. The surgical approach should be planned carefully and must achieve the prescribed appropriate margins. While intralesional removal may be associated with excellent outcomes for many patients with benign latent tumors and benign active tumors, more aggressive surgery is indicated for some locally aggressive benign tumors and many malignant tumors.

Management of malignant spinal tumors is more complex and requires a multidisciplinary approach. Early detection of the tumor followed by complete excision is advisable [61]. Advances in chemotherapy and techniques for resection and reconstruction have expanded the role of local surgical management. For optimal surgical treatment, oncological staging of lesion is essential. Local control of the malignant pediatric spinal tumor can only be achieved with a well-planned wide resection. However, wide en bloc excision procedure may be impossible in some cases because of the location and the extent of the tumor.

Three different en bloc resection surgeries have been defined: vertebrectomy, sagittal resection, and resection of the posterior arch. Vertebrectomy implies removal of all the elements of the vertebra, which may be total, or hemi in the sagittal plane. These procedures can be performed in staged, sequential, or simultaneous anterior and posterior approaches or in a single stage through posterior approach [5, 51, 61, 57, 64]. Our limited experience of 11 cases using these resection techniques has yielded very promising results. Lesions involving the posterior elements of the spine can be managed with posterior approaches for excision as well as postexcision stabilization with promising results [7] (Fig. 11.3 a–g).

11.3 Specific Spinal Column Tumors

11.3.1 Benign Tumors

11.3.1.1 Eosinophilic Granuloma (Langerhans Cell Histiocytosis)

This lesion is a reactive proliferation of langerhans cells forming granulomas and may produce focal destruction because of this essentially inflammatory character. Clinical manifestations range from a single bony lesion to multiple granulomas in bones and soft tissues to systemic forms of disease. The incidence of spinal involvement ranges from 7 to 25% [10, 18, 41, 53, 56, 66]. It is commonly seen in children less than 10 years of age and is more common in males [20, 36, 54]. The most common presenting symptoms is pain [20, 37, 47, 68]. Vertebra plana is the typical radiological appearance caused by the partial or complete collapse of the vertebral body. An important point in the differential diagnosis between eosinophilic granuloma and infection in the presence of a totally collapsed vertebral body is to note the completely normal neighbouring discs in the former whereas infection always starts from and/or involves at least one of them. Asymmetrical vertebral collapse can lead to the scoliosis or severe kyphosis but the most common deformity is mild to moderate kyphosis [11]. These lesions are the most common pathologic conditions causing vertebra plana and are usually solitary and affect the body, most commonly in the thoracic spine [10] (see Fig. 11.2). Neurological symptoms due to vertebral collapse may rarely be seen.

A skeletal survey or bone scan should be done to rule out other lesions of eosinophilic granuloma, which is associated with multifocal disease. MRI is helpful for the differential diagnosis from malignancy. However, diagnosis is usually confirmed by biopsy performed with the principles delineated earlier. Histology of these lesions has three main components that are lipid-containing histiocytes with "coffee-bean" appearance, eosinophils, and langerhans giant cells.

Solitary lesions are usually a self-limited disease. Treatment is somewhat controversial, but it is clear that many patients heal their lesions without any treatment, or for that matter, any treatment other than biopsy. Observation with or without spinal immobilization with cast, body jacket, orthosis, or collar can be used for few months to several years has been the standard modality of treatment. This conservative treatment allows the load sharing of the anterior column and may produce an enhancement in the growth plate activity leading to a possible restoration of vertebral height [29]. Raab et al. [47] have reported that 18.2–97% vertebral body height restoration was possible in conservatively treated patients. It appears that the age of the patient is an important factor in this context. If the lesion had been identified at least 4 years before skeletal maturity, remaining growth capacity is usually enough for adequate remodeling regardless of location at the cervical, thoracic, or lumbar regions. Radiotheraphy, chemotherapy (only for disseminated form), and steroid injections have been advocated with no proven benefits over observation for solitary lesions. Operative treatment is only necessary in the rare

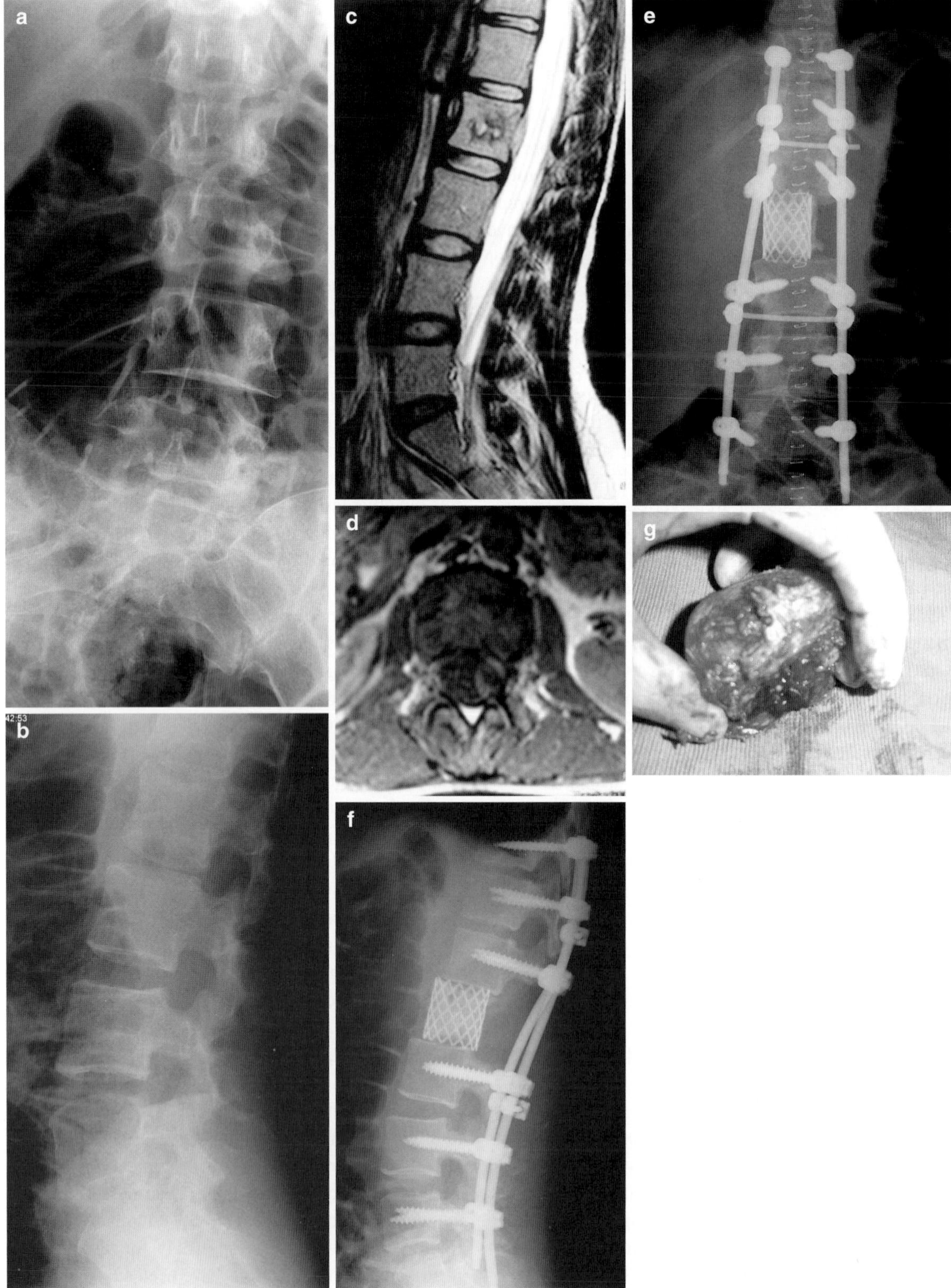

Fig. 11.3 A 15-year-old female presenting with back pain. (**a**, **b**) AP and lateral plain radiographs negative for any significant finding. (**c**, **d**) T2-weighted sagittal and axial MRI demonstating the tumor located within the body of L2. Oncologically staged as IIB, surgically (Weinstein, Boriani, Biagnini) [63] staged as zones 4 to 10 from B to D because of the epidural component. Needle biopsy under CT guidance confirmed the diagnosis as Ewing's Sarcoma. (**e**, **f**) Postoperative radiographs following enbloc excision. (**g**) Resected vertebral body

instance such as neurological involvement secondary to vertebral collapse, compression of the spinal cord, extraosseous extension and instability of spine, or persistent pain.

11.3.1.2 Osteoid Osteoma and Osteoblastoma

These lesions are most frequently seen in the first two decades of life and show a propensity for the posterior elements. They may be located in the pedicles, transverse processes, laminae, and spinous processes. Osteoblastoma shows an even greater predisposition for the spine. The overall rate of being located in the spine ranges from 10 to 41% for osteoid osteoma and 30–50% for osteoblastoma [64]. Pain is the predominant symptom and is usually worse at nights and activity. It may resolve with the use of nonsteriodal antiinflammatory drugs (NSAID). Night pain and dramatic response to NSAID should evoke the clinical suspicion for osteoid osteoma, almost automatically. On the other hand, osteoblastoma pain has a low response to NSAIDs. These tumors often produce pain before they become visible on plain radiographs. A CT scan is often required to diagnose the lesions, which have the typical appearance of osteosclerosis surrounding a radiolucent nidus of less than 2 cm in diameter for osteoid osteoma and greater than 2 cm for osteoblastoma (Fig. 11.4). Technetium bone scan can be useful in establishing the diagnosis, while roentgenograms are still negative, and the pain definition by the patient is vague and nonlocalizing by showing a nonspecific but intense, well-defined focal uptake of activity [49, 58, 65]. Osteoid osteoma is typically a benign latent self-limiting lesion that has a tendency to spontaneously regress over several years, whereas osteoblastomas are usually locally aggressive tumors.

Painful scoliosis is another fairly well-recognized presentation of osteoid osteoma and osteoblastoma [1, 31, 48], the incidence of being the initial symptom of spinal osteoid osteoma and osteoblastoma ranges from 25 to 63% [40, 45]. Lesions with scoliosis are more common in thoracolumbar spine than cervical spine and have been identified as the most common cause of pain provoked reactive scoliosis [39]. Saifuddin et al. [52] have reported on the typical findings associated with scoliosis in osteoid osteoma and osteoblastoma, based on a series in which 63% of patients had scoliosis overall. Lesions were mostly located on the concave side near the apex. Asymmetrical location of lesion within the vertebral body or neural arc appeared to be the most significant factor for the development of scoliosis, whereas a lesion at the center of vertebral body (e.g., spinous process) had the least likelihood. It was postulated that asymmetrical inflammatory effect of the lesion caused asymmetrical muscle spasm and secondary scoliosis. Cervical lesions were associated with a minor chance of developing scoliosis, predominantly at the lower cervical spine, but asymmetrical inflammation may lead to torticollis.

If the patient's symptoms can be managed with NSAIDs without any significant side effects, a trial of medical treatment may be prescribed. Long-term medical treatment was found to be as effective as surgical treatment [33]. However, such prolonged use of drugs is often associated with at least gastrointestinal irritation and may lead to severe hemorrhage. Surgical treatment should be considered if medical treatment cannot be used or is not successful, that of osteoid osteoma being intralesional excision. There is no need for the removal of the entire sclerotic reaction; however, the nidus should be completely removed to insure pain relief and to prevent recurrences. As pain is usually radically improved after complete resection of the nidus, it can attest to the completeness of the excision as well. Spinal deformity improves in almost all patients within 15 months [31, 45, 64].

Contrary to osteoid osteomas, treatment of osteoblastomas consists of complete surgical excision. Curettage has been advocated in the past, but with an unacceptable rate of recurrence. Even marginal excisions carry a recurrence risk of about 10% [59]. Radiotherapy has been advocated in the past because of these relatively high rates of recurrence after surgery but has been mostly abandoned now in the era of modern spinal surgery as it may be associated with the danger of malignant transformation of these lesions.

11.3.1.3 Aneurysmal Bone Cyst

Aneurysmal bone cysts are benign and highly vascular bony lesions that are relatively rare. In total, 3–20% of lesions are located in the vertebral column [3, 11, 67]. These lesions usually occur in the second decade of life and have a tendency to be located at the posterior elements of vertebra [13, 15, 42, 62, 64]. Aneurysmal bone cysts may occasionally be seen in association with langerhans cell histiocytosis, chondroblastoma, osteosarcoma, and giant cell tumors.

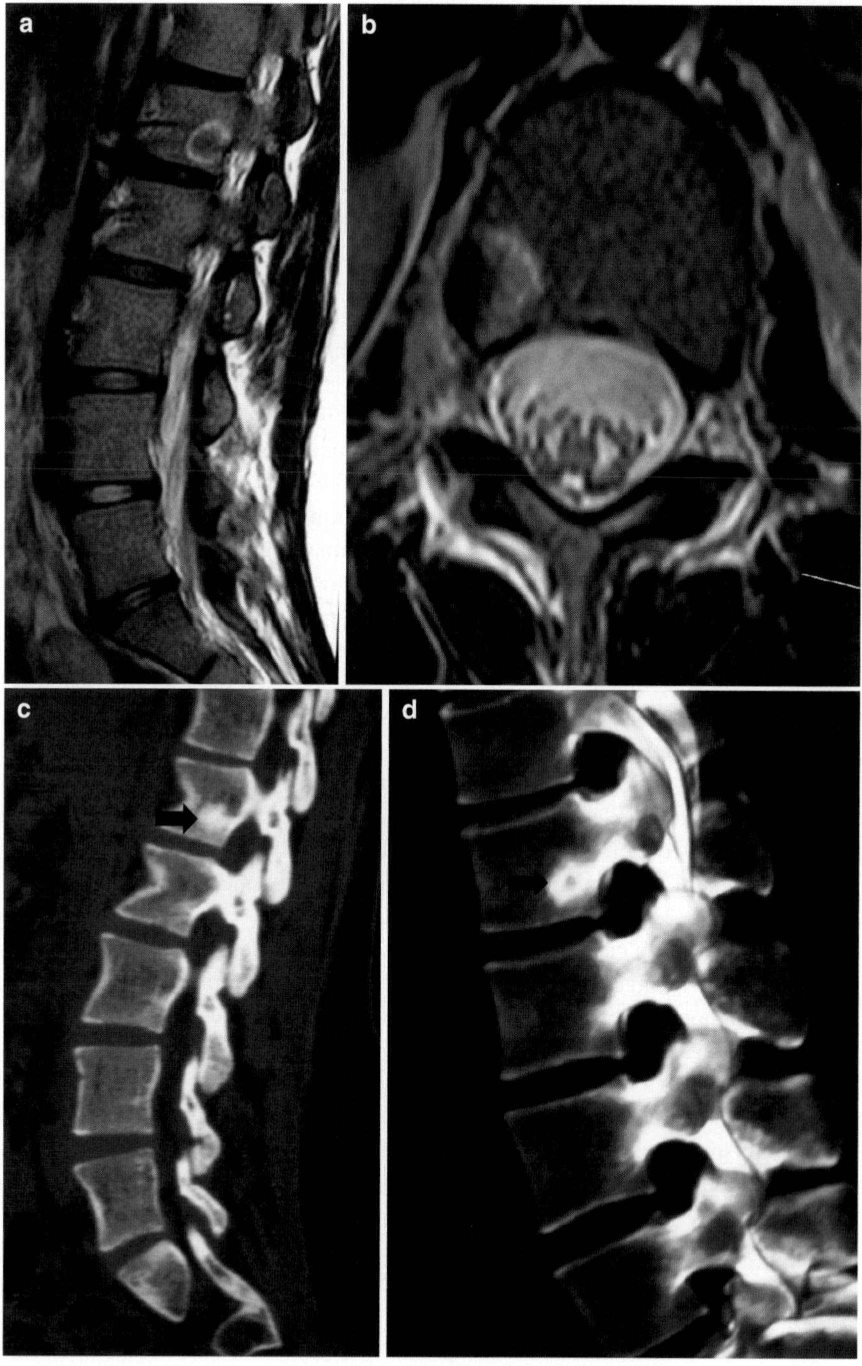

Fig. 11.4 A 14-year-old female presenting with back pain that is worse at night time and reasonably responsive to salicylates. MRI was prescribed, revealing a completely hypointense nucleus surrounded by a relatively hyperintense zone on sagittal (**a**) and axial (**b**) T2-weighted images. (**c**, **d**) Sagittal and 3D reconstructions of CT images demonstrating a sclerotic zone surrounding a relatively lytic nidus typical for osteoid osteoma

They are mostly located in the cervical and thoracic spine, they also involve the lumbar spine and sacrum, although a predilection has been reported for the lumbar spine and female patients in one report [13, 43, 62]. Aneurysmal bone cyst is a benign but locally aggressive lesion [8, 24]. The most common complaints are pain and neurological symptoms as a result of spinal cord or nerve root compression both of which usually, almost immediately, regress with surgical decompression [38, 43]. Radiography reveals an expansile, lytic lesion with bubbly appearance surrounded by a thin shell of reactive bone. Fine bony septations give the lesion a soap-bubble appearance. Occasionally, they may involve three or more adjacent vertebra. CT and MRI provide optimal evaluation of lesion content and expansion of tumor. MRI reveals multiloculated, septated, expansile lesions with fluid–fluid levels, whereas CT is important in demonstrating the intact bony shell as a telltale sign of a benign lesion. Definitive diagnosis may be established with CT-guided needle biopsy, trocar biopsy, or open biopsy and/or frozen section at the time of the resection procedure. A thorough histological study coupled with clinical and radiographic data is essential for a correct diagnosis, as the differential diagnosis includes tumors with similar histological appearances such as giant cell tumors as well as osteosarcoma [43]. Angiography may also be helpful in the surgical planning of these lesions. Selective embolization can be used as a stand-alone treatment or to reduce the intraoperative bleeding if performed before the surgery. Radiotherapy has been advocated in the past but it is now established that lesions treated with radiotherapy have a risk of malignant transformation [11, 38, 43]. Early surgical intervention with intralesional curettage of all affected bone is recommended after the diagnosis has been established by biopsy. Intraoperative excessive bleeding may be a problem that can be solved with selective arterial embolization before surgery or early removal of the thin bony wall of the lesion before the resection of the cystic lesion itself, thereby shortening the period of surgery with significant blood loss. Recurrence rates of 10–50% have been reported with intralesional excision [8, 11, 24, 43]. As a real danger of recurrence after simple intralesional curettage exists, cauterization of the osseous cysts wall, extended curettage with high-speed diamond burrs, and administration of dilute (5%) phenol and absolute alcohol administration have been advocated in order to decrease this rate [21]. More aggressive resection margins should be reserved for cases in which it is feasible without creating any iatrogenic instability or recurrent cases in which intralesional surgery has definitely failed. Spinal fusion should be performed when the lesion or the surgical procedure has rendered the spine unstable.

11.3.1.4 Hemangioma

These lesions are usually clinically silent and found incidentally. Symptomatic hemangioma of bone is a relatively uncommon entity. On the other hand, spine is the most commonly affected part of the skeleton. Hemangiomas are predominantly located at the anterior elements of vertebra and especially in thoracic region. Cases of soft tissue extension with nerve root or spinal cord compression have been documented [63, 64]. Patients' main symptom may be pain which may or may not be associated with pathological fractures in large lesions. CT scan and MRI are diagnostic. Axial CT views demonstrate the typical honeycomb pattern that is diagnostic, whereas MRI reveals the fluid content and increased vascular blood flow. Most patients do not require treatment as long as they remain symptom free. Fairly large lesions may be considered as candidates of treatment because of the possibility of a fracture but specific guidelines regarding the size and location of the lesion in regard to the risk of impending fracture have not been established. Embolization may be used in painful lesions as a stand-alone treatment or in conjunction with surgery. Vertebroplasty or kyphoplasty are becoming increasingly popular and have the potential of rendering any open surgery unnecessary [12, 23]. Open surgery with resection of the lesion should be reserved for those patients with pathologic fractures and neurological compromise.

11.3.1.5 Osteochondroma

Osteochonromas (exostoses) are the most common benign bone tumors. They occasionally occur in the spine, especially in the pediatric population. Multiple hereditary exostosis is more likely to involve spine. Posterior elements of cervicothoracic spine are the most frequent location. A simple painless mass may be the only presenting symptom. They may as well be diagnosed incidentally or, very rarely, may cause neurological symptoms. Plain radiographs are usually adequate in demonstrating the sessile or pedinculated mass. CT may be used to understand the exact location of the lesions, whereas MRI may be necessary to evaluate the thickness of the cartilage cap. There has always been a debate on the importance of the thickness of the cartilage cap, most current information suggesting that a cap thicker than 2 cm may be associated with malignant degeneration [14]. Osteochondromas of spine tend to grow fairly slowly until skeletal maturity and remain dormant thereafter. Painful lesions with neurological compromise and those that had been demonstrated to commence growth after skeletal maturity need to be treated operatively. An essential feature of excisional surgery is the necessity of the removal of the entire cartilaginous cap. Recurrence risk is low in children in whom it could completely be excised [14].

11.3.1.6 Other Benign Tumors

Giant cell tumors occur very rarely in the pediatric population. This tumor is composed of a highly vascularized network with numerous multinucleated giant cells. Most giant cell tumors are benign and locally aggressive tumors with a predilection for the vertebral body. Pain, local tenderness, swelling, and neurological problems are the usual presenting symptoms [62, 64]. Sacrum is the most commonly affected area. As occasional pulmonary metastases have been reported, chest radiograms or CT should be performed in oncological staging [30, 50]. Pediatric patients with giant cell tumors should be managed with wide resection whenever possible. If obtaining wide margins is not possible, a marginal resection can be performed but the patient and family should be warned on the possibility of recurrence. Recurrence rates are high in adult population but little is known for the pediatric population because of the rarity of the tumor. Adjuvant surgical treatments like phenol, polymethylmethacrylate, or liquid nitrogen may be used. For large giant cell tumors or tumors with critical locations that would render them virtually unresectable (e.g., sacrum), repeated arterial embolizations has been reported as a useful stand-alone treatment modality with favorable results but our experience in a limited number of cases has not been very promising so far [27, 64]. Radiotherapy is the last resort because of the potential for increased malignant transformation and should be reserved for those uncontrollable lesions with multiple recurrences.

Another uncommon lesion is fibrous dysplasia of the spine. Some cases of fibrous dysplasia have been reported. Pain is usually the main complaint. Monostotic and polyostotic forms may be seen in children with the most common site of location at the lumbar and the thoracic spine. The possibility of neurological involvement has also been reported [36, 46]. Scoliosis has also been reported in extensive fibrous dysplasia and may require management with standard scoliosis surgery [22].

11.3.2 Malignant Tumors

11.3.2.1 Osteosarcoma

Osteosarcoma is the most common primary malignant bone tumor [64]. Primary osteosarcomas are relatively uncommon in the spine consisting of 3% of all osteosarcomas and often affect the thoracic and lumbar spine [28, 62]. Vertebral body is predominantly involved. Most osteogenic sarcomas of spine in children are metastatic. They are most frequently encountered in the second decade of life. Pain is the most common and earliest presenting symptom [64]. Night pain will be present in approximately 25% of patients and up to 40% will be expected to have neurological symptoms [14, 28]. Laboratory findings usually are not helpful except for the possibility of elevated serum alkaline phosphatase levels. Osteosarcomas are locally and systemically aggressive, high-grade malignancies. They radiographically present with a lytic, blastic, or mixed lesion with an ossifying matrix. All patients in whom a primary or metastatic osteosarcoma is included in the differential diagnosis should be evaluated with an MRI of the involved region so as to define the lesion and extension. Osteosarcomas have a very high tendency to metastasize, almost exclusively to the lung, rarely to the other bones. Pulmonary CT and bone scans (or total body MRI) are essential requirements for staging the disease.

For those highly malignant lesions, biopsy should be performed at the center and by the surgical team who will assume the definitive responsibility for the treatment. A diagnosis of osteosarcoma on biopsy is usually followed by neoadjuvant chemotherapy so as to achieve the best results in regards to oncological outcome, followed by the definitive resection of the tumor whenever possible. Primary osteosarcomas of spine present complex therapeutic problems in management, mainly because of the difficulties posed by surgical resection. Every effort should be made to remove the tumor en bloc excision with clear margins. It has to be understood and relayed to the patients and families that spinal osteosarcomas have a very poor prognosis. Median survival of spinal osteosarcomas has been reported to be for 6–10 months; however, new surgical techniques and technologies and modern treatment regimens may improve this outcome [28, 42, 62].

11.3.2.2 Ewing's Sarcoma

Ewing's sarcoma is the most common primary malignancy of the childhood to be located in the spinal column. It is most frequently seen in the first two decades of life but is uncommon under 5 years of age. Approximately 8% of all Ewing's sarcomas occur in the spinal column, with sacrum being the most common site. The tumor histologically consists of uniform, small, round, and highly undifferentiated cells [64]. These may resemble neuroblastomas, rhabdomyosarcomas, and lymphomas; and malignant tumors with similar small round cells. Pain and neurological deficits are the most common presenting symptoms. Unlike osteosarcoma, Ewing's sarcoma may present with systemic symptoms such as fever and weight loss and may be mistaken as a systemic infection at the early stages. It is very common to have the systemic inflammatory signs such as ESR and CRP elevated.

Plain radiographs reveal lesions with a moth-eaten appearance, a shadow of the soft tissue mass and aggressive periosteal reaction. The occurrence of vertebra plana is also possible and may lead to a misdiagnosis of eosinophilic granuloma. As the lesion usually starts at the bone of the vertebral body, disk spaces are usually preserved until late disease. Like osteosarcoma, MRI is mandatory to evaluate the soft tissue extension and the spinal canal. Ewing's sarcoma's staging strategy is similar to osteosarcoma and necessitates chest CT and bone scans (or total body MRI) so as to detect lung and bone metastases. Although specific staging systems have been advocated and commonly used in the past, the use of the SSS is getting to be more popular and accurate because of the advances in the general understanding of tumor behavior and in treatment. The traditional treatment of Ewing's sarcoma consists of neoadjuvant chemotherapy followed by local control with radiation therapy or surgery or both. There has been an ongoing debate on the usefulness of ablative surgery for such tumors that are reasonably responsive to radiotherapy but recent studies have demonstrated clearly better results in favor of surgical resection [34] (see Fig. 11.3). It is advisable to use neoadjuvant chemotherapy for a better treatment outcome and especially to decrease the volume of the tumor mass for easier and safer surgical resection [62]. In our experience radiotherapy is only recommended if the lesion could not be resected with adequate margins (wide), which has been relatively frequent but becoming less so. Spinal metastases of Ewing's sarcoma have poorer prognosis compared to primary Ewing's sarcoma of the spine [14] (Fig. 11.5).

11.3.2.3 Leukemia

Leukemia is the most common cancer in young children. Peak incidence is between 2 and 5 years of age. All organ systems may be affected, the skeleton being one of the most frequent diagnostic sites of the acute form of the leukemia. Bone pain may be the presenting symptom in 25% of patients. The others symptoms are lethargy, anemia, and fever. Changes in laboratory tests such as increased WBCs and decreased platelet count are characteristics of leukemia when present. Elevated ESR and CRP levels may also be seen. Plain radiograms often do not have any definitive diagnostic appearance. Diffuse osteopenia, osteosclerosis, osteolysis, and periosteal reaction may be seen in and around the vertebral bodies of leukemia patients. Pathologic fractures with or without vertebral body collapse also may occur. Definitive treatment is specific to the type of leukemia but in some cases surgery may be needed for the treatment of spinal instability or pain associated with pathologic fractures [19, 26, 42].

11.3.2.4 Other Malignant and Metastatic Lesions

Metastatic involvement of the spine in children may occur in rhabdomyosarcomas, neuroblastomas, Wilms tumor, lymphomas, and teratomas. Pain is the main symptom because of micro- or macro-pathologic fractures. Vast majority of metastatic tumors are sarcomas with varying levels of radioresistance. Treatment depends on the definitive diagnosis of the primary tumor as well as the stage of the disease and the general condition of the patient. In cases of instability, spinal stability should be reinstituted with segmental spinal instrumentation [35, 62].

11.4 Summary

Tumors of the spinal column in pediatric age group have distinct features in regards to diagnosis and management. Primary lesions are far more common compared to adults. Some tumors such as leukemia may be almost specific to this age group as well. On the other hand, the general principles of evaluation, staging, biopsy, and

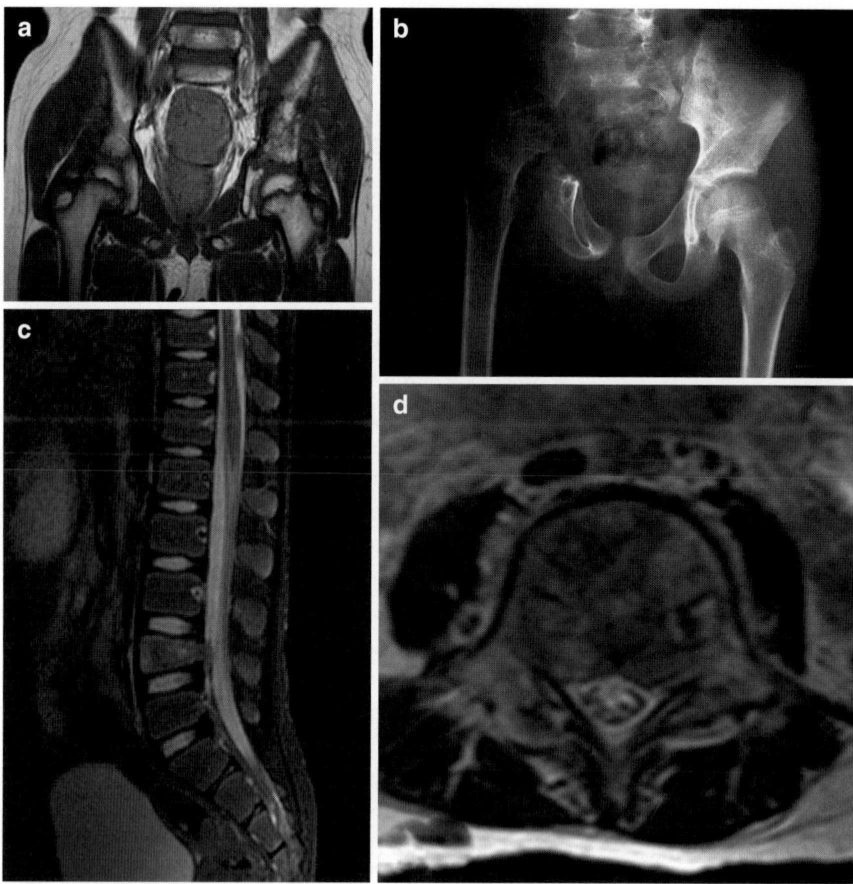

Fig. 11.5 A 8-year-old male presenting with right-sided hip and buttock pain. (**a**) T1-weighted MR image demonstating a mass located at the iliac wing, infiltrating the surrounding muscle. Oncologically staged as IIB, biopsy revealed a Ewing's sarcoma. (**b**) Plain AP pelvis view following wide excision of the tumor after neoadjuvant chemotherapy. Developed mild back pain 1 year after index surgery. (**c**–**e**) Lateral plain radiograph and STIR axial and sagittal MRI demonstrating metastatic lesion at L4. Oncological staging III, surgical (WBB) [63] staging zones 4 to 9, B and C. Patient was not referred to surgery at this stage, received radiotherapy followed by another episode of chemotherapy.

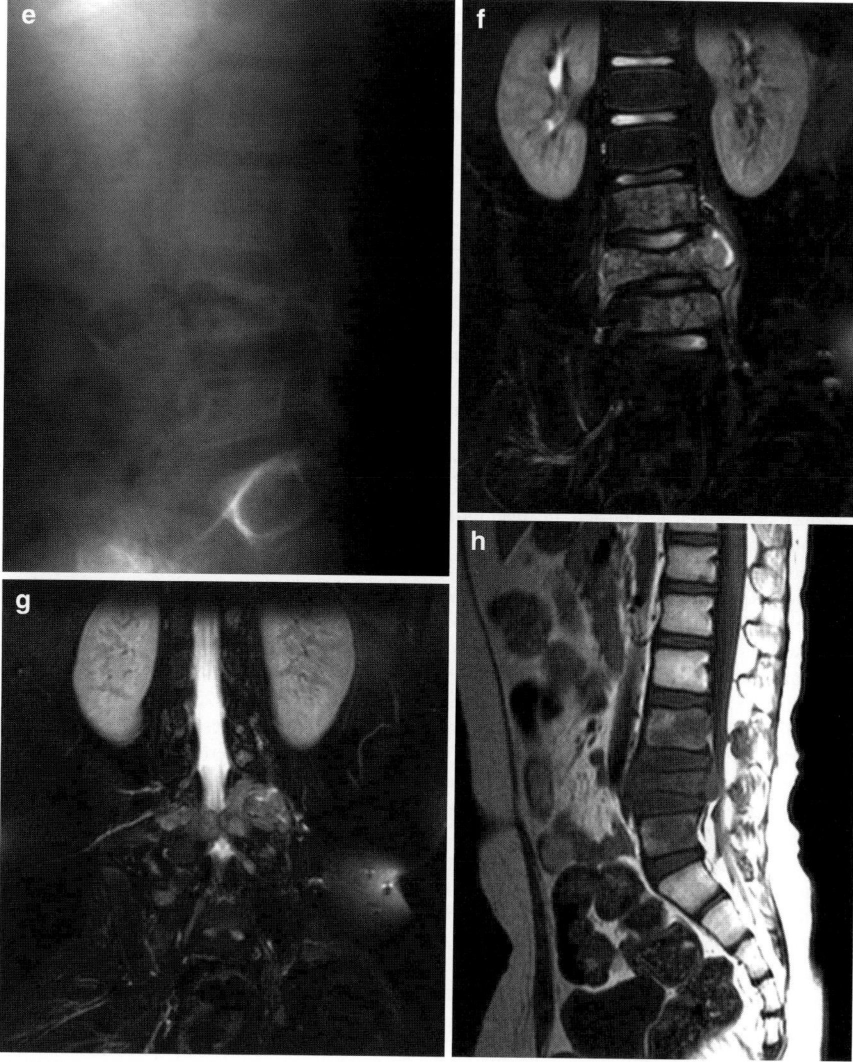

Fig. 11.5 (continued) (**f, g**) STIR coronal MRI at 6 months after the radiotherapy. Note that the the lesion has spread not only both of the neighboring levels but also completely surrounds the dural sac at his point. (**h**) T1-weighted sagittal MR image confirming the involvement of additional levels as well as the epidural space (WBB staging [63] 3 levels, 1 to 12, B to D). This patient was considered to have become in-operable at this stage, became paraplegic soon after and expired 3 months later

treatment are not different from the guidelines established for the general population. Profound knowledge of the principles of musculoskeletal tumor surgery as well as an understanding of the specific difficulties of oncological surgery in the spinal column is essential.

References

1. Akbarnia BA, Rooholamini SA (1981) Scoliosis caused by benign osteoblastoma of the thoracic or lumbar spine. JBJS Am 63:1146–1155
2. Beer SJ, Menezes AH (1997) Primary tumors of the spine in children. Natural history, management, and long term follow-up. Spine 22:649–658; discussion 658–659
3. Biesecker JL, Marcove RC, Huvos AG, Mike V (1970) Aneurysmal bone cysts: a clinicopathologic study of 66 cases. Cancer 26:615–625
4. Boriani S, Capanna R, Donati D et al (1992) Osteoblastoma of the spine. Clin Orthop 278:37–45
5. Boriani S, Biagini R, De lure F et al (1994) Lumbar vertebrectomy for the treatment of bone tumors: surgical technique. Chir Organi Mov 79: 163–174
6. Boriani S, Chevalley F, Weinstein JN et al (1996) Chordoma of the spine above sacrum: treatment and outcome in 21 cases. Spine 21:1569–1577
7. Boriani S, Weinstein JN, Biagini R (1997) Primary bone tumors of the spine: terminology and surgical staging. Spine 22(9):1036–1044
8. Boriani S, De Iure F, Campanacci L et al (2001) Aneurysmal bone cyst of the mobile spine. Spine 26(1):27–35
9. Campanacci M, Boriani S, Glunti A (1990) Giant cell tumors of the spine. In: Sundaresan SN, Schmidek HH, Schiller AL,

Rosenthal DL (eds) Tumors of the spine: diagnosis and clinical management. W.B. Saunders, Philadelphia, pp 163–172
10. Canadell J, Villas C, Martinez-Denegri J et al Imizcoz A (1986) Vertebral eosinophlic granuloma. Spine 11: 767–769
11. Capanna R, Albisinni U, Picci P et al (1985) Aneurysmal bone cyst of the spine. JBJS Am 67:527–531
12. Chiras J, Barragan-Campos HM, Cormier E et al (2007) Vertebroplasty: state of the art. J Radiol 88(9 Pt 2): 1255–1260
13. Cottalorda J, Kohler R, Sales de Gauzy J et al (2004) Epidemiology of aneurysmal bone cyst in children: a multicenter study and literature review. J Pediatr Orthop B 13:389–394
14. Cronen GA, Emery SE (2006) Benign and malignant lesions of the spine. In: Spivak JM, Connilly JP (eds) Orthopaedic knowledge update. The American Academy of Orthopaedic Surgeons, Rosemont
15. de Kleuver M, van der Heul RO, Veraart BE (1998) Aneurysmal bone cyst of the spine: 31 cases and the importance of the surgical approach. J Pediatr Orthop B7: 286–292
16. Enneking WF (1983) Musculoskeletal tumor surgery. Churchill Livingstone, New York, pp 69–122
17. Fraser RD, Paterson DC, Simpson DA (1977) Orthopaedic aspect of spinal tumors in children. JBJS Br 59:143–151
18. Fowles JW, Bobecho WP (1970) Solitary eosinophlic granuloma in bone. JBJS Br 52:238–243
19. Gallagher DJ, Phillips DJ, Heinrich SD (1996) Orthopaedic manifestations of acute pediatric leukemia. Orthop Clin North Am 27:635–644
20. Garg S, Metha S, Dormans JP (2004) Langerhans cell histiocytosis of the spine in children. Long term follow-up. JBJS Am 86:1740–5170
21. Garg S, Mehta S, Dormans JP (2005) Modern surgical treatment of primary aneurysmal bone cyst of the spine in children and adolescents. J Pediatr Orthop 25:387–932
22. Guille JT, Bowen JR (1995) Scoliosis and fibrous dysplasia of the spine. Spine 20(2):248–251
23. Hadjipavlou A, Tosounidis T, Gaitanis I et al (2007) Balloon kyphoplasty as a single or as an adjunct procedure for the management of symptomatic vertebral haemangiomas. JBJS Br 89(4):495–502
24. Hay MC, Paterson D, Taylor TK (1978) Aneurysmal bone cysts of the spine. JBJS Br 60:406–411
25. Healey JH, Ghelman B (1986) Osteoid osteoma and osteoblastoma. Current concepts and recent advances. Clin Orthop Relat Res 204:76–85
26. Heinrich SD, Gallagher D, Warrior R et al (1994) The prognostic significance of the skeletal manifestations of acute lymphoblastic leukemia of childhood. J Pediatr Orthop 14:105–111
27. Hosalkar HS, Jones KJ, King JJ et al (2007) Serial arterial embolization for large sacral giant-cell tumors: mid- to long-term results. Spine 32(10):1107–15
28. Ilaslan H, Sundaram M, Unni KK, Shives TC (2004) Primary vertebral osteosarcoma: imaging findings. Radiology 230: 697–702
29. Ippolito E, Farsetti P, Tudisco C (1984) Vertebra plana long-term follow up in five patients. JBJS Am 66:1364–1368
30. Kay RM, Ecjkart JJ, Seeger LL et al (1994) Pulmonary metastasis of benign giant cell tumors of bone: six histological confirmed cases, including one of spontaneous regression. Clin Orthop 302:219–230
31. Keim HA, Reina EG (1986) Osteoid-osteoma as a cause of scoliosis. JBJS Am 68:159–163
32. Kirwan EO, Hutton PA, Pozo JL (1984) Osteoid osteoma and benign osteoblastoma of spine. Clinical presentation and treatment. JBJS Br 66:21–26
33. Kneisl JS, Simon MA (1992) Medical management compared with operative treatment for osteoid osteoma. JBJS Am 74:179–815
34. Lawrence W (1998) Ewing's sarcoma. In: Simon MA, Springfield D (eds) Surgery for bone and soft tissue tumors. Lippincott-Raven, New York
35. Leeson MC, Makley JT, Carter JR (1985) Metastatic skeletal disease in the pediatric population. J Pediatr Orthop 5: 261–267
36. Leet AI, Magur E, Lee JS et al (2004) Fibrous dysplasia in the spine: prevalence of lesions and association with scoliosis. JBJS Am 86(3):531–537
37. Levine SE, Dormans JP, Meyer JS, Corcoran TA (1996) Langerhans cell histiocystosis of the spine in children. Clin Orthop Relat Res 323:288–923
38. Marcove RC, Sheth DS, Takemoto S et al (1995) The treatment of aneurysmal bone cyst. Clin Orthop 311:157–163
39. Metha MH, Murray RO (1977) Scoliosis provoked by painful vertebral lesions. Skeletal Radiol 1:223–230
40. Nemoto O, Moser RP, Van Dam BE et al (1990) Osteoblastoma of spine: a review of 75 cases. Spine 15:-1272–1280
41. Nesbit ME, Kieffer S, D'Angio GJ (1969) Reconstruction of vertebral height in histiocytosis X: a long term follow-up. JBJS Am 51:1360–1368
42. Ozaki T, Flege S, Liljenqvist U et al (2002) Osteosarcoma of the spine: experience of the Cooperative Osteosarcoma Study Group. Cancer 94: 1069–1077
43. Papagelopoulos PJ, Currier BL, Shaughnessy WJ et al (1998) Aneurysmal bone cyst of the spine. Management and outcome. Spine 23: 621–628
44. Parikh SN, Crawford AH (2003) Orthopaedic implication in the management of pediatric vertebral and spinal tumors: a retrospective review. Spine 28(20):2390–2396
45. Pettine KA, Klassen RA (1986) Osteoid-osteoma and osteobalstoma of the spine JBJS Am 68:354–356
46. Przybylski GJ, Pollack IF, Ward WT (1996) Monostotic fibrous dysplasia of the thoracic spine. A case report. Spine 21(7):860–865; review
47. Raab P, Hohmann F, Kühl J, Kraupse R (1998) Vertebral remodelling in eosinophilic granuloma of the spine: a long term follow-up. Case report. Spine 23(12):1351–5134
48. Ransford AO, Pozo JL, Hutton PAN et al (1984) The behavior pattern of scoliosis associated with osteoid osteoma or osteoblastoma of the spine. JBJS Br 66:16–20
49. Rinsky LA, Goris M, Bleck EE et al (1980) Intraoperative skeletal scintigraphy for localization of osteoid osteoma in the spine. Case report. JBJS Am 62: 143–144
50. Rock MG, Pritichard DJ, Unni KK (1984) Metastases from histologically benign giant-cell tumors of bone. JBJS Am 66:269–274
51. Roy-Camille R, Mazel CH, Saillant G, Lapresle PH (1990) Treatment of malignant tumors of the spine with posterior instrumentation. In: Sundaresan N, Schmidek HH, Schiller AL, Rosenthal DI (eds) Tumors of the spine: diagnosis and clinical management. W.B. Saunders, Philadelphia, pp 473–847

52. Saifuddin A, White J, Sherazi Z et al (1998) Osteoid osteoma and osteoblastoma of the spine: Factors associated with the presence of scoliosis. Spine 23(1):47–53
53. Schajowicz F, Slullitel J (1973) Eosinophilic granuloma of bone and its relationship to Hand-Schuller-Christian and Letter-Siwe syndrome. JBJS Br 55:545–565
54. Silberstein MJ, Sundaram M, Akbarnia B et al (1985) Eosinophilic granuloma of the spine. Orthopaedics 8:267–724
55. Simon MA, Biermann JS (1993) Biopsy of the bone and soft-tissue lesions. JBJS Am 75(4):616–621
56. Slatter JM, Swarm OJ (1980) Eosinophlic granuloma of bone. Med Pediatr Oncol 8:151–164
57. Sundaresan N, DiGiacinto GV, Krol G, Hughes JEO (1990) Complete spondilectomy for malignant tumors. In: Sundaresan N, Schmidek HH, Schiller AL, Rosenthal DI (eds) Tumors of the spine: diagnosis and clinical management. W.B. Saunders, Philadelphia, pp 438–445
58. Swee RG, Mcleod RA, Beabout JW (1977) Osteoid osteoma. Detection, diagnosis and localization. Radiology 130: 117–123
59. Sypert WG (1990) Osteoid osteoma and osteoblastoma of the spine. In: Sundaresan N, Schmidek HH, Schiller AL, Rosenthal DI (eds) Tumors of the spine: diagnosis and clinical management. W.B. Saunders, Philadelphia, pp 258–261
60. Tachdjian M, Matson D (1965) Orthopaedic aspect of intraspinal tumors in infants and children. JBJS Am 17: 223–248
61. Tomita K, Kawahara N, Baba H et al (1997) Total en bloc spondylectomy: a new surgical technique for primary malignant vertebral tumors. Spine 22(3):324–333
62. Tomita T (1990) Special consideration in surgery for pediatric surgery of spine tumors. In: Sundaresan N, Schmidek HH, Schiller AL, Rosenthal DI (eds) Tumors of the spine: diagnosis and clinical management. W.B. Saunders, Philadelphia, pp 258–261
63. Weinstein JN (1994) Primary tumors. In: Weinstein S (ed) The pediatric spine. Raven Press, New York
64. Weinstein JN, Boriani S, Phillips FM, Wetzel FT (1998) Management of benign tumors of the spine. In: Simon MA, Springfield D (eds) Surgery for bone and soft tissue tumors. Lippincott-Raven, New York
65. Winter PF, Johnson PM, Hilal SK, Feldman F (1977) Scintigraphic detection of osteoid osteoma. Radiology 122: 177–178
66. Wroble RR, Weinstein SL (1988) Histiocytosis X with scoliosis and osteolysis. J Pediatr Orthop 8:213–218
67. Vergel De Dios AM, Bond JR, Shives TC et al (1992) Aneurysmal bone cyst. A clinicopathologic study of 238 cases. Cancer 69:2921–2931
68. Yeom JS, Lee CK, Shin HY et al (1999) Langerhans cell histiocytosis of the spine. Spine 24: 1740–1749

12 Pediatric Spine Trauma

John P. Dormans, Ejovi Ughwanogho, and Jaimo Ahn

Key Points

- A majority of pediatric spine injuries occur at the cervical spine, with most fractures occurring at the upper cervical spine.
- Ligamentous laxity, horizontal orientation of vertebral facets, wedge shaped vertebral body, and underdeveloped paraspinal muscles in the immature spine result in a relatively high incidence of cervical spine injuries.
- The clinician should be cognizant of normal anatomic variants of the immature spine when interpreting pediatric spine radiographs.
- Unfused physeal lines, pseudosubluxation, and absence of cervical lordosis may be normal findings in the developing spine.
- Odontoid fracture, a common injury pattern in the immature cervical spine, typically occurs at the synchondrosis and can be managed conservatively with immobilization.
- Atlanto-axial rotatory subluxation is managed conservatively if diagnosed early. Chronic cases may require manual reduction under anesthesia, or fusion.
- SCIWORA is a very common injury in the pediatric population
- Thoracolumbar injuries are more prevalent in the adolescent population and most commonly occurs at T4–T12 then T12–L2.
- Thoracolumbar spine injuries result from significant trauma, and the presence of extraspinal injuries is the norm.
- In a flexion-distration injury, the anterior column fails in compression, while the middle and posterior columns fail in tension.
- Stable injuries of the thoracolumbar spine can be treated conservatively with brief bed rest, spasmolytics, thoracolumbosacral orthosis, and mechanically unstable fractures with neurological deficits should be managed surgically.

12.1 Introduction

Incidence of pediatric spinal fractures is relatively low and ranges from 1 to 10% in all traumas. They often result from motor vehicular accidents, falls, athletics, and occasionally child abuse. Unique features of the pediatric spine results in specific injury patterns. The ligaments, discs, and soft tissue of the pediatric spine are laxer in comparison with the adult spine. This laxity, however, also accounts for the increase incidence of spinal cord injuries without radiographic abnormalities (SCIWORA) [9, 22, 49].

Of note is the different pattern of injuries in a young child and an adolescent patient. Increased elasticity, a large head-to-torso ratio in the child of 8 years of age and less, results in preponderance of upper cervical spine pathology in this cohort. In contrast, the adolescent patient, with more mature structures, present with injury patterns similar to that of the adult. Nitecki and Moir [35] showed an 87% incidence of upper cervical spine

J. P. Dormans (✉)
Department of Orthopaedic Surgery, Children's Hospital of Philadelphia, University of Pennsylvania, Philadelphia, PA 19104-4399, USA
e-mail: dormans@email.chop.edu

B. A. Akbarnia et al. (eds.), *The Growing Spine*,
DOI: 10.1007/978-3-540-85207-0_12, © Springer-Verlag Berlin Heidelberg 2011

injuries in patients younger than 8 years of age in a series of 227 consecutive C-spine fractures in children.

Fractures commonly seen in the pediatric population include atlanto-occipital dissociation, upper cervical spine injuries, SCIWORA, and the thoracolumbar compression fractures.

12.2 Cervical Spine Trauma

12.2.1 Epidemiology

The overall incidence of cervical trauma in the pediatric patient has been estimated to range from 1 to 2%. However, a majority of pediatric spine injuries (60–80%) occurs at the C-spine. A difference in the pattern of cervical spine injury has been established in patients below and above 8 years of age. In children presenting with spinal injuries, cervical injuries appear to be more common in younger children compared with adolescents. In addition, upper cervical injuries appear to be more prevalent in the younger population. Osenbach and Menezes [38] reported a 79% incidence of cervical spine trauma in children 8 years of age or less presenting with spinal trauma. In contrast, the incidence of cervical trauma in those 8 years of age or older was 54%. They also demonstrated higher rate of upper cervical spine injury in children 8 years of age or less. Subluxations and neurological injuries were more common in the younger population. SCIWORA injuries were also more common in the younger population. Hadley et al. [21] corroborated the above findings in their study of 122 cases of vertebral column injuries in adolescent patients. Brown et al. [3] reported a 68% prevalence of upper cervical spine injuries in children. Cervical spine injury, especially upper cervical spine, SCIWORA, and neurologic injuries were more common in patients <9 years of age. SCIWORA is also a common finding in the abused child presenting with C-spine trauma. Other patterns of injury reported in the abused child include epidural and subdural hematoma of the spinal cord at the cervicomedulary junction and ventral spinal contusion in the upper C-spine [3, 21, 25, 38, 41].

Motor vehicle crashes (MVC), athletics, and falls are the most common causes of injuries in the pediatric population. Brown et al. [3] attributes 52% of cervical trauma to MVC; 27% to sports-related injuries and 15% to falls. Mortality after pediatric spine trauma has been estimated at 18.5–28% [3, 41].

12.3 Cervical Spine Anatomy

The atlas is formed by three ossification centers, located at the anterior arch and each neural arch. Ossification of the anterior arch is often absent at birth and may not appear before the first year. Union of the anterior ossification center and the lateral centers occurs by 7 years of age. The posterior arch results from posterior fusion of the neural arch and occurs by 3 years of age.

The axis is formed by four ossification centers, located within the central mass, the neural arches and the dens. These centers are present at birth. Two ossification centers, fused in utero at 7 months, form the odontoid process and are separated from the body by a cartilaginous physes. Often the two odontoid ossification centers may persist after birth. The dentocenral basilar synchondroses, located below the atlanto-axial facet joint fuse between 3 and 6 years of age. Knowledge of the location of the odontocentral physeal line, which may be present radiographically until 11 years of age, prevents erroneous diagnoses of a transverse dens fracture. The ossiculum terminali, a secondary ossification center at the apex of the dens appears between 3 and 6 years of age. The neural arches fuse with the body between 3 and 6 years of age, and fuse posteriorly to form the posterior arch by age 2–3 years (Fig. 12.1). C3–C7 have similar patterns of development with three ossification centers: one located within the vertebral bodies and two within the neural arches. Union of the neurocentral synchondrosis occurs between 2 and 6 and the posterior arches fuse between 2 and 4 [9, 13].

Distinctive anatomic features in the immature C-spine account for the pattern of injuries seen in this population. The horizontal orientation of the vertebral facet joints in the pediatric cervical spine and the relative ligamentous laxity results in a relatively high incidence of upper cervical subluxation and cervical injuries in this population. Before 8 years of age, the articular facets have an orientation of ~30° and progressively become more vertical. By adolescence, the orientation is similar to that of an adult at 55–70° [9]. Furthermore, the relatively high head-to-body ratio of the pediatric patient localizes the fulcrum of spinal

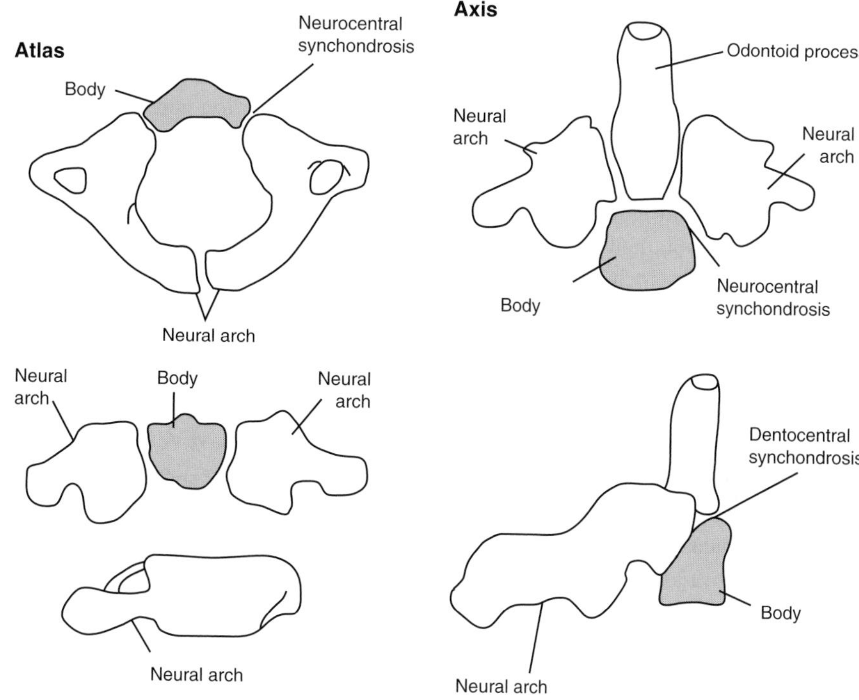

Fig. 12.1 Ossification centers of the atlas and axis. (Reprinted with permission from Dormans [32])

flexion at C2–3 as opposed to C5 and C6 in the adult [11]. Other anatomic features contributing to the pattern on injuries seen in this population include delayed ossification of the uncinate process (a stabilizer in the adult spine), anterior wedge of the immature vertebral body and underdevelopment of cervical para-spinal muscles. These factors contribute to the relatively high incidence of upper cervical instability/injuries in the pediatric patient [17].

12.3.1 Clinical Evaluation

Cervical spine injury in the pediatric patient often results from considerable trauma such as motor vehicular accidents, fall from height, and penetrating injuries. Athletic injuries and child abuse are also potential causes of trauma in the pediatric spine. Patients may be unconscious at presentation [58]. When conscious, they report neck pain or spasm. Signs of trauma to the head and face, bruising caused by seat or shoulder belts, may also be present. Often these findings are absent in the young child, and instead, the child may report occipital headaches.

In addition to strict adherence to ATLS protocol, a comprehensive neurological examination should be performed on all patients with suspected spinal injuries, the patient should also evaluated for other associated injuries [32].

The child presenting with a suspected cervical spine injury should be immobilized in a spine board. Indications for immobilization include loss of consciousness (GCS,13), altered mentation, fall from height, mechanism of injury suggestive of spinal injury, head or facial trauma, neck pain, or guarding [13]. Because of the relatively large head of children <8 years of age, there is a tendency for flexion of the head, when these patients are immobilized in a traditional spine board. This can be prevented by elevating the torso relative to the head with a thin mattress or using a board with a recess [23]. A halo ring and vest is also a viable method of immobilizing the pediatric cervical spine. The construct requires the use of 8–12 pins applied with low insertional torques (1–5 in-lbs). A CT scan of the head obtained prior to application of the halo can help identify cranial sutures and thin areas of the skull. These areas should be avoided when inserting halo pins. Advantages of a halo vest immobilization include relative ease of application, earlier mobilization of the patient, access to wounds of the neck and scalp, and freedom of mandibular motion. Pin site infection is the most common complication associated with halo vest immobilization [8, 14].

12.3.2 Radiologic Evaluation

The standard trauma series, including an AP, lateral, and odontoid views of the cervical spine, including the T1 level, can be obtained when a C-spine injury is suspected. In the lucid and older patient without neurologic deficits, flexion and extension views of the C-spine should also be obtained if instability is suspected. Indices of instability include segmental kyphosis, anterior soft tissue swelling and equivocal subluxation in the standard radiographic views [9, 46]. In small infants, odontoid views and lateral views may be difficult to interpret because of the overlapping skull. In these instances, a lateral view of the skull may be utilized to evaluate the upper cervical spine [9].

Radiographic parameters used for the evaluation of upper cervical stability include the atlanto-dens interval (ADI), Powers ratio, and the basion-axis distance. The ADI describes the distance between the anterior surface of the dens and the posterior surface of the anterior arc of the atlas and should be <5 mm. The powers ratio defines the ratio between the distance of the basion and the posterior arc of the atlas and the distance between the opisthion and the anterior arc of the atlas. This ratio averages 0.77 and a value exceeding 1 or <0.55 is indicative of atlanto-occipital dislocation. The basion-axis distance is the distance between the basion and a vertical line extended cephalad from the posterior border of the dens. This line should be 12 mm or less in children 13 years of age or less (Fig. 12.2) [32, 59].

Normal anatomic variants in the developing spine should be recognized and differentiated from pathologic findings. For example, on the lateral view, there may be physiologic displacement between C2 and C3, and less often C3 and C4. Cattell et al. demonstrated a 46% prevalence of C2 and C3 pseudosubluxation on lateral dynamic views in patients <8 years of age. That said, a displacement of >4 mm is an abnormal fiding [4].

Absence of cervical lordosis, a pathologic finding in the adult patient, may be normal variant in some pediatric patients younger than 16. In these patients, an intraspinous distance of 1.5 times the distance of the adjacent intraspinous distances or less confirms stability [4, 50].

Differentiation of true fractures from un-fused physeal line is essential in the evaluation of the pediatric spine. Secondary ossification centers in the spinous processes and unfused ring apophyses of vertebral bodies may mimic fractures on radiographs. Normal physeal plates are smooth, regular areas of radiolucency with underlying subchondral sclerotic lines and occurring at predictable locations. In contrast, acute fractures are irregular, without sclerosis, and occur at any location within the C-spine [32, 50].

12.4 Specific Injury Patterns

12.4.1 Atlanto-Occipital Dislocations

A historically fatal injury, current management protocols have decreased the mortality associated with these injuries. These protocols include improved resuscitation at the scene of injury, early immobilization, high index of suspicion, and improved diagnostic modalities. These injuries often result from a rapid deceleration during an MVA. The head is hyperflexed relative to the torso resulting in dislocation of the atlanto-occipital joint. The lack of inherent bony stability of the atlanto-occipital joint, and ligamentous laxity of the pediatric cervical spine, predisposes the young child to this injury. Three types of atlanto-occipital dislocation (AOD) have been described. Type 1 involves anterior displacement of the occiput relative to the atlas, type 2 describes longitudinal displacement of the occiput from the atlas and type 3 describes a posterior displacement [59].

The paired semilunar occipital condyles located at the inferior surface of the cranium articulate with the concave lateral masses of C1. At birth, the surfaces of the lateral masses are relatively flat and progressively become more concave with age. This absence of bony articular congruence contributes to the increased risk of atlanto-occipital instability in the young pediatric patient.

Numerous ligaments provide atlanto-occipital stability. The tectorial membrane, a cranial extension of the posterior longitudinal ligament, attaches C1 to the anterior surface of the foramen magnum. Deep to the tectorial ligament are the paired alar and apical ligaments. These ligaments originate from the dens, with the former attaching to the medial aspects of the occipital condyles and the latter attaching to the foramen magnum. The tectorial, alar, and apical ligaments constitute the major stabilizers of the atlanto-occipital joint. The tectorial membrane limits extension, while odontoid impaction on the basion limits flexion. The

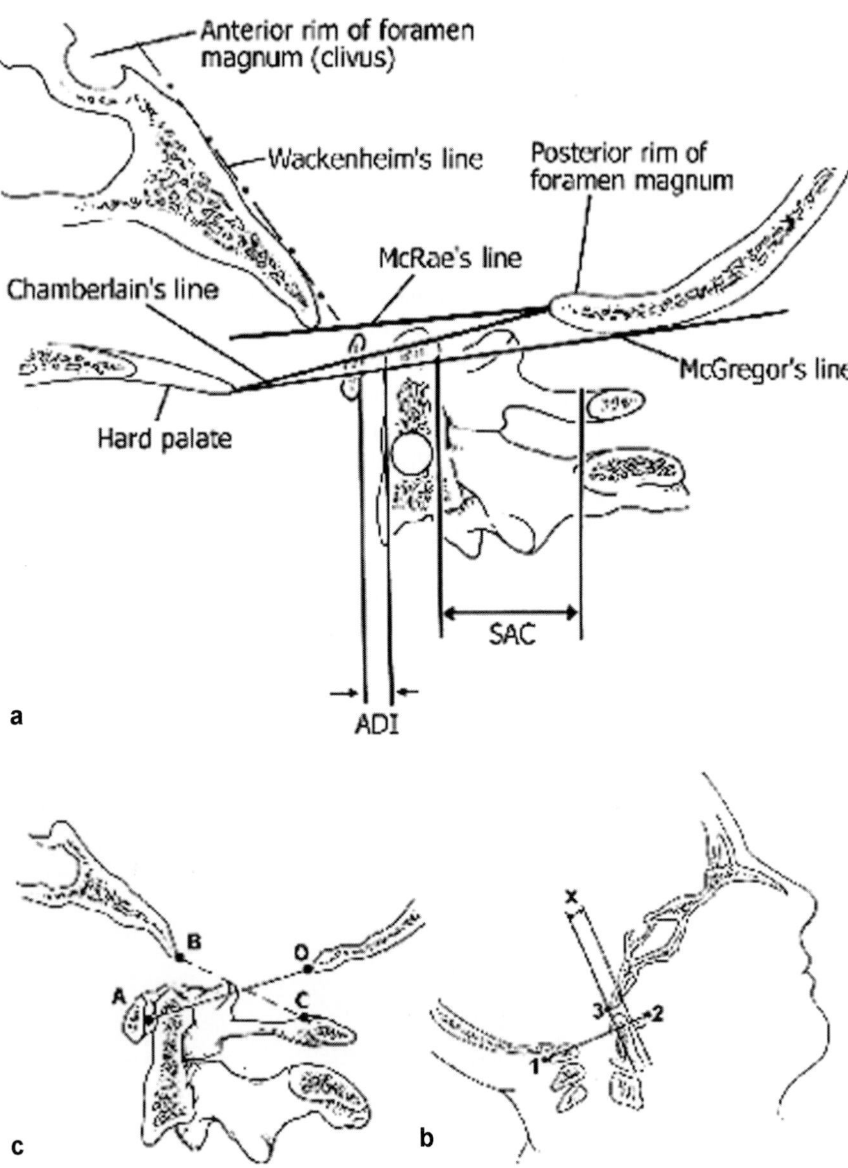

Fig. 12.2 Lateral craniometry. (**a**) The lines commonly used to determine basilar impression and the measurements for determining atlantoaxial instability. *ADI* atlanto-odontoid interval; *SAC* space available for cord. (**b**) Method of measuring atlanto-occipital instability according to Wiesel and Rothman. [61] The atlantal line joins points 1 and 2. A line perpendicular to the atlantal line is made at the posterior margin of the anterior arch of the atlas. The distance (*x*) from the basion (3) to the perpendicular line should not vary by 1 mm or more in flexion and extension. (**c**) The ratio of powers is determined by drawing a line from the basion (B) to the posterior arch of the atlas (C) and a second line from the opisthion (O) to the anterior arch of the atlas (A). The length of line BC is divided by the length of line OA. A ratio of 1.0 or greater is diagnostic of anterior occipitoatlantal dislocation. (Reprinted with permission from Dormans [32])

alar ligaments limit lateral bending. Both the alar ligaments and tectorial membranes limit distraction [57].

The patient with AOD is often polytraumatized with numerous associated injuries including head injuries. Hemodynamic instability, often secondary to neurogenic shock, is a common finding. On presentation, the patients may be intubated and on pressors. The earlier clinical state often conceals the presence of an AOD and prevents a comprehensive neurological examination. High clinical suspicion is therefore needed to diagnose AODs and optimize management. Patients often present with quadriplegia or quadraparesis. In addition, cranial nerve palsies, especially the 6, 9–12th is often present. The lower CN palsies may be secondary to stretch injury, while the 6th palsy may result from head injury. The vertebral arteries may also be injured [6, 24, 44].

Plain radiographs are the mainstay in the evaluation of patients with AOD. Powers ratio, the Wackenheim line, and the occipitocondylar distance are radiographic parameters used in the evaluation of atlanto-occipital instability. On the lateral view, the Wackenheim line is drawn along the clivus and tangentially intersects the tip of the odontoid. Anterior or posterior displacement of this line relative to the odontoid signifies a corresponding displacement of the occiput on the axial spine. The occipital condylar distance defines the distance between the occipital condylar facet and the C1 facet. A distance greater than 5 mm signifies disruption of the atlanto-occipital joint (see Fig. 12.2) [32, 50, 59].

CT scan is a sensitive method of evaluating atlanto-occipital instability. Fine-cut CT with coronal and sagittal reconstruction clearly demonstrates malalignment of the atlanto-occipital joints. MRI has also been utilized to evaluate atlanto-occipital instability. It provides excellent visualizations of the ligaments and soft tissue structures above the atlanto-occipital joint. Visualization of a complete defect of the tectorial membrane on MRI is diagnostic of AOD. Furthermore, injuries to the spinal cord can be visualized on MRI [57].

As with all polytraumatized patients, ventilation should be optimized and hemodynamic stability maintained. The C-spine should be immobilized in a neutral position. Use of cervical traction remains controversial with some advocating its utility in type 1 and type 3 injuries. That said, cervical traction has no role in the management of type 2 injuries because alignment is adequate [16, 24, 44, 57].

Definitive management of AOD is controversial with many authors advocating early posterior fusion. Techniques described in the literature include contoured loop fixation, atlantoaxial transarticular screw placement, and wire fixation with bone grafting. Two techniques using wire fixation and autologous iliac crest graft or rib grafts have been described. Both the procedures require the use of cables or wires affixed to two burr holes drilled on the occiput. In the former, a single shaped iliac graft is attached to a trough prepared at the base of the occiput and to the spinous process of the axis. In the latter procedure, paired autologous rib grafts, with a natural curve resembling the spinal anatomy are harvested, and fixed to the occiput and axis with sub-laminar wires (Fig. 12.3a–d) [6, 13, 24].

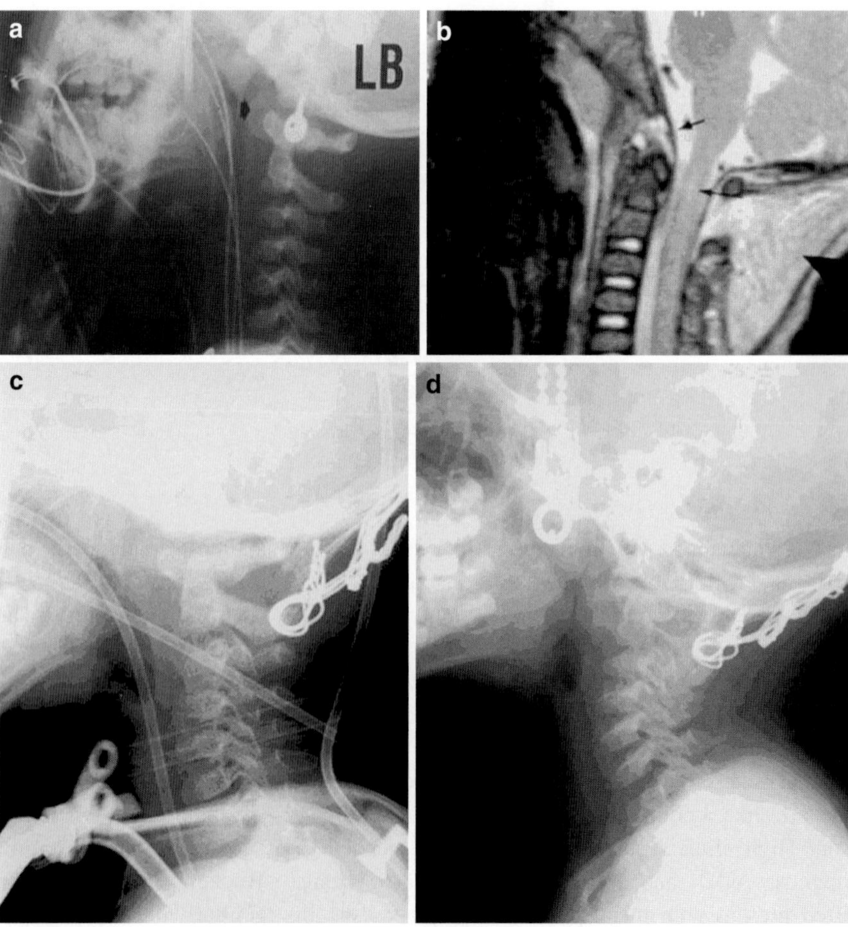

Fig. 12.3 A 1-year-old male pedestrian stuck presenting with the AOD. (**a**) Lateral C-spine radiographs showing an AOD and atlanto-axial disruption. (**b**) T2 MRI demonstrating spinal cord contusion. (**c** and **d**). Post op (12 weeks and 55 weeks after posterior fusion) radiographs showing normal alignment and graft consolidation. (Reprinted with permission from Hosalkar [24])

Factors favoring a decision to proceed with immediate posterior fusion include 3 years of age or later, and a complete AOD with neurological deficits. Some have, however, recommended initial nonoperative management with an orthosis as it is believed that the pediatric spine has a higher repair capacity. Healing can thus be obtained without instrumentation. Because of the technical difficulties involved in instrumentation of the very immature spine, and the high healing capacity of very young children, non-operative management is often a viable option in this population. Nonoperative management may also be indicated in patients with incomplete injuries [6, 13, 20, 24, 37, 57].

12.4.2 Fractures of the Atlas

Fractures of the atlas, classically the Jefferson fracture, are uncommon injuries in the pediatric population. It is usually secondary to an axial compression load resulting from a fall onto the top of the head or after a motor vehicular crash. Force is transmitted from the occiput to the lateral masses, resulting in a fracture at the weakest point of the atlas. This is usually the anterior or posterior arch. Diastasis of the lateral masses can also result in avulsion of the transverse ligament, leading to atlantoaxial instability. Current studies show a 6.9-mm displacement of the lateral masses, suggest a transverse ligament rupture, which result in instability [7, 31, 56].

Pediatric patients with a fracture at the atlas usually present with neck pain, cervical muscle spasm, torticolis, and reduction in range of motion. Neurologic deficits are uncommon with C1 fractures. Though the earlier mentioned signs and symptoms are nonspecific, they should raise the index of suspicion and prompt assessment for the presence of this fracture pattern [1].

Isolated fractures of C1 is often absent on plain radiographs. Findings suggestive of these fractures include a prevertebral hematoma on the lateral cervical spine views, or separation of the lateral masses on an odontoid view. A CT scan of the C-spine and MRI is needed for accurate diagnosis of these fractures (Fig. 12.4a, b) [27, 31, 56].

There are few reports of isolated pediatric C1 ring fractures in the literature and conservative management of these fractures with external immobilization seem to be the consensus recommended treatment. Successful use of soft cervical color, halo vest, and rigid cervical collar for varied duration has been documented. Recovery of full function and return to activities is expected with conservative management [1, 26, 27, 29, 54].

12.4.3 Odontoid Fractures

Odontoid fractures are common in the pediatric population. Like most cervical spine injuries in this population, the cause of injury often involves an MVC or a fall from height. Odontoid fractures usually occur at the base of the dens at the synchondrosis. The weak synchondrosis and the relatively large head size of the young pediatric patient predispose this location to injury.

The clinical presentation of patients with odontoid fractures can range from neck pain to significant spinal cord injuries. Fasset et al. [18] demonstrated 33% incidence of neurologic deficits in patients presenting with odontoid fractures. When present, spinal cord injuries

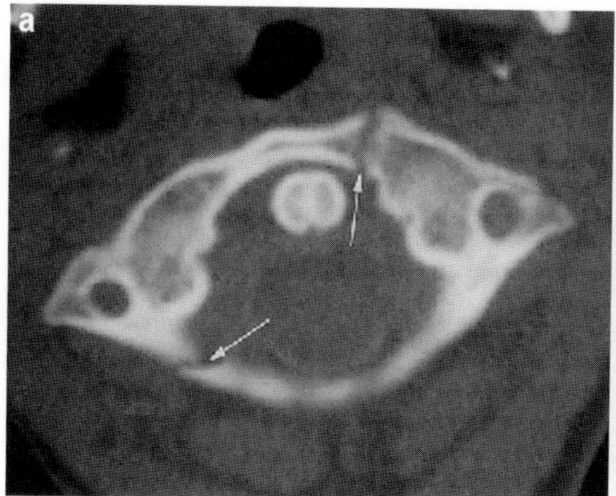

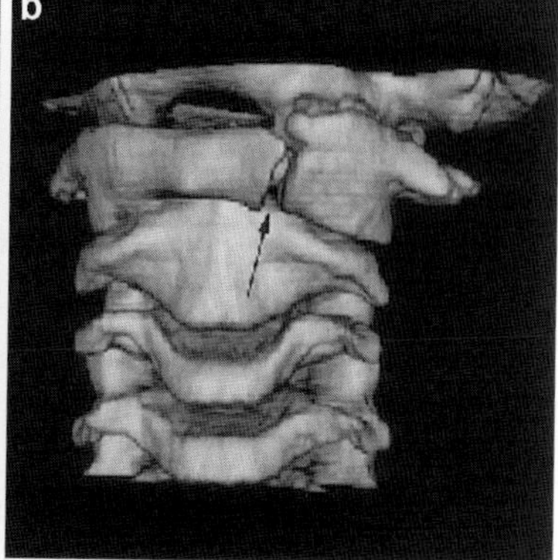

Fig. 12.4 Axial CT scan through C1 (**a**) and three-dimensional reformatted CT scan of the upper cervical-spine (**b**) obtained in a 6-year-old boy showing anterior and posterior ring fractures of C1 (*arrows*). (Reprinted with permission from Lustrin et al. [32])

(SCI) tend to occur at the cervicothoracic junction. It has been proposed that this may be secondary to a traction injury of the cord resulting from hyperflexion [36]. In the Fasset et al. series [18] series, 53% of SCIs occurred at the cervicothoracic level.

Radiographic evaluation of odontoid fractures begins with a plain radiograph of the C-spine. On the lateral view, anterior angulation or displacement of the dens is often apparent. A CT scan with a sagittal and 3-D reconstruction may be needed to further delineate the fracture site and demonstrate diastasis of the synchondroses. In equivocal cases, MRI imaging can be useful. Soft tissue changes at the C1 and C2 levels combined with a high signal at the synchondroses in the appropriate clinical setting suggest a fracture [18, 32, 52].

Odontoid fractures can be managed nonoperatively. Closed reduction can be obtained with extension or hyperextension of the C-spine (Fig. 12.5). Fifty percent apposition of the fracture segment is usually sufficient for healing. The C-spine is subsequently immobilized in a halo vest or pinless halo for 6–8 weeks. Frequent radiographic follow-up is required to insure stability is maintained. Fasset et al. showed a fusion rate of 93% with conservative management. Operative management is indicated in fractures where reduction is not obtained with external immobilization, or with nonunion (no evidence of healing after 3–6 months). Viable surgical options include posterior C1 and C2 fusion with bone grafting and wiring. Motion-sparing procedures have not been proven to be efficacious in the pediatric population [18].

12.4.4 Hangman's Fracture

Traumatic spondylolisthesis is extremely rare in the pediatric population with only a few cases reported. It occurs most commonly in children 2 years of age and or less. Various factors account for this pattern of injury in the developing spine. As indicated earlier, the relatively large head-to-body ratio of the young child localizes fulcrum of flexion over the upper cervical spine. This is further compounded by relative ligamentous laxity and weak neck muscles of the young child. That said, injury results from cervical hyperextension [47, 59].

Radiological diagnosis of pediatric Hangman's fracture is complicated by unique features of the pediatric spine, as discussed earlier. Hangman's fractures involve fractures of the pars interarticularis and anterolisthesis of C2 on C3. Evaluation of the pediatric Hangman's fracture begins with standard plain radiographic views, with CT and MRI reserved for more detailed evaluation. On radiographs, a radiolucent line can be observed anterior to the pedicles of the axis. Pathologic anterior displacement of C2 is likely, if the tip of the spinous process of C2 is greater than 2 mm anterior to a line (Swischuk's line) connecting the spinous processes of C1–C3 (see Fig. 12.2) [13, 59].

The Levine classification system for traumatic spondylolisthesis can be extrapolated to the pediatric population. Type 1 injury describes 3 mm or less translation between C2 and C3 without angulation. In type 2 injuries, there is greater than 3 mm of translation between C2 and C3 and greater than 10° angulation.

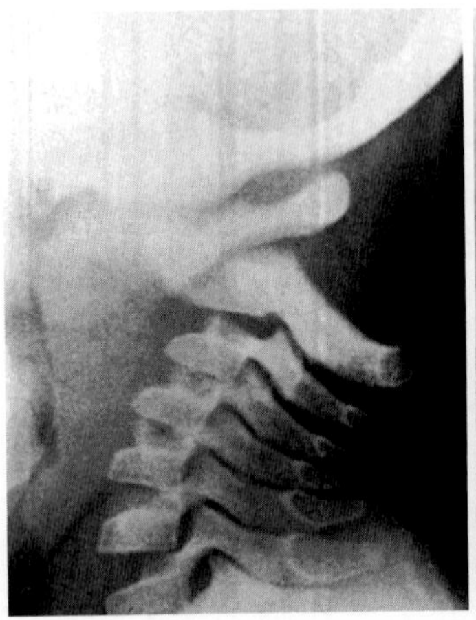
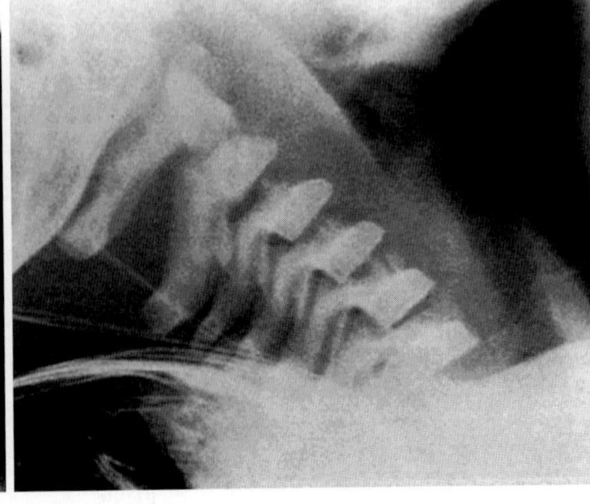

Fig. 12.5 Lateral C-spine radiographs of a young child with a severely displaced odontoid fracture after a fall. The second image shows a reduced fracture with hyperextension. (Reprinted with permission from Sherk et al. [53])

Type 3 fractures include the characteristics of type 2 fractures as well as bilateral facet dislocation and have greater angular components [30].

Management of nondisplaced Hangman's fracture is conservative with immobilization in a halo ring and vest or pinless halo. Levine type 3 fractures are managed surgically with open reduction and posterior fusion [59].

12.4.5 Atlanto-axial Subluxation

Injuries of the atlanto-axial joint include ligamentous disruptions resulting in instability and odontoid fractures. The atlanto-axial joint is a relatively mobile joint with 50% of cervical rotation occurring at this joint. Furthermore, its diameter, one-third occupied by the dens, one-third by the spinal cord, and one-third by sub-arachnoid space allows for significant cervical motion before cord injury [32, 42].

Atlanto-axial subluxation is most often secondary to infection or trauma. Upper respiratory infections, retropharyngeal abscesses are common causes of atlanto-axial instability. However, it also results from trauma in ~20–45% of the patients [9, 59].

Children with atlanto-axial subluxation present with torticollis, with the chin rotated to one side and head extended to the contralateral side. In addition, there is spasm of the sternocleidomastoid muscle opposite to the side of chin rotation. They will typically report headaches and neck pain. In a fixed subluxation, rotation of the atlanto-axial joint is prevented or limited by impingement of the C1 facet joint on C2. An attempt at manual reduction of the deformity is usually painful. Neurological deficits are the exception [9, 42, 44].

Radiographic assessment of patients presenting with suspected atlanto-axial dislocation include standard cervical spine series complemented with a CT scan. In the absence of neurological findings, MRI have minimal role in the evaluation of these patients. Findings indicative of subluxation on lateral radiographs include absence of a defined craniocervical junction and lack of orientation of the anterior arch in a true lateral plane. On the AP plane, the anteriorly subluxated lateral mass may appear wider and more proximal to the mid line, while the opposite mass appears farther and smaller. Significant displacement is however unlikely in the presence of a normal ADI. Plain radiography is often difficult to interpret because of the malaligned position of the head (Fig. 12.6a–d) [32, 59].

Fielding and Hawkins [19] classified atlanto-axial rotatory *subluxation* (AARS) into four categories. Type 1, the most common shows no displacement of C1 and a normal ADI. It results from unilateral facet subluxation without disruption of the transverse ligament. Type 2 demonstrates a greater than 3–5 mm anterior displacement with compromise of the transverse ligament. Type 3 describes bilateral facet dislocation associated with complete rupture of the transverse ligament. It is manifested by a >5 mm ADI. Type 4 demonstrates posterior displacement of C1 and is rare.

Atlanto-axial rotatory *fixation* (AARF) can be demonstrated with a dynamic CT. A fixated C1 and C2 unit rotates as one on a CT obtained at rest, and with attempted neck rotation. It results from an untreated AARS [32].

Management of atlanto-axial rotatory subluxation may involve conservative management or in rare instances surgical stabilization. Often, mild subluxations may reduce spontaneously and patients do not present for formal intervention. Patients presenting with symptoms of <1 week duration can be treated with a soft cervical collar, NSAIDS and muscle relaxants. If symptoms have persisted for >1 week, patients may be treated with head halter traction, supplemented with muscle relaxants and analgesics. Conservative therapy is unlikely to be successful in patients presenting with symptoms persisting for >1month. In this setting, reduction can be attempted with a halo traction or manual manipulation under anesthesia. If successful, the patient can be immobilized in a halo vest for 6 weeks. If this modality is unsuccessful surgery may be indicated. Surgery is also indicated in the presence of persistent instability, neurological deficits and may include bilateral facet reduction with fusion. The atlanto-axial joint may also be fused in a subluxated position [45, 59].

12.4.6 Spinal Cord Injury Without Radiographic Abnormalities

Spinal cord injury without radiological abnormalities is a relatively prevalent injury in the pediatric population. Its incidence has been estimated from 4% to as high as 67% of all pediatric spinal traumas [3, 39]. Anatomic and biomechanical features already described earlier predispose the developing spine to SCIWORA. The

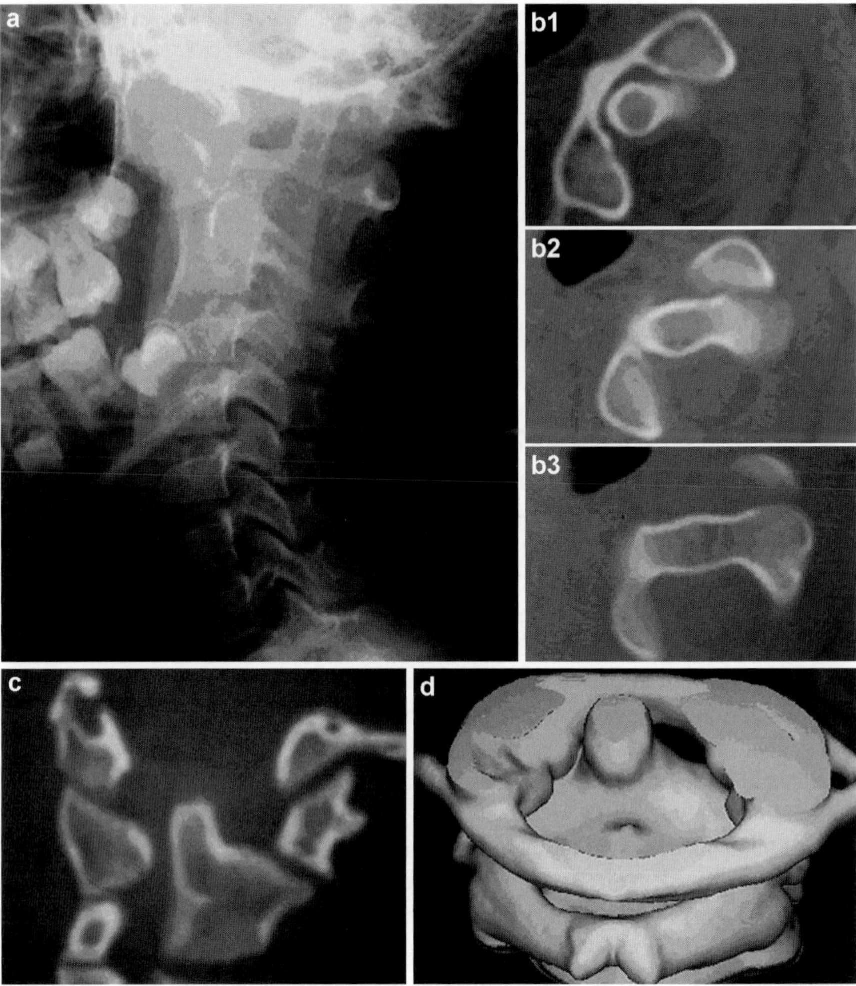

Fig. 12.6 Lateral radiograph of the cervical spine (**a**), axial CT scans (**b**), coronal CT scan (**c**), and 3D reformatted CT scan (**d**) through C1 and C2 in a 12-year-old girl with atlantoaxial rotatory subluxation. (Reprinted with permission from Lustrin [32])

osseous and ligamentous structures of the spinal column are laxer than the spinal cord. Consequently, these structures can undergo significant deformation without failure. The underlying spinal cord may however be injured in these settings. Biomechanical studies have shown the bony and soft tissue structures can stretch for ~2 inches before failure. The cord however can be ruptured after 0.25 inches of displacement. SCIWORA results from transient traction or compression of the spinal cord resulting from cervical hyperextension or hyperflexion. Hyperextension of the spine results in compression of the cord by the ligamentum flavum, while flexion results in a traction injury to the spinal cord [32, 59].

MRI is the study of choice for the patient presenting with spinal cord injury without evidence of trauma on plain radiograph and CT. Cord edema or hemorrhage, soft tissue or ligamentous injury, and apophyseal endplate translation are radiographic findings indicative of SCIWORA. However, MRI may also be negative [59].

In the absence of osseous abnormalities, or mechanical instability, management of SCIWORA involves prolonged rigid immobilization for 2–3 months. If instability is noted, surgical stabilization may be necessary. Prognosis following SCIWORA is dependent on status at presentation. Younger children with high energy injuries typically present with more significant cord injuries as compared to the adolescent patient with injuries secondary to athletic activities [3, 59].

12.5 Cervical Spine Injuries Outcomes

Platzer et al. [43] reported a 66% incidence of neurologic deficits in a study of 56 pediatric patients with cervical spine injury over a 25-year period. Complete recovery of neurological function occurred in 68% of these patients. A 75% mortality rate was reported in patients with complete spinal injuries. The overall mortality rate in this series was 27%. In their series of 103 consecutive C-spine injuries, Brown et al. [3] reported a mortality of 18.5%. In this series, 18% of patients required operative intervention with the most common indication being instability. Closed head injuries were often associated with cervical spine injury and were a significant adverse prognostic factor. In the same series, Brown et al. reported a mortality rate of 49% in the presence of closed head injuries.

In a large multicenter review of cervical spine injuries, n = 1,098, Patel et al. [41] noted a 35% incidence of spinal cord injury. Of these, 50% were SCIWORAs, and 76% of these patients had incomplete injuries with 24% suffering complete neurologic injuries. Complete neurologic injury was a significant predictor of mortality; 53% of patients with complete neurologic injuries died. In contrast, a 15% mortality rate was noted in patients without neurological deficits, and 16% for those patients with incomplete deficits. Overall mortality was 17% [41].

12.6 Thoracolumbar Fractures

12.6.1 Epidemiology

Thoracolumbar injuries in the pediatric population occur primarily in children between the ages of 14 and 16. The most common location is T4–T12 and then T12–L2. In a retrospective review of 610 cases of pediatric spine injuries in adolescents, the majority (63%) of injuries occurred in males [5]. Most of the injuries occurred during sporting activities (53%), and then MVC (26%). Falls accounted for 13% of the injuries. Fractures occurred in 67% of these cases with 26% incidence of neurological injuries. Child abuse also accounts for some thoracolumbar fractures in infants and younger children. Types of injuries associated with battering and shaking include fractures of the spinous processes, pars, pedicles, or compression fractures of multiple vertebral bodies [5].

12.6.2 Anatomy

Anatomic differences between the immature thoracolumbar spine and the adult spine result in different patterns of injury. As with the subaxial cervical spine, each thoracolumbar spine has three centers of ossification, one centrum and two neural arches. Fusion typically occurs between the ages of 2 and 6. The facet joints of the thoracolumbar spine are more horizontally oriented and incompletely ossified resulting in increased intervertebral mobility. The articular facets begin to attain a mature configuration at the age of 8 with complete adult orientation occurring at the age of 15 [5].

The developing vertebral body consists of two physes located at the superior and inferior end plates. The physes becomes apparent radiographically between the ages of 8 and 12 when apophyseal ossification begins to occur at the cartilaginous end plates. At this time, the end plate is bordered superiorly by hyaline cartilage subjacent to the overlying nucleus and inferiorly by physeal cartilage. Fusion begins at the age 14–15, and physeal lines may be misinterpreted as fractures until the age of 15–21 when complete fusion occurs. Before 12 years of age, the pediatric vertebra has significant remodeling potential after compression fractures. If the wedging deformity is <30°, physeal injury is avoided and complete reconstitution of vertebral morphology can occur. However, a more significant deformity causing physeal injury may result in a deformed vertebral body during the adolescent growth spurt [5].

12.6.3 Mechanisms of Injury

Three main mechanisms of injury, flexion with or without compression, distraction, and shear occur in children, with hyperflexion being the most common. Hyperflexion results in failure of the anterior column with preservation of the middle column. Although the posterior column may remain intact, a distraction injury may occur with greater degrees of flexion. Fractures resulting from hyperflexion most commonly occur at LI. More significant forces may result in a burst fracture. A burst fractures involves failure of the anterior and middle columns as a result of axial loading. The posterior cortex of the vertebral body is fractured with retropulsion of fragments into the spinal canal. An increase in the interpedicular distance on plain radiograph typifies this fracture pattern [11, 54].

Distraction injuries usually occur during rapid automobile deceleration in a restricted patient (seat belt injury). In this injury pattern, the posterior and middle columns are distracted as the torso is hyperflexed over a lap belt. This results in tension injury to the posterior ligamentous and bony structures. Compression loading may also result in fracture of the vertebral apophysis. This injury is common in the adolescent population and is discussed at length in the sports section. That said, it most commonly occurs at the L4 level and is diagnosed with CT and MRI [5, 44, 55].

12.6.4 Clinical Evaluation

Comprehensive evaluation of the pediatric patient presenting with thoracolumbar injuries should include institution of the pediatric ATLS protocols. These injuries are often a result of significant trauma such as motor vehicular accidents and associated extraspinal injuries are frequent. A comprehensive history should be obtained when possible. The lucid pediatric patient with thoracolumbar injury will report back pain and should be able to localize the pain. Mechanism of injury, spinal maturity, time of injury, presence of neurologic complaints, and associated extraspinal symptoms should be ascertained. A systematic physical examination includes assessment of the airway, breathing, circulation, presence of disability, and the ABCDs of ATLS. This prevents omission of associated injuries.

Subtle spinal injuries are often missed or diagnosed late in the polytraumatized patient. Evaluation of the spine begins with a careful neurological examination. Initial evaluation for sensation at all the four extremities includes assessing for perception of light touch. The patient should also be instructed to move his/her fingers and toes. Inspection of the back occurs during the log roll. Bruising, swelling, or deformity over the spine should be noted. The entire spine should be palpated for tenderness and deformity. A rectal examination should also be performed paying particular attention to rectal tone. The bulbocavernosus reflex should be elicited as its absence may indicate the presence of spinal shock. Perianal sensation should be assessed.

A formal neurologic examination should be performed in all the patients with suspected injury to the spine. Perception of pain in a dermatomal fashion should be assessed. Reflex testing of the upper and lower extremities should be performed and strength should be graded in a myotomal fashion. Injury to the spine should be suspected in patients with abdominal seat belt abrasions.

Historically, patients with neurologic deficits have been administered intravenous methylprednisolone to minimize cord edema. Patients presenting within 3 h of injury are given 30 mg/kg bolus over 15 min for the first hour, followed by an infusion of 5.4 mg/kg/h for 23 h. Treatment should be extended for an additional 24 h if treatment is started within 3–8 h from injury [2]. Recent studies have, however, questioned the efficacy of the earlier regiment. Sayer et al. [51] in a systematic review of current literature, found insufficient evidence to support the use of methylprednisolone in acute spinal cord injuries.

12.6.5 Radiographic Evaluation

Most vertebral fractures can be visualized on plain radiographs; however, CT scan may be needed to further define the character of these fractures (Fig. 12.7). CT is especially useful in the evaluation of the spinal canal after a burst fracture. In cases where neurologic deficit is present, an MRI should be obtained to assess the extent of cord injury. On T2 weighed images, a high

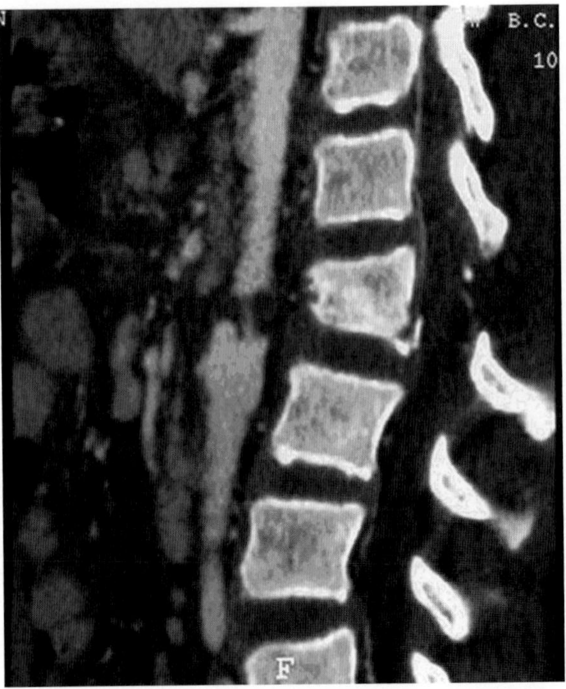

Fig. 12.7 Sagittal CT scan demonstrating a flexiondistraction injury associated with abdominal aortic dissection in a 9-year-old child. (Reprinted with permission from Reilly [48])

signal suggests cord edema, a mixed signal indicates contusion and, a low signal acute hemorrhage [5].

Radiographic studies can be used to assess for stability in the injured thoracolumbar spine. Findings indicative of instability on radiographs include vertebral body collapse with widening of the pedicles, >33% canal compromise by fragments of the lamina or middle column, translation of more than 2.5 mm between vertebral bodies in any plane, bilateral facet dislocation, significant distraction of the posterior components with greater than 50% collapse of the vertebral body. Presence of neurologic deficits also suggests spinal instability. On plain radiographs, disruption of two or more columns indicates instability. However, fractures involving more than 2 columns cephalad to T8 can be stable, if the sternum and ribs are intact. Integrity of the sternocostal joint tends to stabilize the thoracic vertebra. In addition, fractures at L4 and L5 can be stable if the posterior elements are intact and if normal lumbar lordosis is maintained [5, 11, 60].

Absence of neurologic deficits in a patient who is able to ambulate after injury usually suggests a stable fracture. However, it should be noted that even in the absence of neurologic injuries, a fracture may be unstable if there is evidence progression of deformity will occur. These fractures include hyperflexion compression fractures where the posterior ligamentous structures are disrupted. This is reflected on plain radiographs by a greater than 50% deformity of the anterior column, with an intact middle column. Greater than 20° of flexion of L1 on L2 also indicates disruption of the posterior ligamentous structures. In burst type fractures with compromise of the middle column and retropulsed fragments, neurological insult may occur if axial load is applied prematurely before healing. Consequently, these fractures are considered unstable even in the absence of neurological deficits at presentation [5].

12.6.5.1 Management

Stable injuries of the spine in an adolescent can be managed nonoperatively. Nonoperative management in this setting includes bed rest, adequate analgesia, and spasmolytics for muscle spasms. After adequate analgesia is obtained, mobilization in a thoracolumbosacral orthosis is started and continued for 6 weeks. Fractures amenable to this treatment include minor spinous process fractures, transverse process fractures, wedge compression fractures, and chance fractures. Chance fractures require hyperextension casting/bracing for 8–12 weeks [5].

Burst fractures can also be treated conservatively in the absence of neurologic compromise. Integrity of the posterior ligamentous structures especially the posterior longitudinal ligament must be ascertained before nonsurgical management is instituted. Treatment involves early mobilization in a TLSO brace. The disadvantages of conservative management in this setting include protracted immobilization and hospital stay. Rarely when surgery poses a significant risk, unstable fractures maybe managed conservatively. This involves 6–10 weeks of bed rest and subsequent immobilization in a TLSO brace for a similar length. The fracture should be assessed frequently with standing radiographs for change in position [15].

Expeditious surgery is indicated in the presence of mechanical instability or neurological deficits. Ultimate outcome is optimized when surgical intervention is expedited. It is recommended that decompression and reduction should be performed within 12–48 h after injury. The length of instrumentation should be minimized but be adequate for stabilization and correction of the deformity. Pedicle screws, hook, and rod constructs one level above and below the fractured level have been utilized. Indirect reduction of retropulsed fragments is possible with distraction if the posterior longitudinal ligament is intact. In the immature spine, the displaced fragments are often attached to the PLL and can be reduced with traction. Surgical management of unstable chance fractures involve compression fixation of the posterior elements, to facilitate ligamentous healing. Severe burst fractures with >40% canal compromise, >15° of kyphosis may require anterior fusion [5, 15].

12.6.6 Outcome Studies for Thoracic and Lumbar Spine Trauma in Pediatric Patients

As in the adult population, favorable outcomes have been reported for stable fractures of the thoracic and lumbar spine managed nonoperatively [12, 33, 40]. Parisini et al. [40] recently reported the outcomes of 44 pediatric and adolescent patients treated for spinal trauma. Of these, 29 involved the thoracic and lumbar spine; 58% of these fractures were unstable. Of the 12 unstable fractures, 41% had spinal cord injuries. Favorable outcomes, absence of significant deformity, persistent stability, were reported in stable fractures managed conservatively. Likewise, Dogan et al. [12] reviewed the outcomes of 89 pediatric patients treated for thoracic, lumbar, and sacral spine injuries. A majority of these patients (85.4%) were neurologically intact at presentation. Neurological deficits were more common in patients with injuries at the thoracic level (53.8%). A majority of the patients were treated conservatively with a 12.6% average loss of vertebral body height at subsequent follow-up. Moller et al. [34] supported the earlier findings in a long-term outcome of 30 adolescent patients with thoracic and lumbar fractures managed nonoperatively [34].

Contrary to the earlier findings, conservative management of unstable burst fractures, even in the absence of neurological deficits, yielded unfavorable outcomes. In the Parisini et al. series [40], conservative management of unstable fractures without neurological deficits in the thoracic and lumbar spine resulted in significant deformity at 4 months follow-up. An average of 18–20° of global kyphosis was noted in the four patients with unstable fractures of the thoracic and lumbar spine managed conservatively. That said, equivocal outcomes have been reported with surgical management of unstable thoracolumbar fractures. Parisini et al. [40] reported a high incidence of subsequent progressive deformity in unstable fractures managed surgically regardless of neurological status at presentation. Six of the nine patients with unstable thoracic and lumbar spine fractures managed surgically had significant spinal deformity at follow-up. Dogan et al. [12] however showed a low incidence of progressive deformity (8.6%) in patients managed surgically in his series.

Of note is the high incidence of spinal deformity in patients with neurological injury before puberty. In Parisini et al. series, 72% of patients with neurological deficits proceeded to develop significant scoliosis and or kyphosis regardless of management. This is consistent with the >90% incidence of post-SCI deformity reported in the literature. Deformity in this setting has been attributed to impaired muscular function [10, 28, 40].

12.7 Conclusion

In conclusion, spinal trauma though rare in the pediatric population can have devastating consequences. Clinicians treating trauma in the immature spine should be cognizant

Table 12.1 American Academy of Pediatrics Car Safety Seats Guideline for Growing Children

Weight (pounds)	Car safety seat recommendation
0–30	Infant only seat, rear facing, never in front seat with passenger-side air bag. Car bed if medically indicated
5–40	Convertible safety seat, rear facing until child is at least 20 lb, then forward facing to the maximum weight and height allowed by seat
20–80	Combination seat with internal harness that transitions to a belt-positioning booster seat; forward facing only, weight varies.
	Forward facing seat with internal harness; weight varies.
	Integrated child seat: toddler seat with harness (20–40 lb) or some as belt-positioning booster seat with lap/shoulder belt (> 30–50 lb), as long as child fits.
30–80	Belt-positioning booster seat with lap/shoulder belt as long as child fits

of the anatomic and biomechanical features that account for the pattern of injuries seen in this population. Furthermore, the relative high prevalence of SCIWORA in this population underscores the need for comprehensive history and physical examination. Prompt diagnosis of neurologic deficits and expeditious management in the setting of trauma enhances outcomes.

An emphasis should be placed on prevention. As indicated earlier, motor vehicular accidents in the young child (typically unrestrained) and sports injuries in the adolescents are the most common mechanisms of injury in the pediatric population. Attempts at prevention should therefore be mechanism directed. Proper use of seatbelts and child safety seats should be encouraged (Table 12.1) [53]. In the adolescent athlete, use of appropriate sporting equipments such as helmets, as well as rules targeted at safety should be instituted. Furthermore, proper conditioning with attention to strengthening of paraspinal muscle groups should be encouraged. Proper and safe techniques such as avoidance of head-first tackling should also be practiced [57].

References

1. Bayar MA, Erdem Y, Ozturk K et al (2002) Isolated anterior arch fracture of the atlas: child case report. Spine 27:E47–E49

2. Bracken MB, Shepard MJ, Holford TR et al (1998) Methylprednisolone or tirilazad mesylate administration after acute spinal cord injury: 1-year follow up. Results of the third National Acute Spinal Cord Injury randomized controlled trial. J Neurosurg 89:699–706
3. Brown RL, Brunn MA, Garcia VF (2001) Cervical spine injuries in children: a review of 103 patients treated consecutively at a level 1 pediatric trauma center. J Pediatr Surg 36:1107–1114
4. Cattell HS, Filtzer DL (1965) Pseudosubluxation and other normal variations in the cervical spine in children. A study of one hundred and sixty children. J Bone Joint Surg Am 47:1295–1309
5. Clark P, Letts M (2001) Trauma to the thoracic and lumbar spine in the adolescent. Can J Surg 44:337–345
6. Cohen MW, Drummond DS, Flynn JM et al (2001) A technique of occipitocervical arthrodesis in children using autologous rib grafts. Spine 26:825–829
7. Copley LA, Dormans JP (1998) Cervical spine disorders in infants and children. J Am Acad Orthop Surg 6:204–214
8. Copley LA, Dormans JP, Pepe MD et al (2003) Accuracy and reliability of torque wrenches used for halo application in children. J Bone Joint Surg Am 85:2199–2204
9. d'Amato C (2005) Pediatric spinal trauma: injuries in very young children. Clin Orthop Relat Res 432:34–40
10. Dearolf WW III, Betz RR, Vogel LC et al (1990) Scoliosis in pediatric spinal cord-injured patients. J Pediatr Orthop 10:214–218
11. Denis F (1983) The three column spine and its significance in the classification of acute thoracolumbar spinal injuries. Spine 8:817–831
12. Dogan S, Safavi-Abbasi S, Theodore N et al (2007) Thoracolumbar and sacral spinal injuries in children and adolescents: a review of 89 cases. J Neurosurg 106(6 Suppl): 426–433
13. Dormans JP (2002) Evaluation of children with suspected cervical spine injury. J Bone Joint Surg Am 84:124–132
14. Dormans JP, Criscitiello AA, Drummond DS et al (1995) Complications in children managed with immobilization in a halo vest. J Bone Joint Surg Am 77:1370–1373
15. Edwards CC, Levine AM (1986) Early rod-sleeve stabilization of the injured thoracic and lumbar spine. Orthop Clin North Am 17:121–145
16. Eismont FJ, Bohlman HH (1978) Posterior atlanto-occipital dislocation with fractures of the atlas and odontoid process. J Bone Joint Surg Am 60:397–399
17. Farley FA, Hensinger RN, Herzenberg JE (1992) Cervical spinal cord injury in children. J Spinal Disord 5:410–416
18. Fassett DR, McCall T, Brockmeyer DL (2006) Odontoid synchondrosis fractures in children. Neurosurg Focus 20:E7
19. Fielding JW, Hawkins RJ (1977) Atlanto-axial rotatory fixation. (fixed rotatory subluxation of the atlanto-axial joint). J Bone Joint Surg Am 59:37–44
20. Georgopoulos G, Pizzutillo PD, Lee MS (1987) Occipito-atlantal instability in children. A report of five cases and review of the literature. J Bone Joint Surg Am 69:429–436
21. Hadley MN, Zabramski JM, Browner CM et al (1988) Pediatric spinal trauma. Review of 122 cases of spinal cord and vertebral column injuries. J Neurosurg 68:18–24
22. Hamilton MG, Myles ST (1992) Pediatric spinal injury: review of 174 hospital admissions. J Neurosurg 77:700–704
23. Herzenberg JE, Hensinger RN, Dedrick DK et al (1989) Emergency transport and positioning of young children who have an injury of the cervical spine. The standard backboard may be hazardous. J Bone Joint Surg Am 71: 15–22
24. Hosalkar HS, Cain EL, Horn D et al (2005) Traumatic atlanto-occipital dislocation in children. J Bone Joint Surg Am 87:2480–2488
25. Kokoska ER, Keller MS, Rallo MC et al (2001) Characteristics of pediatric cervical spine injuries. J Pediatr Surg 36:100–105
26. Kontautas E, Ambrozaitis KV, Kalesinskas RJ et al (2005) Management of acute traumatic atlas fractures. J Spinal Disord Tech 18:402–405
27. Korinth MC, Kapser A, Weinzierl MR (2007) Jefferson fracture in a child – illustrative case report. Pediatr Neurosurg 43:526–530
28. Lancourt JE, Dickson JH, Carter RE (1981) Paralytic spinal deformity following traumatic spinal-cord injury in children and adolescents. J Bone Joint Surg Am 63:47–53
29. Lee TT, Green BA, Petrin DR (1998) Treatment of stable burst fracture of the atlas (Jefferson fracture) with rigid cervical collar. Spine 23:1963–1967
30. Levine AM, Edwards CC (1985) The management of traumatic spondylolisthesis of the axis. J Bone Joint Surg Am 67:217–226
31. Levine AM, Edwards CC (1991) Fractures of the atlas. J Bone Joint Surg Am 73:680–691
32. Lustrin ES, Karakas SP, Ortiz AO et al (2003) Pediatric cervical spine: normal anatomy, variants, and trauma. Radiographics 23:539–560
33. McPhee IB (1981) Spinal fractures and dislocations in children and adolescents. Spine 6:533–537
34. Moller A, Hasserius R, Besjakov J et al (2006) Vertebral fractures in late adolescence: a 27 to 47-year follow-up. Eur Spine J 15:1247–1254
35. Nitecki S, Moir CR (1994) Predictive factors of the outcome of traumatic cervical spine fracture in children. J Pediatr Surg 29:1409–1411
36. Odent T, Langlais J, Glorion C et al (1999) Fractures of the odontoid process: a report of 15 cases in children younger than 6 years. J Pediatr Orthop 19:51–54
37. Ogden J (ed) (2000) Skeletal injury in the child, 3rd edn. Springer, New York
38. Osenbach RK, Menezes AH (1992) Pediatric spinal cord and vertebral column injury. Neurosurgery 30:385–390
39. Pang D, Pollack IF (1989) Spinal cord injury without radiographic abnormality in children – the SCIWORA syndrome. J Trauma 29:654–664
40. Parisini P, Di Silvestre M, Greggi T (2002) Treatment of spinal fractures in children and adolescents: long-term results in 44 patients. Spine 27:1989–1994
41. Patel JC, Tepas JJ, 3rd, Mollitt DL et al (2001) Pediatric cervical spine injuries: defining the disease. J Pediatr Surg 36:373–376
42. Phillips WA, Hensinger RN (1989) The management of rotatory atlanto-axial subluxation in children. J Bone Joint Surg Am 71:664–668
43. Platzer P, Jaindl M, Thalhammer G et al (2007) Cervical spine injuries in pediatric patients. J Trauma 62:389–396; discussion 394–386

44. Powers B, Miller MD, Kramer RS et al (1979) Traumatic anterior atlanto-occipital dislocation. Neurosurgery 4:12–17
45. Rahimi SY, Stevens EA, Yeh DJ et al (2003) Treatment of atlantoaxial instability in pediatric patients. Neurosurg Focus 15:ECP1
46. Ralston ME, Chung K, Barnes PD et al (2001) Role of flexion-extension radiographs in blunt pediatric cervical spine injury. Acad Emerg Med 8:237–245
47. Ranjith RK, Mullett JH, Burke TE (2002) Hangman's fracture caused by suspected child abuse. A case report. J Pediatr Orthop B 11:329–332
48. Reilly CW (2007) Pediatric spine trauma. J Bone Joint Surg Am 89(Suppl 1):98–107, review
49. Rekate HL, Theodore N, Sonntag VK et al (1999) Pediatric spine and spinal cord trauma. State of the art for the third millennium. Childs Nerv Syst 15:743–750
50. Roche C, Carty H (2001) Spinal trauma in children. Pediatr Radiol 31:677–700
51. Sayer FT, Kronvall E, Nilsson OG (2006) Methylprednisolone treatment in acute spinal cord injury: the myth challenged through a structured analysis of published literature. Spine J 6:335–343
52. Sherburn EW, Day RA, Kaufman BA et al (1996) Subdental synchondrosis fracture in children: the value of 3-dimensional computerized tomography. Pediatr Neurosurg 25:256–259
53. Sherk HH, Nicholson JT, Chung SM (1978) Fractures of the odontoid process in young children. J Bone Joint Surg Am 60(7):921–924
54. Smith WS, Kaufer H (1969) Patterns and mechanisms of lumbar injuries associated with lap seat belts. J Bone Joint Surg Am 51:239–254
55. Sovio OM, Bell HM, Beauchamp RD et al (1985) Fracture of the lumbar vertebral apophysis. J Pediatr Orthop 5:550–552
56. Spence KF, Jr., Decker S, Sell KW (1970) Bursting atlantal fracture associated with rupture of the transverse ligament. J Bone Joint Surg Am 52:543–549
57. Steinmetz MP, Lechner RM, Anderson JS (2003) Atlantooccipital dislocation in children: presentation, diagnosis, and management. Neurosurg Focus 14:ecp1
58. Sullivan J (1994) Fractures of the spine in children. In: Green N, Swiontkowski, MF (eds) Skeletal trauma in children. WB Saunders, Philadelphia
59. Vaccaro AR (ed) (2005) Orthopaedic knowledge update, 8th edn. American Academy of Orthopaedic Surgeons, Rosemont, IL
60. White AA (1978) Clinical biomechanics of the spine. J.B Lippincott, Philadelphia
61. Wiesel SW, Rothman RH (1979) Occipitoatlantal Hypermobility. Spine 4:187–191

13 The Growing Spine and Sports

John M. Flynn, Ejovi Ughwanogho, and Danielle B. Cameron

Key Points

- Injuries to the immature spine are frequent in sports such as gymnastics, wrestling, weightlifting, and football. These injuries can result in significant morbidity and loss of play time.
- Back pain in the pediatric athlete is more likely to be attributed to a specific pathology when compared with an adult patient presenting with back pain with rates of spondylolysis as high as 47% in some series.
- Symptomatic stress reactions of the pars, without frank cortical disruption can be treated conservatively with bracing and rest. Prompt treatment facilitated by early diagnosis of stress reactions with CT or SPECT has resulted in optimal outcomes with conservative management.
- Disc herniation is a rare cause of back pain in the adolescent athlete.
- Apophyseal ring fracture is a rare injury in the pediatric population, occurring primarily in the male adolescent athlete. Surgical treatment is often required.
- Athletes with Down syndrome represent a subset of children with a high risk of spine injury during participation in sports. Current data suggest that 15% of individuals with Down syndrome have atlanto-occipital or atlanto-axial instability.

J. M. Flynn (✉)
The Children's Hospital of Philadelphia,
Division of Orthopaedic Surgery, 2nd Floor, Wood Center,
34th Street and Civic Center Blvd., Philadelphia, PA 19104, USA
e-mail: flynnj@email.chop.edu

13.1 Introduction

Participation in recreational and competitive sports continues to increase among children and adolescents. Predictably, there is an increase in the corresponding incidence of musculoskeletal injuries, including injuries to the spine. Injuries to the immature spine are frequent in sports such as gymnastics, wrestling, weightlifting, and football. These injuries can result in significant morbidity and loss of play time. This chapter reviews specific injuries to the immature spine occurring during sports. These injuries will be discussed in the context of back pain as this is a common manifestation of spinal injuries in this population. Injuries to the cervical spine occurring during sports will also be reviewed briefly as these injuries may result in catastrophic consequences.

13.1.1 Cervical Spine Injuries

Injuries occurring during participation in sports account for a significant proportion of spine fractures in the pediatric population. In an analysis of 610 injuries to the spine and spinal cord in adolescent patients, 53% of the injuries resulted from sports or recreational activities [16]. In a study of 103 spine injuries, Brown et al. [13] demonstrated that 27% of injuries were resulted from participation in sports. These injuries were more common in the adolescent population, and most commonly involved the upper cervical spine. Notably, there was a high prevalence of spinal cord injury without radiographical abnormalities (SCIWORA) in this group. In total, 21 of 28 children in this study were presented with this injury pattern.

Cervical cord neurapraxia (CCN) is a similar, albeit milder, form of SCIWORA occurring in the pediatric

B. A. Akbarnia et al. (eds.), *The Growing Spine*,
DOI: 10.1007/978-3-540-85207-0_13, © Springer-Verlag Berlin Heidelberg 2011

athlete. CCN defines a transient diminution of neurological function involving both the motor and sensory deficits. At its extreme, paralysis may be present for several days, but symptoms are typically brief and mild. Like SCIWORA, CCN may result from hyperextension, hyperflexion or axial loading of the C-spine. In contrast to the adult athlete, current evidence suggests that cervical spinal stenosis is not a risk factor of CCN in the pediatric athlete [11]. It is believed that the relative laxity of the soft tissues about the pediatric C-spine results in hypermobility of the C-spine and predisposes the spinal cord to injury.

Normal ATLS protocol should be instituted in the patient presenting with CCN. In the presence of persistent neurological deficits, these patients should be immobilized with a cervical orthosis at the scene of injury and taken expeditiously to a treatment facility. For those presenting within 6-h postinjury, steroids should be administered as per the National Acute Spinal Cord Injury. After evaluating plain radiographs, Magnetic resonance imaging (MRI) is utilized to evaluate soft tissue structures about the C-spine and to assess for extent of cord injury [11]. In the absence of radiographic evidence of fracture, management consists of immobilization. Immobilization may be discontinued when symptoms completely resolve, and patient has a pain free ROM with normal strength. If pain persists, immobilization in a hard collar should be continued and the patient should be revaluated in 2 weeks. Collar immobilization can be discontinued at this time in the presence of a normal neurological examination, normal dynamic and static cervical spine radiographs, and complete resolution of symptoms. It has been suggested to complete a physical therapy program that includes strengthening of the paracervical muscles before returning to sports [28].

13.1.2 Back Pain in the Pediatric Athlete

13.1.2.1 Introduction

Back pain is common in pediatric athletes. Its prevalence in this population has been estimated at approximately 46%, significantly higher than that of nonathletes (18%) [29]. Furthermore, it appears to be more common in certain sports namely gymnastics, wrestling, football, soccer, and tennis. Incidence of back pain in gymnasts has been estimated at 11–85% in the literature [14]. These sports involve repetitive loading of the lumbar spine. Goldstein et al. [23] showed a higher incidence of lumbar spine abnormalities on MRIs of gymnasts than swimmers. This difference was attributed to the repetitive stress placed on the lumbar spine by the gymnast. That said, a history of previous back pain has been demonstrated to be the best predictor of future complaints of back pain [24].

Back pain in the pediatric athlete is more likely to be attributed to a specific pathology when compared with the adult patient presenting with back pain. This is likely secondary to the lower rate of secondary gain in this population. Micheli et al. [34] demonstrated a higher incidence of identifiable pathology in a population of young athletes presenting with back pain, when compared with adult patients with similar complaints.

Common causes of back pain in the pediatric athlete include muscle strain and stress fractures (spondylolysis and pediculolysis); much less common causes are spondylolisthesis, lumbar Scheuermann's disease, and disc herniation. Fractures of the lumbar vertebra are also a common cause of back pain in the adolescent athlete and are discussed extensively in the pediatric spine trauma chapter.

13.1.2.2 Evaluation

Evaluation of the adolescent athlete with back pain involves obtaining a thorough history and physical examination, complemented by the appropriate radiographic studies. The exact location, onset, duration, and severity of pain should be ascertained. Pain localized to the lower back and gluteal regions are likely secondary to mechanical etiology while leg pain is likely a result of nerve compression or irritation. Aggravating activities and relieving factors should also be determined as these could elucidate the probable cause and direct management. In general, pain exacerbated by flexion suggests discogenic pathology while pain worsened by extension suggests injury to the posterior elements.

Additional important historical information includes the type of sport and level of competition the patient is involved in. The literature has demonstrated an association between certain sports and specific types of injuries. For example, a high incidence of spondylolysis and spondylolisthesis has been associated with weightlifting, diving, wrestling, and gymnastics. These sports involve repetitive hyperextension, a proposed mechanism of injury for spondylolysis. Congeni et al. [17] reported a 47% incidence of spondylolysis in athletes participating in gymnastics and diving.

A comprehensive review of systems should be performed in the adolescent athlete presenting with back pain. The presence of significant weight loss, night pain, fever, and urinary symptoms should spur further investigation of systemic causes of back pain such as tumor, infection, and renal pathology. Finally a history of previous treatments received by the patient should be reviewed.

The examination of the adolescent athlete presenting with back pain begins with inspection of the back. Posture should be assessed for abnormal curvature. A scoliotic or kyphotic spine in the adolescent athlete can result in back pain. Next, the thoracolumbar spinous processes and paraspinal muscles should be palpated for point tenderness or masses. The sacrum should also be palpated. Range of motion should be quantified in the coronal (lateral bending) and sagittal planes (forward flexion/extension). Pain associated with range of motion should be noted. Several provocative maneuvers are useful in the evaluation of back pain in the pediatric athlete. The straight leg raise and single leg hyperextension are the common maneuvers used in the physical examination of the pediatric athlete. A comprehensive neurological examination, including motor strength testing, sensory examination, and reflex testing should also be performed in every athlete presenting with back pain. The tips should also be examined as hip pathology may be manifested as back pain. Bone anatomy about the hips should be palpated and range of motion should be assessed. Finally, gait should be assessed.

As discussed earlier, a majority of pediatric athletes presenting with back pain have an identifiable structural cause of pain. Consequently imaging plays an important role in the evaluation of these patients. Standard plain radiographs, including AP, lateral, and oblique views of the lumbar spine should be obtained. Flexion and extension views may also be warranted if instability is suspected. Additional imaging such as bone scan, single photon emission computed tomography (SPECT), computed tomography (CT) scan, and MRI should be obtained when indicated.

A comprehensive review of the common causes of back pain in the pediatric athlete is mentioned later. The epidemiology, pathogenesis, relevant anatomy, pertinent historical, physical examination, radiographic findings, and management will be discussed.

13.1.3 Stress Fractures

Stress fractures of the spine are a common cause of back pain in the immature athlete (Fig. 13.1). It is particularly common in athletes participating in sports that

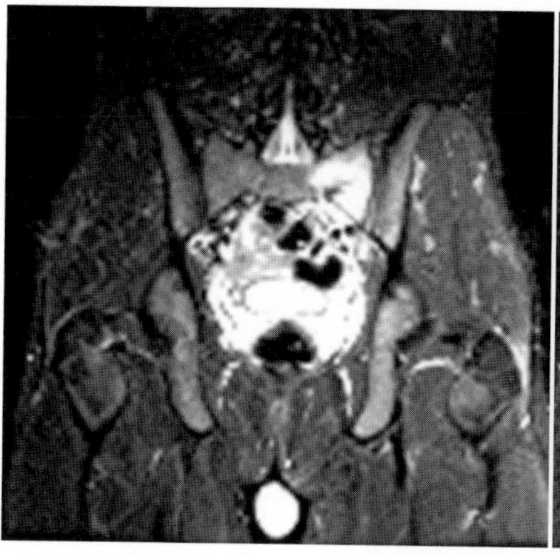

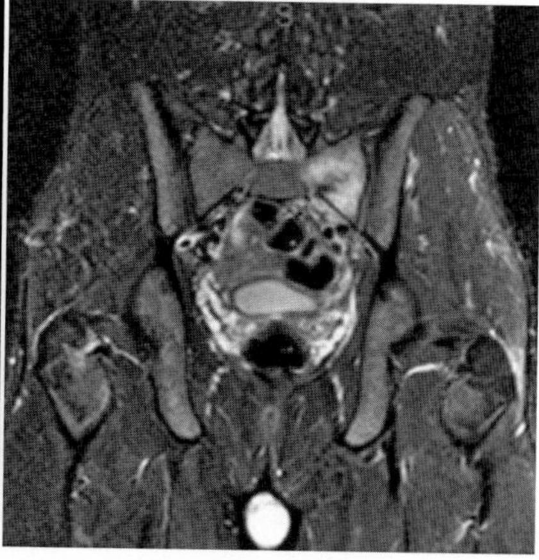

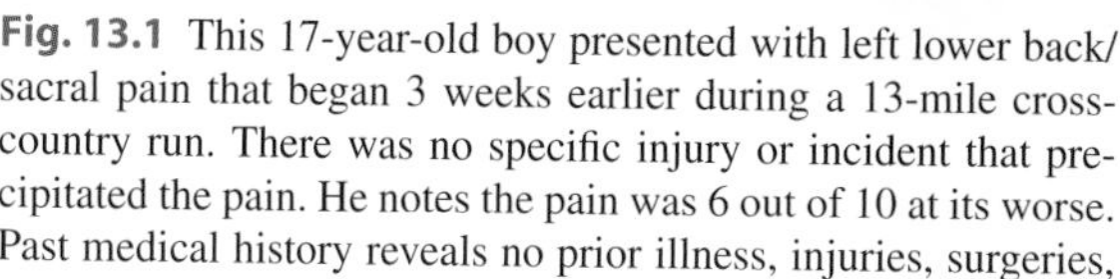

Fig. 13.1 This 17-year-old boy presented with left lower back/sacral pain that began 3 weeks earlier during a 13-mile cross-country run. There was no specific injury or incident that precipitated the pain. He notes the pain was 6 out of 10 at its worse. Past medical history reveals no prior illness, injuries, surgeries, or hospitalization. On physical examination, his pain was localized with palpation along the left posterior superior iliac spine. Radiographs show no evidence of stress fractures or other osseus abnormalities. MRI of the pelvis reveal a left sacral stress fracture with soft tissue edema

require repetitive hyperextension and flexion [19]. Stress fractures are skeletal defects resulting from repetitive load to the bone. Such loads are low in intensity and are typically below the threshold required for fracture. Two theories have been postulated to explain the occurrence of stress fractures. In the overload theory, repetitive rhythmic contractures of muscles result in stress at their osseous insertions, consequently reducing the mechanical resistance of the bone. The muscle fatigue theory attributes stress fractures to diminished shock absorbing properties of a fatigued muscle subjected to repetitive stress. This leads to aberrant loading of bone and subsequent failure [34, 47].

The immature adolescent spine is particularly susceptible to stress fractures because of the absence of complete ossification. Areas of incomplete ossification within the vertebrae are weak points that become susceptible to failure when subjected to repetitive compressive, torsional, or distraction forces [19]. The adolescent athlete participating in sports, such as gymnastics, weightlifting, diving, etc., exposes their spine to such forces; thus, increasing their risks for stress injury. Of note, there is an additional risk seen in competitive female athletes with eating disorders. The relative osteopenic state their bone and their propensity for overexercising puts them at further risks of stress fractures [34].

13.1.4 Spodylolysis/Spondylolisthesis

Spondylolysis is a common cause of back pain in the adolescent athlete (Fig. 13.2). Studies abound on the incidence of spondylolysis in the adolescent athlete in the literature. Notably, Micheli et al. [34] reported 47% incidence of spondylolysis in adolescent athlete presenting with back pain. Rossi [40] reported a much lower incidence of 15% in a review of radiographs of adolescent athletes. Spondylolysis describes a defect in the pars interarticularis of the vertebral arches. It most commonly occurs at the L5–S1 motion segment, though it may also occur at more cephalad levels. Subsequent translation of the cephalad vertebral body on the caudad vertebral body describes spondylolisthesis [15] (Fig. 13.3).

Numerous classification systems have been developed for spondylolysis and spondylolisthesis with the

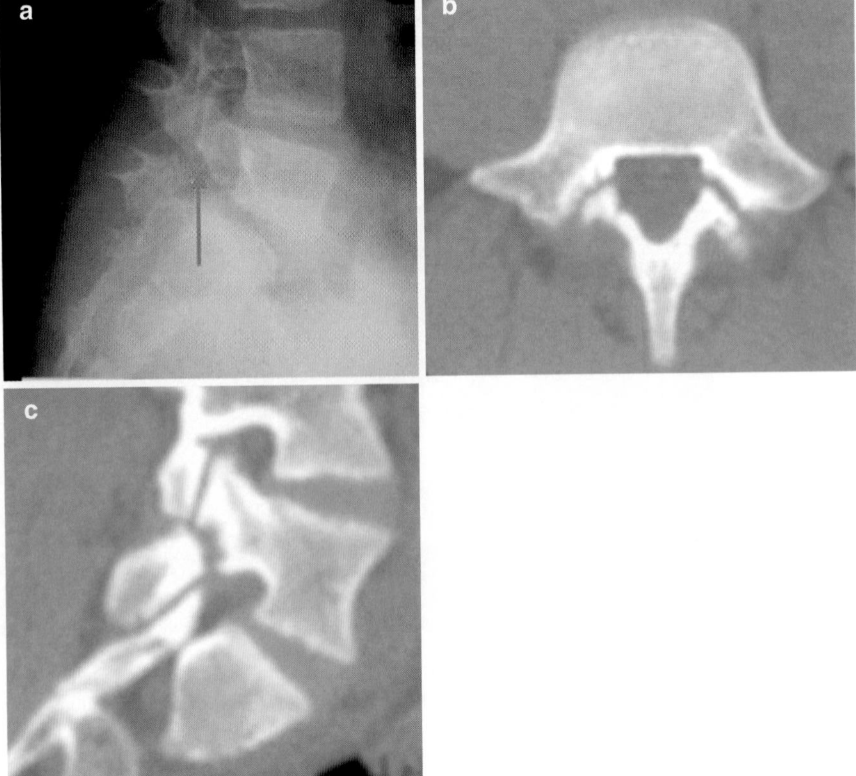

Fig. 13.2 13-year-old elite level gymnast with 2 years of back pain, diagnosed with spondylolysis. (**a**) Lesion visible on lateral radiograph (**b**) and (**c**) CT images further define the stress fracture. Note the sclerotic margins on the transverse cut, typical of a long-standing fracture with failure to heal

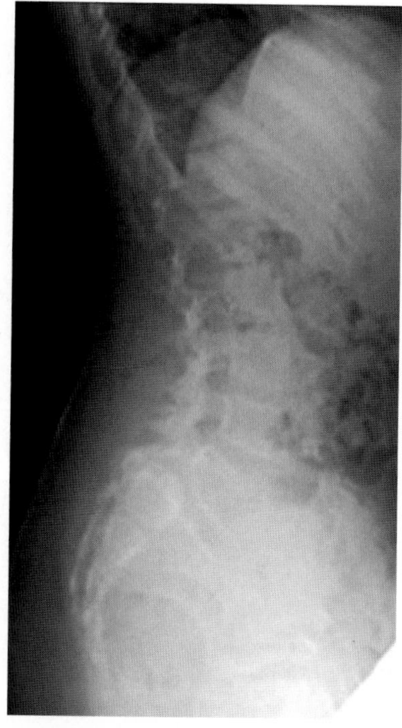

Fig. 13.3 Plain radiograph lateral view of an 8-year-old female with grade 3 spondylolisthesis

Wiltse–Newman system being the most commonly applied [57]. It categorizes spondylolysis/spondylolisthesis into five types, two of which are applicable to the child/adolescent athlete. Type 1 (dysplastic) spondylolysis is a congenital defect in the L5–S1 articular facets and constitutes 14–21% of spondylolysis. In these patients, there is hypoplasia and malrotation of the facet joints. Subsequent repetitive loading of this joint may result in anterolisthesis of L5 on SI. Type 2 (isthmic) spondylolysis/spondylolisthesis results from lesions in the pars interarticularis and is the most common type. It is subclassified into three types. Type 2a is fatigue fracture of the pars interarticularis and is the most prevalent. Type 2b is an elongation of the pars secondary to healed repetitive microfractures. It is often difficult to differentiate type 2b from dysplastic spondylolysis. Type 2c describes an acute fracture of the pars interarticularis.

13.1.4.1 Pathophysiolgy

Isthmic spondylolysis is a fatigue injury resulting from repetitive subclinical load to the pars interarticularis. It has been postulated that an initial microfracture of the pars is caused by a single traumatic event, with eventual failure resulting from subsequent repetitive loads. The high rate of this injury in the adolescent athlete has been attributed to repetitive load the lumbar spine is subjected to in this cohort. Cyron and Hutton [18] demonstrated the susceptibility of the pars to cyclic loading with fractures in 55 of 74 cadaveric lumbar specimens subjected to repetitive shear forces. This finding was corroborated by Dietrich and Kurowski [20] in a study identifying the pars as the region of highest stress during flexion and extension. These findings support existing the evidence indicating a strong association between sports requiring repetitive lumbar motion and spondylolysis.

Low-grade spondylolisthesis is often detectable at presentation in patients with isthmic spondylolysis. Progressive displacement is however unlikely except for in patients diagnosed before their adolescent growth spurt and in those presenting with >50% displacement. Several authors have demonstrated a low risk of slip progression with active participation in sports [22, 33, 37]. Muschik et al. [37] showed only 12% of adolescent patients involved in active sports had a slip progression of >10% after an average follow up of 4.8 years. These patients had an average initial slip of 10.1%.

Dysplastic spondylolysis is a much less common cause of spondylolysis in the pediatric athlete, but is more likely to progress to spondylolisthesis. In these patients, anterolisthesis of L5, with its intact posterior elements, can result in L5 radiculopathy. Bowel and urinary incontinence can also result from sacral nerve root compression. Mcphee et al. [33] demonstrated a higher frequency of progression in dysplastic spondylolysis (32%) when compared with isthmic spondylolysis (4%).

13.1.4.2 Clinical Presentation

Spondylolysis is often asymptomatic. The symptomatic athlete typically reports focal back pain, with occasional radiation to the buttocks or proximal thighs. The pain may be of insidious onset or associated with an inciting traumatic event. Patients may also report a history of mild pain significantly exacerbated by an acute trauma. Pain is often exacerbated by activities requiring repetitive flexion and extension of the lumbar spine [46] Hamstring tightness is also a common complaint of patients with spondylolysis, especially in the presence of advanced spondylolisthesis and may be manifested by a shortened gait stride with flexion at the hips and knees. Radicular symptoms are rare in spondylolysis and low-grade spondylolisthesis, but may be present with high-grade spondylolisthesis [15].

The physical examination of the patient presenting with spondylolysis is often nonspecific. The one-legged hyperextension maneuver is considered by many to be pathognomonic for spondylolysis. In this maneuver, pain is elicited with a one-legged stance and lumbar extension. If the lesion is unilateral, pain is often localized to the ipsilateral side. Masci et al. [32] however recently questioned the utility of this maneuver in the detection of spondylolysis. Other findings include a hyperlordotic thoracolumbar posture, which compensates for loss of lumbar lordosis. Neurological deficits is usually absent unless in the presence of significant spondylolisthesis.

13.1.4.3 Imaging

Radiographic evaluation of the patient with suspected spondylolysis involve the use of multiple imaging modalities including the plain radiograph, bone scintigraphy, CT scans, and MRI. The standard, AP, lateral, and lateral oblique views should be obtained in the patient presenting with suspected spondylolysis. On the lateral oblique view, a radiolucent area is visualized in the pars interarticularis. This has been classically described as the "scotty dog" lesion. It has the appearance of a broken collar on a dog. In addition, the degree of spondylolisthesis can be ascertained from the lateral view. The Meyerding classification system of spondylolisthesis, derived from the lateral X-ray, categorizes spondylolisthesis according to the degree of translation. The slip angle can also be derived from the lateral view. It is the angle subtended by the intersection of a line parallel to the superior endplate of L5 and a line perpendicular to the tangent of the posterior sacral cortex. Current evidence suggests a slip angle >50% or translation of >50% is associated with a greater risk of slip progression and instability [12].

Visualization of spondylolytic lesions on the plain radiograph is often suboptimal, as the defect may not be orthogonal to any of the standard radiological views. Amato et al. showed 84% of pars defect were identified only on the spot lateral view and 19% only on the lateral oblique view. In a study of 60 spondylotic defect using CT scan [3]. Saifuddin et al. [42] demonstrated marked variation in the orientation of the pars lesion with only 32% of the lesions aligned within 15° of the lateral oblique plain. Consequently,

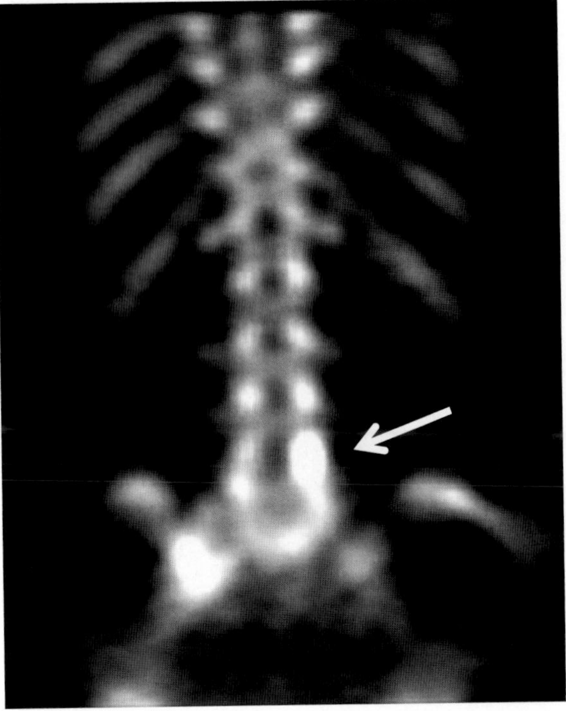

Fig. 13.4 Single photon emission computed tomography

additional imaging is often needed in the evaluation of these patients.

Nuclear radiography has an important role in the evaluation of individuals presenting with spondylolysis. Comparative studies between SPECT, planar bone scans, and radiographs have shown higher sensitivity of SPECT and planar bone scan in the detection of spondylolysis when compared with radiographs (Fig. 13.4). More importantly, current evidence has established the role of nuclear radiography in identifying symptomatic lesions. Nuclear radiography is however limited by its low specificity [9, 27, 30].

Like nuclear radiography, CT scans have demonstrated a higher sensitivity than plain radiographs in the detection of spondylolysis. However, it is more specific than bone scans and has the added advantage of delineating further details of the nature of the lesion. Furthermore, CT scan can also identify other causes of back pain such as disc herniation and osteod osteoma not visualized on bone scan [17, 53].

The use of MRI in the evaluation of young athletes with spondylolysis should be limited to those with neurological findings. Nerve compression, spinal cord abnormalities, and disc pathology can be clearly delineated on MRI in this setting.

13.1.4.4 Management

Symptomatic stress reactions of the pars, without frank cortical disruption can be treated conservatively with bracing and rest. Prompt treatment facilitated by early diagnosis of stress reactions with CT or SPECT has resulted in optimal outcomes with conservative management. Treatment involves the use of a thoracolumbosacral orthosis with or without a thigh extension for 6–12 weeks. Immobilization is discontinued when the patient is asymptomatic and there is evidence of healing on CT scan. Absence of healing on CT scan in an asymptomatic patient suggests the presence of fibrous union which is often stable [49].

Management of isthmic spondylolysis (presence of a cortical defect) differs from a pars stress reaction as the goal of treatment is pain relief, improved mobility, diminished spasm, and not union. These patients can be treated with rest and physical therapy until symptoms resolve. Bracing is only indicated if symptoms persist after adequate rest and physical therapy. In this setting, an anti-lorditic brace that limits extremes of spinal motion can be prescribed and has shown efficacy in pain relief [19, 48]. Duration of treatment is 6–8 weeks with subsequent progression to physical therapy. Physical therapy should involve exercises specifically targeted to improve dynamic stability of the lumbar spine. These exercises include strengthening of the deep abdominal muscles (internal oblique and transverse abdominus) and the lumbar multifidus proximal to the pars defect. Stretching of the hamstrings has also shown efficacy in expediting the resolution of symptoms [15, 38]

The natural course of isthmic spondylolisthesis differs from that of dysplastic spondylolisthesis. Progressive displacement is unlikely in low-grade isthmic spondylolisthesis, thus these patients can be managed conservatively as illustrated earlier. Activities do not need to be restricted in the asymptomatic child. In contrast, the patient with dysplastic spondylolisthesis has a higher likelihood of progression and development of neurological deficits thus should be followed closely even when asymptomatic. Frequent radiographic assessments and physical examinations are needed in these patients [15].

Surgical intervention is indicated in patients with intractable pain from nonhealing stress fractures of the pars, spondylolytic defect, or low-grade spondylolisthesis refractory to a minimum of 6 months of conservative management. Surgery is also indicated in the patient presenting with symptomatic high-grade spondylolisthesis, progressive dysplastic spondylolisthesis, or patients with neurological deficits. Other potential cause of back pain must be ruled out before proceeding with surgery since pars defect may be an incidental finding. Currently, posterior L5–SI fusion, or direct pars repair, is the recommended treatment for L5 spodylolysis or low-grade L5–S1 spondylolisthesis. Pars defect on LI-L4 can be directly repaired. Meyerding grade 3 and above spondylolisthesis should be treated with L4-S1 fusion with reduction of the lumbosacral kyphosis. The patient should also be immobilized for a minimum of 6 weeks [6].

13.1.5 Pedicle Fractures

A component of the neural arch, the pedicles like the pars are also vulnerable to the cyclic loads encountered by the lumbosacral spine during sports. However, pedicle stress fractures are much less common than pars stress fractures [34]. This is partly secondary to the greater intrinsic strength of the pedicles and shorter moment arm from the vertebral body. The pedicles are therefore capable of resisting greater shear forces. In a biomechanical study evaluating the mechanical strength of 74 vertebral units, Cyron and Hutton [18] demonstrated five pedicular stress fractures compared to 55 pars fractures lumbar units subjected to cyclic shear loads. Contralateral pedicular fractures have been associated with isthmic fractures. This phenomenon has been attributed to increased and aberrant loading of the pedicles that result from an unstable neural arch following a pars fracture [1, 4, 44] Ulmer et al. showed a 40% incidence of reactive changes on MRI in pedicles with contralateral spondylolysis [55]

Radiographic evaluation of pedicular fractures involves radiographs and CT scan. As with pars stress reactions, sensitivity of plain radiographs is limited in the evaluation of a pedicular defect. When visible, hypertrophy or sclerosis is seen on the involved pedicle. CT scan has demonstrated higher accuracy in the evaluation of these patients. Pediculolysis is clearly demonstrated as a linear lucency at the base of the involved pedicle on CT. In addition, presence of a concomitant pars defect can also be identified [44, 54]. A significant differential diagnosis of pediculolysis is osteiod osteoma and osteoblastoma. These entities can be differentiated from a pediculolysis by the absence of a nidus, the presence of contralateral pars defect, and the presence of a linear defect in a pedicular stress fracture. Differentiating these lesions is important because excision of a pedicle – a management option for symptomatic tumor – may further destabilize an already unstable neural arch [26, 44]

Early diagnosis of pedicular stress fracture and prompt treatment is necessary to facilitate rapid return to sports. Management of pedicular stress fractures is similar to that of pars stress fracture. Initial management is conservative and involves rest and bracing. Surgery is indicated in the setting of failed conservative treatment. Techniques described in the literature include compression fixation of the defect, excision of the hypertrophic defect with lateral fusion, bone grafting of the pars defect and pedicular defect with subsequent pedicle screw fixation [1, 25, 44].

13.1.6 Other Causes of Back Pain in the Adolescent Athlete

13.1.6.1 Disc Herniation

Disc herniation is a rare cause of back pain in the adolescent athlete (Fig. 13.5); 1% of disc herniations occur in the second decade [51]. As opposed to an incidence, 48% in the adult population, only 11% of adolescent athletes present with symptomatic disc herniation. The most common location of herniation in the young athlete is the L4 and L5 and L5–SI level. In the skeletally immature patient, the disk may be herniated into the end plate with axial loading. This is manifested radiographically as a Schmorl's nodule [5, 56]

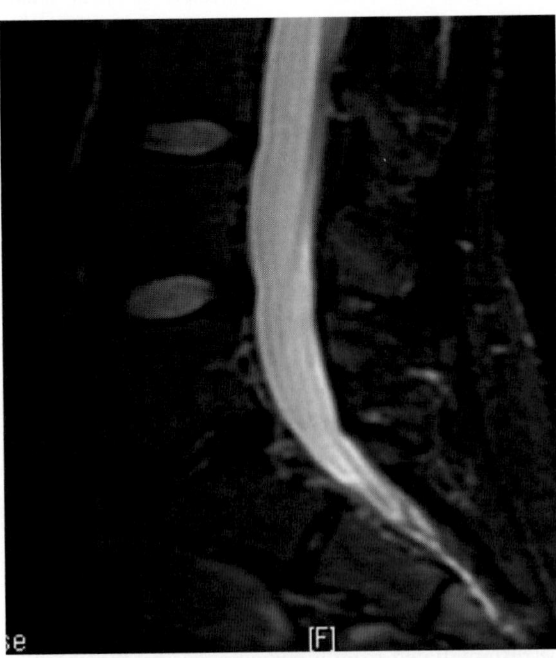

Fig. 13.5 Disc herniation and degenerative changes at L5-S1

Young athletes with disc herniations typically present with localized back pain and paraspinal muscle spasm. Impingement of the nerve roots may result in radicular symptoms. When this occurs, further evaluation with an MRI is warranted. In the absence of neurological compromise, conservative management is recommended for the treatment of these patients. Patients are usually able to return to full participation in sports [56].

13.1.6.2 Lumbar Scheuermann's Disease

Lumbar Scheuermann's disease is also a cause of back pain in the adolescent athlete. It is an overuse injury of the lumbar spine and occurs in sports requiring repetitive flexion and extension such as football, weightlifting and is more common in males. Patients with Scheuermann's disease present with localized back pain exacerbated by forward flexion. Pain may be associated with muscle spasm and loss of lumbar lordosis. Neurologic deficit is however a rare finding.

Radiographic evaluation of Scheuermann's disease includes a plain lateral radiograph of the lumbar spine. Anterior wedging deformity of three consecutive vertebral bodies is required to make the diagnosis. Schmorls nodule may also be seen on plain radiographs [5, 30]

Lumbar Scheuermann's disease can be managed conservatively. Activity modification and lumbar bracing may facilitate pain control. Physical therapy should be directed at pelvic and lumbar stabilization exercises. The patient may return to play when pain subsides and after completion of physical therapy [5]

13.1.6.3 Muscle Strain

Muscle strains are a common cause of back pain in the adolescent athlete. It has been estimated to occur in 27% of adolescent athletes presenting with lower back pain [10, 35] Strains result from disruption in muscle fibers within the muscle belly or musculotendinous junction.

Numerous factors such as acute trauma, repetitive stress, poor technique, obesity, muscle imbalance, and poor footwear contribute to muscle strain. Patients with back strain present with progressively worsening lower back pain that peaks 24–48 h after the onset of pain. Pain is often associated with spasms. Diagnostic testing such as plain radiography, bone scan, and MRI, are usually negative but may be necessary to rule out other ominous causes of back pain in the immature athlete [10].

Many children presenting with "mechanical back pain" are experiencing failure of their core muscles during exertional activities. After a growth spurt, an adolescent athlete often develops transient lower extremity muscle contractures, further altering the stresses at the lumbosacral junction. Treatment should focus on lower extremity stretching and core strengthening exercises.

13.1.6.4 Vertebral Apophyseal Avulsion Fractures

Apophyseal ring fracture is a rare injury in the pediatric population, occurring primarily in the male adolescent athlete [31] (Fig. 13.6). It most frequently affects L4 and L5. It has been suggested that the incidence of apophyseal fractures may be underreported as it is frequently misdiagnosed as lumbar disc herniation in the adolescent population [50].

In the developing lumbar spine, the superior and inferior endplates are bordered by the vertebral ring apophysis. Ossification of the apophysis commences at approximately 5 years and progresses to completion by the age of 18. During the rapid adolescent growth phase, the apophysis is separated from the underlying vertebral body by a physeal zone. This area of weakness is susceptible to avulsion injuries. It has been suggested that hyperextension of the lumbar spine or rapid flexion with axial load may be the causative mechanism.

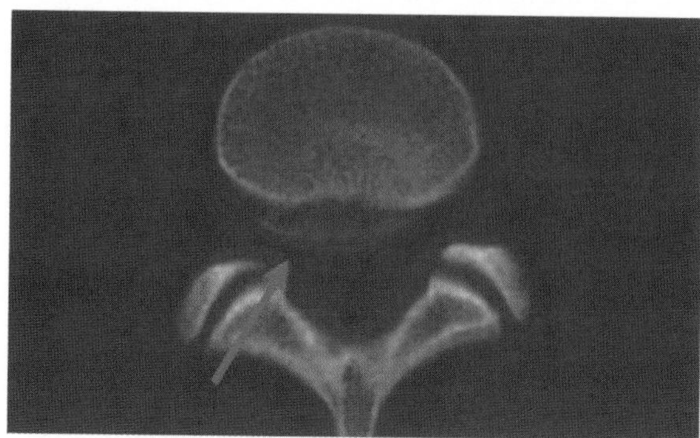

Fig. 13.6 Vertebral apophyseal avulsion fracture

This hypothesis is supported by the relatively high incidence of this fracture in the athletic adolescent population [31].

Takata et al. [50] reported the largest series of apophyseal injury to date and classified these injuries into 3 categories based on CT findings. Type 1 fracture is a separation of the posterior rim of the vertebra body with negligible defect in the vertebra body. This type was noted primarily in patients between the ages of 11 and 13. Type 2 describes an avulsion fracture of the posterior rim of vertebra body including the posterior segment of the overlying annulus fibrosus. It is more prevalent in older patients. Type 3 fracture is a small localized fracture posterior to an irregularity in the cartilaginous endplate.

Clinical presentation includes lower back pain with infrequent reports of radicular symptoms. Neurogenic claudication, paraparesis, and cauda aquina syndromes have also been reported in some series. The most common finding on examination is restricted lumbar range of motion. Some authors have reported the presence of a positive straight leg raise in these patients. That said, neurological deficits are usually rare [36, 43, 50].

Radiographic evaluation involves the use of both the plain radiograph and CT scan. Bone defects can be visualized on the lateral radiograph; however, the CT scan (axial cuts) has been proven to be more sensitive in the evaluation of these patients [7].

In the absence of neurological deficits, initial management is conservative and includes the use of NSAIDs, lumbar bracing, and activity restriction. However, many patients will not improve with the same conservative care given to adults with a herniated lumbar disc. Surgery is indicated for pain refractory to conservative management and the presence of neurological deficits. Surgery includes laminectomy and excision of the fractured fragments. Though an option in the adult population, a discectomy should be avoided in the adolescent patient without evidence of disc degeneration [21, 37].

13.1.7 Return to Sports After Spine Surgery

There is a paucity of level 1 studies in the literature addressing the appropriate timing of return to sports after spinal surgery in the pediatric population. To date, this issue has not been addressed by a formal prospective randomized controlled study.

Rubery and Bradford [41] recently surveyed a number of SRS members on the appropriate timing of return to play after spine surgery. There was no clear consensus in the timing of return to sports after scoliosis surgery. Factors affecting the decision to initiate sports after scoliosis surgery included time of surgery, use of instrumentation, and type of sport. Patient age and clinical progress did not play a critical role in the determination of return to sports. On the contrary, evidence of radiographic union and time from surgery were important determinants of when to return to play in patients undergoing surgery for spondylolisthesis. That said, most practitioners seem to initiate noncontact sports after 6months. Contact sports were typically resumed by most practitioners after 12 months. However, a small percentage prohibited resumption of contact sports permanently. A majority of clinicians discouraged resumption of collision sports such as football.

There was also a lack of consensus in the appropriate timing of resumption of sports after surgery for spondylolisthesis. Most practitioners recommended return to noncontact sports after 6 months and contact sports after 1 year. A minority of practitioners (14% in patients with low-grade spondylolisthesis and 21% with high-grade spondylolisthesis) prohibited their patients from participating in contact sports permanently. About half the practitioners prohibited collision sports [41].

Most surgeons surveyed allowed gym activities and noncontact sports between 6 months to 1 year after deformity correction. Resumption of contact sports was allowed by most surgeons after 1 year, while 11% of surgeons prohibited all contact sports after deformity correction. A majority of surgeons either prohibited or recommended against collision sports such as football. Those (36%) allowing collision sports usually did so 1 year after surgery. Factors such as use of instrumentation, time after surgery, and type of sport most frequently influenced a surgeon's decision to allow resumption of activities [41]. With the advent of pedicle screw fixation, surgeons are increasingly allowing an earlier return to full activity. The authors, and many others, allow swimming and low-impact activities as soon as comfort allows, and impact activities by 6 months after surgery. For most teenage athletes, this allows them to avoid missing their favorite sports season by scheduling surgery as soon as the season ends.

13.1.7.1 Special Olympics and the Disabled Athlete

An increasing number of disabled children currently participate in various sporting activities. Participation in sports in this population enhances physical and mental health in this population. The Special Olympics provides an avenue for disabled individuals to participate in competitive sport. It is held annually in each state, with the best athletes advancing to a yearly national competition. As with other athletes, ensuring the safety of the special Olympian is essential. In this population, there is a higher incidence of abnormalities that may result in significant injuries during certain sporting events [8]. Consequently, it is important to carefully screen these individuals prior to participation in sports.

Athletes with Down syndrome represent a subset of children with a high risk of spine injury during participation in sports. Current data suggests that 15% of individuals with Down syndrome have atlanto-occipital or atlanto-axial instability [2, 39]. As a result, the Special Olympic currently mandates a preparticipation spine evaluation of all patients with Down syndrome. In addition to a thorough history and physical examination, radiographic evaluation of the cervical spine is required to clear a patient with Down syndrome for participation in the Special Olympic events. Dynamic flexion, extension, and neutral lateral radiographs of the cervical spine should be obtained in these patients. In appropriately obtained radiographs, atlanto-dens interval (ADI) greater than 4.5 mm indicates instability in children. Individuals with radiographic evidence of instability are disqualified from participating in high-risk sports such as diving, gymnastics or power lifting. However, this restriction can be waived if the parents/guardians and two physicians acknowledges the risks involved with the earlier mentioned sports and consent to the participation of the minor in a written certification [8, 45].

Although the natural history of atlanto-axial instability in persons with Down syndrome has not been clearly delineated, the Special Olympics does not currently recommend follow up screening cervical radiographs for individuals with normal spine radiographs at initial screening [39]. That said, intervention is not required in those patients with asymptomatic atlanto-axial instability. They should be observed and restricted from participation in high-risk sports as stated earlier. Surgical intervention should be considered in patients with symptomatic atlanto-axial instability [52].

References

1. Aland C, Rineberg BA, Malberg M et al (1986) Fracture of the pedicle of the fourth lumbar vertebra associated with contralateral spondylolysis. Report of a case. J Bone Joint Surg Am 68(9):1454–1455
2. Alvarez N, Rubin L (1986) Atlantoaxial instability in adults with Down syndrome: a clinical and radiological survey. Appl Res Ment Retard 7(1):67–78
3. Amato M, Totty WG, Gilula LA (1984) Spondylolysis of the lumbar spine: demonstration of defects and laminal fragmentation. Radiology 153(3):627–629
4. Araki T, Harata S, Nakano K et al (1992) Reactive sclerosis of the pedicle associated with contralateral spondylolysis. Spine 17(11):1424–1426
5. Baker RJ, Patel D (Mar 2005) Lower back pain in the athlete: common conditions and treatment. Prim Care 32(1):201–229
6. Bartolozzi P, Sandri A, Cassini M et al (2003) One-stage posterior decompression-stabilization and trans-sacral interbody fusion after partial reduction for severe L5-S1 spondylolisthesis. Spine 28(11):1135–1141
7. Beggs I, Addison J (1998) Posterior vertebral rim fractures. Br J Radiol 71(845):567–572
8. Birrer RB (2004 Nov-Dec) The Special Olympics athlete: evaluation and clearance for participation. Clin Pediatr (Phila) 43(9):777–82
9. Bodner RJ, Heyman S, Drummond DS et al (1988) The use of single photon emission computed tomography (SPECT) in the diagnosis of low-back pain in young patients. Spine 13(10):1155–1160
10. Bono CM (Feb 2004) Low-back pain in athletes. J Bone Joint Surg Am 86-A(2):382–396
11. Boockvar JA, Durham SR, Sun PP (2001) Cervical spinal stenosis and sports-related cervical cord neurapraxia in children. Spine 26(24):2709–2712; discussion 2713
12. Boxall D, Bradford DS, Winter RB et al (1979) Management of severe spondylolisthesis in children and adolescents. J Bone Joint Surg Am 61(4):479–495
13. Brown RL, Brunn MA, Garcia VF (2001) Cervical spine injuries in children: a review of 103 patients treated consecutively at a level 1 pediatric trauma center. J Pediatr Surg 36(8):1107–1114
14. Burton AK, Clarke RD, McClune TD et al (1996) The natural history of low back pain in adolescents. Spine 21(20): 2323–2328
15. Cavalier R, Herman MJ, Cheung EV et al (2006) Spondylolysis and spondylolisthesis in children and adolescents: I. Diagnosis, natural history, and nonsurgical management. J Am Acad Orthop Surg 14(7):417–424
16. Clark P, Letts M (2001) Trauma to the thoracic and lumbar spine in the adolescent. Can J Surg 44(5):337–345
17. Congeni J, McCulloch J, Swanson K (1997) Lumbar spondylolysis. A study of natural progression in athletes. Am J Sports Med 25(2):248–253
18. Cyron BM, Hutton WC (1979) Variations in the amount and distribution of cortical bone across the partes interarticulares of L5. A predisposing factor in spondylolysis. Spine 4(2): 163–167
19. d'Hemecourt PA, Gerbino PG, 2nd, Micheli LJ (2000) Back injuries in the young athlete. Clin Sports Med 19(4):663–679
20. Dietrich M, Kurowski P (1985) The importance of mechanical factors in the etiology of spondylolysis. A model analysis of loads and stresses in human lumbar spine. Spine 10(6): 532–542
21. Epstein NE, Epstein JA (1991) Limbus lumbar vertebral fractures in 27 adolescents and adults. Spine 16(8):962–966
22. Fredrickson BE, Baker D, McHolick WJ et al (1984) The natural history of spondylolysis and spondylolisthesis. J Bone Joint Surg Am 66(5):699–707
23. Goldstein JD, Berger PE, Windler GE et al (1991) Spine injuries in gymnasts and swimmers. An epidemiologic investigation. Am J Sports Med 19(5):463–468
24. Greene HS, Cholewicki J, Galloway MT et al (2001) history of low back injury is a risk factor for recurrent back injuries in varsity athletes. Am J Sports Med 29(6):795–800
25. Guillodo Y, Botton E, Saraux A et al (2000) Contralateral spondylolysis and fracture of the lumbar pedicle in an elite female gymnast: a case report. Spine 25(19):2541–2543
26. Gunzburg R, Fraser RD (1991) Stress fracture of the lumbar pedicle. Case reports of "pediculolysis" and review of the literature. Spine 16(2):185–189
27. Jackson DW, Wiltse LL, Dingeman RD et al (1981) Stress reactions involving the pars interarticularis in young athletes. Am J Sports Med 9(5):304–312
28. Kim DH, Vaccaro AR, Berta SC (2003) Acute sports-related spinal cord injury: contemporary management principles. Clin Sports Med 22(3):501–512
29. Kujala UM, Kinnunen J, Helenius P et al (1999) Prolonged low-back pain in young athletes: a prospective case series study of findings and prognosis. Eur Spine J 8(6):480–484
30. Lowe J, Schachner E, Hirschberg E et al (1984) Significance of bone scintigraphy in symptomatic spondylolysis. Spine 9(6):653–655
31. Martinez-Lage JF, Poza M, Arcas P (1998) Avulsed lumbar vertebral rim plate in an adolescent: trauma or malformation? Childs Nerv Syst 14(3):131–134
32. Masci L, Pike J, Malara F et al (2006) Use of the one-legged hyperextension test and magnetic resonance imaging in the diagnosis of active spondylolysis. Br J Sports Med 40(11): 940–946; discussion 946
33. McPhee IB, O'Brien JP, McCall IW et al (1981) Progression of lumbosacral spondylolisthesis. Australas Radiol 25(1): 91–95
34. Micheli LJ, Wood R (1995) Back pain in young athletes. Significant differences from adults in causes and patterns. Arch Pediatr Adolesc Med 149(1):15–18
35. Micheli LJ, Curtis C (2006) Stress fractures in the spine and sacrum. Clin Sports Med 25(1):75–88, ix
36. Molina V, Court C, Dagher G et al (2004) Fracture of the posterior margin of the lumbar spine: case report after an acute, unique, and severe trauma. Spine 29(24):E565–567
37. Muschik M, Hahnel H, Robinson PN et al (1996) Competitive sports and the progression of spondylolisthesis. J Pediatr Orthop 16(3):364–369
38. O'Sullivan PB, Phyty GD, Twomey et al (1997) Evaluation of specific stabilizing exercise in the treatment of chronic low back pain with radiologic diagnosis of spondylolysis or spondylolisthesis. Spine 22(24):2959–2967
39. Pueschel SM, Scola FH, Pezzullo JC (Jun) A longitudinal study of atlanto-dens relationships in asymptomatic individuals with Down syndrome. Pediatrics 89(6 Pt 2):1194–8

40. Rossi F (1978) Spondylolysis, spondylolisthesis and sports. J Sports Med Phys Fitness 18(4):317–340
41. Rubery PT, Bradford DS (2002) Athletic activity after spine surgery in children and adolescents: results of a survey. Spine 27(4):423–427
42. Saifuddin A, White J, Tucker S et al (1998) Orientation of lumbar pars defects: implications for radiological detection and surgical management. J Bone Joint Surg Br 80(2): 208–211
43. Savini R, Di Silvestre M, Gargiulo G et al (1991) Posterior lumbar apophyseal fractures. Spine 16(9):1118–1123
44. Sirvanci M, Ulusoy L, Duran C (2002) Pedicular stress fracture in lumbar spine. Clin Imaging 26(3):187–193
45. Special Olympics. Participation by individuals with Down syndrome who have atlantoaxial instability. Available at: www.specialolympics.org. Accessed 5 December 2006
46. Standaert CJ, Herring SA (2000) Spondylolysis: a critical review. Br J Sports Med 34(6):415–422
47. Stanitski CL, McMaster JH, Scranton PE (1978) On the nature of stress fractures. Am J Sports Med 6(6):391–396
48. Steiner ME, Micheli LJ (1985) Treatment of symptomatic spondylolysis and spondylolisthesis with the modified Boston brace. Spine 10(10):937–943
49. Sys J, Michielsen J, Bracke P et al (2001) Nonoperative treatment of active spondylolysis in elite athletes with normal X-ray findings: literature review and results of conservative treatment. Eur Spine J 10(6):498–504
50. Takata K, Inoue S, Takahashi K et al (1988) Fracture of the posterior margin of a lumbar vertebral body. J Bone Joint Surg Am 70(4):589–594
51. Tall RL, DeVault W (1993) Spinal injury in sport: epidemiologic considerations. Clin Sports Med 12(3):441–448
52. Tassone JC, Duey̆-Holtz A (2008) Spine concerns in the Special Olympian with Down syndrome. Sports Med Arthrosc 16(1):55–60, review
53. Teplick JG, Laffey PA, Berman A et al (1986) Diagnosis and evaluation of spondylolisthesis and/or spondylolysis on axial CT. AJNR Am J Neuroradiol 7(3):479–491
54. Traughber PD, Havlina JM, Jr. (1991) Bilateral pedicle stress fractures: SPECT and CT features. J Comput Assist Tomogr 15(2):338–340
55. Ulmer JL, Elster AD, Mathews VP et al (1995) Lumbar spondylolysis: reactive marrow changes seen in adjacent pedicles on MR images. AJR Am J Roentgenol 164(2):429–433
56. Waicus KM, Smith BW (2002) Back injuries in the pediatric athlete. Curr Sports Med Rep 1(1):52–58
57. Wiltse LL, Newman PH, Macnab I (1976) Classification of spondylolisis and spondylolisthesis. Clin Orthop Relat Res 117:23–29

Spinal Deformity in Metabolic Diseases

14

James O. Sanders, Kerry Armet, and Susan Bukata

Key Points

- Scoliosis is the primary deformity from soft bone diseases in children.
- Bracing has little role in these disorders both because it is ineffective and because it can create significant chest wall deformity.
- Medical treatment of these disorders has assumed a much larger role in both preventing spinal deformity and in providing improved fixation when surgery is necessary.

14.1 General Concepts

14.1.1 Soft Bone and Spinal Deformity

Soft bone disease comes in many forms and may cause or coexist with spinal deformity. The poor bone quality may cause macrofractures or microfractures or plastic bone deformation creating a spinal deformity. Bracing is typically ineffective and the pressure from bracing creates secondary deformities of the chest wall. Surgery is complicated by the soft bone, which makes correction difficult from poor bone purchase and which bleeds if fractured. There are several strategies to minimize these problems, but some appear unavoidable with current knowledge and techniques. This chapter outlines some generalities that are discussed in more detail with the specific diseases.

J. O. Sanders (✉)
Department of Orthopaedics and Rehabilitation, University of Rochester, 601 Elmwood Avenue, Rochester, NY 14642, USA
e-mail: James_Sanders@urmc.rochester.edu

14.1.2 Scoliosis

Unlike adults in whom the primary disorder from soft bone is kyphosis, scoliosis is the primary disorder in children. Although older studies recommend bracing, the evidence for bracing, particularly in this population, is poor. Bracing exerts pressure upon the ribs, which can deform and constrict lung volume. If bracing is attempted, it must be done with great caution and careful evaluation for its effects. Halo traction using multiple halo pins to provide sufficient surface area contact has been used successfully in obtaining preoperative correction in soft bone disease. This is likely because the ligaments are often relatively strong despite the bone abnormality and ligament laxity. Scoliosis correction can be difficult, and most authors recommend operating upon curves before they become large. Patients in early studies had little correction, but this appears improved with modern techniques.

14.1.3 Kyphosis

While rarer than scoliosis, kyphosis still occurs in children with soft bone. When occurring over a short segment, typically from fractures, it can cause spinal cord compression that may require decompression. Kyphoplasty and vertebroplasty are now commonly performed in adults with kyphosis from pathological

B. A. Akbarnia et al. (eds.), *The Growing Spine*,
DOI: 10.1007/978-3-540-85207-0_14, © Springer-Verlag Berlin Heidelberg 2011

compression fractures. Its reported use in osteogenesis imperfecta (OI) is limited to a case report in a middle-aged man [41]. Correction of kyphosis in the young may require an anterior fusion for structural support. This can be difficult because the anterior bone is often substantially weaker than the posterior bone.

14.1.4 Spondylolysis and Spondylolisthesis

Pathologic bone is a separate classification in the major spondylolisthesis classifications [30, 48, 86]. We have only seen it below posterior fusions, but there is no reason to suppose it does not occasionally occur otherwise. It is usually best treated by observation.

14.1.5 Basilar Invagination

Basilar invagination occurs when the heavy skull settles on the upper cervical spine. The foramen magnum is compressed by the dens causing brainstem compression and abnormal CSF flow. Although patients are often asymptomatic, they may present with headache, lower cranial nerve problems, hyperreflexia, quadriparesis, ataxia, and nystagmus [64].

14.1.6 Poor Bone Purchase

Fixation in soft bone can be quite difficult. The basic principles are to purchase the strongest bone possible with the widest surface area possible. This can be achieved with multiple wires, screws, and hooks. The anterior cancellous bone is often quite thin and does not provide good purchase. Screw purchase can be maximized using diameters large enough to engage the pedicular cortex and catching the endplates which are stronger than the vertebral bodies. Polymethylmethacrylate (PMMA) has been used to improve purchase of both hooks and screws. Since the advent of bisphosphonate treatment of soft bone disease in children, we have not used PMMA, but have instead used two or three courses of intravenous pamindronate preoperatively to improve purchase.

14.2 Rickets and Rickets-Like Syndromes

14.2.1 Rickets

The classic metabolic bone disease is rickets. Rickets includes several conditions that lead to abnormal bone mineralization in a growing child. Rickets refers to a failure or delay in mineralization of newly formed osteoid at the growth plates, while osteomalacia is a delay in mineralization of newly formed osteoid as a part of bone remodeling. Children suffer from both problems, while skeletally mature individuals have osteomalacia only. Vitamin D plays a vital role in the development of rickets and osteomalacia. Vitamin D can be consumed in the diet and can also be formed in the skin by UV-B irradiation from sunlight. Vitamin D is transported to the liver where it is hydroxylated to 25(OH) vitamin D, and then to the kidney where it is again hydroxylated by 1-α-hydroxylase to 1,25 (OH)2 vitamin D. This active form of vitamin D increases intestinal absorption of calcium and phosphorus, and renal reabsorption of calcium (and phosphorus) to maintain a supersaturated state of a calcium–phosphorous product in the serum that results in passive mineralization of newly formed osteoid [32]. 1,25 (OH)2, vitamin D also has direct effects on osteoblast activity, increasing expression of several bone proteins [42]. Levels of calcium, phosphorus, and parathyroid hormone (PTH) closely regulate the 1-α-hydroxylase enzyme, allowing for homeostatic balance. There are different forms of rickets, including vitamin D deficiency, vitamin D-dependent and vitamin D-resistant rickets, and hereditary hypophosphatemic rickets.

The most common rickets is vitamin D deficiency rickets, which results from deficient intake, absorption, or production of vitamin D. Diets low in vitamin D (especially the exclusively breast fed infant or the strict vegetarian), dark skin pigmentation, limited sun exposure, or regular strict use of sunscreen are all risk factors as are malabsorptive syndromes, anticonvulsants, and steroids. Children may have failure to thrive, short stature, delayed development, muscular hypotonia, or hypocalcemic seizures. Widening of the wrists and ankles, chest deformities, and bowing of the long bones are common skeletal manifestations. In advanced disease, calcium and phosphorus are both low, AP and

PTH are elevated and 25(OH) vitamin D is low. 1,25 (OH)2 levels are not helpful as they are generally normal or even elevated. Treatment includes vitamin D and calcium. Serum 25(OH) vitamin D levels are the best clinical indicators of nutritional vitamin D status and should be maintained at levels >32 ng/ mL (75–80 nM) [19].

Vitamin D-dependent rickets results from deficient or abnormal function of the renal 1-α-hydroxylase resulting in low 1,25 (OH)2 vitamin D levels vitamin D-resistant rickets are caused by a defect in the vitamin D receptor that prevents 1,25(OH)2 vitamin D binding. Both types are caused by genetic mutations and lead to hypocalcemia, secondary hyperparathyroidism, hypophosphatemia, and the typical skeletal manifestations seen in vitamin D deficiency rickets. Treatment includes pharmacologic doses of vitamin D or 1,25 (OH)2 vitamin D (calcitriol), as well as calcium.

In hereditary hypophophatemic rickets, abnormal renal phosphate reabsorption occurs, and phosphate "wasting" ensues. This is typically X-linked, but rarely, autosomal dominant inheritance occurs. Patients have hypophosphatemia, hyperphosphaturia, and elevated serum alkaline phosphatase, but normal calcium, PTH, and 25(OH) vitamin D levels, and decreased 1,25 (OH)2 vitamin D levels. Skeletal manifestations are similar to those seen with the other forms of rickets; symptoms related to hypocalcemia (seizures and tetany), however, do not occur. Interestingly, there is no evidence of increased osteoclast activity, and in treated patients, bone mass can be normal [67]. Treatment is with large quantities of oral phosphate.

In the late-nineteenth through mid-twentieth century, rickets was considered a common cause of scoliosis [14]. This was supported by experiment evidence from bipedal rats on a rachitogenic diet that produced scoliosis in contrast to either quadrapedial rachitic or bipedal nonrachitic rats [87]. Pehrsson et al. [57] found an increased mortality rate in scoliosis with rickets and an increased incidence of severe scoliosis, but the study is hampered by uncertain diagnosis of the rickets with other dwarfing conditions. Rickets does result in an increased incidence of asymmetric posture [38]; however, human scoliosis in practice is rarely if ever caused by rickets [14]. We have treated a large cohort with familial hypophosphatemic rickets and have not identified any patients with scoliosis, perhaps because their growth spurt is markedly diminished compared to uninvolved children.

14.3 Hypophosphatasia

Hypophosphatasia results from abnormally low activity of tissue nonspecific alkaline phosphatase (TNSALP), which leads to rickets and/or osteomalacia. Several mutations and inheritance patterns are present and depend on the type of hypophosphasia. The different forms of this disorder are classified by the age of onset of skeletal manifestations: perinatal, infantile, childhood, and adult. Two other forms include odontohypophosphatasia and pseudohyphosphatasia. The perinatal form is lethal; those that are stillborn may have bone spurs of the extremities and characteristic radiographic findings – abnormal ossification of bones, round and flattened vertebral bodies. Those that survive birth suffer from respiratory failure. The infantile form may present as failure to thrive, poor feeding, and hypotonia in the first 6 months of life. Craniosynostosis, dolicocephaly, short stature, and fractures may occur. This form carries a 50% mortality rate, usually from rachitic rib changes and subsequent respiratory compromise. The childhood form may present as delayed motor development and early loss of deciduous teeth. Many patients suffer from severe bone pain. The adult form presents in the 4th–5th decade of life with symptoms resulting from stress fractures or joint pain. Premature loss of deciduous teeth also occurs. Odontohypophosphatasia is characterized by premature loss of teeth and no evidence of skeletal disease. Pseudohypophasphatasia is clinically indistinguishable from the perinatal form, except for normal alkaline phosphatase activity. It is thought that although TNSALP functions normally in vitro, it has abnormal activity in vivo. There are three reported cases of scoliosis in hypophosphatasia [2, 84] Whether this was caused or coexisting with the disease is unknown, although Arun et al. [2] suggested a genetic linkage rather than a common etiology. It has also been reported rarely in hepatobiliary rickets [31].

14.4 Lowe's Syndrome

Patients with Lowe's oculocerebrorenal syndrome may have scoliosis or kyphosis, but more commonly have upper cervical abnormalities similar to patients with storage diseases that are discussed later [33].

14.5 Osteogenesis Imperfecta

OI commonly results in spinal deformity. Over the past decade, the molecular mechanisms of these disorders have been increasingly understood. While much of the older literature classified OI into congenita and tarda with divisions into gravis and levis, this older classification is inadequate to incorporate the advances in molecular genetics or to discuss patients with nonorthopaedic colleagues. For surgeons dealing with various severities of spinal deformity, a classification based upon the phenotype and molecular defect is more appropriate.

OI is a disorder of congenital bone fragility, resulting from abnormal type I collagen. It can result from normal but insufficient type I collagen, which is typical of type I OI. Collagen is a triple helix, and more severe forms of OI can result when one abnormal collagen monomer destabilizes the entire triple helix. Mutations in the COL1A1 and COL1A2 genes, coding for type I collagen, can lead to both qualitative and quantitative disturbances of this protein. Types of OI are distinguished by the severity of their manifestations. Type I is the mildest form of OI, where fractures are most common in infancy. Patients have blue sclera and occasionally abnormal dentition. Long bone deformities are typically absent. Type II is often fatal in the perinatal period. In utero fractures are present, and lung hypoplasia and CNS malformations are common causes of death. Type III is considered a severe type of OI with more frequent fractures, including in utero. Long bone deformities are characteristic and muscle weakness and bone pain can be debilitating. Kyphoscoliosis may be severe enough to cause respiratory compromise and basilar invagination may be fatal. Sclera are not typically blue. Type IV's inheritance pattern is not well-defined and has phenotypic similarities to type I, with more severe bone involvement and lack of blue sclera. Types V–VIII similarly overlap with the types I–III, but do not have mutations in the COL1A1/A2 genes; instead, other genetic mutations have been identified. Table 14.1 lists the currently described types of OI, links to the Online Mendelian Inheritance in Man (OMIM), and their known association with spinal deformity.

Pulmonary failure is the leading cause of death in adults with OI, and it is closely associated with thoracic scoliosis. Widmann et al. [85] found a high negative correlation between pulmonary function and thoracic scoliosis and but not with chest wall deformity or kyphosis. They also found diminution in vital capacity below 50% in thoracic curve of 60° or more.

Spinal deformity in OI is directly related to the severity of osseous involvement [7, 16, 21], though body weight is also a factor in bone density [43] While ligamentous laxity, also from type I collagen deficiency, may also contribute, a series of patients with various types of OI found less scoliosis in those with ligamentous laxity [21]. There is a tendency for later development of scoliosis in those with early development of motor milestones, particularly supported sitting [22]. Overall, the worse the osseous involvement in terms of intrinsic vertebral body deformity and decreased Z-scores for bone density [83], the worse the scoliosis and the more difficultly achieving good fixation for correction. The morphology of the vertebral bodies ranges from normal contours to flattened, wedged, and biconcave with the biconcave vertebra more likely to develop severe scoliosis [28, 34]. Six or more biconcave vertebra before puberty appears prognostic of developing scoliosis of greater than 50° [34]. The spine may also become kyphotic particularly in those with more severe involvement [21] (Fig. 14.1). Cervical fractures [51] including spontaneous paraplegia from chiropractic manipulation [89], and thoracic fractures with spinal cord injury [23], and multiple flexion stress endplate fractures of the thoracic and lumbar spine [25] have been reported. Daivajna et al. [17] reported a modified anterolateral approach for decompression of myelopathy from severe cervical kyphosis in a 9-year-old patient with OI.

Bracing has been attempted for spinal deformity from OI. However, the corrective force applied through the pathological ribs only leads to further rib deformity and may contribute to worsening pulmonary function [7, 8, 15]. Current braces cannot achieve this. Patients who are not operative candidates can be fitted with custom seating for comfort and function [62, 88]. Bracing's role in OI is primarily limited to postoperative temporary support, though there is some suggestion that an orthosis can slow the progression of basilar impression [64].

Positioning patients for surgery can be very difficult and must be carefully supervised because of chest wall deformities, fragile extremities, ribs, and frequent contractures. Unpadded blood pressure cuffs can result in fractures. Surgery for these patients should typically occur in institutions accustomed to their care [80]. Fatality has been reported from intraoperative rib fractures [72]. Classically, correcting curves in severely soft

Table 14.1 Metabolic disorders, their location in Mendelian Inheritance in Man (OMIM – available though the National Library of Medicine online or PubMed), and the association with scoliosis

Disorder and OMIM link	Pathophysiology and Inheritance	Typical features	Treatment	Association with spinal deformity
Rickets-like disorders:				
Vitamin D deficient rickets	Vitamin D deficiency from poor dietary intake, often breast fed, dark skinned	Widened physes, lethargy, limb deformities	Physiological doses of vitamin D and calcium	Historically believed to be a strong etiologic factor in scoliosis. Spinal deformity will occur in bipedial rats on a rachetogenic diet [87]. Human scoliosis is rarely if ever caused by dietary deficiency rickets [10]
Vitamin D-dependent rickets #264700 (type I) #277440 (type II)	Type I – AR, 12q13; genetic deficiency of enzyme 1-α-hydroxylase	Type I - low levels 1,25 (OH)2 vitamin D	Type I – calcitriol	Spinal deformity rarely associated, possibly because of decreased growth velocities
%600785 (type II with normal Vitamin-D receptor) #193100 (autosomal dominant type)	Type II – abnormality of calcitriol receptor; end-organ resistance;	Type II - increased levels 1,25 (OH)2 vitamin D; severe hypocalcemia	Type II – calcitriol, calcium	
X-linked hypophasphatemic rickets #307800	X-linked dominant, PHEX gene, Xp22 coding for a protease	Hypophosphatemia, decreased levels 1,25(OH)2 vitamin D; normal calcium	Calcitriol; phosphate	Spinal deformity rarely associated, possibly because of decreased growth velocities
Autosomal dominant #193100	AD, FGF23 gene, 12p13			
Lowe's syndrome #309000	Mutation in OCRL1 gene; Xp26; deficiency of phosphatidylinostitol 4,5-biphosphanate 5-phosphatase	Phosphaturia, hypophosphatemic rickets; aminoaciduria; decreased ammonia production by kidney – acidosis; carnitine wasting; cataracts; MR	Replacement therapy – phosphate, carnitine, alkali; supportive care	May develop increased lordosis and occasionally scoliosis [33]
Hypo phosphatasia #241500 (infantile) #241510 (childhood) #146300 (adult and odonthypophosphatasia forms)	Defect in alkaline phosphatase production	Identified in perinatal, infantile, childhood, adult, and odontohypophosphatasia forms. Perinatal hypophosphatasia lethal. Infantile form has a roughly 50% mortality rate with symptoms appearing within the first 6th months after birth. The other forms are generally nonlethal. Adult form and odontohypophosphatasial form are marked by premature teeth loss. Common symptoms include bone malformations and higher chance of bone fracture		Isolated cases reports of scoliosis in infantile form [2, 84]. Suggested as a genetic linkage rather than a common etiology [2]

(*continued*)

Table 14.1 (continued)

Disorder and OMIM link	Pathophysiology and Inheritance	Typical features	Treatment	Association with spinal deformity
Osteogenesis imperfecta	Over 100 different mutations lead to OI	Incidence 1:10–20,000		
Type I OI 166240 (IA), #166200 (IB)	AD. COL1A1 (chromosome 17) or COL1A2 (chromosome 7) functional null alleles causing reduced amounts of normal collagen I	Mildest and most common form of OI. Blue sclera, conductive hearing loss, with or without dentigenesis imperfecta	Bisphosphonate treatment currently for more sever cases with either pamindronate or alendronate	Occurrence of scoliosis is related to the severity of bone involvement
Type II OI 166210	Typically new mutation in either the COL1A1 gene or the COL1A2 gene	Fatal perinatally with intrauterine fractures, intracranial hemorrhage		Fatal too early for scoliosis
Type III OI #259420	AD, rarely AR. Mutation in most cases lies in one of the genes for type I collagen, COL1A1 or COL1A2	1/8th as common as type I. Severe involvement with progressive deformities, dentigenesis imperfecta, hearing loss, easy bruising, triangular facies	Bisphosphonate treatment currently with either pamindronate or alendronate	Scoliosis is very common. Kyphosis may also occur but is less common
Type IV OI #166220	AD. COL1A1 or COL1A2	Similar to type I without blue sclera and more severe osseous involvement	Bisphosphonate treatment currently with either pamindronate or alendronate	Similar to type III
Type V OI %610967	AD. Rare. Uncertain molecular mechanism	Similar to type 5 but with hyperplastic callus formation at fracture sites, calcification of the interosseous membrane between the radius and ulna, and the presence of a radioopaque metaphyseal band adjacent to the growth plates [27, 15]	Bisphosphonate treatment currently with either pamindronate or alendronate	Similar to type III
Type VI OI %610968	AD with parental mosaicism. Rare. Uncertain molecular mechanism	Similar to type IV [27]	Bisphosphonate treatment currently with either pamindronate or alendronate	Similar to type III
Type VII OI #610682	8 affected individuals in a small consanguineous First Nations community in northern Quebec. Mutation in the CRTAP gene (also cause type IIB)	Bone fragility and low bone mass	Uncertain	Uncertain

Table 14.1 (continued)

Disorder and OMIM link	Pathophysiology and Inheritance	Typical features	Treatment	Association with spinal deformity
Type VIII OI #610915	AR. Mutation in the gene encoding leprecan (LEPRE1)	Lethal	Uncertain	Uncertain
Other osteopenic syndromes				
Bruck syndrome %259450	Rare. Possibly gene encoding bone telopeptide lysyl hydroxylase	Bone similar to type I OI, multiple joint contractures, severe scoliosis [11, 12, 13]	Uncertain	Severe scoliosis similar to OI type III
Osteoporosis-pseudoglioma syndrome #259770	Familial gene encoding low density lipoprotein receptor-related protein-5	Blindness. Brittle bones	Uncertain	Scoliosis is reported
Idiopathic juvenile osteoporosis 259750	Uncertain etiology	Idiopathic osteoporosis which resolves with adolescence	Uncertain. Protect spine	May develop spine compression fractures
Mucopoly saccharidoses	Pathophysiology	Typical features	Treatment	Association with spinal deformity
Type I (Hurler's syndrome) #607014	Gene encoding α-L-iduronidase	Course features are evident early. Bulging fontanels, neurological compression, corneal clouding,; upper airway obstruction; pulmonary edema postoperatively; short stature; carpal tunnel;	Bone marrow transplant Enzyme therapy may help Gene therapy	Gibbus deformity lower spine. Upper cervical instability, odontoid hypoplasia and compression from instability or dural and ligamentous hypertrophy may occur
Type II (Hunter syndrome) +309900	Deficient activity of iduronate 2-sulfatase X-linked; mapped to Xq27–28 Dx: Enzyme assays in cultured fibroblasts/ leukocytes Increased urinary heparan and dermatan sulfate	Two forms exist (type A – severe; type B – mild) Type A – clinical features as in type IH; onset age 1–2 years; death in adolescence, 3rd decade Type B – may be diagnosed in adulthood Course facial features; hearing loss; mental retardation (type A); absence of corneal clouding; upper airway obstruction; pulmonary edema postoperatively; HSM; dysostosis multiplex; short stature; HCP; carpal tunnel; ivory skin lesions; Mongolian spots; hypertrichosis	Bone marrow transplant Enzyme therapy may alter disease progression; not curative Idursulfase ?Gene therapy	Similar to other mucopoly-saccharidosis (MPS)
Type III (Sanfilippo syndrome) #252900	Type A – deficiency of heparan N-sulfatase (17q25.3) Type B – deficiency of α-*N*-acetylg-lucosaminidase (17q21)	Type A – most severe, aggressive Behavioral issues at 2-years, neurologic manifestations at 6 years Death in second decade	Supportive care Not improved by bone marrow transplant	Similar to other MPS

(*continued*)

Table 14.1 (continued)

Disorder and OMIM link	Pathophysiology and Inheritance	Typical features	Treatment	Association with spinal deformity
#252920 #252930 #252940	Type C – deficiency of acetyl-CoA: α-glucosaminide acetyltransferase (14) Type D – deficiency of *N*-acetyl glucosamine-6-sulfatase (12q14) Dx: Increased urinary heparan sulfate	Corneal clouding not a common finding; attentional/behavioral problems; hyperactivity; seizures; diarrhea; URI		
Type IV (Morquio syndrome) numerous types	Type A – deficiency of galactosamine-6-sulfatase (GALNS gene, 16q24.3) Type B – β-galactosidase (GLB1 gene, 3p21.33) Increased urinary excretion of keratin sulfate (cartilage/cornea) Mild may not excrete ELISA Enzyme assay in cultured fibroblasts/leukocytes Genetic testing to detect mutations in GALNS, GLB1	Clinically, both forms may be similar; great variability in severity within both groups Mortality related to atlantoaxial instability, myelopathy and pulmonary compromise For severe, death in 2nd or 3rd decade of life No course facial features; normal intelligence; spondyloepiphyseal dysplasia; ligamentous laxity; odontoid hypoplasia; shortened trunk dwarfism; genu valgus; greater incidence of spinal involvement; bowel/bladder incontinence; OSA; pulmonary infections – chest wall deformity; heart valve thickening/defects; corneal clouding; enamel Less common – hearing loss, hernias	Supportive treatment	Similar to other MPS. These patients survive long enough that orthopaedic treatment, particularly for cervical instability may be necessary
Type VI (Maroteaux–Lamy syndrome) #253200	AR Deficiency of *N*-acetyl-galactosamine 4-sulfatase Accumulation of dermatan sulfate	Acceleration in growth during first year; followed by regression and short stature; course features, HSM, corneal clouding; normal intelligence Other: hearing loss, respiratory infections, valvular disease	Bone marrow transplant reported as successful	Similar to other MPS
Type VII (Sly disease) #253220	Deficiency of β-glucoronidase, required for degradation of dermatan sulfate, heparin sulfate, and chondroitin sulfate Mutation in gene mapped to chromosome 7	Phenotype varies; severe form (subtype 1) present at birth – jaundice, anemia, hydrops; milder forms present later, before (subtype 2) or after (subtype 3) age 4 years; course features; HSM; hernias; MR; dysostosis multiplex	Bone marrow transplant reported as successful in improving daily function but not the mental retardation	Similar to other MPS

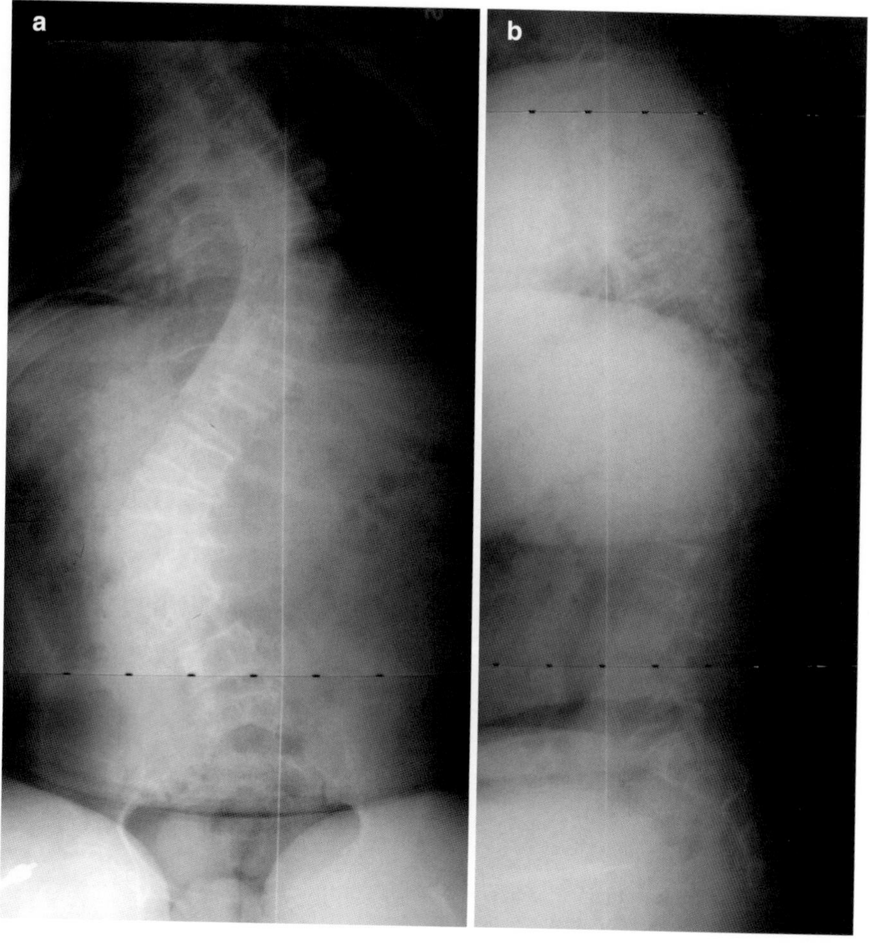

Fig. 14.1 (**a, b**) Sitting AP and lateral in a boy with severe type I OI showing the biconcave vertebrae, osteopenia, and dysplastic scoliosis

bone has been difficult at best with most authors recommending stabilization rather than relying upon correction [15]. The stability of fixation depends upon both the strength of the bone and the quality of the fixation's purchase. PMMA has been used for additional fixation [8, 26, 54]. Historically, has included each new type of fixation has been attempted. As might be expected, the greater the purchase and the more segmental the fixation, the less stress required on any single level and the greater the correction achieved [55] (Fig. 14.2). Preoperative halo gravity traction using multiple pins may be useful [36, 78], though both sixth and fourth nerve palsies have been reported in OI patients [58]. Postoperatively, there is little change from preoperative ambulatory ability or activity [15, 52, 88], thought patients report less pain, fatigue and dyspnea [77], and the improvements gained at surgery are usually maintained into adulthood [36, 77]. Spondylolysis [5] or an elongated pars with spondylolysthesis [6] can occur below a long spinal fusion. Anterior interbody fusion has been described [6], but the disorder may not be symptomatic (Fig. 14.3).

Basilar invagination with the odontiod protruding above Chamberlain's line is often difficult to see in these children with short necks, wide chests, and poor bone quality. If it is suspected, an MRI can be helpful. [37]. Basilar impression from platybasia can be very difficult to treat and shunting may be necessary [54] (Fig. 14.4). The symptoms typically develop in early adolescents and the signs include headache, lower cranial nerve problems, hyperreflexia, quadriparesis, ataxia, and nystagmus, although many patients remain asymptomatic [64]. It occurs primarily in those with more severe involvement and kyphosis, particularly with type III OI [21]. In general, patients with reducible deformities can be treated with instrumentation transferring the weight of the head to the cervical [53] or thoracic spine [29]. When reduction is not feasible, transoral [29] and an extended

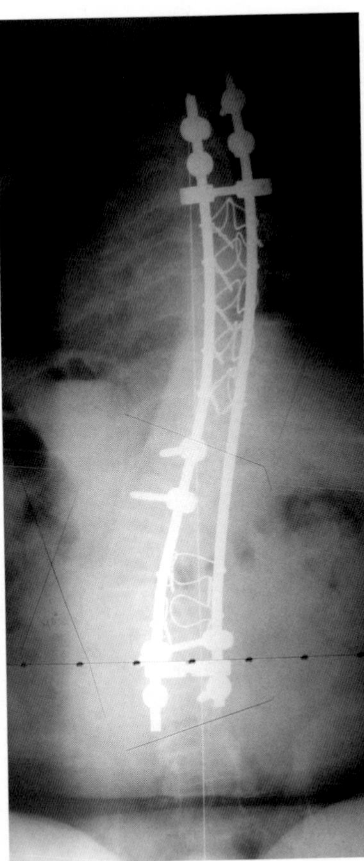

Fig. 14.2 Postoperative sitting AP radiograph showing the use of multiple fixation points for maximum bone purchase

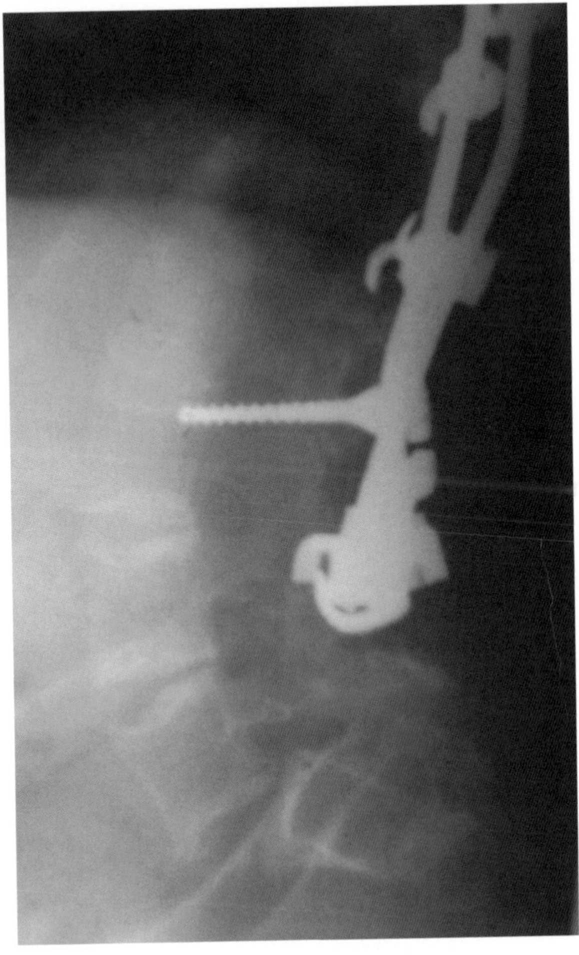

Fig. 14.3 Asymptomatic spondylolisthesis below an instrumented scoliosis spinal fusion in a patient with osteogenesis imperfecta

maxillotomy approach [35] for anterior decompression have both been used. Unfortunately, the basilar invagination can progress despite a solid fusion [64]. Prolonged immobilization, particularly during adolescence, with a custom Minerva may help improve symptoms and slow progression [64].

In our experience, bisphosphonate therapy seems to improve the bone quality for fixation, and certainly seems to improve the patients' bone pain and overall quality of life [27, 47]. Pamindronate may actually help reverse some of the pathological changes of the deformed bone [46] and may prevent scoliosis in some younger children [3]. Postoperative bisphosphontes have been suggested because progression may occur after surgery [77] Bone mineral density continues to improve for up to 2 years after pamidronate discontinuation, but not as much as in those with continued treatment [60]. Bisphosphonates should be continued until skeletal maturity is reached.

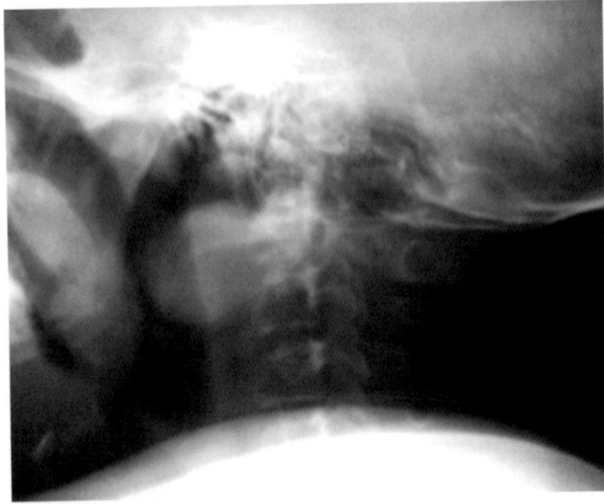

Fig. 14.4 Basilar impression currently managed with an orthosis in a patient with type III osteogenesis imperfecta

14.6 Storage Diseases

The mucopolysaccharidosis constitute a family of storage diseases with spinal abnormalities similar to those seen in spondyloepiphyseal dysplasia. In these disorders, enzymatic abnormalities prevent the normal breakdown of glycosaminoglycans (GAGs) with subsequent accumulation within lysosomes. Mucopolysaccharidoses include a group of disorders that occurs when specific lysosomal enzymes are deficient. Lysosomal enzymes are responsible for the degradation of GAGs, long-chain carbohydrates comprising a major component of connective tissue. The different types of MPS vary in severity, as well as clinical manifestations. Some features that many of the MPS share include course facies, skeletal involvement – dysostosis multiplex and short stature, organomegaly, corneal opacification, and varying degrees of mental retardation. Table 14.1 lists the different types of MPS, as well as their pathophysiology, clinical manifestations, and treatment.

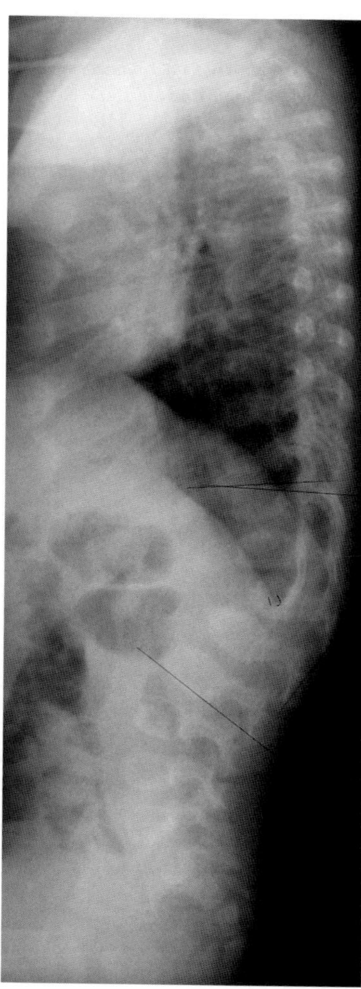

Fig. 14.5 The bullet shaped vertebra classic for storage diseases

The various types are listed in the table. At birth, the children are normal, but the accumulated GAG products produce soft tissue swelling that can cause direct spinal cord compression particularly around the craniovertebal junction and odontoid [4, 39, 45, 56, 70, 73, 74, 75, 76, 77, 81]. They may also have cervical compression from odontoid hypoplasia [40, 61, 75], and atlantoaxial instability [40, 59, 76]. A thoracolumbar gibbus is often present on presentation with a classic bullet shaped vertebra (Fig. 14.5). Occasionally, thoracic or thoracolumbar gibbus can be progressive, cause spinal cord compression, and require decompression and fusion [18, 20, 75]. Despite the improvements in MPS I (Hurlers) from bone marrow transplant, spinal abnormalities may persist because of poor enzymatic penetration of bone and require treatment [24]. These children pose substantial anesthesia risks because of their enlarged pharangeal soft tissues [4, 63, 65, 68].

14.7 Juvenile Osteoporosis

Juvenile osteoporosis is an unusual but self-limiting disease, which may result in pathological kyphosis. The diagnosis is one of the exclusion particularly looking for malignancy. Results of medications including bisphosphonates, calcitriol, fluoride, and calcitonin are equivocal with mixed results reported [1, 10, 44, 50, 66, 71]. Treatment is aimed at protecting the spine until remission [44] and the patients should be referred to an endocrinologist.

14.8 Anorexia Nervosa

Anorexia nervosa can cause decreased bone density and is most frequent in the same population as girls with idiopathic scoliosis and should be considered in patients with a low BMI and osteopenia. It can result in pathological kyphosis from multiple compression fractures [9, 49, 69, 82].

References

1. Allgrove J (2002) Use of bisphosphonates in children and adolescents. J Pediatr Endocrinol Metab 15(Suppl 3):921–928
2. Arun R, Khazim R, Webb JK et al (2005) Scoliosis in association with infantile hypophosphatasia: a case study in two siblings. Spine 30:E471–E476
3. Astrom E, Jorulf H, Soderhall S (2007) Intravenous pamidronate treatment of infants with severe osteogenesis imperfecta. Arch Dis Child 92:332–338
4. Ballenger CE, Swift TR, Leshner RT et al (1980) Myelopathy in mucopolysaccharidosis type II (Hunter syndrome). Ann Neurol 7:382–385
5. Barrack RL, Whitecloud TS, III, Skinner HB (1984) Spondylolysis after spinal instrumentation in osteogenesis imperfecta. South Med J 77:1453–1454
6. Basu PS, Hilali Noordeen MH, Elsebaie H (2001) Spondylolisthesis in osteogenesis imperfecta due to pedicle elongation: report of two cases. Spine 1:26:E506–E509
7. Benson DR, Donaldson DH, Millar EA (1978) The spine in osteogenesis imperfecta. J Bone Joint Surg Am 60:925–929
8. Benson DR, Newman DC (1981) The spine and surgical treatment in osteogenesis imperfecta. Clin Orthop Relat Res 159:147–153
9. Bernstein AE, Warner GM (1983) Onset of anorexia nervosa after prolonged use of the Milwaukee brace. Psychosomatics 24(11):1033–1034
10. Bianchi ML (2005) How to manage osteoporosis in children. Best Pract Res Clin Rheumatol 19:991–1005
11. Blacksin MF, Pletcher BA, David M (1998) Osteogenesis imperfecta with joint contractures: Bruck syndrome. Pediatr Radiol 28:117–119
12. Brenner RE, Vetter U, Stoss H et al (1993) Defective collagen fibril formation and mineralization in osteogenesis imperfecta with congenital joint contractures (Bruck syndrome). Eur J Pediatr 152:505–508
13. Breslau-Siderius EJ, Engelbert RH, Pals G et al (1998) Bruck syndrome: a rare combination of bone fragility and multiple congenital joint contractures. J Pediatr Orthop B 7:35–38
14. Brunk M (1951) The importance of rickets in childhood as a cause of scoliosis in adult age. Acta Orthop Scand Suppl 9:3–114
15. Cheung MS, Glorieux FH, Rauch F (2007) Natural history of hyperplastic callus formation in osteogenesis imperfecta type V. J Bone Miner Res 22:1181–1186
16. Cristofaro RL, Hoek KJ, Bonnett CA et al (1979) Operative treatment of spine deformity in osteogenesis imperfecta. Clin Orthop Relat Res 40–48
17. Daivajna S, Jones A, Hossein Mehdian SM (2005) Surgical management of severe cervical kyphosis with myelopathy in osteogenesis imperfecta: a case report. Spine 1:30: E191–E194
18. Dalvie SS, Noordeen MH, Vellodi A (2001) Anterior instrumented fusion for thoracolumbar kyphosis in mucopolysaccharidosis. Spine 26:E539–E541
19. Dawson-Hughes B, Heaney RP, Holick MF et al (2005) Estimates of optimal vitamin D status. Osteoporos Int 16: 713–716
20. Ebara S, Kinoshita T, Yuzawa Y et al (2003) A case of mucopolysaccharidosis IV with lower leg paresis due to thoraco-lumbar kyphoscoliosis. J Clin Neurosci 10:358–361
21. Engelbert RH, Gerver WJ, Breslau-Siderius LJ et al (1998) Spinal complications in osteogenesis imperfecta: 47 patients 1–16 years of age. Acta Orthop Scand 69:283–286
22. Engelbert RH, Uiterwaal CS, van der HA et al (2003) Scoliosis in children with osteogenesis imperfecta: influence of severity of disease and age of reaching motor milestones. Eur Spine J 12:130–134
23. Ferrera PC, Hayes ST, Triner WR (1995) Spinal cord concussion in previously undiagnosed osteogenesis imperfecta. Am J Emerg Med 13:424–426
24. Field RE, Buchanan JA, Copplemans MG et al (1994) Bone-marrow transplantation in Hurler's syndrome. Effect on skeletal development. J Bone Joint Surg Br 76:975–981
25. Frater CJ, Murray IP, Calligeros D (1995) Multiple flexion-stress vertebral end-plate fractures. An osteogenesis imperfecta presentation. Clin Nucl Med 20:1055–1057
26. Gitelis S, Whiffen J, DeWald RL (1983) The treatment of severe scoliosis in osteogenesis imperfecta. Case report. Clin Orthop Relat Res 56–59
27. Glorieux FH (2000) Bisphosphonate therapy for severe osteogenesis imperfecta. J Pediatr Endocrinol Metab 13 (Suppl 2):989–992
28. Hanscom DA, Winter RB, Lutter L et al (1992) Osteogenesis imperfecta. Radiographic classification, natural history, and treatment of spinal deformities. J Bone Joint Surg Am 74:598–616
29. Harkey HL, Crockard HA, Stevens JM et al (1990) The operative management of basilar impression in osteogenesis imperfecta. Neurosurgery 27:782–786
30. Herman MJ, Pizzutillo PD (2005) Spondylolysis and spondylolisthesis in the child and adolescent: a new classification. Clin Orthop Relat Res 434:46–54
31. Holda ME, Ryan JR (1982) Hepatobiliary rickets. J Pediatr Orthop 2:285–287
32. Holick MF (2003) Vitamin D: a millenium perspective. J Cell Biochem 1:88:296–307
33. Holtgrewe JL, Kalen V (1986) orthopaedic manifestations of the Lowe (oculocerebrorenal) syndrome. J Pediatr Orthop 6:165–171
34. Ishikawa S, Kumar SJ, Takahashi HE et al (1996) Vertebral body shape as a predictor of spinal deformity in osteogenesis imperfecta. J Bone Joint Surg Am 78 :212–219
35. James D, Crockard HA (1991) Surgical access to the base of skull and upper cervical spine by extended maxillotomy. Neurosurgery 29:411–416
36. Janus GJ, Finidori G, Engelbert RH et al (2000) Operative treatment of severe scoliosis in osteogenesis imperfecta: results of 20 patients after halo traction and posterior spondylodesis with instrumentation. Eur Spine J 9:486–491
37. Janus GJ, Engelbert RH, Beek E et al (2003) Osteogenesis imperfecta in childhood: MR imaging of basilar impression. Eur J Radiol 47:19–24
38. Juskeliene V, Magnus P, Bakketeig LS et al (1996) Prevalence and risk factors for asymmetric posture in preschool children aged 6–7 years. Int J Epidemiol 25:1053–1059
39. Kachur E, Del MR (2000) Mucopolysaccharidoses and spinal cord compression: case report and review of the literature with implications of bone marrow transplantation. Neurosurgery 47:223–228

40. Kalteis T, Schubert T, Caro WC et al (2005) Arthroscopic and histologic findings in Morquio's syndrome. Arthroscopy 21:233–237
41. Kaso G, Varju C, Doczi T (2004) Multiple vertebral fractures in osteogenesis imperfecta treated by vertebroplasty. Case illustration. J Neurosurg Spine 1:237
42. Khosla S (2001) Minireview: the OPG/RANKL/RANK system. Endocrinology 142:5050–5055
43. Kok DJ, Uiterwaal CS, Van Dongen AJ et al (2003) The interaction between silence type and BMD in osteogenesis imperfecta. Calcif Tissue Int 73:441–445
44. Krassas GE (2000) Idiopathic juvenile osteoporosis. Ann N Y Acad Sci 900:409–412
45. Kulkarni MV, Williams JC, Yeakley JW et al (1987) Magnetic resonance imaging in the diagnosis of the craniocervical manifestations of the mucopolysaccharidoses. Magn Reson Imaging 5:317–323
46. Land C, Rauch F, Munns CF et al (2006) Vertebral morphometry in children and adolescents with osteogenesis imperfecta: effect of intravenous pamidronate treatment. Bone 39:901–906
47. Lowing K, Astrom E, Oscarsson KA et al (2007) Effect of intravenous pamidronate therapy on everyday activities in children with osteogenesis imperfecta. Acta Paediatr 96: 1180–1183
48. Marchetti PG, Bartolozzi P (1997) Classification of spondylolisthesis as a guideline for treatment. In: DeWald RL, Bridwell KH (eds) The textbook for spinal surgery, 2nd edn. Lippincott-Raven, Philadelphia, pp 1211–12154
49. Mehler PS (2003) Osteoporosis in anorexia nervosa: prevention and treatment. Int J Eat Disord 33:113–126
50. Melchior R, Zabel B, Spranger J et al (2005) Effective parenteral clodronate treatment of a child with severe juvenile idiopathic osteoporosis. Eur J Pediatr 164:22–27
51. Meyer S, Villarreal M, Ziv I (1986) A three-level fracture of the axis in a patient with osteogenesis imperfecta. A case report. Spine 505–506
52. Moorefield WG, Jr., Miller GR (1980) Aftermath of osteogenesis imperfecta: the disease in adulthood. J Bone Joint Surg Am 62:113–119
53. Nakamura M, Yone K, Yamaura I et al (2002) Treatment of craniocervical spine lesion with osteogenesis imperfecta: a case report. Spine 27:E224–E227
54. Oppenheim WL (1995) The spine in osteogenesis imperfecta: a review of treatment. Connect Tissue Res 31:S59–S63
55. Osebold WR, Yamamoto SK, Hurley JH (1992) The variability of response of scoliotic spines to segmental spinal instrumentation. Spine 17:1174–1179
56. Parsons VJ, Hughes DG, Wraith JE (1996) Magnetic resonance imaging of the brain, neck and cervical spine in mild Hunter's syndrome (mucopolysaccharidoses type II). Clin Radiol 51:719–723
57. Pehrsson K, Larsson S, Oden A et al (1992) Long-term follow-up of patients with untreated scoliosis. A study of mortality, causes of death, and symptoms. Spine 17:1091–1096
58. Pinches E, Thompson D, Noordeen H et al (2004) Fourth and sixth cranial nerve injury after halo traction in children: a report of two cases. J AAPOS 8:580–585
59. Pizzutillo PD, Osterkamp JA, Scott CI Jr et al (1989) Atlantoaxial instability in mucopolysaccharidosis type VII. J Pediatr Orthop 9:76–78
60. Rauch F, Munns C, Land C et al (2006) Pamidronate in children and adolescents with osteogenesis imperfecta: effect of treatment discontinuation. J Clin Endocrinol Metab 91: 1268–1274
61. Rigante D, Antuzzi D, Ricci R et al (1999) Cervical myelopathy in mucopolysaccharidosis type IV. Clin Neuropathol 18:84–86
62. Ring ND, Nelham RL, Pearson FA (1978) Moulded supportive seating for the disabled. Prosthet Orthot Int 2:30–34
63. Roberts W, Henson LC (1995) Anesthesia for scoliosis: dwarfism and congenitally absent odontoid process. AANA J 63:332–337
64. Sawin PD, Menezes AH (1997) Basilar invagination in osteogenesis imperfecta and related osteochondrodysplasias: medical and surgical management. J Neurosurg 86:950–960
65. Semenza GL, Pyeritz RE (1988) Respiratory complications of mucopolysaccharide storage disorders. Medicine (Baltimore) 67:209–219
66. Shaw NJ, Boivin CM, Crabtree NJ (2000) Intravenous pamidronate in juvenile osteoporosis. Arch Dis Child 83: 143–145
67. Shore RM, Langman CB, Poznanski AK (2000) Lumbar and radial bone mineral density in children and adolescents with X-linked hypophosphatemia: evaluation with dual X-ray absorptiometry. Skeletal Radiol 29:90–93
68. Sjogren P, Pedersen T, Steinmetz H (1987) Mucopolysaccharidoses and anaesthetic risks. Acta Anaesthesiol Scand 31: 214–218
69. Smith FM, Latchford G, Hall RM et al (2002) Indications of disordered eating behaviour in adolescent patients with idiopathic scoliosis. J Bone Joint Surg Br 84:392–394
70. Sostrin RD, Hasso AN, Peterson DI et al (1977) Myelographic features of mucopolysaccharidoses: a new sign. Radiology 125:421–424
71. Speiser PW, Clarson CL, Eugster EA et al (2005) Bisphosphonate treatment of pediatric bone disease. Pediatr Endocrinol Rev 3:87–96
72. Sperry K (1989) Fatal intraoperative hemorrhage during spinal fusion surgery for osteogenesis imperfecta. Am J Forensic Med Pathol 10:54–59
73. Taccone A, Tortori DP, Marzoli A et al (1993) Mucopolysaccharidosis: thickening of dura mater at the craniocervical junction and other CT/MRI findings. Pediatr Radiol 23:349–352
74. Tamaki N, Kojima N, Tanimoto M et al (1987) Myelopathy due to diffuse thickening of the cervical dura mater in Maroteaux-Lamy syndrome: report of a case. Neurosurgery 21:416–419
75. Tandon V, Williamson JB, Cowie RA et al (1996) Spinal problems in mucopolysaccharidosis I (Hurler syndrome). J Bone Joint Surg Br 78:938–944
76. Thorne JA, Javadpour M, Hughes DG et al (2001) Craniovertebral abnormalities in Type VI mucopolysaccharidosis (Maroteaux-Lamy syndrome). Neurosurgery 48: 849–852
77. Tolboom N, Cats EA, Helders PJ et al (2004) Osteogenesis imperfecta in childhood: effects of spondylodesis on functional ability, ambulation and perceived competence. Eur Spine J 13:108–113
78. Topouchian V, Finidori G, Glorion C et al (2004) Posterior spinal fusion for kypho-scoliosis associated with osteogenesis

imperfecta: long-term results. Rev Chir Orthop Reparatrice Appar Mot 90:525–532
79. Vijay S, Wraith JE (2005) Clinical presentation and follow-up of patients with the attenuated phenotype of mucopolysaccharidosis type I. Acta Paediatr 94:872–877
80. Vitale MG, Matsumoto H, Kessler MW et al (2007) Osteogenesis imperfecta: determining the demographics and the predictors of death from an inpatient population. J Pediatr Orthop 27:228–232
81. Wald SL, Schmidek HH (1984) Compressive myelopathy associated with type VI mucopolysaccharidosis (Maroteaux-Lamy syndrome). Neurosurgery 14:83–88
82. Warren MP, Brooks-Gunn J, Hamilton LH et al (1986) Scoliosis and fractures in young ballet dancers. Relation to delayed menarche and secondary amenorrhea. N Engl J Med 314:1348–1353
83. Watanabe G, Kawaguchi S, Matsuyama T et al (2007) Correlation of scoliotic curvature with Z-score bone mineral density and body mass index in patients with osteogenesis imperfecta. Spine 32:E488–E494
84. Whyte MP, Kurtzberg J, McAlister WH et al (2003) Marrow cell transplantation for infantile hypophosphatasia. J Bone Miner Res 18:624–636
85. Widmann RF, Bitan FD, Laplaza FJ et al (1999) Spinal deformity, pulmonary compromise, and quality of life in osteogenesis imperfecta. Spine 24:1673–1678
86. Wiltse LL, Newman PH, Macnab I (1976) Classification of spondylolisis and spondylolisthesis. Clin Orthop Relat Res 117:23–29
87. Yamamoto H (1966) Experimental scoliosis in rachitic bipedal rats. Tokushima J Exp Med 13:1–34
88. Yong-Hing K, MacEwen GD (1982) Scoliosis associated with osteogenesis imperfecta. J Bone Joint Surg Br 64: 36–43
89. Ziv I, Rang M, Hoffman HJ (1983) Paraplegia in osteogenesis imperfecta. A case report. J Bone Joint Surg Br 65: 184–185

Spinal Manifestations of the Skeletal Dysplasias

15

Michael C. Ain and Eric D. Shirley

Key Points

- When a patient with skeletal dysplasia associated with atlantoaxial instability undergoes any type of surgery, the cervical spine must be evaluated.
- Thoracolumbar kyphosis in infants with achondroplasia usually resolves without treatment.
- The treatment guidelines for scoliosis associated with the skeletal dysplasias are similar to those for idiopathic scoliosis.
- Foramen magnum stenosis may occur in patients with achondroplasia or hypochondroplasia, resulting in snoring, apnea, other signs/symptoms of brainstem compression, or sudden infant death.

15.1 Introduction

Skeletal dysplasias are a heterogeneous group of disorders caused by abnormalities in the growth and development of bone and/or cartilage. Most dysplasias result in short stature, with height more than 2 standard deviations below the population mean for the given age. Spinal manifestations are common in patients with skeletal dysplasias [7]. Dysplasias currently associated with spinal deformity include achondroplasia, chondrodysplasia punctata, diastrophic dysplasia, Kniest dysplasia, Larsen syndrome, metaphyseal chondrodysplasias, metatropic dwarfism, mucopolysaccharidoses, pseudoachondroplasia, spondyloepiphyseal dysplasia congenita and tarda, and spondyloepimetaphyseal dysplasia.

15.2 Spinal Pathology Associated with Skeletal Dysplasias

Several different spinal abnormalities occur in patients with skeletal dysplasias. The most common abnormalities include atlantoaxial instability and odontoid hypoplasia, cervical kyphosis, thoracolumbar kyphosis, scoliosis, foramen magnum stenosis, and spinal stenosis.

15.2.1 *Atlantoaxial Instability and Odontoid Hypoplasia*

When patients with skeletal dysplasias that are associated with odontoid hypoplasia and atlantoaxial instability present for any type of surgery, the cervical spine

[1]The views expressed in this article are those of the author(s) and do not necessarily reflect the official policy or position of the Department of the Navy, Department of Defense, or the United States Government. None of the authors or the department to which they are affiliated has received anything of value from or owns stock in a commercial company or institution related directly or indirectly to the subject of this article.

M. C. Ain (✉)
Department of Orthopaedic Surgery, Johns Hopkins Bayview Medical Center, The Johns Hopkins University, 4940 Eastern Avenue, A665, Baltimore, MD 21224-2780, USA
e-mail: ehenze1@jhmi.edu

B. A. Akbarnia et al. (eds.), *The Growing Spine*,
DOI: 10.1007/978-3-540-85207-0_15, © Springer-Verlag Berlin Heidelberg 2011

must be evaluated. Skeletal dysplasias frequently associated with atlantoaxial instability include Conradi–Hunermann syndrome (subtype of chondrodysplasia punctata), Kniest dysplasia, metaphyseal chondrodysplasia (McKusick and Schmid type), metatropic dwarfism, Morquio syndrome (type of mucopolysaccharidoses), pseudoachondroplasia, and spondyloepiphyseal dysplasia congenita and tarda.

Atlantoaxial instability can result in cervical myelopathy and manifest with a progressive lack of endurance and upper motor neuron signs (hyperreflexia, clonus, positive Babinski sign, and spasticity). However, the presentation of myelopathy caused by atlantoaxial instability in children with skeletal dysplasias may be atypical and may present with general tiredness, vague pains in the extremities, inability to move the limbs on awakening in the morning, failure to develop gait, and unexplained paroxysmal tachypnea. Fatigue generally occurs before the development of neurologic signs. A diagnosis of odontoid hypoplasia or aplasia is made by plain radiographs, and lateral flexion-extension cervical spine radiographs identify the presence of atlantoaxial instability.

C1–C2 arthrodesis is indicated for an atlantodens interval of more than 8 mm or for neurologic compromise. If the translation is between 5 and 8 mm, a magnetic resonance imaging (MRI) scan in flexion and extension is necessary, and arthrodesis is performed if the flexion-extension MRI shows spinal cord compromise. C1–C2 arthrodesis is also considered if the spinal cord space is 14mm or less [3]. C1–C2 laminectomies with enlargement of the foramen magnum are performed as needed. Internal fixation of the cervical spine in patients of small stature can be achieved with cables, lateral mass screws, pedicle screws, or C1–C2 intraarticular screws [3]. For successful arthrodesis, autogenous bone graft is preferred.

15.2.2 Cervical Kyphosis

Cervical kyphosis may occur in patients with diastrophic dysplasia and Larsen syndrome. However, the natural history of the kyphosis in these dysplasias differs markedly, with a greater potential for resolution occurring in patients with diastrophic dysplasia (see subsequent sections on these two disorders for additional information on the natural history of each condition).

In the presence of neurologic signs/symptoms or if the kyphosis continues to progress despite bracing, surgery is indicated. Surgery consists of posterior cervical spinal arthrodesis and, if anterior compression is present, anterior decompression. Severe spinal cord compression or myelopathy requires corpectomy with strut grafting. Instrumentation is used if pedicle size allows. Autogenous bone graft is obtained from the iliac crest. The femurs or tibia may be used as a source if more bone is required.

15.2.3 Thoracic and Thoracolumbar Kyphosis

Thoracic or thoracolumbar kyphosis is a manifestation of several skeletal dysplasias, and it may occur in patients with: achondroplasia, Conradi–Hunermann syndrome, diastrophic dwarfism, metatropic dwarfism, mucopolysaccharidoses, or spondyloepiphyseal dysplasia.

In achondroplasia (see later section), the thoracolumbar kyphosis typically resolves. The natural history of the kyphoses associated with the other dysplasias is not as favorable. Anterior or posterior fusion is required for progressive kyphoses.

15.2.4 Scoliosis

Scoliosis may occur in association with several of the skeletal dysplasias, including chondrodysplasia punctata, diastrophic dwarfism, metatropic dwarfism, Morquio syndrome, pseudoachondroplasia, spondyloepiphyseal dysplasia congenita, and spondyloepimetaphyseal dysplasia.

The curve type and natural history depend on the type of dysplasia with which the scoliosis is associated. In general, treatment guidelines for scoliosis associated with the skeletal dysplasias are similar to those for idiopathic scoliosis. Bracing is indicated for curves between 25° and 45°. Posterior spinal arthrodesis is indicated for curves larger than 50°. Growing rod instrumentation or anteroposterior arthrodesis can be performed in younger patients, with definitive fusion delayed until the patient is older, to prevent the development of crankshaft and curve progression.

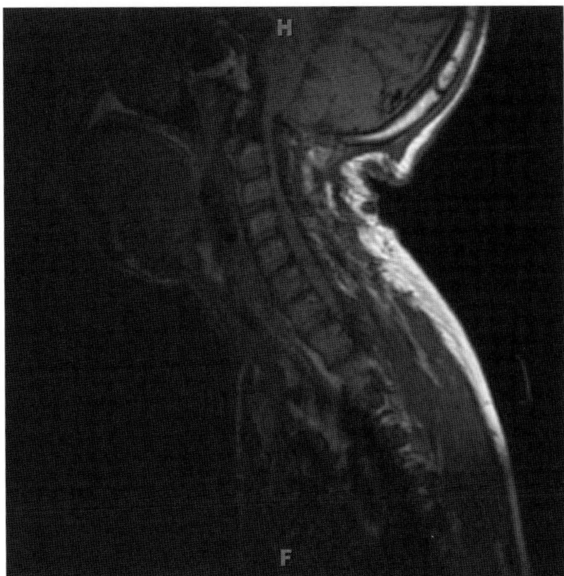

Fig. 15.1 MRI of a patient with achondroplasia and foramen magnum stenosis

15.2.5 Foramen Magnum Stenosis

In addition to spinal deformity and instability, narrowing of the spinal canal may occur in patients with skeletal dysplasias. Stenotic problems are seen along the entire spinal canal. Foramen magnum stenosis may occur in patients with achondroplasia and hypochondroplasia.

The most common symptoms of stenosis at the level of the foramen magnum are excessive snoring and apnea [5]. Stenosis can also result in other signs or symptoms of chronic brainstem compression, including lower cranial nerve dysfunction, hyperreflexia, hypotonia, weakness or paresis, clonus, and swallowing difficulty. Stenosis may also result in developmental delay. Most importantly, foramen magnum stenosis may result in sudden death. Therefore, diagnosis is critical and may be made via a sleep study and MRI (Fig. 15.1). Treatment requires surgical decompression.

15.2.6 Spinal Stenosis

In addition to the stenosis seen at the level of the foramen magnum, patients with skeletal dysplasias may also have spinal stenosis at more distal levels. Spinal stenosis may occur in patients with achondroplasia and Conradi–Hunermann syndrome. The initial treatment of spinal stenosis is nonoperative. Surgical indications include progressive symptoms, urinary retention, severe claudication with symptoms after less than two city blocks, and neurologic symptoms at rest.

15.3 Classification of Dysplasias

There are several methods of classifying skeletal dysplasias. One method is by type of body disproportion: short limb or short trunk. Short-limb types are further divided by the location of the short segment within the limb: proximal (rhizomelic), middle (mesomelic), or distal (acromelic). A second method is to classify the dysplasias by the causative genetic defects. Finally, skeletal dysplasias may be classified by the presence or absence (e.g., multiple epiphyseal dysplasia) of spinal deformity. These dysplasias with spinal manifestations can be further divided into achondroplasia, diastrophic dysplasia, pseudoachondroplasia, dysplasias secondary to mutations in collagen synthesis, the mucopolysaccharidoses, and other skeletal dysplasias.

15.3.1 Achondroplasia

Achondroplasia, the most common skeletal dysplasia, has an incidence of 1 in 30,000 persons [19]. Achondroplasia is caused by a mutation of fibroblast growth factor 3 receptor, which results in defective endochondral bone formation [26]. Inheritance is autosomal dominant. Manifestations include rhizomelic short stature, trident hand, genu varum, and elbow flexion contractures. Medical complications include frequent otitis media, obstructive sleep apnea, decreased respiratory drive, decreased pulmonary function, and hydrocephalus. Spinal manifestations of achondroplasia include thoracolumbar kyphosis, foramen magnum stenosis, and spinal stenosis.

The first spinal manifestation that may occur in achondroplasia is foramen magnum stenosis, which can present during the first 2 years of life. The stenosis is the result of the presence of a comparatively small foramen magnum at birth with defective endochondral ossification, resulting in impaired growth of the foramen magnum in the first year of life. Foramen magnum stenosis is treated with surgical decompression. Although most patients who become symptomatic require decompression during the first 2 years of life, symptoms may also occur in older patients and require treatment at that time. Decompression extends to C1 in younger patients and to T4 in older patients.

Bagley et al. [5] reviewed 43 patients with achondroplasia who underwent cervicomedullary decompression for foramen magnum stenosis (mean age at surgery, 5 years 10 months; range, 2–199 months). Improvement of respiratory symptoms in infants occurred soon after the decompression. Complications included cerebrospinal fluid leaks (seven), recurrent stenosis requiring revision surgery (five), and infection (four) [3, 5].

The second spinal manifestation to occur during development is thoracolumbar kyphosis. Thoracolumbar kyphosis is a common manifestation of achondroplasia, with a frequency of 87% in 1- to 2-year-olds [12]. Thoracolumbar kyphosis in the newborn with achondroplasia is typically 20°. When sitting begins (usually between 6 and 18 months of age), the infant will often slump forward because of trunk hypotonia in combination with a relatively oversized head and protuberant abdomen. Repeated slumping results in an increase of the kyphosis, and anterior vertebral wedging may occur (Fig. 15.2). Most of these kyphoses tend to resolve at 12–18 months of age as trunk strength improves and the child begins to walk. This natural resolution results in a rate of kyphosis of 39% for 2- to 5-year-olds and of 11% for 5- to 10-year-olds [12].

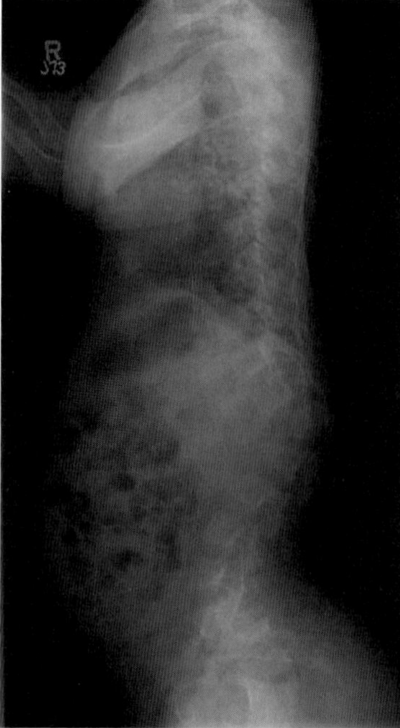

Fig. 15.2 Lateral radiograph of 5-year-old with achondroplasia, thoracolumbar kyphosis, and vertebral wedging

Efforts are made to prevent the development of kyphoses by prohibiting an infant from unsupported sitting and from sitting up more than 60° even with support [21]. Kyphoses that persist can result in deformity progression, hip flexion contractures, and hyperlordosis. In addition, persistent kyphoses can increase the severity of coexisting spinal stenosis.

Bracing is considered for thoracolumbar kyphosis if the kyphosis is progressing and is associated with vertebral wedging. Bracing is continued until wedging resolves and the kyphosis has decreased. In a series of 66 patients treated by Pauli et al. [20] with sitting modifications and bracing as needed, none of the 66 patients developed progressive kyphosis. However, applying a brace to a child with small stature and hypotonia may result in increased falls and decreased mobility. Therefore, bracing is not always used for such patients.

When vertebral wedging or kyphosis persists, surgery is indicated. The natural history of persistent kyphoses is not well described, but kyphoses larger than 50° will most likely develop a rigid angular kyphosis with neurologic symptoms. Therefore, surgery is indicated for patients with kyphoses and neurologic compromise or kyphoses larger than 50° [2]. Surgical treatment consists of posterior arthrodesis alone or combined anterior–posterior arthrodesis. Indications for an anteroposterior surgery include anterior impingement and pedicle size inadequate for pedicle screws. If there is anterior impingement, anterior corpectomy with a strut graft is performed. Laminectomy is performed if spinal stenosis is present. Pedicle screws are preferred for posterior instrumentation because wires and hooks are contraindicated secondary to the preexisting small spinal canal. The arthrodesis is extended to the sacrum with or without iliac fixation if the sacrum is destabilized by the decompression. However, extending the arthrodesis to the sacrum may result in problems with personal hygiene.

Safe insertion of pedicle screws requires technical experience and knowledge of the pedicle morphometry in patients with achondroplasia [30]. In patients with achondroplasia the pedicles have cranial inclination, and the starting points for screw insertion diverge progressively in the lumbar spine [30]. Pedicle lengths are significantly shorter, and screws 20–25-mm long are appropriate for lower thoracic and lumbar pedicles in adult achondroplasts. Pedicle screw diameters of

5–7 mm may be used in most adult patients. Transverse angulation is greatest at L5 and smallest at T12 [30].

Ain and Shirley [2] described four patients who underwent a two-stage anterior and posterior spinal arthrodesis with anterior instrumentation. Correction ranged from 23% to 31%; there were no complications. Ain and Browne [1] reported on 12 patients (mean age, 12 years; range, 4–21 years) who underwent posterior-only spinal arthrodesis (seven patients), anteroposterior arthrodesis with posterior instrumentation (two patients), or anterior instrumentation (three patients). Successful fusion was obtained in all patients; there were no intraoperative or postoperative neurologic complications. The mean preoperative thoracolumbar kyphosis was 64° (range, 43°–88°). The final mean thoracolumbar kyphosis was 29° (range, 16°–48°), representing a mean correction of 50% (range, 17%–73%) [1].

Finally, patients with achondroplasia are at risk for the development of spinal stenosis. Stenosis typically becomes symptomatic in the third or fourth decade, but symptoms may also begin in skeletally immature patients [27]. The incidence of symptomatic spinal stenosis increases from 10% of 10 year-olds to 80% of patients in the sixth decade [9].

Spinal stenosis in achondroplasia occurs as a result of several factors. The endochondral ossification defects result in shortening of both the vertebral bodies and pedicles [17]. The pedicles are also thickened [17]. The interpediculate distance typically decreases from L1 to L5 (Fig. 15. 3), but this decrease does not occur in all patients [15]. The soft-tissue elements are also affected, with hyperplasia of the intervertebral discs and ligamentum flavum. These abnormalities result in a 40% reduction of the sagittal and coronal diameters of the achondroplastic spine [14]. Although the spinal canal is narrowed, the spinal cord and neural elements are of normal size.

Surgical decompression is indicated for symptoms that are progressive or not alleviated by nonoperative measures. Computed tomography myelography (via high cervical puncture) and MRI are obtained preoperatively. To prevent recurrent stenosis and the need for additional surgery, decompression for stenosis in the lower lumbar spine should extend three levels cephalad to the level of stenosis and at least to S2 [21]. Rarely, total craniospinal decompression is required. In one study of spinal decompressions in patients with achondroplasia by Uematsu et al. [33], 13 of 111 (12%) required total craniospinal decompression. If lateral stenosis is evident on preoperative imaging studies, a wide decompression is performed with exploration of the nerve root recesses on both sides.

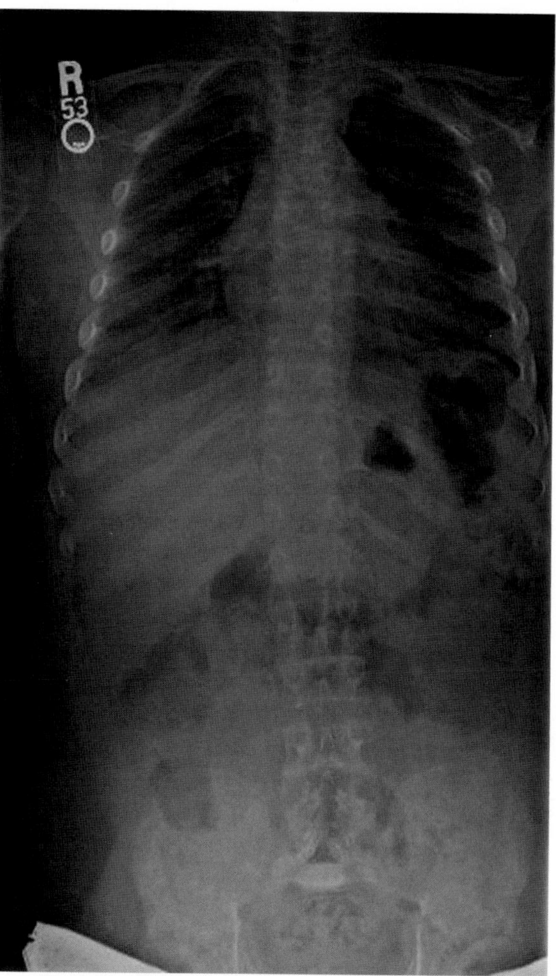

Fig. 15.3 Anteroposterior lumbar spine radiograph of a patient with achondroplasia and decreasing interpediculate distance from L1 to L5

In the skeletally immature patients with achondroplasia, complications of decompression for spinal stenosis include incomplete recovery, dural tears, urinary dysfunction, wound infection, and postlaminectomy kyphosis.

In a study of 20 patients with achondroplasia who underwent laminectomies, Streeten et al. [31] reported that neurologic deficits improved in 14 patients. Severe preoperative deficits, including paraplegia and sphincter dysfunction, did not improve substantially unless treated acutely. In another series of 44 pediatric patients with achondroplasia who underwent a total of 60 decompressive procedures, Sciubba et al. [28] found complications in 11% of cases: four dural tears, two wound breakdowns, and one instrumentation failure. Of those 60 procedures, 11 were revision surgeries. Reasons for revision surgery included progressive deformity in the nonfused spine (five cases), decompression of junctional stenosis (five cases), and repeat decompression at same levels (one case). The dural tear rate is high in the patient with achondroplasia because the dura is especially thin and fragile, although it was as low as 7% in the study by Sciubba et al. [28].

Postlaminectomy kyphosis is a common complication in the skeletally immature, but not the adult, patient with achondroplasia [4, 21]. Ain et al. [4] reviewed ten consecutive skeletally immature patients with achondroplasia who underwent five-to eight-level thoracolumbar laminectomies for symptomatic spinal stenosis during a 10-year period. The mean preoperative kyphosis was 31° (range, 10°–50°). Despite preservation of more than 50% of each medial facet, postlaminectomy thoracolumbar kyphoses (mean, 94°; range, 78°–135°) developed in all patients, and all patients required secondary arthrodesis 10 months to 2.6 years after the initial surgery. Because of the high risk of developing a postlaminectomy kyphosis, concurrent spinal arthrodesis should be performed in the skeletally immature patient with achondroplasia who undergoes thoracolumbar laminectomy [4].

15.3.2 Diastrophic Dysplasia

Diastrophic dysplasia is caused by mutations in the sulfate transporter gene, and it primarily affects cartilage because of the presence of negatively charged sulfate groups in proteoglycan molecules. Inheritance is autosomal dominant. This dysplasia is extremely rare, except in Finland [22, 24, 26]. Manifestations include marked short stature with rhizomelic shortening, hitchhiker thumbs, severe clubfeet, skewfoot, joint contractures, and severe osteoarthritis.

Nonorthopaedic manifestations include cleft palate, trachelomalacia, and cauliflower ear. Spinal manifestations include: cervical kyphosis, cervical spina bifida, scoliosis, and kyphoscoliosis [7].

Cervical kyphosis occurs in up to one-third of patients with diastrophic dysplasia [22]. The kyphosis typically has an apex at C3 or C4, with hypoplasia of the vertebral bodies C3–C5 [22]. Concurrent cervical spina bifida is present in 80% of patients [25]. However, the etiology of the kyphosis is related to vertebral body hypoplasia and not to the presence of the spina bifida.

The natural history of cervical kyphosis in diastrophic dysplasia is favorable. Most kyphoses resolve as the children begin to hold their heads up, which strengthens the extensor muscles and decreases the stress on the vertebrae. The decreased mechanical load also results in the resolution of the vertebral hypoplasia [22]. However, if the kyphosis is larger than 60° and the apical vertebrae is round or triangular and totally displaced posteriorly, then progression is likely [22].

Treatment usually is not required, but bracing is considered if the kyphosis progresses. The Milwaukee brace can be effective in such patients [6]. Surgery is indicated if there are neurologic sign/symptoms or if the kyphosis continues to progress despite bracing.

Scoliosis is extremely common in patients with diastrophic dysplasia (up to 90% of those patients) [23]. The development of scoliosis may be related to abnormal disc structure and rapid degeneration [24]. Three types of curves are found in such patients: mild nonprogressive, idiopathic-like, and early progressive [23]. The early progressive type is similar to the progressive form of infantile scoliosis and is characterized by an age at onset of less than 3 years, severe rotation, and a rapid rate of progression. Kyphosis may also be present [16]. Without treatment, these curves will progress beyond 100° [23]. Treatment consists of growing rod instrumentation in younger patients, or posterior spinal arthrodesis with or without anterior spinal arthrodesis in older patients.

15.3.3 Pseudoachondroplasia

Pseudoachondroplasia is caused by a mutation in the gene for cartilage oligomeric matrix protein, an extracellular matrix glycoprotein found in the territorial matrix surrounding chondrocytes. Inheritance is autosomal dominant. Pseudoachondroplasia is characterized by involvement of the spine, metaphyses, and epiphyses. Manifestations include a short trunk, rhizomelic or mesomelic shortening of the extremities, ligamentous laxity, expanded metaphyses and small/fragmented epiphyses, hip subluxation, lower extremity malalignment, and delicate facies. Severe osteoarthritis of the weight-bearing joints occurs. Spinal manifestations include odontoid hypoplasia and scoliosis.

Of patients with pseudoachondroplasia, 60% have os odontoideum [29]. The presence of inherent ligamentous laxity and the os odontoideum results in atlantoaxial instability in 10%–20% of patients (see Sect. 15.2.1 for discussion on treatment) [8]. Scoliosis in patients with pseudoachondroplasia tends to be mild [11]. Bracing is indicated for scoliosis between 25° and 45°. Curves do not typically progress more than 50°, and surgery is rarely necessary [11]. When surgery is required, preoperative pulmonary evaluation may be necessary because respiratory impairment may be present as a result of progressive respiratory muscle paralysis.

15.3.4 Dysplasias Secondary to Mutations in Collagen Synthesis

Several skeletal dysplasias are secondary to mutations in collagen. These dysplasias, which may be associated with spinal abnormalities, include Kniest dysplasia, spondyloepiphyseal dysplasia congenita/tarda, and the metaphyseal chondrodysplasias.

Kniest dysplasia, an autosomal-dominant disorder caused by mutations in type-II collagen α-1 chain (*COL2A1*), is characterized by short-trunk disproportion. Manifestations include dumbbell-shaped long bones with broad metaphyses and irregular dysplastic epiphyses, joint contractures, genu valgum, and equinovarus feet. Degenerative arthritis may occur as early as the teen years. Associated nonorthopaedic conditions include midface hypoplasia, myopia, retinal detachment, and deafness. Spinal manifestations include odontoid hypoplasia, hypoplasia of the remaining cervical vertebrae, flattening of all vertebrae (platyspondyly), kyphosis, and mild scoliosis. Platyspondyly is seen in many different skeletal dysplasias and does not require treatment (see Sects. 15.2.1, 15.2.3, 15.2.4 for descriptions of treatment of the other conditions). When surgical treatment is required, patients need to be evaluated for the presence of cleft palate or tracheomalacia, which could result in respiratory complications.

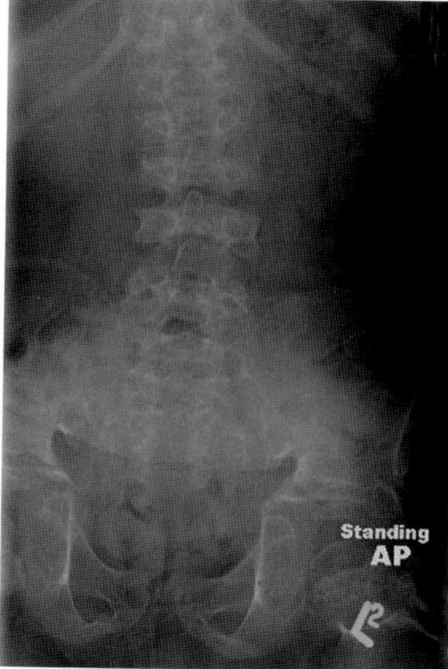

Fig. 15.4 Anteroposterior lumbar spine radiograph of a patient with metatropic dysplasia and platyspondyly

Spondyloepiphyseal dysplasia congenita and tarda are both associated with spinal abnormalities. Spondyloepiphyseal dysplasia congenita is also caused by mutations in type-II collagen (*COL2A1*). Inheritance is autosomal dominant, but most cases occur secondary to new mutations. This extremely rare dysplasia is characterized by a short trunk and short limbs with abnormal formation of the long-bone epiphyses and lower extremity malalignment. Other manifestations include retinal detachment, severe myopia, and sensorineural hearing loss. Spinal abnormalities include atlantoaxial instability, platyspondyly, kyphosis, and scoliosis [32]. Atlantoaxial instability may be the result of odontoid hypoplasia or ligamentous laxity. Scoliosis in such patients occurs early in life and is often resistant to bracing. Treatment is described in the earlier section, with surgery recommended for curves of more than 50° [32]. For larger curves or those with excessive kyphosis, anteroposterior arthrodesis with anterior grafting may be required [18].

Spondyloepiphyseal dysplasia tarda is milder than spondyloepiphyseal dysplasia congenita. X-linked inheritance is the most common type of inheritance. Spondyloepiphyseal dysplasia tarda may result from a mutation in type-II collagen, but the mechanism remains to be shown. Manifestations include odontoid hypoplasia, mild platyspondyly, scoliosis, and osteoarthritis.

Finally, spinal disorders may occur in patients with metaphyseal chondrodysplasias. This group of disorders is characterized by metaphyseal involvement with epiphyseal preservation, short stature, and genu varum. The Schmid type is caused by an α-1 chain of type-X collagen (*COL110A1*) mutation. Inheritance is autosomal dominant. The McKusick type, also known as cartilage-hair hypoplasia, is caused by a mutation of the *RMRP* gene (ribosomal nucleic acid component of mitochondrial ribosomal nucleic acid processing endoribonuclease). Manifestations also include ligamentous laxity, pectus abnormalities, fine hair, impaired T-cell immunity, anemia, Hirschprung disease, and an increased risk of malignancy. Atlantoaxial instability (see description in Sect. 15.2.1) may occur in these two types of metaphyseal chondrodysplasia.

15.3.5 Mucopolysaccharidoses

The mucopolysaccharidoses are a group of lysosomal storage diseases resulting from enzymatic deficiency. Inheritance is autosomal recessive except in type II (Hunter syndrome), which is X-linked. Manifestations vary with each subtype. In general, these dysplasias are characterized by short stature, stiff joints, and capacious acetabuli. The most common subtypes are types I and IV.

Mucopolysaccharidoses type I is subdivided into the Hurler and Scheie forms, which represent the severe and mild types of the disease, respectively. Hurler syndrome is characterized by progressive mental retardation, severe deformities, and organ dysfunction. Death occurs before the age of 10 years. The Scheie form is characterized by joint stiffness, limb malalignment, and a normal life expectancy. Both forms are associated with upper cervical anomalies, including odontoid hypoplasia and atlantoaxial instability.

In type IV, Morquio syndrome, the degradation of keratan sulfate, which is found only in the cornea, cartilage, and nucleus pulposus of the intervertebral discs, is defective. This defective degradation results in the presence of corneal opacities and urinary excretion of keratan sulfate. Manifestations include short-trunk dwarfism, genu valgum, ligamentous laxity, and early hip and knee arthritis. Spinal manifestations include platyspondyly, odontoid hypoplasia/atlantoaxial instability, and scoliosis.

All patients with Morquio syndrome have odontoid hypoplasia. Atlantoaxial instability may result in myelopathy, which can cause delayed motor development. This delay in motor development can be inappropriately attributed to the coexisting genu valgum. When surgery is required for atlantoaxial instability, pulmonary and cardiac evaluations may be necessary to rule out pulmonary hypertension and congenital cardiac anomalies [17]. Restrictive lung disease, sleep apnea, or pulmonary hypertension may be found [17]. Cardiac involvement is the result of aortic insufficiency or cardiac ischemia from infiltration of the coronary arteries with mucopolysaccharides [17]. An anterior hypertrophic soft-tissue mass may be present along with atlantoaxial instability. After successful posterior fusion, the soft-tissue mass typically resolves. Therefore, anterior decompression is not usually performed at the time of the index surgery.

15.3.6 Other Skeletal Dysplasias

Other skeletal dysplasias associated with spinal manifestations include chondrodysplasia punctata, Larsen syndrome, and metatropic dwarfism, and spondyloepimetaphyseal dysplasia.

Chondrodysplasia punctata, also known as congenital stippled epiphysis, has multiple subtypes. The cause is related to defective cholesterol biosynthesis. Manifestations include short stature, facial anomalies, and radiographic stippling. The most common subtype is Conradi–Hunermann syndrome. Spinal manifestations of Conradi–Hunermann syndrome include atlantoaxial instability, scoliosis, kyphosis, and spinal stenosis. Cervical stenosis may occur, but it is rare [34]. Scoliosis occurs in two types: a slowly progressive type without dysplastic vertebrae and a rapidly progressive type with dysplastic vertebrae and kyphoscoliosis. When surgery is required for the slowly progressive type, standard posterior arthrodesis is sufficient [18]. Surgery for the rapidly progressive type often requires anteroposterior arthrodesis to decrease the risk of pseudarthrosis [18]. Hemiepiphysiodesis is not as successful as it might be for congenital deformities with dysplastic vertebrae because all of the vertebrae in such patients are potentially dysplastic [18]. When surgery is required, preoperative cardiac and renal function needs to be evaluated because of potential congenital abnormalities.

Larsen syndrome is characterized by multiple joint dislocations, hypertelorism, and hypotonia. Dislocations commonly involve the elbows, hips, and knees. Inheritance may be autosomal dominant or autosomal recessive. Spinal pathology may also occur, including cervical kyphosis, cervical/thoracic spina bifida, atlantoaxial instability, subaxial instability, spondylolisthesis, and scoliosis. Cervical kyphosis occurs in up to 60% of cases of Larsen syndrome [10, 13]. The kyphosis is associated with hypoplastic vertebral bodies at C4 and C5. Unlike in patients with cervical kyphosis and diastrophic dysplasia, spontaneous improvement of the kyphosis does not occur. Posterior spinal arthrodesis is indicated for kyphoses larger than 40°. After arthrodesis, additional correction can occur as the child grows because the fusion acts as a posterior tether.

Metatropic dwarfism is characterized by a short-limb dwarfism that converts to a short-trunk pattern when kyphosis and scoliosis develops. The condition is associated with enlarged metaphyses and joint contractures (Fig. 15.4). Vertebrae are markedly flattened throughout the spine. In addition to kyphosis and scoliosis, atlantoaxial instability may occur. Scoliosis in patients with metatropic dysplasia is characteristically rigid. Surgical treatment may require anterior release before posterior spinal arthrodesis. When surgery is required, pulmonary evaluation is important because respiratory impairment may occur.

Finally, spondyloepimetaphyseal dysplasia is a rare dysplasia characterized by generalized spine, epiphyseal, and metaphyseal involvement. Severe kyphoscoliosis may occur [35]. The kyphoscoliosis can present within the first 2 years of life and progress rapidly to cause paraplegia or cor pulmonale [35]. Surgical treatment is challenging and often requires anteroposterior spinal arthrodesis.

15.4 Conclusions

In summary, spinal manifestations are common in patients with skeletal dysplasias. These spinal manifestations include atlantoaxial instability, cervical kyphosis, thoracolumbar kyphosis, scoliosis, foramen magnum stenosis, and spinal stenosis. The natural history and treatment of these conditions may differ, depending on the dysplasia with which the spinal pathology occurs.

References

1. Ain MC, Browne JA (2004) Spinal arthrodesis with instrumentation for thoracolumbar kyphosis in pediatric achondroplasia. Spine 29:2075–2080
2. Ain MC, Shirley ED (2004) Spinal fusion for kyphosis in achondroplasia. J Pediatr Orthop 24:541–545
3. Ain MC, Chaichana KL, Schkrohowsky JG (2006) Retrospective study of cervical arthrodesis in patients with various types of skeletal dysplasia. Spine 31:E169–E174
4. Ain MC, Shirley ED, Pirouzmanesh A et al (2006) Postlaminectomy kyphosis in the skeletally immature achondroplast. Spine 31:197–201
5. Bagley CA, Pindrik JA, Bookland MJ et al (2006) Cervicomedullary decompression for foramen magnum stenosis in achondroplasia. J Neurosurg 104:166–172
6. Bethem D, Winter RB, Lutter L (1980) Disorders of the spine in diastrophic dwarfism. A discussion of nine patients and review of the literature. J Bone Joint Surg Am 62:529–536
7. Bethem D, Winter RB, Lutter L et al (1981) Spinal disorders of dwarfism. Review of the literature and report of eighty cases. J Bone Joint Surg Am 63:1412–1425
8. Chang H, Park JB, Kim KW et al (2000) Retro-dental reactive lesions related to development of myelopathy in patients with atlantoaxial instability secondary to Os odontoideum. Spine 25:2777–2783
9. Hunter AGW, Bankier A, Rogers JG et al (1998) Medical complications of achondroplasia: a multicentre patient review. J Med Genet 35:705–712
10. Johnston CE II, Birch JG, Daniels JL (1996) Cervical kyphosis in patients who have Larsen syndrome. J Bone Joint Surg Am 78:538–545
11. Kopits SE (1976) Orthopaedic complications of dwarfism. Clin Orthop Relat Res 114:153–179
12. Kopits SE (1988) Thoracolumbar kyphosis and lumbosacral hyperlordosis in achondroplastic children. Basic Life Sci 48:241–255
13. Laville JM, Lakermance P, Limouzy F (1994) Larsen's syndrome: review of the literature and analysis of thirty-eight cases. J Pediatr Orthop 14:63–73
14. Lutter LD, Langer LO (1977) Neurological symptoms in achondroplastic dwarfs – surgical treatment. J Bone Joint Surg Am 59:87–92
15. Lutter LD, Longstein JE, Winter RB et al (1977) Anatomy of the achondroplastic lumbar canal. Clin Orthop Relat Res 126:139–142
16. Matsuyama Y, Winter RB, Lonstein JE (1999) The spine in diastrophic dysplasia. The surgical arthrodesis of thoracic and lumbar deformities in 21 patients. Spine 24:2325–2331
17. Morgan KA, Rehman MA, Schwartz RE (2002) Case report. Morquio's syndrome and its anaesthetic considerations. Paediatr Anaesth 12:641–644
18. Morita M, Miyamoto K, Nishimoto H et al (2005) Thoracolumbar kyphosing scoliosis associated with spondyloepiphyseal dysplasia congenita: a case report. Spine J 5:217–220
19. Oberklaid F, Danks DM, Jensen F et al (1979) Achondroplasia and hypochondroplasia. Comments on frequency, mutation rate, and radiological features in skull and spine. J Med Genet 16:140–146
20. Pauli RM, Breed A, Horton VK et al (1997) Prevention of fixed, angular kyphosis in achondroplasia. J Pediatr Orthop 17:726–733
21. Pyeritz RE, Sack GH, Jr., Udvarhelyi GB (1987) Thoracolumbosacral laminectomy in achondroplasia: long-term results in 22 patients. Am J Med Genet 28:433–444
22. Remes V, Marttinen E, Poussa M et al (1999) Cervical kyphosis in diastrophic dysplasia. Spine 24:1990–1995
23. Remes V, Poussa M, Peltonen J (2001) Scoliosis in patients with diastrophic dysplasia: a new classification. Spine 26: 1689–1697
24. Remes V, Tervahartiala P, Poussa M et al (2001) Thoracic and lumbar spine in diastrophic dysplasia. A clinical and magnetic resonance imaging analysis. Spine 26:187–195
25. Remes VM, Marttinen EJ, Poussa MS et al (2002) Cervical spine in patients with diastrophic dysplasia – radiographic findings in 122 patients. Pediatr Radiol 32:621–628

26. Rousseau F, Bonaventure J, Legeai-Mallet L et al (1994) Mutations in the gene encoding fibroblast growth factor receptor-3 in achondroplasia. Nature 371:252–254
27. Schkrohowsky JG, Hoernschemeyer DG, Carson BS et al (2007) Early presentation of spinal stenosis in achondroplasia. J Pediatr Orthop 27:119–122
28. Sciubba DM, Noggle JC, Marupudi NI et al (2007) Spinal stenosis surgery in pediatric patients with achondroplasia. J Neurosurg 106:372–378
29. Shetty GM, Song HR, Unnikrishnan R et al (2007) Upper cervical spine instability in pseudoachondroplasia. J Pediatr Orthop 27:782–787
30. Srikumaran U, Woodard EJ, Leet AI et al (2007) Pedicle and spinal canal parameters of the lower thoracic and lumbar vertebrae in the achondroplast population. Spine 32:2423–2431
31. Streeten E, Uematsu S, Hurko O et al (1988) Extended laminectomy for spinal stenosis in achondroplasia. Basic Life Sci 48:261–273
32. Tolo VT, Spinal deformity in skeletal dysplasias. In: Weinstein SL (ed) The pediatric spine: principles and practice. Raven Press, 1994; New York, pp 369–393
33. Uematsu S, Wang H, Kopits SE et al (1994) Total craniospinal decompression in achondroplastic stenosis. Neurosurgery 35:250–257, comments 257–258
34. Violas P, Fraisse B, Chapuis M et al (2007) Cervical spine stenosis in chondrodysplasia punctata. J Pediatr Orthop B 16:443–445
35. Winter RB, Bloom BA (1990) Spine deformity in spondyloepimetaphyseal dysplasia. J Pediatr Orthop 10:535–539

Syndromic Spinal Deformities in the Growing Child

16

Paul D. Sponseller and Justin Yang

Key Points

- Patients with syndromes rarely respond well to bracing.
- Involve a medial specialist or geneticist to help manage patient. The surgeon should be aware of the key medical features and prognosis of the syndrome.
- Imaging of entire spine and complete skeletal examination are key.
- Functional goals and expectations should be set with families.

16.1 Introduction

The term "syndrome" is derived from the Greek, meaning "to run together." By definition, therefore, syndromes are diverse. The term "syndrome" implies that a condition is defined by its evident features and not by a single underlying etiologic principle. Congenital syndromes are often characterized by differences in connective tissue structure and neurological control that affect the spine. However, there are some general principles which govern the management of spinal deformities in children. This chapter will highlight these principles and then discuss in detail several syndromes which present with early onset scoliosis: Marfan, Loeys–Dietz, Shprintzen-Goldberg, Ehlers–Danlos, Prader–Willi, Rett and Down syndromes.

P. D. Sponseller (✉)
Johns Hopkins Medical Institution, 601 N. Caroline Street, Baltimore, MD 21287-0882, USA
e-mail: psponse@jhmi.edu

16.2 General Principles of Syndromic Deformity Management

The general spinal considerations for patients with these and other syndromes are presented in Table 16.1.

16.2.1 Role of Nonoperative Management

Patients with syndromic disorders often present with significant curves at a young age. Therefore, they often require more than simply orthotic treatment or spinal fusion near the age of maturity. Syndromic curves can present as early as infancy. There are virtually no studies showing efficacy of orthotic treatment in syndromic curves. In addition, D'Astous and Sanders [4] have shown that Mehta casting is less effective for infants with scoliosis due to syndromes that is in idiopathic infantile scoliosis. Practically, bracing is commonly recommended in young syndromic patients with curves between 35 and 50°. Orthotic treatment may show in-brace correction but there have been no studies which document an improvement in the expected natural history. The physician should consider refraining from overzealous application of bracing for large curves (over approximately 50°) in young patients at the expense of quality of life.

B. A. Akbarnia et al. (eds.), *The Growing Spine*,
DOI: 10.1007/978-3-540-85207-0_16, © Springer-Verlag Berlin Heidelberg 2011

Table 16.1 General spinal considerations in patients with syndromes

Theme	Specific suggestions
Role of nonoperative management	Curves become large at a young age Brace early or not at all; avoid in low-yield situations
Comprehensive imaging	Image entire spine MRI before surgery in most cases CT to define abnormal bony anatomy Traction films more useful than bending
Medical considerations	Communicate with specialists Consider genetic consultation Consult Online Mendelian Inheritance in Man for information Assess nutrition, respiratory status
Operative considerations	Blood loss likely more Bone density often lower Have appropriate size implants Failure of fixation more likely Do not "fuse short" in syndromes Have ICU available postoperatively Consider rehab needs postoperatively

16.2.2 Comprehensive Imaging

Another principle of treating patients with syndromic curves is that the whole spine is at the risk of developing differently. The cervical, thoracic and lumbar spine should be examined and imaged as indicated. "Coned" films (focal images centered on area of interest) should be obtained of any area that requires further definition. In addition, there is a greater chance for abnormality of the neuraxis. For this reason, whole-spine magnetic resonance imaging (MRI) should be considered prior to surgical intervention. Findings such as dural ectasia, stenosis, spondylolysis, instability, and disc pathology are more likely to be seen than in idiopathic deformity. Computed tomography (CT) with multiplanar or three-dimensional reconstruction may be invaluable in defining dystrophic bony features and pedicle character, if suspected. Flexibility is often best assessed with traction films rather than bending films in young patients with syndromes.

16.2.3 Medical Considerations

Patients mature at different rates; skeletal maturation in syndromic patients may be earlier or later than in idiopathic deformity. Medical comorbidities are more often seen in syndromic patients. The surgeon should take advantage of pediatric consultants in genetics, pulmonary, gastroentrology, and cardiology specialties. A geneticist can be a great help both preoperatively and postoperatively in managing patients with syndromes, tying all of the disparate features together. A good source of genetic information is Online Mendelian Inheritance in Man (OMIM), rapidly available to all on the Entrez Pub Med series of applications. This site allows one to search for diagnoses by listing a series of physical findings. A set of matches, discussion, and references will appear.

Specialists can also provide helpful input in determining the proper role of surgery for a given patient. It is helpful to ask, "what other specialists are you seeing?" so that the orthopaedic management plan can be integrated with that of other specialists. Testing prior to surgery may also include echocardiography or sleep study for patients at risk of cardiac or pulmonary difficulties. Specific cardiovascular manifestations of specific syndromes will be discussed further in the subsequent sections. Finally, nutritional and gastrointestinal issues can affect this group of patients as well. Specifically, severe curvatures can cause abdominal compression, including acid reflux. At least one case of postoperative superior mesenteric syndrome has been reported in the literature following scoliosis surgery of in patient with Marfan syndrome (MFS) [7]. Malabsorption has been reported in Ehlers–Danlos syndrome (EDS) and MFS secondary to bacterial overgrowth in large jejunal diverticula. Feeding problems and indigestion have been reported in most of the syndromic scoliosis disorders. We recommend a gastrointestinal consultation if these issues come to light.

16.2.4 Operative and Postoperative Management

Implant size may be a problem in young patients with poor nutrition, such as infantile Marfan patients. A range of implant diameters should be available. Osteopenia and increased blood loss may affect surgery. Failure of fixation is another complication commonly seen in syndromic patients following spinal instrumentation. The number and types of anchors should be chosen to minimize this risk. Because of balance and connective tissue factors, principles of instrumentation and fusion that apply to idiopathic patients may not apply to syndromic patients. Attempts to "save levels" do not always work as predictably as in idiopathic deformity. Patients with syndromes often require more involved postoperative care. Intensive care stay may be appropriate. Their return to function may be significantly slower than in idiopathic patients. Inpatient rehabilitation may occasionally be indicated after discharge from hospital.

16.3 Specific Syndromes

16.3.1 Marfan Syndrome

MFS is an autosomal dominant disorder of connective tissue that is characterized by cardiovascular, skeletal, and ocular abnormalities. The Ghent Nosology [5] is the most widely accepted diagnostic criteria. Major and minor criteria are listed by organ systems in Table 16.2. For the skeletal system to be involved, at least four major criteria must be present. Major criteria in other systems include ectopic lentis, aortic root dilatation and aortic dissection, dural ectasia, and a positive family history. Some delays in motor milestones are common but intellectual impairment is not typical.

The disorder has been linked to mutations of the FBN1 gene on chromosome 15 that encodes the fibrillin protein. This is an essential component of elastic connective tissue. It also has a role in transforming growth factor beta (TGF-β) binding. Aneurysm of the ascending aorta can cause aortic regurgitation, dissection or rupture [11]. Management of vascular disease in MFS includes regular echocardiography to monitor the aorta, β-adrenergic blockade to decrease arterial pressures, and prophylactic valve or aortic surgery if indicated. Early treatment with Losartan, a blood pressure medication that also antagonizes TGF-β, has shown promise to slow the rate of aortic root dilatation. A randomized trial is under way.

In the skeletal system, scoliosis exists in two-thirds of MFS patients. The curve patterns resemble that of idiopathic curves, but with earlier onset. There is also a tendency for thoracolumbar kyphosis. Bracing for scoliosis in MFS is successful in only 17% of patients [8]. Approximately one-eighth of patients eventually develop a severe curve requiring surgical intervention [8]. Marfan patients with infantile spinal curvature are a special group (Fig. 16.1a–f). They more often have no family history (spontaneous mutation) and more severe phenotypes. For these patients, growing rods are effective. In the experience of the author, one of the two types of constructs can be used. For patients with excessive

Table 16.2 Ghent criteria [5]

Cardiovascular system
Major criteria
Aortic arch dilatation or dissection
Minor Criteria:
Descending thoracic or abdominal aortic aneurysm
Mitral valve prolapse
Pulmonary artery enlargement
Ophthalmologic system
Major criteria
Lens dislocation
Minor criteria
Increased length of the globe
Flattened cornea
Neurological system
Major criteria
Dural ectasia
Skeletal system
Major criteria (need 4 of these for major skeletal involvement)
Pectus carinatum
Pectus excavatum requiring surgery
Reduced upper-segment to lower-segment ratio or arm span to height ratio >1.05
Wrist and thumb signs
Scoliosis of >20° or spondylolisthesis
Reduced extension at the elbows (<170°)
Medial displacement of the medial malleolus, causing pes planus
Protrusio acetabulae of any degree (ascertained on radiographs)
Minor criteria
Pectus excavatum of moderate severity
Joint hypermobility
Highly arched palate with crowding of teeth
Facial appearance (dolichocephaly, malar hypoplasia, enophthalmos, retrognathia, down-slanting palpebral fissures)
Pulmonary system
Minor criteria
Spontaneous pneumothorax or apical blebs
Cutaneous system
Minor criteria
Striae or recurrent inguinal hernia

The index patient requires major criteria in two different organ systems and involvement of a third; if the FBN-1 mutation is present or a risk-degree relative is diagnosed then one major criterion and involvement of a second organ system suffices

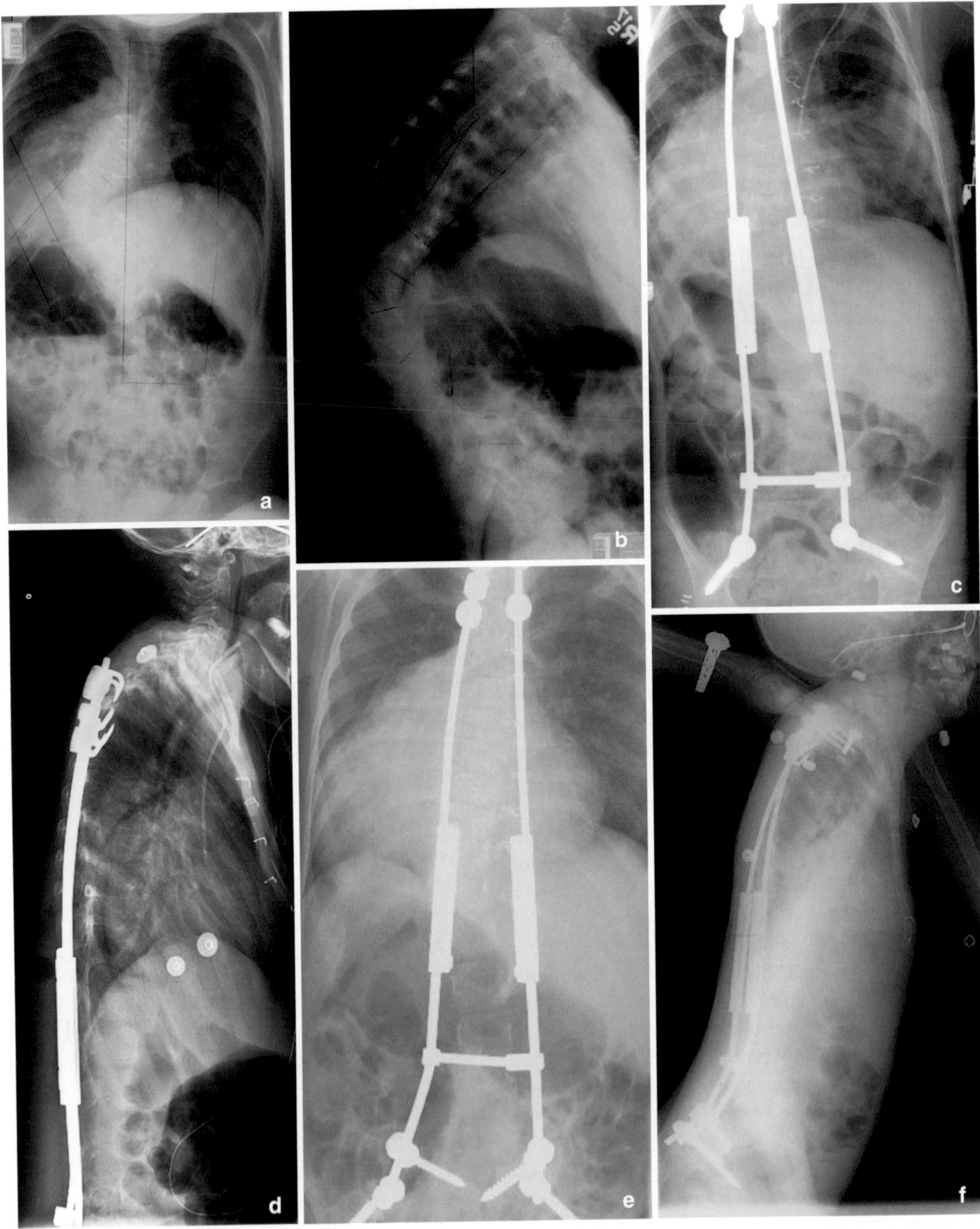

Fig. 16.1 A 2-year-old patient with Marfans with preoperative curve of 72° (**a, b**) underwent placement of growing rods from T2–4 to Ilium with laminar hooks as proximal anchors and screws as distal anchors (**c, d**). The patient's curve at 3-year follow-up was 10° (**e, f**)

thoracolumbar kyphosis or severe lower lumbar curves, the distal anchor may be placed in the pelvis (see Fig. 16.1a–f). For those patients with no significant sagittal abnormality, more "typical" growing rod anchors in the thoracic and lumbar spine may be used. It is critical to have an anesthesiologist expert at managing cardiovascular problems, and to have pediatric intensive care and cardiology available. Outpatient lengthening is advised only in the most stable of patients.

When inserting growing rod anchors in this population, the surgeon should be prepared for fixation challenges. The laminae are often thin, creating a risk of hook dislodgement. For this reason, pedicle fixation is preferred if at all possible. However, if hooks are used, a three-level "claw" is recommended [1]. Pedicles are often thin in MFS, especially proximally. Small-diameter screws and even the use of cervical systems may be necessary. Because of the thin, dysplastic pedicles, the author advises liberal use of fluoroscopy when inserting pedicle screws. Submuscular placement of growing rods is recommended due to problems with implant prominence in this population related to the asthenic habitus. Intraoperative leakage of cerebrospinal fluid occurs with a higher frequency in this population. Due to dural ectasia, the dura in MFS often expands to fill the entire spinal canal and is extremely thin and fragile. This was often seen when dissecting under the lamina or attempting to cannulate the narrow pedicles. Fibrin glue is typically used along with sutures to deal with dural leaks. Sometimes the dura is too friable to hold a suture, but patients virtually always respond to a period of postoperative recumbence. Postoperative bracing is typically not used in this population. Although it is more common to lengthen growing rods approximately every 6 months, patients who are on Coumadin are usually lengthened only yearly, in order to minimize the risks of stopping and restarting the anticoagulation. Complications of rod breakage and implant dislodgement have been low in the experience of the author. This may be due to the fact that patients are restricted from high-impact activities to avoid stress on the aorta or the eye. Bleeding is also more extensive in the MFS population.

16.3.2 Loeys–Dietz Syndrome

Loeys–Dietz syndrome (LDS) is a newly recognized entity that was defined originally in a subset of MFS patients. Though it shares many systemic and skeletal findings with MFS, it is characterized by a triad of findings, (1) hypertelorism, (2) bidfid uvula with or without cleft palate, and (3) generalized arterial tortuoisty with widespread vascular aneurysms [9]. The molecular etiology is an autosomal dominant mutation in the genes encoding TGF-β receptors 1 and 2. Affected patients have a high risk of aortic dissections or ruptures at an early age and at blood vessel sizes that are not associated with risk in other conditions. LDS has been further subdivided into types 1 and 2. LDS type 1 is associated with craniofacial involvement consisting of cleft palate, craniosynostosis, or hypertelorism, whereas type 2 is associated with Ehlers–Danlos syndrome [10]. Typically, vascular involvement is also more progressive in LDS patients than in MFS patients. Motor delays have been reported but intellectual impairment is not typical. Early vascular surgical intervention is recommended and usually successful, which distinguishes LDS from Ehlers–Danlos syndrome, which will be discussed later in this chapter. Because of the phenotypic overlap in these conditions, DNA testing for mutations in TGFβR1 and TGFβR2 is considered the gold standard in diagnosis [10]. Medical management includes 3D CT or MRI scan with contrast from the head to the pelvis to monitor for aneurysms. Routine echocardiograms are also recommended. They should not exercise to the point of exhaustion, do weight lifting, or isometric exercises. Similar to MFS, early treatment with Losartan is advised.

Cervical spine instability has been associated with LDS. The authors recommend obtaining cervical spine films in flexion and extension to assess for this prior to surgery. Other unique skeletal manifestations include atypical club foot deformities and camptodactyly. Scoliosis is seen in approximately 25% of patients with LDS, with either early or late onset. There is no data on the efficacy of bracing.

In the authors' experience, early onset in LDS can be treated similarly to MFS with growing rods if it becomes significant (Fig. 16.2a–d). Osteoporosis is reported with greater frequency in LDS compared to MFS. Dural ectasia is also seen in LDS.

16.3.3 Shprintzen–Goldberg Syndrome

Shprintzen–Goldberg syndrome (SGS) is a disorder of yet undefined etiology comprising craniosynos tosis, tall, slender habitus with skeletal, neurological,

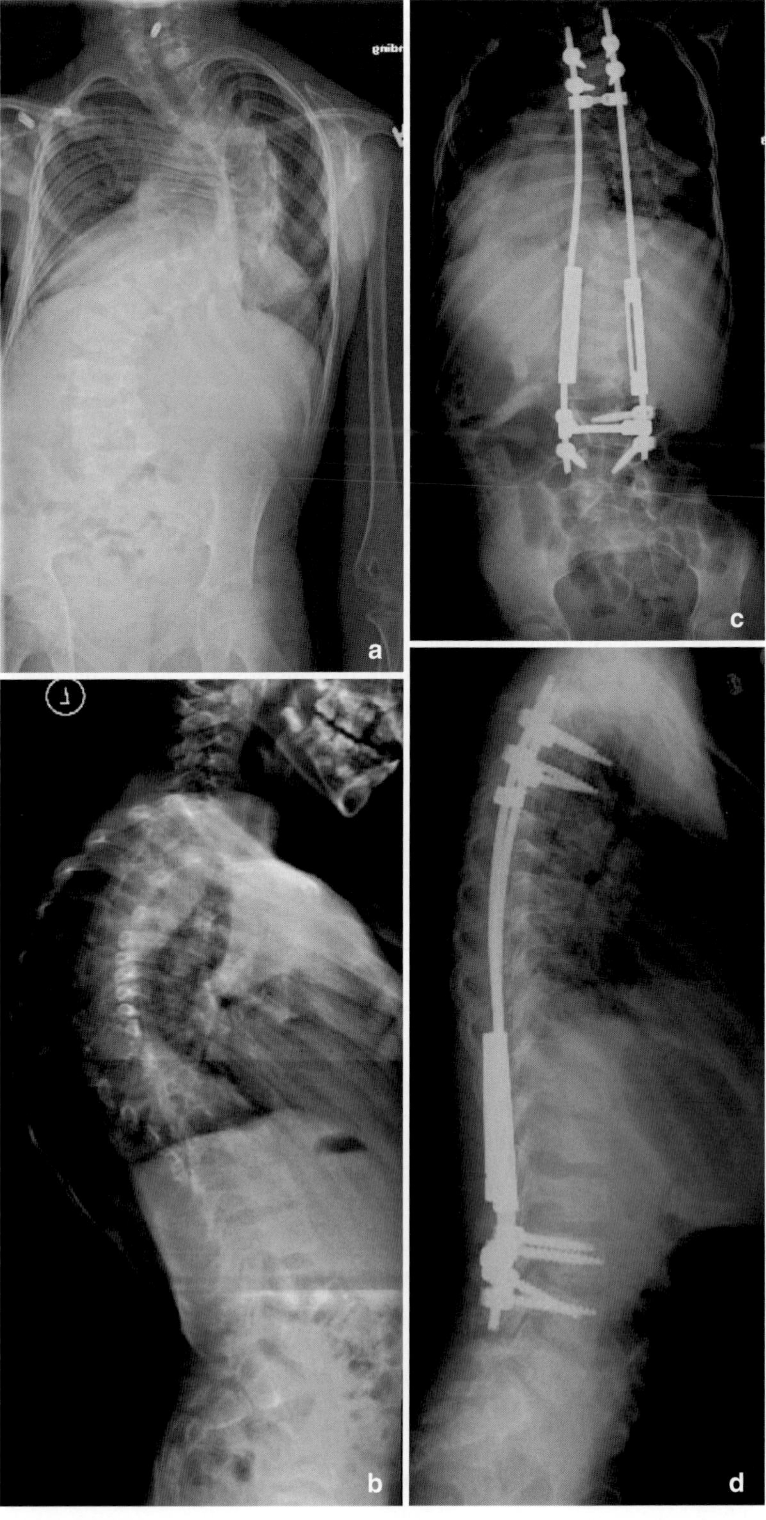

Fig. 16.2 A 6-year-old girl with LDS (preoperative: **a, b**) was treated with growing rods from T3 and T4 to L3 and L4. Pedicle screws were used for both proximal and distal fixation. Rods were inserted below the submuscular layer and autologous bone graft was liberally used. Cross-links were used distally and proximally for stable fixation. A small dural leak was encountered due to dural ectasia. Major curve correction using the growing rods in the patient was significant from 101 to 40°. Postoperative complications included a small superficial wound infection that was successfully treated with antibiotics. At the time of publication, the patient has not yet been followed long enough for considerations in lengthening (latest follow-up: **c, d**)

cardiovascular, and connective tissue anomalies. Unlike MFS or LDS, there are no pathognomonic signs of SGS and diagnosis is dependent on recognitions of examination patterns and molecular anomalies. Craniosynostoses and cognitive delay are thought to be distinguishing features [7]. Facial features include hypertelorism, down-slanting palpebral fissures, high-arched palate, micrognathia, and low-set ears. Other reported features include neonatal hypotonia, and abdominal hernias [15]. In the skeletal system, SGS is associated with arachnodactyly, pectus deformity, camptodactyly, scoliosis, and joint hypermobility [15]. Genetic mutations in both the FBN1 and TGFRβ2 have been associated with SGS [9, 16]. This, along with phenotypic features overlapping with LDS, MFS, and EDS may make the diagnosis challenging.

Scoliosis is common in SGS and can again be treated similarly to MFS. Significant coronal and sagittal imbalance may occur (Fig.16.3a–f).

16.3.4 Ehlers–Danlos Syndrome

Ehlers–Danlos syndrome (EDS) is a class of connective tissue disorder caused by defects in collagen synthesis. It is characterized by distensible and thin skin, easy bruising, hyperextensible joints, facial features, and severe arterial complications. The eye, gastrointestinal, respiratory, and cardiovascular systems can also be affected. EDS is not a homogenous disorder and can be thought of as a group of related entities that share, to varying degrees, the same complex of physical anomalies. Therefore, various subclassifications exist with different clinical presentations and different genetic mutations. Kyphoscoliosis is a hallmark feature of type VI EDS; however, scoliosis also often presents at an early age in patients with other classes of EDS, most notably type I, II and, III (Fig. 16.4a–c). Osseous fragility is often seen in this condition as well.

With scoliosis surgery, it is important to keep in mind the vascular fragility that is inherent in this disease. Although spine surgery in MFS can be associated with increased bleeding, anterior approaches to the spine should be avoided in EDS because such surgery can be catastrophic involving large arteries and veins. Growing procedures in EDS patients, if begun early enough, may allow posterior-only approaches so that the patient never requires an anterior procedure or a complex posterior osteotomy. Measures such as hypotensive anesthesia and careful dissection of segmental arteries are advised [2]. Recently, report of using Factor VIIa to help control massive bleeding following spontaneous large vessel rupture in type IV EDS has been published [6].

16.3.5 Prader–Willi Syndrome

Prader–Willi syndrome is characterized by early hypotonia, developmental and motor delay, small hands and feet, and later hyperphagia resulting in massive obesity. It is caused by a lack of paternal expression of a region of chromosome 15. Pituitary dysfunction results in many of the manifestations [13]. Scoliosis is seen in over 50% of patients [13]. Its onset is often in the infantile or juvenile period. Orthoses have a role if body habitus does not prohibit it. Administration of human growth hormone has been shown to aid in the management of many aspects of this condition [13]. Initially, there was concern that HGH may increase the prevalence and severity of scoliosis [13]. However, it appears to help control many aspects of the disease and does not increase the incidence or severity of scoliosis. Treatment of scoliosis in this condition should follow usual clinical guidelines. If curve size increases beyond orthotic range in the early juvenile period, there may be a role for growth-guiding surgery. At the time of any surgical procedure, monitoring for sleep apnea is important.

16.3.6 Rett Syndrome

Described over a generation ago by an Austrian physician Andreas Rett, this syndrome is often confused with cerebral palsy. Its etiology has been recently defined as a defect in the transcription repressor MECP2 gene [14]. Virtually all patients are female, and manifest stereotypic hand movements, little to no expressive language, seizures, and a neurological picture combining dystonia and spasticity. Approximately half of patients have scoliosis to some degree, often with early onset. Bracing has not been proven to affect curve progression. Growing rod instrumentation is an option to control curves. Because of the profound neurological disorder, pelvic obliquity should be controlled, and

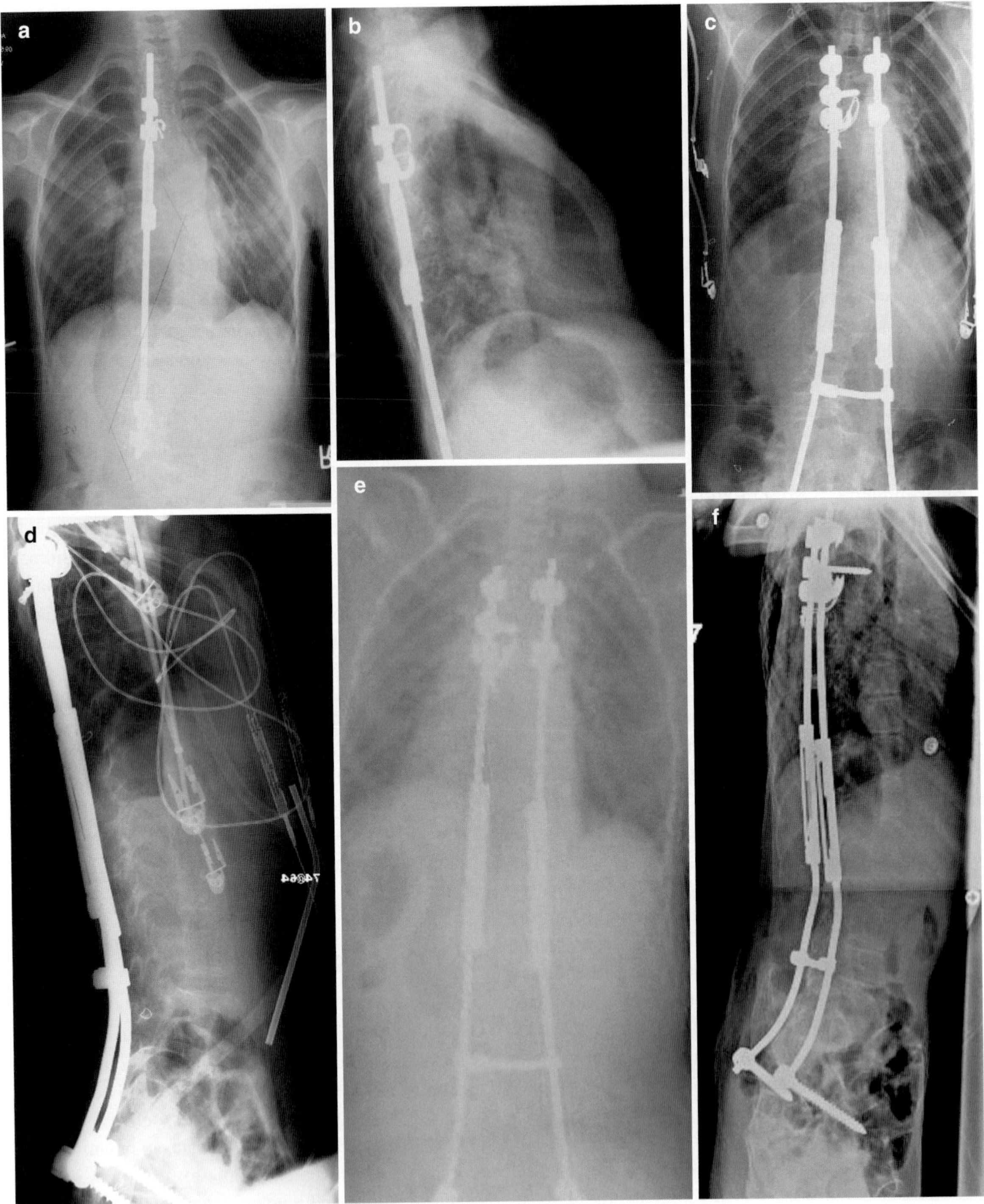

Fig. 16.3 A 9-year-old patient with SGS was initially thought to have clinical features suggestive of LDS but later diagnosed with SGS due to lack of a TGFRβ1 or TGFRβ2 mutation. Growing rod was inserted from T3 and T4 to the pelvis because of significant pelvic obliquity (**a, b**). Pedicle screws were used for proximal and iliac fixation (**c, d**). Rods were inserted below the submuscular layer. Major curve correction using the growing rods in the patient was significant from 60 to 38°. Pelvic obliquity improved to 6.5°s from 23°. In postoperative follow-up, this patient has had three lengthenings in the 3 years with a total increase of 4 cm in T1–S1 length (**e, f**). Complications since initial surgery have included distal screw breakage and rod erosion that required successful revisions

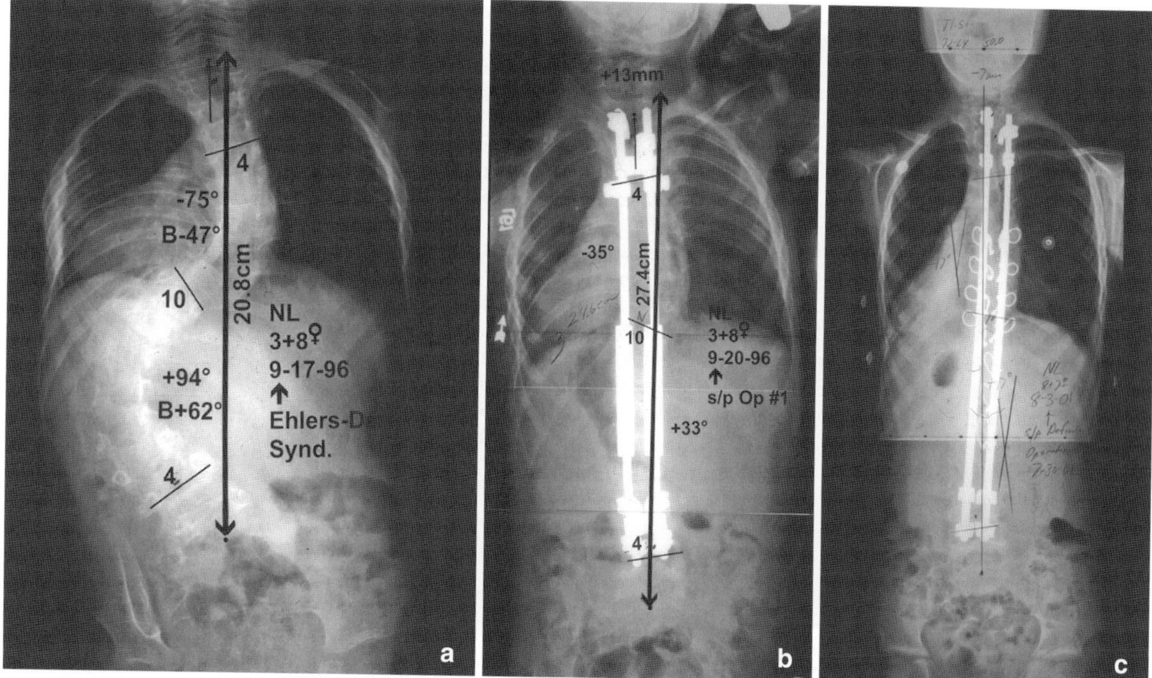

Fig. 16.4 A 3-year-old female with EDS with preoperative curve over 90° (**a**) underwent placement of growing rods from T3–4 to L3–4 with laminar hooks as proximal anchors and claws as distal anchors (**b**). The patient later went on to successful posterior fusion at the age of 8 (**c**) with curve at last follow-up of 25° (case courtesy of Marc Asher)

therefore strong consideration given to pelvic fixation. Osteoporosis is common. Experienced pulmonary backup or support is needed even after simple lengthening procedures.

16.3.7 Down Syndrome

Down syndrome is the most common chromosomal disorder. Most cases involve complete trisomy of the 21st chromosome, but a smaller number are translocations and carry less pronounced manifestations. Scoliosis is seen in a small number of cases; reviews have estimated that 10% of Down patients have scoliosis over 20° [3, 12]. This should be screened for at regular visits to the pediatrician or orthopaedic surgeon. Treatment efficacy is undocumented. For curves of 25–40°, bracing may be offered for compliant patients. Surgical fusion is indicated in curves greater than approximately 55° [3]. Before any surgical procedure, cervical stability should be demonstrated. There is no data on the efficacy of nonfusion options for this population currently.

16.4 Conclusions

Care of children with syndromes is both challenging and rewarding. Many of them present with significant spinal deformities at a young age. They usually have associated medical problems. By building the appropriate care team and skill set, the pediatric spine surgeon can successfully manage deformities that would otherwise cause significant morbidity and even mortality.

Acknowledgements The authors would like to thank Dr. Marc Asher for his contributions of several radiographs in this chapter.

References

1. Akbarnia BA, Marks DS, Boachie-Adjei O et al (2005) Dual growing rod technique for the treatment of progressive early-onset scoliosis. Spine 30:S46–S57
2. Akpinar S, Gogus A, Talu U et al (2003) Surgical management of the spinal deformity in Ehlers–Danlos syndrome type VI. Eur Spine J 12:135–140
3. Caird M, Wills B, Dormans JP(2006) Down Syndrome: the role of the orthopaedic surgeon. J Am Acad Orthop Surg 14(11):611

4. D'Astous JL, Sanders JO (2007) Casting and traction treatment methods for scoliosis. Orthop Clin North Am 38(4):477–484, v. Review
5. De Paepe A, Devereux RB, Dietz HC, et al (1996) Revised diagnostic criteria for the Marfan syndrome. Am J Med Genet. 62(4):417-26.
6. Faber P, Craig WL, Duncan JL et al (2007) The successful use of recombinant factor IIa in a patient with vascular-type Ehlers–Danlos syndrome. Acta Anaesthesiol Scand 51:1277–1279
7. Hutchinson DT, Bassett GS (1990) Superior mesenteric artery syndrome in pediatric orthopaedic patients. Clin Orthop Relat Res 250:250–257
8. Jones KB, Erkula G, Sponseller PD et al (2002) Spine deformity correction in Marfan syndrome. Spine 27:2003–2012
9. Kosaki K, Takahashi D, Udaka T et al (2005) Molecular pathology of Shprintzen–Goldberg syndrome. Am J Med Genet A 140:104–105
10. Loeys BL, Chen J, Neptune ER et al (2005) A syndrome of altered cardiovascular, craniofacial, neurocognitive and skeletal development caused by mutations in GFBR1 or TGFBR2. Nature 37:275–281
11. Loeys BL, Schwarze U, Holm T et al (2006) Aneurysm syndromes caused by mutations in the TGF-β receptor. NEJM 355:788–798
12. Mik G, Gholve PA, Scher DM et al (2008) Down syndrome: orthopaedic issues. Curr Opin Pediatr 20(1):30–36
13. Nabai T, Obata K (2006) Growth hormone therapy and scoliosis in patients with Prader–Willi syndrome. Am J Med Genet A. 140(15):1623–1627
14. Percy AK (2008) Rett syndrome: recent research progress. J Child Neurol 23:543–549
15. Robinson PN, Neumann LM, Demuth S et al (2005) Shprintzen–Goldberg syndrome: fourteen new patients and a clinical analysis. Am J Med Genet A 135:251–262
16. van Steensel MA, van Geel M, Parren LJ et al (2008) Shprintzen-Goldberg syndrome associated with a novel missense mutation in TGFBR2. Exp Dermatol 17: 362–365

Section 

Spinal Deformities in the Growing Child

17 Idiopathic Scoliosis: Infantile and Juvenile

Gregory M. Mundis and Behrooz A. Akbarnia

Key Points

- Careful history and physical examination are imperative to rule out other etiologies of scoliosis in growing children.
- Quality AP and lateral spinal radiographs are imperative to the evaluation and management decision making.
- In infantile scoliosis, curves with an RVAD of 20° or more, Cobb angle of 25° or more, or a phase 2 rib head should be followed closely for progression. Curves with an RVAD of less than 20° and a phase 1 rib head almost certainly do not progress.
- All curves 20° or more should be evaluated with advanced imaging (such as MRI) to rule out brain and spine anomalies.
- Our current recommendation for treatment of infantile and juvenile idiopathic scoliosis is dual growing rods placed subfascial using a two-incision technique with a skin bridge. Lengthening should occur every 6 months.

17.1 Introduction

> It "develops rapidly and relentlessly, causing the severest form of orthopaedic cripple with dreadful deformity, marked dwarfing and shortening of life"
>
> J.I. James, MD on infantile scoliosis, 1959

G. M. Mundis (✉)
San Diego Center for Spinal Disorders, 4130 La Jolla Village Drive, Suite 300, La Jolla, CA 92037, USA
e-mail: gmundis1@gmail.com

Management of spine deformity in children 5 years of age or less presents one of the most challenging tasks in spine surgery. It requires intimate knowledge of normal spine development as well as the etiology, natural history, clinical evaluation, and available nonoperative and operative treatments for infantile scoliosis. Early recognition and diagnosis by both parents and pediatricians is essential. Immediate orthopaedic referral is mandatory as early treatment may ultimately affect patient outcome.

Harrenstein [24] in 1936 coined the term infantile idiopathic scoliosis (IIS). He treated 46 children and noted mixed success treating the curve with bracing, and attributed the deformity primarily to rickets [23]. In 1951, James [28] reported on 33 cases of scoliosis in infants aged 3 years and younger. They were predominantly boys with left-sided thoracic curves. Four cases resolved spontaneously, but the remainder progressed very aggressively. In 1954, he first described scoliosis according to chronologic age at a presentation including infantile from birth to 3 years, juvenile with onset up to 8 years, and adolescent with onset from 10 years to maturity [29]. Interestingly, no reference was made for those between 8 and 10 years [29]. Dickson [12] later recommended that scoliosis in children be classified as early (5 years or less) or late (>5 years) onset. The rationale for this is twofold. As Dimeglio and Bonnel [14] have shown, growth velocity in the spine is highest from birth to 5 years, followed by a deceleration between age 6 and 10 years. From 11 to 18 years, there seems to be another peak in growth velocity but not equal to that of early life. Early onset, therefore, more accurately describes this growth. Similarly, this group is at a higher risk for developing significant cardiopulmonary complications if thoracic curves progress, whereas these complications are rare in the late onset group. Complications include pulmonary hypoplasia, restrictive pulmonary

B. A. Akbarnia et al. (eds.), *The Growing Spine*,
DOI: 10.1007/978-3-540-85207-0_17, © Springer-Verlag Berlin Heidelberg 2011

disease, pulmonary artery hypertension, cor pulmonale, and thoracic insufficiency syndrome.

This chapter aims to equip the spine deformity surgeon with all the relevant knowledge to diagnose, educate, and effectively treat the child with infantile and juvenile scoliosis.

17.2 Natural History

17.2.1 Growth and Development

Dimeglio [15] and Dimeglio and Bonnel [14] very nicely illustrated that spine growth velocity is greatest from birth to 5 years, averaging >2 cm growth per year. From the age of 6 to 10 years, velocity decreases to 0.5 cm per year and increases to 1.3 cm per year from the age of 11 to 18 years. Chest growth is most easily assessed as thoracic volume, which shows a similar trend as spine growth. At birth, it is 5% of adult volume. By 5 years of age, it has reached 30%, a staggering 600% increase in volume [15]. At 10 years of age, lung volume is 50% and reaches adult size at the age of 15, in both males and females. Lung development is best measured by change in alveolar volume and number. It is estimated that 20 million alveoli exist at birth and increase to 250 million by the age of 4 and complete development by 8 years of age. A similar increase in alveolar volume also occurs. Respiratory branches also increase from 20 at birth to 23 by 8 years.

17.2.2 Epidemiology

Several authors have reported the incidence and prevalence of infantile and juvenile idiopathic scoliosis (IIS, JIS) [12, 30, 47]. In the United States, IIS comprises less than 1% of idiopathic cases. A slightly higher incidence has been reported in Europe [30, 47]. Unlike late onset, it is more common in males with a ratio of 3:2, and curves tend to be left sided. It occurs in the mid to lower thoracic spine in 75–90% of cases [12, 30, 60]. Since the initial description by James [29] in 1951, it appears that the incidence has decreased. McMaster [47] most recently reported on a declining prevalence of patients with IIS scoliosis in Edinburgh, a major referral for scoliosis in Scotland. Between 1968 and 1972, they averaged 16.5 new patients per year with a 34% incidence of progressive curves. From 1980 to 1982, there was an average of two referrals per year. On the contrary, referrals for adolescent idiopathic scoliosis increased during this same time period.

JIS accounts for 12–21% of reported idiopathic cases [30, 53]. It is more prevalent in females with a 2:1–4:1 ratio. Between 3 and 6 years of age, the gender difference is neutral, and after 10 years of age, females are affected at a rate of 8:1 [20, 64]. Males are usually diagnosed by 5 years of age and females by 7 years of age. This difference as well as the age of skeletal maturity makes progression more likely in males. Right-sided thoracic and double major curves are the principal curve patterns associated with JIS [20, 42].

17.2.3 Prognosis

James [28] in 1951 reported his initial series of 33 patients, 18 (55%) were progressive, 11 (33%), stationary, and 4 (12%), spontaneously resolved. In 1954, he increased his numbers to include 52 children who were treated with physiotherapy, plaster-of-Paris beds, and orthoses [29]. Curves in 43 patients progressed (83%) with all curves being >70° at the age of 10 and several progressing >100°. In the remaining nine patients (17%), the curves resolved spontaneously without treatment. In 1959, James et al. [30] reported on 212 infantile cases from two separate institutions. Seventy-seven (31%) patients had spontaneous correction and the remainder progressed aggressively (135/212). Of these 135 patients, 47 were between 0 and 5 years, and 23 of these already had a curve >70°. Thirty-seven patients were between 5 and 10 years, and 27 of 37 had a curve >70° and 14, > 100°. Of the 23 children of 11 years and older, 12 had a curve >100°, and two at skeletal maturity had curves in excess of 150°.

Scott and Morgan [60] reported on 28 patients with IIS, of which 14 were followed to skeletal maturity. All had severe scoliosis with a mean of 120°. The remaining 14 were still growing. At 6 years of age, the average Cobb measured 65° with the largest being 112°. Three patients died in the late second and third decades of life from cardiopulmonary complications. All patients in their series had small thoracic cages with reduction in both pulmonary and cardiac function. Younger age at diagnosis and progression were found to be predictors of poorest outcome.

In 1965, Lloyd-Roberts and Pilcher [38] reviewed 100 patients with idiopathic curves who were diagnosed before 12 months of life. Ninety-two of these curves resolved spontaneously. Several other authors have subsequently reported their rates of resolution ranging from 20 to 80% [13, 31, 38]. James [31] followed 90 patients with nonprogressive curves and found that all resolved by the age of 6 years. Diedrich et al. [13] reported 34 patients with resolving curves followed through maturity, and found that none progressed during the adolescent growth spurt. Of the 34, 20 were treated with an orthosis, and no children had significant disabilities related to their spine.

Fernandes and Weinstein [19] reviewed the literature and summarized the data on nonprogressive and progressive infantile idiopathic curves. They identified 573 patients with nonprogressive curves with a male to female ratio close to 3:2. Ninety percent were thoracic curves, 80% apex left with greatest Cobb angle ranging from 20 to 48°. A large majority had associated intrauterine molding features. Perhaps the most significant finding was age at diagnosis that averaged 5.5 months compared to 12 months among the progressive group. Furthermore, the progressive group showed greater variability compared to historic reports. Gender ratio was closer to 1.2:1 (male to female), 81% with thoracic curves and 75% left sided. It is important to recognize that girl infants with right-sided thoracic curves may have a worse prognosis and may not follow the typical rate of spontaneous correction.

Juvenile idiopathic scoliosis differs from IIS in its natural history [36]. The curves progress at a slow to moderate rate [20, 26, 29, 34, 53]. The earlier onset usually leads to more severe deformity than adolescent idiopathic scoliosis. Tolo and Gillespie [64] reported on their series of 59 patients, of which 71% (42) progressed to require surgery. Similarly, Figueiredo and James [20] found that 56% (55) of 98 JIS patients progressed. Mannherz et al. [42] reported on a series of JIS patients who did no progress. All patients presented with curves <25°.

Pulmonary complications are the most morbid results of untreated infantile scoliosis. As previously described, the spine, chest wall, and respiratory system rapidly develop during the first 5 years of life [15]. Alteration in normal development of one of these can have deleterious effects on the others. Scoliosis that presents and progresses during this time period has a higher chance of causing unwanted cardiopulmonary side effects [51]. Infantile scoliosis alters normal development of alveoli and pulmonary vessels resulting in ventilation defects. The severity of pulmonary involvement is directly related to the age of onset of scoliosis. The earlier the onset and progression, the more the disability. Pulmonary dysfunction usually presents as restrictive lung disease with reduced vital capacity (VC), total lung capacity (TLC), and increased residual volume (RV). The loss of compliance of the chest wall and both lungs contributes to the restrictive pattern of disease. Persistence of restrictive lung disease usually results in pulmonary hypertension and cor pulmonale. Hypoxemia is related to reduced tidal volume as gas exchange is normal in these kids. Respiratory failure is a late development as these patients have significant pulmonary reserve. This pattern of disease has been consistently shown in the literature; however, it is a rare finding in curves that present after maturation of the lungs (8 years) [11, 32]. Similarly, it differs from thoracic insufficiency syndrome, which presents with respiratory failure at a very early age [9].

17.2.4 Etiology

Browne [8] in 1956 was the first to suggest that infantile scoliosis was initially attributed to an intrauterine packaging problem. He found in his series that 83% of infants had some form of intrauterine crowding deformity such as plagiocephaly, plagiopelvy, decreased hip abduction, and abnormal rib molding with infantile scoliosis. Mehta [48] later agreed that intrauterine crowding was responsible. In 1965, Lloyd-Roberts and Pilcher [38] termed this association "molded baby syndrome". Further study would refute this theory as scoliosis was not found to be present at birth and did not explain the gender difference or the variance in geographic regions. The difference in incidence in Europe and the United States gave rise to the thought of an environmental theory. Mau [45] in 1968 proposed that infantile scoliosis was linked to how an infant was positioned for sleeping. In the United States, it was more common to place the infant prone in bed which decompresses the spine. This is in contrast to the Europeans who were placing their infants supine. Children, in this position tend to turn to a slight oblique position with a tendency to lie oblique to the right. He also suggested that the molding deformities noted were caused by constant pressure on the soft bones of infants. He also added four other components to the molding theory: unilateral contracture of neck muscles, associated oblique posture of the head, calcaneus foot deformity, and the subsequent development of fixed dorsolumbar kyphosis. These findings aim to raise awareness and prompt intervention for earlier diagnosis of infantile scoliosis.

The geographic differences further influenced Wynne-Davies [67] to analyze 180 medical records from the Edinburgh Scoliosis Clinic. She identified 114 eligible patients and studied the prevalence of scoliosis between first, second, and third-degree relatives. She analyzed these patients in two groupings: early (before age 8) and late onset. In the early group, 88% had left thoracic curves with a slight male predilection. She identified a 2.6% prevalence of scoliosis in the infantile group compared to 0.39% of controls, a 30-fold higher risk. The late/adolescent group had an even stronger association at 6.94%. Plagiocephaly was found in 100% of patients compared to 11% among controls. Mental retardation and epilepsy were found in 13% of patients. Advanced maternal age was also commonly associated with progressive curves.

Ward et al. [65] have made recent advances in genetic testing among the adolescent idiopathic group. Several gene locuses have been identified to strongly predict those patients with progressive curves. The future is very promising to expand this technology to infantile and juvenile scoliosis for early detection and treatment.

17.3 Clinical Evaluation

17.3.1 History

A thorough and systematic history prior to physical examination is imperative in the diagnosis of infantile and juvenile scoliosis. Careful attention to detail in the history will lead the spine surgeon to pursue further diagnostic testing. Idiopathic scoliosis is a diagnosis of exclusion, and therefore all measures need to be exhausted for accurate diagnosis. Differential diagnosis includes: neuromuscular scoliosis, syringomyelia, spinal tumor, congenital spinal deformity, intraspinal anomalies, neurofibromatosis, syndromic, and spinal infection. Patients need to be carefully screened for any other associated anomalies including cardiac defects, history of hip dysplasia, cognitive deficits, congenital muscular torticollis, and other molding abnormalities. This information is often overlooked during an interview, and we recommend having history forms that are conducive to eliciting this information.

During history taking, careful attention should be directed to prenatal history of the mother, including any health problems, previous pregnancies, and medications. Birth history should include length of gestation, delivery type (vaginal or cesarean), weight and any complications. Like developmental dysplasia of the hip (DDH), there has been an association between scoliosis and breech presentation. Unlike DDH, however, infantile scoliosis is more common in premature low birth weight males. Careful attention should be given to developmental milestones and cognitive function. This information can be gleaned from conversation with family or from simple observation in the waiting room and during the examination. Wynne-Davies [67] found mental retardation in 13% of males with infantile scoliosis.

17.3.2 Physical Examination

Physical examination should be performed systematically with special attention given to the skin, head, spine, pelvis, extremities, and neurological examination. Findings in this group of patients are often subtle, and workup is largely dependent on examination findings in order not to miss an underlying cause for scoliosis. The skin examination should include careful inspection for café-au-lait spots and axillary freckling seen in neurofibromatosis. A hairy patch along the spine may indicate spinal dysraphism, and bruising may indicate trauma. The head examination aims primarily to identify any plagiocephaly, where the recessed side of the head is often on the left side of patients. Wynne-Davies [67] found a 100% incidence of plagiocephaly among the infantile idiopathic group.

The spine examination should begin with inspection, palpation, and careful evaluation of the child's posture, head, shoulder, trunk, and pelvic symmetry. Owing to the patients age, an Adam's forward bend test (looking for prominence of ribs in the thoracic spine or transverse processes in the lumbar spine) is not possible, but the test can be simulated by lying the child prone over the examiner's knee with the convex side downward. Lateral pressure in this position will illicit curve flexibility. The more rigid the curve, the higher the likelihood of progression. Chest or flank asymmetry and limitation in chest excursion should make the examiner aware of the association with syndromic scoliosis. Abdominal reflex abnormalities should initiate a more thorough neurological examination. Absence of this reflex has been reported as the only objective finding in patients with Chiari malformations [50]. The abnormal reflex is typically found on the convex side of the curve [69]. Further work-up is appropriate in this setting with total spine magnetic resonance imaging.

Other physical findings that should not be overlooked include plagiopelvy, and developmental hip dysplasia, both with strong associations to idiopathic infantile scoliosis [7, 8, 10, 27, 68]. Hooper [27] found a 6.4% prevalence of congenital hip dislocation among 156 patients with infantile scoliosis. This is approximately ten times higher than the general population. Wynne-Davies [68], similarly reported on four patients among her infantile scoliosis cohort who had DDH. In 1980, Ceballos et al. [10] reported on 113 patients with a 25% prevalence of DDH. Interestingly, the dislocations were found mainly among females and resolving curves. There was no correlation with side of dislocation and direction of curve. Finally, limb length inequality must be ruled out as an etiology for scoliosis. When it is the cause, the lumbar prominence is found on the side of the longer limb. Other means of testing this include a sitting forward bend test or by placing a lift under the short limb to equalize limb lengths.

17.4 Diagnostic Testing

17.4.1 Radiologic Evaluation

Plain radiography is a simple and reliable tool in the work-up of a child with suspected scoliosis. Patients typically are diagnosed in the first 6 months to 1 year of life, and early recognition and treatment are essential for optimal outcomes. Radiographs will help rule out congenital scoliosis as well as establish baseline measurement for future comparisons. Treatment decisions are traditionally based on progression of Cobb angle and rib vertebral angle difference (RVAD) obtained at subsequent visits. Progression has been associated with compensatory curves (including lumbar, double thoracic, and thoracic), greater vertebral rotation, and shorter length of curves.

High-quality radiographs are essential for thorough radiographic analysis. Initial evaluation should include anterior–posterior (AP) and lateral radiographs of the spine (including cervical spine and pelvis). In children too young to stand, films should be obtained supine. Special attention should be paid to the cervical spine for anomalies, as well as to the lumbosacral junction for spinal dysraphism, and the pelvis and hips to ensure a reduced position of the hips. Measurements should include both Cobb angle and RVAD (Fig. 17.1a). Mehta [48] is credited for developing this powerful tool for predicting progression of infantile curves. Out of frustration with the inability to predict progression with Cobb measurements, she evaluated the relationship of the rib attachment to the vertebral body. She noted variability in the takeoff angle of the ribs from the convex vs. the concave side of the curve. The rib vertebral angle measures the angle of a line drawn perpendicular to the apical thoracic vertebra end plate and a line drawn down the center of the concave and convex ribs. The RVAD is calculated by subtracting the convex from the concave angles. An RVAD of less than 20° indicates a curve that is most likely to resolve (85–90%), while an RVAD of 20° or more is frequently associated with progression. She also described a second radiographic parameter to assist in prediction known as the *phase of the rib head* (Fig. 17.1b, c). This radiographic tool uses the relationship of the head and neck of the rib to the vertebral body, at the apex of the convexity of the scoliosis. In phase-1, there is no overlap of the rib head or neck on the apical

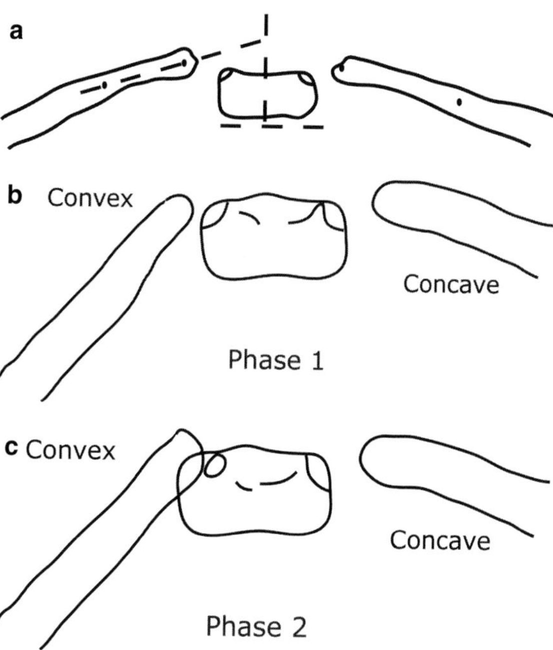

Fig. 17.1 (**a**) Rib vertebral angle difference (RVAD). (**b**) Phase of rib head: phase 1. (**c**) Phase of rib head: phase 2. (Redrawn from reference [48])

vertebra. In this group of patients, the RVAD should be measured to detect progression. In phase-2, the head or neck of the rib is overlapped on the apical vertebra. It has been shown that a phase-2 rib head is a certain predictor for progression and RVAD does not need to be measured. Mehta [48] reported on 46 infantile patients with phase-1 rib heads whose scoliosis resolved. She found that 83% had a RVAD of less than 20°. Of the remaining patients with an RVAD of 20° or more, the angle was found to consistently decrease with follow-up. The decrease in RVAD also preceded the decrease in Cobb angle. Of the group with progressive curves, 84% had an initial RVAD of 20° or more (range 18–30°).

Ceballos et al. [10] corroborated Mehta's findings reporting 92% of their resolving curves having an RVAD of 20° or less. Of the remaining 8% with an RVAD greater than 20° all showed improvement at the 3-month follow-up. Robinson and McMaster [56] in 1996 found that the curves that progressed among their 109 patients had a mean initial RVAD of 31°, while those that resolved had a mean of 9° on initial exam.

Mehta [48] recognized a special radiographic feature among the less common (and more aggressive) double major and lumbar curve patterns. She recognized that the RVAD at the apical thoracic vertebra was frequently less than 20° and found there to be significant asymmetry at the 12th vertebra. Here, she found the rib on the concave side becoming more vertical than the rib on the convex side, making the RVAD negative. The 12th rib is initially part of the upper curve but becomes the apex of a secondary curve developing caudally to the first. Consequently, the rib that is on the concavity of the upper curve drops secondary to the progression of the vertebral rotation and increases in magnitude of the caudal curve.

17.4.2 The Role of Advanced Imaging and Neural Axis Abnormalities

The role of advanced imaging in infantile and juvenile scoliosis is directly related to the presence of neural axis abnormalities. As IIS and JIS are a diagnosis of exclusion, all attempts must be made to identify possible etiologies. The incidence of neurological abnormalities has been reported as high as 20% in patients under the age of 10 [18, 35, 37, 48]. Lewonowski et al. [37] reported an magnetic resonance imaging (MRI) study of 26 consecutive patients with idiopathic scoliosis under the age of 10 years. They found 5 patients (19%) with neuropathology, and only 2 patients with atypical curves. Four of their patients were infantile, and two patients had abnormal findings: a 4-month-old boy with a terminal lipoma and a 3-year-old girl with a syrinx.

Gupta et al. [22] conducted a prospective and retrospective MRI study to evaluate the prevalence of neural axis abnormalities in patients 10 years of age or younger with idiopathic scoliosis and a normal clinical examination. In the prospective arm, he followed 34 patients with a mean age of 9 years and found abnormalities in 6 patients (18%). Within this group, six patients were infantile, and three patients had identifiable neuropathology. Among the 64 retrospective patients, 20% were found to have neural axis pathology.

Most recently, Dobbs et al. [16] in multicenter study identified 11 of 46 infantile scoliosis patients with neural axis abnormalities. All patients were clinically asymptomatic and had curves of 20° or less. Five patients had an Arnold–Chiari type-I malformation, three with syringomyelia, one with a low-lying conus, and one with a brain tumor. Of these 10 patients, 8 required surgical intervention. On the basis of the findings of this paper and other reports, it is our recommendation that all patients with IIS or JIS with a curve of 20° or less have both, a brain and a complete spine magnetic resonance Imaging MRI.

Other imaging modalities exist to aid in management and provide continued relevant information in the care of these children. Computed tomography (CT) scans can be helpful for preoperative evaluation in selected patients where the spine will be instrumented. Pedicular anatomy and bony anomalies are made very clear. CT scans can also be used to assess the three-dimensional lung volumes and can be a marker of treatment.

17.5 Management Themes (Fig. 17.2)

17.5.1 Selecting Surgical Candidates

Management of children with infantile scoliosis is based on anticipated or actual curve progression. Mehta's [48] prognostic criteria, as discussed earlier, are very helpful in identifying curves at risk. Curves with an RVAD of less than 20° and a Cobb angle of less than 25° are at low risk of progression. These patients are safely treated

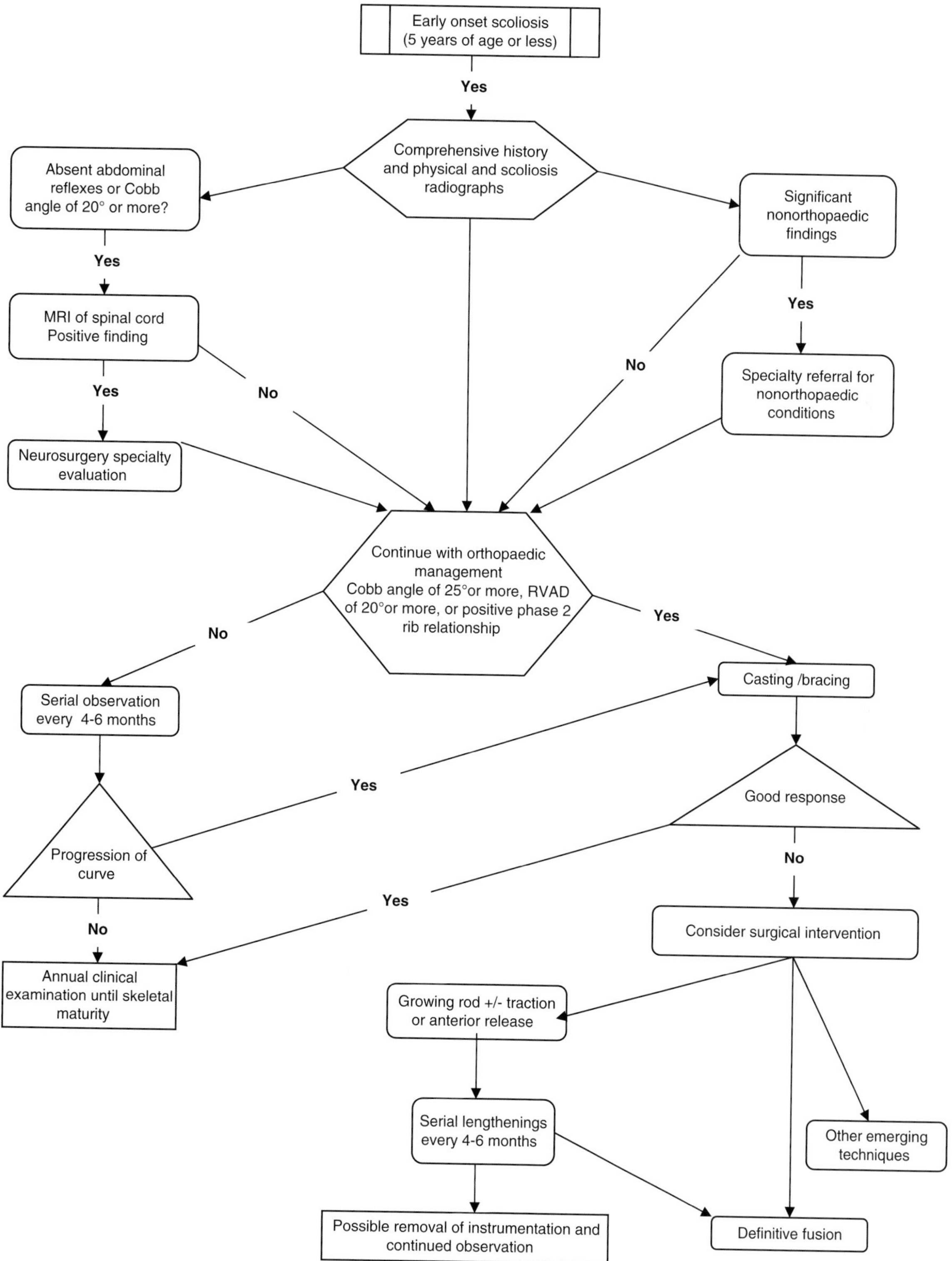

Fig. 17.2 Treatment algorithm for infantile and juvenile idiopathic scoliosis. (Adopted from reference [21])

with observation; however, they should be followed clinically every 4–6 months for progression. Once the curve has resolved, the follow-up interval can be extended to 1–2 years. We recommend following these patients to maturity to ensure that there is no recurrence during the adolescent growth spurt. Diedrich et al. [13] reported on 25-year follow-up of infantile scoliosis, validating the use of RVAD, and demonstrated that there was no advantage to supine plaster bed treatment over physiotherapy, in regard to time to resolution or functional outcome.

Infants with an RVAD of 20° or more or a phase 2 rib–vertebral relationship and a Cobb angle between 20 and 35° have a higher risk of progression. This group of patients should be followed closely at 4–6 month intervals for clinical and radiographic evaluation. Active treatment should be initiated when progression of Cobb angle of 5° or more is documented over 1 year [3]. Active treatment at this point is usually in the form of casting or bracing, which will be discussed thoroughly in separate chapters.

17.5.2 Surgical Treatment: Historic Perspective

The goals of surgical treatment of infantile scoliosis are multifold: To stop curve progression and allow for maximum growth of the spine, lungs, and thoracic cage. Surgery is recommended in children with Cobb angle of 45° or more and documented curve progression. This statement reflects the current trend toward more aggressive operative management since the techniques for fusion-less surgery have become refined, and the natural history of this disease, more clearly understood.

Historically, the goals of surgery were a straight shortened spine rather than a deformed spine of near normal length. Isolated posterior spinal fusion in this age group quickly went out of favor, after Dubousset et al. [17] described the crankshaft phenomenon. This phenomenon seen in skeletally immature patients describes progression of deformity following posterior spinal fusion due to continued anterior growth of the spine. Sanders et al. [58] further correlated open triradiate cartilage and Risser 0 to high risk of crankshaft in light of an isolated posterior spinal fusion. Anterior arthrodesis was therefore recommended, in addition to posterior to prevent crankshaft. Anterior and posterior fusion, however, results in a significant amount of height loss and thoracic development. As discussed earlier, Dimeglio [15] very nicely outlined spinal growth throughout childhood with two noticeable peaks of growth (0–5 years and 10–15 years). Using his formula for calculating normal growth, expected loss of height can be determined in lieu of an anterior–posterior fusion. Winter [66] similarly described a formula for calculating amount of projected height loss. To calculate it in centimeters, you multiply 0.07 by the number of segments fused and the number of growth years remaining. This data is very valuable in educating family and caretaker, of the potential ramifications of fusion in this very young patient population. It should also be noted that the effect of fusion on the spine could have morbid effects on lung and thoracic cage development. This has been a motivating factor over many decades to devise other surgical methods that avoid circumferential fusion.

Over 45 years ago, Roaf [55] attempted to modulate spine growth, much like one would modulate an angular deformity in a pediatric lower extremity with hemiepiphysiodesis. He proposed that the spinal deformity was the result of asymmetric growth between the convex (faster growing) and concave (inhibited) side of the curve. His technique of modulation involved ablation of the convex epiphyseal cartilage and adjacent discs at the vertebrae near the apex of the curve. Only 23% of his treated patients showed improvement of Cobb angle, while 40% showed little or no improvement (Cobb angle <10° change). Marks et al. [44] built upon this idea and used hemiepiphysiodesis and simultaneous Harrington internal fixation. No significant improvement was measured in 13 consecutive patients with 12 demonstrating progression of deformity.

Harrington, [25] in 1962, described a fusion-less technique in 27 idiopathic and postpolio patients, placing a single distraction rod on the concavity of the curve connected to hooks at both ends. The hooks and rods were placed after a subperiosteal approach to the spine. The idea was to instrument the spine without arthrodesis in an attempt to preserve spinal growth, correct deformity, and control the residual deformity. Although no longitudinal results were reported, he believed that children under 10 years could be managed with instrumentation alone, and those, 10 years and older required arthrodesis.

Moe et al. [49] modified the technique described by Harrington and limited subperiosteal exposure to the site of hook placement and passed the rod subcutaneously. Furthermore, they modified the rod to have a smooth, thicker central portion to prevent scare formation to the threads and allow for sagittal contouring. Patients were lengthened when a loss of Cobb angle >10° occurred. Of the two patients treated with idiopathic infantile scoliosis, both were reported as having a notable decrease in curve magnitude. They furthermore reported a complication rate of 50%, including rod breakage and hook dislodgement from the rod or the lamina.

In 1997, Klemme et al. [33] reported on 20-year experience of the Moe technique. Sixty-seven patients were followed from initial instrumentation to final fusion, with an average of 6.1 procedures per patient. Curve progression was arrested or improved in 44 of 67 patients with an average curve reduction of 30%. Of the remaining 23 patients, 12 were neuromuscular, and the curves progressed on average 33%.

In 1977, Luque and Cardosa [39] described their technique of fusion-less treatment of scoliosis with segmental spinal instrumentation. In 1982, Luque [40] modified this technique by adding sublaminar wires and replacing the Harrington rod with L-shaped rods, later to be known as the Luque trolly. His initial series included 47 paralytic patients who grew by an average of 4.6 cm over the immobilized segment with an average curve correction of 78%. This system became less favored after reports that subperiosteal exposure and sublaminar wire passage created scar tissue and weakened the lamina, which made revision and later definitive fusion difficult. There were also several reports of spontaneous fusion and substantially less growth preservation than predicted. These findings were attributed to the exposure that was required at each level to pass wires.

Patterson et al. [52] combined segmental spinal instrumentation with anterior apical convex growth arrest and fusion in 9/13 patients who had previously undergone surgery at an average age of 5 years and 5 months. Curve correction averaged 46% at 2-year follow-up. Less curve deterioration was identified in those patients who had anterior apical growth arrest compared to those who had segmental instrumentation alone.

In 1999, Pratt et al. [54] performed a retrospective review of patients treated with Luque trolley instrumentation with and without convex epiphysiodesis in 26 patients. Eight were treated with Luque trolley alone and all showed significant curve deterioration. Of those treated with combined convex epiphysiodesis and Luque instrumentation, the Cobb angle worsened in 7 of 13, remained unchanged in 4 and improved for 2. Growth was found to be 49% of predicted in the Luque trolley alone group and 32% among those undergoing combined surgery.

Blakemore et al. [6] further reported periodic lengthening with a submuscular rod with and without apical fusion. Apical fusion was performed on curves 70° or more and in those whose curves were stiff on bending radiographic testing. The rod was placed within the muscle above the spine periosteum, placing the rod closer to the spine for better contour and alignment without inducing spontaneous fusion. He reported on 29 children, 10 idiopathic, all treated in a Milwaukee brace postoperatively. Mean Cobb angle improved from 66 to 38° immediately postoperatively with most recent follow-up showing a slight deterioration to 47°. Complication rate was 24% including hook dislodgement (5), rod breakages (3), and superficial wound infection (1).

17.5.3 Current Approaches to Surgical Management

Once the decision for surgery has been made, several factors have to be considered before choosing the correct surgical approach. The rigidity of the curve plays an important role in decision making, as curves that have little flexibility will not likely be as amenable to a growing construct alone. In this situation, there may be a role for anterior release prior to posterior fusion-less surgery. Marks, [43] in unpublished results, discusses the use of annulectomy vs. nucleotomy as anterior release options. No long-term results exist, however, to make any definitive recommendations.

The next decision to make is which lengthening procedure is ideal for the patient. Salari et al. [53] recently reported on the results of a survey sent to 40 qualified surgeons on ideal treatment of 11 different case scenarios of infantile scoliosis. Seventeen surgeons responded with a wide variation in treatment recommendations for each patient scenario. The most common treatment selected was a dual growing-rod construct (56.7%) followed by nonoperative management (16.6%), SHILLA (15.5%), VEPTR (7%), and fusion or resection, and immediate fusion (4%). This study is important to highlight the lack of standardized treatments offered to our patients by highly qualified surgeons [57].

The next two sections briefly describe the various fusion-less surgeries. They are subdivided into two categories. Distraction-based growing rods and growth directed surgery. VEPTR, a form of distraction-based growing rod will be discussed in a separate chapter.

17.5.4 Distraction-Based Growing Rods

The unpredictability and high implant associated complication rate associated with single rod distraction techniques led Akbarnia and Marks [1] to develop a dual growing rod technique, building on concepts formulated by Asher (Fig. 17.3a–d). This is the current technique preferred by the authors. Subperiosteal dissection is limited to the proximal and distal foundations (anchor sites). Hooks or pedicle screws are placed on both ends over two or three spinal levels. Foundation sites are fused using local bone graft supplemented with synthetic graft. Upper and lower contoured 3/16 in.-diameter rods are placed submuscularly on both sides of the spine. The rods are joined on each side with extended tandem connectors placed at the thoracolumbar junction to avoid disturbing sagittal balance. The first lengthening is typically performed at the index procedure. A distractor designed to fit within the longitudinal opening in the tandem connector is used at time of lengthening that typically occurs at 6-month intervals starting with the index surgery. The intent of the original lengthening is to obtain modest correction of the scoliotic curve without unduly stressing the foundations. We have found approximately 50% correction of coronal Cobb angles at the original surgery. More aggressive lengthening can be performed starting with the first lengthening after fusion. Somatosensory evoked potential monitoring is performed during each lengthening. Lengthening can be performed as outpatient surgery with appropriate anesthesia and nursing support. Bracing is utilized until fusion is achieved at the foundation sites.

Akbarnia et al. [4] reviewed 13 patients with no previous surgery and noncongenital curves who were followed to final fusion. They found a mean spinal growth of 5.7 cm during a 4.4-year treatment period. The curve improved from 81 to 36° after initial surgery and to 28° at final fusion. T1–S1 length improved from 24 to 29 cm after initial surgery to 35 cm at final fusion. Those patients lengthened at 6-month or less intervals experienced significantly more growth and curve correction than those lengthened less frequently [4].

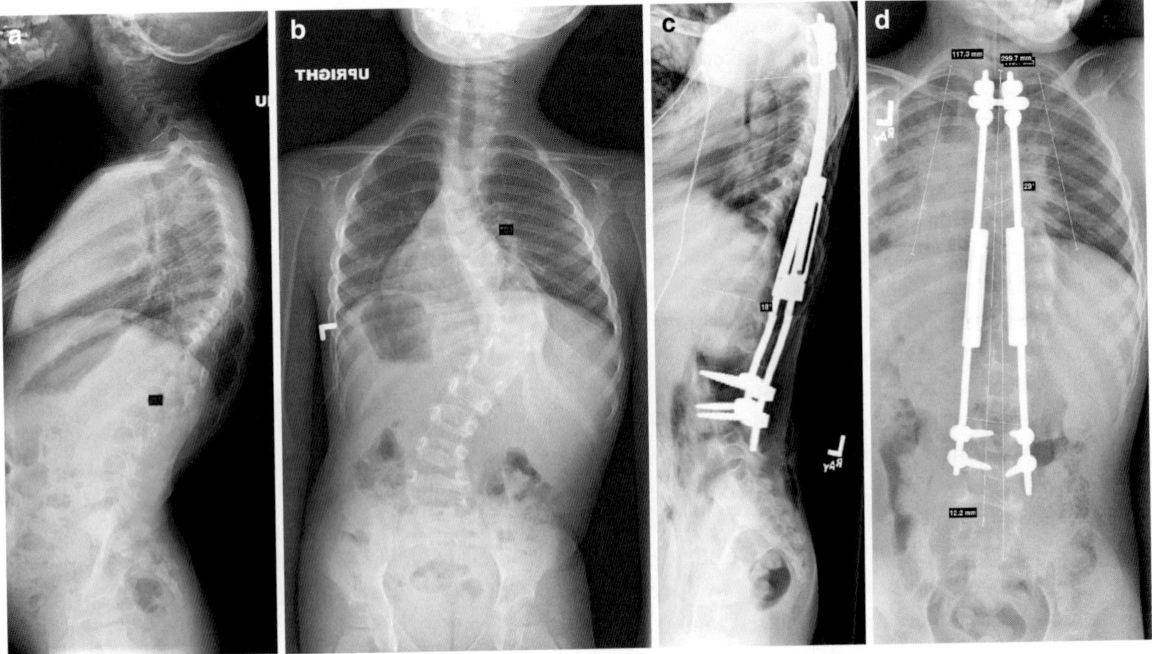

Fig. 17.3 (**a, b**) Severe progressive scoliosis in a 4-year-old patient with idiopathic infantile. (**c, d**) Post initial surgery radiographs

A recent report by Sankar et al. [59] reviewed 782 growing rod surgeries in 252 patients where neuromonitoring was performed. Surgeries included 252 primary rod implantations, 168 implant exchanges, and 362 lengthenings. Neuromonitoring changes occurred in two primary implant surgeries (0.8%), in one implant exchange (0.6%), and one lengthening (0.3%). The change noted in the case of implant exchange also resulted in a clinical deficit, which resolved within 3 months. The monitoring change that occurred in the lengthening was in a child with an intracanal tumor that also had a change during the primary surgery. The final recommendation was that the overall rate of neuromonitoring change seen in primary and implant exchange surgeries justifies its use. No definitive recommendations could be made for lengthenings because of sample size.

Akbarnia et al. [2] reported on a multicenter study with 2-year follow-up (24–111 months) of 23 patients, 7 of which had idiopathic infantile scoliosis. The average age at initial surgery was 5 years and 5 months, with an average of 6.6 lengthenings. Mean Cobb angle improved from 82 to 38° following initial surgery and 36° at latest follow-up. Growth averaged 1.21 cm per year as calculated by T1–S1. Seven patients completed treatment and averaged 11.8 cm of total growth (T1–S1) from preoperative to postfinal fusion (1.66 cm per year). Among 14 patients with thoracic curves, the space available for lung as described by Campbell et al., improved from 0.87 preoperatively to 1.00 at latest follow-up or final fusion. Complications occurred in 11 of 23 patients between initial surgery and final fusion. They included three anchor (hook or screw) displacements, two rod breakages, two deep wound infections, four superficial wound problems, one crankshaft, and one junctional kyphosis requiring an extension of instrumentation. Although the complication rate is high, the authors contested that it is safe and effective, and carried with it a lower complication rate than single rod systems.

Thompson et al. [62] compared the results of single and dual growing rod systems in 28 patients followed to definitive surgery. Five had a single rod construct with anterior and posterior apical fusion, 16 had single rod without apical fusion, and 7 had dual rod without fusion. Mean Cobb angle, respectively, improved from 85 to 65°, 61 to 39°, and 92 to 26°. Spinal growth, respectively, was 0.3 1.0, and 1.7 cm per year. The authors concluded that the improved results seen in dual rod systems are likely attributable to its greater strength and more frequent lengthening.

Mahar et al. [41] recently published results of a biomechanical study investigating the construct of the foundation in a porcine model. They investigated four constructs: (1) hook-hook with cross-link, (2) hook-screw with cross-link, (3) screw-screw with cross-link, and (4) screw–screw without cross-link. They found that a four-screw construct in adjacent vertebral bodies provides the strongest construct in pullout testing. A cross-link did not provide any additional strength to the all screw construct. They also found that the hook construct had significantly higher pullout strength in the lumbar spine compared to the thoracic spine.

In a multicenter study, Bess et al. [5] (Growing Spine Study Group) reported on complications in 910 growing rod surgeries in 143 patients with minimum 2-year follow-up. They divided the group as single (n = 73 patients) or dual rod (n = 70 pts) and subcutaneous (n = 54) or submuscular (n = 89). Complication rate per surgery was <20%. Complication rates were equivalent among single and dual rod constructs. Significance was found in number of implant-related complications requiring unplanned return to the operating room for single rod constructs compared to dual. The subcutaneous group had more complications per patient (1.6 vs. 0.99) and more wound problems (13 vs. 4 patients). Furthermore, subcutaneous placement of dual rods had higher overall complication rate, higher wound problems, prominent implants and patients undergoing implant-related unplanned return to the operating room. The conclusion was that the overall complication rate is comparable to historic reports; dual rods reduce unplanned trips to the operating room and submuscular position of implants is preferred over subcutaneous.

17.5.5 Growth Directed Surgery

Growth directed surgery is the phrase used to describe procedures where reduction of the spinal deformity relies on the remaining growth available. The classic example of this is the Shilla procedure described by McCarthy et al. This surgery involves limited instrumentation and reduction of the apical segment with specialized polyaxial Shilla screws that house two rods and allow those rods to glide within the construct. The concept is to improve the deformity of the spine by naturally directed growth along a new path (the rods that are placed).

McCarthy et al. [46] recently reported on 10 patients with 2-year follow-up. Three of these patients were either infantile or juvenile idiopathic scoliosis. Initial curve correction went from 70.5 (40–86°) to 27° (5–52°) at 6 weeks, and 34° (18–57°) at 2-year follow-up. Two patients had a staged anterior apical release. Complications included rod revision for growth off the end of the rods, rod exchange for a shorter one due to prominence, one broken rod, and two wound infections for a total of five surgeries among all ten patients beyond the index procedure. It was predicted that this same group of patients would have required 49 additional surgeries in a distraction-based growing rod model. For more details regarding this technique, please see Chap. 48.

17.6 On the Horizon and Conclusion

Significant strides have been made in the last decade regarding understanding and management of infantile and juvenile scoliosis. This unique disease entity, however, still leaves many areas undiscovered including genetic etiology, accurate scientific predictability of progression, ideal treatment for individual curves, and refinement in surgical technique.

The ideal surgery would include a minimally invasive approach with a durable and inert implant that rarely requires reoperation. Takaso et al. [61] in 1998, reported on the development of a rod containing a direct-current motor attached to a radio-controlled receiver. They performed successful correction of experimental scoliosis in beagles. The main issues with this device were its size (16 mm) and the placement of the receiver in the abdominal cavity. Akbarnia has recently explored the idea of remote lengthening, and animal studies are under way investigating this promising technology.

Ward et al. [65], as discussed in another chapter, are currently studying this very unique patient population to identify any markers for progression and the genetic basis of IIS and JIS. It is the hope of all treating physicians that success in this arena will be as productive as it has been in identifying these markers in adolescent idiopathic scoliosis.

In conclusion, idiopathic infantile and juvenile scoliosis is a disease entity that if left untreated can result in devastating and life-threatening complications. Early recognition and timely treatment are essential to management and for good outcome. Exciting new technology and improved surgical technique will result in lower complication rates, avoidance of natural history, and ultimately improved patient outcome [62].

References

1. Akbarnia BA, Marks DS (2000) Instrumentation with limited arthrodesis for the treatment of progressive early-onset scoliosis. Spine: State Art Rev 14(1):181–189
2. Akbarnia BA, Marks DS, Boachie-Adjei O et al (2005) Dual growing rod technique for the treatment of progressive early-onset scoliosis: a multicenter study. Spine 30(17 Suppl): S46–S57
3. Akbarnia B (2007) Management themes in early onset scoliosis. J Bone Joint Surg Am 89(Suppl 1):42–54
4. Akbarnia BA, Breakwell LM, Marks DS, et al (2008) Dual growing rod technique followed for three to eleven years until final fusion. Spine 33(9): 984–990
5. Bess R, Akbarnia BA, Thompson GH et al (2010) Complications in 910 growing rod surgeries: use of dual rods and submuscular placement of rods decreases complications. J Bone Joint Surg Am: In Press
6. Blakemore LC, Scoles PV, Poe-Kochert C et al (2001) Submuscular Isola rod with or without limited apical fusion in the management of severe spinal deformities in young children: preliminary report. Spine 26(18):2044–2048
7. Browne D (1936) Congenital deformities of mechanical origin. Proc R Soc Med 49:1409–1431
8. Browne D (1956) Congenital postural scoliosis. Proc R Soc Med 49(7):395–398
9. Campbell R, Smith MD, Mayes, TC et al (2003) The characteristics of thoracic insufficiency syndrome associated with fused ribs and congenital scoliosis. JBJS 85-A: 399–408
10. Ceballos T, Ferre-Torrelles M, Castillo F et al (1980) Prognosis in infantile idiopathic scoliosis. J Bone Joint Surg Am 62(6):863–875
11. Davies G, Reid L (1971) Effect of scoliosis on growth of alveoli and pulmonary arteries and on right ventricle. Arch Dis Child 46(249):623–632
12. Dickson R (1994) Early-onset idiopathic scoliosis. In: Weinstein S (ed) The pediatric spine: principles and practice. Raven, New York, pp 421–429
13. Diedrich O, von Strempel A, Schloz M et al (2002) Long-term observation and management of resolving infantile idiopathic scoliosis a 25-year follow-up. J Bone Joint Surg Br 84(7):1030–1035
14. Dimeglio A, Bonnel F (1990) Le rachis en croissance. Springer, France, pp 392–394
15. Dimeglio A (1993) Growth of the spine before age 5 years. J Pediatr Orthop 1-B:102–107
16. Dobbs M, Lenke L, Szymanski DA et al (2002) Prevalence of neural axis abnormalities in patients with infantile idiopathic scoliosis. J Bone Joint Surg Am 84-A(12):2230–2234
17. Dubousset J, Herring JA, Shufflebarger H (1989) The crankshaft phenomenon. J Pediatr Orthop 9(5):541–550

18. Evans S et al (1996) MRI of 'idiopathic' juvenile scoliosis. A prospective study. J Bone Joint Surg Br 78(2):314–317
19. Fernandes P, Weinstein SL (2007) Natural History of Early Onset Scoliosis. J Bone Joint Surg Am 89(Suppl 1): pp 21–33
20. Figueiredo UM, James JI (1981) Juvenile idiopathic scoliosis. J Bone Joint Surg 63-B(1):61–66
21. Gillingham BL, Fan RA, Akbarnia BA (2006) Early Onset Idiopathic Scoliosis. J. Am. Acad. Ortho. Surg. 14(2): 101–112
22. Gupta P, Lenke LG, Bridwell KH (1998) Incidence of neural axis abnormalities in infantile and juvenile patients with spinal deformity. Is a magnetic resonance image screening necessary? Spine 23(2):206–210
23. Harrenstein R (1930) Die Skoliose bei Saueglingen und ihre Behandlung. Z Orthop Chir 52:1–40
24. Harrenstein RJ (1936) Sur la scoliose des nourrissons et des jeunes enfants. Revue d'Orthopedie (23):289
25. Harrington PR (1962) Treatment of scoliosis. Correction and internal fixation by spine instrumentation. J Bone Joint Surg Am 44-A:591–610
26. Hefti F, McMaster M (1983) The effect of the adolescent growth spurt on early posterior spinal fusion in infantile and juvenile idiopathic scoliosis. J Bone Joint Surg Br 65(3): 247–254
27. Hooper G (1980) Congenital dislocation of the hip in infantile idiopathic scoliosis. J Bone Joint Surg Br 62-B(4): 447–449
28. James JI (1951) Two curve patterns in idiopathic structural scoliosis. J Bone Joint Surg Br 33-B(3):399–406
29. James JI (1954) Idiopathic scoliosis; the prognosis, diagnosis, and operative indications related to curve patterns and the age at onset. J Bone Joint Surg Br 36-B(1): 36–49
30. James JI, Lloyd-Roberts GC, Pilcher MF (1959) Infantile structural scoliosis. J Bone Joint Surg Br 41-B:719–735
31. James J (1975) The management of infants with scoliosis. J Bone Joint Surg Br (57):422–429
32. Kafer ER (1976) Idiopathic scoliosis. Gas exchange and the age dependence of arterial blood gases. J Clin Invest 58(4): 825–833
33. Klemme WR, Francis D, Winter RB et al (1997) Spinal instrumentation without fusion for progressive scoliosis in young children. J Pediatr Orthop 17(6):734–742
34. Koop S (1988) Infantile and juvenile idiopathic scoliosis. Orthop Clin North Am 19(2):331–337
35. Kristmundsdottir F, Burwell R, James J (1985) The rib-vertebra angles on the convexity and concavity of the spinal curve in infantile idiopathic scoliosis. Clin Orthop Relat Res 201:205–209
36. Lenke LG, Dobbs MB et al (2007) Management of juvenile idiopathic scoliosis. J Bone Joint Surg – Am Vol 89 (Suppl 1):55–63
37. Lewonowski K, King JD, Nelson MD (1992) Routine use of magnetic resonance imaging in idiopathic scoliosis patients less than eleven years of age. Spine 17(6 Suppl): S109–S116
38. Lloyd-Roberts GC, Pilcher MF (1965) Structural idiopathic scoliosis in infancy: a study of the natural history of 100 patients. J Bone Joint Surg Br 47:520–523
39. Luque E, Cardosa A (1977) Segmental spinal instrumentation in growing children. Orthop Trans 1:37
40. Luque ER (1982) Paralytic scoliosis in growing children. Clin Orthop (163):202–209
41. Mahar A, Bagheri R, Oka R et al (2007) Biomechanical comparison of different anchors (foundations) for the pediatric dual growing rod technique. Spine J 8(6):933–939
42. Mannherz RE, Betz RR, Clancy M et al (1988) Juvenile idiopathic scoliosis followed to skeletal maturity. Spine 13(10):1087–1090
43. Marks D, (2009) Personal communication
44. Marks D, Iqbal M, Thompson AG et al (1996) Convex spinal epiphysiodesis in the management of progressive infantile idiopathic scoliosis. Spine 21(16):1884–1888
45. Mau H (1968) Does infantile scoliosis require treatment? J Bone Joint Surg Am 50B:881
46. McCarthy R, McCulough FL, Luhmann SJ et al (2008) Shilla growth enhancing system for the treatment of scoliosis in children: greater than two year follow up. In: Scoliosis Research Society Annual Meeting. Salt Lake City, UT
47. McMaster MJ (1983) Infantile idiopathic scoliosis: can it be prevented? J Bone Joint Surg Br 65(5):612–617
48. Mehta MH (1972) The rib-vertebra angle in the early diagnosis between resolving and progressive infantile scoliosis. J Bone Joint Surg Br 54(2):230–243
49. Moe JH, Khalil K, Winter RB et al (1984) Harrington instrumentation without fusion plus external orthotic support for the treatment of difficult curvature problems in young children. Clin Orthop (185):35–45
50. Muhonen MG, Menezes AH, Swain PD et al (1992) Scoliosis in pediatric Chiari malformations without myelodysplasia. J Neurosurg 77(1):69–77
51. Muirhead A, Conner AN (1985) The assessment of lung function in children with scoliosis. J Bone Joint Surg Br 67(5):699–702
52. Patterson JF, Webb JK, Burwell RG (1990) The operative treatment of progressive early onset scoliosis. A preliminary report. Spine 15(8):809–815
53. Ponseti IV, Friedman B (1950) Prognosis in idiopathic scoliosis. J Bone Joint Surg Am 32A(2):381–395
54. Pratt RK et al (1999) Luque trolley and convex epiphysiodesis in the management of infantile and juvenile idiopathic scoliosis. Spine 24(15):1538–1547
55. Roaf R (1963) The treatment of progressive scoliosis by unilateral growth-arrest. J Bone Joint Surg Br 45: 637–651
56. Robinson C, McMaster M (1996) Juvenile idiopathic scoliosis. Curve patterns and prognosis in one hundred and nine patients. J Bone Joint Surg Am 78(8): 1140–1148
57. Salari PA, Oliveira D, Akbarnia BA et al (2009) Infantile idiopathic scoliosis; variations in preferred treatment options: In: 16th International Meeting on Advanced Spine Techniques (IMAST), Vienna Austria, July 15–18
58. Sanders JO, Herring JA, Browne RH (1995) Posterior arthrodesis and instrumentation in the immature (risser-grade-0) spine in idiopathic scoliosis. J Bone Joint Surg Am 77(1): 39–45
59. Sankar WN, Skaggs DL, Emans JB et al (2009) Neurologic risk in growing rod spine surgery in early onset scoliosis: is neuromonitoring necessary for all cases. Spine 34(18): 1952–1955
60. Scott JC, Morgan TH (1955) The natural history and prognosis of infantile idiopathic scoliosis. J Bone Joint Surg Br 37-B(3):400–413
61. Takaso M, Moriya H, Kitahara H et al (1998) New remote-controlled growing-rod spinal instrumentation possibly

applicable for scoliosis in young children. J Orthop Sci 3(6):336–340
62. Thompson GH, Akbarnia BA, Kostial P et al (2005) Comparison of single and dual growing rod techniques followed through definitive surgery: a preliminary study. Spine 30(18):2039–2044
63. Thompson G, Lenke L, Akbarnia BA et al (2007) Early onset scoliosis: future directions. J Bone Joint Surg Am 89(Suppl 1):163–166
64. Tolo VT, Gillespie R (1978) The characteristics of juvenile idiopathic scoliosis and results of its treatment. J Bone Joint Surg 60-B(2):181–188
65. Ward K, Nelson LM, Chettier R et al (2008) Genetic profile predicts curve progression in adolescent idiopathic scoliosis. In: Scoliosis Research Society Annual Meeting. Salt Lake City, UT
66. Winter R (1977) Scoliosis and spinal growth. Orthop Rev (6):17–20
67. Wynne-Davies R (1968) Familial (idiopathic) scoliosis- a family survey. J Bone Joint Surg Am 50-B(1):24–30
68. Wynne-Davies R (1975) Infantile idiopathic scoliosis. Causative factors, particularly in the first six months of life. J Bone Joint Surg Br. 57(2):138–141
69. Zadeh HG, Sakka SA, Powell MP et al (1995) Absent superficial abdominal reflexes in children with scoliosis. An early indicator of syringomyelia. J Bone Joint Surg Br 77(5):762–767

18 Congenital Scoliosis

Muharrem Yazici and Guney Yilmaz

Key Points

- Congenital scoliosis is caused by vertebral malformations, which interrupt the longitudinal growth of the spine.
- The progression of congenital scoliosis basically depends on the type of the anomaly.
- The evaluation of a patient with congenital scoliosis should include detailed spine and neurological examination, radiographic evaluation and investigation of associated anomalies.
- There are many treatment alternatives for congenital scoliosis. The age of the patient, type of anomaly, limitations of the surgeon and surgery room should be considered to choose the most appropriate way of treatment.

18.1 Introduction

Congenital scoliosis is a lateral curvature of the vertebral column. It is caused by vertebral malformations, which interrupt the longitudinal growth of the spine. Congenital malformation is always present at birth; however, scoliosis develops in some patients as the spinal column grows longitudinally.

Congenital scoliosis is caused by early embryologic development failure of vertebral column. Failure of formation, segmentation, or both can cause anomalous development [3]. Either these malformations can be a benign anomaly that results in mild curvatures and does not affect spinal balance, or they can be one with high potential to deteriorate and affect spinal balance [21].

The exact incidence of congenital scoliosis is unknown [25], while the prevalence rate of congenital scoliosis is thought to be approximately 1 in 1,000 live births [16]. It occurs more often in girls than in boys, with a ratio of 2.5–1 [23].

18.2 Etiology

The causes of congenital scoliosis have not yet been investigated in detail. The etiology is thought to be multifactorial. It is believed that the genetic and teratogenic factors play a role in the development of congenital scoliosis. Vertebral malformations may be an isolated finding or, in some cases, may occur with other cardiac, renal, and intraspinal malformations. They may also occur as part of an underlying chromosome abnormality or syndromes such as Alagille, Jarcho-Levin, Klippel–Fiel, Goldenhar, Trisomy 18, diabetic embryopathy, and VACTERL (vertebral, cardiac, renal, limb anomalies, anal atresia, tracheo-esophageal fistula) association [1, 14]. Ingestion of antiepileptic drugs during pregnancy has also been accused as a possible cause [43].

Carbon monoxide (CO) and hypoxia are the two most common teratogenic factors believed to be possible causes of congenital vertebral malformations. CO is a well-known teratogen [37]. It is a colorless and odorless gas and has 200–300 times greater affinity for hemoglobin than oxygen. Therefore, CO binds to hemoglobin in the lungs easily, while it does not unbind in peripheral tissues, thus interfering with tissue

M. Yazici (✉)
Department of Orthopaedics and Traumatology, Hacettepe University, Faculty of Medicine, 06100 Sihhiye, Ankara, Turkey
e-mail: yazioglu@hacettepe.edu.tr

B. A. Akbarnia et al. (eds.), *The Growing Spine*,
DOI: 10.1007/978-3-540-85207-0_18, © Springer-Verlag Berlin Heidelberg 2011

oxygenation [13]. CO crosses the placenta. Even though how the CO leads to spinal malformations is unknown, the relation between CO exposure and spinal malformations has been shown in different studies. Studies of maternal carbon-monoxide exposure have demonstrated vertebral and rib malformation in offsprings of mice and rabbits. Loder et al. found spinal malformations in 70% of offsprings of mice exposed to 600 ppm CO on gestation day 9 [27]. The dose and the timing of CO exposure seem critical. Maximum effect is seen on day 9 of gestation, which corresponds to fourth week in human embryonic fetal life, with an exposure to 600 ppm of CO [13]. Hypoxia was shown to be an etiologic factor in experimental animal models. These reports showed a relation between time and dosage of hypoxia and vertebrae and rib malformations. The malformations were segmentation and formation defects, similar to those found in man [22, 36].

Based on mouse studies, a series of candidate genes, known to cause vertebral malformations has been identified [4, 15]. *Wnt3a, PAX1, DLL3, Sim2 genes* have been proposed to be responsible for vertebral malformation in mouse models. Mutations of these genes may disrupt early somite development, leading to rib fusion and deficient development of the anterior vertebral elements and failure of formation of the dorsal neural arches [15, 17, 18, 29].

18.3 Classification

A congenital scoliosis is often rigid, while some forms are inclined to deteriorate, and others do not disturb spinal balance. Therefore, it is crucial to anticipate when a congenital scoliosis is at risk for rapid progression. A proper classification system of the malformations is mandatory, for an accurate estimation of the progression risk. Congenital scoliosis is mostly classified under three main categories: failure of formation, failure of segmentation and complex malformations. MacEven described a classification system for congenital spinal malformations, which was modified by Winter et al. [44] in 1968, and was later accepted by Scoliosis Research Society.

Winter et al. classification (44)

I. Unclassifiable: There is a collection of many types of segmentation defects. There is no dominating type.

II. Fusion of ribs.

III. Unilateral failure of formation of a vertebra, partial: This produces a wedge or trapezoid-shaped vertebra. A vestigial pedicle may be present.

IV. Unilateral failure of formation of a vertebra, complete: This produces a hemivertebra.

V. Bilateral failure of segmentation: This refers to the condition in which there is absence of the disc space between adjacent vertebral bodies.

VI. Unilateral failure of segmentation: This produces an unsegmented bar and may involve, two or more vertebrae and only the bodies or only the posterior elements.

Failure of formation arises as a result of an absence of a part of vertebra. Anterior, anterolateral, posterior, posterolateral and lateral region of the vertebral ring may be affected [26]. Failure of formation may be incomplete or complete. A wedge vertebra is an incomplete formation defect. The anomalous vertebra has two pedicles, but one side of the vertebrae is hypoplastic. Hemivertebra is a complete formation defect. The anomalous vertebra has one pedicle, and there is only half of the vertebra. There are three types of hemivertebra: fully segmented, partially segmented and unsegmented. Fully segmented hemivertebra has growth plates, both cranially and caudally. In this way, a fully segmented hemivertebra continues to grow longitudinally both cranially and caudally and has great effect on spinal balance. Alternatively, a nonsegmented hemivertebra is not separated from cranial and caudal vertebra; thus, it has lower growth potential and less effect on spinal balance. A partially segmented hemivertebra has functional disc only on one side and fusion on the other side. In hemimetameric shift, a hemivertebra is counterbalanced by contralateral hemivertebra on the other side of the spinal column. They are separated by at least one normal vertebra and are most commonly seen in thoracic region [38].

Segmentation defects present an abnormal connection between vertebras. The bar stops the growth on the affected side and causes a tethering effect. If the bar is bilateral (block vertebra) it has much less effect on spinal balance [21].

Complex malformations contain segmentation and formation defects in the same patient. These patients have a great risk for rapid progression. Since only 30%

of the spinal column is ossified at birth, it is difficult to diagnose these kinds of malformations at the beginning of life.

Generally, posterior element anatomy is neglected in classification systems of congenital scoliosis. Understanding the posterior anatomy is especially helpful for planning the surgery. Posterior elements may be totally normal; however, there may also be fused laminas or bifid areas with exposed neural structures. Therefore, knowledge about posterior anatomy prior to surgery via three–dimensional computed tomography (CT) is very valuable.

Nakajima et al. [32] emphasized the importance of three-dimensional analysis of the congenital scoliosis in a group of patients. They examined the anterior and posterior anatomy of congenital scoliosis patients with formation failure. They classified the posterior anatomy in patients with solitary malformed vertebra into bi-pedicle and hemi–pedicle group, which were further grouped according to malformation of lamina. In some of the patients with multiple malformations, they observed union between the vertebral arches. They concluded that observation of formation failure with three-dimensional CT can demonstrate various morphologic abnormalities in posterior elements of malformed vertebrae.

18.4 Natural History

Longitudinal spine growth basically comes from superior and inferior end plates. Curve progression is caused by unbalanced growth of one side of the spine. Well formed and normal appearing discs suggest healthy growth plates and potential for asymmetric growth. On the other hand, the presence of bar or fused ribs are signs of restricted growth on this side and may cause progressive deformities [21]. Therefore the progression of congenital scoliosis basically depends on the type of the anomaly. The location of vertebral malformation and the growth potential of the patient are the other two most important factors in predicting the deterioration potential of the curve.

The two most important natural history studies were published by Winter et al. [44] in 1968 and McMaster and Ohtsuka [30] in 1982:

Winter et al. [44] followed 234 patients with congenital scoliosis and found that thoracic and thoracolumbar curves progressed more than cervico-thoracic and lumbar curves. A mild cervicothoracic curve might cause serious cosmetic deformity because of head tilt, prominence of the neck, and drooping of one shoulder. It was also found that the rate of progression was not related to the severity of the curve, since some of the mild curves progressed more rapidly than the severe ones. Progression was most likely to occur when there were multiple unilateral anomalies in the thoracic spine. It was also reported that most severe deterioration of the curve was seen during preadolescence and infancy period. McMaster and Ohtsuka [30] followed 216 patients for an average period of 5.1 years and reported that the rate of curve deterioration was found to depend on both the level and type of the malformation. For each type of deformity, the deterioration of the curve was less severe in upper thoracic regions, more severe in mid-thoracic region, and worst in thoracolumbar region. Block vertebra and bilateral failure of segmentation are the most benign forms of anomaly and the progression rate is less than 2° per year. Wedge vertebra, hemivertebra and unilateral bar cause more severe deformities, respectively. A unilateral bar and contralateral hemivertebra were the most severe anomalies and has a progression rate of 5–10° per year.

18.5 Patient Evaluation

The evaluation of a patient with congenital scoliosis focuses on physical examination including detailed spine and neurological examination, radiographic evaluation and investigation of associated anomalies.

Since the spinal growth is a major concern in congenital scoliosis, physical examination should start with recording the sitting and standing height, and weight. The growth of the child should be monitored, as there is a close relationship between growth and curve progression, as discussed in natural history part.

Congenital spinal deformities may cause spinal imbalance, therefore sagittal and coronal spinal imbalance should be recorded. Spinal balance in sagittal and coronal plane, and pelvic balance, head tilt, and shoulder balance must be keenly recorded. The rigidity of the curve is assessed.

Rib cage deformities can be seen with vertebral malformation; therefore any anomaly of rib cage should be recorded. Inspiratory and expiratory capacity of lungs should be evaluated by pulmonary function tests to detect any restrictive lung disease.

A detailed neurological examination including muscle forces, sensation of the skin, abdominal and deep tendon reflexes should be recorded to rule out any spinal dysraphism. Patient's back should be examined carefully for any hair patches, lipomata, dimples and abnormal pigmentation, which can be the first signs for intraspinal pathology. Physical findings such as asymmetrical calves, cavus feet, clubfeet, and vertical talus can also be the manifestations of spinal dysraphism, so a detailed lower extremity examination is mandatory.

18.6 Imaging

Appropriate imaging techniques should be used during patient evaluation in order to define the pathologic anatomy, classify the malformation and make a logical surgery plan.

Routine radiographs are essential to evaluate the deformity. Radiographs in infants can be taken supine. As the child becomes older and can stand independently, standing posterior–anterior (PA) and lateral views should be obtained [21]. Measurement of Cobb angle is often more difficult in patients with congenital scoliosis, because of the distorted end plates and the malformed pedicles. However, with high quality radiographs, it is possible to determine the type of the malformation, the magnitude of the curve and the growth potential of the vertebral anomaly. It is also a reliable method for follow-up of curve progression [12].

In a study investigating intra- and inter-observer variability in measurement of the Cobb angle in congenital scoliosis, Loder et al. [26] found a variability of ±9.6° and ±11.8°, respectively. According to the authors, to ensure with 95% confidence that the increase in the curve is not due to error of measurement, at least 23° of change is necessary. Facanha-Filho et al. [12] stated that the variability in Loder et al. study was very high and performed another study to assess variability in measurement of the Cobb angle. They found a mean intraobserver variance with an average of 2.8° and the interobserver variance was 3.35°.

It is possible to estimate the growth potential of malformed vertebrae from disc spaces and their relative sizes on direct radiographs. If they are narrow and poorly defined, they do not have much growth potential. On the other hand, visible, wide, normal appearing discs associate a high potential for growth and curve progression. Even though the conventional method of evaluating congenital scoliosis is direct roentgenograms, these images can be difficult to interpret in patients with small size, overlying structures obscuring the deformity, and in complex deformities. In patients, who are candidates for surgery, more detailed imaging techniques are necessary.

New improvements in computed tomography (CT) and magnetic resonance imaging (MRI) technology made both of these modalities indispensable, especially in patients undergoing spinal stabilization, and with complex deformities.

Three dimensional computed tomography (3D-CT) is the best modality for defining the osseous anomalies and their relationships [33]. It is mostly recommended for complex deformities, but not for routine observation or serial follow-up. Hedequist et al. [20] compared the findings in direct radiogram and 3D-CT of congenital scoliosis patients with the findings in surgery. In all patients, anterior and posterior anatomy correlated with the CT findings.

MRI is the standard diagnostic tool for assessment of intraspinal pathology because it is noninvasive and sensitive [8]. Specific indications for MRI include the presence of neurological signs such as weakness, sensory loss, bowel or bladder dysfunction, a skin abnormality over the spine like dimple, hairy patch or nevus, leg or back pain, lumbosacral kyphosis, interpedicular widening. MRI is also very important in any patient undergoing spinal correction and stabilization.

Since the genitourinary system abnormalities are found in 18–40% of congenital scoliosis patients, screening renal ultrasonography is recommended to all patients [28, 10]. The incidence of congenital heart disease in patients with congenital spine deformity was found to be 26% in a recent study of Basu et al. [6] revealing the high importance of detailed cardiac examination and an echocardiography for a thorough examination.

18.7 Associated Anomalies

The development of vertebral column is closely associated with the spinal cord; therefore the neural and vertebral malformations often coexist. These malformations may cause neurological findings. However, absence of any neurological finding does not rule out intraspinal pathology [21]. Mesoderm, which is responsible for the formation of vertebra, is also responsible for the formation of urogenital, pulmonary and cardiac systems. Malformation of these systems can also accompany congenital vertebral malformations [24]. Therefore, systemic evaluation of the patients with proper imaging techniques is mandatory.

In a study using direct radiogram and myelogram, McMaster et al. [31] found intraspinal pathology in 18.3% of 251 congenital scoliosis patients. When MRI was used as diagnostic tool for evaluation of the congenital scoliosis, neural axis abnormalities rises up to 30–38% [8, 34].

The most common malformation of spinal cord is diastematomyelia (split cord), which is defined as partial or complete split of spinal cord or cauda equina with a bony or fibrous spur [31]. Diastematomyelia is found in approximately 20% of patients with congenital scoliosis [19]. In patients with diastematomyelia, the normal movement of spinal cord is restricted. While the spinal column grows longitudinally, the spinal cord stretches. Any corrective manipulation of spine may cause more stretching of the cord, and this may result in neurological deterioration. Therefore, it is very important to evaluate the whole spine before any corrective surgery. Other congenital intraspinal anomalies associated with congenital scoliosis are epidermoid cysts, dermoid cysts, neuroenteric cysts, tethered cord, lipomas and teratomas [31].

Evidence from a number of retrospective studies shows diminished pulmonary function in patients with congenital scoliosis. Because of the complex interconnections between spine, sternum and ribs, the displacement and rotation of the vertebrae in scoliosis have profound effects on the shape of the thorax. Individuals with congenital scoliosis and chest wall deformities are believed to have a thoracic deformity which limits lung growth, and rib deformities leading to thoracic instability and alteration in respiratory mechanics. The expansion of the thoracic cavity is limited as the movement of the ribs is impeded, which in turn decreases chest wall compliance and makes breathing significantly harder despite the absence of any lung disease. Altered development and morphology in patients with scoliosis can lead to measurable changes in lung function most consistent with restrictive lung defect.

Renal system abnormalities may be found in 18–40% of congenital scoliosis patients. Anomalies may affect the kidneys, ureters, bladder and urethra. Unilateral renal agenesis, duplicated kidneys and ureteral obstruction are the most common renal abnormalities associated with congenital scoliosis [10, 28].

Congenital heart disease is present in 10–26% of patients Atrial and ventricular septal defects are the most common cardiac abnormalities. More complex cardiac malformations like tetralogy of fallot and transposition of great vessels can also be seen in congenital scoliosis patients [6, 35].

Musculoskeletal anomalies like clubfeet, Sprengel's deformity, Klippel-Feil syndrome, developmental dysplasia of the hip, may all be seen in these patients [21].

18.8 Treatment Alternatives

Once the congenital scoliosis is diagnosed in a patient, it is very important to note the patient's age, spinal balance and to classify the anomaly. Treatment should be started regardless of age, if the patient has vertebral anomaly with high potential to deteriorate such as unilateral hemivertebra and contralateral unsegmented bar. Patients with anomalies less inclined to deteriorate should be carefully followed with serial radiograms, and Cobb angle of the curve should be measured in each visit to detect any progression.

There are many treatment alternatives for congenital scoliosis. The age of the patient, type of anomaly, limitations of the surgeon and surgery room should be considered to choose the most appropriate way of treatment. As all these methods are discussed in the following chapter separately, they were briefly summarized here:

18.8.1 Observation

Patients with balanced spine and vertebral malformations, less prone to deteriorate like hemimetameric shift or block vertebra can be followed with serial plain radiograms at 4–6-month intervals. It is important to note the spinal balance of the patient and the Cobb angle of curve. Most recent radiograms should be compared with the earliest radiograms of the patient in order to detect any progression.

18.8.2 Bracing

Short and rigid curves rarely respond to brace treatment. Bracing can be considered for long, flexible curves and for compensatory curves, proximal or distal to anomalous segment.

18.8.3 Growth Inhibition

Spine fusion via posterior exposure with or without instrumentation remains the basic treatment method for congenital scoliosis. Adding instrumentation for stabilization helps to obtain better correction; meanwhile risk of neurological complications should always be taken into consideration during surgery and follow-up. It is possible to obtain significant levels of reconstruction via instrumented fusion on congenital spinal deformities, provided surgical methods increasing the spinal column flexibility are employed, and manipulations to elongate the vertebral column are avoided during the reconstructive maneuvers [5]. (Fig. 18.1a–k).

18.8.4 Growth Modulation

Growth inhibition on the convex side of the deformity by means of insitu fusion (convex growth arrest) without instrumentation, or by pedicle screws or staples is another option, especially for deformities with normal growth potential on concave side. Patients 5 years of age or less with scoliosis 70° or less and without any lordosis or kyphosis are ideal candidates for growth modulating surgical treatment [45]. Convex growth arrest appears to be an effective procedure to halt the progression of the curve with an expected correction over time in scoliosis patients without signs of advanced skeletal maturity. The overall main problem seems to be the unpredictability of the results [42].

18.8.5 Growth Preservation/Stimulation

- *Growing rod*

The growing rod technique, which is principally described for idiopathic or idiopathic-like deformities where the vertebral anatomy is normal, is based on reconstructing the deformity via a distraction maneuver. However, detailed examination of the growing spine series, published in the past few years, revealed that the method has also been applied in patients with congenital deformities [2, 41]. A recent multicentric study, where 19 congenital scoliosis patients were treated with growing rod technique and were followed for at least 2 years, reports 31% correction in scoliosis angle and 12 mm yearly elongation of T1-S1 segment [11]. Also, space available for lungs ratio increased from 0.81 preoperative to 0.94 postoperative. The fact that none of the patients presented a neurological complication should be attached importance. The growing rod technique is a safe and reliable method for young children, who present some flexibility in the anomalous segment, or when the congenital anomaly involves a vertebral segment too long for resection, or with compensating curve with structural pattern concomitant to the congenital deformity (Fig. 18.2a–i).

- *Thoracic expansion*

Growing rod technique is a spinal instrumentation method addressing to the deformity in the spine and therefore should be used in patients where the primary problem is at the vertebral column. If the patient has rib fusions, and/or thoracic insufficiency syndrome, in other words, if the primary problem involves the thoracic cage, it would be a preferable approach to employ the treatment method addressing to the thorax deformity, which is the thoracic expansion [9].

18.8.6 Reconstruction

- *Hemivertebrectomy*

Since the scoliosis due to hemivertebrae present bone excess on the convex side (or shortfall in concave side), the most reasonable and ideal treatment method is the resection of this bone (hemivertebrae). Although hemivertebrectomy has been technically defined as a procedure long time ago, in the beginning it has not been frequently applied, since it involved a long and challenging surgery on young children, who face other comorbidities. Because of the developments in anesthesia and postoperative care, today surgery has become the standard treatment method for the single hemivertebrae of the thoracolumbar and lumbar regions [7] (Fig. 18.3a–e).

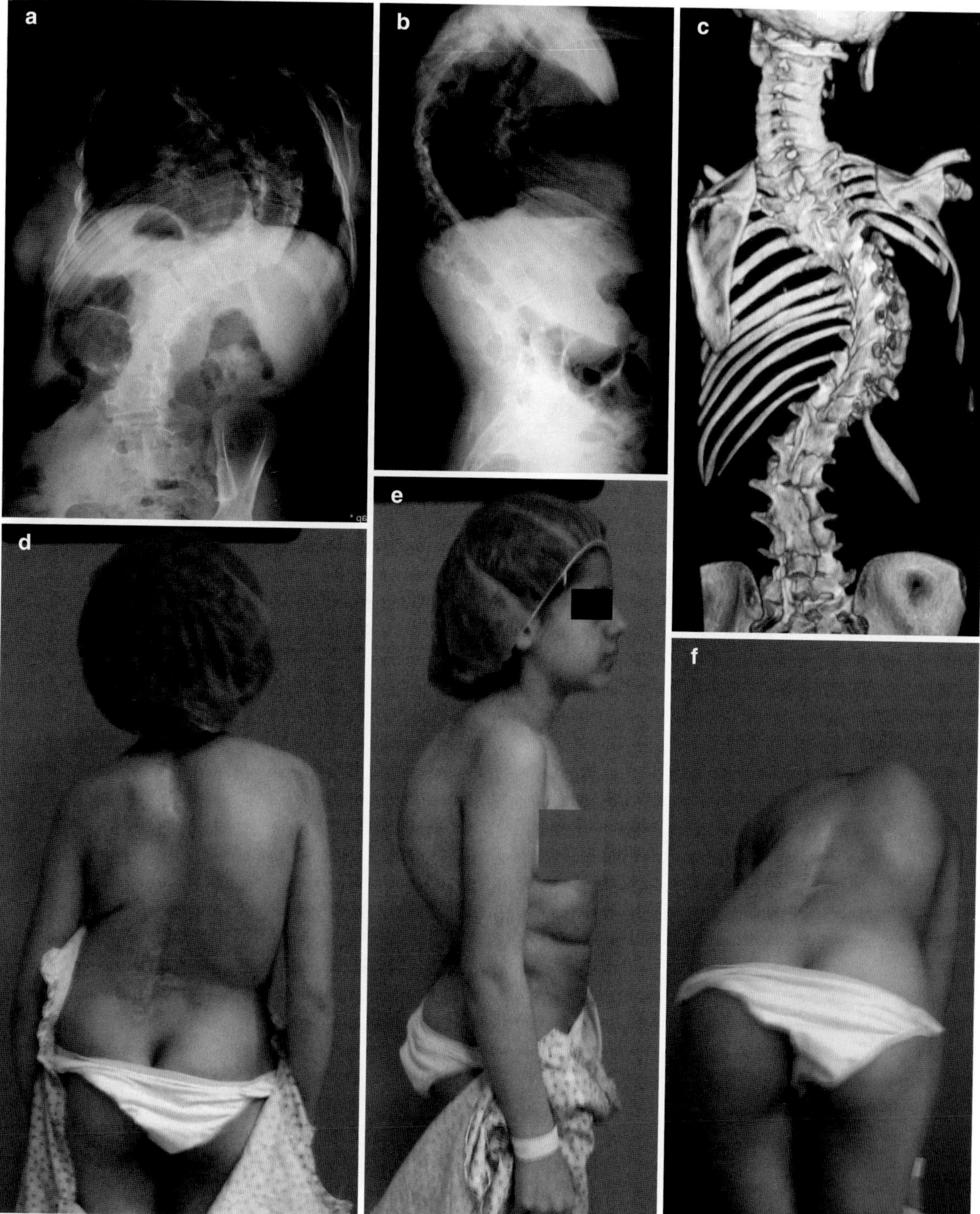

Fig. 18.1 Twelve-year-old girl with congenital spinal deformity (**a–f**)

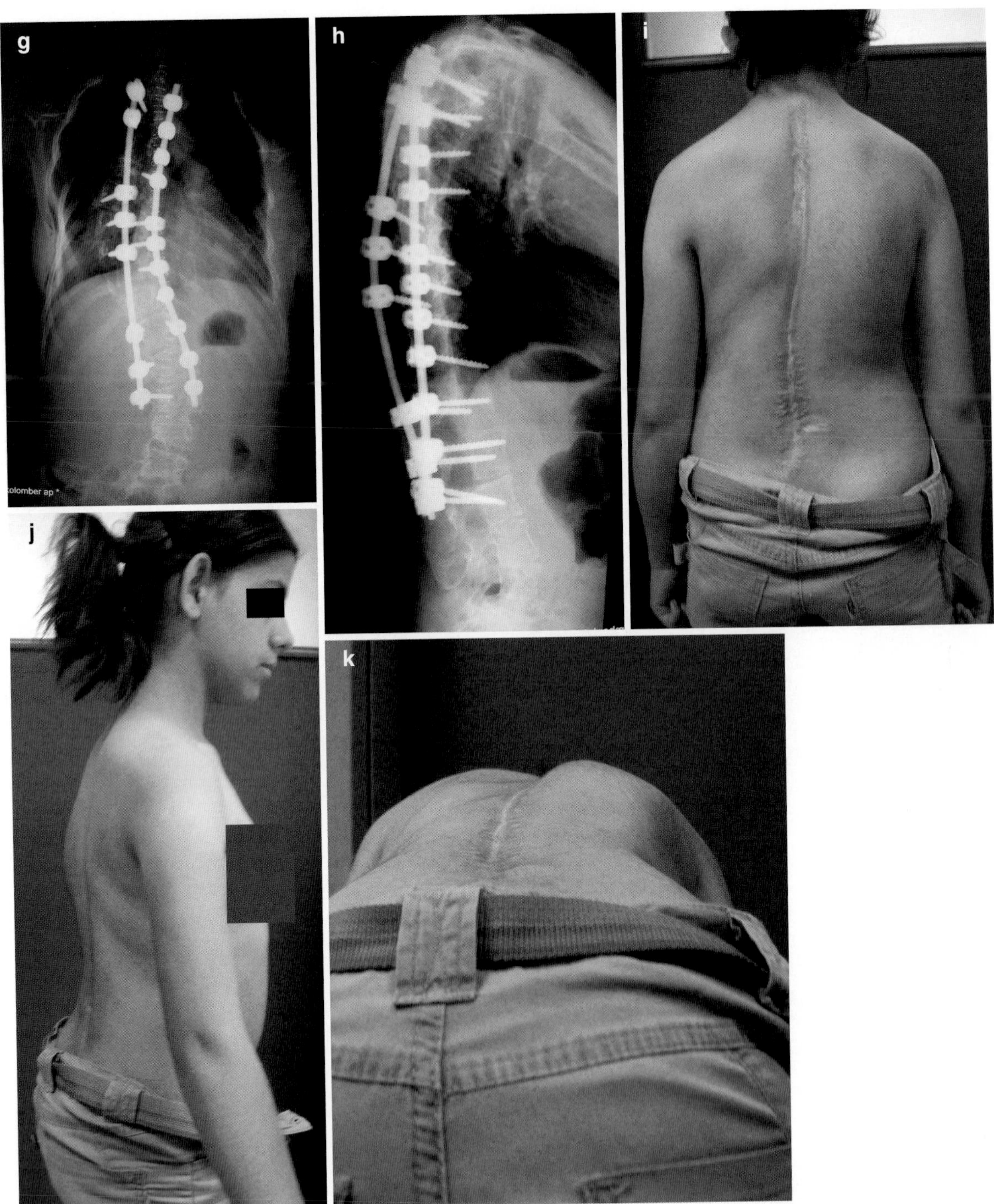

Fig. 18.1 During the posterior instrumentation and fusion, additional multiple Chevron osteotomies and concave rib osteotomies were performed (**g–k**)

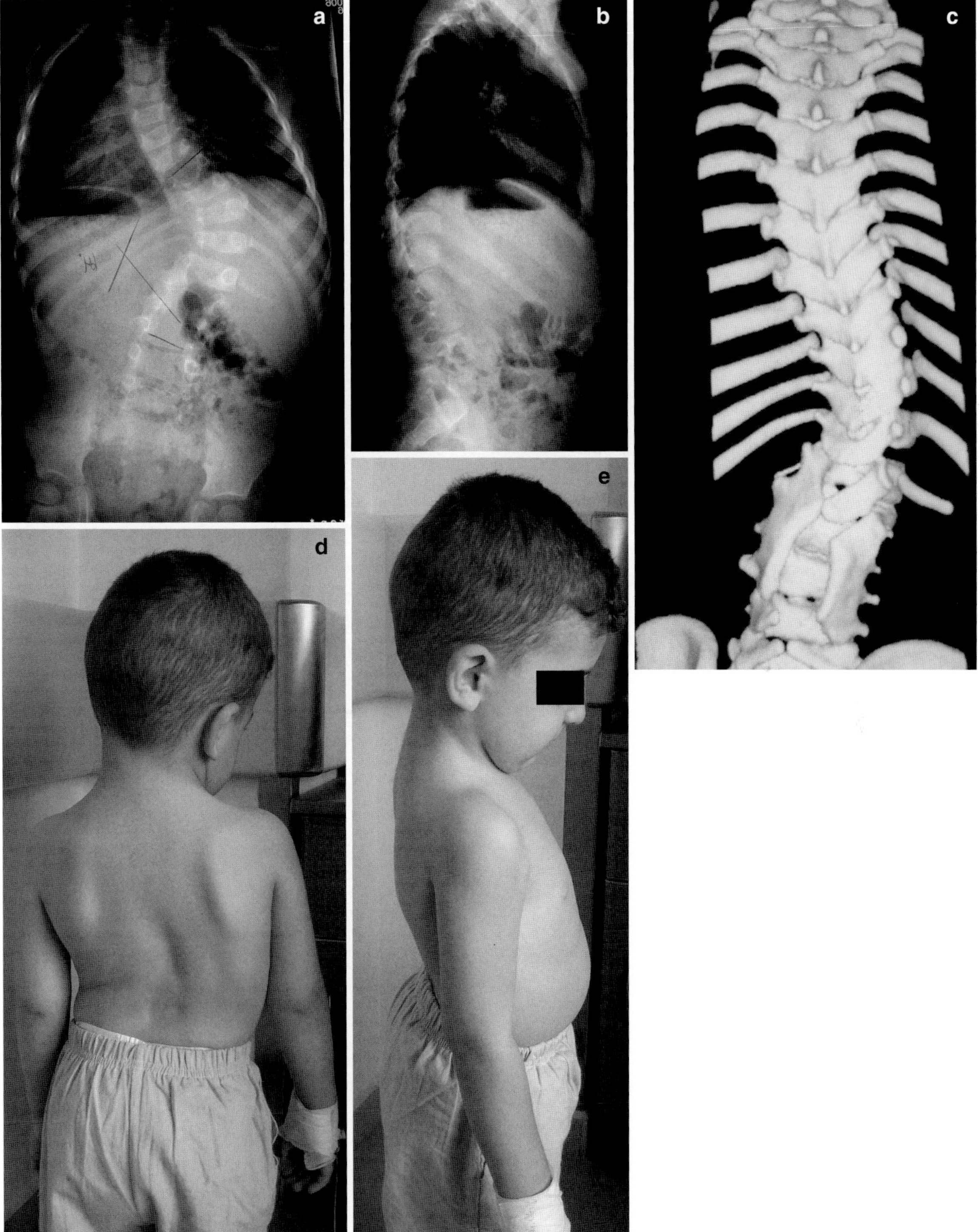

Fig. 18.2 Three and half-year-old boy. He presented with thoracolumbar deformity. He had unsegmented bar and contralateral hemivertebrae (**a–e**)

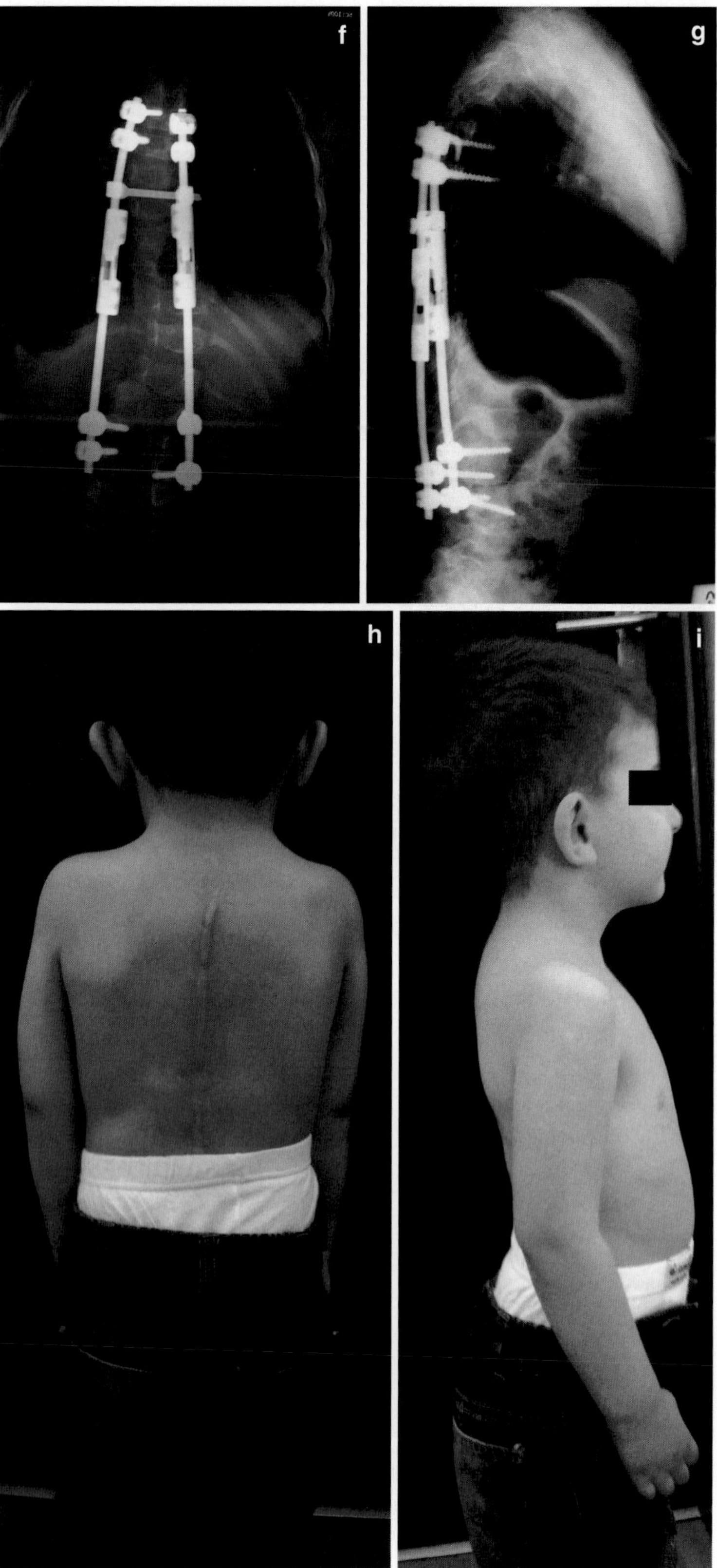

Fig. 18.2 His deformity improved after growing rod instrumentation (**f–i**)

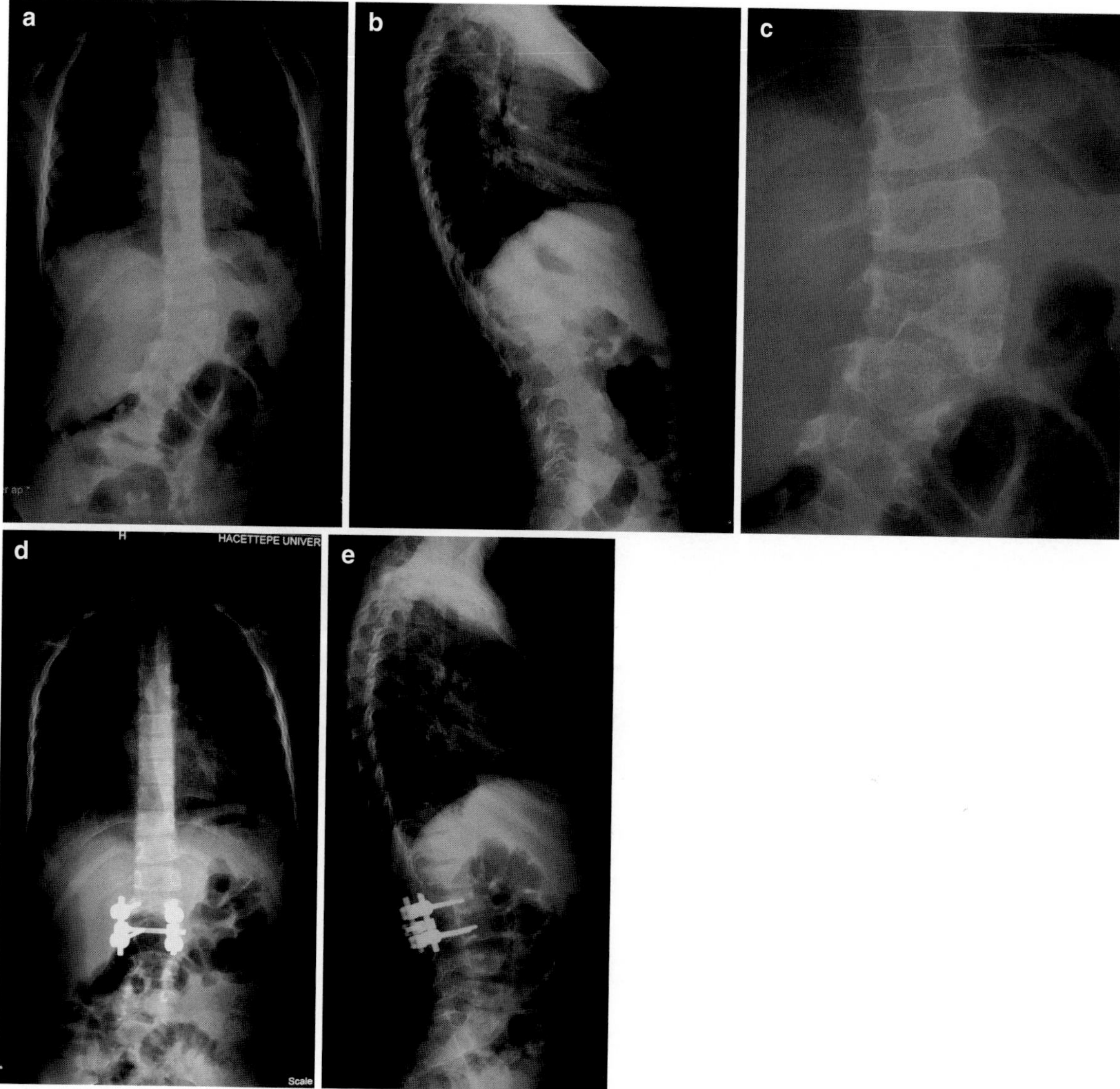

Fig. 18.3 Four-year-old girl (**a–c**). Single hemivertebra at L1 was treated with hemivertebrectomy and posterior instrumented fusion (**d, e**)

- *Vertebral column resection*

Sometimes, congenital spinal deformity may emerge due to an anomaly much more complicated than a simple hemivertebrae. Simple hemivertebrectomy would definitely not suffice for the treatment of multiplanar complex deformities (mostly) occurring in case of multiple hemivertebrae and unsegmented bars. Vertebral column resection is a technically challenging procedure [39, 40]. This operation takes a long time and involves excessive bleeding. Moreover, it is open to severe complications, including serious neurological deficits [40]. Despite all these risks, it is being widely practiced in experienced centers. It is turning into a standard procedure for the complex spinal deformities leading to serious trunk imbalance (Fig. 18.4a–i).

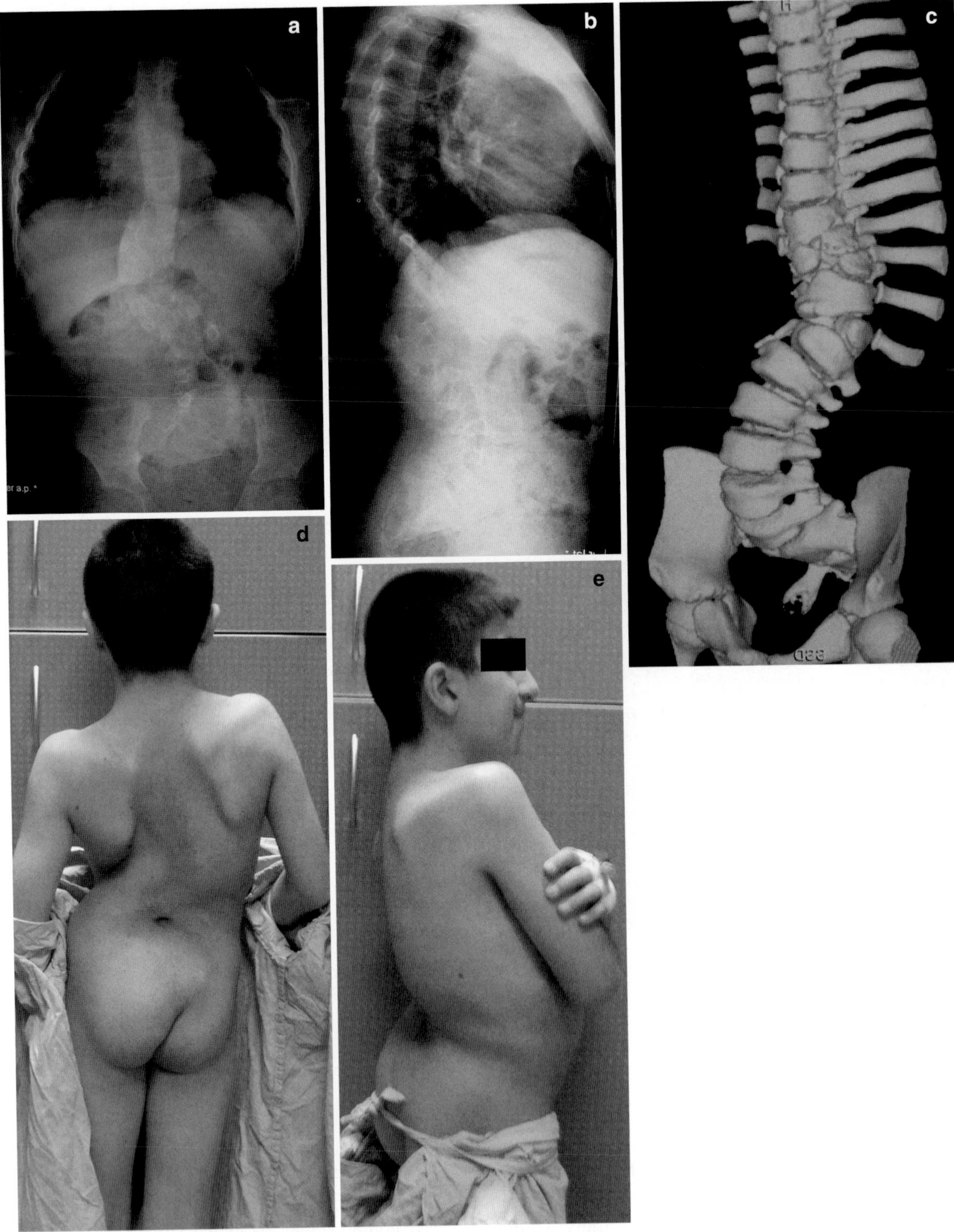

Fig. 18.4 Eleven-year-old boy with congenital scoliosis (**a–e**)

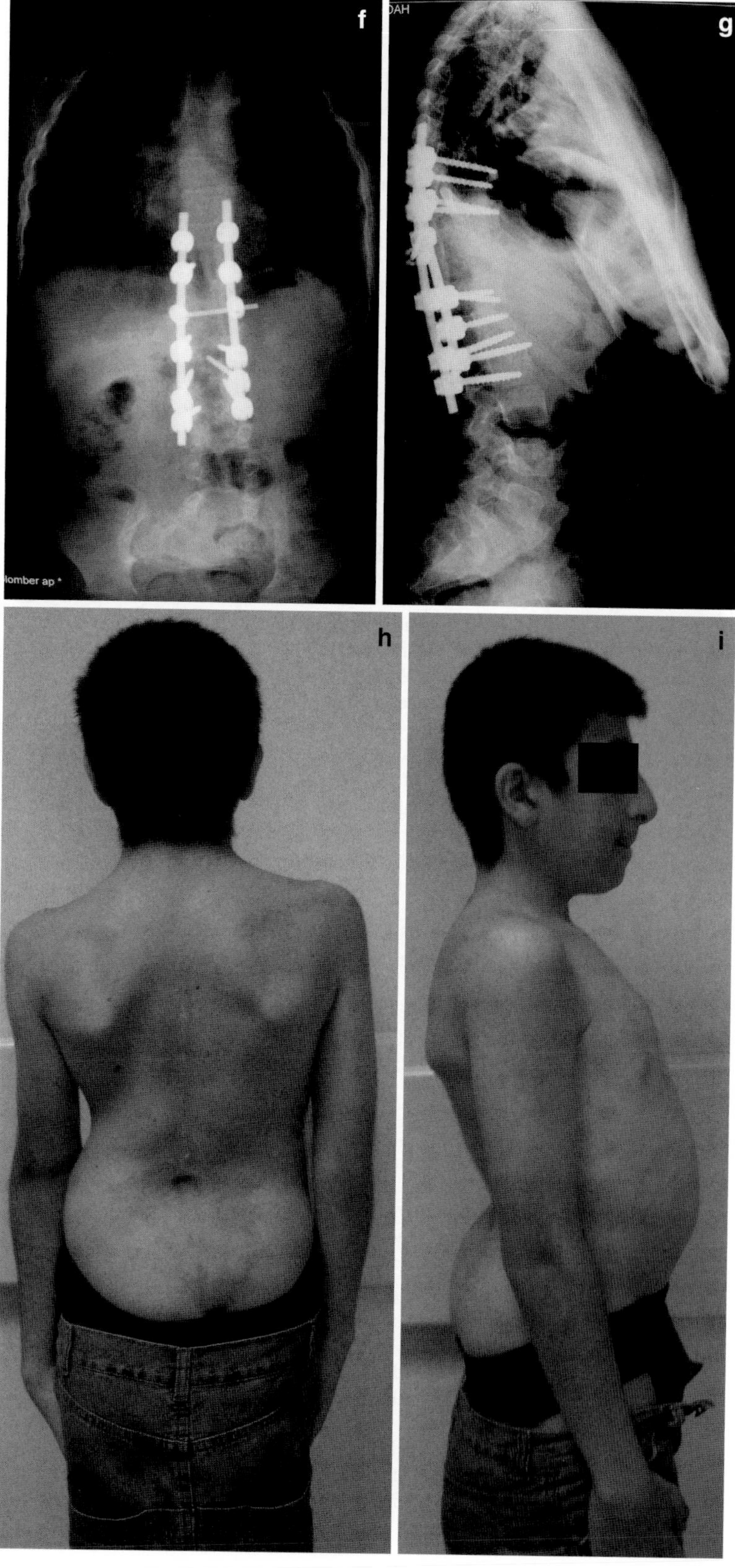

Fig. 18.4 He underwent a neurosurgical intervention previously for diastematomyelia. After vertebral column resection, his deformity was improved, both clinically and radiologically (**f–i**)

References

1. Aberg A, Westbom L, Källén B (2001) Congenital malformations among infants whose mothers had gestational diabetes or preexisting diabetes. Early Hum Dev 61:85–95
2. Akbarnia BA, Marks DS, Boachie-Adjei O et al (2005) Dual growing rod technique for the treatment of progressive early-onset scoliosis: a multicenter study. Spine 30:S46–S57
3. Arlet V, Odent T, Aebi M (2003) Congenital scoliosis. Eur Spine J 12:456–463
4. Aulehla A, Wehrle C, Brand-Saberi B et al (2003) Wnt3a plays a major role in the segmentation clock controlling somitogenesis. Dev Cell 4:395–406
5. Ayvaz M, Alanay A, Yazici M et al (2007) Safety and efficacy of posterior instrumentation for patients with congenital scoliosis and spinal dysraphism. J Pediatr Orthop 27:380–386
6. Basu PS, Elsebaie H, Noordeen MH (2002) Congenital spinal deformity: a comprehensive assessment at presentation. Spine 27:2255–2259
7. Bollini G, Docquier PL, Viehweger E et al (2006) Thoracolumbar hemivertebrae resection by double approach in a single procedure: Long-term follow-up. Spine 31:1745–1757
8. Bradford DS, Heithoff KB, Cohen M (1991) Intraspinal abnormalities and congenital spine deformities: a radiographic and MRI study. J Pediatr Orthop 11:36–41
9. Campbell RM Jr, Hell-Vocke AK (2003) Growth of the thoracic spine in congenital scoliosis after expansion thoracoplasty. J Bone Joint Surg 85A:409–420
10. Drvaric DM, Ruderman RJ, Conrad RW et al (1987) Congenital scoliosis and urinary tract abnormalities: are intravenous pyelograms necessary? J Pediatr Orthop 7:441–443
11. Elsebaie HB, Yazici M, Thompson GH et al (2007) Safety and efficacy of growing rod technique for pediatric congenital spinal deformities. 1st International Congress of Early Onset Scoliosis and Growing Spine, 2–4 November, Madrid, Spain
12. Facanha-Filho FA, Winter RB, Lonstein JE et al (2001) Measurement accuracy in congenital scoliosis. J Bone Joint Surg 83A:42–45
13. Farley FA, Loder RT, Nolan BT et al (2001) Mouse model for thoracic congenital scoliosis. J Pediatr Orthop 21:537–540
14. Ghebranious N, Raggio CL, Blank RD et al (2007) Lack of evidence of WNT3A as a candidate gene for congenital vertebral malformations. Scoliosis 23:2–13
15. Giampietro PF, Raggio CL, Blank RD (1999) Synteny-defined candidate genes for congenital and idiopathic scoliosis. Am J Med Genet 83:164–177
16. Giampietro PF, Blank RD, Raggio CL et al (2003) Congenital and idiopathic scoliosis: clinical and genetic aspects. Clin Med Res 1:125–136
17. Giampietro PF, Raggio CL, Reynolds CE et al (2005) An analysis of PAX1 in the development of vertebral malformations. Clin Genet 68:448–453
18. Giampietro PH, Raggio CL, Reynolds C et al (2006) DLL3 as a candidate gene for vertebral malformations. Am J Med Genet 140A:2447–2453
19. Hall JE, Herndon WA, Levine CR (1981) Surgical treatment of congenital scoliosis with or without Harrington instrumentation. J Bone Joint Surg 63A:608–619
20. Hedequist DJ, Emans JB (2003) The correlation of preoperative three-dimensional computed tomography reconstructions with operative findings in congenital scoliosis. Spine 28:2531–2534
21. Hedequist D, Emans J (2004) Congenital scoliosis. J Am Acad Orthop Surg 12:266–275
22. Ingalls TH, Curley FJ (1957) Principles governing the genesis of congenital malformations induced in mice by hypoxia. N Engl J Med 257:1121–1127
23. Jaskwhich D, Ali RM, Patel TC, Green DW (2000) Congenital scoliosis. Curr Opin Pediatr 12:61–66
24. Kaplan KM, Spivak JM, Bendo JA (2005) Embryology of the spine and associated congenital abnormalities. Spine J 5: 564–576
25. Kose N, Campbell RM (2004) Congenital scoliosis. Med Sci Monit 10:104–110
26. Loder RT, Urquhart A, Steen H et al (1995) Variability in Cobb angle measurements in children with congenital scoliosis. J Bone Joint Surg 77B:768–770
27. Loder RT, Hernandez MJ, Lerner AL et al (2000) The induction of congenital spinal deformities in mice by maternal carbon monoxide exposure. J Pediatr Orthop 20:662–666
28. MacEwen GD, Winter RB, Hardy JH et al (2005) Evaluation of kidney anomalies in congenital scoliosis.1972. Clin Orthop Relat Res 434:4–7
29. Maisenbacher MK, Han JS, O'Brien ML et al (2005) Molecular analysis of congenital scoliosis: a candidate gene approach. Hum Genet 116:416–419
30. McMaster MJ, Ohtsuka K (1982) The natural history of congenital scoliosis. A study of two hundred and fifty-one patients. J Bone Joint Surg 64A:1128–1147
31. McMaster MJ (1984) Occult intraspinal anomalies and congenital scoliosis. J Bone Joint Surg 66A:588–601
32. Nakajima A, Kawakami N, Imagama S et al (2007) Three-dimensional analysis of formation failure in congenital scoliosis. Spine 32:562–567
33. Newton PO, Hahn GW, Fricka KB et al (2002) Utility of three-dimensional and multiplanar reformatted computed tomography for evaluation of pediatric congenital spine abnormalities. Spine 27:844–850
34. Prahinski JR, Polly DW Jr, McHale KA et al (2000) Occult intraspinal anomalies in congenital scoliosis. J Pediatr Orthop 20:59–63
35. Reckles LN, Peterson HA, Weidman WH et al (1975) The association of scoliosis and congenital heart defects. J Bone Joint Surg 57A:449–455
36. Rivard CH (1986) Effects of hypoxia on the embryogenesis of congenital vertebral malformations in the mouse. Clin Orthop Relat Res 208:126–130
37. Schwetz BA, Smith FA, Leong BK et al (1979) Teratogenic potential of inhaled carbon monoxide in mice and rabbits. Teratology 19:385–392
38. Shawen SB, Belmont PJ Jr, Kuklo TR et al (2002) Hemimetameric segmental shift: A case series and review. Spine 27:E539–E544
39. Shimode M, Kojima T, Sowa K (2002) Spinal wedge osteotomy by a single posterior approach for correction of severe and rigid kyphosis or kyphoscoliosis. Spine 27: 2260–2267

40. Suk SI, Kim JH, Kim WJ et al (2002) Posterior vertebral column resection for severe spinal deformities. Spine 27:2374–2382
41. Thompson GH, Akbarnia BA, Kostial P et al (2005) Comparison of single and dual growing rod techniques followed through definitive surgery: a preliminary study. Spine 30:2039–2044
42. Uzumcugil A, Cil A, Yazici M et al (2004) Convex growth arrest in the treatment of congenital spinal deformities, revisited. J Pediatr Orthop 24:658–666
43. Wide K, Winbladh B, Källén B (2004) Major malformations in infants exposed to antiepileptic drugs in utero, with emphasis on carbamazepine and valproic acid: a nation-wide, population-based register study. Acta Paediatr 93:174–176
44. Winter RB, Moe JH, Eilers VE (1968) Congenital scoliosis a study of 234 patients treated and untreated. J Bone Joint Surg 50A:1–15
45. Winter RB, Lonstein JE, Denis F et al (1988) Convex growth arrest for progressive congenital scoliosis due to hemivertebrae. J Pediatr Orthop 8:633–638

19 Treatment of Spinal Deformity in Cerebral Palsy

Suken A. Shah

Key Points

- Scoliosis in cerebral palsy is related to the severity of neurological involvement; dependent sitters with poor head control have a very high rate of scoliosis. Curve progression leads to subsequent deformity and trunk imbalance with associated loss of function.
- The goals of surgery for the higher functioning patient are to provide a more normal spinal balance and alter the progression of disease, and to preserve function with respect to ambulatory potential; in the wheelchair-bound patient, the aim is to maintain independence in sitting and facilitate care.
- Although it is generally accepted that in the cerebral palsy patient with scoliosis bracing likely will not alter the progression of the curve, it is reasonable to utilize an orthosis to improve muscle balance and sitting while closely following the curve. Improved sitting may correlate with attentiveness in class, easing of care, improvement of self-image, and decrease in the rate of decubitus ulcers.
- In general, surgical intervention is considered for curve magnitude greater than 40 or 50° and significant deterioration in function.
- Anterior fusion for the so-called "crankshaft phenomenon" is not necessary, even for young patients, when rigid, segmental instrumentation, such as a unit rod, is used posteriorly.
- The unit rod is the preferred method of instrumentation and offers a powerful mechanism of correction in both the coronal and sagittal plane. Iliac screws provide rigid fixation to the pelvis, and pedicle screws allow powerful correction of deformities in multiple planes.
- The risk of complications, both perioperatively and postoperatively, is substantial but manageable with a careful preoperative workup, multidisciplinary care, and attention to detail.
- Caregiver satisfaction is high after this procedure and affords a good long-term outcome with a positive impact on the patient's sitting ability, physical appearance, comfort, and ease of care

19.1 Introduction

A scoliotic deformity arising in the clinical setting of muscle imbalance secondary to an underlying neuropathic or myopathic disease can be classified as neuromuscular scoliosis. The associated muscle imbalance in neuromuscular disease causes abnormal biomechanical loading of the spine. According to the Heuter–Volkmann principle, abnormal biomechanical loading secondary to this muscle imbalance and spinal collapse results in asymmetric vertebral body growth in a skeletally immature individual. Progressive deformity is believed to be the result of both progressive muscle imbalance and anatomic deformity.

S. A. Shah
Department of Orthopaedics, Alfred I. duPont Hospital for Children, 1600 Rockland Rd., PO Box 269, Wilmington, DE 19899, USA
e-mail: sshah@nemours.org

B. A. Akbarnia et al. (eds.), *The Growing Spine*,
DOI: 10.1007/978-3-540-85207-0_19, © Springer-Verlag Berlin Heidelberg 2011

Table 19.1 Neuromuscular disorders associated with scoliosis and their classification

Neuropathic
Upper motor neuron
Cerebral palsy
Spinocerebellar degeneration
Friedreich ataxia
Charcot–Marie–Tooth
Roussy–Levy
Syringomyelia
Spinal cord tumor
Spinal cord trauma
Lower motor neuron
Poliomyelitis and other viral myelitides
Traumatic
Spinal muscle atrophy
Werdnig–Hoffmann
Kugelberg–Welander
Dysautonomia
Myopathic
Arthrogryposis
Muscular dystrophy
Duchenne
Limb-girdle
Facioscapulohumeral
Fiber-type disproportion
Congenital hypotonia
Myotonia dystrophica

Of the neuropathic and myopathic disorders associated with scoliosis (Table 19.1), cerebral palsy is the most prevalent. This chapter will mainly focus on the operative treatment of scoliosis due to cerebral palsy. Cerebral palsy (CP) has an estimated incidence of 7 per 100,000 live births, with an incidence of scoliosis estimated between 6.5 and 38% [2, 24, 30]. More severe forms of CP such as spastic quadriplegia are associated with a higher incidence; Madigan and Wallace [24] found a 64% incidence in the institutionalized CP population. Lonstein and Akbarnia [22] classified scoliotic curves as a result of CP into two groups: Group I curves, which are double curves with thoracic and lumbar components (S-curves), and Group II curves with more lumbar or thoracolumbar curves that extended into the sacrum with associated pelvic obliquity (C-curves.) (Fig. 19.1).

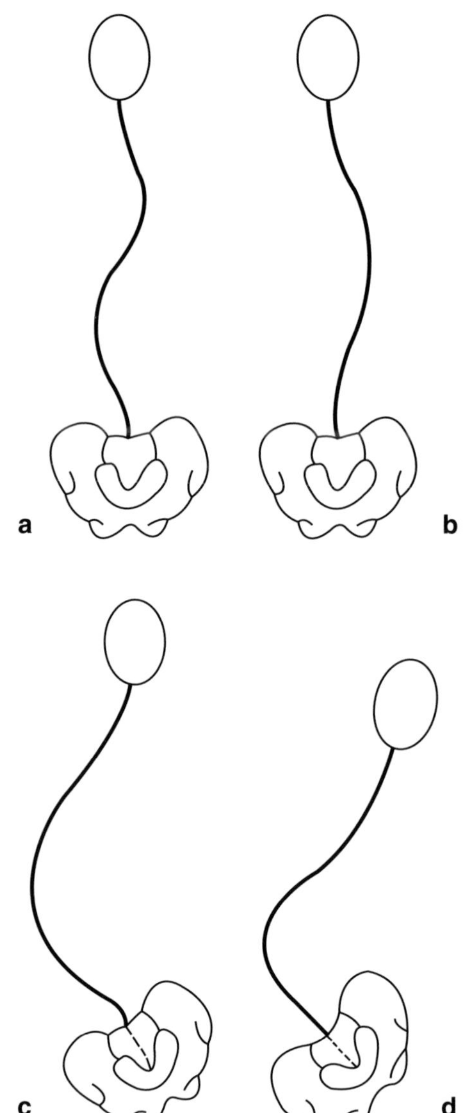

Fig. 19.1. Curve patterns in cerebral palsy scoliosis. Group I curves are double curves with little pelvic obliquity that may be balanced (**a**) or unbalanced (**b**). Group II curves (**c** and **d**) are large lumbar or thoracolumbar curves with marked pelvic obliquity. Adapted from Lonstein and Akbarnia [22], p 800

19.2 Clinical Presentation and Evaluation

Neuromuscular scoliotic curves generally develop at a younger age than idiopathic scoliosis, and the flexible, postural curve tends to develop into a torsional structural deformity with growth and finally, a stiff curve of considerable magnitude before growth is complete. CP has a broad spectrum of severity; in general, there is a proportional relation between the severity of involvement of CP and curve severity. Dependent sitters with poor head control have a rate of scoliosis approaching 90%. While the rate of curve progression is highly variable, the average progression cited in one report is 0.8° a year in curves less than 50° and 1.4° a year in curves more than 50° [39], and during periods of rapid growth, much more severe progression can occur. Curve progression leads to subsequent deformity and trunk imbalance with associated loss of function. CP scoliosis may also be associated with significant pain due to sitting difficulties, especially with pelvic obliquity and pressure sores; however, many of these patients are unable to articulate their symptoms.

Initial evaluation should consist of clinical monitoring by physical examination and when a curve is identified, standing position (when possible) 36-inch posterior-anterior (PA) and lateral radiographs of the spine should be obtained. Radiographs in sitting position may be obtained if the patient is unable to stand; it may be necessary to support the head and trunk in severely affected children with poor truncal control. At our center, we use a standardized sitting frame with lateral support straps to obtain films in the sitting position with minimal external support. Supine bending films can be obtained to assess curve flexibility. Curve magnitude, spinal balance (sagittal and coronal), pelvic obliquity, curve flexibility, and curve progression need to be assessed. (Fig. 19.2a, b) A magnetic resonance imaging (MRI) should be obtained if there is any suspicion of intraspinal pathology, such as very rapid progression at a young age or a change in neurologic status, which could be harbingers of a tethered cord. The patient with established scoliosis due to CP requires at least yearly follow-up examination to assess curve progression, but with severe curves or during periods of rapid growth, biannual follow-up is desirable.

In the global planning of disease management, several factors need to be considered. Of paramount importance are the preservation of function, facilitation of daily care, and the alleviation of pain. Given the universal progressive nature of neuromuscular scoliosis, early diagnosis of deformity is essential. Curve progression increases the magnitude of deforming forces on the apex of the curve and may lead to progressive muscle imbalance. As the patient's trunk falls forward and there is progressive pelvic obliquity, ambulatory function is compromised. In the wheelchair-bound patient, progressive deformity may compromise sitting.

The role of bracing in CP scoliosis is questionable. It is generally accepted that bracing is ineffective, in significantly altering the ultimate disease progression in the patient with spastic quadriplegia [27], but some physicians will still recommend a rigid TLSO for a patient with neuromuscular scoliosis. Although it may not alter the final disposition, a soft (polypropylene foam) TLSO can provide seating support and augment function.

Operative intervention in CP scoliosis is controversial. Given the wide spectrum of disease presentation and progression as well as the concomitant variability in functional status of the patient, the decision to proceed with operative correction and stabilization is based, in large part, on patient-specific factors. For the higher functioning patient, operative intervention aims

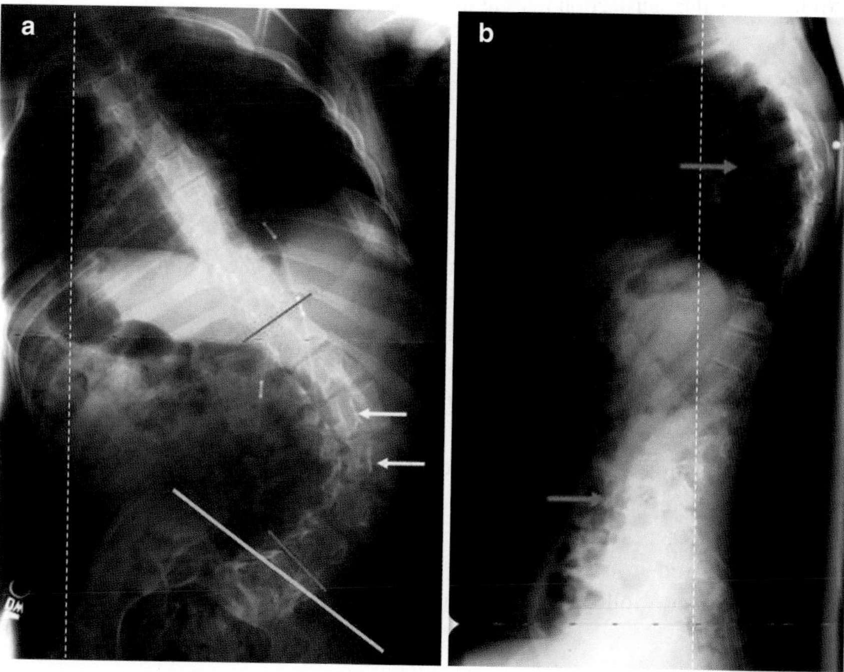

Fig. 19.2. When evaluating a patient with CP scoliosis, there are other radiographic parameters in addition to the Cobb angle (*red lines*). Note the severe apical rotation (*white arrows*), pelvic obliquity (*yellow line*) (**a**), hyperkyphosis, and hyperlordosis (*red arrows*) (**b**) and coronal and sagittal imbalance (*dashed lines*)

to provide a more normal spinal balance and alter the progression of disease with the goal to preserve function with respect to ambulatory potential. Similarly, in the wheelchair-bound patient the aim is to maintain independence in sitting and facilitate care.

In the highly functioning child with CP, it is intuitively desirable to intervene to halt the progression of deformity and associated loss of function, and the parents or caretakers can make an informed decision weighing the risks and benefits for their child. Problematically, as observed by Madigan and Wallace [24] the severity of scoliosis is directly proportional to severity of involvement of CP. In the spastic quadriplegic, nonambulatory patient, concern has been raised regarding the risk of an extensive surgical procedure in a medically compromised patient is warranted. Comstock et al. [11] assessed both patient and caregiver satisfaction in a cohort of 100 patients with total-body-involvement spastic CP that underwent spinal fusion. The satisfaction of both caregivers and patients was assessed via interview responses to standardized questions, and physical examination was used to assess functional status. Eighty five percent of the parents interviewed indicated that they were satisfied with the results and would repeat the surgery again. There was an impression by caregivers that the patients had an improved self-image, and patients that were able to respond to questions confirmed this. Both parents and caregivers felt that the surgery had a positive impact on the patient's sitting ability, physical appearance, comfort, and ease of care. Bulman et al. [10] and Sussman et al. [36] found similar satisfaction rates in their studies.

19.3 Nonoperative Care

Nonoperative management of patients with neuromuscular spinal deformities should be directed at maximizing sitting ability and postural control to facilitate motor and cognitive function. Initial close observation of curves that are 20° or less is reasonable; if progression occurs initial intervention with a brace may be an option. Bracing is felt to be largely ineffective in stopping curve progression, but may slow the rate. Miller et al. found no impact on scoliosis curve, shape, or rate of progression in spastic quadriplegic patients that were braced 23 h per day over a mean period of 67 months compared to a similar cohort that were not braced and were followed to spinal fusion [27]. Terjesen et al. [38] retrospectively examined a cohort of 86 patients with spastic quadriplegic CP and found a mean rate of progression per year of 4.2° with a custom-molded polypropylene thoracolumbosacral orthosis. Interestingly, 25% of the patients had no progression or progression of less than 1° per year. The degree of curve correction in the orthosis appeared to correlate with nonprogression of the curve. Of note, Terjesen's study had a mean initial Cobb angle of 68.4°.

The bracing studies to date on both neuromuscular and idiopathic scoliosis have had a wide range of inclusion criteria, undefined endpoints, methods of assessment, and follow-up periods [29]. While it is generally accepted that in the CP patient with scoliosis bracing likely will not alter the progression of the curve, it is reasonable to utilize an orthosis to improve muscle balance and sitting while closely following the curve. Improved sitting may correlate with attentiveness in class, ease of care, improved self-image, and decreased rate of decubitus ulcers.

Another option for patients with flexible curves in need of seating support is the adjustment of offset lateral chest supports and modular seating systems on the wheelchair. This three-point control of the coronal deformity will prop up the child and address sitting balance; the wheelchair should be the primary seating device. Therapeutic stretching, electrical stimulation, or botulinum toxin are lacking scientific validity and should have no role in the management of deformity.

19.4 Operative Care

As discussed, the decision to proceed with operative intervention is complex and each patient has unique factors to be considered. In general, surgical intervention is considered for curve magnitude greater than 40 or 50° and significant deterioration in function [11, 23, 28]. There is sufficient evidence that these curves will progress, even if the child has completed his growth. The goals of surgery are to correct the spinal deformity, reestablish coronal and sagittal balance, restore pelvic obliquity and achieve a solid fusion mass.

Managing growth in young children with neuromuscular deformities is challenging, as the scoliosis can be quite progressive during the prepubescent growth spurt. For curves 60–90°, surgery is considered when the deformity becomes stiff by physical examination, and this combination of increasing magnitude and stiffness is an indication for surgery, even if substantial growth remains. Growth assessment in these children can be difficult, as many children with CP and other upper motor neuron diseases can have delayed onset of puberty and delayed bone age. In addition to serial height and weight measurements in the clinic, assessment of the triradiate cartilage status and digital skeletal age has been useful in our CP clinic to assess remaining growth. If the spine displays continued flexibility on physical examination during growth, surgery can be delayed until 90°, and can still be performed with a posterior-only procedure. There is limited experience with growing rods in children with spastic quadriplegic CP, and the literature does not currently support their use. There may be a role for growing rod instrumentation in children with hypotonic CP or syndromic scoliosis, however.

For stiff curves, or those 90° or greater anterior release of the apical levels of the curve is indicated, since it is necessary to gain flexibility to obtain correction. Anterior surgery increases the complication rate and morbidity of spinal surgery in these patients, and it is unclear whether to stage the anterior and posterior procedures separately (1 week apart) or to do both the procedures on the same day. Evidence exists to support both the strategies, and it is our practice to stage surgeries for patients with severe involvement and multiple medical comorbidites and problems. For relatively healthy patients, we usually perform both stages on the same day, provided that the time under anesthesia or blood loss is not too substantial after the anterior release. Anterior fusion for the so-called "crankshaft phenomenon" is not necessary, even for young patients, when rigid, segmental instrumentation such as a unit rod is used posteriorly [13, 15, 42].

Sagittal plane deformities such as pathological hyperkyphosis or lordosis may develop in patients with neuromuscular disorders, either with or without scoliosis. Flexible, postural deformities may be addressed in younger patients with tight hamstrings by lengthening the posterior thigh musculature and address the associated posterior pelvic tilt in these patients, or by appropriate modifications to the wheelchair or shoulder harness, but in older children, these adaptations do not work as well. Patients who have undergone a previous dorsal rhizotomy can be at particular risk for developing a pathologic hyperlordosis. Fusion and segmental spinal instrumentation is indicated for collapsing deformities and painful sitting when no other alternatives exist [12].

Historically, fusions with Harrington instrumentation had an unacceptably high rate of pseudarthrosis occurring in 18–27% of the cases [7, 11, 22, 34]. The advent of Luque rod segmental instrumentation yielded improved results over the Harrington system [6, 9, 17, 35, 36] and obviated the need for postoperative casting. Comstock et al. [11] found a mean correction of 51% in a posterior-only instrumentation cohort and in an anterior–posterior cohort 57%. Multiple authors have noted progression of pelvic obliquity if the fusion is not extended to the pelvis [11, 31, 36]. An increased incidence of proximal curve progression, especially proximal junctional kyphosis has been observed if the proximal level of instrumentation does not extend to at least T2 [9], since most of these children lack sufficient head control.

The Galveston technique to extend the fusion across the pelvis by placing each Luque rod between the pelvic tables [1] has demonstrated acceptable fusion rates across the L5-S1 segment, and appears to provide good control of pelvic obliquity. While the impaction of two Luque rods into the pelvis with associated segmental fusion via sublaminar wires provides a strong construct in the sagittal plane, there exists a moment arm of rotation about the two rods allowing for rod translation with respect to one another, loss of torsional control and subsequent progression of pelvic obliquity, pseudarthrosis, and implant failure [4]. The use of Luque rods smaller than ¼ inch diameter may increase the incidence of implant failure [9, 18, 31], but the intraoperative bending of ¼ inch diameter steel rods to the optimal geometry for pelvic implantation presents a technical challenge. Rigid fixation is essential for surgical success. Sanders et al. [31] found in their retrospective study of Luque rod instrumentation that a postoperative curve greater than 35°, preoperative curves greater than 60°, crankshaft deformity, and not fusing to the pelvis were the factors associated with postoperative curve progression.

Historically, there has been debate regarding when to extend the posterior spinal fusion to the pelvis. Pelvic obliquity has been noted to progress in neuromuscular scoliosis if the pelvis is not fused [8, 14, 31], and traditionally many authors have recommended fusion to the pelvis in nonambulatory patients. In the ambulatory patient with pelvic obliquity, fusion to the pelvis has been traditionally avoided due to the belief that it will adversely affect ambulatory function [3, 26]. A recent retrospective study by Tsirikos et al. [41] demonstrated preserved ambulatory function in ambulatory patients with CP that were fused with unit rod instrumentation. They hypothesized that the conventional assumption that ambulatory potential is limited by fusion to the pelvis arose from early attempts at pelvic fixation with Harrington rods that removed lumbar lordosis, and possibly from the confounding variable of prolonged immobilization and bed rest in earlier segmental systems that did not provide sufficient rigidity for immediate postoperative mobilization and ambulation therapy.

The unit rod developed by Bell et al. [4] addresses some of the potential limitations of dual Luque rod instrumentation. The implant design of a proximally connected, precountored rod provides for better rotational control, as the degree of rotational freedom between two independent Luque rods is eliminated. Initial mean curve corrections with the unit rod were reported to be 54.6% [4], with a mean loss of correction of 6.5% at 2-year-follow-up; Westerlund et al. [42], more recently, found a mean scoliosis correction with the unit rod of 66 and 75% correction of pelvic obliquity. In total, 27 of the 28 patients in Westerlund's cohort were Risser 2 or less, with preoperative Cobb angles ranging from 45 to 94°. At an average follow-up of 58 months there was a mean loss of correction of 3°. Dias et al. [13] noted similar results in a large group of patients with CP scoliosis managed with unit rod instrumentation and curve correction approaching 80%.

Iliac screws perform better in pullout strength than smooth Galveston rods for pelvic fixation, and the use of segmental pedicle screw constructs have shown substantial correction and fusion rates, while accomplishing the goals of leveling pelvic obliquity and addressing seating problems. These newer, modular systems can navigate some of the substantial challenges in these patients, such as abnormal pelvic anatomy, osteoporotic bone, and hyperlordosis, and avoid some of the risk in early instrumentation failure, but they come at a substantial monetary expense.

19.5 Preoperative and Perioperative Concerns

The individual with CP scoliosis is medically complex and may have significant preoperative risk. For a family that is intent on providing maximal medical treatment for a severely involved child, with the intent of caring for the child at home and keeping the child involved in school and other outside, community activities, surgical treatment of the spinal deformity will accomplish this goal with the greatest ease and comfort. The risk and complications of a procedure of this magnitude are directly related to the severity of neurological impairment. Lipton et al. [21] have reported that a child who is not fed orally, is severely mentally retarded, cannot speak, has seizures and who cannot sit independently, by far, has the highest rate of complications. Medical management of seizures, respiratory problems, gastroesphageal reflux and motility issues, and nutrition should be addressed before surgery. Standard preoperative laboratory work including hematology, metabolic profile, urinalysis, and a coagulation panel should be obtained as well as an assessment of nutrition, but we have found the laboratory values are not always a reliable assessment of the preoperative status of the child. Blood loss can be substantial, and a type and crossmatch of 1–1.5 times the patient's blood volume should be available prior to the start of surgery [12]. Coagulation factor replacement and core body temperature maintenance is also important if substantial bleeding is encountered, since coagulopathy may develop. The use of antifibrinolytics such as aprotinin or Amicar can be an important adjunct in decreasing blood loss during surgery.

Many parents and caretakers have noted that they were not prepared for the complexity of the patient's postoperative course [11]. Preoperative counseling of the family and caretakers should stress the potential of a prolonged intensive care unit stay, as well as the significant possibility of postoperative complications, which can prolong the hospitalization.

Intraoperatively, the surgeon must maintain constant communication with the anesthesia staff. Intraoperative hypotension is frequently secondary to inadequate volume replacement. Correction of a kyphotic deformity can impede venous return to the heart with resultant hypotension [12]. In the event of hypotension during curve correction, an attempt to release pressure on the spine should be made and an increase in the rate of intravenous fluid and/or blood replacement should be performed; after the blood pressure has been stable for 5–10 min it may be safe to proceed with a gradual correction to allow time for the soft tissues to stretch.

Spinal cord monitoring with intraoperative transcranial motor-evoked potentials and somatosensory-evoked potentials should be used. While it is common for the severely involved child to have weak or absent signals at baseline, and thus intraoperative neurophysiologic monitoring would be unreliable, those children that can stand or ambulate or have some purposeful lower extremity movement can and should be monitored intraoperatively to protect function.

19.6 Surgical Technique

After intubation, appropriate monitoring leads and establishment of large bore IV access, arterial and central venous catheterization, the patient, should be placed prone on a radiolucent table or four post frame. Care should be taken to ensure that all bony prominences are well padded to avoid skin breakdown, especially in thin patients and that the abdomen hangs free. The hips can be allowed to gently flex with knee and thigh support to passively correct lumbar hyperlordosis. Intraoperative traction has been described to correct pelvic obliquity, but this is rarely necessary.

A standard posterior exposure of the spine from T1 to the sacrum is done, subperiosteally, out to the transverse process with the use of Cobb elevators and electrocautery for hemostasis. An aggressive posterior release with facetectomies and ligamentum flavum resection is important in creating flexibility in the rigid apical portion of the curve and in all but the largest, stiff curves makes a posterior-only approach sufficient for correction of the scoliosis.

At the inferior margin of the incision, the outer wing of the ilium is subperiosteally exposed down to the sciatic notch. The right and left drill guides for the unit rod are placed in the respective sciatic notch; care should be taken to ensure that the drill guide is as inferior as possible along the posterior superior iliac spine. The handles of the drill guide are the reference points for alignment: the lateral handle should be parallel with the pelvis and the axial handle parallel with the sacrum. The drill hole is next made utilizing the guide using a 3/8" drill to the predetermined depth; the hole is palpated with a ball-tipped feeler to confirm that there has been no breach of the cortical bone of the inner or outer pelvic table. Gelfoam should be inserted into the drill holes and sponges packed out over the pelvis to maintain hemostasis.

When placing iliac screws in lieu of smooth Galveston pelvic fixation, the starting point is similar – just below the posterior superior iliac spine. A notch is cut out with an osteotome to avoid screw head prominence, and the cancellous bone between the inner and outer table is cannulated with a drill or pedicle gearshift. We have found that successful iliac screw fixation is possible with a mini-access approach to avoid extensive muscle dissection of the paraspinal muscle at the lumbosacral junction and outer table of the pelvis by using intraoperative fluoroscopy. By tilting the image intensifier obliquely in the plane of the iliac wing and cephalad so that it is parallel to the cortical bone of the sciatic notch, the "teardrop" of the ilium can be visualized (Fig. 19.3c). Iliac screw placement in this area ensures excellent fixation in strong cancellous bone, adequate length to extend past the pivot point of the lumbosacral junction, and safe avoidance of the sciatic notch and acetabulum (Fig. 19.4a–c). The iliac screw can then be connected to the longitudinal members of the thoracolumbar construct to level the pelvis (Fig. 19.5a–c).

The spinous process of each level is removed to expose the ligamentum flavum. Care must be taken to preserve the lamina as they are key to the strength of fixation, especially the supralaminar cortex, which even in osteoporotic bone, can be strong. After the removal of the spinous processes and exposure of the sublaminar space the sublaminar wires are passed at each level. A 16-gauge double Luque wire is passed at each level from T2 to L4, and two wires are placed at T1 and L5. The wire is passed from inferior to superior. After passing the wire it is contoured back over the lamina and the ends of the wire are contoured to the edges of the incision; this will maintain the intraspinal portion of the wire against the undersurface of the lamina as the remaining levels are instrumented. While passing the wire care must be taken to avoid levering off the lamina and impinging against the cord; the diameter of the contoured bend should approximate the length of the lamina.

For unit rod fixation, the length of the rod is measured from T1 to the pelvis. Note that the correction of a kyphotic deformity will shorten the spine and the correction of a lordotic deformity will lengthen the spine. This can be confirmed by placing the rod upside down with the top of the rod at T1 and confirming that the corner of the rod is at the level of the pelvic drill holes [12]. Intraoperatively, if the rod is noted to be too long

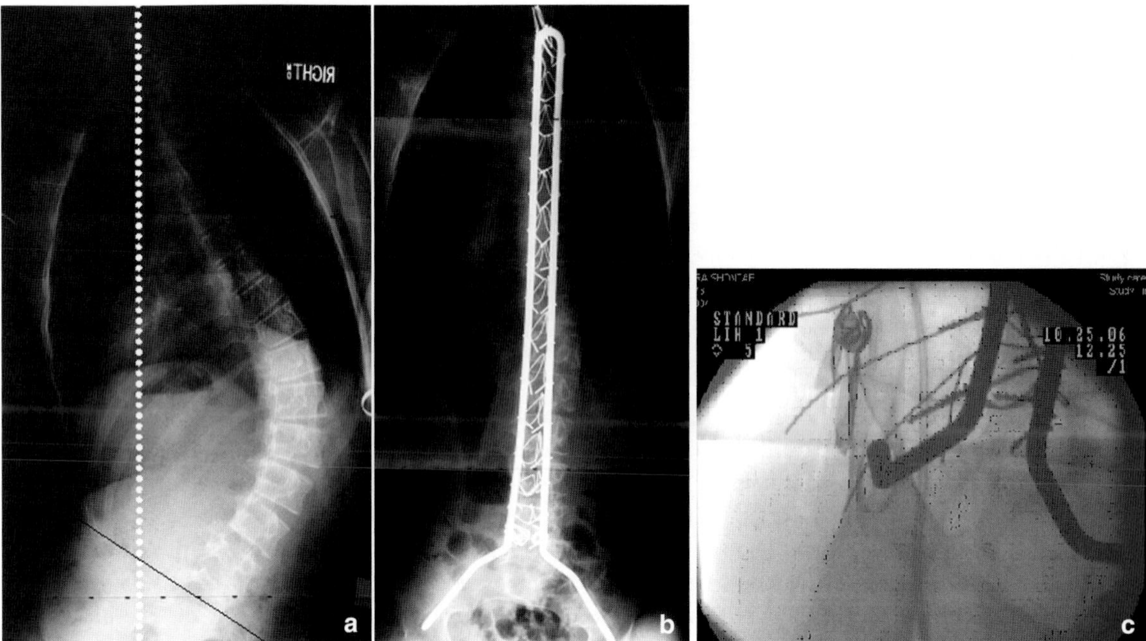

Fig. 19.3 (**a, b**) Preoperative and postoperative PA sitting radiographs of an ambulatory child with cerebral palsy scoliosis after posterior spinal fusion with the unit rod. Note the restoration of truncal balance and pelvic obliquity. (**c**) Intraoperative view of a pelvic limb of the unit rod placed between the inner and outer table of the ilium, in the "teardrop"

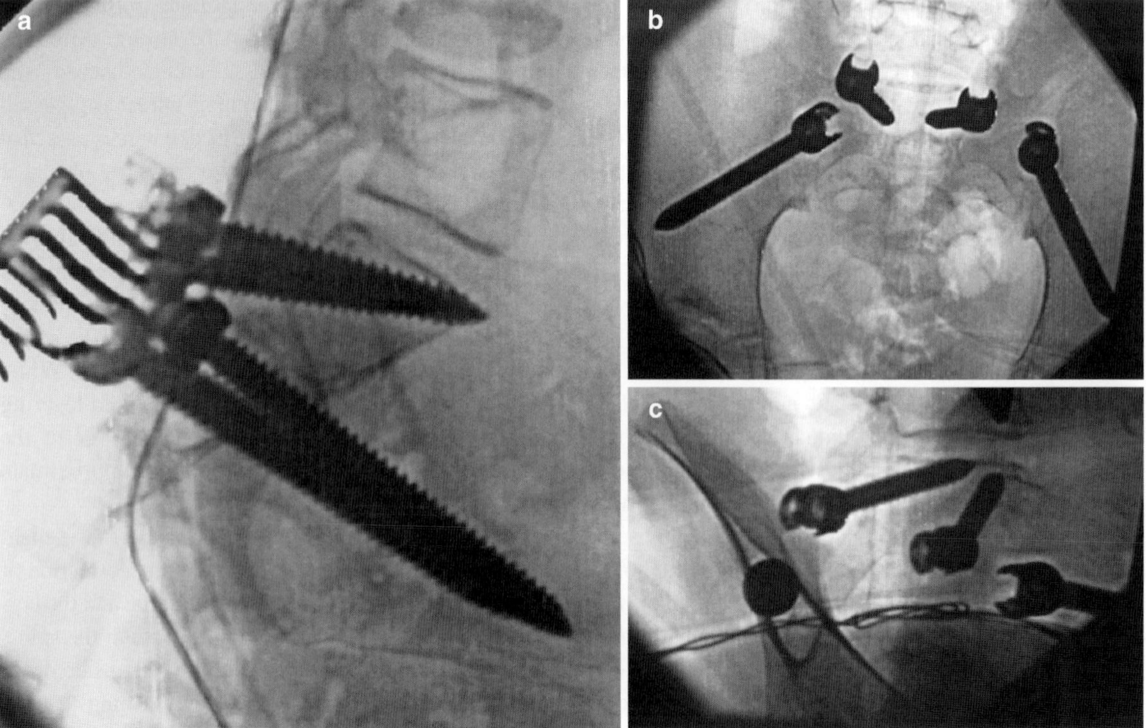

Fig. 19.4 (**a–c**) Lateral, AP, and oblique views showing satisfactory placement of pedicle screws in S1 pedicle and iliac screws

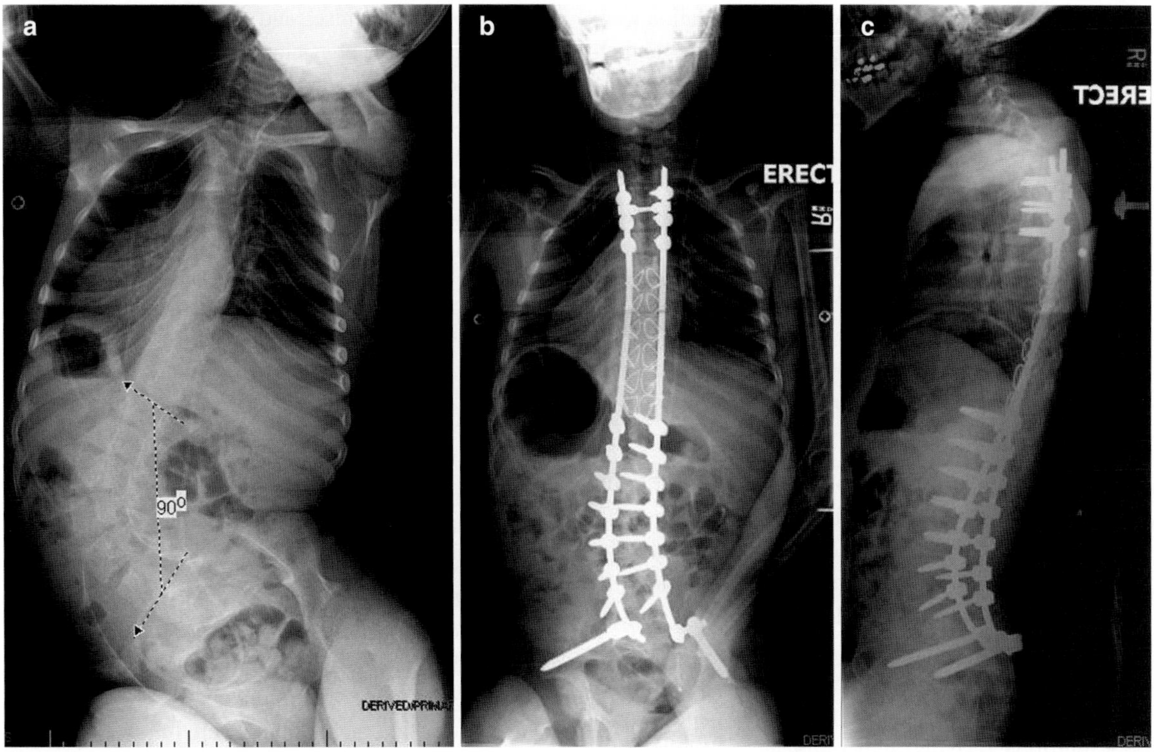

Fig. 19.5 (**a–c**) Radiographs of a 12-year-old male with quadriplegic cerebral palsy and scoliosis with a 90° curve, lumbar hyperlordosis, 30° pelvic obliquity, and seating difficulties. Wide posterior releases were used to make the curve more flexible, and the spine was corrected with modular segmental instrumentation using pedicle screws, sublaminar wires, and iliac screws

(i.e., superior to T1) the limbs at T1 can be secured with cross connectors and the excess rod cut. If the rod is noted to be too short the end may be cut and a piece of another rod joined with rod-to-rod connectors to achieve the necessary length. Both scenarios, however, will weaken the unibody construction of the rod and decrease the ability to generate sufficient cantilever moment.

Facetectomies and decortication are performed and a preliminary grafting of the area under the rod is performed. The pelvic limbs of the rod are crossed and inserted into their respective drill holes. Each limb should be advanced alternatively in 1-cm increments with an impactor. Care must be taken to maintain control of the rod and insure that it does not penetrate either table of the pelvis. In the setting of hyperlordosis, the marked anterior inclination of the pelvis increases the risk of the pelvic limb perforating the inner cortex during insertion. The pelvic ends of the rod need to be directed in a more posterior direction to accommodate this angulation; rod placement is facilitated by manual correction of the lordosis prior to rod insertion. In instances of marked lordosis, the pelvic limbs of the rod may be cut and inserted separately and then attached to the rod with rod-to-rod connectors. (Alternatively, iliac screws may be used with modular connectors.) (See Fig. 19.5).

The spine is manually corrected to the rod and the wires are tightened sequentially. Pushing the rod to the spine can generate substantial force at the lever arm of the pelvic insertion with subsequent fracture, so a few of the lumbar levels should be wired prior to generating substantial cantilever forces. After tightening and retightening the wires, the wires are cut 1-cm long and bent down to the lamina to avoid implant prominence. Copious crushed cancellous allograft is packed and the wound is meticulously closed. A drain is generally not used.

Dabney et al. [12] noted that, in incidences of marked lordotic deformity, better fixation and correction was achieved with pedicle screws in the lordotic segment. A cadaveric biomechanical study has confirmed that the use of L5 pedicle screws significantly increases the lateral and oblique stiffness of the unit rod construct [16]. McCall and Hayes [25] retrospectively examined a cohort of patients with neuromuscular scoliosis in whom those with a stable lumbosacral articulation were instrumented with a “U-rod” (unit rod without the pelvic limbs) with L5 pedicle screw fixation. The L5-S1 interspace mobility was assessed on the basis of L5 tilt; patients with more than 15° of L5 tilt were instrumented with a standard unit rod construct. McCall and Hayes [25] found that in follow-up the patients that were instrumented to L5 with the U-rod had similar results to those fused with the standard unit rod construct.

19.7 Postoperative Care

Postoperatively, the patient should be maintained, intubated, in an intensive care setting for 24–48 h and volume status and urine output closely monitored. The hemoglobin should be maintained over 9 gm/dL to ensure adequate perfusion, and the coagulation parameters and platelet count should be corrected as needed, as these patients are frequently coagulopathic. Prophylactic antibiotics are continued for 24 h. In patients with poor nutritional status, hyperalimentation should be started postoperatively intravenously or via a J-tube. There is no need for immobilization postoperatively, and the patient should be mobilized out of bed and into a wheelchair as soon as medically appropriate. The child’s personal wheelchair should be readjusted to accommodate his new trunk proportions and pelvic alignment. Children can return to school in 3–4 weeks, when sitting tolerance is attained, and no postoperative restrictions or orthoses are employed.

19.8 Complications

As previously discussed, a patient undergoing spinal fusion for neuromuscular scoliosis frequently has significant associated medical comorbidities, and postoperative complications are prevalent and should be anticipated. The incidence of postoperative complication has been noted to range from 18 to 68% [5, 6, 9, 11]. Curves 70° or greater, severity of neurologic involvement, and severity of recent history of medical problems have been shown to increase the risk of postoperative complications [21]. Respiratory complications are frequent, namely atelectasis, or more severe problems requiring prolonged ventilatory support. Postoperative ileus, pancreatitis, superior mesenteric artery syndrome, pulmonary compromise, and cholelithiasis can occur [19, 20, 32] and the physician must be vigilant in evaluating any clinical abnormalities. Postoperative wound infections are of particular concern [33]. Infection rates have been reported from 2 to 15% [13, 17, 37]. Most deep infections in the early postoperative period respond well to drainage and irrigation with delayed wound closure over drains or a vacuum-assisted device with intravenous antibiotic therapy and retention of the instrumentation.

19.9 Outcomes

Correction of neuromuscular scoliosis with the unit rod is typically 75–80% with leveling of the pelvis and excellent sagittal alignment. With proper surgical technique and the rigidity of the instrumentation, fusion rates are superior, and pseudarthrosis can be avoided. The parent and caregiver satisfaction is very high for this procedure, and over 85% of the caregivers noted benefits beyond sitting and facilitation of care for the child postoperatively [11, 13]. In a group of children that included even the most severely involved, there was a predicted 70% survival rate at 11 years following surgery [40].

In summary, scoliosis is common in this group of children with neuromuscular disorders. The majority of these children have progressive spinal deformities that interfere with sitting and other functions and will require surgical stabilization to address these problems and facilitate care. The unit rod is the preferred method of instrumentation and offers a powerful mechanism of correction in both the coronal and sagittal plane. The risk of complications both perioperatively and postoperatively is substantial, but manageable. Caregiver satisfaction is high after this procedure and affords a good long-term outcome.

References

1. Allen BL Jr, Ferguson RL (1982) The Galveston technique for L rod instrumentation of the scoliotic spine. Spine 7:276–284
2. Balmer GA, MacEwen GD (1970) The incidence and treatment of scoliosis in cerebral palsy. J Bone Joint Surg Br 52:134–137
3. Banta JV, Drummond DS, Ferguson RL (1999) The treatment of neuromuscular scoliosis. Instr Course Lect 48: 551–562
4. Bell DF, Moseley CF, Koreska J (1989) Unit rod segmental spinal instrumentation in the management of patients with

progressive neuromuscular spinal deformity. Spine 14: 1301–1307
5. Benson ER, Thomson JD, Smith BG et al (1998) Results and morbidity in a consecutive series of patients undergoing spinal fusion for neuromuscular scoliosis. Spine 23:2308–2317; discussion 18
6. Boachie-Adjei O, Lonstein JE, Winter RB et al (1989) Management of neuromuscular spinal deformities with Luque segmental instrumentation. J Bone Joint Surg Am 71:5 48–562
7. Bonnett C, Brown JC, Grow T (1976) Thoracolumbar scoliosis in cerebral palsy. Results of surgical treatment. J Bone Joint Surg Am 58:328–336
8. Bradford D (1987) Neuromuscular spinal deformity. In: Bradford D, Lonstein J, Ogilvie J et al (eds) Moe's textbook of scoliosis and other spinal deformitites. WB Saunders, Philadelphiapp 271–305
9. Broom MJ, Banta JV, Renshaw TS (1989) Spinal fusion augmented by Luque-rod segmental instrumentation for neuromuscular scoliosis. J Bone Joint Surg Am 71:32–44
10. Bulman WA, Dormans JP, Ecker ML et al (1996) Posterior spinal fusion for scoliosis in patients with cerebral palsy: a comparison of Luque rod and unit rod instrumentation. J Pediatr Orthop 16:314–323
11. Comstock CP, Leach J, Wenger DR (1998) Scoliosis in total-body-involvement cerebral palsy. Analysis of surgical treatment and patient and caregiver satisfaction. Spine 23: 1412–1424; discussion 24–5
12. Dabney KW, Miller F, Lipton GE et al (2004) Correction of sagittal plane spinal deformities with unit rod instrumentation in children with cerebral palsy. J Bone Joint Surg Am 86-A(Suppl 1):156–168
13. Dias RC, Miller F, Dabney K et al (1996) Surgical correction of spinal deformity using a unit rod in children with cerebral palsy. J Pediatr Orthop 16:734–740
14. Dias RC, Miller F, Dabney K et al (1997) Revision spine surgery in children with cerebral palsy. J Spinal Disord 10:132–144
15. Dubousset J, Herring JA, Shufflebarger H (1989) The crankshaft phenomenon. J Pediatr Orthop 9:541–550
16. Erickson MA, Oliver T, Baldini T et al (2004) Biomechanical assessment of conventional unit rod fixation versus a unit rod pedicle screw construct: a human cadaver study. Spine 29:1314–1319
17. Gersoff WK, Renshaw TS (1988) The treatment of scoliosis in cerebral palsy by posterior spinal fusion with Luque-rod segmental instrumentation. J Bone Joint Surg Am 70:41–44
18. Herndon WA, Sullivan JA, Yngve DA et al (1987) Segmental spinal instrumentation with sublaminar wires. A critical appraisal. J Bone Joint Surg Am 69:851–859
19. Korovessis PG, Stamatakis M, Baikousis A (1996) Relapsing pancreatitis after combined anterior and posterior instrumentation for neuropathic scoliosis. J Spinal Disord 9: 347–350
20. Leichtner AM, Banta JV, Etienne N et al (1991) Pancreatitis following scoliosis surgery in children and young adults. J Pediatr Orthop 11:594–598
21. Lipton GE, Miller F, Dabney KW et al (1999) Factors predicting postoperative complications following spinal fusions in children with cerebral palsy. J Spinal Disord 12:197–205
22. Lonstein JE, Akbarnia A (1983) Operative treatment of spinal deformities in patients with cerebral palsy or mental retardation. An analysis of one hundred and seven cases. J Bone Joint Surg Am 65:43–55
23. Lonstein JE (2001) Spine deformities due to cerebral palsy. In: Weinstein SL (ed) The pediatric spine: principles and practice. Lippincott Williams & Wilkins, Philadelphia, pp797–807
24. Madigan RR, Wallace SL (1981) Scoliosis in the institutionalized cerebral palsy population. Spine 6:583–590
25. McCall RE, Hayes B (2005) Long-term outcome in neuromuscular scoliosis fused only to lumbar 5. Spine 30: 2056–2060
26. McCarthy RE (1999) Management of neuromuscular scoliosis. Orthop Clin North Am 30:435–449, viii
27. Miller A, Temple T, Miller F (1996) Impact of orthoses on the rate of scoliosis progression in children with cerebral palsy. J Pediatr Orthop 16:332–335
28. Renshaw T (2001) Cerebral palsy. In: Morrisy R (ed) Lovell and Winter's pediatric orthopaedics. Lippincott Williams & Wilkins, Philadelphia pp563–599
29. Richards BS, Bernstein RM, D'Amato CR et al (2005) Standardization of criteria for adolescent idiopathic scoliosis brace studies: SRS Committee on Bracing and Nonoperative Management. Spine 30:2068–2075; discussion 76–77
30. Robson P (1968) The prevalence of scoliosis in adolescents and young adults with cerebral palsy. Dev Med Child Neurol 10:447–452
31. Sanders JO, Evert M, Stanley EA et al (1992) Mechanisms of curve progression following sublaminar (Luque) spinal instrumentation. Spine 17:781–789
32. Shapiro G, Green DW, Fatica NS et al (2001) Medical complications in scoliosis surgery. Curr Opin Pediatr 13: 36–41
33. Sponseller PD, LaPorte DM, Hungerford MW et al (2000) Deep wound infections after neuromuscular scoliosis surgery: a multicenter study of risk factors and treatment outcomes. Spine 25:2461–2466
34. Stanitski CL, Micheli LJ, Hall JE et al (1982) Surgical correction of spinal deformity in cerebral palsy. Spine 7: 563–569
35. Sullivan JA, Conner SB (1982) Comparison of Harrington instrumentation and segmental spinal instrumentation in the management of neuromuscular spinal deformity. Spine 7: 299–304
36. Sussman MD, Little D, Alley RM et al (1996) Posterior instrumentation and fusion of the thoracolumbar spine for treatment of neuromuscular scoliosis. J Pediatr Orthop 16: 304–313
37. Szoke G, Lipton G, Miller F et al (1998) Wound infection after spinal fusion in children with cerebral palsy. J Pediatr Orthop 18:727–733
38. Terjesen T, Lange JE, Steen H (2000) Treatment of scoliosis with spinal bracing in quadriplegic cerebral palsy. Dev Med Child Neurol 42:448–454
39. Thometz JG, Simon SR (1988) Progression of scoliosis after skeletal maturity in institutionalized adults who have cerebral palsy. J Bone Joint Surg Am 70:1290–1296
40. Tsirikos AI, Chang WN, Dabney KW et al (2003) Life expectancy in pediatric patients with cerebral palsy and neuromuscular scoliosis who underwent spinal fusion. Dev Med Child Neurol 45:677–682
41. Tsirikos AI, Chang WN, Shah SA et al (2003) Preserving ambulatory potential in pediatric patients with cerebral palsy who undergo spinal fusion using unit rod instrumentation. Spine 28:480–483
42. Westerlund LE, Gill SS, Jarosz TS et al (2001) Posterior-only unit rod instrumentation and fusion for neuromuscular scoliosis. Spine 26:1984–1989

20 Myelodysplasia

Lawrence I. Karlin

Key Points

- Myelodysplasia is a complex multisystem disorder with an extremely variable clinical presentation. Most involved children have some degree of spinal deformity, which will be present at birth or develop within the first 10 years of life.
- The curvatures have a variable etiology and some causes, such as syringomyelia, hydrocephalus, and spinal cord tethering, can be treated and curve progression prevented.
- The type and timing of treatment will depend upon the consequences of the deformity and will be affected by the age and ambulatory status of the patient and the severity of the deformity.
- Treatment is usually surgical, and is fraught with difficulty given the anatomic abnormalities and numerous associated orthopaedic, neurological and medical comorbidities. Present-day technology has addressed many of the problems of the past, and provides a wide range of options, including segmental instrumentation systems and growth preserving techniques. Surgical techniques can be tailored to the needs of the individual.

20.1 Myelodysplasia

By definition, all children with myelodysplasia have some form of spinal abnormality at birth, and most will develop some degree of spinal deformity by 10 years of age. The clinical presentation of the affected individuals is extremely variable with pathology ranging from occult inconsequential bony defects to significant abnormalities in the osseous and neurological components of the spine, brain and brain stem, as well as orthopaedic deformities of the extremities, and disturbances in the urologic and endocrine systems. Problems may occur at any time from birth through skeletal maturity, and the varied combinations of pathologic anatomy in each patient demands individualized treatment. The goal of the clinician is to maximize function by both the appropriate treatment of existing deformities, and the avoidance of preventable deformities, such as progressive scoliosis due to tethered spinal cord, unique to this population. The most common and severe form of myelodysplasia is myelomeningocele. It is the form most likely to produce significant spinal deformities and is the subject of this chapter.

Myelodysplasia has likely been present since antiquity. By the seventeenth century, it was being described in the literature. Nicolaus Tulp, the prosector in Rembrandt's *The Anatomy Lesson of Dr. Tulp* included an engraving of an autopsy specimen of a child with myelomeningocele in his *Observationum Medicarum* in 1641 (Fig. 20.1) [75]. He admonished against surgical treatment as did Morgagni who theorized the etiology of spina bifida in 1761, and wrote of a clinical experience: "I cautioned the parents not to have the tumor opened. The surgeon, however, being ignorant of its nature, promised to cure the disease. He was permitted to thrust a knife into the middle of the tumor from whence it burst a considerable quantity of limpid fluid and toward the last some bloody fluid escaped.

L. I. Karlin
Department of Orthopaedic Surgery, Children's Hospital Medical Center, 300 Longwood Avenue, Boston, MA 02115, USA
e-mail: lawrence.karlin@childrens.harvard.edu

B. A. Akbarnia (eds.), *The Growing Spine*,
DOI: 10.1007/978-3-540-85207-0_20, © Springer-Verlag Berlin Heidelberg 2011

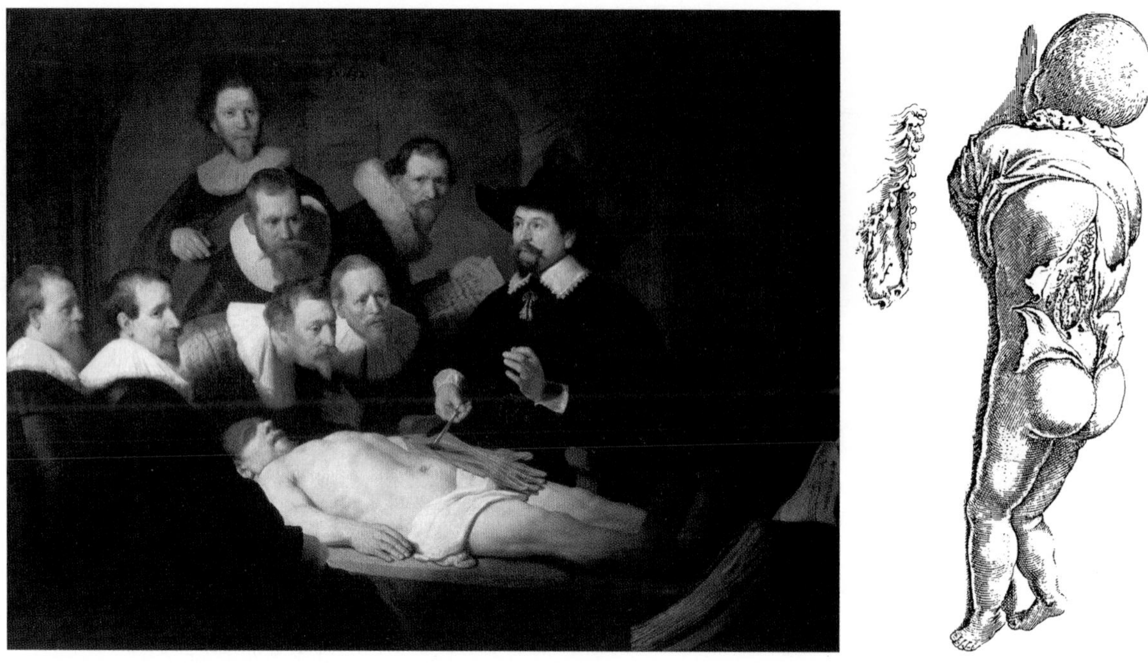

Fig. 20.1 Nicholas Tulip, immortalized in Rembrandt's *The Anatomy Lesson of Dr. Tulip* (**a**) the Hegue ([75], p 469), included an engraving of the autopsy findings in spina bifida in his book, circa 1630 (**b**) [108]

…. The child did not cease to cry, the body trembled, the face became pale and wrinkled, and death followed on the third day" [108].

The uniformly fatal prognosis of open neural tube defects (NTDs) continued until advances of the second half of the twentieth century. Antibiotic therapy, urologic, and neurosurgical care played a significant role in the improved survival. A seminal event, and an example of the remarkable commitment seen in the families of children with myelomeningocele, is the development of a shunt for the treatment of hydrocephalus. In 1955, John Holter was working as a technician in a hydraulics factory when his first son, Casey, was born with spina bifida and hydrocephalus. With encouragement of Dr. Eugene Spitz, a neurosurgeon, Holter dedicated himself to improve the current treatment options. Using Silastic, he produced a safe and functional shunt, and revolutionized the treatment of children with myelomeningocele [7].

20.2 Classification

Myelodysplasia is one, though perhaps not the best, term used to describe a number of congenital anomalies characterized by an abnormality in the formation of the neural tube. An investigation on a search engine will yield more than you may want to know about blood, because the Greek root myelo means marrow as well as spinal cord [86]. Other general terms are spinal dysraphism and spina bifida.

Spina bifida occulta in the orthopaedic literature refers to a lack of fusion of a spinous process without neurological abnormality. In the neurosurgical literature, the term implies some risk of an occult intraspinal lesion, and refers to lesions involving a spinous process or laminar defect with intact overlying skin, and in some cases, dimples, sinuses, hypertrichosis, or hemangiomata [69, 110, 121].

A *meningocele* presents as a skin-covered cystic distention of the meninges protruding through a dorsal defect of one or more vertebrae. The sac contains cerebral spinal fluid (CSF). Ganglion cells have been identified, but the spinal cord and cauda equina are confined to the spinal canal and are usually normal. Though there is some association with hydrocephalus, major central nervous system abnormalities are not present, and the prognosis is excellent [110, 121]. In a *lipomeningocele*, the sac contains a lipoma intimately involved with the sacral nerves. Neurological function is usually normal at birth but may deteriorate over time.

The most severe form of spinal bifida compatible with life is *myelomeningocele* (Fig. 20.2). Again, there is a midline defect of the posterior bony elements, but

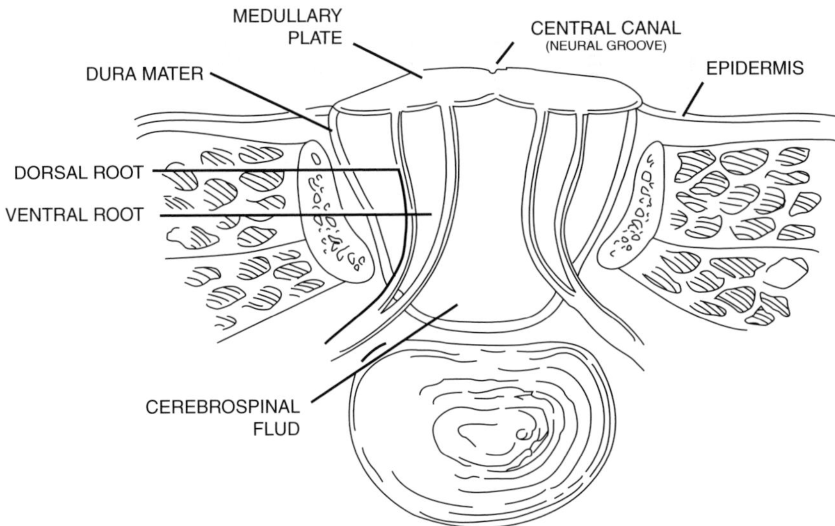

Fig. 20.2 The basic lesion of most children with myelomeningocele is the open neural placode. The dorsal surface is the interior of the neural tube, while the ventral surface is what would have been the entire outside of the neural tube had it closed. There is no skin overlying the defect and the placode is covered by an extremely thin arachnoid, which will breakdown shortly after birth allowing infection, meningitis, and death if closure is not performed. Passing down the center of the placode is a narrow groove, which is continuous with the central canal of the closed spinal cord. CSF passing down the central canal is discharged through a small opening at the upper end of the placode and bathes the external surface of the neural tissue (with permission [69])

here the protruding meningeal sac is not skin covered and contains the spinal cord and cauda equina. A portion of the neural tube remains open with the neural folds attached to the adjacent ectoderm and the neural plate or placode exposed. CSF accumulating in the subarachnoid space displaces the overlying placode to the dorsal surface of the sac. Children with a myelominingocele will have the Arnold–Chiari malformation and most of them will have hydrocephalus. There will be motor and sensory loss to the lower extremities associated with a neuropathic bladder, and orthopaedic deformities. This is the form most associated with spinal deformities [95, 110]. The term *myeloschisis* refers to the condition in which CSF fails to accumulate beneath the placode, which then lies flat on the dorsal surface.

Rachischisis is a condition of complete failure of ectodermal and mesodermal closure over the brain and spinal cord and is incompatible with life.

20.3 Incidence, Etiology

Myelodysplasia is the most common congenital birth defect [69]. Each day 12 babies are born with myelomeningocele or anencephaly [14]. The worldwide incidence varies by geographic location [121]. In the United States the incidence is 0.15% in whites and 0.04% in African Americans [29, 72, 117]. Recently, a definite decrease in the incidence of spina bifida has occurred presumably due to improved prenatal care, terminated pregnancy following prenatal diagnosis and perinatal folic acid administration [12, 86, 108].

Most NTDs are thought to occur through the pattern of multifactorial inheritance. These are isolated malformations caused by a variety of inherited and acquired factors. There may be a number of associated anomalies (Table 20.1). In families with an affected individual the recurrence rate is increased [27, 66]. In the U.S., the occurrence of a NTD in a first-degree relative of an affected member is 3.2%, in a second-degree relative is 0.5%, and in a third-degree relative is 0.17% [137].

Occasionally, NTDs may occur as part of a syndrome involving chromosomal or single-gene abnormalities. In these cases, the NTD is found in combination with other nonrelated congenital abnormalities [73]. Autosomal dominant, autosomal recessive, and sex-linked recessive patterns have been reported [36]. NTD can also be associated with syndromes of nongenetic origin (Table 20.2), or be caused by environmental factors such as prenatal exposure to teratogenic agents such as valproic acid [63].

Table 20.1 Systemic anomalies associated with pina bifida

Skeletal	Gastrointestinal	Pulmonary	Craniofacial	Cardiovascular	Genitourinary
Clubfeet, vertical talus + other foot deformities	Inguinal hernia	Tracheoesophageal fistula	Synostosis	Ventriculo-septal defect	Hydronephrosis
Lower extremity contractures	Mickel's diverticulum	Situs inversus	Cleft palate	Atrialseptal defect	Hydroureter
Hip dislocation	Malrotation		Stabismus	Patent ductus	Horseshoe kidney
Scoliosis	Omphalocele		Low-set ears	Coarctation	Undescended testes
Kyphosis	Imperforate anus		Hypertelorism		Hydrocele
Spondylolysthesis					Malrotation
Pectus Excavatum					Exstrophy
Syndactaly					
Rib anomalies					
Charcot arthropathy					

Adapted from Reigel with permission [110]

Table 20.2 Recognized syndromes including a neural tube defect

Genetic syndromes
Meckel
Median cleft face
Robert's
Anterior sacral meningomyelocele and anal stenosis
Trisome-13
Trisomy-18
Triploidy
Others including unbalanced translocation and ring chromosome
Nongenetic syndromes
Syndrome of the amnios rupture sequence
Oculoauriculovertebral dysplasia

Adapted from Luciano and Velardi with permission [73]

The role of folic acid in NTDs deserves further discussion. Since 1991, 50% of the cases of NTD have been found to be related to nutritionally based deficiency of folate [117]. Supplemental folate diets will reduce the incidence of NTD in populations both with [126] and without involved children [49, 152]. The U.S. Food and Drug Administration recommends that all woman of childbearing age receive 0.4 mg of folate before conception and during early pregnancy. Uniform compliance is estimated to decrease the incidence of NTD by up to 70% reducing the overall incidence from 2 to 0.6 per 1,000 pregnancies, and to prevent disease in approximately 2,000 babies per year [25]. Woman in the high-risk group should take 4 mg per day [49].

Despite recommendations to do so, many woman of childbearing age do not take folate [133]. In 1998, to address this unprotected group, the FDA required folic acid fortification of enriched grain products. Since then, the incidence of spina bifida has decreased 24–46% [33]. Additionally, folate fortified populations may exhibit a reduced severity and improved survivorship of children that are born with spina bifida [17, 30].

20.4 Prenatal Diagnosis

Alpha fetoprotein (AFP) is present in fetal tissue. Once the abdominal wall and neural tube close, AFP is no longer released into the amnionic fluid, but if either structure remains open, amnionic AFP levels will remain high. It was the finding of increased AFP concentrations in the amniotic fluid of mothers that gave birth to children with anencephaly or myelomeningocele that, in 1972, ushered in the era of prenatal diagnosis for NTD [19, 20].

Population screening at present is performed between 16–18 weeks of gestation by the analysis of maternal serum AFP. This test will detect 75–80% of open spina bifida [147]. It is not specific for NTDs and will be elevated for underestimated gestational age, multiple pregnancy, missed or threatened abortion, abdominal wall defects, and congenital nephroses. It will not detect skin-covered spinal malformations such as meningocele. If the levels are elevated the test is repeated, and if both are increased an ultrasound examination is performed. When questions still exist, amniocentesis for AFP should be performed keeping in mind the test's 10% miscarriage risk [46]. Acetylcholinesterase levels in amnionic fluid are also elevated in NTDs and the test is 14% more sensitive than amnionic AFP [32]. Accuracy of diagnosis is increased when both the amnionic AFP and AChE are performed together. Woman who have had a previous child with a NTD are at high enough risk of recurrence to merit amniocentesis if an ultrasound is negative [95].

20.5 In Utero Surgery

In utero surgery has been used to treat life-threatening conditions such as diaphragmatic hernia and obstructive uropathy. Its use in fetuses with myelomeningocele is based on the assumption that the intervention will diminish future morbidity [22, 64, 84].

At present, in utero surgery for known myelomeningocele fetuses is being performed in designated centers as part of a prospective study. Hysterotomy and repair are performed at 24-week gestational age. The surgery seems to be successful in defect closure and decreases the incidence of hydrocephalus and Arnold–Chiari malformation and the need for ventriculo-peritoneal (VP) shunting [22, 135, 144]. Neurodevelopmental outcomes may be improved [58], but improvements in lower limb motor function and bladder function have not been substantiated [54, 58, 135].

20.6 Associated Abnormalities: Factors Responsible for Progressive Spinal Deformities

At birth, most children with myelomeningocele will have a neurological deficit for which little can be done. What can be done is to carefully monitor the child with myelodysplasia for the preventable neurological deterioration and related spinal deformity progression that may be caused by hydrocephalus, Arnold–Chiari malformation, and the tethered spinal cord (Table 20.3).

20.6.1 Arnold–Chiari Malformation

In 1891 and 1896, Chiari described various anatomic patterns of herniation of the cerebellum and brain stem through the foraman magnum [35]. The Chiari II malformation, also known as the Arnold–Chiari malformation, is characterized by the displacement of the medulla oblongata into the cervical canal and an upward course of the cervical roots [69]. Almost all children born with myelomenigocele will have the Chiari II malformation, which can cause periodic stridor, apnea, swallowing difficulties, upper extremity paresis, hypertonia, nystagmus, and opisthotonis. The symptoms are worse in early childhood. In most of the affected children, treatment of hydrocephalus with a ventriculoperitoneal shunt will alleviate the symptoms, but in some a decompression of the posterior fossa will be necessary.

Table 20.3 Delayed neurological complications of spina bifida

Seizure Disorder
Hydrocephalus
±Shunt malfunction
Arnold–Chiari malformation
Tethered spinal cord
Tethered spinal cord with tumor
Lipoma
Dermoid
Neurenteric cyst
Fibroma
Diastematomyelia
Arachnoiditis
Hydromyelia
Dermal sinus and stalks

Adapted from Reigel [110] with permission

20.6.2 Hydrocephalus

The Chiari II malformation obstructs the CSF circulation. At birth, the open communication between the fourth ventricle and the central canal allows for decompression of the cerebrospinal fluid into the myelomeningocele sac. Once the sac is closed, this avenue of decompression is lost and hydrocephalus occurs. A ventriculoperitoneal shunt is the treatment of choice.

Unfortunately, the shunts frequently fail and hydrocephalus recurs. In children, the clinical signs of acute hydrocephalus are bulging fontanelles, altered mental status, nausea, vomiting, and severe headaches [57]. Hydrosyringomyelia may occur when the CSF pressure within the central canal increases secondary to untreated hydrocephalus. Symptoms include increasing lower extremity weakness, spasticity, back pain, rapid progressive of scoliosis, and upper extremity weakness. Early correction of hydrocephalus by shunt revision is usually curative. Shunt function must be evaluated prior to cordotomy or intraoperative spinal cord manipulation to avoid catastrophic complications [45, 150].

20.6.3 Tethered Spinal Cord

The spinal cord is considered tethered when the conus medullaris is located at an abnormal level and fixed there by an inelastic structure. In the 20-week embryo, the conus medullaris terminates at the L4–5 level, and by 2 months of postnatal age is at the adult level of L1–2 [12]. In general, the caudal end of the spinal cord below the L2–3 interspace and the diameter of the filum terminale greater than 2 mm are considered abnormal [98]. When neurological findings consistent with spinal cord tethering are present, the cauda below the L1–2 interspace, a filum diameter of greater than 1 mm, or thickening of the filum alone may be considered sufficient diagnostic criteria.

The pathophysiology of the tethered spinal cord and its treatment in the occult dysraphic states is described elsewhere in this book. In the child with myelomeningocele, the spinal cord is tethered not only by an expendable and easily resected thickened filum terminale, but also by adherence between the neural placode, the surrounding tissues, and the repaired dural layer. Most, if not all, children who have undergone operative closure of a myelomeningocele will demonstrate a low-lying tethered spinal cord on magnetic resonance imaging (MRI) examination. In these individuals, the diagnosis of the tethered spinal cord syndrome is a clinical one based upon the presence of both tethering and neurological deterioration, and the exclusion of other causes of deterioration such as hydromyelia, shunt malfunction, and symptomatic Chiari II malformation. An MRI assessment will define the nature of the tether and assess the presence of possible associated pathologies including diastematomyelia, lipomas, dermoids, granulomas, inclusion cysts, and teratomas [52, 110].

Neurological deterioration due to a tethered spinal cord will occur in up to 30% or more of children with repaired myelomeningocele [52, 131]. Release should be performed before major functional loss occurs. Although the conus level does not significantly change after de-tethering [21], the procedure can be expected to produce improvement or stabilization in most cases as illustrated by a comparison of outcomes in two long-term studies of sacral level myelomeningocle populations. In one study of patents that had detethering procedures, none of the 62 lost ambulatory ability and 61 were community ambulators [136]. In another similar study of 36 patients who did not have routine untethering one-third had gait deterioration, 11 became wheelchair dependent, and spinal deformities and lower extremity contractures developed in 44% [18].

Results from untethering seem to vary with respect to the symptoms. Cochrane et al. demonstrated improvement or stabilization in motor findings, but only 2 of 7 with alterations in bladder capacity and continence improved, while 2 deteriorated [28]. McClone [80] reviewed the results of untethering procedures from several series. Motor deficits improved in 72%, stabilized in 25%, and worsened in 3%. Pain improved in 92% and stabilized in 8%. Urologic function improved in 44% and stabilized in 56%. Unfortunately, symptomatic retethering occurs in 30–55% [13, 36].

In properly selected myelomeningocele patients, tethered spinal cord release can stabilize a progressive scoliosis. Pierz et al. evaluated the effect of tethered spinal cord release on scoliosis in 21 myelomingocele patients. Three had improvement in the curvatures, and 6 stabilized. Twelve patients progressed greater that 10°. Eighty-six percent of patients with initial curvatures over 40° and 100% of those with a thoracic level required spinal fusion [105]. McLone et al. reported on 30 patients with myelomeningocele and scoliosis. In patients with curvatures greater than 50°, 1 out of 6 improved, while 14 of 23 with less-severe curvatures stabilized [81].

20.7 Other Associated Abnormalities

20.7.1 Latex Allergy

As many as 28% of individuals with myelomeningocele have a known allergy to latex rubber, and many others will test positive [10, 31, 61, 78, 83, 87, 138, 153]. These are IgE-mediated reactions that include urticaria, bronchospasm, rhinoconjunctivits, laryngeal edema, and systemic anaphylaxis. Especially, worrisome is intraoperative anaphylaxis that is characterized by hypotension, tachycardia, flushing, and bronchospasm and usually, but not always, begins 30–45 min after the onset of the procedure. Risk factors for intraoperative anaphylaxis are the number of operations and atopic predisposition [47, 48, 56, 61, 92].

The best screening tool for latex allergy seems to be a careful history that questions previous reactions to catheters, rubber gloves, balloons, and dental cofferdams. The absence of a positive history does not assure safety. Gold et al. reported that of 15 patients with intraoperative anaphylactic reactions only 7 had a previous history of latex allergy [48].

Tests for allergy to latex are skin-prick, intradermal, and serum radioallergosorbent (RAST). Skin prick is 100% sensitive [24, 47, 48, 68, 103, 125, 134] but not risk free. In a series by Kelly et al. [62], 9 of 118 patients with known latex allergy had allergic reactions to the testing including 4 with anaphylactic reactions. RAST testing has sensitivities reported of 53–100% [47, 48, 68, 87, 123–125, 134, 145].

Preoperative prophylactic management with diphenhydramine, cimetidine or ranitidine, and corticosteroids has been used successfully for those with known allergy [37, 132, 141], but allergic reactions have occurred despite prophylaxis [37, 65, 120].

Given the large pool of patients that are sensitive to latex but have no history of allergy, and the risk and insensitivity of testing, it seems reasonable to assume all myelomeningocele patients are allergic to latex, and to treat them in a latex-free environment. Holzman, [55] Gerber et al. [47], and others have reported successful reoperation in patients that had previous anaphylactic reoperation by perioperative latex avoidance alone. Gentili et al. [46] noted no allergic reactions during surgery in 26 allergic patients treated with latex precautions alone. Birmingham and Suresh [15] compared surgical results in myelomeningocel patients before and after the initiation of a latex avoidance protocol. Before the protocol, 18 of 473 demonstrated an allergic reaction, while after the protocol 7 of 552 had a reaction. In 3 of these, there was a breakdown in the protocol. Additionaly, a latex-free environment may diminish the number of myelomeningocele patients that become sensitized [84]. In one study, the latex sensitization rate fell from 26.7 to 4.5% following the initiation of a latex-free environment [93].

20.7.2 Short Stature and Precocious Puberty

Short stature for age is present in 47–60% of children with myelomeningocele [65, 127, 140, 141], and is affected by neurological level, ambulatory status, skeletal deformity, and endocrine function [140]. Trollman et al. [141] demonstrated that arm span could be used to screen the subgroup of patients in whom short stature was due to growth hormone deficiency. Serum insulin-like growth factor 1 and insulin-like growth factor binding protein levels were normal in 10 of 12 short statured patients with normal arm span and low in 8 of 11 with reduced arm span. Growth hormone replacement seems to produce increased stature and mobility [114, 142]. Trollman et al. [143] also demonstrated early and increased activation of adrenal androgen secretion in prepubertal girls.

Precocious puberty in girls is common. Proos et al. noted breast development by age 9 and related the risk of precocious puberty to increased intracranial pressure and shunt malfunction [107]. Furman and Mortimer [43] noted that girls with myelomeningocele began menstruation on average at 10 years, 3 months earlier than their mothers and siblings.

20.8 Spinal Deformity

Spinal deformity occurs commonly in children with myelodysplasia. Piggott noted a 90% incidence of some form of spinal deformity by age 10. In half the patients, the curvature was significant enough to merit surgical treatment [106]. The principle deformities are scoliosis and hyperkyphosis and these are often classified by causative mechanism as congenital and developmental, though often the deformity may be due to a combination of both. Congenital deformities include scoliosis and rarely kyphosis due to failure of formation or segmentation, and the rather unique form of kyphosis found in the myelomeningocele population due to dysplastic posterior elements. Developmental curvatures were originally defined as those occurring without vertebral malformation presumably due to muscle paralysis, muscle malposition, or hip deformity and pelvic obliquity [106, 109]. The category must now include the more recently appreciated causative factors such as hydrocephalus, syringomyelia, and spinal cord tethering from a variety of causes. Additionally, an increased incidence of spondylolisthesis has been reported [60, 129].

Problems caused by spinal deformity include recalcitrant ulcerations over the gibbus in individuals with kyphosis or of the ischium or sacrum in wheelchair sitters with scoliosis and trunk imbalance. Pulmonary compromise can occur with significant scoliosis or kyphosis.

Those with trunk imbalance in either the sagittal or frontal plane may need to use their hands for support and in so doing lose upper extremity function [5, 53, 59, 116]. The goal of management is to maximize function and prevent progression. This will involve periodic evaluations of spinal alignment as well as careful monitoring of neurological function and orthopaedic deformities.

20.8.1 Scoliosis

Scoliosis of 10° or more will occur in 50–80% of myelomeningocele children by age 10 years [8, 88, 106, 122]. The risk for progression is related to age and severity. Muller et al. [91] reported progression of 12° per year in curvatures over 40° and a maximum rate of progression in the 11–15-year age group.

Congenital scoliosis is present in 7–38% of individuals with myelodysplasia [88, 106, 109, 115]. This will progress when growth is unbalanced and may be associated with intraspinal pathology. Treatment is similar to that of congenital scoliosis, which is not associated with spinal dysraphism [84], but in the myelomeningocele group posterior fusion alone in the dysplastic portion of the spine is likely to fail due to the deficient bone stock and should be supplemented by anterior fusion [70, 71].

Developmental scoliosis is the more common variety, and its incidence relates to the neurological and anatomic levels. Trivedi et al. [139] defined scoliosis in this group as a curvature greater than 20° and noted the three most predictive factors for the development of scoliosis to be motor level, ambulatory status, and last intact laminar arch (LILA). The scoliosis prevalence was 93, 72, 43, and 7% in patients with thoracic, upper lumbar, lower lumbar, and sacral motor levels respectively and 89, 44, 12%, and 0° respectively at similar LILA. In Mackel and Lindseth's [76] study, 85% of thoracic neurological level patients had a curvature of greater than 45°, while 60% of those with a L4 neurological level had a scoliosis and of these 40% required surgery.

Lindseth [69] has identified several curve patterns in developmental scoliosis that seem related to etiology. Long-sweeping C-shaped curvatures often associated with kyphosis are typically due to muscle weakness, asymmetric levels of paralysis, or spasticity due to hydrocephalus. Progression is anticipated if growth remains or the curvature is greater than 50° [91]. An S-shaped thoracic or thoracolumbar curve resembling an idiopathic pattern and frequently associated with pelvic obliquity is often seen in association with syringomyelia. Spinal cord tethering results in a lumbar or thoracolumbar deformity with excessive lordosis [69].

20.8.1.1 Orthotic Treatment

Progressive curvatures over 20° may be treated with an orthosis. Muller and Nordwell [89] reported that the Boston brace arrested progression if initiated before the curvature reached 45°, but most believe bracing in this population is at best a temporizing method [42, 50, 69, 95, 112]. Although it may not prevent progression, an orthosis can improve function by providing improved support for seating. The rigid "active" control braces utilized in idiopathic deformities are often associated with skin irritation, but total contact "soft" orthoses seem to be well tolerated. Letts et al. [67] reported on the use of the "soft Boston orthosis" in the management of neuromuscular scoliosis. The brace is constructed of "Aliplast," a material similar to Styrofoam, and reinforced with polyethylene. While the improvement of the scoliosis averaged 15°, postural position or seating stability was enhanced 90%. Orthoses may be modified to accommodate individual needs (Fig. 20.3).

20.8.1.2 Surgical Indications, Complications, and Planning

The absolute indication for surgical treatment is functional loss generated by the deformity. Another indication is a curvature over 50° based on the assumption that these will progress and that function will deteriorate. Better to deal with the deformity when it is manageable than to wait for the extra morbidity involved with the surgical treatment of a dramatic deformity. This philosophy assumes functional loss with progression though there are essentially no large studies of the natural history of untreated scoliosis in myelomeningocele.

Surgical treatment has many benefits. Mazur et al. [79] reported improved sitting balance in 70% of the patients following anterior/posterior procedures on patients with developmental scoliosis, and Schoenmakers et al. [118] noted significant improvement in scores for self-care. Others have noted

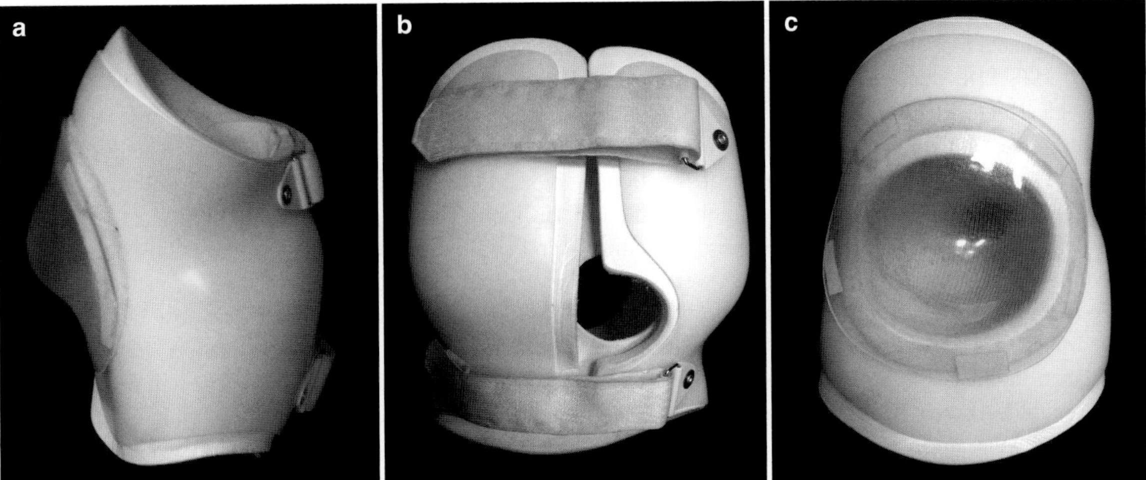

Fig. 20.3 Spinal orthoses may not prevent deformity progression, but may improve function. Here a "soft" brace has been reinforced with polypropylene and adapted to accommodate a rigid kyphotic deformity associated in this child with skin ulceration. The removable clear plastic bubble over the gibbus protects the skin, while allowing for its easy inspection (**a**, **c**). The orthosis is further modified (**b**) to allow for drainage catheters. The device allowed this child to maintain full function during treatment of the skin ulceration

improved pulmonary function despite anterior procedures following deformity correction [9, 25]. Ajeena et al. [1] reported significant improvement in self-esteem following deformity correction, but Wai et al. [146] noted no relationship of self-perception to spinal deformity.

Enthusiasm for correction of spinal deformity must be tempered by the considerable con side of the equation. Surgery for myelomingocele spinal deformity has rates of complications, including infection, pseudarthrosis and instrumentation failure, and neurological deterioration, that are among the highest of all deformity surgery [6, 14, 30, 72, 77, 79, 82, 90, 118, 119, 132, 148]. In defense of surgery, it must be realized that some of these studies relate to methods no longer used. Improved spinal instrumentation, earlier mobilization, attention to urosepsis, nutritional support, neurosurgical evaluation, prophylactic antibiotic treatment, and proper tissue handling have combined to decrease the complications. Nevertheless, this particular population continues to be a difficult one to treat despite the use of modern surgical techniques. Even when compared to the neuromuscular population, a group known to have high complication rates, the myelomeningocele patients stand out as the most risky to treat. Stevens and Beard [132] reported on 76 patients with neuromuscular spinal deformity undergoing segmental spinal instrumentation. A preponderance of the serious complications

Table 20.4 Segmental Spinal instrumentation for neuromuscular spinal deformity – complications by diagnosis

Complication	Myelodysplasia (30 patients)	Other (46 patients)
Deep infection	10	1
Skin breakdown	6	1
Neurological deficit	6	4
Permanent	4	4
Temporary	2	0
Inadequate correction	3	6
Minor revision rod/wire	2	8
Broken rod	1	4
Mechanical failure	1	4
Curve progression	0	3
Pseudarthrosis	0	3

In this study, a notable preponderance of serious complications occurred in the myelodysplasia sub-group. Ninety percent of the myelodysplasia patients had one or more complications. Of 27 patients that had an unplanned procedure half were in the myelodyusplasiqa group. From Stevens and Beard [132]. With permission

occurred in the 30 patients with myelodysplasia. Ninety percent of the myelodysplasia patients had a complication and half of the unplanned reoperations were in this group (Table 20.4). In a similar series, Benson et al. [14] noted that the 13 patients with myelodysplasia in a study group of 50 had over half the complications.

A number of reports have demonstrated loss, rather than improvement in function following surgery [115–117, 126, 127]. In series by Mazur et al. [79]

Schoenmaker et al. [118] and Muller et al. [90], 50% or more of patients lost ambulatory ability following surgery [79, 90, 118]. Only rarely was this attributed to neurological deterioration. Most of these individuals were at best borderline community ambulators requiring KAFO support. One possible cause of functional loss was the increased difficulty in swing through gait following fusion across the lumbosacral junction. Probably, more importantly, these patients were immobilized for prolonged periods of time following surgery. In the Mazur et al. [79] series, plaster body jackets were used for 6 months, and in Schoenmaker et al. [118], pantaloon spica braces were used for 3 months. It is hypothesized that upper extremity weakness prevented subsequent crutch utilization. Lower extremity contractures also contributed to the morbidity. In the Mazur et al. [79] series, the mean hip flexion contracture was 15.2° before surgery and 38.4° after. The increased deformity may be due to change in lumbar lordosis secondary to the surgery, contractures secondary to immobilization, or a combination of the two. It must be remembered that some loss of ambulation is always anticipated with or without surgery as the borderline ambulators age.

Skin ulceration due to seating imbalance is an indication for surgical correction of deformity, yet the problem can be exacerbated following surgery. A rigidly fused lumbosacral junction with significant residual obliquity is problematic. In the Mazur et al. [79] series, the average pelvic obliquity at follow-up was 15° and the average lordosis was reduced from 63 to 40°, with a range of 0–70. Of those with lordosis below the normal range, 80% developed sacral pressure sores [39, 96]. These results were obtained with Harrington instrumentation. It is assumed that newer generation systems will obviate the complication due to immobilization and sagital malalignment. Nevertheless, prior to surgery, families should receive a balanced discussion of risks as well as benefits of these large undertakings.

20.8.1.3 Preoperative Evaluation

The preoperative assessment begins with a thorough history and physical examination. This is a multisystem disease and the evaluation must be inclusive; associated abnormalities may not only adversely affect the outcome, but may in fact be at least partially responsible for the curvature. The patient should be questioned for the symptoms of cord tether, hydrocephalus, and syringomyelia. Latex allergy should be documented.

The skin in the area of the surgery must be assessed for scarring, fragility, and suppleness. The large correction and bulky spinal instrumentation will make closure difficult. The magnitude and flexibility of the sagittal and coronal plane deformities and pelvic obliquity are evaluated. The gait and method of active transfers should be observed to determine just how the lumbosacral motion affects mobilization. Hip motion is measured. A hip flexion contracture will be aggravated if the lordosis is decreased, thus making ambulation more difficult. Limited hip flexion, which may have been accommodated by relative lumbar hypolordosis will make sitting more difficult if the lumbar spine is fixed in normal lordosis. A thorough neurological examination is carried out as a change in neurological function may be indicative of the known associated neurological abnormalities. Laboratory assessment must include a urine culture and nutritional evaluation. Growth and maturity should be evaluated to determine the amount of future growth and to predict the possibilities of crankshaft and trunk height loss. The bone age will help determine the appropriate timing of surgery as chronological age is a less accurate maturity determinant in this population known to have precocious puberty. Shunt function must be assessed as altered CSF dynamics generated intraoperatively may produce acute neurological deterioration [45, 150].

The radiographic assessment should include full-length views of the spine in the position of function, standing for ambulators and sitting for nonambulators. A sitting upright will eliminate the affect of hip contractures on the spinal alignment. This view when performed in the anterior/posterior as opposed to the posterior/anterior fashion affords better assessment of the lumbosacral articulation and pelvic obliquity. Flexibility is assessed with side bends, traction, or fulcrum bends as needed to determine the need for releases and the extent of the fusion. An MRI should be performed to evaluate for syringomylia and intraspinal tumors as well as the position of the cord. The conus will essentially always be further distal than the norm, and this finding must be put in context with the other findings to determine if there is symptomatic tethereing. If needed the head should be included to evaluate for hydrocephalus and Arnold–Chiari malformation. A spinal CT scan is helpful to better analyze the three-dimensional anatomy. It is especially useful in determining the size and orientation of the pedicles in the dysplasitic portion of the spine when pedicular fixation is planned.

20.8.1.4 Surgery

The surgical treatment of spinal deformity in children with myelomeningocele is arguably the most challenging type of spinal surgery. The deformities are often long, severe, and rigid. There is poor soft tissue coverage and the skin is often insensate, scarred, and fragile. The posterior elements are deficient and dysplastic, offering a poor mass for fusion and difficult instrumentation purchase and placement. There may be tenuous neurological status and associated urologic abnormalities.

The surgical options for the treatment of spinal deformity in the myelomeningocele population are increasing as new technologies develop. While introduction of spinal instrumentation dramatically improved the treatment of spinal deformities, first-generation implants were less than ideal in the myelomeningocele as they were intended for placement into intact posterior elements. Certainly, segmental spinal instrumentation has been a significant improvement allowing a secure fixation to the dysraphic portion of the spine, and perhaps altering the standard of treatment. The improved fixation allows for dramatic deformity correction in multiple planes and reduces or eliminates the need for postoperative immobilization. The menu now includes definitive long fusions and instrumentation via combined anterior and posterior approaches, anterior- or posterior-only instrumentation and fusion, and instrumentation without fusion. Caution must be exercised in analysis of the literature supporting one or another form of instrumentation as the studies for the most part are of small numbers and do not have the power to statistically support one or another method. Neither the studies nor the patient populations are homogeneous. The individuals studied usually have a wide range of curvature patterns, severity, flexibility, deformity levels, and posterior element dysplasia, and the studies often combine different instrumentation techniques, and types of deformities such as scoliosis and kyphosis.

The choice of surgical methods must be individualized based on the patient's needs and function, and the curve characteristics. Attempts to spare mobile lumbar segments seem appropriate in ambulatory patients. More rigid and severe curvatures with extensive dysplastic segments will require more secure posterior fixation obtained through increased segmental anchors and, perhaps, the inclusion of the pelvis. The stresses on those fixation anchors can be lessened through anterior releases. Fusion rates may be improved when anterior fusion is performed especially when there is significant posterior bone deficiency.

The timing of surgery is another matter for consideration. These deformities are by definition early onset. There is little data, though, on the consequences of early spinal fusion in the myelomeningocele population. Frequently, the surgery involves anterior and posterior fusions that addresses the crankshaft phenomenon, and any adverse effect on pulmonary function would be difficult to determine on clinical grounds given the wheel chair status of most undergoing early surgery. Clearly, many factors must be considered in the clinical decision making process.

Combined Anterior Posterior Instrumentation and Fusion

In the myelomeningocele population, combined anterior and posterior spinal procedures have been the standard of surgical treatment. A review of deformity correction techniques in the era of spinal instrumentation (Table 20.5) illustrates the dramatic improvement in surgical results when anterior surgery was combined with posterior nonsegmental instrumentation. With Harrington instrumentation, the dysraphic posterior elements necessitated hook placement in the sacrum and lengthy postoperative immobilization was required. The relative instability of the instrumentation and the deficient bone stock for the fusion mass resulted poor correction, a high pseodarthorosis and instrumentation failure rate, and complications secondary to the immobilization. It is no surprise that fusion rates increased when the posterior procedure was combined with anterior fusion with or without instrumentation of the relatively normal vertebral bodies. Osebold et al. [97] reviewed the Twin Cities Scoliosis Center experience with five fusion techniques. All fusions extended to the pelvis and the posterior instrumentation was Harrington. The average scoliosis correction was 23% with posterior-only procedures and 56% when anterior fusion and either Dwyer or Zielke instrumentation was combined with posterior Harrington instrumentation and fusion.

Table 20.5 Myelomeningocle scoliosis surgical correction: a comparison of instrumentation techniques

	Reference	Scoliosis correction (%)	Pelvic obliquity (%)	Infection	Pseudo/ instrument failure
Post nonsegmental	Osebold et al. [97]	23	29	33%	46%
	Mazur [79]	32	39	7%	33%
	Parisini et al. [11]	17	50	30%	70%
Post nonsegmantal anterior fusion	Ward et al. [148]	57	60		
	Osebold et al. [97]	48	46	50%	100%
Post nonsegmental and anterior instrumentation	Osebold et al. [97]	56	47	18%	23%
	DeWald and Faut [34]	55		0	31%
	Mayfield [77]	75		11%	11%
	Mazur [79]	42	41		
	McMaster [82]	63	72		
Anterior only	Mazur et al. [79]	48	14		29%
	Sponseller et al. [128]	57	44	7% (superficial)	36% revision
	Basobas et al. [13]	59	64.3	5%	24% revision
	Stark et al. [130]	37	62	0	87% revision
Posterior segmental and anterior fusion	Ward et al. (Luque) [148]	51	56		
	Banta (Luque) [6]	53		11%	16%
	Parsch et al. (CD) [100]	37			33%
	Geiger et al. (CD) [45]	52			33%
	Yazici et al. (Isola) [151]	68	96		
Posterior segmental and anterior instrumentation	Ward et al. (Luque) [148]	63	71		18%
	Geiger et al. (CD) [45]	59			
	Parsch et al. (CD) [100]	57			18%
	Wild (without pelvic fixation) [149]	56	81	27% (superficial)	
Posterior segmental	Geiger et al. [45]	52			
	Parsch et al. [100]	41			40%
	Banit [11]	40	29	8%	20%
	Rodgers et al. 14/24 [112]	58	64	0	14%
	Parisini et al. [101]	47	40	10%	10%
	Yazici et al. [151]	69	50		

The pseudoarthrosis rate was 23% with the combined method and 46% with posterior Harrington instrumentation and fusion. Mazur et al. [79] compared results of anterior fusion and Dwyer instrumentation, posterior fusion and Harrington instrumentation, and a combination of the two. The best corrections were 42% and were obtained with the combined procedure. The pseudarthrosis rate was 33% with Harrington instrumentation, 29% with Dwyer instrumentation, and 11% with the combination. Improved results were observed with combined anterior posterior procedures reported by others [34, 77, 97, 132].

Although good results in terms of correction and fusion rates can be obtained with nonsegmental posterior instrumentation combined with anterior surgery, the limited stability provided requires prolonged postoperative immobilization and recumbency. In the myelomengocele patient, this is more consequential than just inconvenience. Insensate skin leads to pressure sores beneath casts or braces. Contractures develop and children with limited strength may lose function by increased weakness [79, 118]. Additional complications may occur secondary to the immobilization. DeWald and Faut [34] reported excellent corrections in a group of 23 patients with paralytic scoliosis. Postoperative care included prolonged support using halo-hoop apparatus, plaster casts, or plastic jackets, and 3 of the 7 myelomenigocle patients developed complications secondary to the immobilization. Significant rates of instrumentation failure such as hook dislodgment are also problematic. Both prolonged immobilization and recumbency and instrumentation dislodgement were addressed with the development of segmental spinal instrumentation.

The use of contoured rods and sublaminar wires as introduced by Luque provided a more stable correction of multiplanar complex deformities and decreased the extent of postoperative immobilization [3, 74]. The Galveston technique provided a secure and low profile method of pelvic fixation [4]. Banta [6] reviewed his results of segmental instrumentation in a myelomeningocele population. Various techniques were used, but most had combined anterior Dwyer instrumentation with either posterior Harrington or Luque segmental instrumentation using sublaminar and, in the dysplastic portion of the spine, pedicle wiring. The mean preoperative curvature was 73° and this was reduced to 34°, a correction of 53%. Eighteen of thirty-eight patients with scoliosis developed complications including four deep infections. There were 6 pseudarthroses cases, of which 3 required revision surgery. These patients were mobilized early in clam shell orthoses for 6 months. Using Luque–Galveston technique combined with anterior surgery, Parisini et al. [100] and Benson et al. [14] reported 57 and 66% scolisiosis deformity corrections and 70 and 54% complication rates, respectively. Ward et al. [148] compared single-stage surgeries with combined anterior/posterior methods using anterior fusion with and without instrumentation and posterior Harrington and Luque methods. They noted a 55% correction of scoliosis and 56% correction of pelvic obliquity using anterior release and posterior segmental instrumentation with the Luque technique and 68 and 71% corrections, respectively, when anterior instrumentation was used with similar posterior technique. He noted a 50% success rate with posterior only vs. 92% with combined anterior/posterior, but found no statistical difference in fusion rate, curve correction, or pelvic obliquity correction between the various combinations of the two-stage anterior and posterior procedures. They and others concluded that superior results were obtained when anterior surgery was combined with posterior, but noted anterior instrumentation did not provide additional benefits [41]. In this series, postoperative immobilization did not vary between groups and consisted of 3 months bed rest with trunk and hip immobilization and a total of 12 months in either a plaster jacket or clam shell orthosis.

Pedicle screw fixation seems especially suitable to the dysraphic section of the spine, which lacks adequate lamina but does have pedicles. The improved fixation may allow less immobilization and eliminate the need for pelvic fixation when that is being preformed just for the improved anchorage (Fig. 20.4). Parsch et al. [102] reported a series of posterior pedicle screw constructs and compared three instrumentation patters; posterior only, anterior release and posterior instrumentation and anterior and posterior instrumentation. Final correction was 43, 37, and 57%. Pseudarthrosis and instrumentation problems occurred in 40% of group 1, 33% of group 2, and 18% of group 3, though these differences were not statistically significant. For those patients with thoracic level lesions, statistically improved results did occur when anterior instrumentation was employed. The patients were mobilized postoperatively with an orthotic utilized for 6 months. Rodgers et al. [113] studied a group of myelomenigocele patients all of whom had pedicle screw fixation. Of 24 patients, 22 had scoliosis as either the only deformity or in association with kyphotic deformity. Ten patients had anterior release. The scoliosis corrections averaged 58% with an 8.2% pseudarthrosis rate. There were no acute wound infections and in most cases postoperative immobilization was not utilized. The authors emphasized the need to visualize the pedicle during screw placement in the severely dysraphic segment of the spine (Fig. 20.5).

Wild et al. [149] studied a series of patients fused short of the pelvis with anterior instrumentation and posterior pedicular segmental instrumentation (Fig. 20.6). The hypothesis here is that the greater stability obtained with pedicle fixation does not require fixation into the pelvis. The mean curvature prior to surgery was 81.8 and 34.7° at last follow-up. The pelvic obliquity was corrected from 32 to 4.8°. There were no skin ulcerations postoperatively despite minimal correction in one patient, due, perhaps, to seating modifications permitted by the more mobile lumbosacral area.

Anterior Only and Posterior Only Instrumentation and Fusion

Improved fixation permitted by newer segmental systems has lead to a renewed interest in anterior- and posterior-only procedures with their associated diminished morbidity. Banit et al. [11] reviewed 50 myelomeningocele patients with posterior only and anterior only instrumentation and fusion. Six of the 50 had Harrington instrumentation and the remainder CD segmental techniques, which included sublaminar wires. Thirty-two of 50 were fused to the pelvis. The

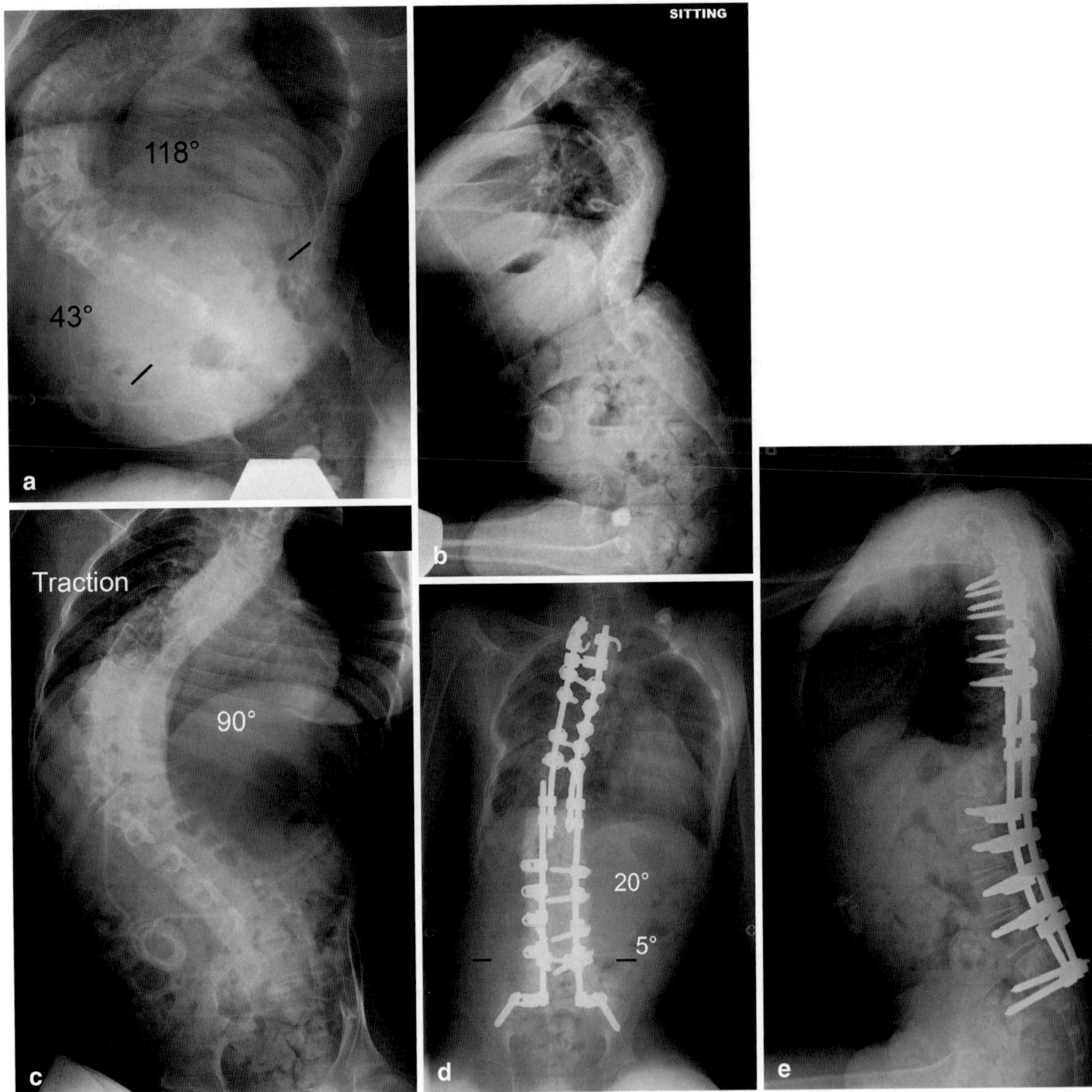

Fig. 20.4 This patient has a dramatic scoliosis of 118° and a pelvic obliquity of 43° (**a, b**). This is a rigid deformity that corrects at best on supine traction to 90° (**c**). The scoliosis and pelvic obliquity were corrected more than 80% through a combination of spinal destabilization procedures, which included anterior releases, vertebral column resection, and rib osteotomies, and rigid segmental instrumentation provided by pedicle fixation (**d, e**). Multiple spinal rods were utilized allowing fixation through many anchors and maximum distribution of the forces generated by the manipulation. A cantilever manipulation then brings the two limbs of the deformity into alignment. Permitting a deformity to progress to this severity is not recommended. The example is intended to show the corrections possible with present generation techniques

correction at follow-up was 40% and there were 8 cases of pseudarthrosis, of which 5 required treatment. These authors noted the results were better than Harrington instrumentation but not as good as those obtained with combined procedures. Twenty-four of 50 were not braced postoperatively. They questioned if these results were sufficient enough to avoid the extra morbidity of a two-stage procedure (Fig. 20.7).

In the report of pedicle screw fixation by Rodgers et al. [113], 14 of 24 patients had posterior only surgery and 11 were fused short of the pelvis. There were two lumbo-sacral pseudarthoroses. These authors concluded

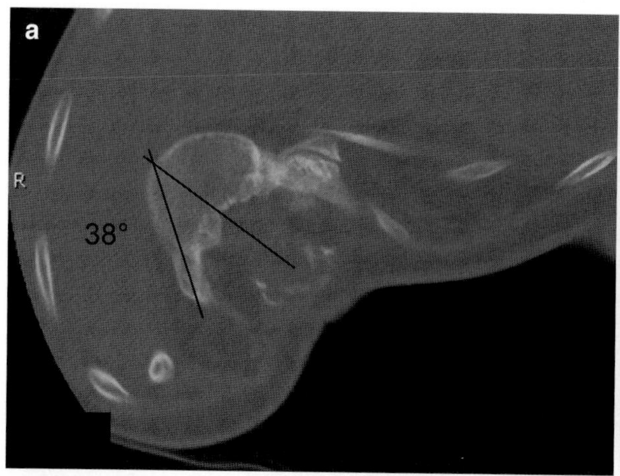

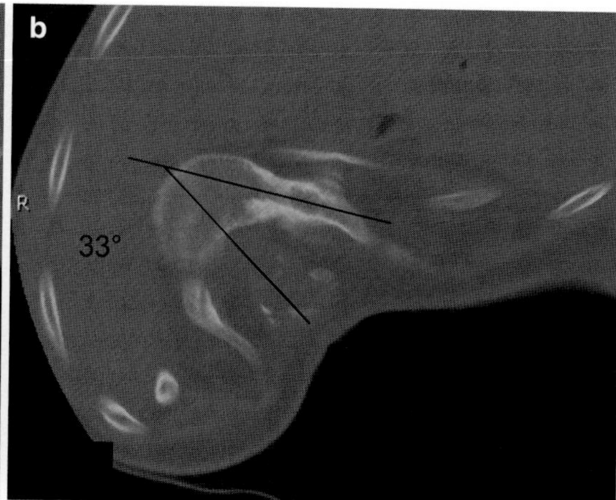

Fig. 20.5 Although pedicle screws offer superior fixation in the dysplasic portion of the spine, placement can be challenging. The pedicle position, orientation, and size may vary within (**a**, **b**) and between levels. Also, note how placement of the left-sided screw is hindered by the paraspinal structures, and how the right-sided screw may be overly prominent

that pedicle fixation produced results from posterior-only surgery that were comparable to those obtained with combined anterior/posterior techniques. Additionally, they felt that in some cases the method obviated the need for inclusion of the sacrum or pelvis. Parisini et al. [101] compared anterior instrumentation combined with posterior Luque fixation to posterior only pedicular fixation. In the combined group, an average scoliosis curvature of 101° was corrected at final follow-up 57%, while in the posterior only group an average preoperative curvature of 85° was corrected 47%. Pelvic obliquity correction averaged 43% and 40%, respectively. The posterior only group had a 30% complication rate compared to the 70% reported in the combined group. Yazici et al. [151] reviewed a series of 47 patients with neuromuscular scoliosis treated with Isola–Galveston technique utilizing pedicular screw fixation. There were 9 patients with myelomeningocle, and of these, 5 had posterior only surgery. There was very little difference between the curvatures and the corrections between the group that had anterior and posterior vs. posterior only surgery. These relatively mild curvatures were 60° and were corrected 68–69%. Pelvic obliquity correction average 96% in the group that had anterior releases as compared to 50% in the posterior only group. Others have also noted improved pelvic obliquity correction when anterior releases are performed [16].

Anterior-only instrumentation would seem well suited to a group of patients with deficient posterior, but essentially normal anterior spinal elements, but historically has been problematic both due to its kyphosing tendency and the adding-on of segments above and below the end-instrumentated vertebrae (Fig. 20.8). Newer more rigid systems have addressed some of these concerns. They provide superior rigidity and avoid the kyphosis produced by the older systems. Anterior-only techniques avoid the soft tissue problems encountered with posterior approaches and have a much lower infection rate [79], (Fig. 20.9).

Basobas et al. [13] reported their results of anterior-only instrumentation and fusion in 21 patients with neuromuscular scoliosis of which 12 were children with myelomeningocle. The mean primary curvature of 60.4° was reduced to 19.9° and was 24.6° at final follow-up. The pelvic obliquity was corrected from 15.1 to 3.2°. It was 5.4° at final follow-up. The mean number of segments preserved below the fusion mass was 3.2. There was no loss of lumbar lordosis. There was one infection and one pseudarthrosis. Four of the twenty-one patients required subsequent extension of the fusion. Sponseller et al. [128] reviewed 14 myelomeningocle patients that had anterior-only instrumentation and fusion. At 40 months, the mean curvature correction was 57% and the mean pelvic obliquity improved from 16 to 9°. Poor results occurred in 2 patients with neurological deterioration, 2 with proximal decompensation, and 1 with screw pull-out. All poor results were in patients with either syringomyelia or curvatures greater than 75°. Stark and Saraste [130] concluded that anterior

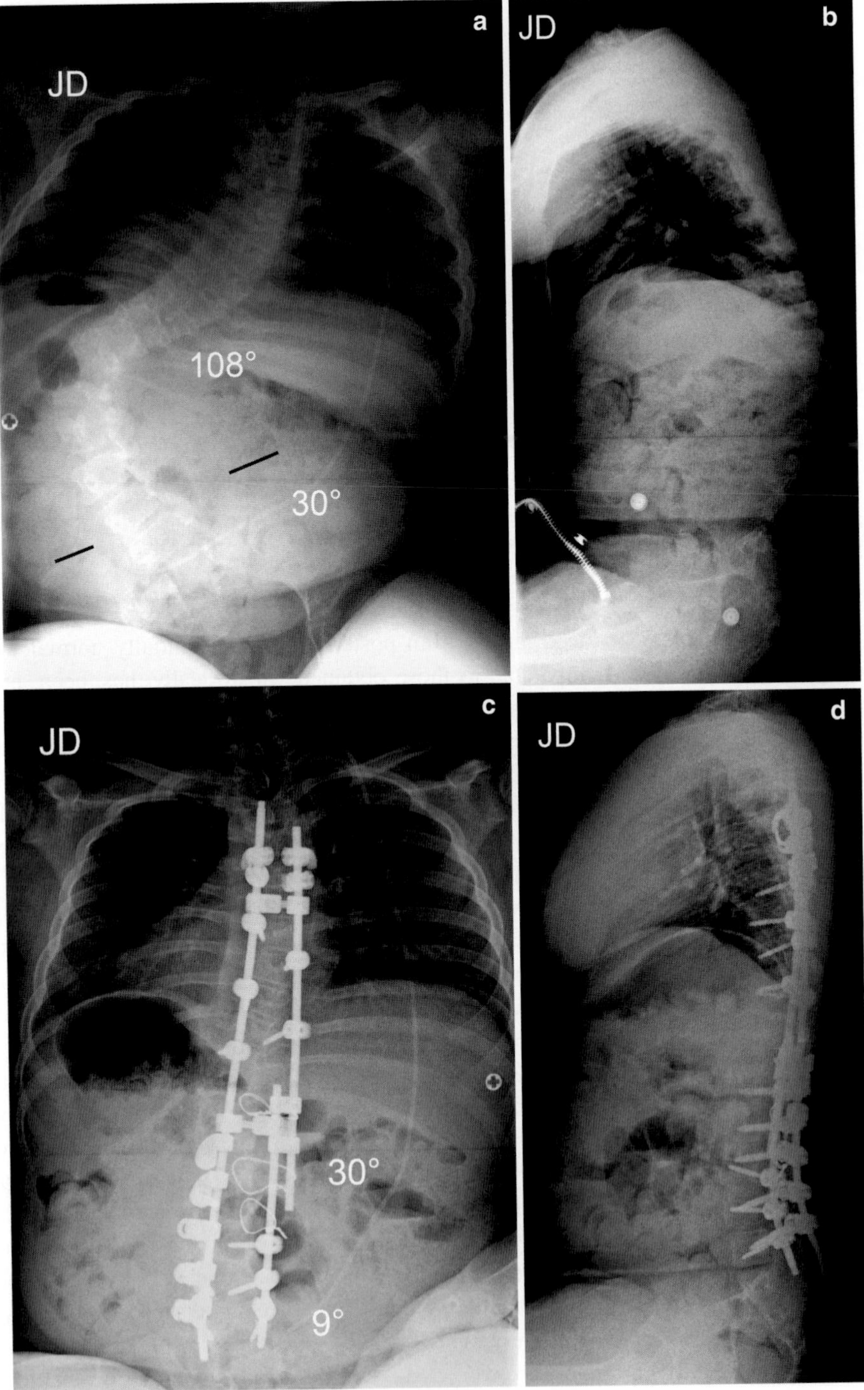

Fig. 20.6 JD has scoliosis, pelvic obliquity, and thoracolumbar kyphosis (**a**, **b**). Corrections of approximately 70% were possible with anterior releases and fusion coupled with posterior spinal segmental instrumentation (**c**, **d**). The pelvis was not felt to be part of the major curvature and the pedicle fixation in the lumbar spine provided excellent stability. Accordingly, the instrumentation and fusion did not cross the lumbosacrum and flexibility through that area was maintained. The child was mobilized without external support immediately following the procedure. Although some pelvic obliquity persists, there have been no seating or skin irritation problems

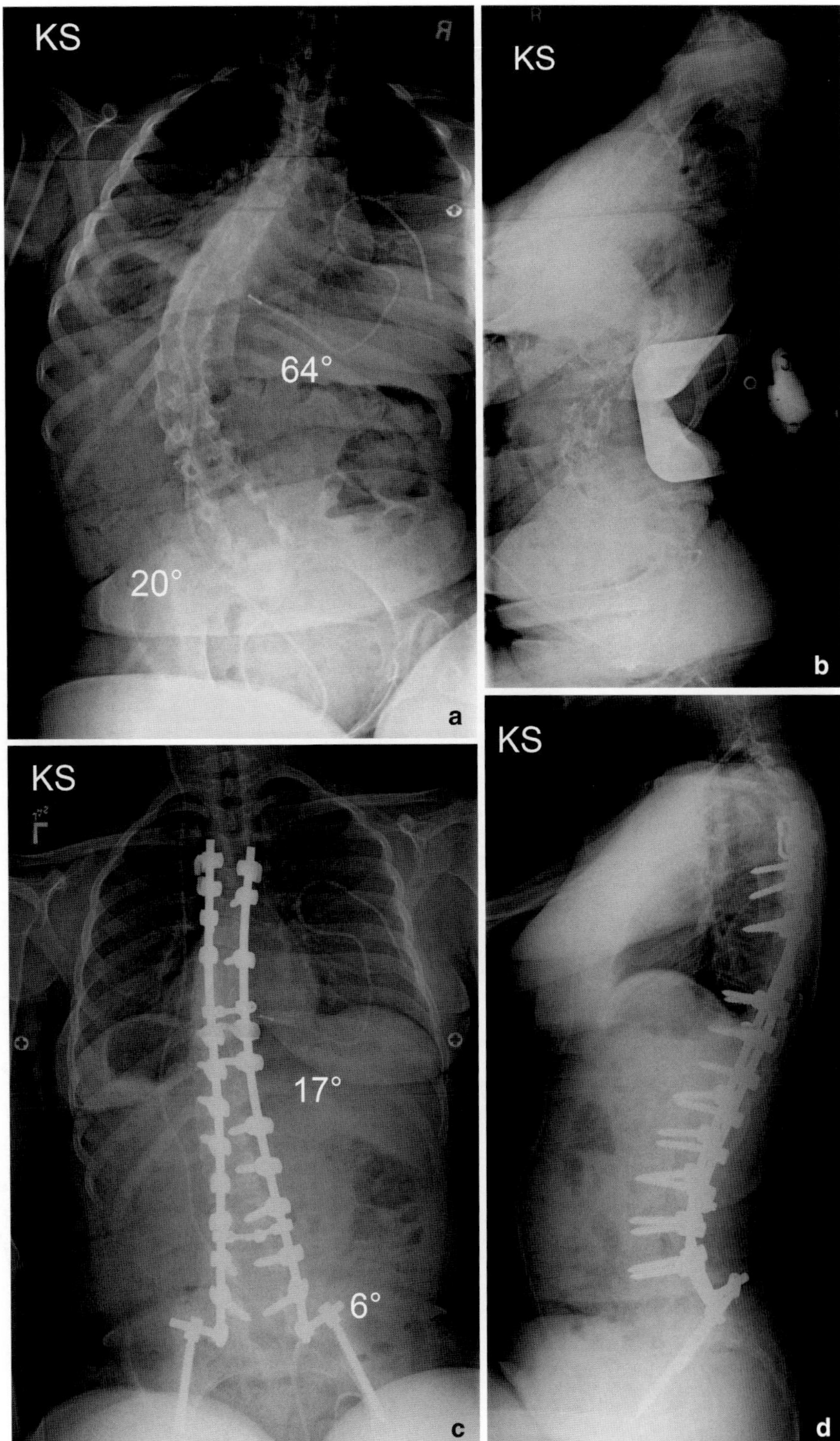

Fig. 20.7 *KS* has a moderate deformity with a 64° scoliosis and a 20° pelvic obliquity (**a**, **b**). Segmental fixation allowed excellent correction and stabilization without the need for an anterior procedure (**c**, **d**). The youngster was mobilized immediately following the procedure without a spinal orthoses. These children, with their dysplastic posterior lumbar spinal elements, do present deficient bone mass for fusion and only long-term follow-up will determine if late instrumentation failure and pseudarthroses will occur (courtesy of Dr. John Emans)

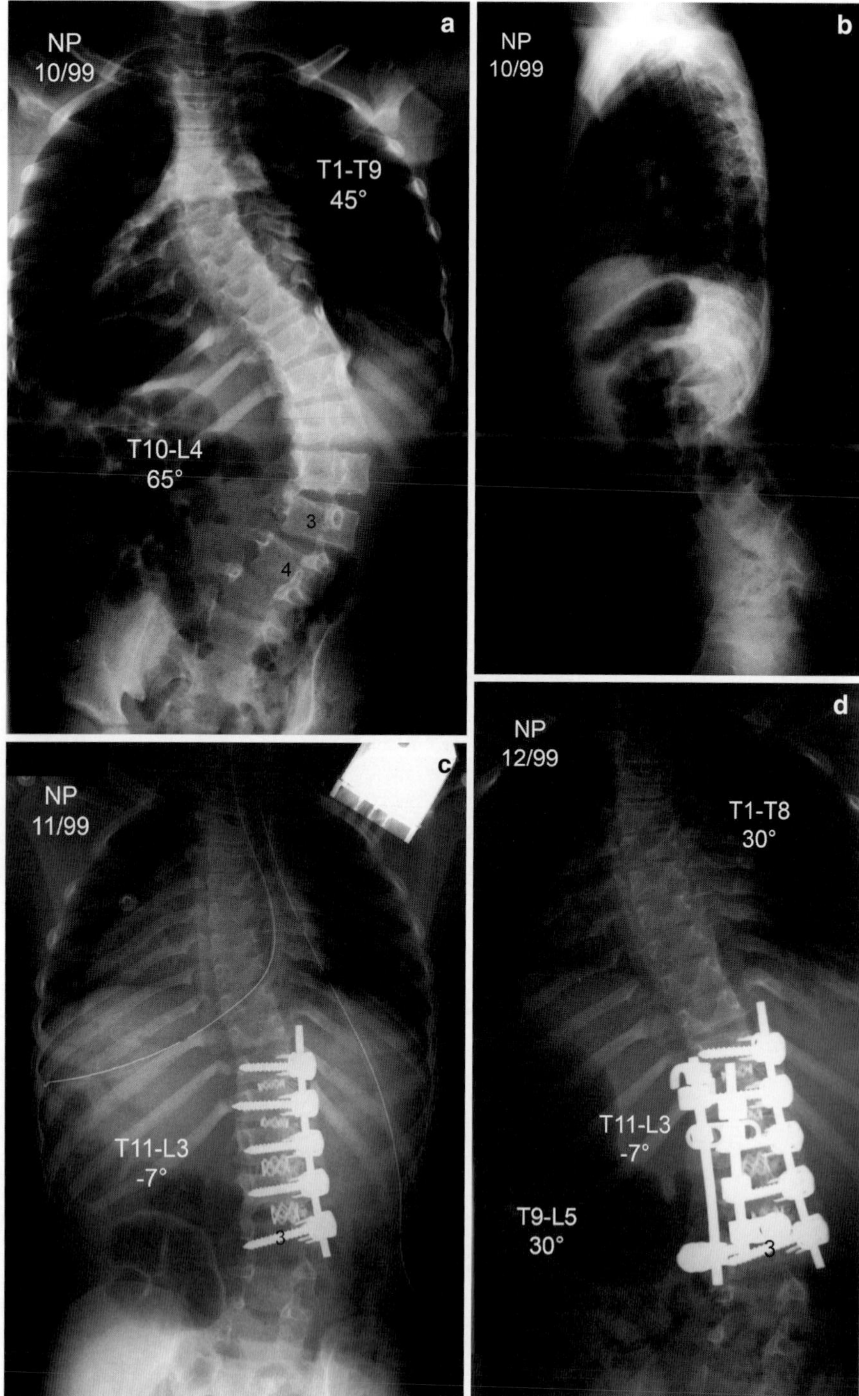

Fig. 20.8 Although not a "pure" anterior only procedure, the clinical course of N.P. illustrates the pitfalls of anterior only instrumentation and fusion for skeletally immature individuals with neuromuscular curvatures (**a, b**). At 8 years of age, the most rigid portion of the major deformity was overcorrected with the anterior technique (**c**). Posterior instrumentation of the same levels was performed as supplemental fixation due to concerns about the strength of the vertebral bodies (**d**)

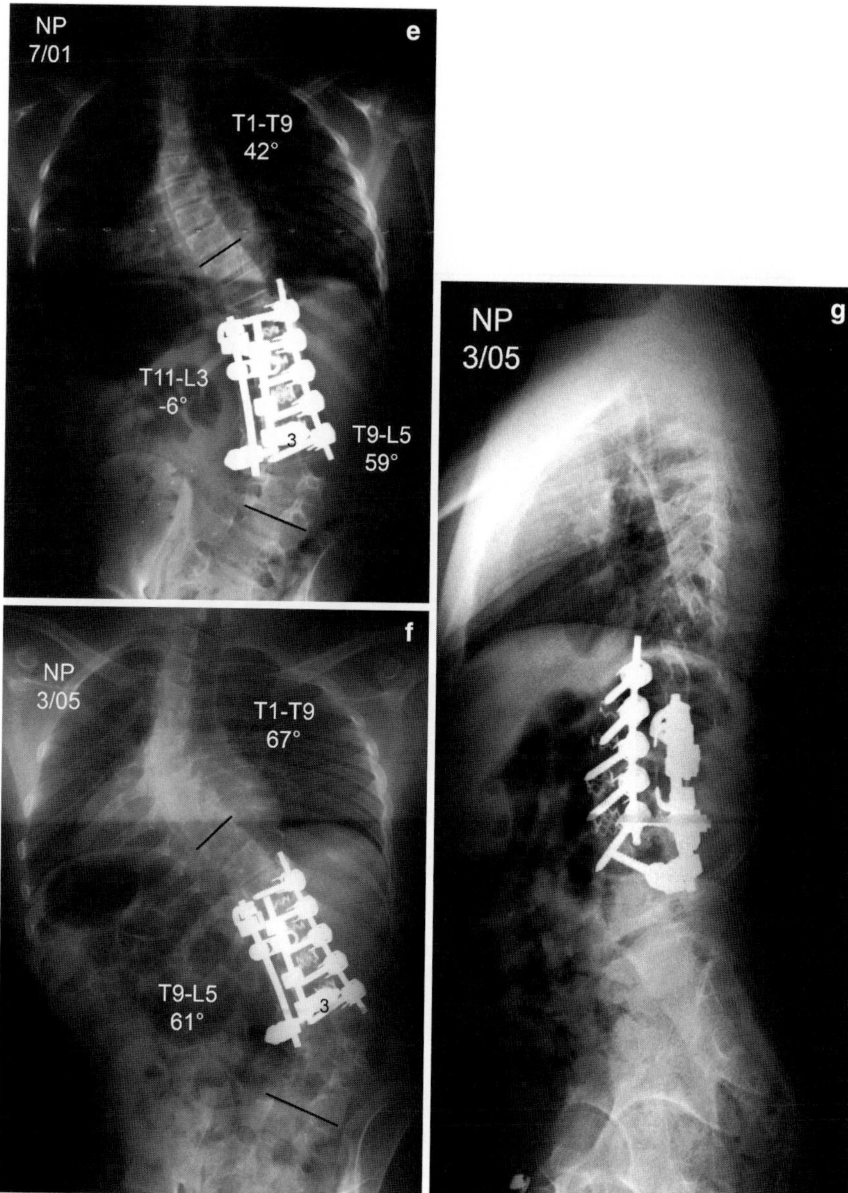

Fig. 20.8 The procedure stopped short of the Cobb terminal and did not include the thoracic curvature. Over time, there was an increase in the magnitude of the lumbar curvature, adding-on of levels in the lumbar spine, and progression of the thoracic curvature (**e**, **f**, **g**). Addressing these long, sweeping deformities from an anterior approach can be difficult. In this case, the original plan was to perform a fusion of minimal length, allow spinal growth, and then to perform a definitive procedure in the future. Despite the curve progression the child's function remains excellent and unchanged. He is fully ambulatory with AFO's and his family does not want to jeopardize that function with further surgery

instrumentation and fusion was insufficient treatment for patients with myelomeningocele. Six patients had anterior only instrumentation and fusion and of these 5 had increase in the deformity above the instrumentation sufficient to merit repeat surgery. The instrumented area ended below the cephalic terminal of the curvature in 4 patients that had an average 34° increase in the curvature. In the 2 patients who had instrumentation that included the entire Cobb curvature, one had no increase and the other only 10°, indicating that the technique might be applicable when the entire curvature was included. There were no infections or pseudarthroses.

20.8.1.5 Posterior Instrumentation Techniques

The unique charactreristics of myelomeningocele spinal deformity is the tenuous skin, deficient soft tissue, and the dysplastic bone as well as the complex deformities, which are a combination of neuromuscular and congenital etiology. The surgical technique must address these elements. If the midline skin is scarred or tenuous, consideration should be given to a triradiate incision. This will avoid the midline skin and minimize the chance for myelomeningocele sac penetration, while affording excellent exposure of the lateral bony masses

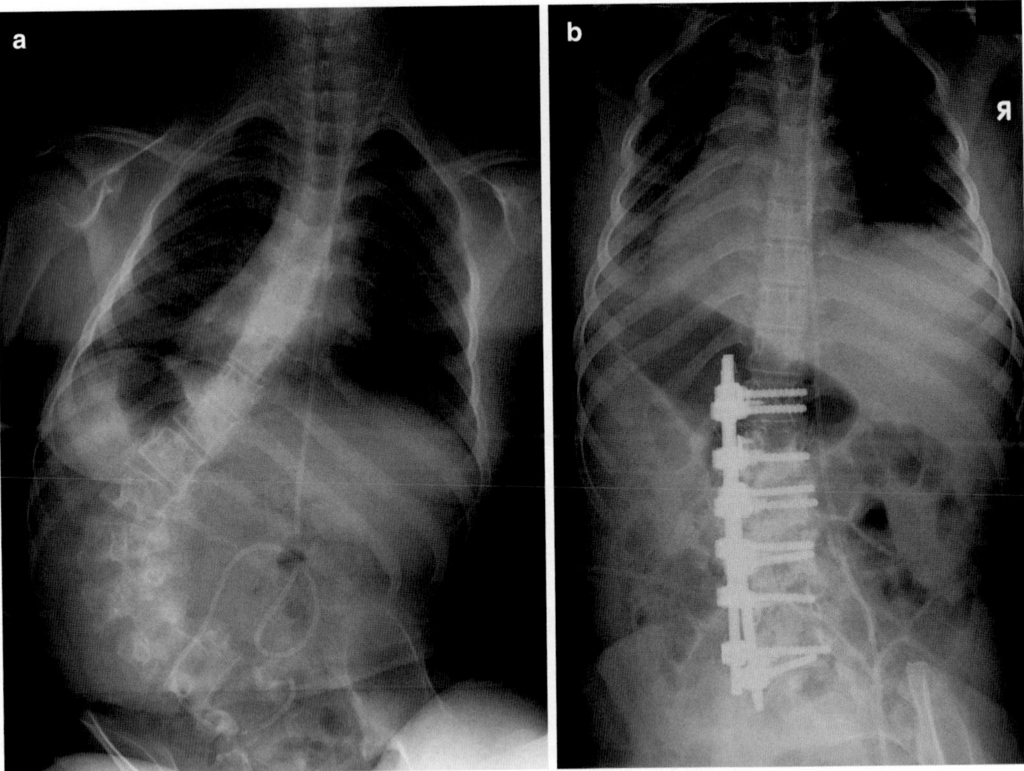

Fig. 20.9 This young woman, a wheelchair ambulatory, was having increasing difficulty with seating due to a progressive scoliosis and pelvic obliquity. The deformity was fairly rigid, improving at best to 64° on corrective radiographs. (**a**) Anterior releases, fusion, and instrumentation with dual rods, allowed very satisfactory correction and resolution of seating difficulties. (**b**) The anterior approach makes use of the relatively normal anterior bone stock for fixation and fusion and avoids the poor skin and deficient posterior soft tissues; ulceration over prominent instrumentation and wound infections are rare. The approach leaves more motion segments to accommodate slight pelvic obliquity and perhaps avoid difficulty in transfers, self catheterization, and other requirements of self-care, which can be adversely affected by a long posterior instrumentation

of the dysraphic spinal elements. Ward et al. [148] noted that 6 of 15 cases with this incision had wound necrosis, but only 2 had a significant clinical problem. They felt that its advantages merited its use and cautioned against undermining the skin and subcutaneous tissues between the two inferior limb and advised that the inferior limbs subtend as large an angle as possible.

When there is soft tissue deficiency, tissue expanders used preoperatively may be helpful in allowing better soft tissue coverage, though reported experience is limited [51, 94, 99]. Dissection of the dural sac is most easily accomplished by proceeding from the portion of the spine with intact posterior elements toward the deficient area.

In the portion of the spine with intact neural arches any anchor system may be used, but due to the osteopenic bone, multiple fixation points are needed to distribute the forces. In the dysraphic portion, a number of options for segmental fixation exist. At present, pedicle screws offer superior fixation, though, placement is challenging as the dysraphic segments present dramatically altered pedicle size, position and orientation. Direct visualization by dural retraction and medical wall dissection allows proper insertion. The relatively nonharmonious orientation of adjacent pedicles may be addressed by using polyaxial screws or adjustable transverse connectors. When pedicle anatomy precludes placement alternatives for segmental instrumentation are Drummond (Wisconsin) wires placed with the button medially [38] and Luque wires placed through the neuroforamina beneath the pedicles. Another technique involves placement of bone screws, which can be of smaller diameter, with wires looped around the screw head [132] or the use of specially designed screws with a hole in the head for wire placement (Depuy Spine).

Cross links are utilized for extra stability but most be contoured to avoid pressure of the sac.

Sacro-pelvic fixation is often required for the extra stability afforded by instrumentation anchorage and for pelvic obliquity correction, especially when the lumbosacral segment is part of the curvature. The Galveston method will provide good coronal plane stability and has the benefit of being low profile in an area of soft tissue deficiency [4, 6, 44, 148]. Visualization of the lateral cortex is advisable as the iliac orientation is variable and the bone stock deficient. Iliac and ilio-sacral screws provide excellent anchorage points and unlike the Galveston method may be left in place to allow for the complex rod contouring maneuvers often necessary for proper seating of the rods in the dysraphic spinal area [85]. When compared to Galveston technique, iliosacral screws demonstrate improved pelvic obliquity correction and less loosening [104].

20.8.1.6 Growth Preserving Instrumentation

The dilemma of early onset scoliosis is well covered in this text and certainly pertains to the child with myelomeningocele. When determining if the amount of spine growth sacrificed with early definitive surgery in the myelomeningocele population is sufficient to merit a growing technique, it must be remembered that many of these children have precocious puberty and chronological age cannot be used to determine the growth remaining.

There is at present only limited experience with growth preserving techniques in the myelodysplasia population. Instrumentation without fusion in a population with paralytic scoliosis secondary to poliomyelitis was studied by Eberle [40]. In 15 out of 16 patients treated with segmental instrumentation without fusion the implant failed to control the deformity. There is a single report in the literature of vertebral wedge osteotomies for the treatment of neuromuscular spinal deformity. The correction is maintained by instrumentation, which is removed 12 weeks after the initial procedure. There were 14 patients with paralytic scoliosis; 4 had myelomeningocele. The initial correction was 86% and at follow-up of between 6 and 29 months, 10 patients maintained some correction [59].

At present, very promising results have been obtained with instrumentation without fusion utilizing third-generation segmental instrumentation and repeated lengthenings [2]. Fusion is limited to the area of instrumentation, which is placed at the cephalic and caudal extent of the deformity and lengthening performed usually at 6-month intervals via a limited approach. Single and dual rod methods have been reported (Fig. 20.10). Additionally, the VEPTR and Shilla techniques are being utilized as well. In the myelomeningocele, population problems anticipated with growth rod techniques are difficult in obtaining fixation in the dysplastic posterior elements subjected to the stress of instrumentation without fusion and wound complications related to repeated incisions through tenuous scarred skin. Most studies to date involve heterogenous populations and a study limited to myelomeningocele patients has not been published (Figs. 20.11 and 20.12). Campbell et al. [23] reported 10 patients with myelomeningocele who had thoracic insufficiency syndrome, spine deformity,

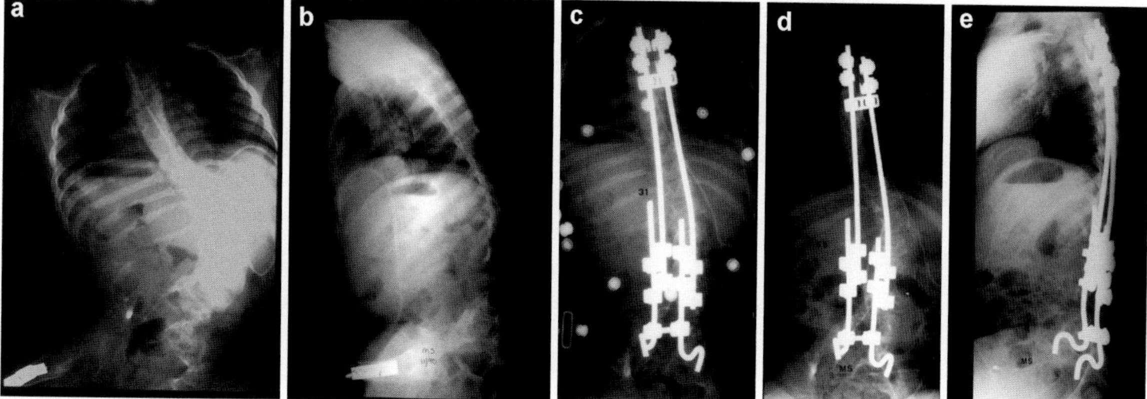

Fig. 20.10 This curvature has been stabilized and growth preserved by use of growing spinal instrumentation (**a-e**). In preliminary studies, myelodysplasia patients do not seem to be more prone to infections or skin problems than others (courtesy of Dr. Richard McCarthy)

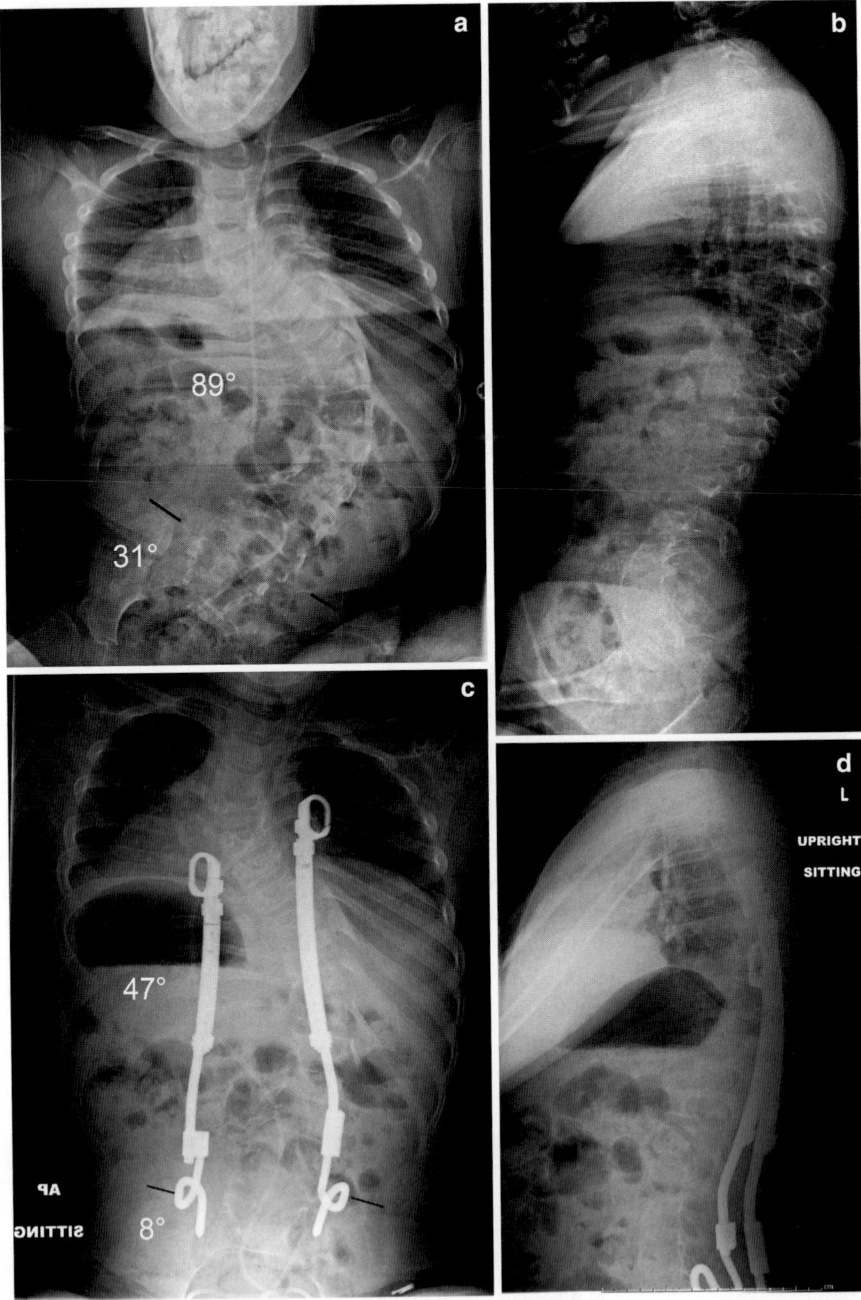

Fig. 20.11 This patient has a significant deformity at age 7. (**a**, **b**) A growth preserving technique was utilized to improve seating and avoid spinal fusion at an early age. (**c**, **d**) The VEPTR technique was selected in part because it could be performed away from the midline scarred tissues. To date, there have been no major complications. If the correction can be maintained, definitive surgery may be less involved than it would have been had the curvature been allowed to progress

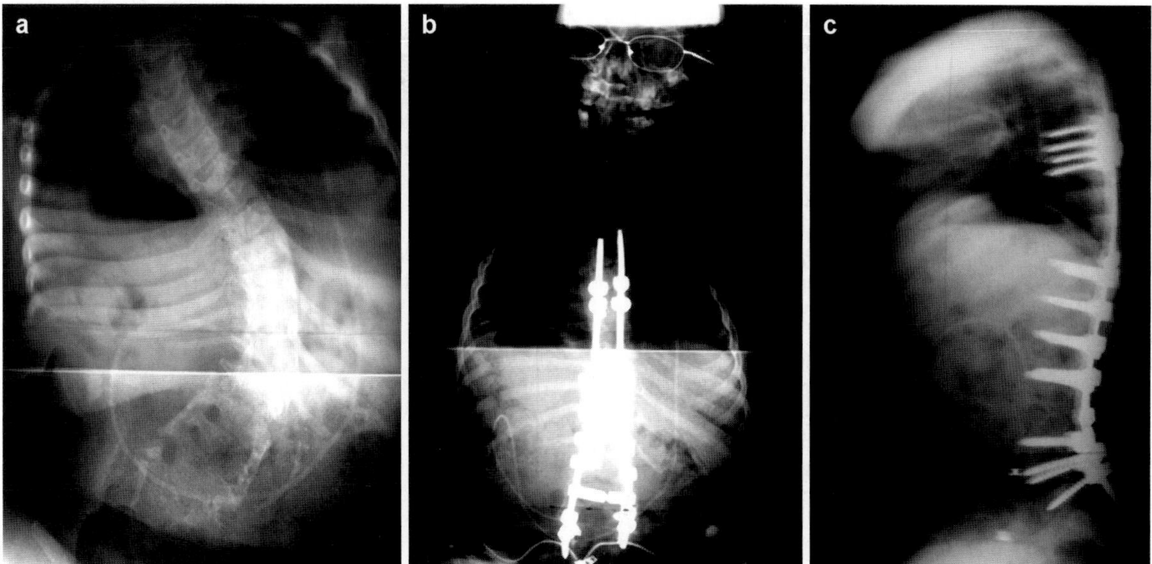

Fig. 20.12 The Shilla procedure allows continued growth without the need for repeated lengthening. The central portion of the deformity is corrected and fused and the "ends" grow under "guidance" of the attached instrumentation (courtesy of Dr. Richard McCarthy)

and pelvic obliquity treated with a hybrid VEPTR construct with s-hook iliac crest fixation. The average follow-up was 5.75 years. The pelvic obliquity improved from 34 to 11, the scoliosis from 73 to 46, and the lumbar kyphosis from 43 to 26. There were three s-hook migrations, two rib cradle migrations, one skin slough, and four wound infections.

20.8.2 Congenital Kyphosis

Kyphosis at the lumbar or thoracolumbar spine is either present at birth or develops over time in up to 15% of children with myelomeningocele [8, 26, 57]. In nearly all cases, the deformity progresses 8–12° per year due to bony and soft tissue abnormalities [42, 100]. The subject is well covered elsewhere in this volume.

References

1. Ajeena AW, Hall IE, Emans JB (1993) Functional outcomes in myelodysplasia following spinal fusion. Orthop Transac 17:107
2. Akbarnia BA, Marks DS, Boachie-Adjei O et al (2005) Dual growing rod technique for the treatment of progressive early-onset scoliosis: a multicenter study. Spine 30:S46–S57
3. Allen BL Jr, Ferguson RL (1979) The operative treatment of myelomeningocele spinal deformity – 1979. Orthop Clin North Am 10:845–862
4. Allen BL Jr, Ferguson RL (1982) The Galveston technique for L rod instrumentation of the scoliotic spine. Spine 7: 276–284
5. Asher M, Olson J (1983) Factors affecting the ambulatory status of patients with spina bifida cystica. J Bone Joint Surg Am 65:350–356
6. Banta JV, Hamada JS (1976) Natural history of the kyphotic deformity in myelomeningocele. J Bone Joint Surg Am 58:279

7. Banta JV, Park SM (1983) Improvement in pulmonary function in patients having combined anterior and posterior spine fusion for myelomeningocele scoliosis. Spine 8: 765–770
8. Banta JV (1990) Combined anterior and posterior fusion for spinal deformity in myelomeningocele. Spine 15:946–952
9. Banta JV, Bonanni C, Prebluda J (1993) Latex anaphylaxis during spinal surgery in children with myelomeningocele. Dev Med Child Neurol 35:543–548
10. Banta JV (1996) The orthopaedic history of spinal dysraphism. I: the early history. Dev Med Child Neurol 38:848–854
11. Banit DM, Iwinski HJ Jr., Talwalker V et al (2001)Posterior spinal fusion in paralytic scoliosis and myelomingocele. J Pediatr Orthop 21:117-25
12. Barson AJ (1970) The vertebral level of termination of the spinal cord during normal and abnormal development. J Anat 106:489–497
13. Basobas L, Mardjetko S, Hammerberg K et al (2003) Selective anterior fusion and instrumentation for the treatment of neuromuscular scoliosis. Spine 28:S245–S248
14. Benson ER, Thomson JD, Smith BG et al (1998) Results and morbidity in a consecutive series of patients undergoing spinal fusion for neuromuscular scoliosis. Spine 23:2308–2317; discussion 2318
15. Birmingham PK, Suresh S (1999) Latex allergy in children: diagnosis and management. Indian J Pediatr 66:717–724
16. Boachie-Adjei O, Lonstein JE, Winter RB et al (1989) Management of neuromuscular spinal deformities with Luque segmental instrumentation. J Bone Joint Surg Am 71:548–562
17. Bol KA, Collins JS, Kirby RS (2006) Survival of infants with neural tube defects in the presence of folic acid fortification. Pediatrics 117:803–813
18. Brinker MR, Rosenfeld SR, Feiwell E et al (1994) Myelomeningocele at the sacral level. Long-term outcomes in adults. J Bone Joint Surg Am 76:1293–1300
19. Brock DJ, Scrimgeour JB (1972) Early prenatal diagnosis of anencephaly. Lancet 2:1252–1253
20. Brock DJ, Sutcliffe RG (1972) Alpha-fetoprotein in the antenatal diagnosis of anencephaly and spina bifida. Lancet 2:197–199
21. Brophy JD, Sutton LN, Zimmerman RA et al (1989) Magnetic resonance imaging of lipomyelomeningocele and tethered cord. Neurosurgery 25:336–340
22. Bruner JP, Tulipan N, Paschall RL et al (1999) Fetal surgery for myelomeningocele and the incidence of shunt-dependent hydrocephalus. JAMA 282:1819–1825
23. Campbell R Jr, Smith M, Allen W et al (1980) The treatment of secondary thoracic insufficiency syndrome of myelomeningocele by a hybrid VEPTR"Eiffel Tower" construct with s-hook iliac crest pedestal fixation. Pediatric Orthopaedic Society of North America Annual Meeting, Albuquerque, NM
24. Carrillo T, Cuevas M, Munoz T et al (1986) Contact urticaria and rhinitis from latex surgical gloves. Contact Dermatitis 15:69–72
25. Carstens C, Paul K, Niethard FU et al (1991) Effect of scoliosis surgery on pulmonary function in patients with myelomeningocele. J Pediatr Orthop 11:459–464
26. Carstens C, Koch H, Brocai DR et al (1996). Development of pathological lumbar kyphosis in myelomeningocele. J Bone Joint Surg Am 78: 945–950
27. Carter CO, Roberts JA (1967) The risk of recurrence after two children with central-nervous-system malformations. Lancet 1:306–308
28. Cochrane DD, Finley C, Kestle J et al (2000) The patterns of late deterioration in patients with transitional lipomyelomeningocele. Eur J Pediatr Surg 10(Suppl 1):13–17
29. Copp AJ (1993) Neural tube defects. Trends Neurosci 16: 381–383
30. Cotter AM, Daly SF (2005) Neural tube defects: is a decreasing prevalence associated with a decrease in severity? Eur J Obstet Gynecol Reprod Biol 119:161–163
31. Cremer R, Hoppe A, Kleine-Diepenbruck U et al (1998) Longitudinal study on latex sensitization in children with spina bifida. Pediatr Allergy Immunol 9:40–43
32. Cuckle H (1994) Screening for neural tube defects. In: Brock G, Marsh J (eds) Neural tube defects, CIBA Foundatiion Symposium. Wiley, Chichester, pp 253–269
33. De Wals P, Tairou F, Van Allen M et al (2007) Reduction in neural-tube defects after folic acid fortification in Canada. N Engl J Med 357:135–142
34. DeWald RL, Faut MM (1979) Anterior and posterior spinal fusion for paralytic scoliosis. Spine 4:401–409
35. Di Rocco C, Rende M (1989) Chiari malformations. In: Raimondi AJ, Choux M, DiRocco C (eds) The pediatric spine: developmental anomalies. Springer, New York, pp 57–90
36. Dirks PB (1995) The genetic basis of neurosurgical disorders. In: Youmans JR (ed) Neurological surgery. WB Saunders, Philadelphia, pp 811–828
37. Dormans JP, Templeton J, Schreiner MS et al (1997) Intraoperative latex anaphylaxis in children: classification and prophylaxis of patients at risk. J Pediatr Orthop 17:622–625
38. Drummond D, Guadagni J, Keene JS et al (1984) Interspinous process segmental spinal instrumentation. J Pediatr Orthop 4:397–404
39. Drummond D, Breed AL, Narechania R (1985) Relationship of spine deformity and pelvic obliquity on sitting pressure distributions and decubitus ulceration. J Pediatr Orthop 5:396–402
40. Eberle C (1988) Failure of fixation after segmental spinal instrumentation without arthrodesis in the management of paralytic scoliosis. J Bone Joint Surg Am 70: 696–703
41. Ferguson RL, Allen BL Jr (1983) Staged correction of neuromuscular scoliosis. J Pediatr Orthop 3:555–562
42. Flippin MA, Canale S, Akbarnia BA (2008) Spinal deformity in myelomeningocele. In: Kim D, Betz R (eds) Surgery of the pediatric spine. Thieme, New York, pp 467–477
43. Furman L, Mortimer JC (1994) Menarche and menstrual function in patients with myelomeningocele. Dev Med Child Neurol 36:910–917
44. Gau YL, Lonstein JE, Winter RB et al (1991) Luque–Galveston procedure for correction and stabilization of neuromuscular scoliosis and pelvic obliquity: a review of 68 patients. J Spinal Disord 4:399–410
45. Geiger F, Parsch D, Carstens C (1999) Complications of scoliosis surgery in children with myelomeningocele. Eur Spine J 8:22–26
46. Gentili A, Lima M, Ricci G et al (2006) Secondary prevention of latex allergy in children: analysis of results. Pediatr Med Chir 28:83–90

47. Gerber AC, Jorg W, Zbinden S et al (1989) Severe intraoperative anaphylaxis to surgical gloves: latex allergy, an unfamiliar condition. Anesthesiology 71:800–802
48. Gold M, Swartz JS, Braude BM et al (1991) Intraoperative anaphylaxis: an association with latex sensitivity. J Allergy Clin Immunol 87:662–666
49. Green N (2002) Folic acid supplementation and prevention of birth defects. J Nutr 132 (8 Suppl):2356S–2360S
50. Guille JT, Sarwark JF, Sherk HH et al (2006) Congenital and developmental deformities of the spine in children with myelomeningocele. J Am Acad Orthop Surg 14:294–302
51. Gullestad HP, Bretteville G, Lundar T et al (1993) Tissue expansion for the treatment of myelomeningocele. Case report. Scand J Plast Reconstr Surg Hand Surg 27: 149–151
52. Herman JM, McLone DG, Storrs BB et al (1993) Analysis of 153 patients with myelomeningocele or spinal lipoma reoperated upon for a tethered cord. Presentation, management and outcome. Pediatr Neurosurg 19: 243–249
53. Hoffer MM, Feiwell E, Perry R et al (1973) Functional ambulation in patients with myelomeningocele. J Bone Joint Surg Am 55:137–148
54. Holmes NM, Nguyen HT, Harrison MR et al (2001) Fetal intervention for myelomeningocele: effect on postnatal bladder function. J Urol 166:2383–2386
55. Holzman R S, Sockin S (1990) Hypotension, flushing, and bronchospasm in myelodysplasia patients (abstract). Anesthesiology 73:1123
56. Holzman RS (1993) Latex allergy: an emerging operating room problem. Anesth Analg 76:635–641
57. Hoppenfield S (1967) Congenital kyphosis in myelomeningocele. J Bone Joint Surg 49:276
58. Johnson MP, Gerdes M, Rintoul N et al (2006) Maternal-fetal surgery for myelomeningocele: neurodevelopmental outcomes at 2 years of age. Am J Obstet Gynecol 194: 1145–1150; discussion 1150–1142
59. Kahanovitz N, Duncan JW (1981) The role of scoliosis and pelvic obliquity on functional disability in myelomeningocele. Spine 6:494–497
60. Karlin L, Zimbler S (1990) The association of spondylolisthesis and myelomeningocele. The Pediatric Orthopaedic Society of North America, Annual Meeting, San Francisco, CA
61. Karol LA, Richards BS, Prejean E et al (1993) Hemodynamic instability of myelomeningocele patients during anterior spinal surgery. Dev Med Child Neurol 35:261–267
62. Kelly KJ, Kurup V, Zacharisen M et al (1993) Skin and serologic testing in the diagnosis of latex allergy. J Allergy Clin Immunol 91:1140–1145
63. Kennedy D, Koren G (1998) Valproic acid use in psychiatry: issues in treating women of reproductive age. J Psychiatry Neurosci 23:223–228
64. Korenromp MJ, van Gool JD, Bruinese HW et al (1986) Early fetal leg movements in myelomeningocele. Lancet 1: 917–918
65. Kwittken PL, Becker J, Oyefara B et al (1992) Latex hypersensitivity reactions despite prophylaxis. Allergy Proc 13: 123–127
66. Lawrence K (1967) Clinical and ethical considerations of alpha-fetoprotein for early prenatal diagnosis of neural tube malformations. Dev Med Child Neurol 16 (Suppl 32): 117
67. Letts M, Rathbone D, Yamashita T et al (1992) Soft Boston orthosis in management of neuromuscular scoliosis: a preliminary report. J Pediatr Orthop 12:470–474
68. Leynadier F, Pecquet C, Dry J (1989) Anaphylaxis to latex during surgery. Anaesthesia 44:547–550
69. Lindseth RE GG (1988) One stage anterior transpedicular and unilateral fusion for congenital scoliosis. Orthop Trans 12:184
70. Lindseth RE (1994) Myelomeningocele spine. In: Weinstein W (ed) The pediatric spine: principles and practice. Raven, New York, pp 1043–1067
71. Lindseth R (2001) Myelomeningocele. In: Morrissy RT, Weinstein SL (eds) Lovell and Winter's pediatric orthopaedics. Lippincott Williams & Wilkins, Philadelphia, pp 601–632
72. Locke MD, Sarwark JF (1996) Orthopaedic aspects of myelodysplasia in children. Curr Opin Pediatr 8:65–67
73. Luciano R, Velardi F (1989) Epidemiology and clues to the etiology of neural tube defects. In: Raimondi A, Choux M, DiRocco C (eds) The pediatric spine I: development and the dysraphic state. Springer, New York, pp 126–147
74. Luque ER (1982) Segmental spinal instrumentation for correction of scoliosis. Clin Orthop Relat Res 163: 192–198
75. Lyons A, Petrucelli, RJ (1978) Medicine, an illustrated history. Harry N. Abrams, New York
76. Mackel JL Lindseth RE (1975) Scoliosis and myelodysplasia. J Bone Joint Surg Am 57:1031
77. Mayfield JK (1981) Severe spine deformity in myelodysplasia and sacral agenesis: an aggressive surgical approach. Spine 6:498–509
78. Mazon A, Nieto A, Estornell F et al (1997) Factors that influence the presence of symptoms caused by latex allergy in children with spina bifida. J Allergy Clin Immunol 99: 600–604
79. Mazur J, Menelaus MB, Dickens DR et al (1986) Efficacy of surgical management for scoliosis in myelomeningocele: correction of deformity and alteration of functional status. J Pediatr Orthop 6:568–575
80. McLone DG, Herman JM, Gabrieli AP et al (1990) Tethered cord as a cause of scoliosis in children with a myelomeningocele. Pediatr Neurosurg 16:8–13
81. McLone DG (2003) Tethered cord in spina bifida. In: Lipotak G (ed) Evidence-based practice in spina bifida: developing a research agenda. Spina Bifida Association of America, Washington, D.C
82. McMaster MJ (1987) Anterior and posterior instrumentation and fusion of thoracolumbar scoliosis due to myelomeningocele. J Bone Joint Surg Am 69:20–25
83. Meeropol E, Kelleher R, Bell S et al (1990) Allergic reactions to rubber in patients with myelodysplasia. N Engl J Med 323:1072
84. Meuli M, Meuli-Simmen C, Hutchins GM et al (1997) The spinal cord lesion in human fetuses with myelomeningocele: implications for fetal surgery. J Pediatr Surg 32: 448–452
85. Miladi LT, Ghanem IB, Draoui MM et al (1997) Iliosacral screw fixation for pelvic obliquity in neuromuscular scoliosis. A long-term follow-up study. Spine 22:1722–1729
86. Mish M (ed) (1997) Merriam webster's collegiate dictionary. Merriam-Webster, Springfield

87. Moneret-Vautrin DA, Laxenaire MC, Bavoux F (1990) Allergic shock to latex and ethylene oxide during surgery for spinal bifida. Anesthesiology 73:556–558
88. Muller EB, Nordwall A (1992) Prevalence of scoliosis in children with myelomeningocele in western Sweden. Spine 17:1097–1102
89. Muller EB, Nordwall A, von Wendt L (1992) Influence of surgical treatment of scoliosis in children with spina bifida on ambulation and motoric skills. Acta Paediatr 81:173–176
90. Muller EB, Nordwall A (1994) Brace treatment of scoliosis in children with myelomeningocele. Spine 19:151–155
91. Muller EB, Nordwall A, Oden A (1994) Progression of scoliosis in children with myelomeningocele. Spine 19: 147–150
92. Nguyen DH, Burns MW, Shapiro GG et al (1991) Intraoperative cardiovascular collapse secondary to latex allergy. J Urol 146:571–574
93. Nieto A, Mazon A, Pamies R et al (2002) Efficacy of latex avoidance for primary prevention of latex sensitization in children with spina bifida. J Pediatr 140:370–372
94. Nolden MT, Sarwark JF, Vora A et al (2002) A kyphectomy technique with reduced perioperative morbidity for myelomeningocele kyphosis. Spine 27:1807–1813
95. Noonan K (2006) Myelominingocele. In: Morrissy RT, Weinstein SL (eds) Lovell and Winter's pediatric orthopaedics. Lippincott Williams and Wilkins, Philadelphia, pp 605–647
96. Okamoto GA, Lamers JV, Shurtleff DB (1983) Skin breakdown in patients with myelomeningocele. Arch Phys Med Rehabil 64:20–23
97. Osebold WR, Mayfield JK, Winter RB et al (1982) Surgical treatment of paralytic scoliosis associated with myelomeningocele. J Bone Joint Surg Am 64:841–856
98. Pang D, Wilberger JE Jr (1982) Tethered cord syndrome in adults. J Neurosurg 57:32–47
99. Paonessa KJ, Zide B, Errico T, Engler GL (1991) Using tissue expanders in spinal surgery for deficient soft tissue or postirradiation cases. Spine 16:S324–S327
100. Parasini P, Greggi T, DiSilvestre M (eds) (2002) Surgical treatment of scoliosis in myelomingocele. IOS Press, Amsterdam
101. Parisini P, Greggi T, DiSilvestre M et al (2002) Surgical treatment of scoliosis in myelomeningocele. In: Griv TB (ed) Research into spinal deformities 4. IOS Press, Amsterdam
102. Parsch D, Geiger F, Brocai DR et al (2001) Surgical management of paralytic scoliosis in myelomeningocele. J Pediatr Orthop 10:10–17
103. Pecquet C, Leynadier F, Dry J (1990) Contact urticaria and anaphylaxis to natural latex. J Am Acad Dermatol 22:631–633
104. Peelle MW, Lenke LG, Bridwell KH et al (2006) Comparison of pelvic fixation techniques in neuromuscular spinal deformity correction: Galveston rod versus iliac and lumbosacral screws. Spine 31:2392–2398; discussion 2399
105. Pierz K, Banta J, Thomson J et al (2000) The effect of tethered cord release on scoliosis in myelomeningocele. J Pediatr Orthop 20:362–365
106. Piggott H (1980) The natural history of scoliosis in myelodysplasia. J Bone Joint Surg Am 62-B:54–58
107. Proos LA, Dahl M, Ahlsten G et al (1996) Increased perinatal intracranial pressure and prediction of early puberty in girls with myelomeningocele. Arch Dis Child 75:42–45
108. Rang M (2000) The story of orthopaedics. W.B. Saunders, Philadelphia
109. Raycroft JF, Curtis B (1972) Spinal curvature in myelomeningocele: natural history and etiology. Symposium on myelomeningocele. C.V. Mosby, Hartford
110. Reigel D (1982) Spina bifida. In: Section of Pediatric Neurosurgery of the American Association of Neurological Surgeons (ed) Pediatric neurosurgery: surgery of the developing nervous system. Grune and Stratton, New York, pp 23–47
111. Reigel D (1983) Tethered spinal cord. In: Humphrey R (ed) Concepts in pediatric neurosurgery. Karger, Basil, p 142
112. Rodgers WB, Frim DM, Emans JB (1997) Surgery of the spine in myelodysplasia. An overview. Clin Orthop Relat Res:19–35
113. Rodgers WB, Williams MS, Schwend RM et al (1997) Spinal deformity in myelodysplasia. Correction with posterior pedicle screw instrumentation. Spine 22:2435–2443
114. Rotenstein D, Reigel DH (1996) Growth hormone treatment of children with neural tube defects: results from 6 months to 6 years. J Pediatr 128:184–189
115. Samuelsson L, Eklof O (1988) Scoliosis in myelomeningocele. Acta Orthop 59:122–127
116. Samuelsson L, Skoog M (1988) Ambulation in patients with myelomeningocele: a multivariate statistical analysis. J Pediatr Orthop 8:569–575
117. Sarwark JF (1996) Spina bifida. Pediatr Clin North Am 43:1151–1158
118. Schoenmakers MA, Gulmans VA, Gooskens RH et al (2005) Spinal fusion in children with spina bifida: influence on ambulation level and functional abilities. Eur Spine J 14:415–422
119. Schut L, Bruce DA, Sutton LN (1983) The management of the child with a lipomyelomeningocele. Clin neurosurg 30:464–476
120. Setlock MA, Cotter TP, Rosner D (1993) Latex allergy: failure of prophylaxis to prevent severe reaction. Anesth Analg 76:650–652
121. Shurtleff DB, Goiney R, Gordon LH et al (1976) Myelodysplasia: the natural history of kyphosis and scoliosis. A preliminary report. Dev Med Child Neurol Suppl: 126–133
122. Shurtleff DB, Lemire RJ (1995) Epidemiology, etiologic factors, and prenatal diagnosis of open spinal dysraphism. Neurosurg Clin N Am 6:183–193
123. Slater JE (1989) Rubber anaphylaxis. N Engl J Med 320:1126–1130
124. Slater JE, Mostello LA, Shaer C et al (1990) Type I hypersensitivity to rubber. Ann Allergy 65:411–414
125. Slater JE (1992) Allergic reactions to natural rubber. Ann Allergy 68:203–209
126. Smithells RW, Nevin NC, Seller MJ et al (1983) Further experience of vitamin supplementation for prevention of neural tube defect recurrences. Lancet 1:1027–1031
127. Sockin SM, Young MC (1991) Preoperative prophylaxis of latex anaphylaxis (Abstract). J Allergy Clin Immunol 87: 269

128. Sponseller PD, Young AT, Sarwark JF et al (1999) Anterior only fusion for scoliosis in patients with myelomeningocele. Clin Orthop Relat Res 364:117–124
129. Stanitski CL, Stanitski DF, LaMont RL (1994) Spondylolisthesis in myelomeningocele. J Pediatr Orthop 14: 586–591
130. Stark A, Saraste H (1993) Anterior fusion insufficient for scoliosis in myelomeningocele: 8 children 2–6 years after the Zielke operation. Acta Orthop Scand 64:22–24
131. Steinbok P, Irvine B, Cochrane DD et al (1992) Long-term outcome and complications of children born with meningomyelocele. Childs Nerv Syst 8:92–96
132. Stevens DB, Beard C (1989) Segmental spinal instrumentation for neuromuscular spinal deformity. Clin Orthop Relat Res:164–168
133. Stoll C, Alembik Y, Dott B (2006) Are the recommendations on the prevention of neural tube defects working? Eur J Med Gen 49:461–465
134. Sussman GL, Tarlo S, Dolovich J (1991) The spectrum of IgE-mediated responses to latex. JAMA 265:2844–2847
135. Sutton LN, Adzick NS, Bilaniuk LT et al (1999) Improvement in hindbrain herniation demonstrated by serial fetal magnetic resonance imaging following fetal surgery for myelomeningocele. JAMA 282:1826–1831
136. Swank M, Dias L (1992) Myelomeningocele: a review of the orthopaedic aspects of 206 patients treated from birth with no selection criteria. Dev Med Child Neurol 34:1047–1052
137. Toriello HV, Higgins JV (1983) Occurrence of neural tube defects among first-, second-, and third-degree relatives of probands: results of a United States study. Am J Med Genet 15:601–606
138. Tosi LL, Slater JE, Shaer C et al (1993) Latex allergy in spina bifida patients: prevalence and surgical implications. J Pediatr Orthop 13:709–712
139. Trivedi J, Thomson JD, Slakey JB et al (2002) Clinical and radiographic predictors of scoliosis in patients with myelomeningocele. J Bone Joint Surg Am 84-A:1389–1394
140. Trollmann R, Dorr HG, Strehl E et al (1996) Growth and pubertal development in patients with meningomyelocele: a retrospective analysis. Acta Paediatr 85:76–80
141. Trollmann R, Strehl E, Wenzel D et al (1998) Arm span, serum IGF-1 and IGFBP-3 levels as screening parameters for the diagnosis of growth hormone deficiency in patients with myelomeningocele – preliminary data. Eur J Pediatr 157:451–455
142. Trollmann R, Strehl E, Wenzel D et al (2000) Does growth hormone (GH) enhance growth in GH-deficient children with myelomeningocele? J Clin Endocrinol Metab 85:2740–2743
143. Trollmann R, Langhans B, Strehl E et al (2001) A cross-sectional study of dehydroepiandrosterone sulfate in prepubertal children with myelomeningocele. Horm Res 56:19–24
144. Tulipan N, Sutton LN, Bruner JP et al (2003) The effect of intrauterine myelomeningocele repair on the incidence of shunt-dependent hydrocephalus. Pediatr Neurosurg 38:27–33
145. Turjanmaa K, Reunala T, Rasanen L (1988) Comparison of diagnostic methods in latex surgical glove contact urticaria. Contact Derm 19:241–247
146. Wai EK, Young NL, Feldman BM et al (2005) The relationship between function, self-perception, and spinal deformity: Implications for treatment of scoliosis in children with spina bifida. J Pediatr Orthop 25: 64–69
147. Wald NJ, Cuckle H, Brock JH et al (1977) Report of UK collaborative study of alpha-fetoprotein in relation to neural tube defects: maternal serum-alpha-fetoprotein measurement in antenatal screening for anencephaly and spina bifida in early pregnancy. Lancet 1:1323–1332
148. Ward WT, Wenger DR, Roach JW (1989) Surgical correction of myelomeningocele scoliosis: a critical appraisal of various spinal instrumentation systems. J Pediatr Orthop 9: 262–268
149. Wild A, Haak H, Kumar M et al (2001) Is sacral instrumentation mandatory to address pelvic obliquity in neuromuscular thoracolumbar scoliosis due to myelomeningocele? Spine 26:E325–E329
150. Winston K, Hall J, Johnson D et al (1977) Acute elevation of intracranial pressure following transection of non-functional spinal cord. Clin Orthop Relat Res:41–44
151. Yazici M, Asher MA, Hardacker JW (2000) The safety and efficacy of Isola–Galveston instrumentation and arthrodesis in the treatment of neuromuscular spinal deformities. J Bone Joint Surg Am 82:524–543
152. Yen IH, Khoury MJ, Erickson JD et al (1992) The changing epidemiology of neural tube defects. United States, 1968–1989. Am J Dis Child 146:857–861
153. Zerin JM, McLaughlin K, Kerchner S (1996) Latex allergy in patients with myelomeningocele presenting for imaging studies of the urinary tract. Pediatr Radiol 26:450–454

Spinal Dysraphism

21

Nejat Akalan

Key Points

- The term "spinal dysraphism" covers two types of spinal congenital malformations, traditionally grouped as "open" and "closed forms. These two groups have almost no features in common, including their embryological origin, presentation, natural history, and treatment algorithm.
- Open spinal dysraphism or myelomeningocele is primarily a neural tube closure defect, resulting with more or less very sereotypic lesion and clinical presentation. The aim of treatment is to preserve the neurological and clinical status of the newborn.
- Closed spinal dysraphism is far more complicated and is represented by various forms of different combinations of mesodermal structures. While the neurological impairment in myelomeningocele is straightforward related to the incomplete differentiation of the neural tissue, the mechanism of neurological impairment in closed dysraphisms are far more complex and controversial. This complexity, in turn, generates an ongoing controversy in establishing universal algorithms for treatment.

N. Akalan
Department of Neurosurgery, Institute of Neurological Sciences, Hacettepe University, 06100 Ankara, Turkey
e-mail: nakalan@hacettepe.edu.tr

Congenital spinal disorders that interfere with neurological function result from imperfect development of either the neural tissue itself or tissues which are designated to cover and support the spinal cord. In current terminology, the terms "spina bifida" and "spinal dysraphism" are used interchangeably to cover all spinal malformations derived from neuroectodermal and mesodermal origin. Those that are believed to be of neuroectodermal maldevelopment form the "open dysraphism" subgroup: "open = appert" implying a visible, exposed lesion of the neural tissue. This group is also called "neural tube defects" along with "anencephaly," which results from failure of fusion of the cranial neural tube. Mesodermal tissue derived embryological anomalies that directly or indirectly hamper normal neurological function form the "closed dysraphism" group with the assumption of the maldevelopment occurring over a normal neuroectodermal differentiation period. The term "closed = occult" describes an obscured lesion covered with intact skin unlike the open counterpart (Fig. 21.1). Although such a simplified classification scheme of spinal dysraphism, according to the embryological origin, may help in understanding and standardizing the diagnostic and therapeutic measures, the diverse clinical manifestations, natural course, and treatment protocols do not necessarily provide prescribed algorithms. Moreover, normal development of the spinal cord and its surroundings is far more complicated and intermingled rather than a consecutive differentiation of neuroectoderm and mesoderm. The insult at certain point of differentiation may contribute to both neural and adjacent tissue maldevelopment resulting with open and closed type of dysraphism exhibited in the same patient.

The aim of this chapter is to discuss the contemporary treatment protocols of this heterogeneous group with emphasis on changing concepts due to accumulating data on their embryogenesis, natural course, and therapeutic alternatives.

B. A. Akbarnia et al. (eds.), *The Growing Spine*,
DOI: 10.1007/978-3-540-85207-0_21, © Springer-Verlag Berlin Heidelberg 2011

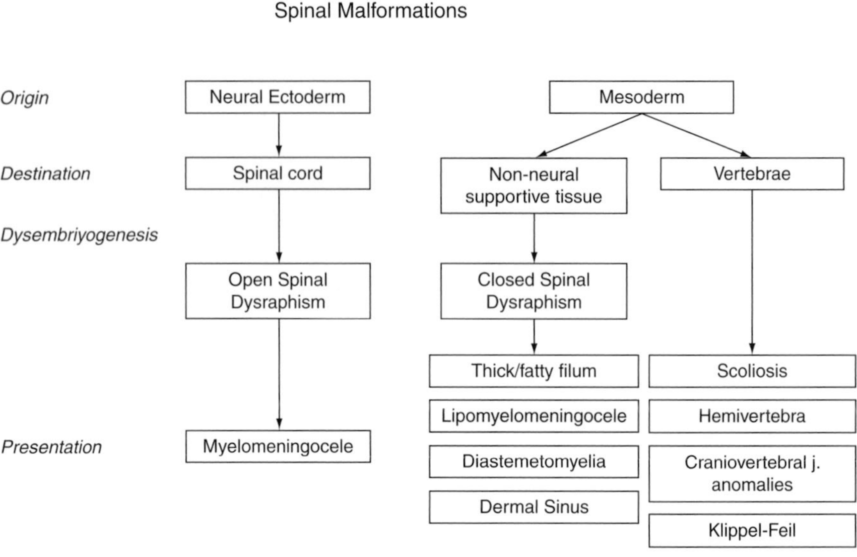

Fig. 21.1 Congenital spinal malformations; disordered embryogenesis during formation of neural tube from neural ectoderm results with myelomeningocele, while different forms of occult dysraphism may occur due to mesodermal disarrangement

21.1 Open Spinal Dysraphism (Myelomeningocele) (also see Chapter 20)

Formation of the spinal cord is identified as primary neurulation in classical embryology, wherein ectoderm of the bilaminar embryo undergoes a series of complex differentiation, yet not through a fully understood mechanism, to form the neural tube. This process requires molecular, biochemical, and mechanical interactions between neuroectodermal cells and adjacent ectodermal derivatives [6, 7, 14, 23]. Although primary neurulation itself represents neural tissue formation, it is closely dependent on the ongoing mesodermal activity that is responsible for the differentiation of the nonneuronal surrounding tissue. While notochordal induction is essential for initiating primary neurulation, a completed neurulation is required for appropriate differentiation of the surrounding tissue.

21.1.1 Pathogenesis

Neural tube formation starts at the 17th day of gestation during which the notochord induces the overlying ectoderm to differentiate into neuroectoderm to form the neural grove in the dorsal midline of the embryo. Neural folds on either side of the groove elevate and meet, the cells fuse dorsally, and primitive spinal cord is formed as a hollow cylinder. This process is completed by day 27 to 28 of gestation. Interruption of the neural tube formation dorsally at a particular segment(s) prevents normal neural tissue differentiation at that level. While this maldevelopment of the spinal cord structure causes a more or less complete neurological impairment below the affected level, additional abnormalities appear as a result of altered induction of the neural tube to the surrounding tissues [2, 7]. The consequence is a visible spinal cord segment, placode, representing an unclosed primitive neural tube remnant without meningeal, bony, or cutaneus enclosures dorsally. The term "spina bifida," although denotes only the missing posterior bony elements over the unclosed neural tissue, is confusingly used to describe the whole anomaly. Likewise, myeloschisis, spina bifida cystica, and myelomeningocele are terms attributive to the different morphological appearance of the same pathology contributing no practical purpose in terms of decision making, surgical technique, or outcome other than confusion. The term "myelomeningocele" is currently preferred to represent almost all variations of open spinal dysraphism that results from a common mechanism of maldevelopment [6, 16, 19].

Disordered embryogenesis of the segmental neural tube formation in myelomeningocele is attributed to either primary failure of neural tube closure or secondary opening after appropriate tube formation. The nonclosure theory is probably for the majority of human myelomeningoceles; however, overdistension may contribute to some experimental neural tube defect models

[7, 16]. Regardless the causative mechanism, unclosed neural tube triggers a cascade of events concerning the nonneural tissue that is designated to cover spinal cord dorsally. The cutaneus ectoderm remains attached to the open neural tube segment and fails to form the future skin over the lesion. Moreover, the normal mechanism in which the cutaneus ectoderm detaches from the dorsal side of the neural tube to allow paraxial mesoderm to move in between to give rise to bone and soft tissue is also distorted. The final pathological anatomy is an exposed lesion at birth, representing the inner surface of the spinal cord on the dorsal midline covered with membranous tissue as the epidermal remnants or exudate, with a groove continuous with the central canal of the unaffected segments. Immature laminar remnants and paraspinal muscles occupy lateral border of the widened spinal canal and can be palpated under the border of the skin defect (Fig. 21.2).

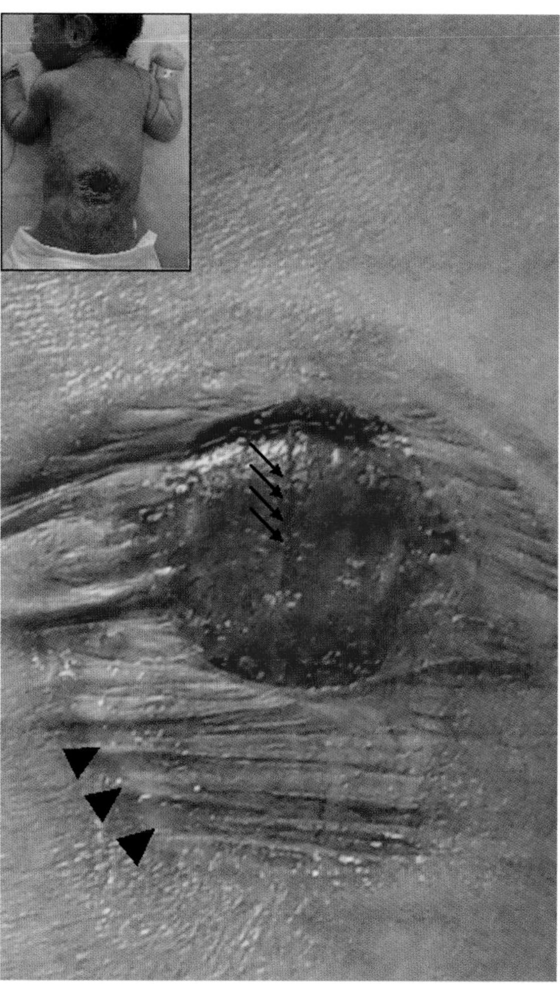

Fig. 21.2 A newborn with myelomeningocele (*upper left*), unclosed primitive neural tube remnant, placode, is exposed without any dorsal covering expect for membranes of epidermal remnants or exudate. The groove (*arrows*) represents the central canal. The healthy skin border (*arrow heads*) denotes the lateral edges of the widened spinal canal segment

21.1.2 Etiology and Epidemiology

Current hypotheses suggest that complex interactions between extrinsic and intrinsic variables are responsible for myelomeningoceles. Clinical and epidemiological data in humans implies maternal illnesses, medications, environmental toxins, and dietary factors such as folic acid that play causative or at least contributing roles in myelomeningocele development. On the other hand, increased incidence demonstrated in certain families situates neural tube defects into complex genetic disorders in which genes and the environment interact through an unknown relationship [7, 14, 23].

The incidence of myelomeningocele is generally accepted as 1/1,000 live births regardless the ethnic and geographic variability. Although several studies demonstrate a variation in different parts of the world depending on the geographic region, seasons at conception, gender of the affected infants, ethnicity, and socioeconomic status of the parents, maternal age and parity, and population-based surveillance studies fail to confirm a definitive correlation with the incidence [22]. A decrease in myelomeningocele frequency has been reported recently in some areas, while the incidence has been stable elsewhere [18]. Although this decrease has been attributed to increased prenatal diagnosis, selective terminations, genetic counseling, and mostly folic acid supplementation during pregnancy, there is no hard data to indicate that the decrease is due to a single factor [9, 13].

21.1.3 Presentation

Myelomeningocele represents one of the most devastating congenital malformations that are compatible with life. This is due to the fact that neurological impairment is inevitable for a myelomeningocele patient and the severity is proportional to the affected level of the spinal cord. As far as 80% of the disclosure takes place at the thoracolumbar spine, the child is practically born paraplegic. The level of neurological deficit descends as the lesion level moves caudally, at best chances; sacral localization avoids a major motor disturbance but ends up with a neurogenic bladder [4, 19, 27].

The neurologic deficit in myelomeningocele is thought to be due to not only incomplete differentiation of the neural tube but also exposure of the uncovered neural tissue to amniotic fluid, as well. Furthermore, associated anomalies extending to 63% as reported in fetal autopsy series contribute to the disability of the myelomeningocele cases [14]. Besides morphological abnormalities of the adjacent vertebral elements, almost all cases with myelomeningocele have associated Chiari II hindbrain malformation. The simplest representation of Chiari II malformation is herniation of the cerebellar tonsils and vermis to the cervical spinal canal through a tight foramen magnum. Additionally, medullary kinking, low-lying tentorium, tectal beaking, brain stem nuclei changes, polimicrogyria, gray matter heterotopias may be associated with the Chiari malformation. Main contribution of the tonsil herniation to the clinical picture of myelomeningocele is hydrocephalus. Hydrocephalus is present in almost 90% of myelomeningocele patients either during delivery or becoming apparent after surgical treatment [4, 6]. Hydrocephalus is one of the major coexisting factors that is responsible for morbidity and overall unfavorable outcome in myelomeningocele cases. Craniolacunae, a mesodermal self-limiting skull abnormality is also a frequent finding in the newborn.

From the practical viewpoint, a myelomeningocele case is born with signs of functional cord transection at the lesion level, neurogenic bladder and being a very close candidate for hydrocephalus. The open lesion carries a substantial risk of getting infected; cerebrospinal fluid exposure to external environment through incomplete dural barrier initiates meningitis and ventriculitis. Meningitis not only complicates a probable treatment for hydrocephalus but also adds the potential risk of seizures and further neurological impairment in terms of intellectual outcome.

21.1.4 Surgical Treatment

The aim of surgical treatment for myelomeningocele is to stabilize the clinical and neurological status of the newborn and prevent the potential risks of deterioration. This is best achieved by reconstructing the open neural tube and its coverings at the earliest possible convenience after birth. The initial management aims to stabilize the infant, avoiding contamination of the lesion and excluding the associated malformations. First, important concern at this point is the decision to treat. This has medical, ethical, and legal grounds to be discussed among two parties, parents and the physicians. In cases with a prenatal diagnosis, the parents have already been acknowledged for the consequences of a congenital anomaly and treatment options. Otherwise, the anticipated problems in myelomeningocele with the limited role of surgical repair in final outcome may result with refusal of surgical treatment. From the physicians' side, severe forms with multisegment, large lesions complicated with associated vertebral anomalies and hydrocephalus may create hesitation for treatment. Unless there is a life-threatening coexisting malformation, current ethico-legal opinion is to provide surgical treatment to all cases [4, 16, 19]. Once treatment has been decided, the second concern is the timing of the surgical procedure. Risks of immediate repair in a newborn should be weighed against the risk of contamination at delayed closure. Surgical repair within 48–72 h after birth is universally accepted and does not necessarily carry increased risk of contamination compared to very early treatment within first 24 h. Furthermore, the time interval provides sufficient postnatal evaluation and stabilization of the infant. Surgical technique by the simplest description is to mimic the normal embryological pattern of development. This is to isolate the nonfused segment, establish the original tube shape for the placode, and recreating and closing the dural envelope followed by approximation and closure of the skin over the lesion (Fig. 21.3). Even very large defects can be closed by relaxation incisions along the axis, avoiding complex muscle and skin flaps once advocated but proved to have major consequences. Almost 10% of cases would exhibit hydrocephalus during birth, which requires treatment simultaneously with the repair. Operative mortality is nearly zero and major morbidity is progressive hydrocephalus, wound infection, breakdown, and cerebrospinal fluid leakage.

Following myelomeningocele repair, the treatment of the other conditions may range from simple observation to extensive surgical procedures. Vast majority will require shunts for hydrocephalus before being

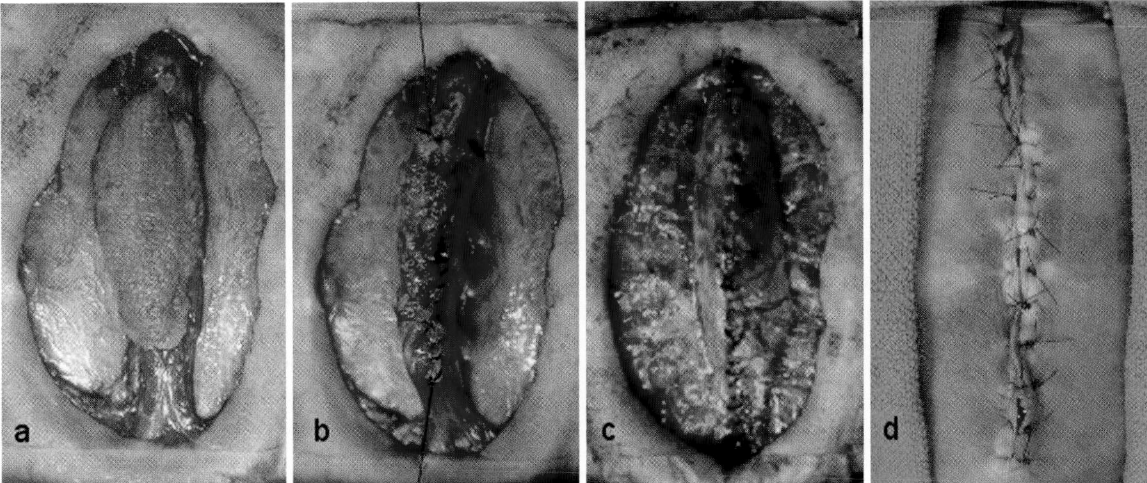

Fig. 21.3 Basic steps of myelomeningocele closure (**a**) Removing membranes and debris and exposure of the placode, (**b**) reapproximation of the flat placode to a tubular form with fine sutures for an easy closure, (**c**) detaching the dural layer from paravertebral fascia and watertight closure over the exposed neural tube, and (**d**) primary closure of the skin defect

discharged; future treatment might be required for associated kyphosis, Chiari malformation, foot deformities, and secondary tethering of the spinal cord for CM-II, syringomyelia, and/or TCS. While myelomeningocele may be regarded a static and nonprogressive defect, clinical worsening is caused by associated problems. Owing to the fact that myelomeningocele is located at thoracolumbar segments in almost 80% of the cases the child is committed to lifetime complications of paraplegia and neurogenic bladder. Therefore, the initial closure is just the beginning and outcome and long-term results greatly depend on the management of the associated conditions [4, 19]. At least 75% of children born with an open spina bifida can be expected to reach their early adult years. Survivors have a high incidence of problems related to pressure sores, obesity, severe renal disease, hypertension, depression, and visual impairment. Mortality is mostly related to shunt dysfunction and infection, urinary complications of neurogenic bladder, or respiratory tract infection [27].

Fetal myelomeningocele repair: fetal surgery is routinely performed for various conditions and myelomeningocele is also a good candidate for in utero repair since it is associated with considerable morbidity after postnatal care; it is compatible with life and can be detected before the 20th week of gestation. Furthermore, there is enough experimental evidence that some function of the placode is preserved initially but can be deteriorated during gestation or at birth. Fetal closure of the open neural tube can prevent secondary damage and preserve neurological function, while existing fetal potential for wound healing and axonal regeneration might reverse preexisting injuries to a certain degree. Since 1994, more than 330 cases of intrauterine repair have been performed by standard multilayer reconstruction through a hysterotomy between 19 and 25 weeks' gestation in certain centers worldwide. Preliminary findings suggest that intrauterine myelomeningocele repair lessens the degree of Chiari malformation and reduces the incidence of shunt-dependent hydrocephalus, but it does not statistically improve lower extremity or bladder function. Therefore, a multicenter randomized controlled trial was initiated in the USA to compare intrauterine with conventional postnatal care, in order to establish the procedure-related benefits and risks and no data from the trial will be published before the final analysis has been completed by the end of 2008 [29].

21.2 Closed (Occult) Spinal Dysraphism

Occult spinal dysraphisms represent a wide spectrum of malformations within congenital spinal disease, the only common feature being a mesodermal developmental error covered with normal skin [10]. Unlike the neuroectoderm that is designated to initiate the spinal cord, embryonic mesoderm gives rise to a variety of structures. Any disarrangement during the differentiation of this pluripotent layer triggers diverse forms of disease with regard to anatomy, clinical presentation, and treatment options. While the neurological impairment in open dysraphism is straightforward related to the incomplete differentiation of the neural tissue, the mechanism of neurological consequences in closed forms are far more complex and controversial. This complexity, in turn, generates an ongoing controversy in establishing universal algorithms for treatment.

21.2.1 Pathogenesis

Neurulation is responsible for the formation of the spinal cord till the future second sacral segment, and the most distal segment of the spinal cord develops by a process called secondary neurulation from the neural ectoderm cell mass caudal to the neural tube, the caudal eminence. Caudal eminence is formed from pluripotent cells derived from the regressing primitive streak. The mesenchymal neural cord then becomes an epithelial cord, acquires a lumen by canalization and regression process, attaches to the primary neural tube, and forms the remaining sacral and coccygeal segments of the spinal cord including the terminal filum [6, 12, 14]. Developmental errors during secondary neurulation, besides several anomalies, lead to the formation of fatty and short/thick filum, a classical representative of occult spinal dysraphism. Other major occult forms of dysraphism; split cord malformations (SCMs) (diastematomyelia), lipomyelomenigoceles, and dermal sinuses represent disordered mesodermal differentiation belonging to different stages during primary neurulation, before secondary neurulation begins [28]. The setoff time for the mesodermal maldevelopment and the stage of neurulation at that instance are critical for the neurological consequences. The more the primary neurulation is disrupted, the chances are higher to be born with a neurological compromise. This is one of the main reasons why, in different forms of occult dysraphism, resultant neurological status ranges from normal to severe impairment, sometimes compatible to myelomeningocele. Segmental, asymmetrical involvement of neurulation results with lower extremity changes; leg or buttock asymmetry, hip and knee problems, and foot deformities that typically worsen due to the muscle imbalance, weight bearing, and gravity as the child grows [16].

21.2.2 Diastematomyelia (SCMs)

SCMs represent a mesodermal anomaly belonging to the earliest stages of embryogenesis. The terms diastematomyelia and diplomyelia refer to a segment formed in two separate hemicords either in individual dural sleeves separated by a bony-cartilaginous septum in between (SCM type I) or hemicords separated by fibrous septa in a single dural sac (SCM type II). Pang et al. [25] introduced this new nomenclature and a new theory for the formation of these anomalies. An adhesion between the ectoderm and endoderm leads to an endomesenchymal tract that divides the spinal cord. In the first weeks of gestation, the primitive neurenteric canal temporarily connects the yolk sac of endodermal origin with the amnion, which is ectodermal in origin. While the primitive neurenteric canal regresses, a second endodermal–ectodermal communication, the accessory, neurenteric canal appears. The persistence of the anterior end of the accessory neurenteric canal causes intestinal duplication, the formation of a fibrous band that interferes with intestinal rotation, or the development of a neurenteric cyst and the persistence of the posterior end results in cutaneous abnormalities such as angiomas, umbilical lesions, and hypertrichosis. The notochord is forced to develop in two separate pieces by the persistence of the intermediate part at that level. The neural ectoderm over the separated notochord is forced to form two separate neural tubes, in return. The duplication of the notocord further initiates abnormal vertebral body formation, like hemivertebrae, bifid, hypertrophic or hyperplastic vertebrae, fusion of adjacent vertebral bodies comprising associated congenital spinal deformity. In this context, a hairy patch marking the level of the malformation mostly at the thoracolumbar area and scoliosis occasionally with lower extremity changes are the hallmarks of classical SCM.

21.2.3 Spinal Lipoma (Lipomyelomeningocele)

Often used as a general term for all lumbosacral lipomas, lipomyelomeningocele refers to a malformation in which a subcutaneous mass of fat extends through a deficient dorsolumbar fascia and lamina to attach to an open neural placode similar to a myelomeningocele. In this most frequently encountered form of occult dysraphism, the lipoma often tethers the cord asymmetrically, leading to

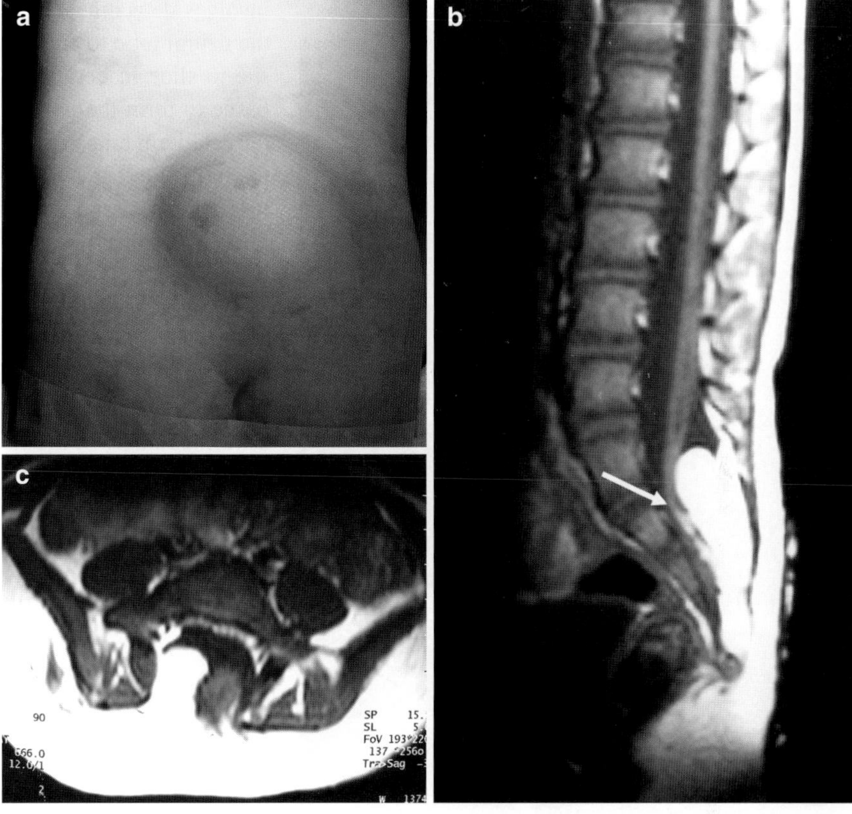

Fig. 21.4 (**a**) Lipomyelomeningocele in a 2-year-old girl. (**b**) Sagittal T1-weighed image reveals a fatty mass attached to conus where conus (*arrow*) lies at almost S1 level instead of L1–2 (**c**) Axial view demonstrates intimate fat-conus interface with a marked torsion of conus and the roots due to lipoma

rotation of the cord and the unequal development of nerve roots. Among various speculative theories, a current theory that accounts for the surgical anatomy is that of McLone et al. [20] and Naidich et al. [21]. It is proposed that the separation of the neural tube from the surrounding ectoderm, disjunction, occurs prematurely, leaving the neural plate open posteriorly and allowing mesenchymal cells to enter this cleft, where they are induced by the primitive ependyma to form fatty tissue, while the remaining anterior half of the neural tube induces the development of normal meningeal and vascular structures. The resulting anatomy is a skin-covered lumbosacral mass continuous through a defective bone and muscular tissue to adhere a partially open spinal cord segment (Fig. 21.4). Subsequent neurological picture at birth varies from normal to asymmetrical lower extremity involvement with neurogenic bladder, similar to SCM.

21.2.3.1 Thick/Fatty Filum

Thick/fatty filum represents a true defective secondary neurulation process where normally the caudal mass, upon completion of the neural tube – primary neurulation – undergoes a canalization and retrogressive differentiation process to form the spinal cord below the lumbar enlargement including the filum terminale. Development of thick/fatty filum is a poorly understood process. Current theories on the maldevelopment of filum terminale with lipomatous lesions center on faulty retrogressive differentiation, with differentiation of pluripotent caudal mass cells into adipocytes. Such a theory is consistent with the observations that these lesions are less frequently associated with cutaneous stigmata, as secondary neurulation occurs after the closure of the overlying ectoderm, and that they often occur in conjunction with other malformations of the caudal cell mass, such as sacral agenesis and VATER syndrome. The consistent finding is a low-lying conus ending well below the level of L1–2 vertebral segments, attached to a thickened, short and fatty filum terminale (Fig. 21.5). This is also reflected to the clinical presentation as almost all cases present with exclusively neurological signs and symptoms of conus involvement apparently at late childhood, without any orthopaedic or vertebral deformity [10, 11, 15]. Fatty filum is also referred to as filum terminale lipoma and included as a subgroup of

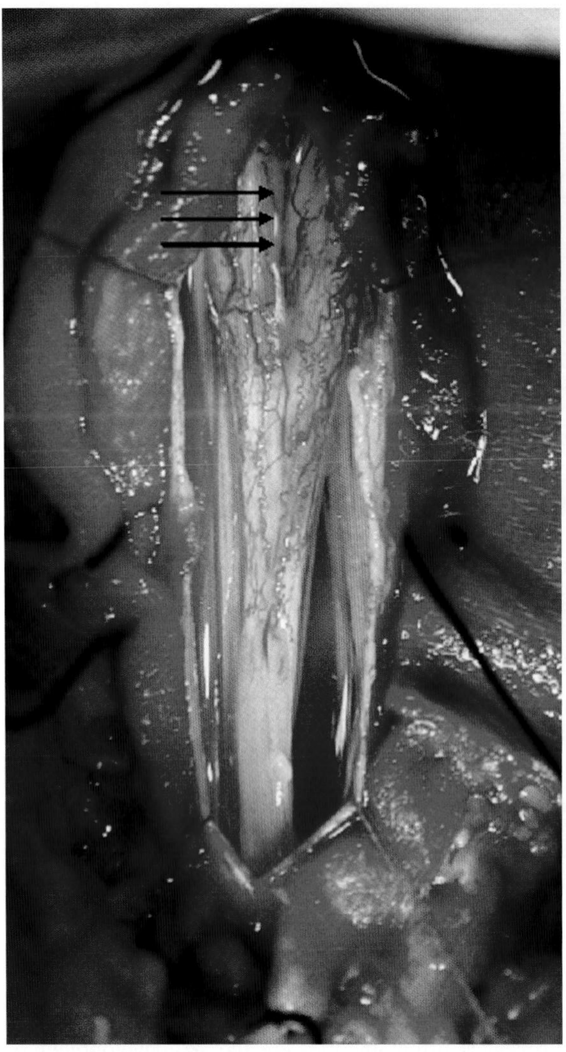

Fig. 21.5 Thick/fatty filum with an additional type II split cord malformation where two hemicords separated by fibrous bands lying within a single dura (*arrows*)

spinal lipomas along with lipomyelomenigoceles and believed to be of common embryological origin.

21.2.3.2 Spinal Dermal Sinus

Spinal dermal sinuses are believed to occur due to incomplete disjunction of the cutaneous ectoderm from the underlying neural ectoderm following the dorsal closure of the neural tube. Disjunction process involves detachment of the cutaneous ectoderm from the neural tube to enable the paraxial mesodermal tissue to slide in between to give rise to bone and soft tissue to form the dorsal aspect future spinal canal. If the ectoderm fails to detach at a given point, most often the future lumbar area, an elongated, the resulting malformation is skin-derived tract connecting the skin surface to the dura through a bony opening and fascia defect [12].

Besides the earlier mentioned common occult dysraphic states, meningocele manqué, neurenteric cysts, terminal syrinx, and caudal regression syndrome are other forms that occur with disordered embryogenesis at various stages of mesodermal differentiation. Although these pathologies may occasionally have a similar pattern in terms of neurological insult, they usually require a different algorithm for treatment and will not be encountered here.

21.2.4 Epidemiology

The true incidence of occult dysraphism is very difficult to assess. Unlike open dysraphisms, closed defects may be asymptomatic throughout the life and diagnosed with the onset of symptoms or incidentally found during workup of unrelated problems. Unlike the reported decline of the incidence of myelomeningocele, the incidence of closed dysraphisms has been increasing due to greater clinical awareness and incidental detection provided by MRI [1].

21.2.5 Presentation

Although malformations within the occult dysraphism group exhibit diverse pathological and clinical properties due to the different embryological step involved, there is a general tendency to unite all these malformations due to a similar pathophysiological mechanism by which symptoms arise. Almost all of the described malformations have a high rate of associated anomalies that would initiate a set of events as scoliosis, lower extremity deformities, and genitourinary anomalies apparent at birth but a substantial number of cases are born with no sign at all except for some cutaneous lesions in some. The existing neurological symptoms or a potential for developing neurological symptoms in time is attributed in a great extent to cord tethering, a term which is interchangeably used as a synonym to occult spinal dysraphism.

The theory of the tethered spinal cord is based on the pathological fixation and mechanical stretching of the lumbosacral cord. During embryogenesis, spinal column elongates and grows much faster than the neural tissue. While neural and corresponding vertebral levels lie on the same plane until the end of third gestational month, the different rate of growth results with conus medullaris to ascend and move to almost L2 vertebral level at term. Mesodermal disarrangement during secondary neurulation in which spinal cord tissue lies adjacent to the same vertebral segments prevents the conus to ascend and remain at its original low-lying position (see Fig. 21.1). Within this context, it is postulated that any inelastic structure like a thick and fatty filum, bony septum, or lipoma anchoring the caudal end of the spinal cord that prevents cephalad movement causes chronic and progressive ischemic spinal cord injury. The resulting clinical outcome includes lower limb motor and sensory deficits, incontinence, and musculoskeletal deformities of various degree and combination [7, 30, 31]. Although tethered spinal cord concept and its pathophysiology are universally accepted, there is major controversy on certain aspects, especially in treatment algorithms of this syndrome [8, 26, 32].

21.2.6 Treatment

There are different clinical presentations in a given type of occult dysraphisms. Appert spinal dysraphisms, where underlying embryological disarrangement, pathological anatomy, and the clinical consequence is almost identical for any case, the algorithm for surgical treatment is straightforward. Unlike the Appert forms, occult dysraphic states present within a wide spectrum of clinical findings from asymptomatic to severe neurological dysfunction. The true incidence and natural course is not clear, which further perplex the decision-making process.

As far as the surgical intervention for occult dysraphism is more or less surgery for the tethered spinal cord, the ultimate goal should be to improve or stabilize deficits in the a symptomatic patient and to prevent future deficits in the asymptomatic ones by detethering the spinal cord. Within this context, decision making is straightforward in those with significant dysraphic abnormality and clear clinical deterioration. Potential benefits of surgery are expected to outweigh the risks. For those with normal neurological finding or stable deficit and in those with incidentally discovered abnormality, the decision-making process becomes less clear and more controversial [3, 8]. While it has been commonly accepted that clinical deterioration is inevitable in asymptomatic cases and therefore prophylactic surgery should be undertaken, conflicting data exists in this regard. Certain forms of disease like thick/fatty filum can be prophylactically treated with a high level of confidence, especially the complex malformations such as lipomyelomenigoceles carry a significant neurological morbidity (Fig. 21.6). Complications in patients with preexisting deficits might be more tolerable, while neurologically normal patients are particularly distressing to surgeons as well as patients [5, 8, 17, 24]. A common scenario is a child with coexisting malformations of different patterns of maldevelopment. Split cord malformations and coexisting vertebral segmentation with scoliosis and urogenital malformations in caudal regression syndrome require different specialties to work simultaneously. There is no evidence-based treatment algorithm that exists in staging or precedence of approach by different surgical teams. While there is no conflict on removing a bony spur and dural reconstruction of a type 1 SCM before correction of scoliosis at the corresponding segments; it is questionable that the benefit gained by removing those remote and neurologically intact SCM either type 1 or 2 or other forms of radiologically diagnosed dysraphisms just for the sake of safe scoliosis correction.

No clear diagnostic or treatment strategy based on basic research and prospective clinical trials exists for occult dysraphism and tethered spinal cord. Until the results of such research are available, indications for treatment remain to be confined to personal experience, expertise, and complexity of the lesion, with the substantial risk of over- and under-treatment.

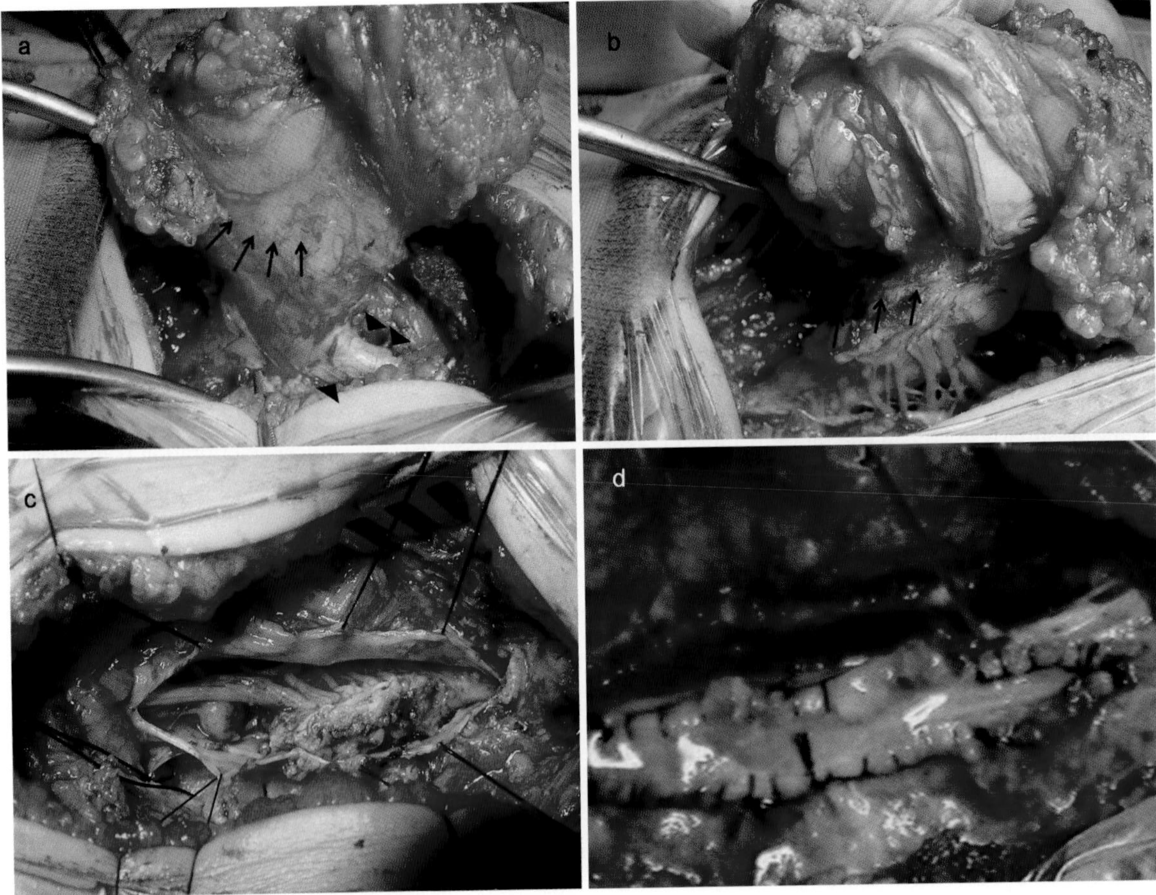

Fig. 21.6 Lipomyelomeningocele, basic steps for excision and untethering. (**a**) Subcutaneous part is freed from surrounding soft tissue and subcutaneous fat and followed to the entrance into intraspinal compartment through the enlarged multilevel spina bifida (*arrowheads*) and dural defect (*arrows*). (**b**) Intradural component is removed from the spinal cord tissue leaving a layer of fat at the cord-lipoma interface (*arrows*). (**c**) Final appearance following resection, note the transverse orientation of the roots unlike the normal longitudinal arrangement of cauda equina due to ascendence of conus during embryogenesis. (**d**) Dural closure should be done with a generous dural patch to prevent cerebrospinal fluid leakage and retethering

References

1. Bui CJ, Tubbs RS, Oakes WJ (2007) Tethered cord syndrome in children: a review. Neurosurg Focus 23(2):E2
2. Campbell LR, Dayton DH, Sohal GS (1986) Neural tube defects: a review of human and animal studies on the etiology of neural tube defects. Teratology 34:171–187
3. Chapman P, Stieg PE, Magge S et al (1999) Spinal lipoma controversy. Neurosurgery 44:186–193
4. Cohen AR, Robinson S (2001) Early management of myelomeningocele. In: McLone DG (ed): Pediatric neurosurgery: surgery of the developing nervous system, 4th edn. WB Saunders, Philadelphia, pp 241–260
5. Cochrane DD (2007) Cord untethering for lipomyelomeningocele: expectation after surgery. Neurosurg Focus 23(2):E9
6. Dias MS, McLone DG (2001) Normal and abnormal early development of the nervous system. In McLone DG (ed) Pediatric neurosurgery: surgery of the developing nervous system, 4th edn.WB Saunders, Philadelphia, pp 31–71
7. Dias MS, Partington M (2004) Embryology of myelomeningocele and anencephaly. Neurosurg Focus 16(2):E1
8. Drake JM (2006) Occult tethered cord syndrome: not an indication for surgery. J Neurosurg 104:(5 Suppl): 305–308
9. Eurocat Working Group (1991) Prevalence of neural tube defects in 20 regions of Europe and impact of prenatal diagnosis, 1980–1986. J Epidemiol Community Health 45:52–58
10. Finn MA, Walker ML (2007) Spinal lipomas: clinical spectrum, embryology, and treatment. Neurosurg Focus 23:(2):E10
11. Hoffman HJ, Taecholarn C, Hendrick EB et al (1985) Management of lipomyelomeningoceles. Experience at the Hospital for Sick Children, Toronto. J Neurosurg 62:1–8

12. Iskandar BJ, Oakes WJ (1999) Occult spinal dysraphism. In Albright AL, Pollack IF, Adelson PD (eds): Principles and practice of pediatric neurosurgery. Thieme, New York, pp 321–351
13. Lemire RJ (1988) Neural tube defects. JAMA 259:558–562
14. Kaplan KM, Spivak JM, Bendo JA (2005) Embryology of the spine and associated congenital abnormalities. Spine J 5:564–576
15. Kanev PM, Bierbrauer KS (1995) Reflections on the natural history of lipomyelomeningocele. Pediatr Neurosurg 22: 137–140
16. Kaufman BA (2004) Neural tube defects. Pediatr Clin North Am 51:389–419
17. Kulkarni AV, Pierre-Kahn A, Zerah M (2004) Conservative management of asymptomatic spinal lipomas of the conus. Neurosurgery 54:868–875
18. McDonnell R, Johnson Z, Doyle A et al (1999) Determinants of folic acid knowledge and use among antenatal women. J Public Health Med 21:145–149
19. McLone DG (1983) Results of treatment of children born with a myelomeningocele. Clin Neurosurg 30:407–412
20. McLone DG, La Marca F (1997) The tethered spinal cord: diagnosis, significance, and management. Semin Pediatr Neurol 4:192–208
21. Naidich TP, McLone DG, Mutluer S (1983) A new understanding of dorsal dysraphism with lipoma (lipomyeloschisis): radiologic evaluation and surgical correction. AJR Am J Roentgenol 140:1065–1078
22. Nikkila A, Rydhstrom H, Kallen B (2006) The incidence of spina bifida in Sweden 1973–2003: the effect of prenatal diagnosis. Eur J Public Health 6:660–662
23. Padmanabhan R (2006) Etiology, pathogenesis and prevention of neural tube defects. Congenit Anom 46:55–67
24. Palmer LS, Richards I, Kaplan WE (1998) Subclinical changes in bladder function in children presenting with nonurological symptoms of tethered cord syndrome. J Urol 159: 231–234
25. Pang D, Dias MS, Ahab-Barmada M (1992) Split cord malformation. Part I: a unified theory of embryogenesis for double spinal cord malformations. Neurosurgery 31: 451–480
26. Pierre-Kahn A, Zerah M, Renier D et al (1997) Congenital lumbosacral lipomas. Childs Nerv Syst 13:298–335
27. Talamonti G, D'Aliberti G, Collice M (2007) Myelomeningocele: long-term neurosurgical treatment and follow-up in 202 patients. J Neurosurg 107(5 Suppl):368–386
28. Tortori-Donati P, Rossi A, Cama A (2000) Spinal dysraphism: a review of neuroradiological features with embryological correlations and proposal for a new classification. Neuroradiology 42:471–491
29. Tubbs RS, Chambers MR, Smyth MD, Bartolucci AA, Bruner JP, Tulipan N, Oakes WJ (2003) Late gestational intrauterine myelomeningocele repair does not improve lower extremity function. Pediatr Neurosurg 38: 128–32
30. Yamada S, Iacono R, Yamada B (1996) Pathophysiology of the tethered spinal cord. In: Yamada S (ed) Tethered cord syndrome. American Association of Neurological Surgeons, Park Ridge, pp 29–45
31. Yamada S, Won DJ, Yamada SM (2004) Pathophysiology of tethered cord syndrome: correlation with symptomatology. Neurosurg Focus 16(2):E6
32. Warder DE, Oakes WJ (1993) Tethered cord syndrome and the conus in a normal position. Neurosurgery 33: 374–378

22 Other Neuromuscular Diseases

Burt Yaszay

Key Points

- Progressive neurological and muscle diseases can cause progressive and severe scoliosis.
- These diseases commonly affect the pulmonary and cardiac systems, which need to be considered when managing the scoliosis.
- Early intervention in Duchenne's muscular dystrophy is recommended to optimize cardiac and pulmonary function.
- Pelvic obliquity is commonly associated with the scoliosis, and in many cases, pelvic fixation is recommended.
- Segmental fixation is recommended in the osteopenic bone, which is commonly found in patients with neuromuscular scoliosis
- New methods of treating early onset neuromuscular scoliosis are being evaluated including growing rods, VEPTR, and Shilla procedure.

22.1 Duchenne's Muscular Dystrophy

Duchenne's muscular dystrophy (DMD) is an X-linked inherited disorder isolated to the dystrophin gene causing an absence in the protein dystrophin [69]. DMD is usually first diagnosed at the age of 5. Initial complaints by parents include delayed walking, clumsiness, or flat feet. It has been suggested to screen any boy not walking by 18 months for DMD [135]. A later concern by parents, usually at age 4 or 5, is their son's inability to keep up with his peers or increased difficulty climbing up stairs. Other clinical findings seen on exam include pseudohypertrophy of the calves, proximal muscle weakness, Achilles and iliotibial band contractures, and a positive Gowers sign.

In suspecting the diagnosis of DMD, the initial laboratory test is evaluating serum levels of creatine phosphokinase (CK). The diagnosis is then confirmed by genetic testing. In the remaining one-third of patients, a muscle biopsy is needed to specifically assess the quantity and quality of dystrophin present.

22.1.1 Spinal Deformity

Spinal deformity is the most critical orthopaedic issue for the patient with DMD. The incidence of scoliosis is about 95%. The onset of spinal deformity usually occurs between the ages of 10 and 14 years, at the same time when patients lose the ability to walk. The risk of progression of scoliosis is also very high. Smith et al. [130] reviewed the natural history of 51 patients with DMD and scoliosis who had no surgical treatment and were followed until their death. Seventeen of these patients had curves greater than 90°. The average rate of progression was 2.1° per month. In many cases, the curves continued to progress until the rib cage contacted the ilium.

The spinal deformity associated with DMD differs from the deformity seen in adolescent idiopathic scoliosis (AIS). The rate of progression is greater in muscular dystrophy patients [61, 70]. Unlike the typical hypokyphotic or lordotic patient with AIS, most progressive scoliosis in DMD patients is kyphotic in the sagittal

B. Yaszay
Pediatric Orthopaedics and Scoliosis Center, Rady Children's Hospital, San Diego, 3030 Children's Way, Suite 410, San Diego, CA 92123, USA
e-mail: byaszay@rchsd.org

B. A. Akbarnia et al. (eds.), *The Growing Spine*,
DOI: 10.1007/978-3-540-85207-0_22,

plane. Wilkins and Gibson [44, 141] suggested two types of spinal deformity in DMD. The more stable deformity is associated with an extended position, whereas the unstable pattern is characterized by a progressive kyphosis. Oda et al. [102] also utilized sagittal alignment to help differentiate the deformity in DMD into three types, recommending surgery for the kyphotic deformities.

Considering that scoliosis develops once the patient becomes wheelchair bound, screening is not needed while the patient is ambulatory. However, once the patient is unable to walk, radiographic screening should occur every 6 months.

22.1.2 Medical Considerations

In addition to the orthopaedic manifestations, there are considerable medical complications associated with DMD. The problem that is most concerning for the spine surgeon is the progressive worsening of pulmonary function. The muscle weakness, contractures and spinal deformity result in a restrictive disease pattern. This progressive decline typically occurs in the second decade of life, worsens with increasing age, and ultimately leads to the patient's death [53, 63, 64].

Kurz et al. [70] strongly suggested that age and curve severity negatively affect pulmonary function. Forced vital capacity peaked when the patient became unable to stand. Each year of age following, this then resulted in a forced vital capacity decline of 4%. If the patient developed scoliosis, an additional decline of 4% occurred for every 10° of thoracic scoliosis. A study by Yamashita et al. [142] also supported the relationship of scoliosis and pulmonary function.

Since age and thoracic scoliosis were the best predictors of pulmonary decline in their study, Kurz et al. [70] recommended early surgical intervention in the Duchenne's patient. Others have also made similar recommendations. Galasko et al. [42] demonstrated slightly improved survival and maintenance of forced vital capacity for the first 36 months in those patients who underwent surgery before progression occurred. Rideau et al. [111] found static vital capacity at 2 years in 5 surgically treated Duchenne patients. Recently, Velasco et al. [137] supported spinal stabilization, demonstrating a significant decrease in the rate of respiratory decline postsurgery compared with presurgery rates.

Some authors have contradicted the positive effects of surgery on pulmonary function. Their studies found no significant difference between the surgical and nonsurgical group in terms of declining respiratory function [93, 94, 125]. Kennedy et al. [65] demonstrated a similar decline in forced vital capacity of 3–5% per year in both operative and nonoperative patients. The criticism of this study was that the surgical patients had severe scoliosis with pulmonary function too poor to benefit from surgery [49]. A recent Cochrane review by Cheuk et al. [27] was unable to give an evidence-based recommendation regarding the effect of surgery on pulmonary function since no randomized controlled clinical trials have been performed.

Prior to any spinal surgery, preoperative pulmonary function tests should be performed. Typical problems encountered included prolonged intubation and the need for permanent tracheotomy. Recently, studies have suggested that with aggressive postoperative pulmonary management, patients with low forced vital capacity could successfully undergo spinal fusion [55, 86]. Of the 45 patients prospectively collected, Harper et al. found no difference in outcomes between patients with a forced vital capacity greater than 30% compared with those less than 30%. We recommend that if spinal fusion is contemplated, then early intervention be performed before further decline in pulmonary function. Short ventilatory assistance followed by early extubation and aggressive pulmonary management minimize the risk of atelectasis and pneumonia.

Patients with Duchenne's should also undergo a cardiac evaluation including echocardiogram. Cardiac involvement includes cardiomyopathy and conduction abnormalities [37, 109, 125]. In those patients with severely reduced cardiac function that cannot be controlled pharmacologically, surgery may not be an option.

Similar to other myopathies, there is an increased risk of malignant hyperthermia in DMD [57, 139]. In extreme cases, patients have died intraoperatively from sudden cardiac arrest. Typically, anesthesiologists refrain from using anesthetics that trigger malignant hyperthermia. Awareness of the risk will maximize the preparedness of the entire team for these medically complicated patients.

22.1.3 Nonsurgical Management of Scoliosis

Spinal deformity in the DMD patient rarely develops in the ambulatory patient. Therefore, close screening of these patients should begin when the patient begins using the wheelchair fulltime. In those rare cases when scoliosis develops in the ambulatory patients, bracing should not be utilized. It has been suggested that bracing is ineffective and may end the ability to walk [50]. For the nonambulatory scoliosis patient, bracing has also been discouraged. Multiple published reports have shown that while there is a decrease in the rate of progression, orthotics does not prevent the development of severe scoliosis [122, 135].

Since Drachman et al. [32] demonstrated positive outcome in the use of steroids for the treatment of DMD, there has been increasing work in investigating the effects on scoliosis. Corticosteroids have been found to stabilize muscle strength for a period of time [5]. A recent Cochrane Review found evidence to support the use of steroids to improve muscle strength and function in the short term (6–24 months) [84]. However, it is not completely clear whether this will have any change in the management of scoliosis. Some studies have suggested that similar to bracing steroids can delay the progression of scoliosis [3, 68, 143]. Alman et al. [3] prospectively compared 30 DMD patients treated with deflazacort with 24 similar control patients. Although they suggested that steroids slowed the progression of scoliosis, they were unable to demonstrate the prevention of spinal deformity. Kinali et al. [68] demonstrated that while steroids delayed the onset of scoliosis, it did not alter the severity at age 17. Currently, there is no data to support corticosteroids as a long-term option for the management of scoliosis. In addition, the use of steroids has to be balanced with the potential complications including weight gain, behavioral problems, fracture, glucose intolerance, gastrointestinal symptoms, skin changes, and cataracts [42, 84].

22.1.4 Surgical Management of Scoliosis

Posterior spinal instrumentation and fusion is the gold standard for the surgical treatment of DMD. For the patient with documented progressive scoliosis that can tolerate surgery there is little controversy for the need for surgical stabilization. The goal is to maintain sitting balance and patient mobility and minimize the effect of scoliosis on pulmonary function. Due to the high likelihood of developing scoliosis, some authors have suggested performing procedures when patients lose the ability to ambulate [130]. These are when patients have maximized their lung function and are most fit to withstand surgery from a pulmonary standpoint. Most authors, however, recommend surgery with radiographic evidence of scoliosis at about 20 – 30° [50, 59, 95, 134].

With the development of segmental instrumentation by Luque, there have been major improvements in the surgical stabilization of Duchenne's patients [82, 83]. Segmental instrumentation has improved the fixation in otherwise osteopenic bone and has minimized the need for prolonged immobilization. Currently, surgeons continue to effectively use the more traditional sublaminar wires with unit rods, whereas others have equal success with more modern instrumentation such as hooks or pedicle screws [119].

There is little controversy where the fusion should begin. It is recommended that the instrumentation should extend into the upper thoracic spine, typically, at T2 [50, 64, 95]. Stopping short of this may allow for cephalic progression of the curve due to progressive trunk and neck muscle weakness, causing the patient to lose head control.

The caudal extent of the fusion, however, continues to have some controversy. Specifically, should the instrumentation end at L5 or the pelvis? Fixation to the pelvis is technically more demanding, increasing both operative time and the potential risk of complications [1, 123]. Sussman [134] suggested that spinal fixation to L5 was sufficient in the early treated patients. Mubarak et al. [95] similarly concluded that instrumentation to L5 was sufficient if treatment was early when there was minimal pelvic obliquity (< 15°). They prospectively followed 12 patients with fusion to the sacrum and 10 patients with fusion to L5 only. The average follow-up was 7 years. Fusions to the pelvis took an additional 30 min longer. Review of the patients' sitting balance and postoperative pelvic obliquity demonstrated only minor differences between the groups.

Sengupta et al. [123] evaluated fixation to L5 utilizing modern pedicle screws and compared them to standard Galveston fixation or L-rod configuration to the pelvis. The minimum follow-up was 3 years. The pedicle screw group had a mean preoperative Cobb angle of 19.8° and pelvic obliquity of 9°. The pelvic group had a mean preoperative Cobb angle of 48° and pelvic obliquity of 19.8°. The pelvic group was on average about 2.5 years older at the time of surgery. The authors documented improved correction of the Cobb angle and pelvic obliquity in both groups. They also acknowledged the difference in deformity between the two groups. Their conclusion was that pedicle screw fixation to L5 provided a solid foundation for those patients who undergo surgery when performed early with minimal pelvic obliquity.

Other studies have recommended fusing to the pelvis at the initial time of surgical intervention [2, 13, 18, 41, 108]. Patients are healthiest at the first surgery. Any attempts to later fuse to the pelvis in those that have progressive pelvic obliquity will pose a greater risk with their worsening medical condition. Alman and Kim [2] reported on 48 Duchenne's patients who underwent spinal fusion. Thirty-eight patients with less than 10° of pelvic obliquity and 40° curvature underwent fusion and instrumentation to L5. Of these patients, 32 had progression of their pelvic obliquity. They found that curves with an apex below L1 were at the greatest risk of progression. Therefore, Alman and Kim recommended fusion to the pelvis for all curves with an apex below L1.

Gaine et al. [41] evaluated 85 patients who underwent spinal fusions to either L4, L5, sacrum, or ilium. They demonstrated that the more proximal the implant ended, the worse the correction of Cobb angles and pelvic obliquity. Intrapelvic fixation maintained the best correction in pelvic obliquity. Interestingly, they found no difference in correction of the pelvic obliquity between instrumentation and fusion that terminated at L5 compared with those that ended at S1.

Brook et al. [18] reported on the results of ten patients who underwent fusion above the pelvis with an L-rod and seven patients who had Galveston fixation to the pelvis. Six of the L-rod patients experienced some curve progression and sitting imbalance. The criticism of this study is that eight of the ten patients had curves greater than 40° and that preoperative pelvic obliquity was not recorded [50]. In addition, four of the ten patients had their fixation end at either L3 or L4.

Segmental instrumentation in the thoracic and lumbar spine has traditionally been with the use of sublaminar wires. With advancements made in instrumentation, some have chosen to use hooks or pedicle screws for the stabilization of the deformity. All have been shown to be effective in the treatment of scoliosis including those associated with DMD. Selection of implants is related to surgeon preference, cost, deformity, and patient anatomy and is beyond the scope of this chapter. Currently, my preferred technique is to utilize pedicle screws in the lumbar spine as well as at the cephalad portion of the construct. Depending on the deformity as well as bone quality I will utilize either sublaminar wires or pedicle screws in between in the thoracic spine (Fig. 22.1).

There are similar choices for instrumentation to the pelvis. Options include the Galveston techniques with either Luque or unit rods, Dunn-McCarthy technique with an s-rod, sacral screw, and iliac screw fixation [1, 18, 85, 89, 105]. Each has its own advantages and disadvantages. Galveston technique is subject to loosening and migration of the rod [64]. In addition, the Galveston technique sometimes requires complex three-dimensional contouring to fit the altered pelvic anatomy. Iliac screws, on the hand, are placed individually into each iliac wing and then connected to the rod through connectors. A recent study by Peelle et al. [105] demonstrated equal effectiveness in controlling pelvic obliquity between the Galveston technique and iliac screw fixation. My preferred method is to utilize iliac screws when instrumenting to the pelvis in Duchenne's patients.

Another important consideration in the preoperative planning for scoliosis is the risk of blood loss during surgery. Of all pediatric spine surgeries, DMD has demonstrated on average to have the highest mean level of blood loss [98, 128]. This is important considering their poor cardiac reserve. These patients require a large exposure from the upper thoracic spine to the lower lumbar spine or pelvis. The paraspinal muscles are difficult to elevate subperiosteally. Dysfunction of vascular smooth muscle as well as decreased platelet adhesion are thought to contribute to increased blood loss [98, 136]. Besides diligent hemostasis intraoperatively, the use of antifibrinolytics may help to minimize the blood loss. Shapiro et al. [129] retrospectively evaluated the use of tranexamic acid in 20 Duschenne's patients and compared them with 36 control patients. Tranexamic acid was found to reduce intraoperative blood loss and the need for homologous transfusions. Other options that have been published for AIS but not Duschenne's muscular dystrophy include the use aminocaproic acid or aprotinin [28, 39, 67]. We currently work with anesthesia preoperatively to insure that each patient is administered an antifibrinolytic during surgery. Intraoperative blood loss is also collected in a cell saver and given back to the patient. Postoperatively, hematocrits are monitored closely to insure that cardiac function is not overly stressed.

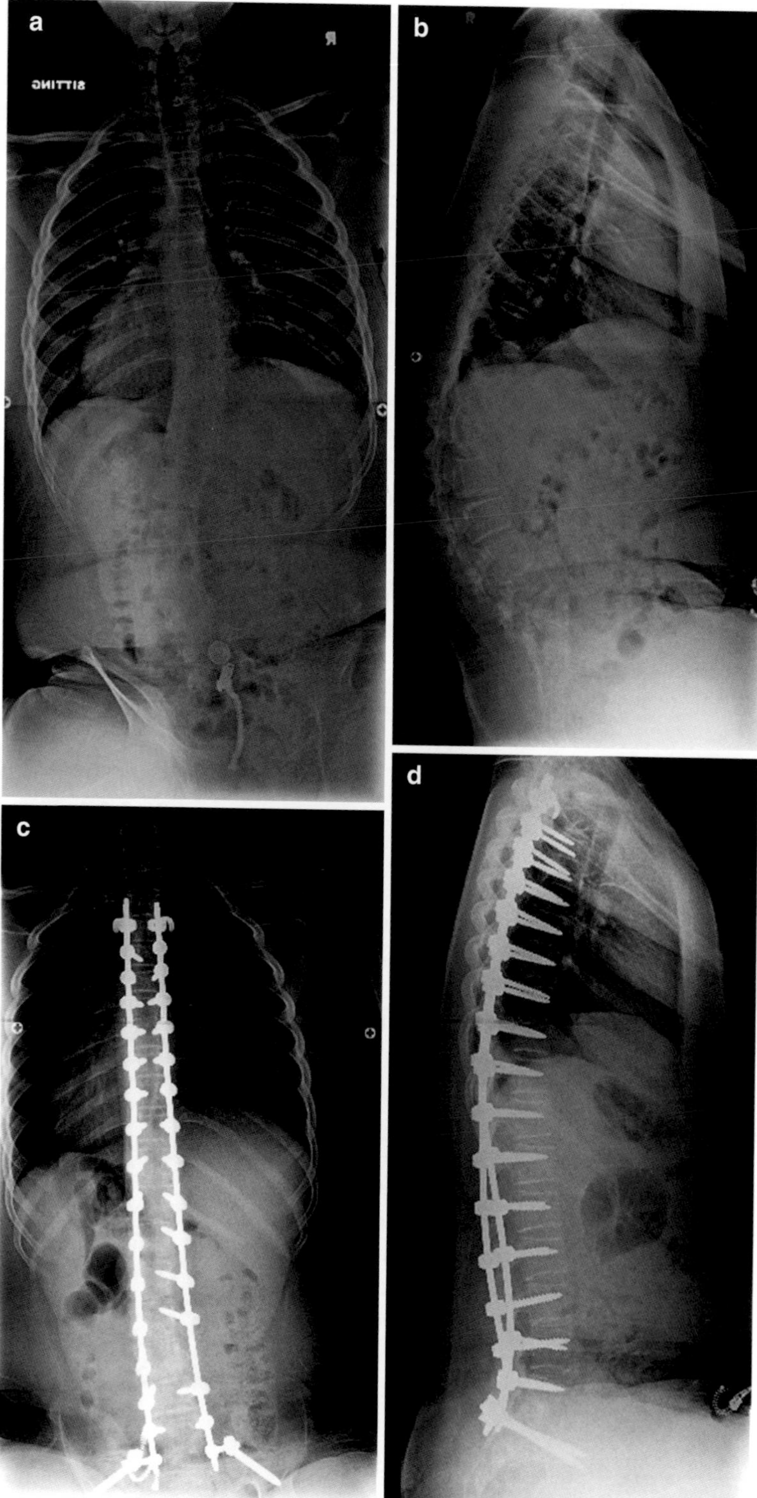

Fig. 22.1 (**a, b**) A 15-year-old male with DMD and progressive kyphoscoliosis. His lumbar curve is 40° and his kyphosis 51°. (**c, d**) Patient underwent posterior spinal instrumentation and fusion from T3 to the pelvis with iliac screws

22.1.5 Long-term Outcomes

As previously discussed there is controversy whether scoliosis surgery improves pulmonary function in the Duchenne's patient. A recent Cochrane Review by Cheuk et al. [27] was unable to provide an evidence-based recommendation for scoliosis surgery in DMD. Their reasoning was the lack of randomized clinical trials. Of the 36 relevant studies addressing the outcomes of scoliosis surgery, none met the inclusion criteria for review.

Studies have suggested that scoliosis surgery does benefit patients beyond pulmonary function [17, 25, 47]. Bridwell et al. [17] sent questionnaires to 33 patients with DMD evaluating function, self image, cosmesis, pain, quality of life, and satisfaction. Patients reported benefits in all the categorizes with the highest ratings in cosmesis, quality of life, and satisfaction. Granata et al. [47] found that sitting position, aesthetic improvement, and quality of life were all improved following spinal fusion. More than 90% of their patients/parents would give there consent again for surgery.

22.1.6 Conclusion

Spinal deformity commonly affects the male patient with DMD. Treatment of this deformity is complicated by the progressive muscle weakness and deteriorating pulmonary function. Current literature suggests that surgical management of the deformity can maintain upright sitting posture, improve quality of life and positively affect short-term pulmonary function. Unfortunately, a lack of randomized controlled trials has prevented any formal evidence-based recommendation from being made by a Cochrane Review. If surgery is contemplated, however, it should be performed early when the patient is at their maximal health. In addition, if there is more than mild pelvic obliquity, one should consider including the pelvis in the instrumentation and fusion.

22.2 Spinal Muscular Atrophy

Initially described by Werdnig, spinal muscular atrophy (SMA) is a rare autosomal recessive disorder characterized by degeneration of the anterior horn cells of the spinal cord and the neurons of the lower bulbar nuclei [114, 132]. Two genes are associated with this disease, the survival motor neuron gene and the neuronal apoptosis inhibitory protein gene [74]. SMN protein appears to interact with RNA-binding proteins and is found in both the nucleus and cytoplasm of cells [75]. It is considered the most common fatal neuromuscular disease of infancy and the most common neuromuscular disease in children below the age of 18 [132].

22.2.1 Classification

Common to all SMA patients is a symmetric muscular weakness predominantly affecting the lower limbs and proximal muscles compared with the upper limbs or distal muscles. Patients usually have normal intelligence with no effect on sensibility. The age of onset and clinical course can have a variable presentation. Owing to this heterogeneity, SMA is most commonly divided into three types [22, 104, 115].

22.2.1.1 Type I, Acute Werdnig–Hoffman Disease

Type I SMA is the most severe form of the disease, usually presenting at birth or within the first 2–6 months of the life. These patients do not meet early motor milestones with the inability to gain head control, to roll over, or sit up. It has been suggested that in utero osteoporosis from decreased movement is responsible for postnatal pathologic fractures [21]. Patients with type I SMA usually do not survive beyond the age of 3 years. Respiratory failure from intercostal weakness and rib collapse is responsible for their mortality. Due to their early mortality, orthopaedic intervention is rarely indicated in these children.

22.2.1.2 Type II, Chronic Werdnig–Hoffman Disease

The clinical onset of type II SMA occurs between the ages of 6 and 24 months. Patients reach early motor milestones, but are never able to walk independently. Weakness usually starts in the lower extremities, affecting the gluteal and quadricep muscles initially. Life expectancy is variable from adolescence to adulthood with some patients living into their fourth decade [62, 132]. The cause of mortality is respiratory failure.

22.2.1.3 Type III, Kugelberg–Welander Disease

The clinical onset of type III SMA occurs following the age of 18 – 24 months. In nearly all cases the diagnosis is made before the age of 10 years. As expected, children attain greater motor milestones compared with type II SMA. Patients are able to walk independently until early adolescence. Russman et al. reported that 50% of those children with an age of onset before 2 years lost their ability to walk without assistance by age 12 [116]. Those children that presented after age 2 typically were ambulating into the fourth decade. Patients who never reached independent ambulation lost their ability to walk at the age of 7.

22.2.1.4 Functional Classification

Evans et al. [36] described a functional classification based on the maximum physical function achieved. The purpose was to give insight into the patient's prognosis. Group I patients never sit independently, have poor head control and develop early progressive scoliosis. Group II children have head control and ability to sit but cannot walk or stand. Group III patients can stand by themselves and are able to walk with external support. Group IV children can walk and run independently.

22.2.2 Diagnosis

For those patients that do not present at birth, presenting concerns by families are a delay in reaching motor milestones. Depending on the age of the patient, these include an inability to gain head control, roll over, sit, stand, or walk independently. Physical examination should then assess motor strength as well as deep tendon reflexes. For those patients who present early (type I or II), gross fasciculations of the tongue or tremors of the finger are commonly present [92, 132].

Once SMA is suspected, further diagnostic work-up includes laboratory studies, nerve conduction studies, electromyography (EMG), and DNA testing. Creatine phosphokinase and aldolase are usually normal or slightly elevated in type III patients [127]. Motor and sensory nerve conduction velocities are normal. EMG findings demonstrate fibrillation potentials associated with denervation as well as large polyphasic motor units associated with renervation [127, 132]. DNA testing is highly sensitive for SMA with PCR, the diagnostic procedure of choice [138] Muscle biopsy is also highly diagnostic. Histologic finding include muscle fiber degeneration and atrophy with no evidence of primary myopathy [127].

22.2.3 Spinal Deformity

Scoliosis is the most common orthopaedic problem in patients with SMA [121]. Nearly 100% of type II patients and half of type III patients develop a spinal deformity [36, 46, 106, 110]. The deformity is typically a right-sided C-shaped thoracolumbar curve. Ninety percent of the patients have a single curve. The curve is usually progressive and, in approximately one-third of the cases, associated with a progressive kyphosis [46, 110]. Similar to Duchenne's patients, development of scoliosis in type III SMA occurs with their loss of ambulation [121]. Pulmonary function is similarly compromised in patients with SMA [113]. The worsening of lung function is secondary to the muscle weakness as well as the progressive scoliosis.

As there is a difference in the clinical presentation between the three types of SMA, there is similar heterogeneity in the risk and progression of scoliosis. Evans et al. [36] demonstrated that the age of scoliosis onset correlated with the severity of muscle disease. Type I patients typically had scoliosis by the age of 2 years, whereas type III patients developed scoliosis between the ages of 4 and 14. The rate of progression was also highly associated with the disease severity ranging from 8.3° per year in severe cases to 2.9° in more mild cases.

As for the severity of the scoliosis, a study by Granata et al. [46] reported curves ranging from 10 to 165°. Schwentker and Gibson [121] reported on 50 patients with SMA. Seventy percent had scoliosis, measuring greater than 20° and 40% had curves greater than 60°. The natural history of these large curves suggests that they can be quite disabling [36]. In addition to trouble sitting, patients can lose upper extremity function to maintain trunk balance as well as develop back pain or pain from rib impingement on the pelvis.

22.2.4 Nonsurgical Management of Scoliosis

Orthotics have generally been thought to be ineffective in preventing the development or progression of neuromuscular scoliosis [6, 46, 124]. However, it has been shown to be effective in improving sitting balance. Letts et al. demonstrated an improvement in sitting stability in 80% of patients with a collapsing neuromuscular scoliosis with the use of a soft Boston orthosis [77]. They also thought that a soft brace was more tolerable than a rigid orthosis and resulted in less skin breakdown.

Some studies have suggested that the use of orthotics may slow the rate of progression of scoliosis [6, 90, 110]. Slowing the rate of scoliosis progression has the advantage of allowing patients to get older when they are more suitable for a surgical intervention. This is especially critical in the early onset patients (type I and II). Unfortunately, most of these study report opinions and have not given reliable data to demonstrate that bracing truly slows the progression of spinal deformity. Bracing is also not without its morbidity. Aprin et al. [6] reported on five patients who had to discontinue their brace secondary to respiratory difficulty.

At our institution, we initiate bracing in patients with spinal deformities on sitting films between 30 and 40°. Typically, the curves in SMA are quite flexible and amenable to the orthosis. We find that the brace in addition to wheelchair supports help to maintain sitting balance. This is especially critical in preadolescent patients where attempts are made to delay surgery until the patient is more mature. In some cases, especially in the type I patient where long-term survival or surgical tolerance is not expected, bracing may be the definitive management of the spinal deformity.

22.2.5 Surgical Management of Scoliosis

Similar to other neuromuscular scoliosis, the decision to operate on a SMA patient is dependent on multiple factors. In general, the radiographic parameters for spinal fusion are not controversial and simple to follow. I recommend spinal fusion for curve magnitudes greater than 50° that are refractory to conservative measures and demonstrate progression. These indications for surgical fusion have been recommended by other authors as well [16, 36, 132].

Unfortunately, patient factors may not make the above rules simple to follow. In some patients with SMA type I, their early onset scoliosis and grim long-term survival has made surgical intervention unreasonable. Type II patients may also present with a progressive scoliosis at an early age. Spinal arthrodesis would have a considerable negative effect on trunk growth as well as lung growth. These patients are also at significant risk of developing a crankshaft deformity necessitating an anterior fusion [33]. In these cases, spinal fusion is indicated, but an attempt at delaying surgery with the use of an orthosis is made. The goal is to maintain some control of the curve until a definitive procedure can be done at about the age of ten. Of course, this may mean watching a curve progress to greater than 80°.

There have been some thought about using an expandable or "growing rod" construct in these young patients. There is only one published report using an expandable or "telescoping" device in type II patients [40]. The device was abandoned due to its technical demands and inability to prevent progression of the deformity and crankshafting. They concluded that a brace should be used until the age of ten when a fusion can be performed. Growing rods may be the answer for these patients, but its role has not been clearly defined. The tolerance for multiple anesthetics needed to expand the device on these already pulmonary compromised patients is also not known. To minimize this need for multiple anesthetics, we have utilized a modified Shilla procedure to manage the early severe scoliosis (Fig. 22.2).

In the SMA patient that requires definitive spinal stabilization, the gold standard is posterior fusion and segmental instrumentation. The goal is to prevent progression and obtain an alignment that will improve or maintain balance and sitting ability. In the nonambulatory patient, this typically involves segmental instrumentation from T2 to the pelvis. Many spinal deformity surgeons report good outcomes using sublaminar wires with Luque rods or a unit rod for the treatment of neuromuscular scoliosis [19, 106, 119]. Others are transitioning to the use of pedicle screws

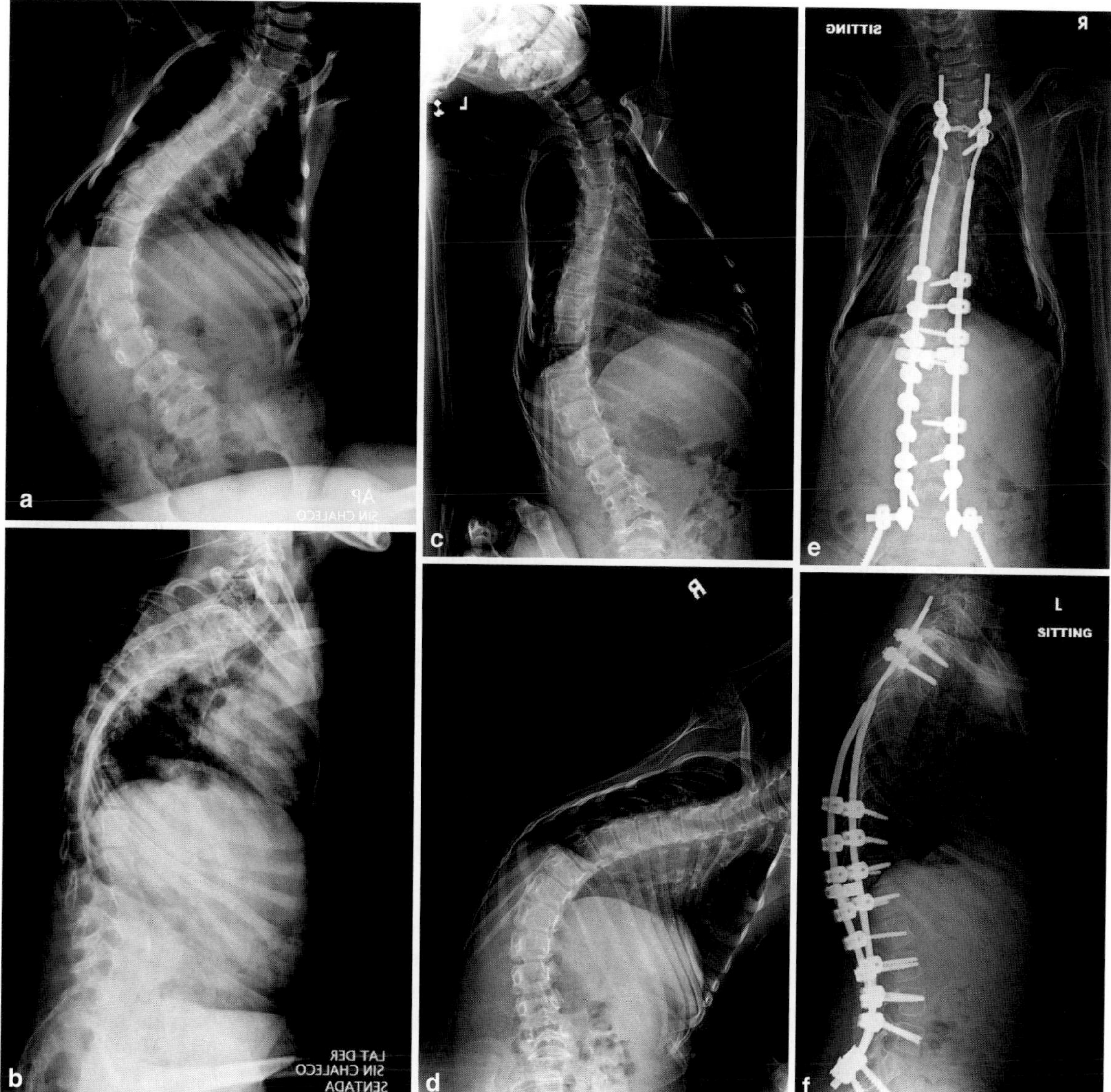

Fig. 22.2 (**a, b**) An 8-year-old female with SMA and progressive kyphoscoliosis. Her coronal Cobb angle measures 90°. (**c, d**) Bending films demonstrate a correction to 41°. (**e, f**) The patient underwent a modified Shilla procedure with instrumentation and fusion from T10 to the pelvis. The instrumentation was extended proximally to pedicle screws at T3 and T4 with fusion across these two levels. The pedicle screws are allowed to slide along the rod as the spine grows. The goal of this procedure is to attain correction with the distal fusion but allow thoracic growth with the Shilla procedure

to provide more rigid fixation [119]. The improved fixation to bone with pedicle screws has decreased the use of postoperative bracing for some neuromuscular patients [132]. I continue to brace all neuromuscular patients for 3 months postoperatively to prevent excessive stress on the osteopenic bone during transfers, including those with all pedicle screw instrumentation. Pelvic instrumentation is recommended to prevent progressive pelvic obliquity and difficulty with sitting [121]. Similar to patients with DMD, options include Galveston technique or iliac screws.

The use of an anterior approach has traditionally been reserved for severe curves or for patients at risk of developing crankshaft deformity. In the case of patients with SMA, other factors need to be considered. These patients typically have poor pulmonary reserve associated with weakness of their respiratory muscles. This places them at increased risk of developing pulmonary complications. The use of segmental fixation may decrease the risk of crankshaft deformity. Smucker and Miller [131] reported on 43 patients with neuromuscular scoliosis and open triradiate cartilage treated with a unit rod. They found no evidence of crankshaft deformity at 2 years follow-up. Some believe that pedicle screws may further decrease the risk by providing three-column fixation. However, this needs to be evaluated. There is also increasing evidence that severe, spinal deformity can be completely managed from a posterior approach. Multilevel posterior osteotomies or single level vertebral column resections stabilized with pedicle screws have been shown to adequately treat the severely deformed, rigid spine [133]. However, this too has not been adequately studied in patients with SMA.

In preparation for spinal fusion, all patients with SMA should be evaluated by a pulmonologist, neurologist and, an anesthesiologist. This will insure that patients are optimized for surgery, especially regarding their pulmonary function. In the immediate postoperative period, patients are most at risk for developing pulmonary complications. Aprin et al. [6] reported a 45% incidence of respiratory problems following surgery. Four of their 22 patients required intubation. Brown et al. [19] reported that tracheostomy was needed in 30% of their patients. The use of preoperative traction has been suggested to increase spinal flexibility and improve pulmonary function, possibly diminishing their risk of respiratory complications [6, 107]. Postoperatively, these patients should have aggressive pulmonary therapy and early mobilization. Ventilatory assistance with the guidance of a pulmonologist may be needed several days following the surgery. Other long-term complications following spinal arthrodesis include crankshafting, pseudoarthrosis, prominent implants, narrowing of the chest, gastric volvulus, and diaphragmatic rupture [6, 17, 80, 110]. Except for crankshafting, these complications were more commonly seen in older patients with larger deformities.

22.2.6 Long-Term Outcomes

In general, the literature supports spinal fusion in SMA patients with progressive scoliosis. Multiple authors have reported improvements in sitting, balance, comfort, and cosmesis [46, 107]. Bridwell et al. [17] evaluated 21 SMA patients with an average follow-up of 7.8 years after surgery. Patients reported benefits in all categorizes with the highest ratings in cosmesis, quality of life, and satisfaction. In contrast, some authors have reported a decline in some functional activities, specifically upper extremity activities. Brown et al. [19] demonstrated a decline in self-feeding, drinking, and self-hygiene at 2 years follow-up with some improvement at 5 years. Furumasu et al. reported similar findings suggesting that the lack of spinal flexibility diminished gross upper extremity motor function due to a change in trunk position. What is unclear in these patients is the influence of a progressive muscle disease in the diminished functional activities.

Pulmonary function also appears to benefit from stabilization of the scoliosis. Robinson et al. [113] demonstrated a significant improvement in lung function in the patients who underwent spinal fusion. They also demonstrated a significant inverse linear relationship between curve magnitude and percentage of predicted vital capacity.

22.2.7 Conclusions

Spinal muscle atrophy is a heterogeneous disease commonly affected by progressive scoliosis. Depending on the severity of the disease, patients can have significant deformity at a very early age. Although ineffective at preventing scoliosis, bracing is utilized to delay surgery. The gold standard for spinal stabilization remains to be posterior spinal instrumentation and fusion. Current literature suggests that surgical management of the deformity can maintain upright sitting posture, improve quality of life, and positively affect pulmonary function. Whether this improvement in pulmonary status improves life expectancy is still unclear.

22.3 Arthrogryposis

Arthrogryposis or "arthrogryposis multiplex congenital" is a heterogeneous group of diseases with the similar phenotype of multiple congenital joint contractures

[14, 52]. Currently, there are more than 150 subtypes that result from a failure of normal movement in utero. The etiology for this lack of movement may be myopathic, neurological, or secondary to connective tissue abnormalities [9]. Amyoplasia is the term used to describe the more classic disease entity seen in orthopaedics. These patients have a dysgenesis of anterior horn cells resulting in replacement of muscle with adipose and fibrous tissue [51].

Patients with arthrogryposis multiplex congenital have significant musculoskeletal deformities secondary to the contractures. The majority of patients have all 4 limbs involved (84%) [14]. Severe equinovarus feet, hip dislocations (unilateral or bilateral), and scoliosis are commonly seen. Nonorthopaedic abnormalities include hypoplasia of the labial folds, inguinal hernias, abdominal wall defects, cryptorchidism, gastroschisis, and bowel atresia [14].

22.3.1 Spinal Deformity

The incidence of scoliosis in arthrogryposis is reportedly between 30 and 67% depending on the definition used [120, 144]. The deformities are similar to other neuromuscular conditions with lumbar and thoracolumbar curves predominating [29, 60]. The curves are frequently stiff. Progression of the deformity can be rapid, up to 6.5° per year [60]. The earlier the presentation of scoliosis, the more severe the curve may become and be associated with pelvic obliquity. Increased lordosis is frequently seen.

The scoliosis is typically refractory to orthotic management [29, 60]. Posterior spinal instrumentation and fusion appears to be effective in preventing progression of the scoliosis. However, correction of the curves appears to be modest, about 35% [29]. Yingsakmongkol and Kumar reported slightly increased correction (44%) with a combined anterior and posterior fusion [144]. These series are dated, however, and do not assess surgical outcomes with current segmental spinal instrumentation. In some cases, instrumentation was not used. If pelvic obliquity is present, fusion to the pelvis should be attempted. Care should also be taken when positioning patients. Their stiff joints and osteopenia place them at increased risk of developing pathologic fracture.

22.4 Poliomyelitis Scoliosis

Poliomyelitis is caused by the infectious poliovirus that targets the large motor neurons of the anterior horn of the spinal cord. Most infections result in no long-term problems. However, approximately 1% of patients progress to an irreversible paralytic form [26]. Depending on the muscles paralyzed, musculoskeletal deformities from the imbalanced muscles can result in scoliosis, limb length discrepancies, joint contractures, and foot abnormalities.

With the introduction of the vaccine by Salk and Sabin, there has been a near eradication of polio infections in North America and Europe [117, 118]. Outbreaks of poliomyelitis continue to be reported in third-world countries where vaccination programs and sanitary conditions are inadequate. As recently as 1998, it has been reported that in China 60,000 patients require surgery for poliomyelitis scoliosis [26].

22.4.1 Spinal Deformity

The incidence of scoliosis among patients with poliomyelitis is between 17 and 65% [26]. Depending on the involved trunk muscles, patients can develop different types and severity of scoliosis. In 1956, Roaf [112] classified the scoliosis into four types: the thoracolumbar C-shaped curve, the lumbar curve with pelvic obliquity, the primary thoracic curve, and the combined thoracic and lumbar curve. The double major thoracic and lumbar curve has been shown to be the most common [88]. Similar to other paralytic scoliosis, patients can develop severe sagittal plane abnormalities as well with both kyphosis and lordosis.

When evaluating patients with spinal deformity, it is necessary to also evaluate the influence of other joint deformities. Both hip contractures and limb length inequalities have been shown to be a factor in producing pelvic obliquity and secondary scoliosis [34, 73]. Whether these need to be addressed in addition to the scoliosis should be determined on an individual basis. It will depend on the patient's ambulatory status and ability to sit.

Similar to other neuromuscular scoliosis, bracing has not been shown to be effective in long-term management [20, 96]. However, for the young patient it has value in delaying the need for surgery to allow for greater spinal growth. The indications for surgical fusion are also similar to other paralytic scoliosis. Patients who demonstrate a progressive spinal deformity greater than 50° are candidates for surgery. The goal of surgery is to improve sitting balance, prevent worsening pulmonary function, and possibly reduce back pain, especially if there is impingement between the ribs and the pelvis.

Since the majority of patients treated with polio scoliosis predate current spinal systems, most published literature report on the use of Harrington rods or Luque segmental wiring [15, 48, 56, 103]. In general, posterior spinal instrumentation and fusion was effective in controlling the deformity. In patients with pelvic obliquity, it was recommended that the pelvis be including in the fusion. O'Brien et al. [100] suggested that progressive pelvic obliquity could lead ultimately to hip dislocation. They, therefore, recommended fusion to the sacrum. The use of anterior releases and halo-gravity traction was also recommended for patients with large, rigid curves [31, 76, 99, 100]. Leong et al. [76] reported on 110 patients treated for polio scoliosis. They found that a combined anterior instrumentation and fusion and posterior fusion gave better results than posterior fusion only. However, it was also associated with a higher morbidity. Depending on curve type, the pseudoarthrosis rate was more than double for the posterior only fusion compared with a combined approach. Unfortunately, there is no information reported in the literature evaluating current spinal instruments and fusion techniques in the polio patient. It is unclear whether similar pseudoarthrosis rates and the need for anterior releases would be required with more modern procedures.

In the young growing spine affected by poliomyelitis, an early progressive scoliosis can be encountered. As already mentioned, an attempt at bracing should be undertaken. However, in some cases, the spinal deformity is not amenable to orthotic treatment. In these cases, a growing construct is recommended. Eberle [35] reported a series of 16 patients between the ages of 5 and 12 that underwent segmental instrumentation without fusion for the treatment of polio scoliosis. Unfortunately, in 15 patients the surgery failed to control the deformity. There were also some cases of spontaneous fusion of the instrumented portion of the spine. Whether the use of a modern growing rod with multiple expansions would be more beneficial has not been evaluated in this patient population.

When considering a spinal fusion in a polio patient, it is important to perform pulmonary function testing. It has been shown that trunk muscle involvement can cause respiratory paralysis and negatively affect a patient's breathing ability [45, 140]. This combined with a large scoliosis can significantly decrease pulmonary function [79]. While this should not preclude surgical intervention, assessment of respiratory status will better prepare the team for the immediate postoperative care.

There has been a significant decrease in the number of patients with poliomyelitis scoliosis in North America and Europe as demonstrated by the lack of recent published reports in the literature. In third-world countries, however, spinal deformity remains to be actively treated in the polio patient. There is currently little data discussing the use of modern surgical techniques and instruments in this population. Therefore, when approaching a patient with poliomyelitis scoliosis, basic treatment principles gained from other neuromuscular conditions should be utilized.

22.5 Rett Syndrome

First described in 1966, Rett syndrome is a progressive neurological disorder that affects 1 in 20,000 females [49, 97]. Patients initially appear normal at birth but then proceed through four stages of deterioration. The first stage typically has an onset between 6 and 18 months with developmental stagnation. The second stage (1–3 years of age) is characterized by lost language skills and autistic behaviors. In stage III (2–10 years of age), patients may have seizures, exhibit some mental retardation, and have repetitive hand motions. In the fourth stage, patients develop spasticity and muscle wasting. Scoliosis is most likely to present in this final stage.

22.5.1 Spinal Deformity

The musculoskeletal manifestations of Rett syndrome include lower extremity contractures, coxa valga, and scoliosis [49, 81]. The spinal deformity is similar to other neuromuscular diseases with a long C-shaped curve being the most common [57, 66]. However, patients can also present with a single thoracic or double major curve. Large curves are frequently associated with pelvic obliquity. As patients get older so does the prevalence of scoliosis. Curve progression has been suggested to be more rapid than idiopathic scoliosis or other neuromuscular scoliosis. Lidstrom et al. demonstrated greater than 15° of progression per year in the final stage of Rett syndrome [78]. For this reason, it has been recommended that patients are evaluated every 6 months following the age of 5 [11].

Bracing has been found to be largely unsuccessful in preventing the progression of scoliosis [11, 57, 66]. However, it can be used to delay the need for surgical intervention to allow for more truncal growth. Posterior spinal instrumentation and fusion is the treatment of choice for the progressive scoliosis. In those patients who are nonambulatory, it is recommended to fuse from the upper thoracic spine to the pelvis to prevent delayed decompensation or pelvic obliquity. Ambulation is possible in patients with Rett syndrome and can be positively affected by surgery. Harrison et al. [57] demonstrated no loss of ambulation in all the five patients who walked preoperatively and improvements in some patients. Overall, spinal fusion is successful in halting curve progression and improving spinal balance in the sitting and walking patient.

22.6 Friedreich's Ataxia

First described by Friedreich in the 1800s, Friedreich's ataxia is a progressive spinocerebellar degenerative disease clinically characterized by a lack of coordination and steadiness. The estimated prevalence of the disease is about 1:50,000 [4]. The essential clinical features for diagnosis include: autosomal recessive inheritance, onset before 25 years of age, progressive ataxia of limbs and gait, absent deep tendon reflexes of the knee and ankle, and evidence of axonal sensory neuropathy [54]. After 5 years from time of onset, patients will exhibit dysarthria, areflexia of all limbs, distal loss of vibration sense, extensor plantar response, and pyramidal weakness of lower limbs [54]. Patients begin to lose the ability to ambulate between 18 and 25 years of age [12, 54]. This is secondary to both the ataxia and lower extremity weakness. Cardiomyopathy is the most common cause of death.

22.6.1 Spinal Deformity

The prevalence of scoliosis is reported to be as high as 100% [23]. The curve patterns of Friedreich's ataxia are more similar to idiopathic scoliosis than to neuromuscular deformities [7, 30]. Labelle et al. reported the distribution of curve types to be 57% double thoracic and lumbar curves, 14% thoracolumbar curves, 7% thoracic and thoracolumbar curves, 4% lumbar curves, and 11% multiple small curves [72]. These authors also reported that not all curves progress. Of the 36 patients evaluated, only 20 had curves greater than 60° and progressed. The other 16 had curves less than 40° and did not progress. Similar to idiopathic scoliosis, if patients had an earlier onset of scoliosis then there was a greater risk of progression especially if continued truncal growth was anticipated. Interestingly, no correlation was found between the overall muscle weakness of the patient and the curve progression [71].

Unlike idiopathic scoliosis, bracing has not been successful in controlling patients with spinal deformity [23, 30]. In addition, bracing may worsen a patient's ability to walk. In cases of early onset, however, temporizing with an orthotic until skeletal maturity is reached so a definitive surgery can be performed is acceptable. The indications for fusion are similar to AIS. Progressive curves greater than 50° should undergo posterior spinal instrumentation and fusion. The use of segmental instrumentation such as sublaminar wires, hooks, or pedicle screws is recommended. The goal is to prevent progression and have a well-balanced spine. All curves should be included as there is no role for selective fusions. The pelvis should not be included in patients who are ambulatory wherein the pelvis is not part of the deformity. Patients who are nonambulatory with a neuromuscular type deformity and pelvic obliquity should have the pelvis included in the fusion. This will insure adequate sitting balance.

When spinal surgery is contemplated, a thorough preoperative assessment is mandatory. Patients are at significant risk of developing cardiomyopathy, which could complicate the anesthesiologist intraoperative management. Patients should undergo preoperative pulmonary function testing. The combination of muscle weakness and scoliosis can diminish a patient's pulmonary reserve. Friedreich's ataxia patient's also have a higher incidence of diabetes requiring insulin and therefore should have their glucose levels screened [4].

Postoperatively, patients should be placed in a TLSO. They are at increased risk of implant failure early on secondary to their ataxia and poor balance. Early mobilization should be encouraged to minimize pulmonary complications. Patients with any evidence of cardiomyopathy or poor pulmonary function testing should be monitored closely during the immediate postoperative period. Those patients who were ambulatory before surgery should be expected to ambulate following surgery.

22.7 Congenital Myopathies

Congenital myopathies are a heterogeneous group of disorders characterized by weakness and hypotonia from birth [10]. Typically, the diseases have similar clinical findings but are classified based on histologic and microscopic findings. Central core disease, nemaline myopathy, and myotubular myopathy are just a few of the multiple congenital myopathies that scoliosis has been described [24, 43, 87, 91, 126]. They are genetically transmitted and can have variable penetrance.

22.7.1 *Spinal Deformity*

The musculoskeletal abnormalities associated with these disorders include congenital hip instability, foot deformities, other joint contractures, as well as scoliosis [126]. The curves are similar to other neuromuscular curves with a long, thoracolumbar shape. Kyphosis can also be associated with the deformity. As the scoliosis progresses it often becomes rigid. Rigid spine syndrome as described by Dubowitz has often been associated with these diseases and other congenital muscular dystrophies [7, 38].

If the patients present early and have flexible curves, the scoliosis may be amenable to management with an orthosis. Those patients who fail bracing or present with large, rigid curves should undergo spinal fusion. Similar consideration as with other neuromuscular scoliosis must be given to the health and age of the patient. Poor pulmonary function has been associated with congenital myopathies [91]. At minimum, patients should undergo preoperative pulmonary function testing. These patients are also at increased risk of developing malignant hyperthermia [43]. The anesthesiologist should be made aware of this before the day of surgery so that adequate preparation can be done.

Depending on the severity of the disease, patients may present with early onset scoliosis. Those that demonstrate progression with the use of an orthosis may require surgical treatment with an expandable device or "growing rod". However, there have been no studies adequately evaluating the use of a "growing rod" in these patients. Those patients who present later in life do well with a posterior spinal instrumentation and fusion. Anterior release can be done for the large rigid curve if the patient can tolerate the exposure. In the nonambulatory patient with pelvic obliquity, the fusion should be extended to the pelvis.

Similar principles to other neuromuscular diseases should be followed when treating patients with congenital myopathies. Posterior fusion is the treatment of choice. The need for traction or fusion to the pelvis should be determined on an individual basis. Depending on bone quality, a brace can be used postoperatively to support the instrumentation. Particular attention, however, has to be made toward the increased risk of hyperthermia.

References

1. Allen BL Jr, Ferguson RL (1984) The Galveston technique of pelvic fixation with L-rod instrumentation of the spine. Spine 9:388–394
2. Alman BA, Kim HK (1999) Pelvic obliquity after fusion of the spine in Duchenne muscular dystrophy. J Bone Joint Surg Br 81:821–824
3. Alman BA, Raza SN, Biggar WD (2004) Steroid treatment and the development of scoliosis in males with duchenne muscular dystrophy. J Bone Joint Surg Am 86-A:519–524
4. Alper G, Narayanan V (2003) Friedreich's ataxia. Pediatr Neurol 28:335–341
5. Angelini C (2007) The role of corticosteroids in muscular dystrophy: a critical appraisal. Muscle Nerve 36:424–435
6. Aprin H, Bowen JR, MacEwen GD et al (1982) Spine fusion in patients with spinal muscular atrophy. J Bone Joint Surg Am 64:1179–1187
7. Arkader A, Hosalkar H, Dormans JP (2005) Scoliosis correction in an adolescent with a rigid spine syndrome: case report. Spine 30:E623–E628
8. Aronsson DD, Stokes IA, Ronchetti PJ et al (1994) Comparison of curve shape between children with cerebral palsy, Friedreich's ataxia, and adolescent idiopathic scoliosis. Dev Med Child Neurol 36:412–418
9. Banker BQ (1985) Neuropathologic aspects of arthrogryposis multiplex congenita. Clin Orthop Relat Res 30–43

10. Barnes MJ (2001) Other neuromuscular deformities. In: Weinstein SL (ed) The pediatric spine principles and practice, 2nd edn. Lippincott Williams & Wilkins, Philadelphia
11. Bassett GS, Tolo VT (1990) The incidence and natural history of scoliosis in Rett syndrome. Dev Med Child Neurol 32:963–966
12. Beauchamp M, Labelle H, Duhaime M et al (1995) Natural history of muscle weakness in Friedreich's Ataxia and its relation to loss of ambulation. Clin Orthop Relat Res 270–275
13. Bentley G, Haddad F, Bull TM et al (2001) The treatment of scoliosis in muscular dystrophy using modified Luque and Harrington–Luque instrumentation. J Bone Joint Surg Br 83:22–28
14. Bernstein RM (2002) Arthrogryposis and amyoplasia. J Am Acad Orthop Surg 10:417–424
15. Bonnett C, Brown JC, Perry J et al (1975) Evolution of treatment of paralytic scoliosis at Rancho Los Amigos Hospital. J Bone Joint Surg Am 57:206–215
16. Bowen JR, Lipton GE (2001) Spinal muscular atrophy. In: Weinstein SL (ed) The pediatric spine principles and practice, 2nd edn. Lippincott Williams & Wilkins, Philadelphia
17. Bridwell KH, Baldus C, Iffrig TM et al (1999) Process measures and patient/parent evaluation of surgical management of spinal deformities in patients with progressive flaccid neuromuscular scoliosis (Duchenne's muscular dystrophy and spinal muscular atrophy). Spine 24:1300–1309
18. Brook PD, Kennedy JD, Stern LM et al (1996) Spinal fusion in Duchenne's muscular dystrophy. J Pediatr Orthop 16:324–331
19. Brown JC, Zeller JL, Swank SM et al (1989) Surgical and functional results of spine fusion in spinal muscular atrophy. Spine 14:763–770
20. Bunch WH (1975) The Milwaukee brace in paralytic scoliosis. Clin Orthop Relat Res 63–68
21. Burke SW, Jameson VP, Roberts JM et al (1986) Birth fractures in spinal muscular atrophy. J Pediatr Orthop 6:34–36
22. Byers RK, Banker BQ (1961) Infantile muscular atrophy. Arch Neurol 5:140–164
23. Cady RB, Bobechko WP (1984) Incidence, natural history, and treatment of scoliosis in Friedreich's ataxia. J Pediatr Orthop 4:673–676
24. Cahill PJ, Rinella AS, Bielski RJ (2007) Orthopaedic complications of myotubular myopathy. J Pediatr Orthop 27:98–103
25. Cervellati S, Bettini N, Moscato M et al (2004) Surgical treatment of spinal deformities in Duchenne muscular dystrophy: a long term follow-up study. Eur Spine J 13:441–448
26. Chen P, Shen Y (2001) Poliomyelitis scoliosis. In: Weinstein SL (ed) The pediatric spine principles and practice, 2nd edn. Lippincott Williams & Wilkins, Philadelphia
27. Cheuk DK, Wong V, Wraige E et al (2007) Surgery for scoliosis in Duchenne muscular dystrophy. Cochrane Database Syst Rev CD005375
28. Cole JW, Murray DJ, Snider RJ et al (2003) Aprotinin reduces blood loss during spinal surgery in children. Spine 28:2482–2485
29. Daher YH, Lonstein JE, Winter RB et al (1985) Spinal deformities in patients with arthrogryposis. A review of 16 patients. Spine 10:609–613
30. Daher YH, Lonstein JE, Winter RB et al (1985) Spinal deformities in patients with Friedreich ataxia: a review of 19 patients. J Pediatr Orthop 5:553–557
31. Dewald RL, Ray RD (1970) Skeletal traction for the treatment of severe scoliosis. The University of Illinois halo-hoop apparatus. J Bone Joint Surg Am 52:233–238
32. Drachman DB, Toyka KV, Myer E (1974) Prednisone in Duchenne muscular dystrophy. Lancet 2:1409–1412
33. Dubousset J, Herring JA, Shufflebarger H (1989) The crankshaft phenomenon. J Pediatr Orthop 9:541–550
34. Eberle CF (1982) Pelvic obliquity and the unstable hip after poliomyelitis. J Bone Joint Surg Br 64:300–304
35. Eberle CF (1988) Failure of fixation after segmental spinal instrumentation without arthrodesis in the management of paralytic scoliosis. J Bone Joint Surg Am 70:696–703
36. Evans GA, Drennan JC, Russman BS (1981) Functional classification and orthopaedic management of spinal muscular atrophy. J Bone Joint Surg Br 63B:516–522
37. Finsterer J (2006) Cardiopulmonary support in duchenne muscular dystrophy. Lung 184:205–215
38. Flanigan KM, Kerr L, Bromberg MB et al (2000) Congenital muscular dystrophy with rigid spine syndrome: a clinical, pathological, radiological, and genetic study. Ann Neurol 47:152–161
39. Florentino-Pineda I, Thompson GH, Poe-Kochert C et al (2004) The effect of amicar on perioperative blood loss in idiopathic scoliosis: the results of a prospective, randomized double-blind study. Spine 29:233–238
40. Fujak A, Ingenhorst A, Heuser K et al (2005) Treatment of scoliosis in intermediate spinal muscular atrophy (SMA type II) in childhood. Ortop Traumatol Rehabil 7:175–179
41. Gaine WJ, Lim J, Stephenson W et al (2004) Progression of scoliosis after spinal fusion in Duchenne's muscular dystrophy. J Bone Joint Surg Br 86:550–555
42. Galasko CS, Delaney C, Morris P (1992) Spinal stabilisation in Duchenne muscular dystrophy. J Bone Joint Surg Br 74:210–214
43. Gamble JG, Rinsky LA, Lee JH (1988) Orthopaedic aspects of central core disease. J Bone Joint Surg Am 70:1061–1066
44. Gibson DA, Wilkins KE (1975) The management of spinal deformities in Duchenne muscular dystrophy. A new concept of spinal bracing. Clin Orthop Relat Res 41–51
45. Gilchrist JM (2002) Overview of neuromuscular disorders affecting respiratory function. Semin Respir Crit Care Med 23:191–200
46. Granata C, Merlini L, Magni E et al (1989) Spinal muscular atrophy: natural history and orthopaedic treatment of scoliosis. Spine 14:760–762
47. Granata C, Merlini L, Cervellati S et al (1996) Long-term results of spine surgery in Duchenne muscular dystrophy. Neuromuscul Disord 6:61–68
48. Gui L, Savini R, Vicenzi G et al (1976) Surgical treatment of poliomyelitic scoliosis. Ital J Orthop Traumatol 2: 191–205
49. Guidera KJ, Borrelli J Jr, Raney E et al (1991) Orthopaedic manifestations of Rett syndrome. J Pediatr Orthop 11:204–208
50. Hahn GV, Mubarak SJ (2001) Muscular dystrophy. In: Weinstein SL (ed) The pediatric spine principles and practice, 2nd edn. Lippincott Williams & Wilkins, Philadelphia

51. Hall JG, Reed SD, Driscoll EP (1983) Part I. Amyoplasia: a common, sporadic condition with congenital contractures. Am J Med Genet 15:571–590
52. Hall JG (1997) Arthrogryposis multiplex congenita: etiology, genetics, classification, diagnostic approach, and general aspects. J Pediatr Orthop B 6:159–166
53. Hapke EJ, Meek JC, Jacobs J (1972) Pulmonary function in progressive muscular dystrophy. Chest 61:41–47
54. Harding AE (1981) Friedreich's ataxia: a clinical and genetic study of 90 families with an analysis of early diagnostic criteria and intrafamilial clustering of clinical features. Brain 104:589–620
55. Harper CM, Ambler G, Edge G (2004) The prognostic value of pre-operative predicted forced vital capacity in corrective spinal surgery for Duchenne's muscular dystrophy. Anaesthesia 59:1160–1162
56. Harrington PR (1973) The history and development of Harrington instrumentation. Clin Orthop Relat Res 110–112
57. Harrison DJ, Webb PJ (1990) Scoliosis in the Rett syndrome: natural history and treatment. Brain Dev 12:154–156
58. Heiman-Patterson TD, Natter HM, Rosenberg HR et al (1986) Malignant hyperthermia susceptibility in X-linked muscle dystrophies. Pediatr Neurol 2:356–358
59. Heller KD, Wirtz DC, Siebert CH et al (2001) Spinal stabilization in Duchenne muscular dystrophy: principles of treatment and record of 31 operative treated cases. J Pediatr Orthop B 10:18–24
60. Herron LD, Westin GW, Dawson EG (1978) Scoliosis in arthrogryposis multiplex congenita. J Bone Joint Surg Am 60:293–299
61. Hsu JD (1983) The natural history of spine curvature progression in the nonambulatory Duchenne muscular dystrophy patient. Spine 8:771–775
62. Iannaccone ST (1998) Spinal muscular atrophy. Semin Neurol 18:19–26
63. Inkley SR, Oldenburg FC, Vignos PJ Jr (1974) Pulmonary function in Duchenne muscular dystrophy related to stage of disease. Am J Med 56:297–306
64. Karol LA (2007) Scoliosis in patients with Duchenne muscular dystrophy. J Bone Joint Surg Am 89 Suppl 1:155–162
65. Kennedy JD, Staples AJ, Brook PD et al (1995) Effect of spinal surgery on lung function in Duchenne muscular dystrophy. Thorax 50:1173–1178
66. Keret D, Bassett GS, Bunnell WP et al (1988) Scoliosis in Rett syndrome. J Pediatr Orthop 8:138–142
67. Khoshhal K, Mukhtar I, Clark P et al (2003) Efficacy of aprotinin in reducing blood loss in spinal fusion for idiopathic scoliosis. J Pediatr Orthop 23:661–664
68. Kinali M, Main M, Eliahoo J et al (2007) Predictive factors for the development of scoliosis in Duchenne muscular dystrophy. Eur J Paediatr Neurol 11:160–166
69. Kunkel LM, Hejtmancik JF, Caskey CT et al (1986) Analysis of deletions in DNA from patients with Becker and Duchenne muscular dystrophy. Nature 322:73–77
70. Kurz LT, Mubarak SJ, Schultz P et al (1983) Correlation of scoliosis and pulmonary function in Duchenne muscular dystrophy. J Pediatr Orthop 3:347–353
71. Labelle H (2001) Spinal deformities in Friedreich's ataxia. In: Weinstein SL (ed) The pediatric spine principles and practice, 2nd edn. Lippincott Williams & Wilkins, Philadelphia
72. Labelle H, Tohme S, Duhaime M et al (1986) Natural history of scoliosis in Friedreich's ataxia. J Bone Joint Surg Am 68:564–572
73. Lee DY, Choi IH, Chung CY et al (1997) Fixed pelvic obliquity after poliomyelitis: classification and management. J Bone Joint Surg Br 79:190–196
74. Lefebvre S, Burglen L, Reboullet S et al (1995) Identification and characterization of a spinal muscular atrophy-determining gene. Cell 80:155–165
75. Lefebvre S, Burlet P, Liu Q et al (1997) Correlation between severity and SMN protein level in spinal muscular atrophy. Nat Genet 16:265–269
76. Leong JC, Wilding K, Mok CK et al (1981) Surgical treatment of scoliosis following poliomyelitis. A review of one hundred and ten cases. J Bone Joint Surg Am 63:726–740
77. Letts M, Rathbone D, Yamashita T et al (1992) Soft Boston orthosis in management of neuromuscular scoliosis: a preliminary report. J Pediatr Orthop 12:470–474
78. Lidstrom J, Stokland E, Hagberg B (1994) Scoliosis in Rett syndrome. Clinical and biological aspects. Spine 19: 1632–1635
79. Lin MC, Liaw MY, Chen WJ et al (2001) Pulmonary function and spinal characteristics: their relationships in persons with idiopathic and postpoliomyelitic scoliosis. Arch Phys Med Rehabil 82:335–341
80. Linson M, Bresnan M, Eraklis A et al (1981) Acute gastric volvulus following Harrington rod instrumentation in a patient with Werdnig-Hoffman disease. Spine 6:522–523
81. Loder RT, Lee CL, Richards BS (1989) Orthopaedic aspects of Rett syndrome: a multicenter review. J Pediatr Orthop 9:557–562
82. Luque ER (1982) Segmental spinal instrumentation for correction of scoliosis. Clin Orthop Relat Res 192–198
83. Luque ER (1982) The anatomic basis and development of segmental spinal instrumentation. Spine 7:256–259
84. Manzur AY, Kuntzer T, Pike M et al (2004) Glucocorticoid corticosteroids for Duchenne muscular dystrophy. Cochrane Database Syst Rev CD003725
85. Marchesi D, Arlet V, Stricker U et al (1997) Modification of the original Luque technique in the treatment of Duchenne's neuromuscular scoliosis. J Pediatr Orthop 17:743–749
86. Marsh A, Edge G, Lehovsky J (2003) Spinal fusion in patients with Duchenne's muscular dystrophy and a low forced vital capacity. Eur Spine J 12:507–512
87. Martinez BA, Lake BD (1987) Childhood nemaline myopathy: a review of clinical presentation in relation to prognosis. Dev Med Child Neurol 29:815–820
88. Mayer PJ, Dove J, Ditmanson M et al (1981) Postpoliomyelitis paralytic scoliosis. A review of curve patterns and results of surgical treatments in 118 consecutive patients. Spine 6:573–582
89. McCarthy RE, Bruffett WL, McCullough FL (1999) S rod fixation to the sacrum in patients with neuromuscular spinal deformities. Clin Orthop Relat Res 26–31
90. Merlini L, Granata C, Bonfiglioli S et al (1989) Scoliosis in spinal muscular atrophy: natural history and management. Dev Med Child Neurol 31:501–508
91. Mertz KD, Jost B, Glatzel M et al (2005) Progressive scoliosis in central core disease. Eur Spine J 14:900–905

92. Miles JM, Gilbert-Barness E (1993) Pathological cases of the month. Type 1 spinal muscular atrophy (Werdnig-Hoffman disease). Am J Dis Child 147:907–908
93. Miller F, Moseley CF, Koreska J et al (1988) Pulmonary function and scoliosis in Duchenne dystrophy. J Pediatr Orthop 8:133–137
94. Miller RG, Chalmers AC, Dao H et al (1991) The effect of spine fusion on respiratory function in Duchenne muscular dystrophy. Neurology 41:38–40
95. Mubarak SJ, Morin WD, Leach J (1993) Spinal fusion in Duchenne muscular dystrophy – fixation and fusion to the sacropelvis? J Pediatr Orthop 13:752–757
96. Nash CL Jr (1980) Current concepts review: scoliosis bracing. J Bone Joint Surg Am 62:848–852
97. Newton PO, Faro F, Wenger D et al (2006) Neuromuscular scoliosis. In: Herkowitz HN, Garfin SR, Eismont FJ, Bell GR, Balderston RA (eds) The spine, 5th edn. Saunders Elsevier, Philadelphia
98. Noordeen MH, Haddad FS, Muntoni F et al (1999) Blood loss in Duchenne muscular dystrophy: vascular smooth muscle dysfunction? J Pediatr Orthop B 8:212–215
99. O'Brien JP, Yau AC, Hodgson AR (1973) Halo pelvic traction: a technic for severe spinal deformities. Clin Orthop Relat Res 179–190
100. O'Brien JP, Dwyer AP, Hodgson AR (1975) Paralytic pelvic obliquity. Its prognosis and management and the development of a technique for full correction of the deformity. J Bone Joint Surg Am 57:626–631
101. O'Brien JP, Yau AC, Gertzbein S et al (1975) Combined staged anterior and posterior correction and fusion of the spine in scoliosis following poliomyelitis. Clin Orthop Relat Res 81–89
102. Oda T, Shimizu N, Yonenobu K et al (1993) Longitudinal study of spinal deformity in Duchenne muscular dystrophy. J Pediatr Orthop 13:478–488
103. Pavon SJ, Manning C (1970) Posterior spinal fusion for scoliosis due to anterior poliomyelitis. J Bone Joint Surg Br 52:420–431
104. Pearn J (1980) Classification of spinal muscular atrophies. Lancet 1:919–922
105. Peelle MW, Lenke LG, Bridwell KH et al (2006) Comparison of pelvic fixation techniques in neuromuscular spinal deformity correction: Galveston rod versus iliac and lumbosacral screws. Spine 31:2392–2398; discussion 2399
106. Phillips DP, Roye DP Jr, Farcy JP et al (1990) Surgical treatment of scoliosis in a spinal muscular atrophy population. Spine 15:942–945
107. Piasecki JO, Mahinpour S, Levine DB (1986) Long-term follow-up of spinal fusion in spinal muscular atrophy. Clin Orthop Relat Res 44–54
108. Ramirez N, Richards BS, Warren PD et al (1997) Complications after posterior spinal fusion in Duchenne's muscular dystrophy. J Pediatr Orthop 17:109–114
109. Reid JM, Appleton PJ (1999) A case of ventricular fibrillation in the prone position during back stabilisation surgery in a boy with Duchenne's muscular dystrophy. Anaesthesia 54:364–367
110. Riddick MF, Winter RB, Lutter LD (1982) Spinal deformities in patients with spinal muscle atrophy: a review of 36 patients. Spine 7:476–483
111. Rideau Y, Glorion B, Delaubier A et al (1984) The treatment of scoliosis in Duchenne muscular dystrophy. Muscle Nerve 7:281–286
112. Roaf R (1956) Paralytic scoliosis. J Bone Joint Surg Br 38-B:640–659
113. Robinson D, Galasko CS, Delaney C et al (1995) Scoliosis and lung function in spinal muscular atrophy. Eur Spine J 4:268–273
114. Russman BS, Melchreit R, Drennan JC (1983) Spinal muscular atrophy: the natural course of disease. Muscle Nerve 6:179–181
115. Russman BS, Iannacone ST, Buncher CR et al (1992) Spinal muscular atrophy: new thoughts on the pathogenesis and classification schema. J Child Neurol 7:347–353
116. Russman BS, Buncher CR, White M et al (1996) Function changes in spinal muscular atrophy II and III. The DCN/SMA Group. Neurology 47:973–976
117. Sabin AB (1985) Oral poliovirus vaccine: history of its development and use and current challenge to eliminate poliomyelitis from the world. J Infect Dis 151:420–436
118. Salk D (1980) Eradication of poliomyelitis in the United States. III. Poliovaccines – practical considerations. Rev Infect Dis 2:258–273
119. Sarwark J, Sarwahi V (2007) New strategies and decision making in the management of neuromuscular scoliosis. Orthop Clin North Am 38:485–496
120. Sarwark JF, MacEwen GD, Scott CI Jr (1990) Amyoplasia (a common form of arthrogryposis). J Bone Joint Surg Am 72:465–469
121. Schwentker EP, Gibson DA (1976) The orthopaedic aspects of spinal muscular atrophy. J Bone Joint Surg Am 58:32–38
122. Seeger BR, Sutherland AD, Clark MS (1984) Orthotic management of scoliosis in Duchenne muscular dystrophy. Arch Phys Med Rehabil 65:83–86
123. Sengupta DK, Mehdian SH, McConnell JR et al (2002) Pelvic or lumbar fixation for the surgical management of scoliosis in duchenne muscular dystrophy. Spine 27: 2072–2079
124. Shapiro F, Bresnan MJ (1982) Orthopaedic management of childhood neuromuscular disease. Part I: Spinal muscular atrophy. J Bone Joint Surg Am 64:785–789
125. Shapiro F, Sethna N, Colan S et al (1992) Spinal fusion in Duchenne muscular dystrophy: a multidisciplinary approach. Muscle Nerve 15:604–614
126. Shapiro F, Specht L (1993) The diagnosis and orthopaedic treatment of inherited muscular diseases of childhood. J Bone Joint Surg Am 75:439–454
127. Shapiro F, Specht L (1993) The diagnosis and orthopaedic treatment of childhood spinal muscular atrophy, peripheral neuropathy, Friedreich ataxia, and arthrogryposis. J Bone Joint Surg Am 75:1699–1714
128. Shapiro F, Sethna N (2004) Blood loss in pediatric spine surgery. Eur Spine J 13(Suppl 1):S6–17
129. Shapiro F, Zurakowski D, Sethna NF (2007) Tranexamic acid diminishes intraoperative blood loss and transfusion in spinal fusions for duchenne muscular dystrophy scoliosis. Spine 32:2278–2283
130. Smith AD, Koreska J, Moseley CF (1989) Progression of scoliosis in Duchenne muscular dystrophy. J Bone Joint Surg Am 71:1066–1074

131. Smucker JD, Miller F (2001) Crankshaft effect after posterior spinal fusion and unit rod instrumentation in children with cerebral palsy. J Pediatr Orthop 21:108–112
132. Sucato DJ (2007) Spine deformity in spinal muscular atrophy. J Bone Joint Surg Am 89(Suppl 1):148–154
133. Suk SI, Kim JH, Cho KJ et al (2007) Is anterior release necessary in severe scoliosis treated by posterior segmental pedicle screw fixation? Eur Spine J 16:1359–1365
134. Sussman M (2002) Duchenne muscular dystrophy. J Am Acad Orthop Surg 10:138–151
135. Sussman MD (1984) Advantage of early spinal stabilization and fusion in patients with Duchenne muscular dystrophy. J Pediatr Orthop 4:532–537
136. Turturro F, Rocca B, Gumina S et al (2005) Impaired primary hemostasis with normal platelet function in Duchenne muscular dystrophy during highly-invasive spinal surgery. Neuromuscul Disord 15:532–540
137. Velasco MV, Colin AA, Zurakowski D et al (2007) Posterior spinal fusion for scoliosis in duchenne muscular dystrophy diminishes the rate of respiratory decline. Spine 32:459–465
138. Vezain M, Saugier-Veber P, Melki J et al (2007) A sensitive assay for measuring SMN mRNA levels in peripheral blood and in muscle samples of patients affected with spinal muscular atrophy. Eur J Hum Genet 15:1054–1062
139. Wedel DJ (1992) Malignant hyperthermia and neuromuscular disease. Neuromuscul Disord 2:157–164
140. Werner AY, Zumeta GR, Newman RW et al (1951) Comparison of vital capacity in normal and poliomyelitic subjects. J Bone Joint Surg Am 33-A:628–632
141. Wilkins KE, Gibson DA (1976) The patterns of spinal deformity in Duchenne muscular dystrophy. J Bone Joint Surg Am 58:24–32
142. Yamashita T, Kanaya K, Yokogushi K et al (2001) Correlation between progression of spinal deformity and pulmonary function in Duchenne muscular dystrophy. J Pediatr Orthop 21:113–116
143. Yilmaz O, Karaduman A, Topaloglu H (2004) Prednisolone therapy in Duchenne muscular dystrophy prolongs ambulation and prevents scoliosis. Eur J Neurol 11:541–544
144. Yingsakmongkol W, Kumar SJ (2000) Scoliosis in arthrogryposis multiplex congenita: results after nonsurgical and surgical treatment. J Pediatr Orthop 20:656–661

23 Neurofibromatosis

Alvin H. Crawford and Viral V. Jain

Key Points

- Progressive early onset scoliosis in young children with neurofibromatosis does not respond to bracing, and growing rods should be considered to control the deformity prior to skeletal maturity.
- Early onset scoliosis in NF1 patients would more likely be dystrophic.
- Modulation, as we know it, may be the result of unrecognized intra and extra spinal tumors. Total spinal and brain MRIs are mandatory in all NF1 patients with spinal deformities.
- Dural ectasia and paraspinal tumors may erode the anchor purchase sites. Preoperative contrast-enhanced CT is indicated for all dystrophic spinal deformities to asses potential anchor sites.
- The distorted anatomy of the posterior elements in these patients may require the use of hooks, screws, and sublaminar wires to establish anchors.
- In severe early dystrophic deformities, we have limited but successful experience performing annulotomies for anterior release, traction, and posterior growing rod stabilization. This allows us to achieve further spinal length before the subsequent anterior discectomy and fusion at maturity.

23.1 Introduction

Neurofibromatoses (NF) are a group of genetic multisystem disorders involving products of all three germ lines: Neuroectoderm, mesoderm, and endoderm. Four varieties of this disorder have been described. The most common form is Neurofibromatosis Type-1 (NF1), previously known as von Recklinghausen disease, which involves predominantly peripheral nervous system, though it involves cells of mesodermal origin as well. Neurofibromatosis Type-2 (NF2) is the second most common form of the disorder involving central nervous system and is associated with bilateral vestibular schwannomas and multiple spinal schwannomas. Segmental neurofibromatosis is considered to be a mosaic form of NF1 with features of NF1 present in single body segment [7]. Schwannomatosis is the most recently described form manifesting itself as multiple deep painful schwannomas and is thought to represent a mosaic form of NF2 [26]. As NF1 is the only form associated with the disorders of the spine, all the discussion in this chapter focuses on NF1.

23.2 Epidemiology and Genetics

NF1 is one of the most common autosomal dominant disorders with a prevalence rate of 1:4,000 [14]. It occurs almost equally in all ethnic groups [16]. Approximately, 50% of all cases of NF-1 are due to new mutations. The NF1 gene mutations have variable expression – the clinical manifestations of NF-1 range from subclinical to severe. However, it has nearly 100% penetrance in adult individuals; therefore, an adult carrying the mutation will eventually exhibit some clinical feature of the disease [15]. The NF1 gene is located on the long arm of

A.H. Crawford (✉)
Cincinnati Children's Hospital, 3333 Burnet Avenue, MLC 2017, Cincinnati, OH 45229, USA
e-mail: Alvin.crawford@cchmc.org

B. A. Akbarnia et al. (eds.), *The Growing Spine*,
DOI: 10.1007/978-3-540-85207-0_23, © Springer-Verlag Berlin Heidelberg 2011

chromosome 17 (17q) and is of relatively large size (350,000 base pairs). This may explain the large rate of new mutation associated with this disorder. The gene product neurofibromin acts as a tumor suppressor gene [30]. Direct sequencing of the NF1 gene is now available for genetic testing. In contrast to the previously used protein truncation assay which only detected 60–70% of NF1 mutations, it detects the mutation in 95% and is considered as the gold standard [28, 34]. Animal models such as knockout mouse are now available that will greatly increase our understandings of the disease and help in development of therapeutic strategies.

23.3 Clinical Features

The most characteristic clinical features of NF1 are multiple hyperpigmented areas (*café au lait* macules) and neurofibroma. The Consensus Development Conference of the National Institutes of Health has published diagnostic criteria of NF1 in 1988 (Table 23.1). The presence of two or more of the criteria is essential for establishing the diagnosis of NF1 [1]. Since the consensus panel meeting, specific kinds of learning disabilities and MRI abnormalities (especially in children) have been associated specifically with NF-1. These are useful even during early life [31]. More recently, anterolateral bowing of the tibia has been considered as one of the criterion for the diagnosis of NF1 [45]. Axillary freckling and especially, *café au lait* spots occur very early and may be the only easily noticeable manifestations of the disease in very young children. Other conditions presenting with similar pigmented macules include Watson's syndrome, McCune-Albright syndrome, LEOPARD syndrome (lentigines, electrocardiogram [EKG] abnormalities, ocular hypertelorism, pulmonary stenosis, abnormalities of genitalia, retardation of growth, and deafness), and Noonan's syndrome.

There are two peaks of severe clinical problems in NF1 patients: one peak from 5 to 10 years of age, and a second from 36 to 50 years of age. At the second peak, 75% of the clinical problems are related to malignant neoplasms [39].

Genetic testing should be utilized to confirm or rule out the diagnosis of NF1 in uncertain cases especially in young children with the presence of *café au lait* spots only. For individuals who meet clinical diagnostic criteria for NF1, molecular testing is generally not felt to be necessary for diagnostic purposes.

Table 23.1 Diagnostic criteria of NF1 [1]

≥6 café au lait macules >5 mm in children >15 mm in adults
≥2 neurofibroma or one plexiform neurofibroma
Axillary or inguinal freckling
Optic glioma
≥2 pigmented iris hamartoma
A distinctive osseous lesion – sphenoid dysplasia, cortical thinning, vertebral scalloping
A first-degree relative with NF1

Presence of two or more criteria is essential for the diagnosis of NF1

23.4 Spinal Abnormalities

23.4.1 Spinal Deformities

Spinal deformities are the most common orthopaedic manifestation of NF1. True incidence of spinal deformities in NF1 is not known. It is quoted as from 2 to 36% in the literature [2, 22]. In the NF clinic at our institution, it is 23% [14]. In a report in 1988, Winter et al. [51] found only 102 patients having NF1 by clinical criteria in a pool of approximately 10,000 patients with scoliosis. Functional scoliosis resulting from limb hypertrophy or long-bone dysplasia leading to limb length inequality must be ruled out in patients with NF1. Rarely, unrecognized extra-pleural thoracic tumors can present as focal scoliosis. These lesions are usually plexiform neurofibroma and are not visible on plain radiographs [41]. The spinal deformities tend to develop early in the life, therefore, all preadolescent children with NF1 should be evaluated by scoliosis screening or the Adam forward-bend test to rule out the presence of a spinal deformity.

Traditionally, two forms of spinal deformities are described in NF1: Dystrophic and Nondystrophic. The distinctions between these two varieties of spinal deformities are clearer in the thoracic and thoracolumbar regions. Nondystrophic curves are similar to idiopathic curves with some exceptions. The dystrophic changes in NF1 are described in Table 23.2. The cause of dystrophic changes may be intrinsic bone dysplasia or associated with anomalies of the spinal canal secondary to abnormalities of the spinal cord/dura mater such as tumors, meningoceles, and/or dural ectasia. Dystrophic changes may also occur even if the intraspinal contents

Table 23.2 Characteristics of dystrophic spine

Rib penciling
Posterior vertebral scalloping
Vertebral wedging
Spindling of transverse processes
Anterior vertebral scalloping
Widened interpedicular distance
Enlarged intervertebral foramina
Lateral vertebral scalloping

are normal. Several investigators have suggested that there is no standard pattern of spinal deformity in NF1 and that the types of curvature are variable [18, 42].

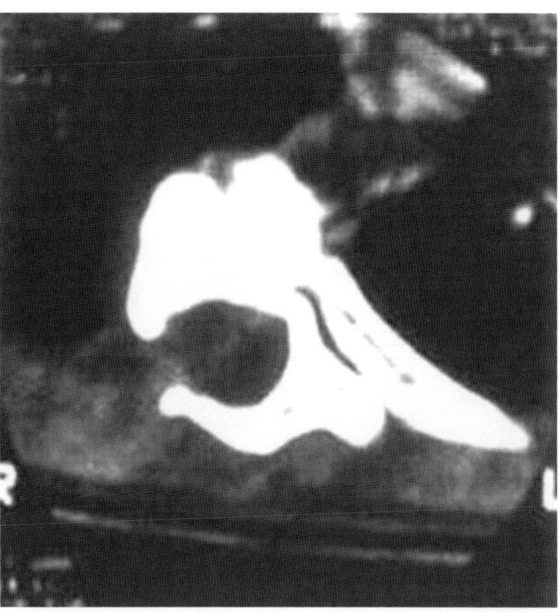

Fig. 23.1 CT scans of the vertebra with the neurofibroma in situ. A soft tissue shadow depicts neurofibroma exiting through the spinal canal. The constriction of the Neurofibroma from the neuroforamminae gives it the appearance of a dumbbell. (Reprinted, with permission, from Crawford and Gabriel [11])

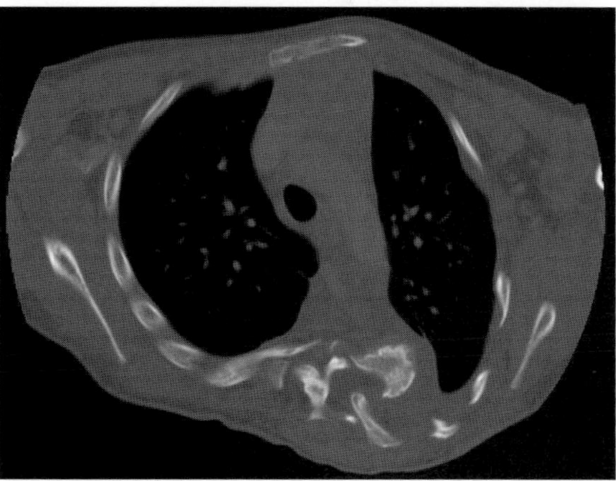

Fig. 23.2 Dislocation of rib head in the spinal canal in a severe dystrophic thoracic curve. Careful evaluation of the preoperative imaging including CT scan is essential to identify this pathology. Decompression prior to correction is essential to prevent intraoperative neurological complications

23.4.2 Dural Ectasia

Dural ectasia is a circumferential dilatation of the dural sac which is filled with proteinaceous fluid. The slow expansion of the dura results in erosion of the surrounding osseous structures resulting in widening of the spinal canal, thinning of the laminae, and ultimately destabilization of the spine. Dural expansion through the neural foramina can cause meningoceles giving the radiographic dumbbell appearance. However, enlargement of a single neural foramen on an oblique radiograph is usually caused by neurofibroma exiting from the spinal canal rather than dural ectasia (Fig. 23.1). Similar lesions are seen in other connective tissue disorders, e.g., Marfan's syndrome and Ehler Danlos syndrome, although cause of these lesions in NF1 is not known.

During this process, the neural elements are not affected. As a result of slow nature of this process andenormous widening of the spinal canal, the neural elements have adequate room for accommodation, and there may be severe angular deformity and distortion without neurological deficit. The patients remain neurologically intact until later in the course of the disease process when destabilization of the vertebral column jeopardizes the neural elements. Dislocation of the vertebral column due to dural ectasia has been reported in the literature [46]. The destabilization at the costovertebral junction can result in penetration of the rib head into the spinal canal with neurological compromise (Fig. 23.2) [19, 32]. The presence of rib head or the neurofibroma in the spinal canal can result in intraoperative neurological deficit if instrumentation is used for correction of the curve without adequate decompression.

Dural ectasia can be readily seen on high-volume computed tomographic (CT) myelography or contrast-enhanced magnetic resonance imaging (MRI) and is recommended before surgical intervention is undertaken for dystrophic curves. Higher imaging studies help to demonstrate extremely thin laminae; in which case, dissection by electocautery rather than by periosteal elevators are recommended during surgical exposure to avoid direct injury to the neural elements/dura by plunging into the spinal canal. Surgical spinal stabilization and fusion does not alter the course of dural ectasia. Dural ectasia can result in failure of the primary fusion or the expanding dura ultimately can destroy a solid fusion leaving behind the instrumentation (Fig. 23.3).

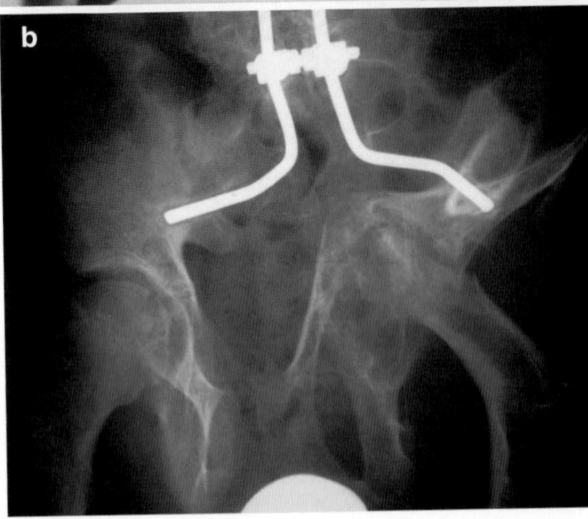

Fig. 23.3 (**a**) Neurofibromatosis in the lumbosacral spine. This patient was treated by fusion and instrumentation extending to the pelvis. (**b**) A few years later, the fusion mass and the vertebrae are eroded completely by expanding dural ectasia leaving behind the instrumentation. Also, note the destruction of the left hip joint by tumor

Spinal affections in NF1 can be described under following regions: cervical, thoracic/thoracolumbar, lumbosacral, and spinal canal.

23.5 Cervical Spine Abnormalities

The cervical spine abnormalities in NF-1 have not received enough attention in the literature [9, 21]. Usually, the cervical lesion is asymptomatic. When the lesion is symptomatic, pain is the most common presenting symptom [37]. Cervical abnormalities are likely to be missed in presence of scoliosis or Kyphosis in lower regions of the spine where the examiner's attention is focused on the more obvious deformity. In a study of 56 patients with NF1, Yong-Hing et al. [52] reported that 17 patients (30%) had cervical spine abnormalities. Out of these, seven patients were asymptomatic, whereas the rest had limited motion or pain in the neck. Four patients had neurological deficits that were attributed to cervical instability. Four of the 17 patients required fusion of the cervical spine. Curtis et al. [17] described eight patients who had paraplegia and NF-1. Four of these patients had cervical spine instability or intraspinal pathology in the cervical spine. The upper cervical spine should also be examined carefully. Isu et al. [25] described three patients with NF-1 who had C1–C2 dislocation with neurological deficit. All patients improved after decompression and fusion. We recommend that the cervical spine should be evaluated at the initial scoliosis assessment.

A lateral radiograph of the cervical spine is the initial screening tool. The NF1 can be manifested on a plain radiograph in the form of dystrophic changes or mal-alignment [12]. If any suspicious area is noted on plain radiographs, right and left oblique views should be obtained to look for widening of the neuroforamina which may represent dumbbell lesions. MRI is the definitive study to evaluate these lesions.

The most common spinal abnormality in the cervical spine is a severe cervical kyphosis (Fig. 23.4), which is often seen following a decompressive laminectomy without stabilization for an intraspinal lesion and is highly suggestive of the disorder [23]. Ogilvie [37] reported on the surgical treatment of cervical kyphosis by anterior fusion with iliac-crest or fibular bone graft or both. He considered halo traction to be a useful preoperative step if the kyphosis was greater than 45°. In the presence of progressive cervical kyphosis, we recommend preoperative halo traction only if the deformity is flexible as judged by the radiographs. This should be

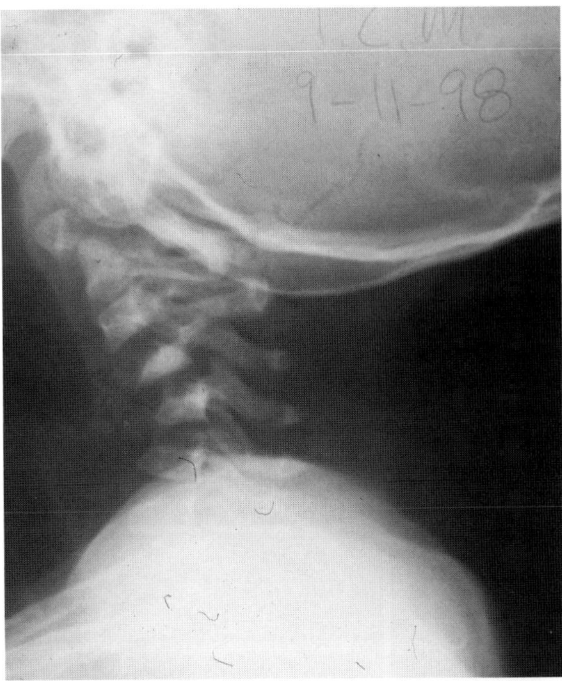

Fig. 23.4 Lateral radiograph of the cervical spine 6 months following laminectomy and excision of the neurofibroma, demonstrating marked kyphosis of the entire cervical spine. Note the dystrophic appearance of the vertebrae

followed by posterior fusion. If the deformity is rigid, then an anterior soft-tissue release followed by traction is safer. If sufficient bone stock is present, internal fixation with rods, wires, screws, or hooks may be used along with posterior fusion. If there is osteolysis with poor bone stock of the vertebral body, combined anterior and posterior fusion is needed, and postoperative immobilization with the use of a halo vest is recommended.

23.6 Thoracic/Thoracolumbar Spinal Abnormalities

The two varieties of spinal deformity are well distinguished in these regions of the spine as mentioned earlier. Also, the natural history of spinal deformities is well studied for thoracic/thoracolumbar region.

23.6.1 Non-Dystrophic Scoliosis

This is the common variety of spinal deformity observed in NF1. These curves behave similar to idiopathic curves with some differences [8, 10, 50]. This form usually involves eight to ten spinal segments. Most often, the deformity is convex to the right. However, these curves usually present earlier than the idiopathic curves and are more prone to progression. Furthermore, the rate of pseudoarthrosis following a fusion surgery is higher in these patients [9].

23.6.2 Dystrophic Scoliosis

This is an uncommon but malignant form of spinal deformity. It is characterized by early-onset, rapid progression, and is more difficult to treat [24, 44]. Typically, the dystrophic curve is a short-segmented, sharply angulated type that includes fewer than six spinal segments. Dystrophic curves may be associated with kyphosis and have a higher incidence of neurological injury [16, 44].

Dystrophic vertebral changes develop over time; on plain films, they are manifested by vertebral scalloping, rib penciling (rotation of the rib about 90°), spindling of the transverse processes, severe apical rotation, severe vertebral wedging, and wide nerve root foramina (see Table 23.2). Dystrophic curves are found most commonly in the thoracic region (Figs. 23.5–23.10) [13].

23.7 Natural History

The onset of spinal deformities may occur early in patients with NF1. Usually, early onset scoliosis is associated with kyphosis giving rise to kyphoscoliotic deformities. Calvert et al. [6] presented a series of treated ($n = 34$) and untreated ($n = 32$) patients who had NF-1 and scoliosis. Seventy-five percent of patients in the nontreated group had kyphoscoliosis. The investigators reported that patients, who had severe anterior vertebral scalloping noted on the lateral view, progressed an average of 23° per year for scoliosis and kyphosis. All other patients had an average rate of scoliosis progression of 7° and kyphosis progression of 8° per year.

Some of the nondystrophic curves exhibit a phenomenon of modulation. Durrani et al. [18] defined modulation as a process by which a nondystrophic curve acquires the features of a dystrophic curve and behaves as a dystrophic curve. They reported that modulation occurred in about 65% of their patients.

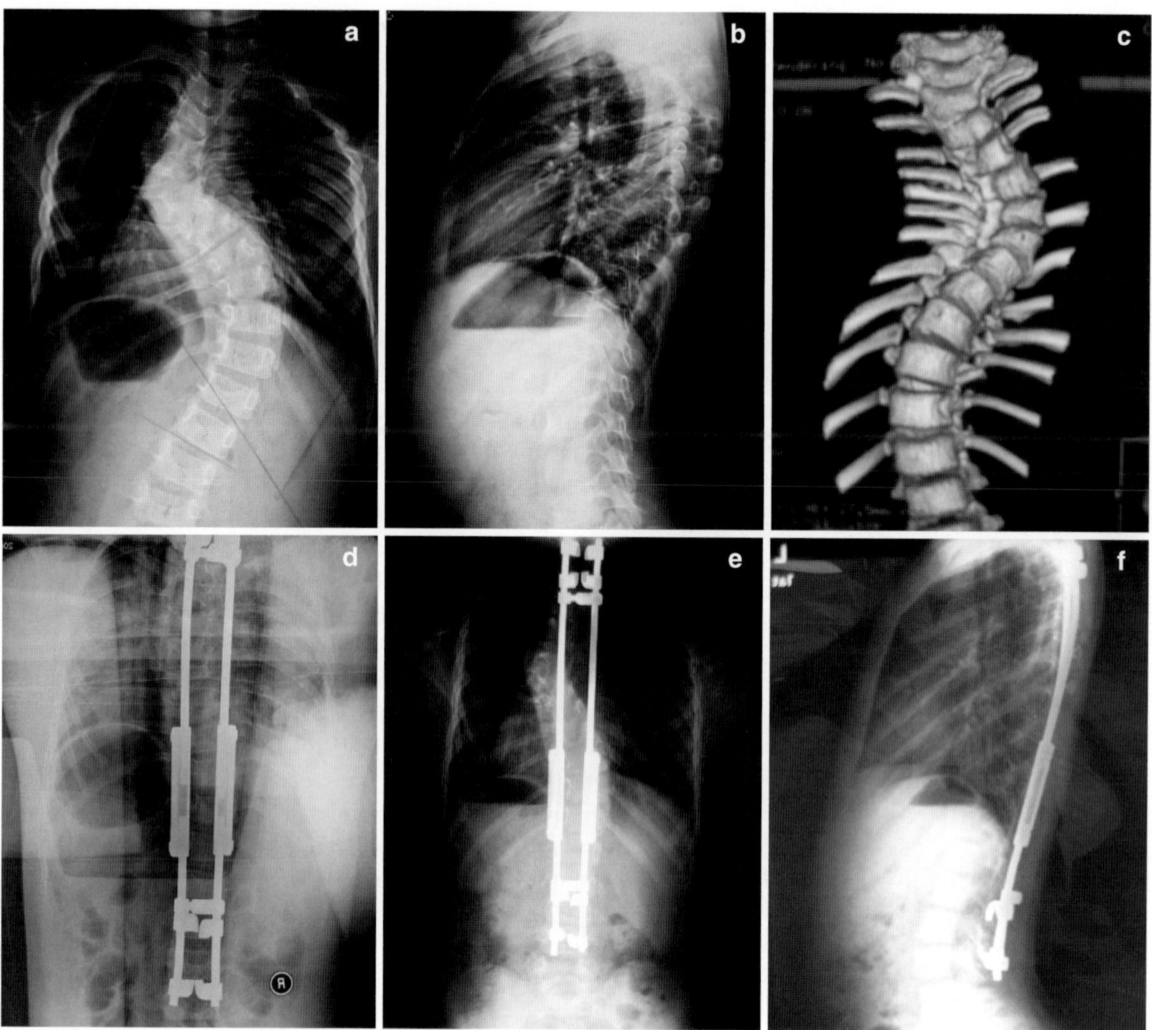

Fig. 23.5 A 6-year-old female with 80° thoracic scoliosis which was untreated. Preoperative 3D CT scan and radiographs (**a-c**) show the presence of typical radiological features of dystrophic vertebral bodies. She underwent a growing rod instrumentation with hook anchors (**d**). At 2-year follow-up, the correction has remained stable and spinal length has increased following serial lengthenings at every 6 month intervals (**e**, **f**)

Modulation occurred in 81% of patients who presented with scoliosis before 7 years of age and in 25% of those diagnosed after 7 years of age. In this study, rib penciling acquired through the modulation period was the only factor that was statistically significant in influencing the progression of the deformity. The rate of progression for "modulated" scoliosis and kyphosis was 12 and 8°, respectively, vs. 5 and 3° for nonmodulated spines. These authors based their report on plain radiographic findings. Some of the recent reports with the use of MRI of spine have shown the presence of dystrophic findings in the spine before they are apparent on the plain radiographs. Based on these reports, it can be speculated that true modulation may be rare, and many of the apparent nondystrophic curves are actually dystrophic curves which subsequently present themselves with radiographic changes of dystrophic curve giving an impression of "modulation."

It is well known that despite apparent solid fusion, some dystrophic curve shows progression. This tendency is more noted in patients with kyphosis (>50°). The vertebral subluxation, disc wedging, and dystrophy of peripheral skeleton are other factors associated with progression of the deformity after fusion [48].

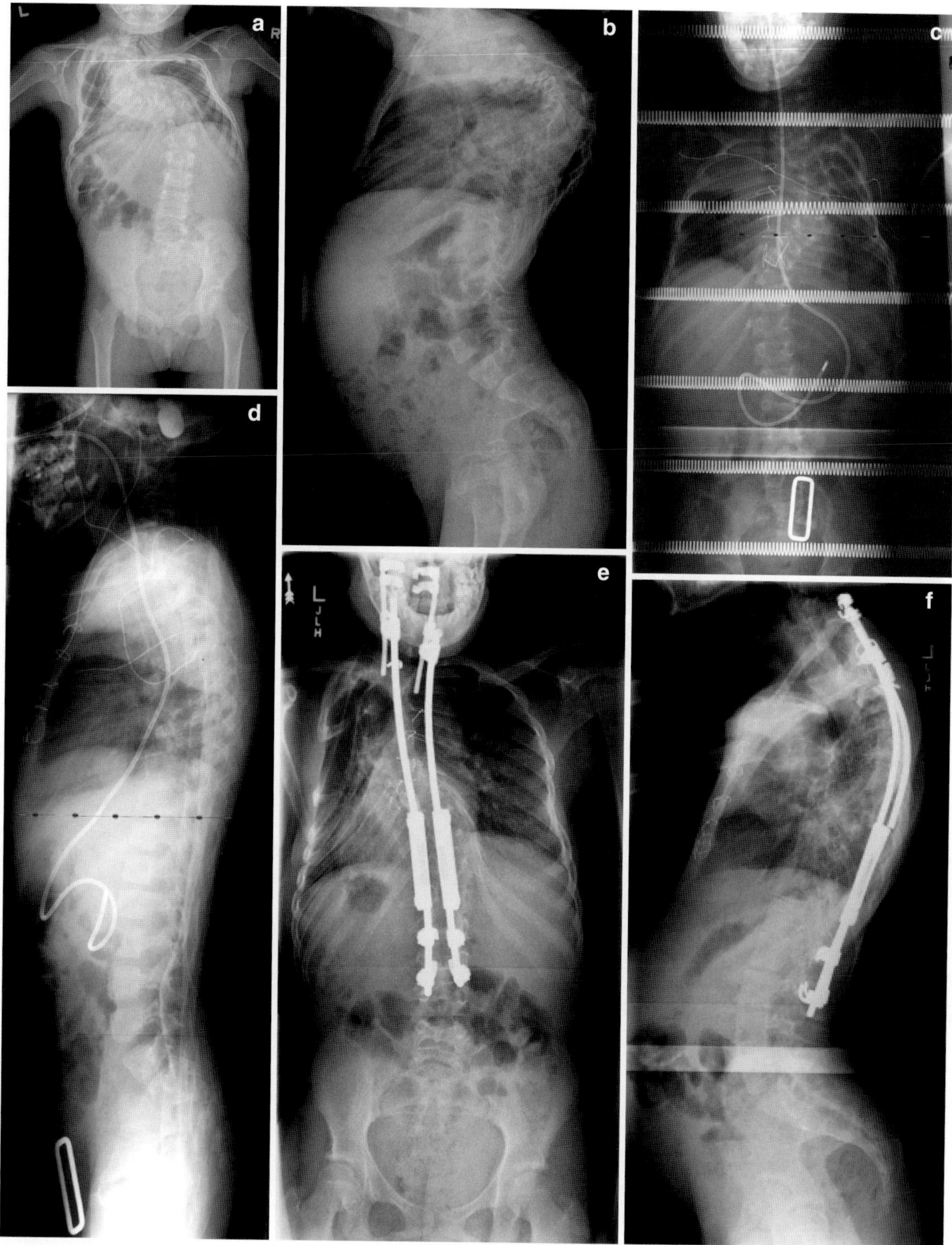

Fig. 23.6 (**a**, **b**) A 6-year-old female with severe thoracic dystrophic kyphoscoliosis. The deformity involves mid and upper thoracic spines. The curvature measures more than 100° in both the planes (**c**, **d**). She underwent an anterior release (annulotomies) through a double "trap door" approach for her upper thoracic and mid thoracic curve followed by a period of 2 weeks of halo-femoral traction. Anterior release with gradual traction alone resulted in significant correction of the deformity. (**e**, **f**) After the traction, the patient underwent growing rod instrumentation with proximal anchors in her lower cervical spine. At 5 years of follow-up, although one rod is broken, her correction is well maintained and her spinal height has increased as measured by digital radiograph

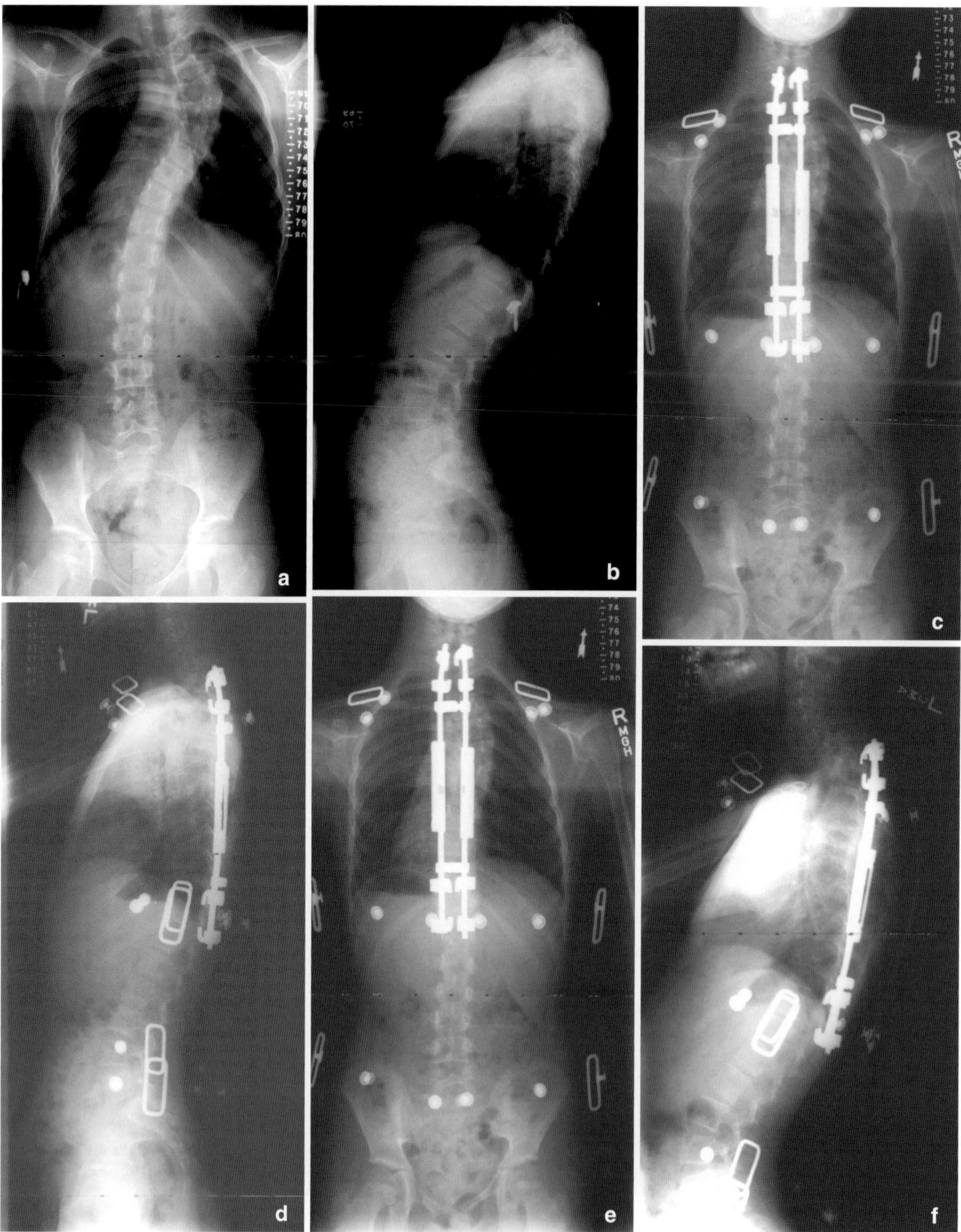

Fig. 23.7 (**a**, **b**) A 7-year-old female with high thoracic dystrophic scoliosis. The brace is usually ineffective in controlling the high thoracic curves (**c**, **d**). The patient underwent a growing rod instrumentation with brace. Moderate correction of the curve was achieved with the index procedure. Note that the proximal hook is at T1 (**e**, **f**). After 1-year post-op, the correction is well maintained after two lengthenings. On the lateral radiograph, gradual development of juctional kyphosis is evident at both proximal- and distal-end instrumented segments. Patient has been asymptomatic at this point in time

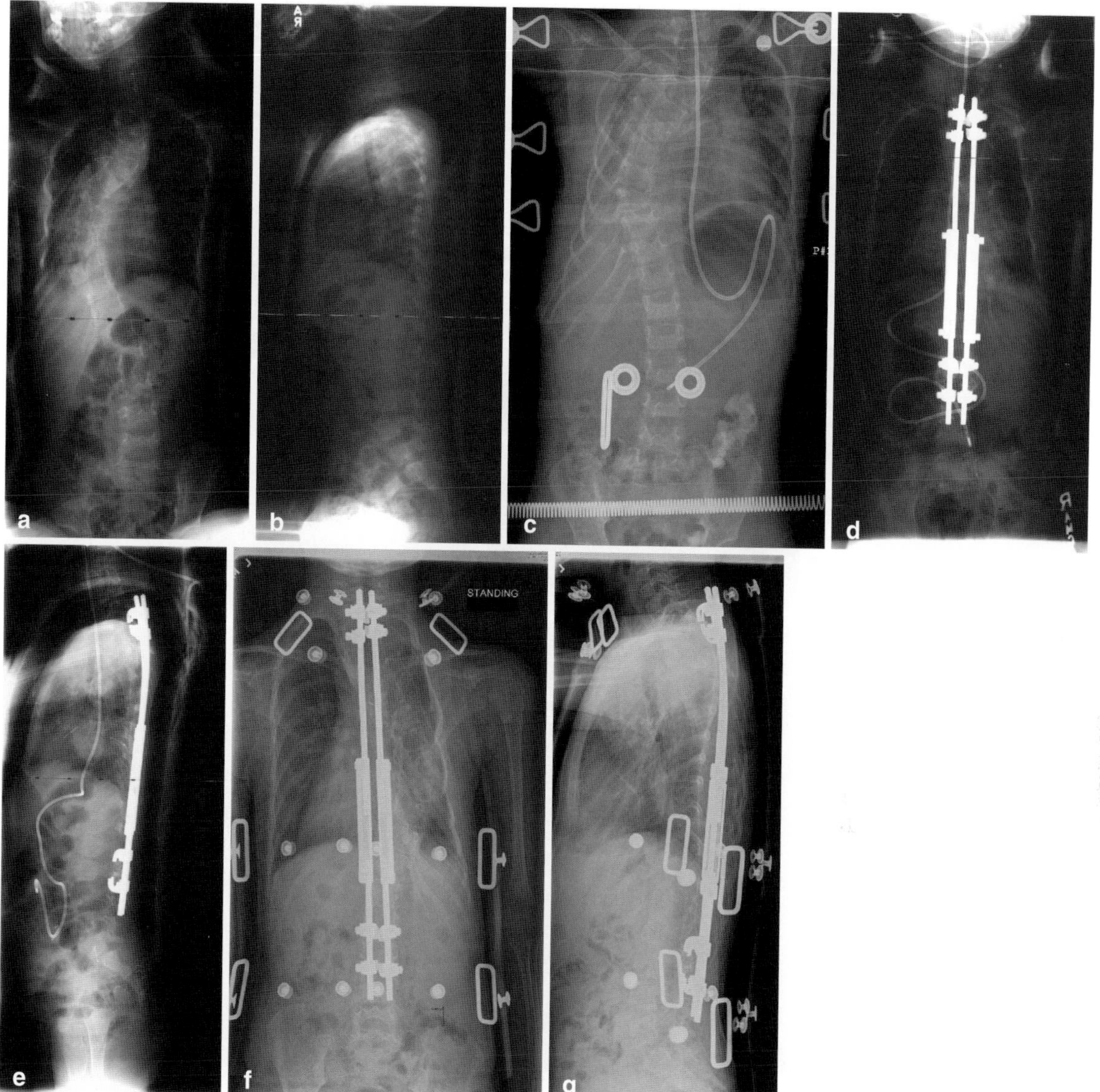

Fig. 23.8 (**a**, **b**) A 4-year-old female with thoracic dystrophic scoliosis who failed cast-brace treatment (**c**-**e**). She underwent anterior annulotomies at the thoracic apex by thoracoscopic procedure followed by traction for 10 days. This was followed by growing rod instrumentation (**f**, **g**). At 2-year follow-up, the correction has remained stable and spinal length has increased following two lenghtenings. Development of proximal juctional kyphosis at this point in time is asymptomatic

23.8 Treatment

The treatment of nondystrophic curvatures is very similar to idiopathic scoliosis. The curve of less than 25° should be observed. Curves between 25 and 40° can be treated with brace successfully [27]. Once beyond 40°, surgery by posterior spinal fusion is usually indicated [5]. Curves >55–60° are treated with anterior release with bone-grafting, followed by an instrumented posterior spinal fusion [9]. This is necessary because the curve is usually more rigid than is a similar-sized curve in idiopathic scoliosis. We recommend postoperative orthotic immobilization, although others have managed these patients without postoperative immobilization, with good early results [42].

Dystrophic curvatures of less than 20° should be treated by observation. Serial spinal radiographs at

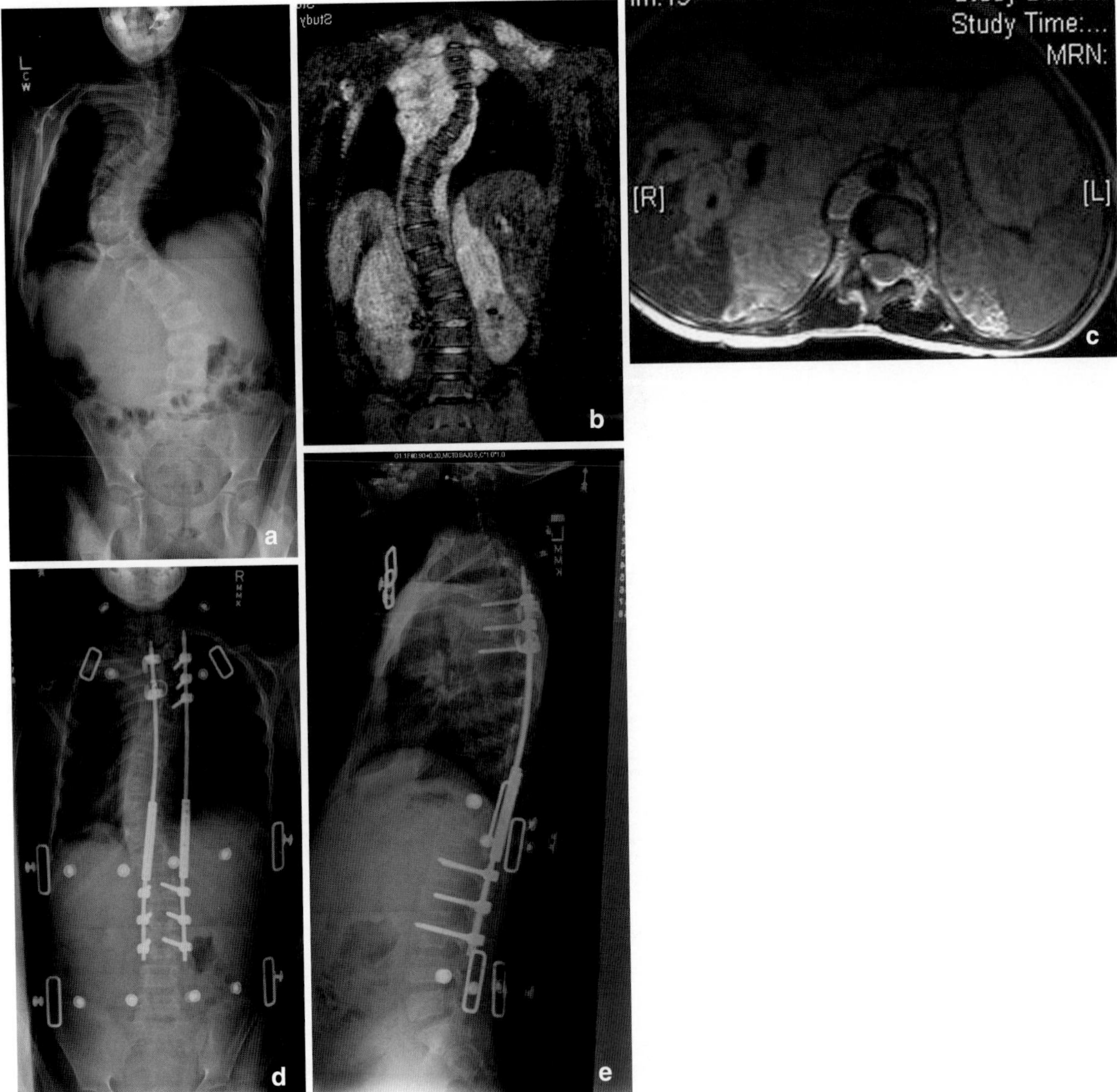

Fig. 23.9 (**a-c**) A 9-year-old female with dystrophic thoracic scoliosis. The MRI examination shows extensive involvement of the thoracic cavity with the tumor (**d**, **e**). This patient underwent single-stage growing rod instrumentation. As the posterior elements were involved by the tumor, pedicle screws were used as an anchor point for the growing rods. At 5-month follow-up, the correction is well maintained and there are no complications. Note the presence of sublaminar wires and hooks to augment pedicle screw fixation

6-month intervals should be obtained to check for progression of the deformity [9]. Bracing of progressive dystrophic curvatures is ineffective and surgery is usually recommended [22, 27, 50]. For adolescent patients with dystrophic curvature greater than 20–40° of angulation, a posterior spinal fusion with segmental spinal instrumentation is recommended [16, 22]. In more severe dystrophic scoliosis, anterior fusion should be performed in addition to posterior fusion, to increase the fusion rate and to reduce the risk for progression despite solid posterior fusion. Preoperative halo traction may be beneficial for the treatment of severe curves, including those with kyphoscoliosis [22, 33, 40, 51]. It allows gradual and controlled soft tissue relaxation and curve correction before surgery or between staged surgeries; however, it is contraindicated in patients who

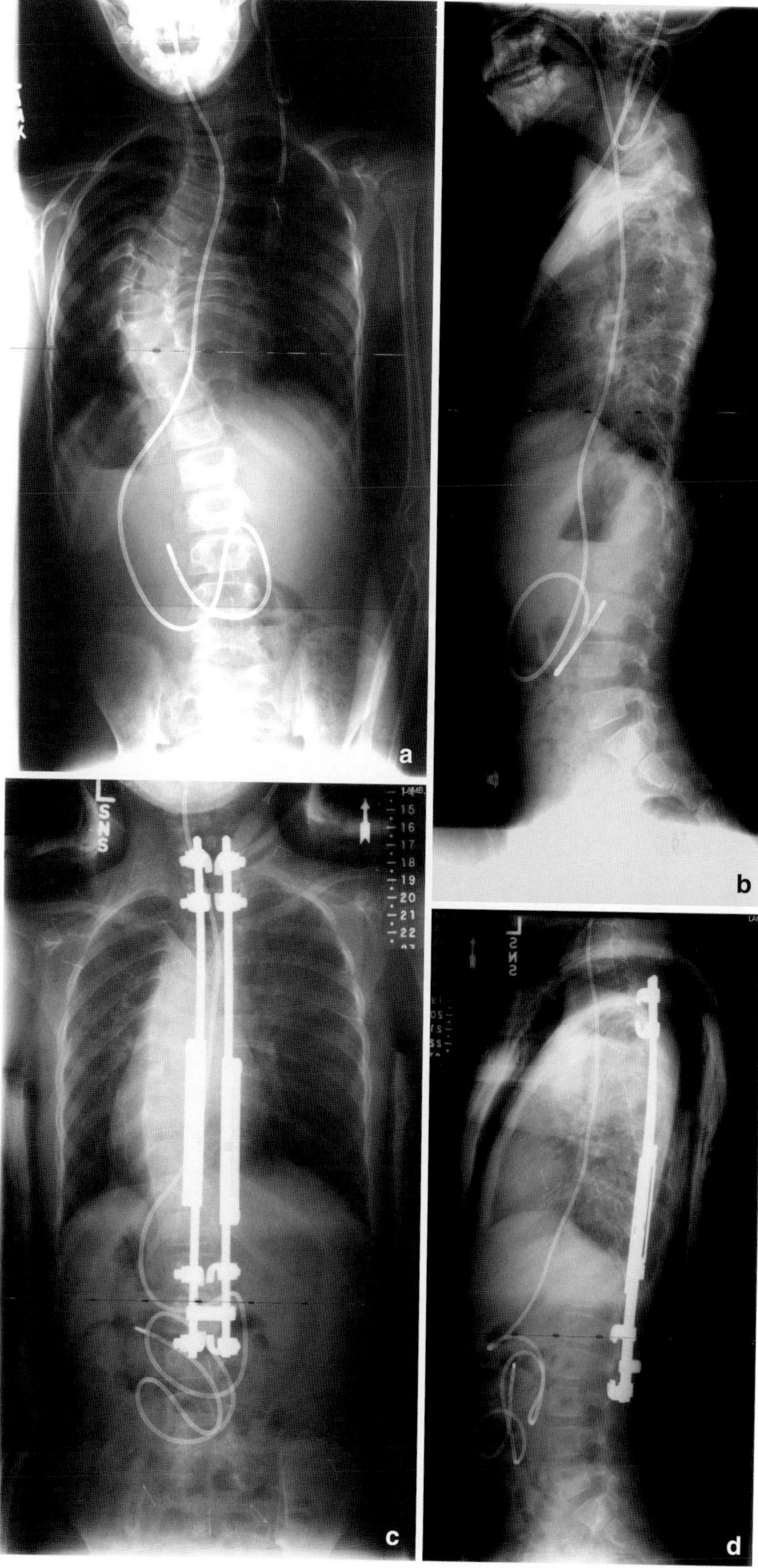

Fig. 23.10 (**a**, **b**) This is a 8-year-old male patient with thoracic scoliosis and dystrophic NF1. Patient also had feeding difficulty requiring preoperative alimentation to increase his BMI (**c**, **d**). He underwent a growing rod instrumentation

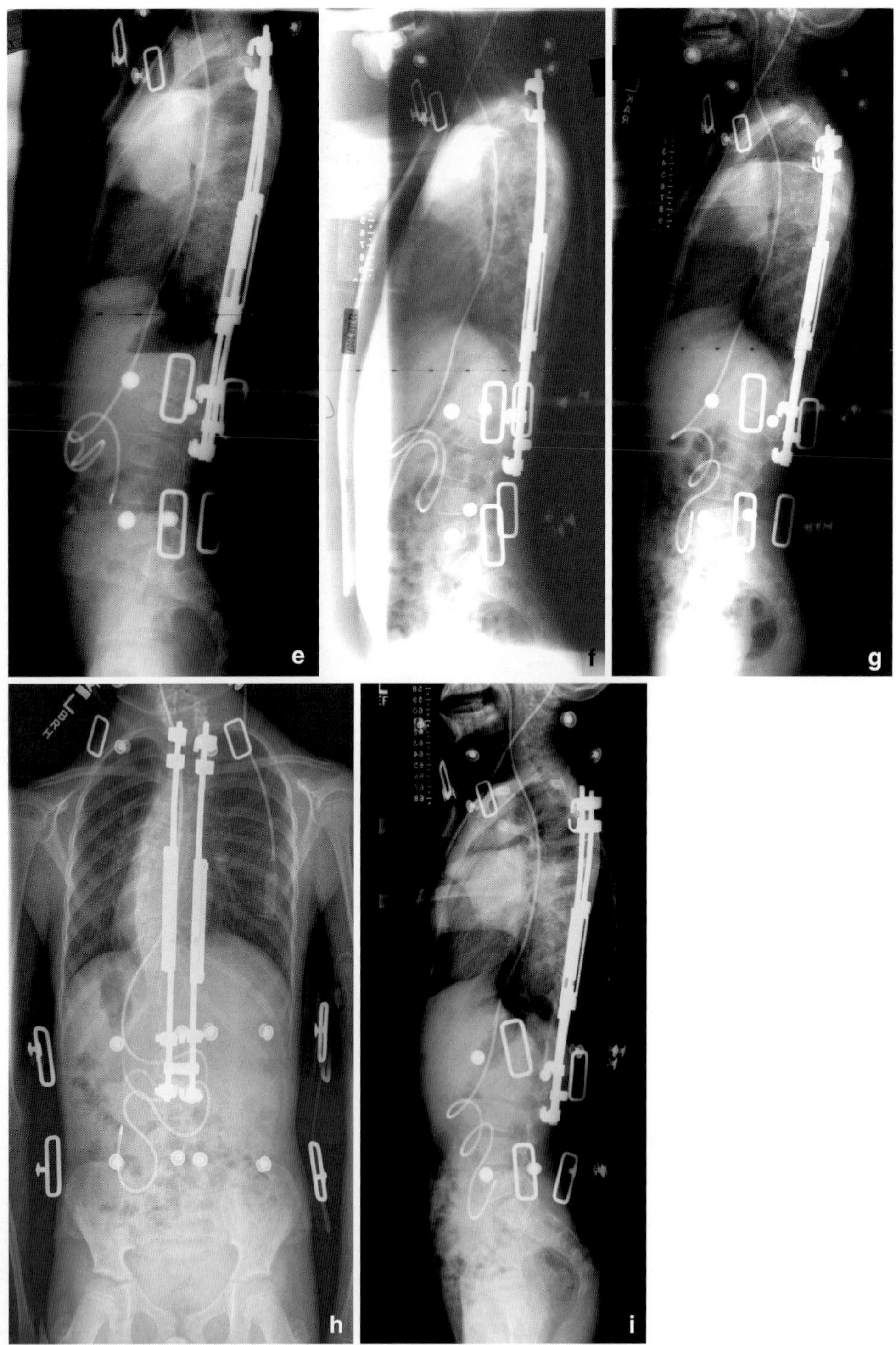

Fig. 23.10 (continued) (**e-g**). During the subsequent follow-ups after a few lengthenings, he was noted to have proximal juctional kyphosis with progressive pulling out of the proximal hooks. He therefore was revised at his proximal end and the encore point was moved more distal leaving his kyphosis alone (**h**, **i**) Following his last lengthening, he developed an abscess at his proximal anchor site which could be attributed to his poor nutritional state. This was treated by removal of the anchors, washout, and reinsertion of the anchors. Patient responded well to this treatment and is currently asymptomatic. At 2-year follow-up, his correction is well maintained, although the increase in spinal length is negligible

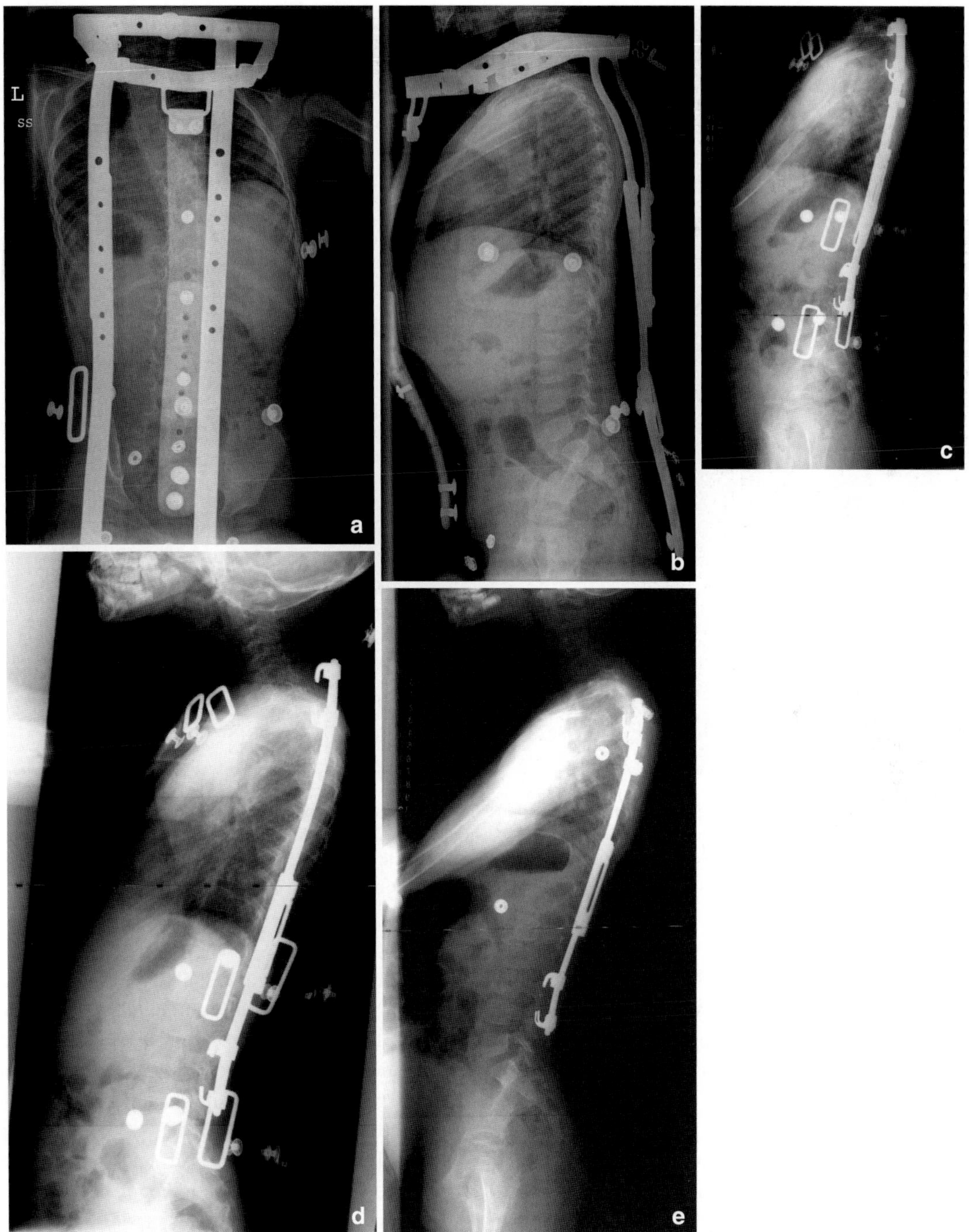

Fig. 23.11 (**a**, **b**) A 6-year-old female with thoracic dystrophic NF1. Patient was earlier treated in a Risser cast followed by a CTLSO for two cycles. Despite in cast and brace, her curve progressed (**c**) She ultimately underwent a growing rod instrumentation (**d**). Following first few lengthenings, she was noted to develop proximal juctional kyphosis with gradual pulling out of her top hooks. There are two options at this time. First is to extend the instrumentation to the cervical spine or (**e**) second is to extend the instrumentation down one segment in order to allow the junctional segment to remain free from the stress and prevent further kyphosis

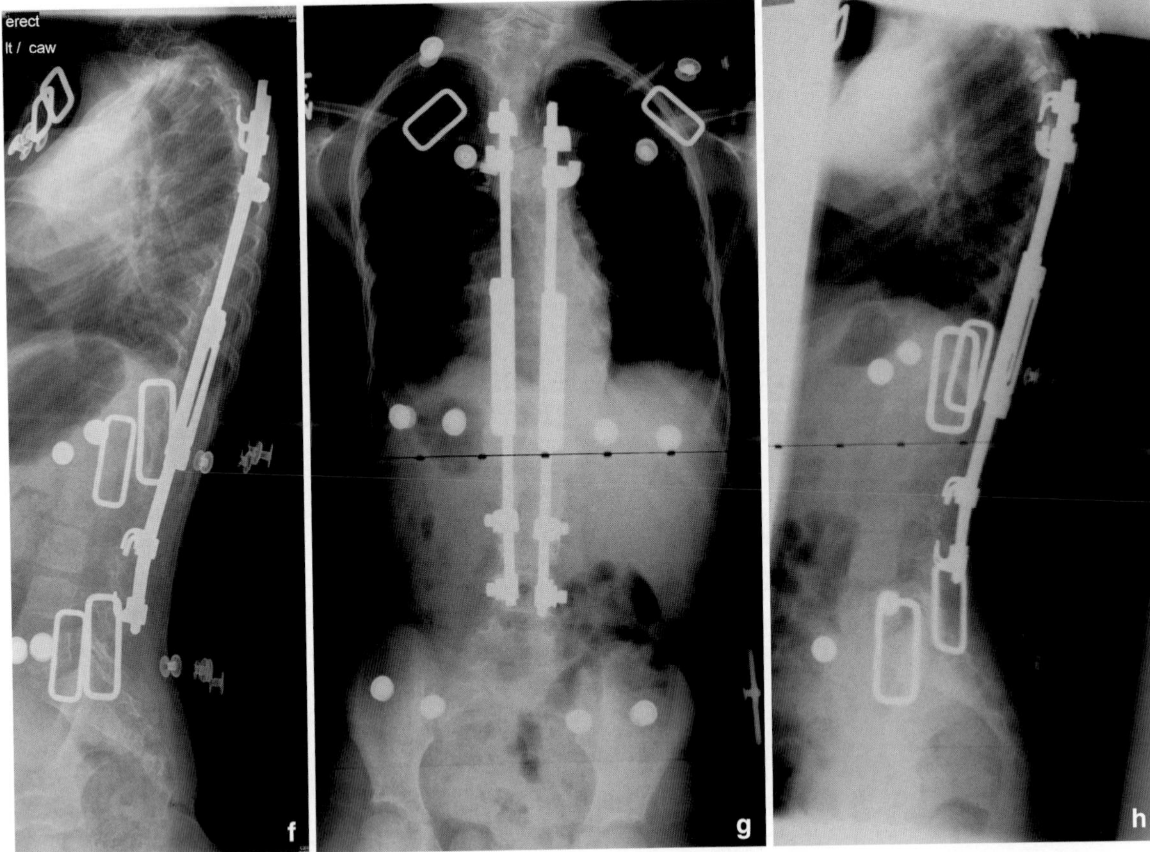

Fig. 23.11 (continued) (**f–h**) The patient developed further kyphosis resulting in the pulling out of the proximal hook. At that point in time, her entire proximal construct was revised and she was given a CTLSO. After a total of 3 years of follow-up, her curve has remain stable and there are no further complications at this time. Furthermore, patient has shown an increase in her spine length as measured on the digital radiography

have additional cervical kyphosis. Daily neurological evaluations are mandatory to avoid spinal or cranial nerve injuries. Nutrition is also paramount during this time. We use supplemental nasojejunal feeding in between the stages to decrease the protein depletion that is seen in staged patients [20, 29]. We recommend anterior release, nasojejunal tube alimentation, and craniofemoral traction for rigid curves of >90°. For curves >100° in any plane, anterior as well as posterior release followed by nasojejunal tube alimentation and craniofemoral traction is recommended (see Fig. 23.6).

The dystrophic curves that are present in late juvenile and early adolescent period pose a challenge to the surgeon. These curves have a high rate of pseudoarthrosis following a posterior spinal fusion [5, 9, 44]. A combined anterior and posterior spinal fusion has been recommended in these patients to decrease the rate of pseudoarthrosis and crank-shaft [4, 35, 38, 43]. We also recommend the use of segmental instrumentation to reduce the rate of curve progression after arthrodesis. In our experience, an early fusion of the spine in this age group does not significantly alter the final height and its benefit outweighs the risk of severe progression. Furthermore, the dystrophic segments have very limited growth potential to begin with [13].

Dystrophic curves in infants, toddlers, and early juvenile patients present even more of a challenge. In this age group, a spinal fusion can certainly have a significant effect on the overall height as well as the size of the thoracic cage. Smaller size of the vertebrae can pose difficulty in the instrumentation. On the other hand, progression of the curve itself can significantly distort the thoracic cage which can lead to cardiothoracic decompensation.

23.8.1 *Trapdoor Procedure*

A few of the NF1 patients develop very high thoracic curve extending in the cervicothoracic junction. These patients need circumferential fusion and instrumentation in the lower cervical and upper thoracic spine. This group of patients may benefit from a "trap door" sternal split approach if anterior fusion is needed (see Fig. 23.6) [35, 36]. This approach allows anterior exposure of the lower cervical and upper thoracic spine. Bracing may need to be extended to the cervical region in cases of severe dystrophic curves that are instrumented into the upper thoracic and cervicothoracic region. Cervical bracing, halo vest, or Minerva casting may help to prevent the possibility of screw/hook pullout. This is especially true for dystrophic curves that have low bone mineral density [30].

23.9 Growing Rod Instrumentation

The so-called "growing rods" have been used successfully in the treatment of early onset idiopathic curves. These devices have been shown to prevent the progression of the curve while preserving the longitudinal growth of the spine [3]. The currently available dual growing rods have been shown to be superior to the previous versions of submuscular single growing rods [47]. We have used dual growing rods on early-onset dystrophic curves with a great deal of optimism [6].

We have used the growing rods directly with fusion of the cranial and caudal anchors only in the patients with flexible curves less than 60° (see Fig. 23.7). Traditionally, this is followed by a period of bracing and lengthening every 6 months. In larger and stiffer curves, we recommend anterior annulotomies (with or without thoracoscope) without fusion to preserve growth (see Figs. 23.6 and 23.8). Annulotomies should be performed with Bovie dissection and the use of a thin rongeur through the annulus fibrosis instead of sharp dissections of the endplate apophysis. Sharp dissection may cause significant bleeding from the often friable cancellous matrix of the vertebral bodies. Care should be taken to preserve the segmental vessels as much as possible. This is followed by insertion of the growing rods and routine lengthening at 6 months interval.

In certain cases, traditional use of pedicle screws as the anchor point may not be feasible (see Fig. 23.9). In these cases, use of hooks and sublaminar wires as anchor points in the spine is advantageous because of erosion from tumor and Dural Ectasia.

The use of growing rod instrumentation in NF1 is also associated with a high incidence of complications. A high rate of complications has also been reported for idiopathic patients [3]. The most common complication we have encountered with growing rods is proximal junctional kyphosis. This is especially common in patients with high thoracic or cervicothoracic curves (see Figs. 23.7–23.11). We believe that it is the result of excessive stress put on the proximal anchors by routine lengthening. This abnormal stress results from the difficulty in applying adequate proximal kyphosis to the rods above the lengthener because of inadequate length. The subsequent lengthening drives the rod directly vertical as opposed to physiologic mechanics. The proximal anchor places a vertical load on the lamina forcing hinging of the vertebra into kyphosis. This is our experience with proximal hook capture systems. An all screw construct may be less problematic. In these patients, we currently do not perform routine lengthening. Other complications encountered are infection (see Fig. 23.10) and rod breakage (see Fig. 23.6).

Although the use of growing rod instrumentation is associated with higher complication rate, its benefits outweighs the risk in patients with early onset dystrophic scoliosis. Our early results with the use of growing rods remain encouraging. This is a promising technique made especially useful because most dystrophic curves are early onset.

23.10 Other Spinal Deformities

23.10.1 *Kyphosis*

Kyphoscoliosis is defined as scoliosis accompanied by a kyphosis of greater than 50°. It may occur by gradual scoliotic rotation and progression, or it can be found early in the disease with an abrupt angular kyphotic curve [49]. Vertebral bodies may be deformed so severely that they are confused with congenital deformities. Severe kyphosis is the most common cause of neurological deficits in NF-1 [16]. Use of traction in patients with rigid and severe kyphosis can increase the tension on the spinal cord leading to neurological deficits.

Traction following anterior release is safe when monitored appropriately. For curves greater than 50°, anterior surgery (release and fusion) is recommended, followed by posterior segmental instrumentation one or two levels above and below the end vertebrae [9, 13, 48, 51].

23.10.2 *Spondylolisthesis*

Spondylolisthesis in patients with NF1 is rare. Spondylolisthesis is usually secondary to increased anteroposterior diameter of the spinal canal, with elongation and thinning of the pedicles, causing a pathologic forward progression of the anterior elements of the spinal column. The most frequent causes of pathologic instability are dural ectasia, meningocele, and neurofibroma. MRI or CT and/or contrast scans are absolutely necessary for preoperative evaluation. The treatment in severe spondylolisthesis is anterior and posterior spinal fusion. Fusion is difficult to obtain because of the mechanical alignment of the lumbosacral region and poor bone formation. We recommend at least an L4-to-sacrum anterior and posterior fusion with lumbosacral instrumentation. Postoperative immobilization is strongly recommended.

23.11 Conclusion

The management of spinal disorders in young children in NF1 continues to be problematic. The use of growing rods allows more longitudinal growth than fusion and more life freedom than bracing. The problems we have encountered are mechanical and could be expected when proximal and distal fixation is performed over an otherwise completely mobile spinal column. The multiple surgeries increase the potential for complications including infections. We continue to pursue solutions to our problems.

References

1. National Institutes of Health Consensus Development Conference Statement (1988) Neurofibromatosis. Bethesda, Md., USA, July 13–15, 1987. Neurofibromatosis 1(3): 172–178
2. Akbarnia BA, Gabriel KR, Beckman E et al. (1992) Prevalence of scoliosis in neurofibromatosis. Spine 17(8 Suppl):S244–S248
3. Akbarnia BA, Marks DS, Boachie-Adjei O et al (2005) Dual growing rod technique for the treatment of progressive early-onset scoliosis: a multicenter study. Spine 30(17 Suppl):S46–S57
4. Al-Sayyad MJ, Crawford AH, Wolf RK (2004) Early experiences with video-assisted thoracoscopic surgery: our first 70 cases. Spine 29:1945–1951; Discussion 52
5. Betz RR, Iorio R, Lombardi AV et al (1989) Scoliosis surgery in neurofibromatosis. Clin Orthop Rel Res 245:53–56
6. Calvert PT, Edgar MA, Webb PJ (1989) Scoliosis in neurofibromatosis. The natural history with and without operation. J Bone Joint Surg [Br] 71:246–251
7. Calzavara PG, Carlino A, Anzola GP et al (1988) Segmental neurofibromatosis. Case report and review of the literature. Neurofibromatosis 1:318–322
8. Crawford AH (1986) Neurofibromatosis in children. Acta orthop Scand 218:1–60
9. Crawford AH (1989) Pitfalls of spinal deformities associated with neurofibromatosis in children. Clin Orthop Rel Res 245:29–42
10. Crawford AH (1994) Neurofibromatosis. In: Weinstein SL (ed) The pediatric spine: principles and practice. Raven, New York, pp 619–649
11. Crawford AH, Gabriel KR (1997) Dysplastic scoliosis: neurofibromatosis. In: Bridwell KH, DeWald RL (eds). The textbook of spinal surgery, 2nd edn. Lippincott-Raven, Philadelphia, PA, pp 292
12. Crawford AH, Schorry EK (1999) Neurofibromatosis in children: the role of the orthopaedist. J Am Acad Orthop Surg 7:217–230
13. Crawford AH (2001) Neurofibromatosis. In: Weinstein SL (ed) The pediatric spine: principles and practice. Lippincott Williams & Wilkins, Philadelphia, PA, pp 471–490
14. Crawford AH, Schorry EK (2006) Neurofibromatosis update. J Pediatr Orthop 26:413–423
15. Crawford AH, Herrera-Soto J (2007) Scoliosis associated with neurofibromatosis. The Orthop Clin N Am 38:553–562; vii
16. Crawford AH, Parikh S, Schorry EK et al (2007) The immature spine in type-1 neurofibromatosis. J Bone Joint Surg [Am] 89(Suppl 1):123–142
17. Curtis BH, Fisher RL, Butterfield WL et al (1969) Neurofibromatosis with paraplegia. Report of eight cases. J Bone Joint Surg [Am] 51:843–861
18. Durrani AA, Crawford AH, Chouhdry SN et al (2000) Modulation of spinal deformities in patients with neurofibromatosis type 1. Spine 25:69–75
19. Flood BM, Butt WP, Dickson RA (1986) Rib penetration of the intervertebral foraminae in neurofibromatosis. Spine 11:172–174
20. Funasaki H, Winter RB, Lonstein JB et al (1994) Pathophysiology of spinal deformities in neurofibromatosis. An analysis of seventy-one patients who had curves associated with dystrophic changes. J Bone Joint Surg [Am] 76:692–700
21. Haddad FS, Williams RL, Bentley G (1995) The cervical spine in neurofibromatosis. Br J Hosp Med 53:318–319
22. Halmai V, Doman I, de Jonge T et al (2002) Surgical treatment of spinal deformities associated with neurofibromatosis type 1. Report of 12 cases. J Neurosurg 97(3 Suppl):310–316
23. Holt JF, Wright EM (1948) The radiologic features of neurofibromatosis. Radiology 51:647–663

24. Holt RT, Johnson JR (1989) Cotrel-Dubousset instrumentation in neurofibromatosis spine curves. A preliminary report. Clin Orthop Rel Res 245:19–23
25. Isu T, Miyasaka K, Abe H et al (1983) Atlantoaxial dislocation associated with neurofibromatosis. Report of three cases. J Neurosurg 58:451–453
26. Kaufman DL, Heinrich BS, Willett C et al (2003) Somatic instability of the NF2 gene in schwannomatosis. Arch Neurol 60:1317–1320
27. Kim HW, Weinstein SL (1997) Spine update. The management of scoliosis in neurofibromatosis. Spine 22:2770–2776
28. Korf BR (2005) The phakomatoses. Clin Derm 23:78–84
29. Lalueza MP, Colomina MJ, Bago J et al (2005) Analysis of nutritional parameters in idiopathic scoliosis patients after major spinal surgery. Europ J Clin Nutr 59:720–722
30. Lammert M, Kappler M, Mautner VF et al (2005) Decreased bone mineral density in patients with neurofibromatosis 1. Osteoporos Int 16:1161–1166
31. Listernick R, Charrow J (1990) Neurofibromatosis type 1 in childhood. J Pediatr 116:845–853
32. Major MR, Huizenga BA (1988) Spinal cord compression by displaced ribs in neurofibromatosis. A report of three cases. J Bone Joint Surg [Am] 70:1100–1102
33. Mehlman CT, Al-Sayyad MJ, Crawford AH (2004) Effectiveness of spinal release and halo-femoral traction in the management of severe spinal deformity. J Pediatr Orthop 24:667–673
34. Messiaen LM, Callens T, Mortier G et al (2000) Exhaustive mutation analysis of the NF1 gene allows identification of 95% of mutations and reveals a high frequency of unusual splicing defects. Human Mutation 15:541–555
35. Mulpuri K, LeBlanc JG, Reilly CW et al (2005) Sternal split approach to the cervicothoracic junction in children. Spine 30:E305–E310
36. Nazzaro JM, Arbit E, Burt M (1994) "Trap door" exposure of the cervicothoracic junction. Technical note. J Neurosurg 80:338–341
37. Ogilvie JW (1995) Moe's textbook of scoliosis and other spinal deformities, 3rd edn. WB Saunders, Philadelphia, PA
38. Parisini P, Di Silvestre M, Greggi T et al (1999) Surgical correction of dystrophic spinal curves in neurofibromatosis. A review of 56 patients. Spine 24:2247–2253
39. Riccardi VM, Kleiner B (1977) Neurofibromatosis: a neoplastic birth defect with two age peaks of severe problems. Birth Defects Original Article Series 13(3C):131–138
40. Rinella A, Lenke L, Whitaker C et al (2005) Perioperative halo-gravity traction in the treatment of severe scoliosis and kyphosis. Spine 30:475–482
41. Schorry EK, Crawford AH, Egelhoff JC et al (1997) Thoracic tumors in children with neurofibromatosis-1. Am J Med Genet 74:533–537
42. Shufflebarger HL (1989) Cotrel-Dubousset instrumentation in neurofibromatosis spinal problems. Clin Orthop Rel Res 245:24–28
43. Singh K, Samartzis D, An HS (2005) Neurofibromatosis type I with severe dystrophic kyphoscoliosis and its operative management via a simultaneous anterior-posterior approach: a case report and review of the literature. Spine J 5:461–466
44. Sirois JL 3rd, Drennan JC (1990) Dystrophic spinal deformity in neurofibromatosis. J Pediatr Orthop 10:522–526
45. Stevenson DA, Viskochil DH, Schorry EK et al (2007) The use of anterolateral bowing of the lower leg in the diagnostic criteria for neurofibromatosis type 1. Genet Med 9:409–412
46. Stone JW, Bridwell KH, Shackelford GD et al (1987) Dural ectasia associated with spontaneous dislocation of the upper part of the thoracic spine in neurofibromatosis. A case report and review of the literature. J Bone Joint Surg [Am] 69:1079–1083
47. Thompson GH, Akbarnia BA, Kostial P et al (2005) Comparison of single and dual growing rod techniques followed through definitive surgery: a preliminary study. Spine 30:2039–2044
48. Wilde PH, Upadhyay SS, Leong JC (1994) Deterioration of operative correction in dystrophic spinal neurofibromatosis. Spine 19:1264–1270
49. Winter RB, Lovell WW, Moe JH (1975) Excessive thoracic lordosis and loss of pulmonary function in patients with idiopathic scoliosis. J Bone Joint Surg [Am] 57:972–977
50. Winter RB, Moe JH, Bradford DS et al (1979) Spine deformity in neurofibromatosis. A review of one hundred and two patients. J Bone Joint Surg [Am] 61:677–694
51. Winter RB, Lonstein JE, Anderson M (1988) Neurofibromatosis hyperkyphosis: a review of 33 patients with kyphosis of 80 degrees or greater. J Spin Dis 1:39–49
52. Yong-Hing K, Kalamchi A, MacEwen GD (1979) Cervical spine abnormalities in neurofibromatosis. J Bone Joint Surg [Am] 6:695–699

Sagittal Plane Deformities in Growing Children

24

Acke Ohlin

Key Points

- Sagittal plane changes in a child during growth; so it is important to understand the physiologic sagittal alignment during growth.
- In the evolution of primates, the erect posture has created many mechanical spine problems.
- Considering sagittal plane configuration in isolation, kyphosis is not only a problem of elderly but also among children with congenital malformations, metabolic disorders, infections, trauma, and tumors.
- Lordosis is a much less common problem. This sagittal entity may, however, play a key role in the development of coronal plane deformities, as cases with severe idiopathic scoliosis usually have a pronounced lordotic shape in the apical region.

24.1 Introduction

During the fetal period, the sagittal profile of the spine is C-shaped. After birth, the spine straightens and when the child is standing, a lumbar lordosis is formed, which is compensated by the new formation of a thoracic kyphosis. Finally, the cervical lordosis will balance the head on top, so that the head will be balanced over the center of the pelvis. The remaining life is a subsequent struggle to resist all kyphosing forces acting on the spine curvature, eventually bending it forward into a global kyphosis.

Postural kyphosis is a mild form, in which no structural changes can be seen. The prognosis is good and no active treatment is needed.

In cases of structural kyphosis, a reduced height of the anterior part of the vertebrae is observed. The underlying process may be congenital malformation, infection, trauma, idiopathic infantile osteoporosis, and tumor as well as iatrogenic types such as postlaminectomy kyphosis, but many cases are idiopathic. Changes in the sagittal plane are also frequently observed after thoracotomies and sternotomies [8].

The most common type of kyphosis is, however, idiopathic – Scheuermanns kyphosis (Table 24.1).

In a well balanced spine, the plumb line passes through the vertebral bodies of axis and C7 and further intersecting the upper posterior corner of S1 [17]. During the prepuberal growth spurt, the anterior elements of the spine grow earlier than the posterior resulting in a flattening of the normal thoracic kyphosis [18], which may have implications in the development of idiopathic thoracic scoliosis [5].

The foundation or the base of the spinal column – the pelvis – is considered to be of crucial importance to the formation of the normal sagittal profile, *and it is shown that the spinal alignment is changing during growth [3].* During the maturation phase, there is an increasing pelvic incidence, an increased lumbar lordosis, and also a more pronounced thoracic kyphosis until adolescence [12].

Hence, if the sagittal plane of a child's spine is restored using normative data obtained from an adult population, an abnormal loading of the unfused spine will result. On the contrary, if the implants are contoured

A. Ohlin
Department of Orthopaedic Surgery, Malmö University Hospital, Lund University, 205 02 Malmö, Sweden
e-mail: acke.ohlin@med.lu.se

B. A. Akbarnia et al. (eds.), *The Growing Spine*,
DOI: 10.1007/978-3-540-85207-0_24, © Springer-Verlag Berlin Heidelberg 2011

Table 24.1 Classification of sagittal plane deformities

Nonstructural kyphosis	Postural kyphosis
Structural kyphosis	Scheuermanns Kyphosis Congenital kyphosis Post infectious kyphosis (Pott) Post-traumatic kyphosis Infantile idiopathic osteoporosis Secondary types of osteoporosis Tumor Postlaminectomy Post-thoracotomy
Structural hyperlordosis	Neuropathic Congenital

according to normative data obtained from a pediatric population, a normal adulthood posture cannot be expected as a result [3]. The clinical implication of this observation is, however, unclear.

The present view is that under normal conditions the spinal balance is depending on a continuing adaptation to the sagittal orientation of the pelvis, and the pelvic incidence is, therefore, of fundamental importance for the development of the sagittal profile.

24.2 Scheuermann's Kyphosis

24.2.1 Etiology

Idiopathic, but there is evidence of a genetic predisposition. Scheuermanns Kyphosis is usually regarded as idiopathic even if we today know that there is a genetic predisposition for the condition. One can differentiate thoracic, thoracolumbar, and lumbar forms. The latter two show more symptoms with pain. Magnetic resonance imaging (MRI) constantly shows dehydration of discs, and very often Schmorl's nodes are apparent. This disorder typically develops during adolescence.

24.2.2 Symptoms

Pain is the most frequent symptom that leads to an orthopaedic consultation. Lung function is generally not reduced, which is reflected by the fact that during the last decades very prominent sportsmen in swimming and tennis apparently had a typical Scheuermanns profile. Some patients have great concerns regarding the cosmetic appearance.

There are rare reports of spinal cord affection due to stretching of neural tissue.

24.2.3 Nonsurgical Treatment

In most cases, there is no need for treatment. Bracing is sometimes recommended, yet there is no good evidence for its effect.

Given that the natural course is variable, treatment is individualized, and in most cases there is no need for treatment.

24.2.4 Operation

The main indication for surgical treatment is pain, although cosmetic complaints can play a role to an extent.

Surgical methods are classically anterior release and posterior instrumentation. Correction by anterior approach alone using an anterior double rod system has been advocated [6]. A posterior operation only has been proposed by Ponte [14]. With his technique multiple posterior wedge osteotomies are created, and by means of a posterior instrumentation, correction is performed. In rigid cases, we use Ponte's technique having had the apical area released thoracoscopically as a first step.

24.3 Congenital Kyphosis

The most common type is failure of formation of vertebrae (Fig. 24.1) but failure of segmentation and mixed types can also be seen. At birth, the kyphotic deformity is most often not developed thus far, and therefore "congenital" can be considered a misnomer. The structural basis of the deformity is, however, present. Malformations may result in an isolated sagittal plane deformity even though these are most often combined with a scoliosis.

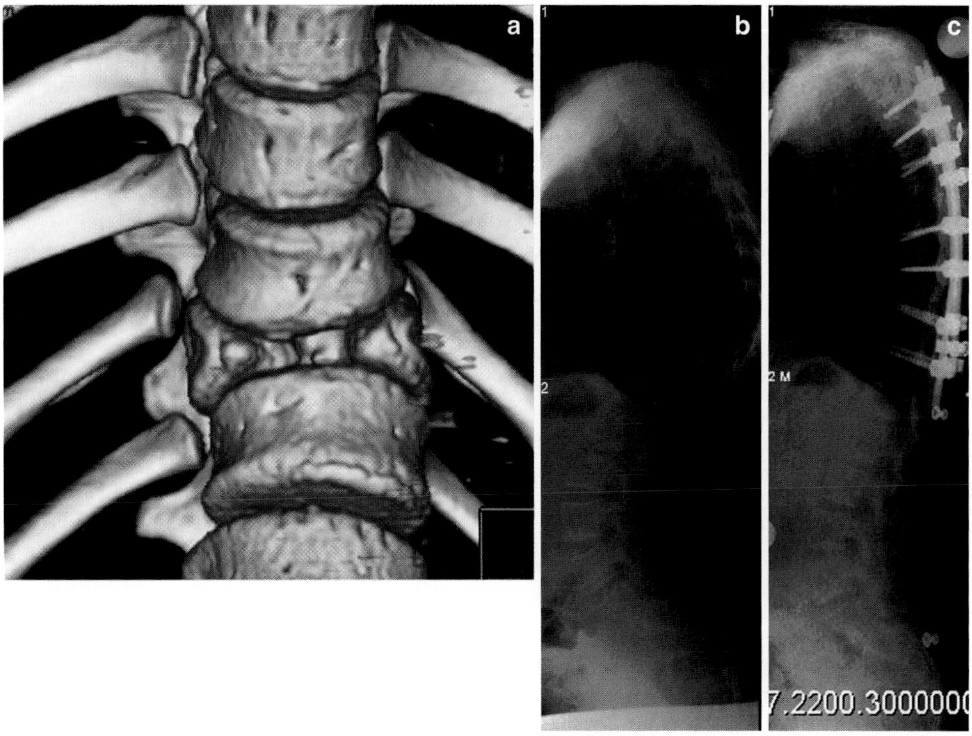

Fig. 24.1 (a) A 3D reconstruction of a case with kyphosis due to failure of formation. (b) Pre-operative lateral view and (c) correction by means of pedicle subtraction osteotomy (PSO) and posterior instrumentation

Other intraspinal pathology is prevalent in 25% of cases, why MRI is mandatory in the evaluation of patients. Malformations of the urogenital tract as well as the heart must be excluded, which a normal ultrasound can outline.

24.3.1 Treatment

24.3.1.1 Nonoperative

A close observation with reassessments at least once a year has to be done, and during periods of rapid growth, investigations should be performed two or three times a year. Standard PA and lateral radiographs, standing or sitting if possible should be obtained.

There is no evidence at all that brace treatment is able to halt the progression [19].

24.3.1.2 Operation

Indication for surgery is a well documented progression for any new neurological symptoms and signs. Historically, noninstrumented posterior fusion and casting was recommended for a kyphosis exceeding 50° in children under the age of 6 years. For older children, a combined anterior and posterior approach was most often recommended. The improved surgical techniques with pedicle subtraction osteotomy (PSO), the "eggshell procedure," and the posterior vertebral column resection (PVCR), in combination with transpedicular screw fixation make the indication for anterior surgery limited at present.

24.4 Myelodysplasia

In myelodysplasia more than 10% of patients with the index diagnosis have kyphosis. This deformity is usually located in the upper or middle part of the lumbar spine. In many cases, the deformity in myelodysplasia is accompanied by skin and soft tissue problem (ulceration) due to a lack of sensitivity, poor blood flow and thin and stretched subcutaneous tissue. The protruding hump is also at the risk of mechanical damage.

Three types of kyphosis in myelodysplasia have been described [2], paralytic, sharp-angled and congenital.

The paralytical type has an almost normal curvature at birth.

The sharp-angled type has a rigid curvature at birth due to the pathological position of the erector spinae muscles, m. quadratus lumborum and the thoracolumbar fascia anterior to the column where they work as flexors, already in utero.

The congenital type is the most severe spinal deformity of all, where also a defect of segmentation occurs anteriorly between vertebrae. This deformity progresses rapidly during the first year of life.

24.4.1 Treatment

24.4.1.1 Nonsurgical

There is no good or really meaningful conservative treatment regimen; however, bracing can theoretically reduce the rate of progression, with skin and respiratory problems as probable or expected side effects, (Fig. 24.2).

24.4.1.2 Operation

Many different techniques have been described. The absence of posterior elements, bad skin, a large thecal sac and a concomitant osteoporosis make this surgery very challenging [11]. Preoperatively, tissue expansion by means of soft tissue expanders can be applied. However, with the shortening of the spine during correction, the "tissue gain" is, in most cases, good enough to provide the surgeon with skin for coverage. A close cooperation with an experienced plastic surgeon is most helpful. Preoperatively, a computed temography (CT) of the brain should be obtained so that any hydrocephalic expansion could be diagnosed if neurological changes occur postoperatively.

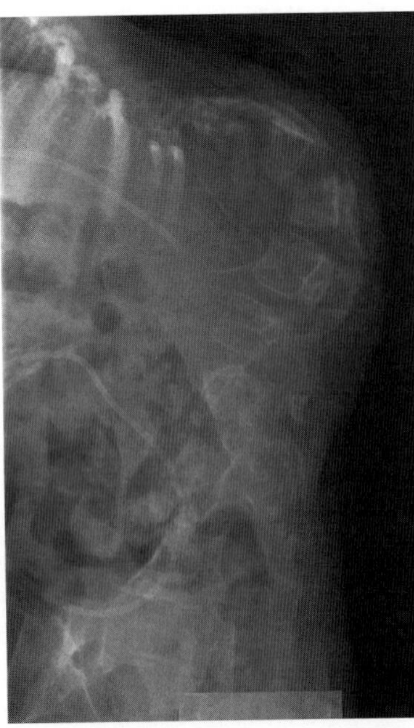

Fig. 24.2 Congenital kyphosis in myelodysplasia, lateral view

As early as 1968 Sharrard [16] described kyphectomy in the neonatal period, by having no other stabilizing techniques than sutures. Recently, Crawford et al. [4] reported a series of kyphectomies, utlizing a sophisticated technique with sutures, at the time of first intervention.

The operation is most often performed at the age of about 6 years. Previously, division of the thecal sac was recommended; however, with modern techniques such as PSO or PVCR, the thecal sac can be left alone. The distal fixation can be performed with various techniques [13]. In such cases, an extension to the upper thoracic region is preferred. Otherwise, problems with adjacent kyphosis is prone to appear. Any growing-rod technique should be considered for the upper part of instrumentation area to prevent a too short torso to develop.

The main problems in kyphosis surgery in myelodysplasia are poor quality of soft tissue, insensitivity, poor vascular supply and the absence of posterior bone elements that make the distal fixation and fusion troublesome (see Chap. 20).

24.5 Post-Infectious Kyphosis

Historically and still today, spinal tuberculosis (TB) is a great problem worldwide, being the main cause of kyphosis in the developing world. Severe kyphosis is a common result of childhood TB. In 2001, Rajasekaran [15] described the natural history of pediatric spinal TB, showing that 15% of cases treated conservatively still had a considerable increase in kyphotic deformity.

He demonstrated that there is a spontaneous remodeling capacity of partially destroyed vertebrae in children under the age of 15 years. He also reported that a child having more than two of the four severe radiographic signs – dislocation of facets, retropulsion of vertebral fragments into the canal, lateral translation, or "toppling" of the superior vertebra, was at significant risk of severe kyphosis development and thus needs surgery. Thoracolumbar TB has the worst prognosis regarding kyphosis.

24.5.1 Treatment

24.5.1.1 Conservative

The primary basic treatment is chemotherapy with a combination of streptomycin, isoniacid and rifampicin. The patients should be braced for at least half a year.

24.5.1.2 Operation

Surgical therapy is indicated with evacuation of pus when having significant paraspinal abscesses. Any neurological sign, as well as kyphosis progression and bony destruction make surgery indicated, at least when fulfilling the criteria of Rajasekaran [15]. In the Western world we often meet these patients after the period of active disease. Surgery is then often considered indicated in cases with sharp kyphosis exceeding 30–40° (Fig. 24.3).

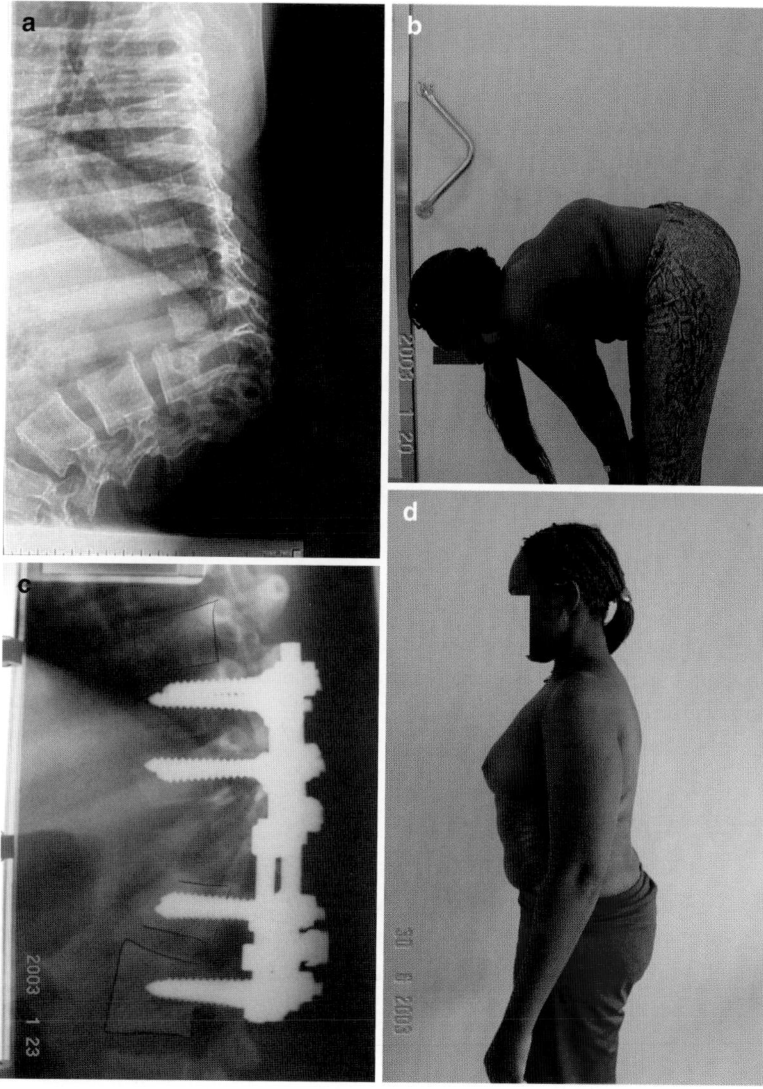

Fig. 24.3 (**a**) Post-tubercular kyphosis. Lateral radiograph. (**b**) The sagittal prophile of the patient. (**c**) After operation with PVCR, lateral radiograph. (**d**) The sagittal prophile of the patient 1 year after surgery

24.6 Post-Traumatic Kyphosis

Young children are not often exposed to high energy trauma, while minor trauma is not infrequent. Spine fractures account for 1–3% of all childhood fractures [10]. In contrast to adolescents and adult patients, fractures in the nonmature children occur more often in the mid-thoracic region. In children the trauma force will, due to the more elastic spine, be transmitted over several segments, resulting in multiple but less severe fractures [7]. There is a great remodeling capacity of vertebral fractures during growth. As a result of a moderate trauma there is no deformity to expect at all when fully grown [9]. Interestingly, this is a similar feature of vertebra remodeling as reported by Rajasekaran [15] in childhood cases of TB.

In the nonmature child, severe kyphosis is rare after trauma. These rare cases usually need a surgical correction and stabilization.

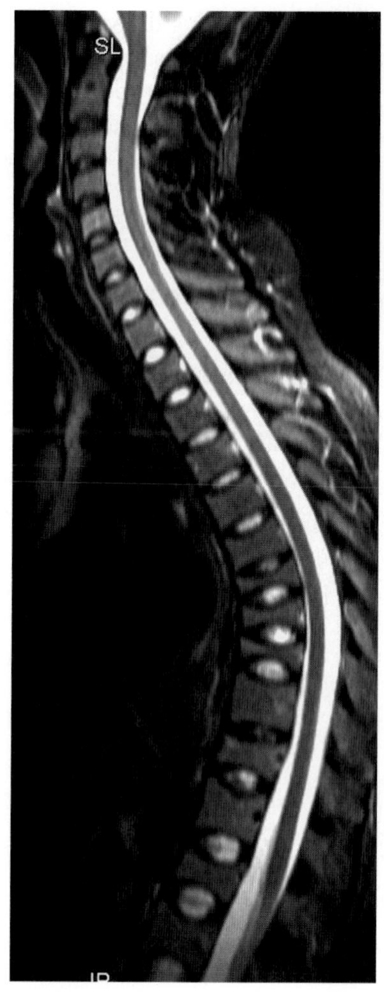

Fig. 24.4 A 17-year old girl with infantile idiopathic osteoporosis. On the sagittal view, T2-weighted MRI, a global kyphosis and multiple vertebral fractures with discs protruding and depressing the vertebral end-plates are observed

24.7 Osteoporosis and Hereditary Disorders

Infantile idiopathic osteoporosis is an extremely rare condition, where intervertebral discs protrude into the vertebral bodies and a kyphosis is formed. Secondary osteoporosis due to metabolic disorders or heriditary conditions such as spondyloepifyseal dysplasia can give rise to a kyphotic spine.

24.7.1 Treatment

Only pharmacological treatment in conjunction with bracing can hopefully be beneficial for this condition today [1], (Fig. 24.4).

24.8 Iatrogenous Kyphosis

In all ages, laminectomy alone in a kyphotic region or the unstable zone (T10–L2) of the spine, without any stabilization and fusion, will inevitably bring the patient to be at risk of kyphosis development. In a pediatric population the risk is much higher as all spinal deformities are most prone to develop during periods of rapid growth.

However, we still observe patients having had laminectomies performed because of spinal cord tumors being successfully treated, though they were left without any posterior support to resist kyphus formation. These patients can present a sharp 90° or more kyphosis from the cervicothoracic region to the upper lumbar part of the spine.

Cardiac surgery, with access through thoracotomy, sternotomy or both, in a child imply a significant higher risk of not only scoliosis but also sagittal plane deformities [8].

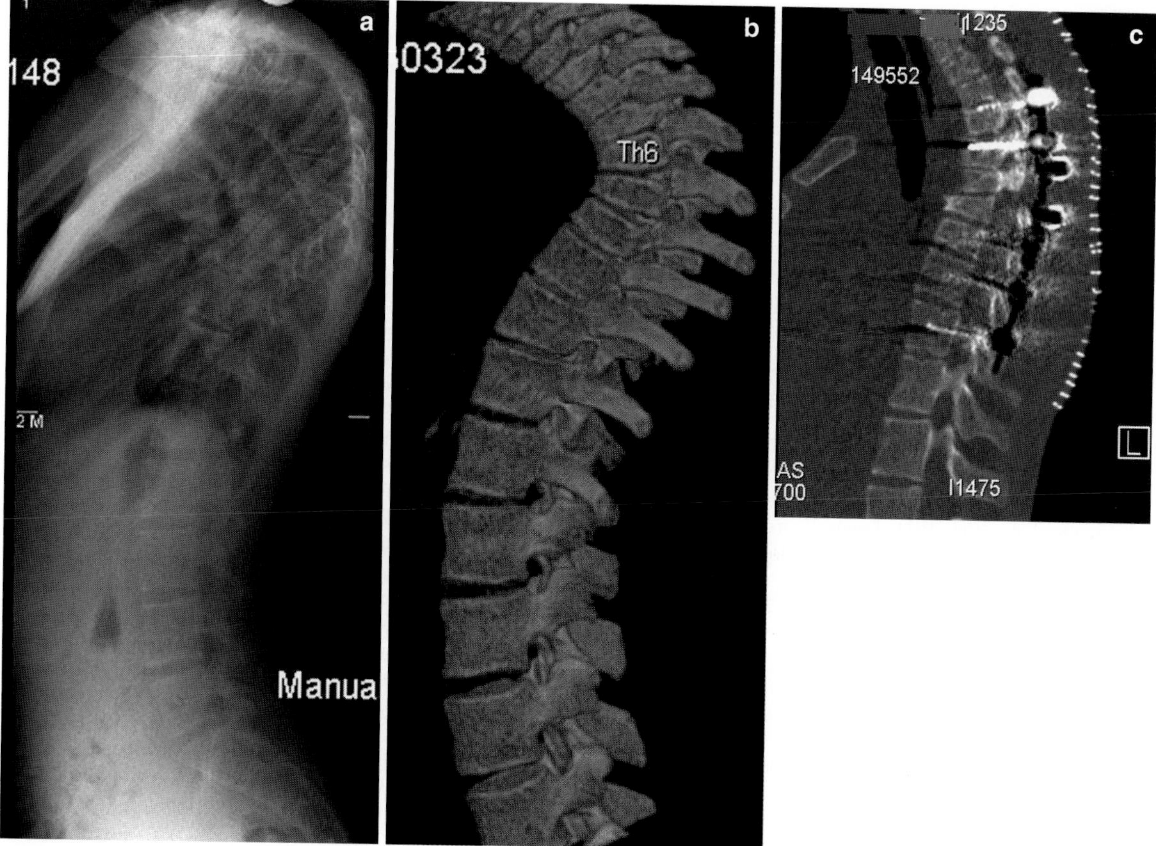

Fig. 24.5 (**a**) At the age of 3 years this boy became paraparetic due to an extradural malignant tumor (embryologic rhabdomyosarcoma) T3–T4. Laminectomy and tumor removal followed by radio- and chemotherapy. No stabilization or fusion was performed. Fifteen years later he was referred due to a progressive kyphosis of almost 100°. (**b**) A 3D CT reconstruction of the spine preoperatively. (**c**) The patient underwent a PVCR and posterior instrumentation at the age of 18 years, a sagittal CT scan

24.8.1 Surgery

Kyphosis correction with PSO or PVCR is recommended. The entire kyphotic part of the spine should be included, otherwise a subsequent junctional kyphosis may occur (Fig. 24.5).

24.9 Hyperlordosis

Neuromuscular hyperlordosis without scoliosis does exist but it is extremely rare.

Hyperlordosis due to failure of segmentation posteriorly in isolation is rare but does exist.

24.9.1 Treatment

Brace treatment might give some effect; there is, however, no scientific evidence of its value.

24.9.2 Operation

Anterior lumbar discectomy, or in case of existing posterior nonsegmented bars division according to

Langenskiöld, and posterior instrumentation and correction are the recommended treatments. Attempts to use a growing-rod technique should be done in the nonmature cases.

References

1. Bianchi ML (2007) Osteoporosis in children and adolescents. Bone 41:486–495
2. Carstens C, Koch H, Brocai DRC et al (1996) Development of pathological lumbar kyphosis in myelomeningocele. J Bone Joint Surg 78-B(6):945–950
3. Cil A, Yazici M, Uzumcusil A et al (2004) The evolution of sagittal segmental alignment of the spine during childhood. Spine 30(1):93–100
4. Crawford A, Strub WM, Lewis R et al (2003) Neonatal kyphectomy in the patient with myelomeningocele. Spine 28(3):260–266
5. Dickson RA, Lawton JO, Archer IA et al (1984) The pathogenesis of idiopathic scoliosis. Biplanar asymmetry. J Bone Joint Surg 66(1)-B:8–15
6. Gaines RW, Marks D, Ohlin A et al (2005) Short segment reconstruction of symptomatic Scheuermann's kyphosis. J Jap Spine Res Soc 16(1):226
7. Hadley MN, Zabrimski JM, Browner CM et al (1988) Pediatric spinal trauma. Review of 122 cases of spinal cord and vertebral column fractures. J Neurosurg 68(1):18–24
8. Herrera-Soto JA, Vander H, Kelly L et al (2007) Retrospective study on the development of spinal deformities following sternotomy for congenital heart disease. Spine 32(18):1998–2007
9. Karlsson MK, Möller A, Hasserius R et al (2003) A modeling capacity of vertebral fractures exists during growth: an up-to-47-year follow-up. Spine 28(18):2087–2092
10. Landin L (1983) Fracture pattern in children. Thesis. Lund University, Lund, Sweden
11. Lintner SA, Lindseth RE (1994) Kyphotic deformity in patients who have myelomeningocele. Operative treatment and long-term follow-up. J Bone Joint Surg-A 76: 1301–1307
12. Mac-Thiong J-M, Berthounnaud E, Dimar IIJR et al (2004) Sagittal alignment of the spine and pelvis during growth. Spine 29(15):1642–1647
13. Nolden MT, Sarwark JF, Vora A et al (2002) A kyphectomy technique with reduced perioperative morbidity for myelomeningocele kyphosis. Spine 27(16):1807–1813
14. Ponte A (2003) Posterior column shortening for Scheuermann's kyphosis: an innovative one-stage technique. In: Haher TR, Merola AA (eds) Surgical techniques for the spine thieme. Stuttgart, New York
15. Rajasekaran S (2001) The natural history of post-tubercular kyphosis in children. J Bone Joint Surg 83-B(7):954–962
16. Sharrard WJW (1968) Spinal osteotomy for congenital kyphosis in myelomeningocele. J Bone Joint Surg-B 50(3): 466–471
17. Vedantam R, Lenke LG, Keeney JA et al (1998) Comparison of standing sagittal spinal alignment in asymtomatic adolescents and adults. Spine 23(2):211–215
18. Willner S (1981) Spinal pantograph – a – non-invasive technique for describing kyphosis and lordosis in the thoracolumbar spine. Acta Orthop Scand 52(5):525–529
19. Winter R, Hall JE (1978) Kyphosis in childhood and adolescence. Spine 3:285–308

25 Spondylolisthesis

Dietrich K. A. Schlenzka

Key Points

- Isthmic lumbar spondylolisthesis occurs in 4.4% of children and about 6% in the adult Caucasian population. In general, it is a benign condition.
- A majority of individuals with a low-grade isthmic lumbar vertebral slip remain free of symptoms for their whole life or get only mild symptoms. Usually, there is no reason for restrictions concerning sports or professional education.
- Slip reduction or the use of instrumentation is not indicated in low-grade slips. Slip reduction in high-grade slips is controversial. It is accompanied by a higher risk of complications. It has not been shown to be superior to in situ fusion.
- Children of preschool age with spondylolysis or spondylolisthesis rarely have back pain symptoms. They are usually diagnosed accidentally or due to gait or posture anomalies. Slip progression is not very common in this age group. Radiologic follow-up is yet necessary.
- Spondylolisthesis in skeletal syndromes has various aspects. It should be assessed and treated according to basic principles considering the underlying condition. Long-term follow-up is mandatory in these rare cases.

D.K.A. Schlenzka
ORTON Orthopaedic Hospital, Invalid Foundation, Tenholantie 10, 00280 Helsinki, Finland
e-mail: dschlenzka@aospine.org

25.1 Introduction

Spondylolisthesis in children – at first glance is a straightforward topic. However, it proves to be difficult if one tries to confine the chapter to children only, i.e., to the age group up to 12 years. Traditionally, an overwhelming majority of sources from the literature dealing with this entity in growing individuals present children and adolescents as one group. In series with a substantial number of young patients, children are represented only as a small minority, the majority being adolescents or young adults [34, 72, 74, 102, 108, 135, 137–140, 152]. There are a few publications reporting on infants or "very young" children [7,13, 61, 63, 73, 82, 91, 109, 158, 164, 174]. To the best of the author's knowledge, there is only one clinical paper published presenting a significant number of patients under the age of 12 years exclusively [136].

According to the present knowledge, there should not be a big difference in the incidence of the condition between preadolescence and adolescence. The explanation for the fact that children are underrepresented in postoperative follow-up series may be that there is a higher probability of becoming symptomatic during adolescence than during childhood. It is impossible to say whether this has to do with the natural history (e.g., influence of the growth spurt), with increasing physical activities during adolescence, or with both of them.

The reader should bear in mind that the information concerning children presented in this chapter is fragmentary due to the poor data situation in the literature. The little information we have does not give any reason to assume that there should be significant differences in the approach to spondylolisthesis in children when compared with adolescents. Despite that, given recommendations should be applied critically and with

B. A. Akbarnia et al. (eds.), *The Growing Spine*,
DOI: 10.1007/978-3-540-85207-0_25, © Springer-Verlag Berlin Heidelberg 2011

great reluctance, especially when dealing with very young patients.

25.1.1 Definitions

Spondylolisthesis means the anterior slip of one vertebra upon the vertebra below. The term was formed from the Greek words "*spondylos*" (= vertebra) and "*olisthesis*" (= the sliding, the slip) and introduced by Kilian [59] in 1853. A slippage of less than 50% of the length of the slipped vertebral body is usually referred to as *low-grade*, a slippage of 50% or more as *high-grade*.

Spondylolysis (Greek "*lysis*" from "*lyein*" = to separate) is the interruption of the pars interarticularis (isthmus) of the vertebral arch [69, 70]. It is a fatigue fracture with the histological characteristics of a fibrocartilaginous pseudarthrosis [26, 104, 110, 134, 166, 175]. Spondylolysis may heal and result in a normal or elongated isthmus.

Spondyloptosis (Greek "*ptosis*" = falling, a fall) is a total slip (100% or more). The vertebral body has lost its contact to the upper endplate of the vertebra below [69].

25.1.2 Etiology

Mechanical and genetical factors have been identified to play a role in the development of spondylolysis and spondylolisthesis.

Owing to the upright position of human beings and the lumbar lordosis, mechanical stress concentrates on the lumbosacral junction. The anterior slope of the upper endplate of the sacrum creates a force vector in anterior–inferior direction acting on the lowest lumbar vertebra. Under normal conditions, the slippage of the vertebra is prevented by posterior bony elements (vertebral arch, facet joints), the intervertebral disc, and the ligaments (Lig. ileolumbalis, Ligg. longitudinale anterior et posterior, Ligg. supra-et interspinalis). The role of the muscles (Ileopsoas, abdominal and back muscles) is not quite clear. The maximum load on the bony structures acts on the pars interarticularis (isthmus) of the vertebral arch, i.e., the part of the vertebral arch between the upper and the lower articular facets.

Farfan et al. [30] analyzed the mechanics of the lumbosacral juction. They alluded to the importance of lumbar lordosis, flexion overload, unbalanced shear forces, and forced rotation. They also proposed the separation of the epiphyseal plate as one explanation for slip progression during adolescence. This mechanism has been further elucidated by Japanese scientists using animal models and three-dimensional finite element analysis. It has been demonstrated that in the presence of a pars defect, the stress on the anulus and the endplate increases with increasing vertebral slip [57, 64, 100, 124–126].

Antoniades et al. [2] could show that sacral kyphosis is related positively to the degree of slip. Marty et al. [88] found that individuals with spondylolisthesis have a higher pelvic incidence, a steeper sacral slope and a greater sacral kyphosis than control persons. The concept of abnormal pelvic morphology and disturbed spino-pelvic balance in spondylolisthesis is supported also by other authors [43, 66]. However, Huang et al. [51] could not confirm increased pelvic incidence as a predictor of slip progression. On the basis of an anthropological study, Whitesides et al. [163] stated that increased pelvic incidence in spondylolisthesis appears to be secondary to changes in the sacral table angle (i.e., the angle between the superior endplate and the posterior wall of S1) caused by the slip.

The importance of mechanical stress as an etiological factor is supported by the high incidence of this condition in individuals practising sports with repeated hyperextension and rotational movements of the lumbar spine or lifting (e.g., gymnasts, divers, javelin throwers, tennis players, weight lifters, ballet dancers) [54, 92, 98, 121, 142, 151].

The condition is also inherited [1, 34, 61, 72, 141, 158, 166, 173]. The primary site of the "inborn error" has not been identified yet. It may be in the bony structures (isthmus, facet joint morphology), in the soft tissues (ligaments, disc, cartilaginous endplate), or in both of them [25, 39, 102, 122, 161, 165, 176].

25.1.3 Classification

Traditionally, spondylolisthesis is classified according to Wiltse, Newman, and Macnab [168] (Table 25.1).

According to their classification, the majority of slips belongs to the *isthmic* type in which an interruption (spondylolysis) or elongation of the pars interarticularis (isthmus) of the vertebral arch is present.

Table 25.1 Classification of spondylolisthesis according to Wiltse, Newman and Macnab [168, 171]

I	Dysplastic
II	Isthmic
	Spondylolysis
	Isthmus elongation
	Acute fracture
III	Traumatic
IV	Degenerative
V	Pathologic
VI	Iatrogenic

The *dysplastic* spondylolisthesis develops due to congenital changes of the upper part of the sacrum and the vertebral arch of L5. Subluxation of the facet joints is always present in this form. True dysplastic spondylolisthesis is rare. Further types are *traumatic* spondylolisthesis in acute fractures, *degenerative* spondylolisthesis as a result of disc and facet joint degeneration in elderly people, and *pathologic* spondylolisthesis caused by infection or tumor destruction of parts of the vertebral arch [102, 168]. *Iatrogenic* spondylolisthesis may occur after excessive resection of posterior vertebral elements [168]. This classification has been critisized rightly for being inconsistent and mixing etiologic (e.g., dysplastic) and anatomic (e.g., isthmic) terms. As its inventors already realized, the distinction between isthmic and dysplastic forms is not always possible. And no specific treatment guidelines are derived. To overcome these shortcomings, recently improved classification systems have been proposed [83, 85].

The Marchetti-Bartolozzi [85] classification (Table 25.2) has gained much popularity especially in North America [87]. It breaks spondylolisthesis down into two main etiologic groups: *developmental* and *acquired*. For all developmental forms, the authors assume a more or less severe congenital dysplasia (i.e., weakness) in the posterior elements ("bony hook") of the vertebra leading with time under physiologic loads to spondylolysis or spondylolisthesis. The developmental form is subdivided into *high dysplastic* and *low dysplastic*, each with spondylolysis or elongation of the pars. The acquired forms of spondylolisthesis are: *traumatic*, *post-surgery*, *pathologic*, and *degenerative* with their respective subgroups.

Table 25.2 Classification of spondylolisthesis according to Marchetti and Bartolozzi [85]

Developmental	Acquired
High dysplastic	*Traumatic*
With lysis	Acute fracture
With elongation	Stress fracture
Low dysplastic	*Post-surgery*
With lysis	Direct surgery
With elongation	Indirect surgery
	Pathologic
	Local pathology
	Systemic pathology
	Degenerative
	Primary
	Secondary

The classification proposed by Mac-Thiong and Labelle [83] has its roots in the Marchetti-Bartolozzi classification. It was refined by adding criteria concerning the sagittal spino-pelvic balance and recommendations for operative treatment based on current practice.

A drawback of these newer classifications is that they are rather complex in view of daily clinical use. The distinction between different types is partly arbitrary and not always clear-cut. There are still "gray zones" [85], and the real benefit for clinical decision making is not obvious. The patient's age, a very important factor, is neglected. And the treatment recommendations given for the different types of spondylolisthesis have not been verified yet prospectively in a sufficient number of patients.

Another new classification designed especially for children and adolescents was proposed by Herman and Pizzutillo [49]. It includes prespondylolytic stress reactions of the isthmus seen in single photon emission computed tomography (SPECT) and in magnetic resonance imaging (MRI). It focuses on nonoperative treatment. According to the inventors, its validation concerning treatment recommendations will take several years.

In the author's experience, for practical decision making at present, the essential factors are the degree of slip, the sagittal alignment (lordosis/kyphosis) at the level of the slip, patient's age, and symptoms. In this context, it is of secondary interest whether a slip is to classify e.g., as dysplastic or not.

25.1.4 Epidemiology

Spondylolisthesis affects only humans. It seems to be extremely rare in nonambulatory individuals [20, 86, 119]. Spondylolisthesis has never been described in animals except in experimental models [107, 127]. It has never been found in newborn. The youngest patient with spondylolisthesis reported in the literature was 15 weeks old [13]. Laurent and Einola [73] published a case of unilateral spondylolysis with 4 mm slip in a 10-month-old girl. In caucasians the prevalence of spondylolysis is 4.4–5% at early school age [3, 32, 61]. It increases during growth being 6.0–7.2% in adult caucasians [96, 133, 160].

In certain ethnic groups the prevalence is much higher (Alaskan inuit: 32.9%, Ainnos in Japan: 41%) [93, 150]. Isthmic spondylolisthesis is more common in males but severe slips occur more frequently in females. Lumbar spondylolysis affects the fifth lumbar vertebra in 90%, the fourth in 5%, and the third in 3% of cases. The risk to get symptoms during adulthood is higher if the changes are located in the segments above L5 [46, 128].

25.1.5 Natural History and Risk of Progression

The natural history of isthmic spondylolisthesis is benign in the majority of cases due to a tendency toward self-stabilization of the affected segment [137, 160]. Despite that, isthmic spondylolisthesis is the most important cause of low-back pain and radiating leg pain in children and adolescents [74]. The average prognosis of the adult individual with isthmic spondylolisthesis concerning low-back problems and working ability does not differ from the rest of the population [10, 33, 46, 159]. There is no explanation yet why some people with spondylolysis or isthmic spondylolisthesis become symptomatic while the majority remains symptomfree. As sources of pain the lytic defect itself, the intervertebral disc, the nerve roots, and the ligaments are under discussion [15, 94, 104, 169].

Spondylolysis may be present without vertebral slip. If the slipping occurs it happens mainly during the growth period and is usually mild [10, 139]. Participation in competetive sports does not seem to increase the risk for progression [98]. Risk factors for progression in young individuals are high degree of slip (>20%) at admission and age before growth spurt [51, 139]. The trapezoid shape of the slipped vertebral body and rounding of the upper endplate of the sacrum in more severe slips are frequently interpreted as "dysplastic" changes or predictors of progression. They are, however, in most cases secondary changes. They express the severe slip, they do not predict it [10, 14, 32, 50, 73, 111, 139].

25.2 Clinical Presentation

25.2.1 Symptoms

Preschool children are usually pain-free. In this young age group, the condition is mostly detected by chance or due to posture changes or gait abnormalities (see Section 25.4.4). In elder children, the onset of the symptoms is often spontaneous. A history of sports activities is very common. Sometimes acute trauma is reported.

The leading symptom is low back pain during physical activities as well as while standing or sitting for a longer period of time. The pain may radiate to the buttocks and to the posterior or lateral aspect of the thigh, seldom more distally to the lower leg, ankle or foot. In the severe slip (>50%), gait disturbances, numbness, muscle weakness, and symptoms of cauda equina compression may be present. There is, however, no direct relationship between severity of subjective symptoms and the amount of slip.

25.2.2 Physical Examination

In a low-grade slip (<50%), the patient's gait and posture are usually normal unless radicular symptoms are present. The mobility of the lumbar spine is free or decreased due to muscle spasm and pain. Maximal extension may induce pain at the lumbo–sacral junction. There is local tenderness during palpation, and in many cases a step can be felt between the spinous processes at the level of the slip. Tightness of the ischiocrural muscles (hamstrings), typical for high-grade spondylolisthesis, is sometimes seen also in the symptomatic patients with a low-grade slip. Muscle strength, reflexes, and skin sensation of the lower extremities are normal in the majority of patients.

In a high-grade slip, the clinical picture is very variable despite the severe local malalignment of the spine seen in the radiograph. In many cases, the patient's posture is disturbed in a typical way (Fig. 25.1): The sacrum is in vertical position due to retroversion of the pelvis. There is a short kyphosis at the lumbosacral

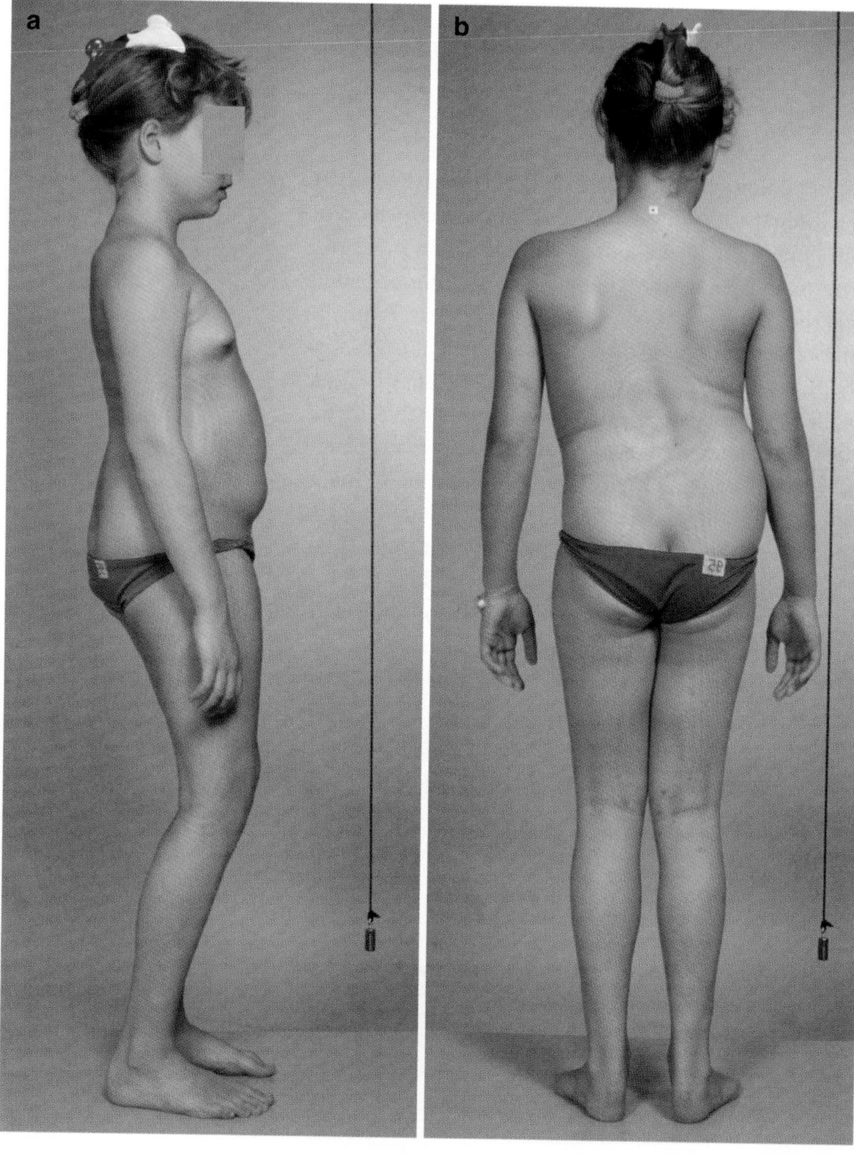

Fig. 25.1 Typical clinical appearance of a symptomatic 11-year-old girl with high-grade isthmic spondylolisthesis. (**a**) Vertical position of the sacrum due to retroversion of the pelvis, the patient is forced to stand with hips and knees flexed. (**b**) The spine is out of frontal balance, there is a secondary "sciatic" lumbar scoliosis

junction and a compensatory hyperlordosis of the lumbar spine usually reaching up into the thoracic region [88]. The spine is scoliotic and often out of balance in the frontal as well as in the sagittal plane. The patient is unable to fully extend hips and knees during standing, and she/he walks with a typical pelvic waddle. In those patients the hamstrings are always extremely tight [112]. Signs of neural impairment (muscle weakness, disturbances of skin sensation, incontinence) may be present. Some patients look clinically normal and show e.g., only some milder hamstrig tightness. Astonishingly, even in severe slips objective neurologic findings are rare. Many patients are subjectively almost free of symptoms despite significant posture changes and hamstring tightness.

In some patients, lumbar or thoracolumbar scoliosis is seen as a secondary phenomenon to spondylolisthesis. "Sciatic" forms (mainly in high-grade slips) are due to pain and muscle spasm and disappear usually after relief of symptoms. Structural ("olisthetic") curves caused by rotational displacement of the slipped vertebra have to be followed closely and lumbosacral fusion operation is indicated if progression occurs [135]. Thoracic scoliosis in a patient with lumbar spondylolisthesis is assessed as a separate entity and treated according to the guidelines of scoliosis management.

25.3 Imaging

25.3.1 Plain Radiographs

Plain radiographs (posterior–anterior and lateral) of the lumbar spine in standing position spine focused on the lumbo–sacral junction should be taken primarily. The images show the alignment of the lumbar spine and the true amount of vertebral slip if there is any. In most cases, the lateral projection also reveals the spondylolysis (Fig. 25.2). The use of traditional oblique plain radiographs to verify a lysis not visible in the standing lateral view is obsolete. The slip is measured according to Laurent and Einola [73] as the quotient between the sagittal slip and the sagittal length of the slipped vertebral body expressed in percent (Fig. 25.3). The sagittal lumbosacral alignment (lordosis/kyphosis) is assessed from the same radiograph and measured as the angle between the posterior border of the first sacral vertebral body and the anterior or posterior border of the fifth vertebral body (Fig. 25.4). Long standing films of the whole spine in two planes are taken if the spine is clinically significantly out of balance or if scoliosis is present.

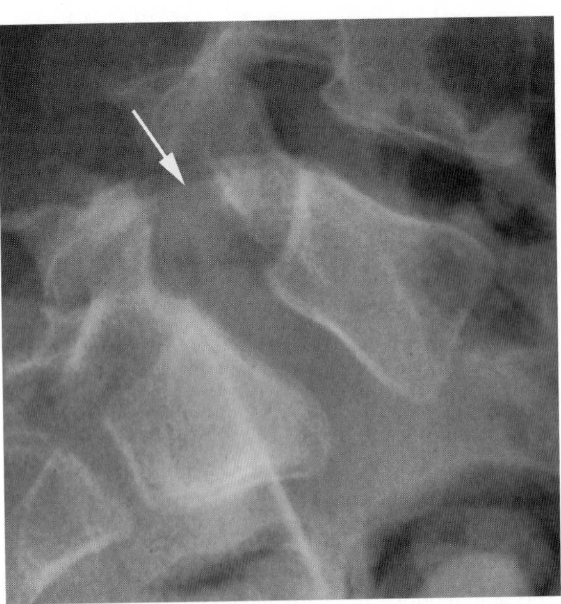

Fig. 25.2 Spondylolysis (*arrow*) and a low-grade L5 slip on a lateral radiograph in standing position

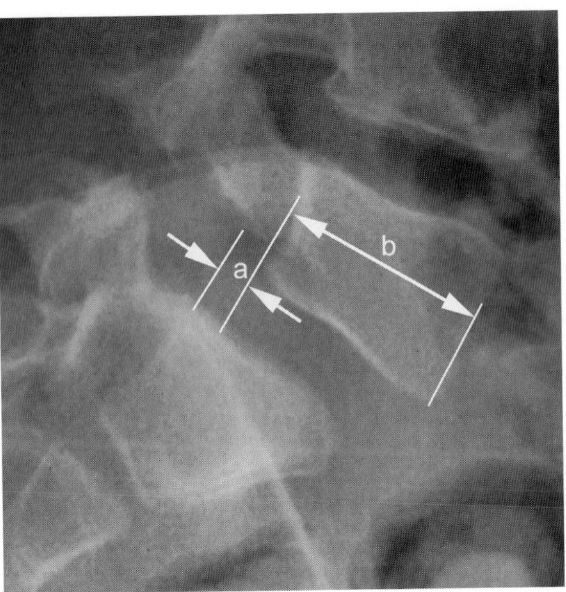

Fig. 25.3 Calculation of the percentage of vertebral slip according to Laurent and Einola [73]. Slip [%] = a/b × 100

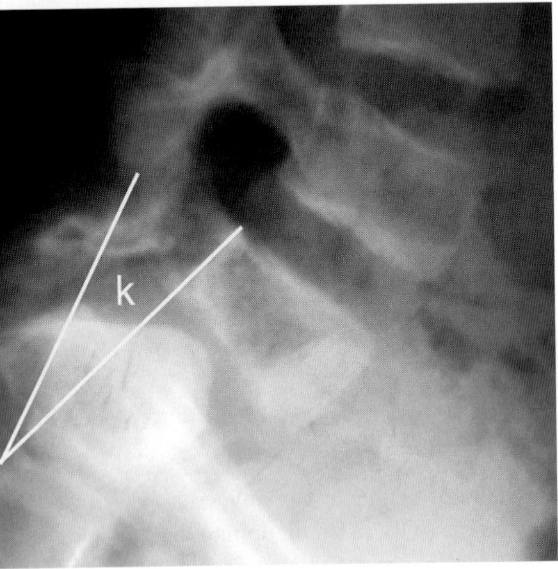

Fig. 25.4 Measurement of lumbosacral kyphosis as the angle (K) between the posterior border of S1 and the posterior (or anterior) border of L5

25.3.2 Functional Radiographs

Flexion–extension radiographs have been traditionally used to detect possible "instability" in the olisthetic segment. They are not in use anymore as we

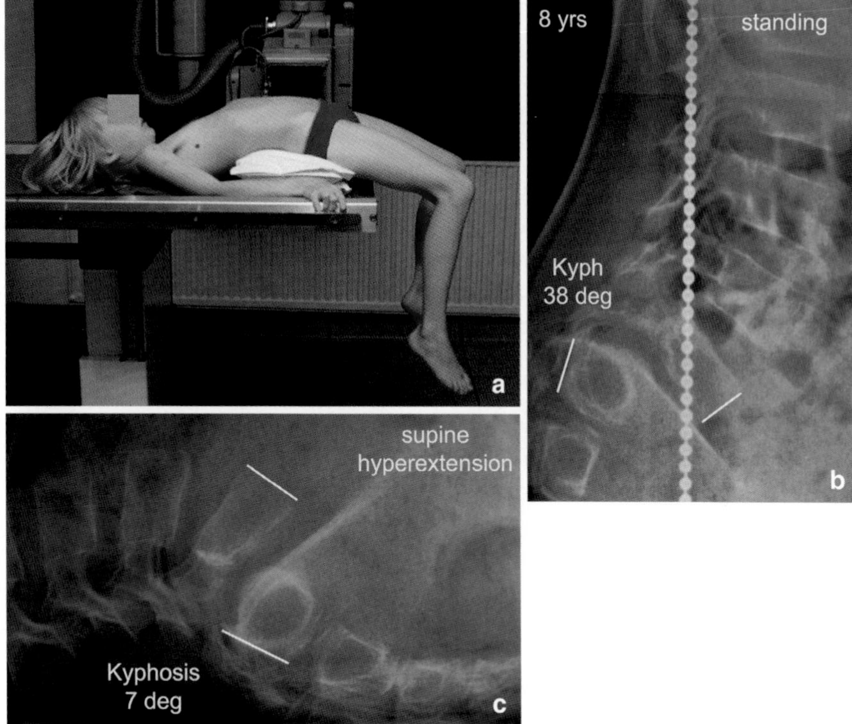

Fig. 25.5 (**a**) Patient positioning for the lateral supine hyperextension radiograph of the lumbosacral junction, (**b**) Standing lateral radiograph shows significant lumbosacral kyphosis, (**c**) On the supine hyperextension radiograph of the same patient, a marked decrease of the kyphosis is visible

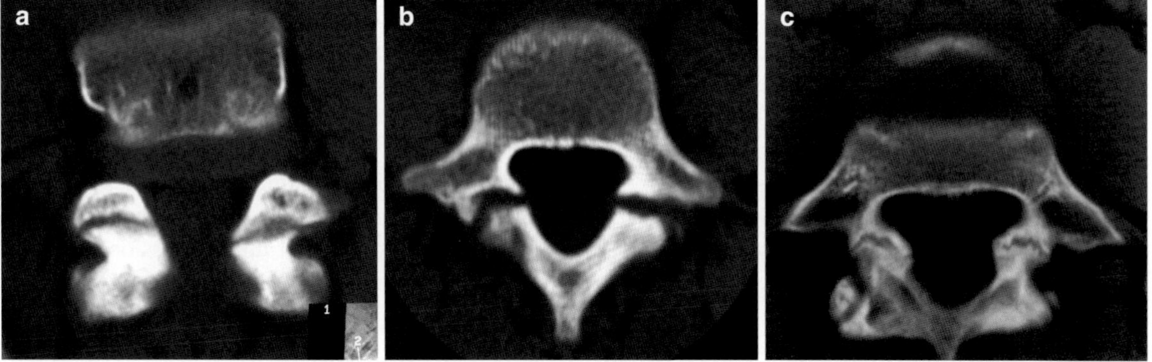

Fig. 25.6 Different appearance of the spondylolysis on isthmus ct-image. (**a**) 10-year-old boy, "early-traumatic." (**b**) 11-year-old girl, "atrophic." (**c**) 14-year-old boy, "hypertrophic"

could not see any value for decision making concerning the patient's treatment. In high-grade slips with lumbo–sacral kyphosis, a lateral hyperextension radiograph in supine position is taken preoperatively (Fig. 25.5). It demonstrates the reducibility of the slipped vertebra to judge whether the disc space below the vertebra will be accessible during a planned anterior procedure without the need for instrumented reduction.

25.3.3 Computed Tomography (CT)

In most cases, the lysis can be easily seen from the standing lateral radiograph. If in doubt, a CT image with the gantry tilted to obtain slices in the longitudinal direction of the isthmus should be taken. It is the most reliable imaging mode for demonstrating the spondylolysis (Fig. 25.6a–c). CT is also very valuable to assess possible healing of the defect [8, 44].

25.3.4 Magnetic Resonance Imaging (MRI)

Increasingly, MRI is used as a primary imaging mode for children with low-back pain. Especially in young athletes increased signal intensity is seen frequently in the area of the isthmus or the pedicles. This is interpreted as a stress reaction. Its importance and natural history are unclear so far. There are difficulties to distinguish these stress reactions from true spondylolysis in MRI. Prospective studies are needed to clarify this phenomenon.

In low-grade slips without neurological signs, there is no rational indication for magnetic resonance imaging (MRI). MRI is indicated in cases with neurological symptoms, cauda equina syndrome, or if disc herniation is suspected. It is helpful to demonstrate the shape of the spinal canal, the intervertebral foramina, and possible compression of neural structures (Fig. 25.7).

MRI also allows to assess the condition of the intervertabral discs at and adjacent to the olisthetic segment. The disc below the slipped vertebra is often pathologic already in young individuals regardless of whether they do have pain symptoms or not. Dehydration of the adjacent disc above the slipped vertebra is relatively common in symptomatic patients [130, 131]. As the clinical relevance of disc dehydration seen on MRI of young persons is unclear, MRI is not of value for clinical decision making in spondylolisthesis in this respect [117].

Symptomatic disc herniation at the level of the slip is very rare in patients with isthmic spondylolisthesis [113].

25.3.5 Single-Photon Emission Computed Tomography (SPECT)

The SPECT technique is nowadays often used for evaluation of low-back pain especially in young athletes. It shows increased uptake in stress reactions, microfractures, and fractures. It allows to differentiate chronic spondylolysis (pseudarthrosis) from fresh, active lesions, which theoretically should have a higher healing potential. However, its predictive value concerning healing of the spondylolysis has not been established yet [11, 21, 27, 92, 150].

25.4 Treatment

The benign natural history of the condition should always be kept in mind when weighing the necessity for treatment and the treatment options. The parents are usually very worried after learning that there is something "broken" in the lower back of their child. In every case, it is very important to explain the basically benign nature of the course to the patient and to the parents. Yet in many cases symptoms resolve after several months without any special treatment. At the same time it should be made clear that the condition may not be ignored either. Follow-up for a certain period of time is necessary to act appropriately if significant progression occurs. The parents should also be informed that effective treatment is at hand if prolonged severe subjective symptoms are present or marked slip progression is seen.

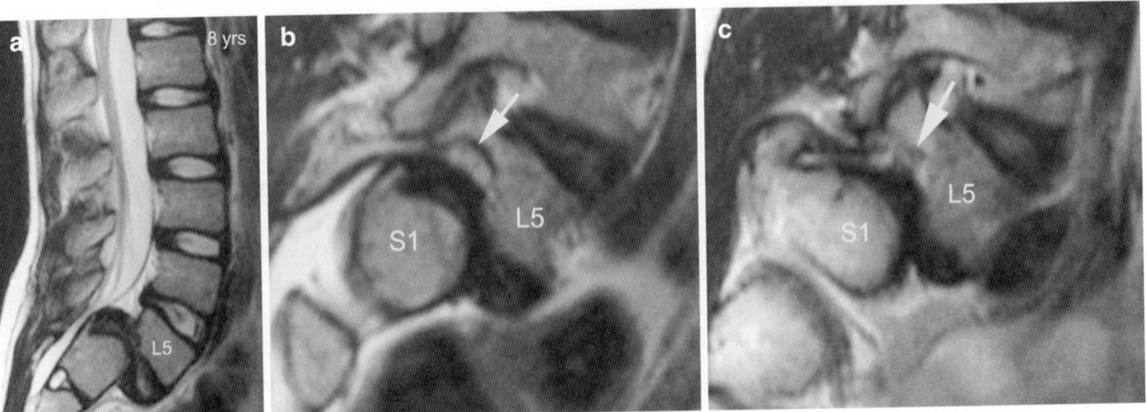

Fig. 25.7 Typical MRI findings in a high-grade spondylolisthesis. (**a**) The central spinal canal is narrowed, the L5–S1 disc is severely damaged. (**b**, **c**) The L5 roots (*arrow*) are caught between the pedicle and the disc

The only case for immediate decision toward active intervention is a high-grade slip with lumbosacral kyphosis or a significant neurological deficit.

25.4.1 Observation

Rapid growth and a slip of more than 20% have been identified as risk factors for progression [51, 139]. Therefore, children before or during the growth spurt have to be checked at regular intervals until the rapid growth is over [139, 167]. Plain lateral standing radiographs of the lumbar spine are taken every 6–12 months depending on the degree of slip at admission and the age of the patient. There is no need for restriction of physical activities during follow-up. At the end of the observation period, the patient and the parents should be assured that there are no restrictions in view of future sports activities or choice of occupation.

25.4.2 Nonoperative Treatment

Symptomatic spondylolysis or low-grade spondylolisthesis (slip <50%) is primarily always treated nonoperatively by decreasing the level of physical activities, strengthening of back and abdominal muscles, and sometimes a brace [9, 84, 149]. Sportsmen are advised to modify their training program to avoid pain-causing exercises. But there is no reason to stop all physical activities. According to the literature, the functional outcome after brace treatment of spondylolysis in young athletes is good or excellent in 80% or more. Healing of the defect could be demonstrated radiologically in 16–57%. Unilateral defects seem to heal more often than bilateral defects as do defects at L4 in comparison with L5 defects. No correlation could be found between healing and good clinical outcome. Neither the efficacy of bracing nor the predictive value of increased activity of the lysis in SPECT scans could be demonstrated definitely as there are no prospective comparative studies available [9, 27, 35, 92, 121, 149, 151].

25.4.3 Operative Treatment

The data on operative treatment of spondylolysis and spondylolisthesis in children (up to 12 years of age) is very sparse because of the fact that in the vast majority of reports children and adolescents are treated as one group. The impact of patients' age at operation on the results is usually not analyzed. No randomized trials comparing operative treatment to natural history are available so far. In his retrospective long-term follow-up study, Seitsalo [137] investigated 149 patients with low-grade slips after a mean follow-up time of 13.3 years. Seventy-two patients (mean age 13.8 years, mean slip 16.2%) had conservative treatment or no treatment at all, 77 patients (mean age 14.6 years, mean slip 16.6%) were treated by uninstrumented posterior or posterolateral fusion. At follow-up, 75% of the conservatively treated patients and 87% of the operatively treated patients were free of pain. None of the primarily conservatively treated patients had an operation at a later date. In the conservative group, 6/72 (8.3%) patients and in the operative group 4/77 (5.2%) patients reported decreased working ability.

The indication for operation in children and adolescents depends on the amount of slip (high grade or low grade), the age of the patient (before, during, or after the growth spurt), and the clinical signs and symptoms. Neurological symptoms (cauda equina syndrome, peroneus paresis) are a clear indication for operation. However, those occur very rarely even in severe slips. The most common reason for operation in low-grade slips is pain not responding to nonoperative measures. In children with a slip of 50% or more, operation is recommended also to prevent further progression even if the patient has only minor symptoms or no symptoms at all. Operation should also be considered in a very young patient with a slip of over 20% if progression occurs during follow-up.

The choice of the operative technique depends on the amount of slip or lumbosacral kyphosis and on the personal experience and preferences of the surgeon. Table 25.3 represents the author's policy. It can be used as a guideline for decision making. The listed numbers for slip percentages and degrees of lumbosacral kyphosis are not based on scientific evidence. They mark a smooth transition, which cannot be defined with mathematical accuracy. The final decision is always made according to the individual situation of the patient taking into consideration patient's stage of sceletal maturity, gender, individual anatomic features of the slip, ability to cooperate, patient's and parents' hopes and desires, and, last but not least, the surgeons personal experience.

Table 25.3 Management of isthmic spondylolisthesis in children[a]

Slip (%)	Symptoms	Treatment
0–25	No	Follow-up
0–25	Yes	Non-operative Posterolateral fusion Direct repair
25–50	Yes/No	Posterolateral fusion
>50 L-s kyphosis <20°	Yes/No	Anterior fusion
50–90 L-s kyphosis > 20°	Yes/No	Combined fusion
90–100 (ptosis)	Yes/No	Partial reduction or Resection + Combined instrumented fusion

[a]The listed values for slip percentages and degrees of lumbosacral kyphosis are not based on scientific evidence. They mark a smooth transition, which cannot be defined with mathematical accuracy. The final decision has to be made after assessing the overall picture of the individual patient

25.4.3.1 Spondylolysis and Low-Grade Slip (≤50%)

Uninstrumented segmental posterolateral fusion in situ using autogenous bone from the posterior iliac crest is the method of choice for cases with an amount of slip up to 50% (Fig. 25.8). The operation is performed through the bilateral paraspinal muscle split approach as recommended by Wiltse et al. [167, 170]. The segment above the slipped vertebra is usually not included into the fusion even if the disc shows signs of dehydration in MRI. The patient is mobilized 1–2 days after the operation wearing a soft brace for 3 months time. Sports activities are forbidden for 6–12 months depending on the radiologic development of the fusion. There are no restrictions of physical activities after solid bony healing. The method is very safe and effective. There are no specific complications. In this young age group it leads to bony fusion in 80–90%. Subjective results and functional outcome are good or satisfactory in 82–96% of the patients [74, 76, 132, 144]. A recent long-term study in 107 children and adolescents with a mean age at operation of 15.9 (range 8.1–19.8) years and a mean follow-up of 20 years has proven the lasting effectiveness and reliability of this method [67]. The mean Oswestry Disability Score [29] was 7.6 (range, 0–68) at last follow-up. It was in the normal range (0–20) in 100 out of 107 patients (93%). Six (6%) out of 107 patients had an Oswestry score of 20–40 (= "moderate disability"), one patient had a score of 68 (= "crippled"). Pseudarthrosis (17% after posterolateral fusion) and adjacent disc degeneration on plain radiographs (12%) did not correlate with poor outcome. The Scoliosis Research Society [41] outcome instrument yielded on average 94.0 (range, 44–114) points at follow-up [47]. Degenerative changes in MRI at follow-up did not have any significant influence on patients' outcome [117].

In low-grade slips, decompressive laminectomy is indicated in young patients only in rare cases with true impingement of neural structures. However, this has not been seen by the author in a low-grade slip during a period of over 30 years. Pseudoradicular symptoms (radiating pain to the posterior aspect of the thigh) and hamstring tightness resolve without laminectomy due to stabilization of the segment by fusion. If decompression is performed during growth segmental fusion has to be added always to prevent subsequent progression of the slip [106].

The use of instrumentation has not been shown to give any advantages in low-grade slips in this age group. Nor is there any reason for reduction of low-grade slips. The author agrees fully with this statement published by Wiltse and Jackson [167] in 1976. Internal fixation, with or without reduction, is connected with longer operation time, more severe muscle trauma, an increased risk of complications, and higher costs. It would probably increase the fusion rate. But the disadvantages mentioned earlier would not countervail this, as pseudarthrosis does not have a measurable negative effect on the outcome in this group of patients [67, 76, 137, 140].

In cases of spondylolysis without a slip or with a slip of less than 25%, the direct repair of the isthmic defect is recommended by some authors reporting favorable results using different methods of internal fixation (screws, cerclage wire, butterfly plate, hook plate, pedicle srews and rods) [18, 38, 55, 60, 79, 97, 103]. Several authors reported favorable outcome especially in younger patients [16, 45, 53, 103]. There are no series published dealing exclusively with children. At the author's institution Scott's wiring technique with autologous bone grafting has been used [103]. For postoperative treatment a plastic TLSO was applied for 3–6 months. In a comparative study in children and adolescents, the results after mid-term and long-term follow-up were very good in the majority of cases, but not better than the results of uninstrumented segmental fusion. Thus, the benefit from saving the lytic–olisthetic motion segment

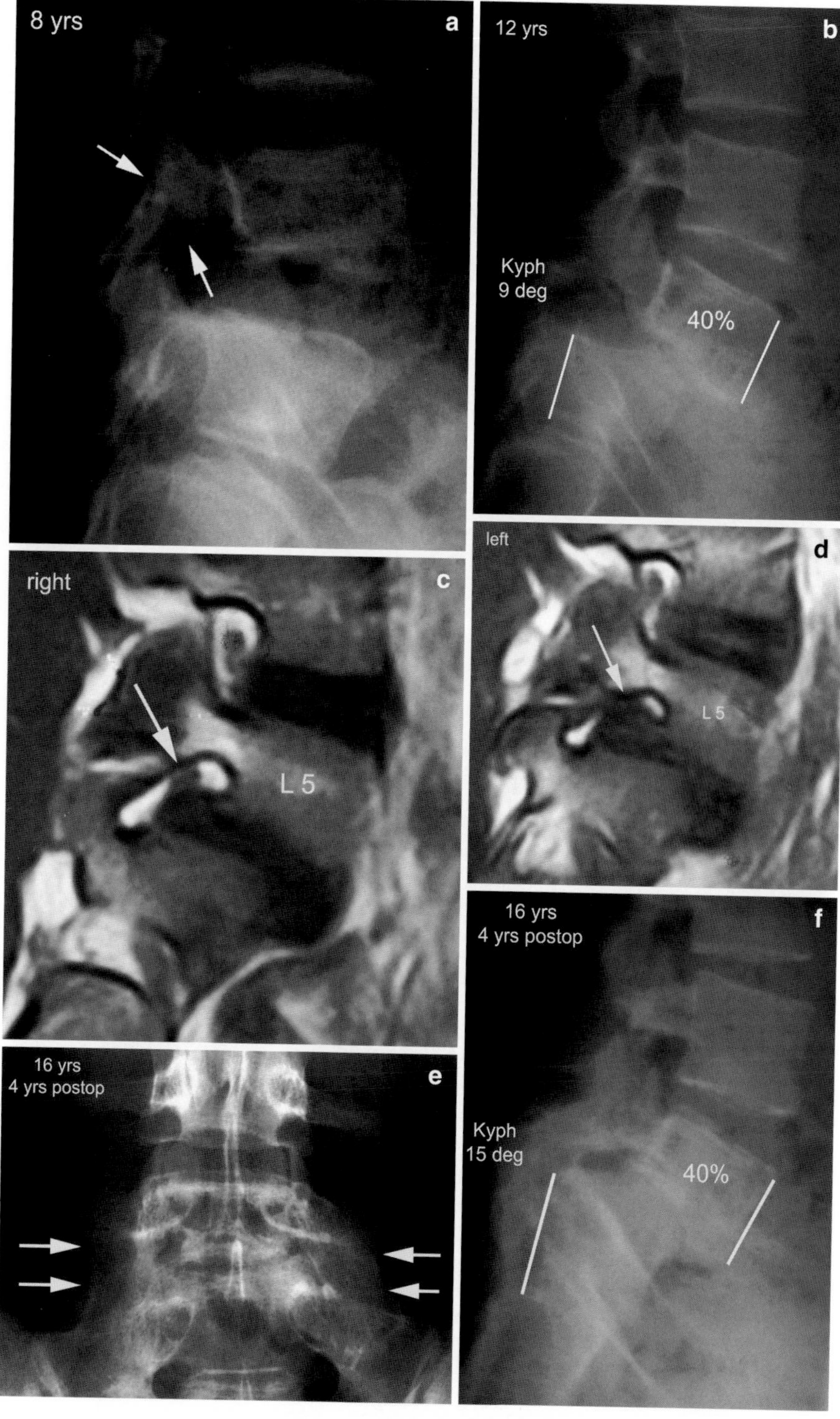

Fig. 25.8 Uninstrumented posterolateral fusion for symptomatic low-grade slip in a 12-year-old boy. (**a**) L5 spondylolysis at the age of 8 years. (**b**) After slip progression low-back pain and left leg pain at the age of 12 years. (**c**) The right L5 root (*arrow*) is free on MRI. (**d**) Compression of the left L5 root (*arrow*). (**e**) Plain ap radiograph 4 years after posterolateral fusion without decompression. Note bilateral mature fusion mass (*arrows*). (**f**) Lateral radiograph 4 years postoperatively. Minimal progression of the kyphosis. The patient is free of symptoms

could not be demonstrated so far [132, 133]. At present, the direct repair is used by the author only in cases of spondylolysis or minimal slips in the segments above L5.

25.4.3.2 High-Grade Slip (>50%)

If the slip approaches 50% of the biomechanical situation changes profoundly with far reaching consequences for the sagittal alignment of the entire spine [78]. The physiologic lumbosacral lordosis decreases and, dependant of the amount of displacement, a kyposis develops owing to the absence of anterior support for the slipping vertebra (Fig. 25.9). In the growing patient, this kyphotic deformity has a risk of progression is almost 100%. Operation should be considered even in patients with minimal subjective symptoms or no symptoms at all [167]. There is no data showing that nonoperative measures (exercises, bracing) or restriction of sports activities would stop the progression. One should not wait and see too long. Proceeding progression makes the necessary operation technically more difficult, increases the risk of complications, and leads possibly to an inferior result. It has, however, to be noted that in some cases even patients with high-grade slips or even spondyloptosis remain subjectively symptomfree. The author agrees with Bridwell that there is no "right way"

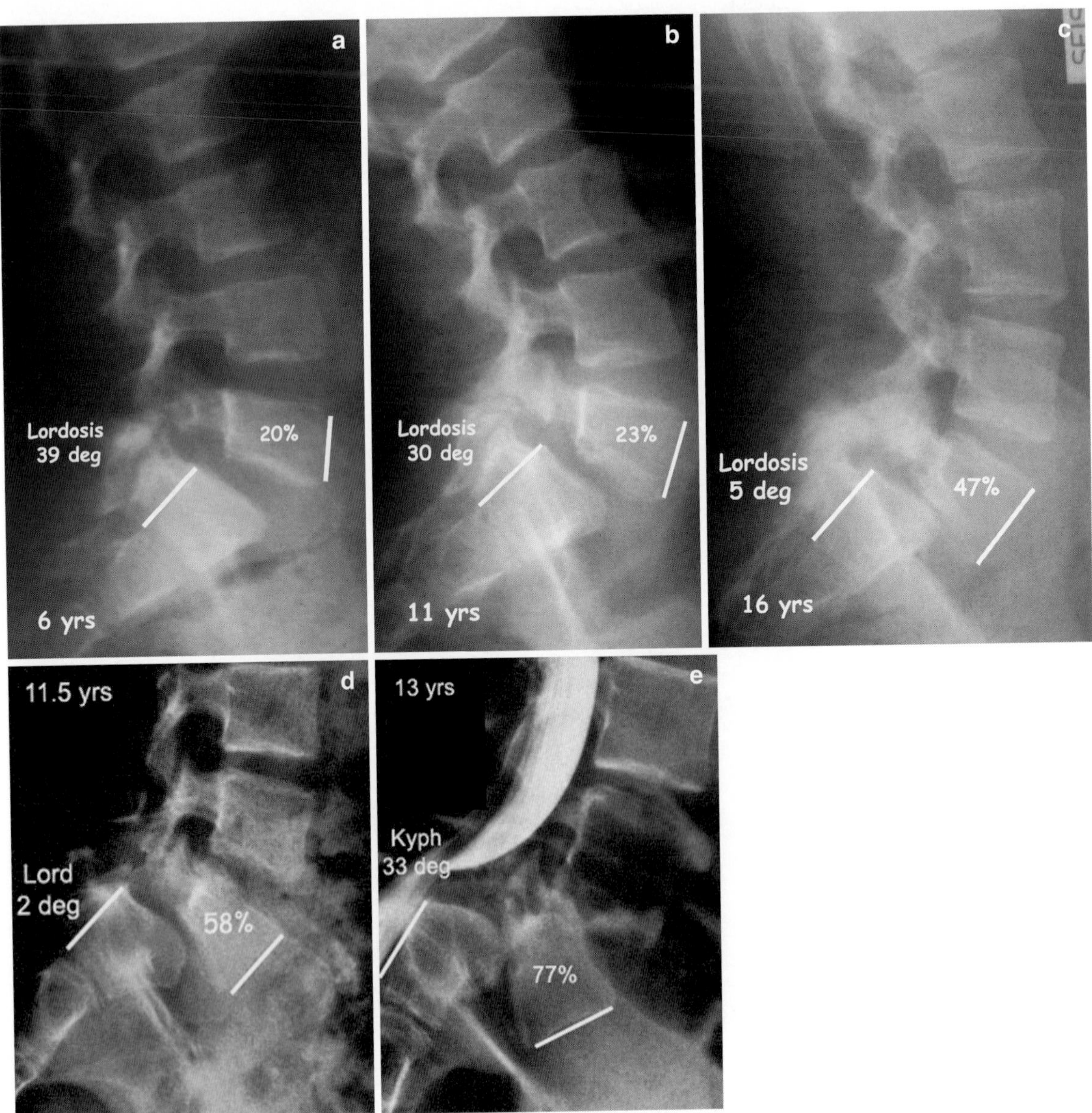

Fig. 25.9 Standing lateral radiographs of a female patient at the age of 6 (**a**), 11 (**b**), and 16 (**c**) years show marked loss of the physiologic lumbosacral lordosis during slip progression. In another female patient, rapid deterioration of the sagittal alignment from 2° of lordosis (**d**) to 33° (**e**) of lumbosacral kyphosis within 18 months time

to treat all high-grade slips [17]. But overtreatment for the sake of radiologic correction should be avoided. The methods applied should be assessed critically for their benefit for the patient in the long run in terms of clinical outcome and function.

A considerable variety of methods for operative treatment of high-grade slips has been published: uninstrumented posterior or posterolateral fusion from L3 or L4 to S1 [40, 48, 52, 71, 77, 118, 138, 167], uninstrumented anterior interbody fusion [48, 114, 115, 154], uninstrumented combined fusion [48, 68], unistrumented posterolateral fusion L4–S1 and anterior fusion L5–S1 with cast immobilization after preoperative gradual conservative reduction [71, 157], uninstrumented posterolateral fusion L3 or L4 to S1 with postoperative cast reduction [19], reduction by preoperative traction followed by posterior instrumentation and posterior fusion from L2 or L3 to the sacrum [118], anterior reduction with anterior screw fixation and interbody fusion, posterior pedicle screw reduction with or without decompression and posterior or combined fusion using bone graft or cages [28, 89, 95, 99, 114, 115, 120, 123] or the Bohlman technique utilizing a transsacral fibular strut graft [42, 146], or a special titanium cage [5, 145], and anterior and posterior reduction with decompression, and double-plating [158].

According to Bradford [15], the goals of treatment for high-grade spondylolisthesis are: to prevent progression, to relieve pain, to improve function, and to reverse the neurological deficit if there is any. These goals can be achieved in the vast majority of cases safely by in situ fusion, which is wrongly is of bad repute. The reason for the negative attitude of many surgeons toward in situ fusion seems to be that many of them have seen symptomatic adult patients with a high-grade slip up to spondyloptosis who had a posterior or posterolateral "in situ" fusion of a more or less severe slip as teenagers. Usually, in the early years after the primary operation, they were symptomfree. But with time, posture deteriorated and symptoms reappeared, sometimes even worse than before the operation. When analyzing the radiographs, one sees that slow progression of the slip and the kyphosis happened over the years despite a solid-looking fusion mass. Retrospectively, one can say that although in situ fusion was attempted, it was not achieved. Several of such cases with slow progression after posterior or posterolateral so-called in situ fusion L4 to S1are are shown in the very instructive papers by Taillard [152] and Burkus et al. [19]. The cause for the failure is misunderstanding of the biomechanics of a high-grade slip, which in fact is a progressive kyphosis. Anterior bony support is insufficient or missing totally. The disc below the significantly slipped vertebra is always severely damaged. It will degenerate further and atrophy due to loss of functional motion after fusion. This all together induces increasing flexion moments on the posterior fusion mass, which will bend and elongate. It must be stressed here that in the author's language successful in situ fusion does mean that a solid bony fusion is achieved and even after long-term follow-up the position of the fused vertebra is not significantly worse than before the operation.

Biomechanically, the most reasonable procedure to stop the progression of a kyphotic deformity is to provide anterior support. This is the rationale for anterior fusion. At the author's institution, uninstrumented anterior interbody fusion in situ without decompression is the method of choice for high-grade slips with no ore minimal (up to 10–20°) lumbosacral kyphosis (Fig. 25.10). The operation is performed through a transperitoneal or retroperitoneal approach using two to three autogenous tricortical iliac crest grafts. Uninstrumented combined anterior and posterolateral fusion in situ without decompression is preferred for slips with greater lumbosacral kyphosis (more than 20°). Combined fusion has been shown to be more effective in preventing the postoperative progression of the lumbosacral kyphosis, i.e., to achieve a true and lasting in situ fusion without late deterioration [48, 118]. Using this technique, there is no need to include more than the olisthetic segment into the fusion. After anterior or combined procedures the patient is mobilized at the second or third postoperative day wearing a plastic TLSO for 3–6 months. Hamstring tightness disappears and spinal balance is regained within a few weeks although no decompression has been performed (Fig. 25.11–25.13). The clinical short- and mid-term results of anterior and combined fusion in the severe slip are comparable with the results of posterior or posterolateral fusion [56, 76, 138, 143, 154]. In a recent long-term follow-up study (67 patients, slip 50–100%, age at operation 8.9–19.6, mean 14.4 years, follow-up time 10.7–26 years.), the outcome after three uninstrumented in-situ fusion techniques (posterolateral, anterior, combined) without decompression was compared. At final follow-up, 14% in the posterolateral and in the anterior fusion group reported low-back pain at rest often or very often, but none in the circumferential

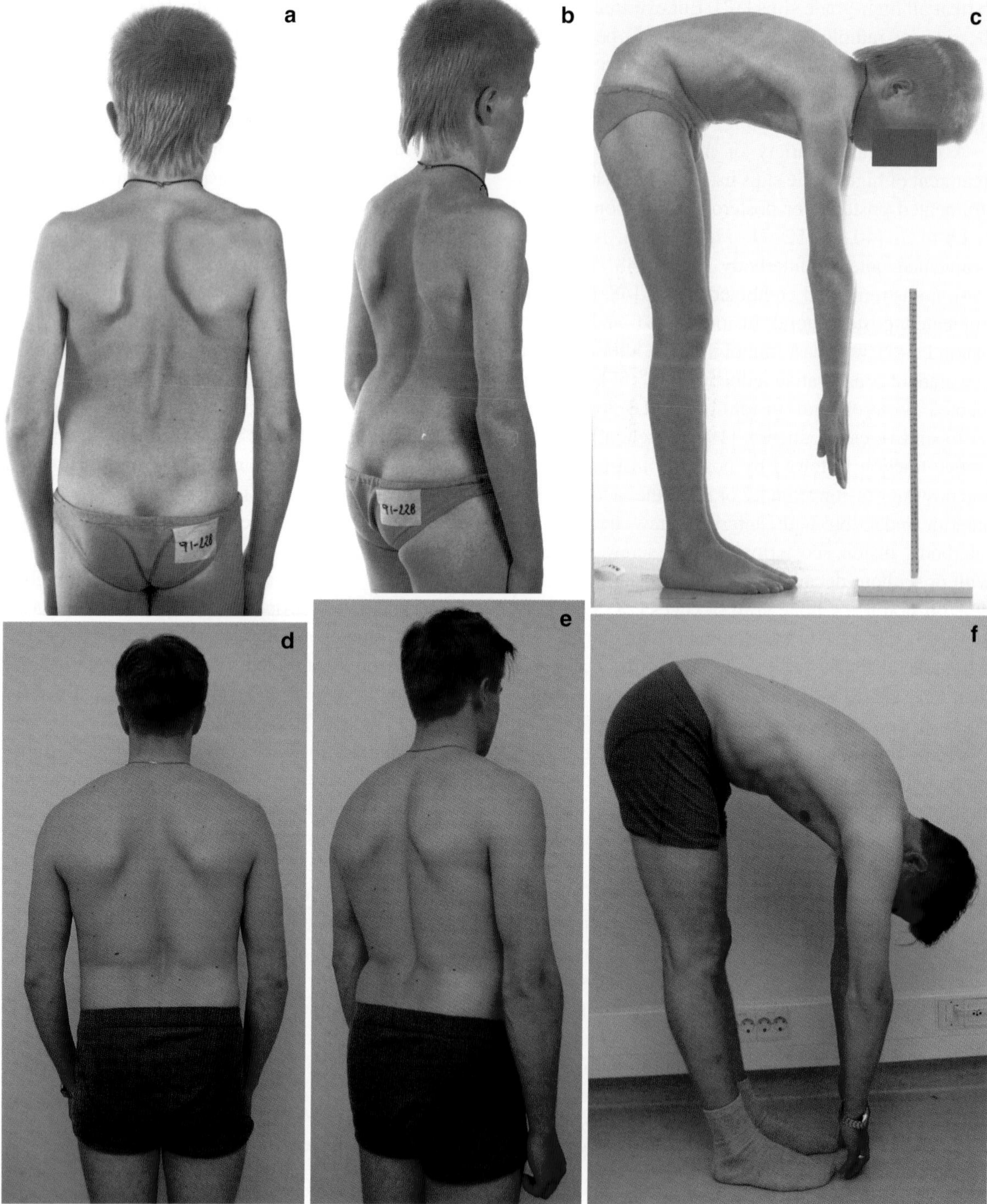

Fig. 25.10 (**a**–**h**) Uninstrumented anterior in situ fusion without decompression for high-grade slip in an 11-year old boy. (**a**–**c**) Preoperative photographs show typical posture changes. (**d**–**f**) Photographs 11 years after the operation, the patient is free of symptoms

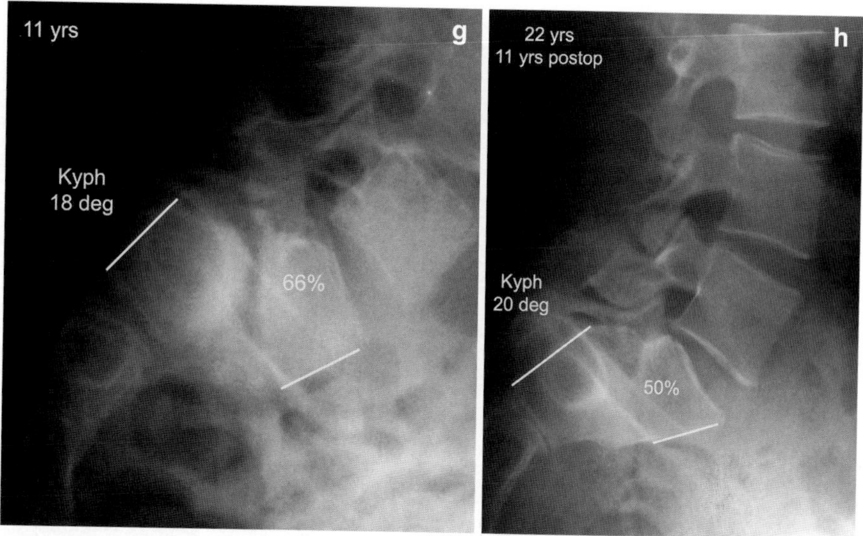

Fig. 25.10 (continued) (**g**) Preoparative radiograph. (**h**) Follow-up radiograph shows stable fusion after 11 years

fusion group. The mean Ostwestry index was 9.7 (0–62), 8.1 (0–32), and 2.3 (0–14) respectively, indicating combined fusion being slightly superior. Radiographs showed some progression of the mean lumbosacral kyphsis during follow-up in the posterolateral and in the anterior only fusion group. No progression of the lumbosacral kyphosis was detected after combined fusion [118]. A comparison of the three groups using the Scoliosis Research Society questionnaire yielded the same kind of results with a slightly better outcome in the circumferential fusion group [48, 67]. It has, however, to be noted that those patients are still in their 30s. And no data is available showing what happens when they reach midlife and seniority.

The risk of complications is obviously higher if using the anterior approach. Massive intraoperative bleeding, postoperative thrombosis, and retrograde ejaculation in male patients may occur. However, in experienced hands these complications are very rare [154]. The anterior approach can be avoided by performing a posterior interbody fusion (PLIF) or by utilizing the Bohlman transsacral strut graft technique. These procedures, however, make it necessary to resect the posterior structures to open the spinal canal with all its drawbacks like exposing the neural structures, significant muscle trauma, and loss of interspinous ligament continuity. In contrast, the direct anterior interbody fusion in combination with a posterolateral fusion through the paraspinal muscle split approach without touching the midline structures causes only very limited soft tissue damage and does not lead to additional destabilization.

Reduction of the slipped vertebra is technically possible [12, 14, 19, 28, 89, 95, 99, 105, 114, 120, 123, 129]. It includes a considerable risk of neurological complications. Although it is a controversial issue, it is recommended by several authorities [22, 77, 87].

The question is, whether reduction is necessary. There are no prospective randomized controlled trials available comparing in situ fusion with reduction and fusion. Five retrospective comparative studies failed to show any measurable benefit from reduction in clinical outcome [19, 95, 99, 114, 115, 155]. The numerous publications on high-grade slip reduction do show that patient's outcome will be good if solid fusion is achieved and no complications occur. Partial reduction is less dangerous than full reduction. But not a single study so far was able to prove that the reduction itself, i.e., the improvement of the position of the slipped vertebra in terms of slip percentage or lumbosacral kyphosis is in anyway related positively to the outcome concerning pain or function. The very satisfactory results of in situ fusion in young patients are mainly due to stabilization. Additionally, there is a significant capacity for remodellation [156]. Possibly, we underestimate the adaptive

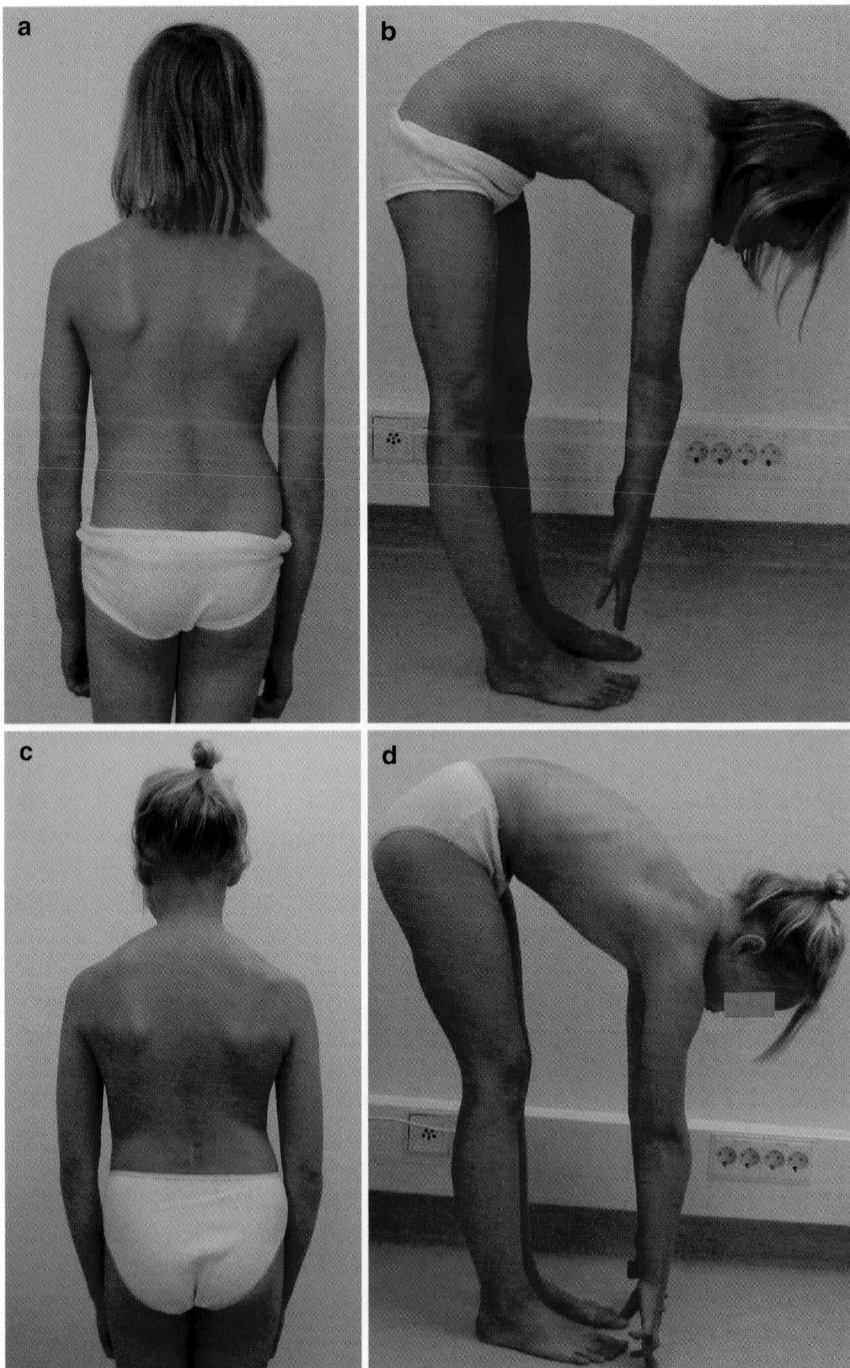

Fig. 25.11 Uninstrumenetd combined in situ fusion without decompression for a high-grade L5 slip in a 9-year-old athlete. The patient was subjectively free of symptoms. A scoliosis was detected by the school nurse. (**a**) C-shaped left convex secondary scoliosis. (**b**) Mild hamstring tightness prevents maximal forward bending. (**c**) One year after operation. The scoliosis has resolved. (**d**) Free forward bending 1 year after fusion

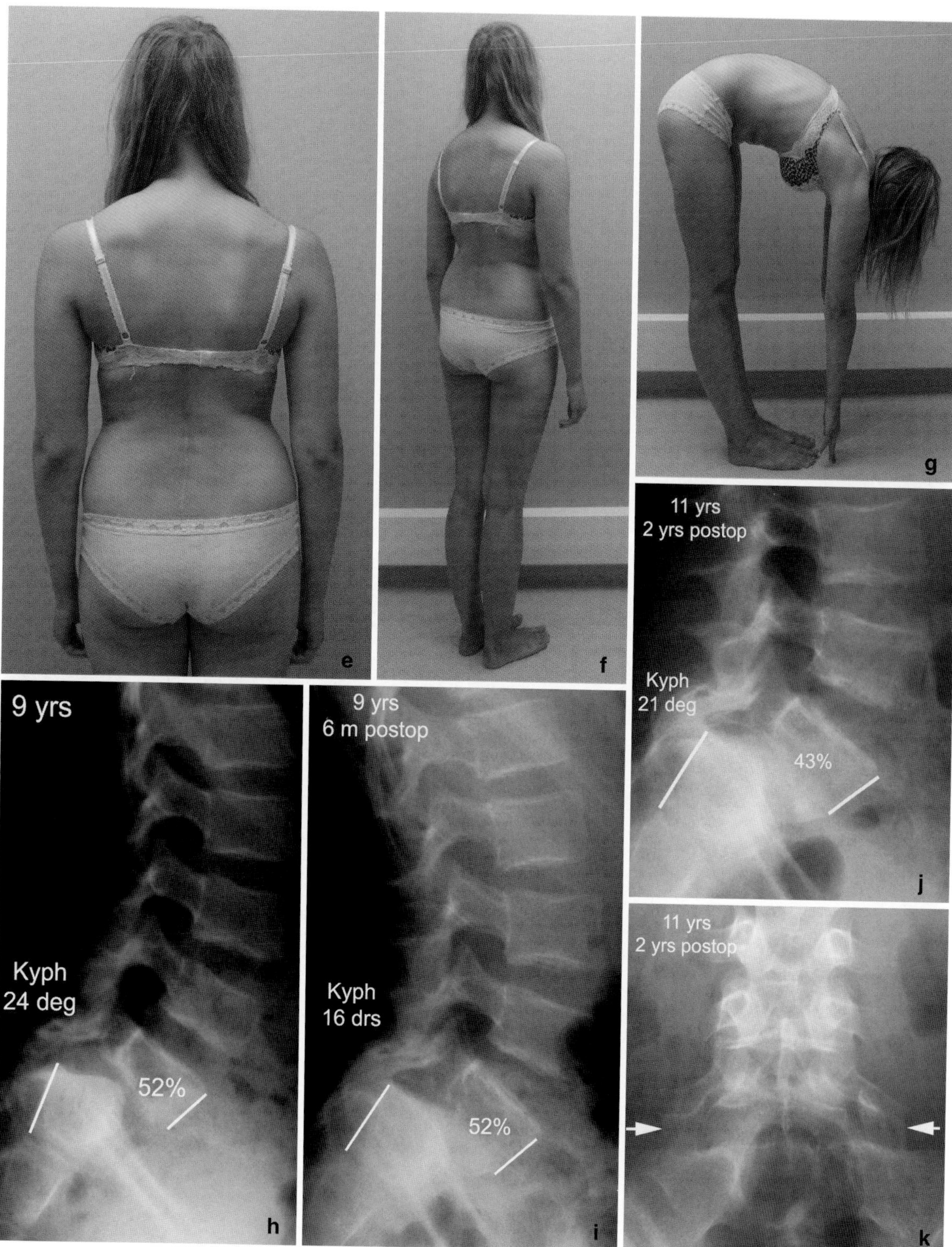

Fig. 25.11 (continued) (**e–g**) Clinical appearance of the patient 4 years after operation. (**h**) Preoperative lateral radiograph. (**i**) Lateral radiograph 6 months after surgery. (**j–k**) Solid anterior and posterolateral fusion on radiographs 2 years after the operation

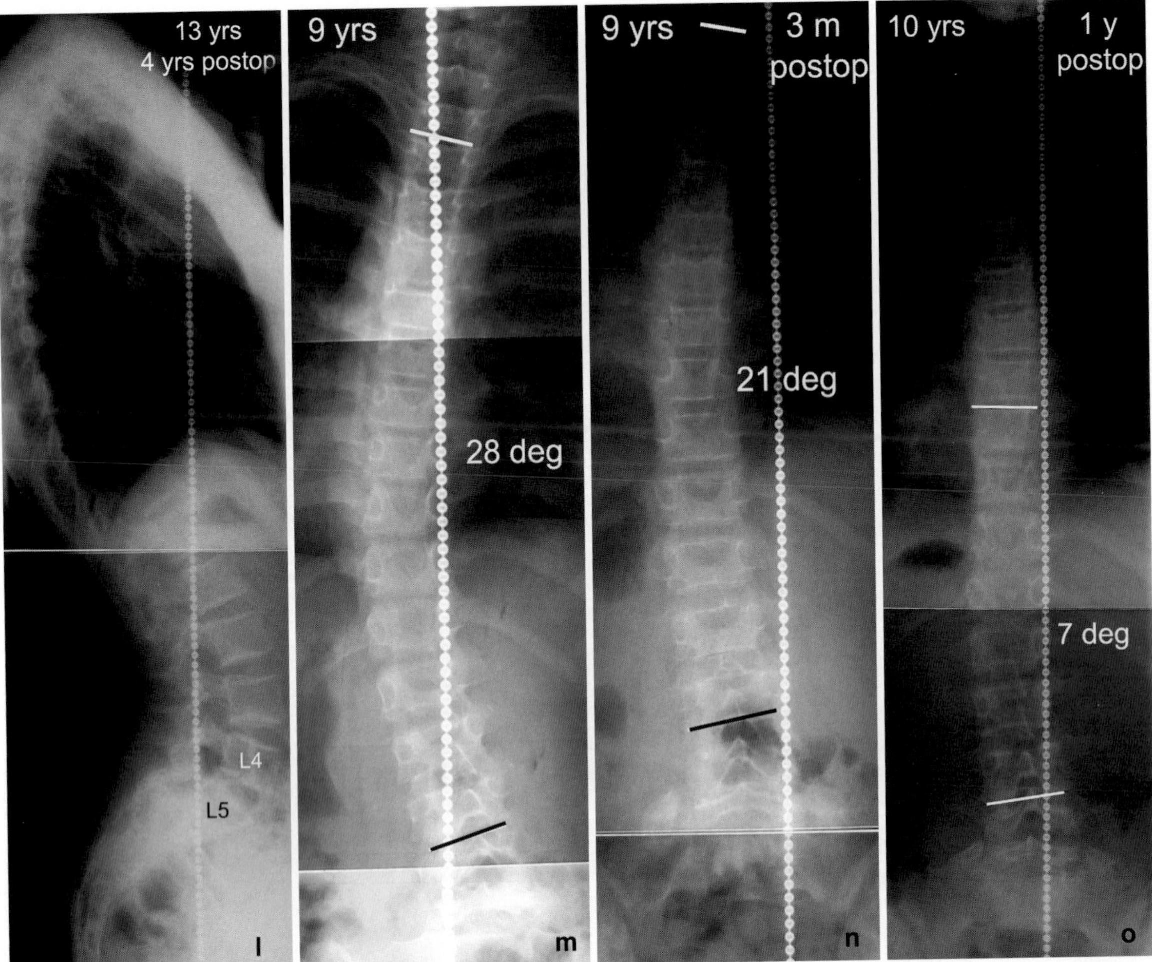

Fig. 25.11 (continued) (**l**) Whole spine lateral radiograph 4 years after surgery shows satisfactory sagittal alignment. (**m**) Secondary scoliosis preoperatively. (**n**) Improvement of the scoliosis after 3 months. (**o**) Unimportant residual curve 1 year after fusion

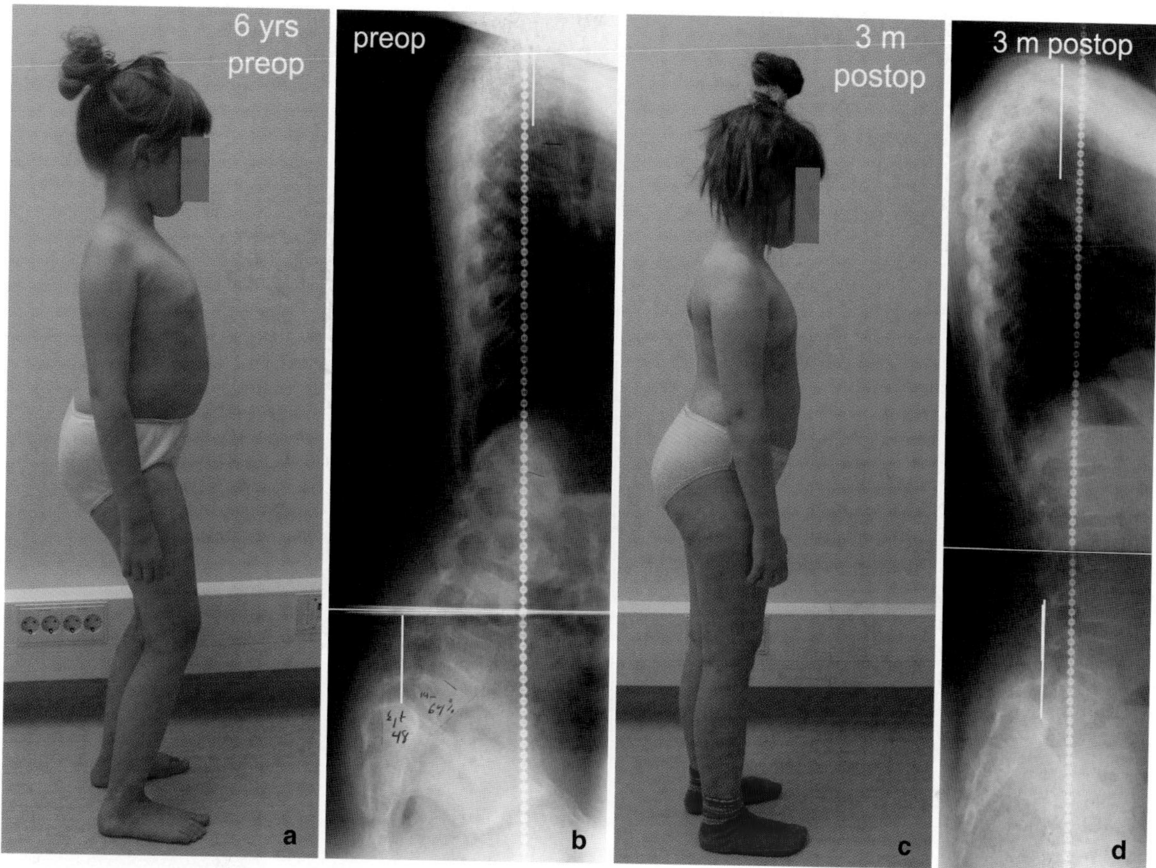

Fig. 25.12 Sagittal rebalancing of the spine in a 6-year-old girl with a high-grade slip after combined uninstrumented in situ fusion without decompression. (**a**) Preoperatively the patient can stand upright only by flexing her hips and knees (**b**). The preoperative lateral radiograph was taken with the patient's hips and knees straight (**c**). Three months after surgery, marked improvement of the sagittal balance clinically (**d**) as well as in the radiograph

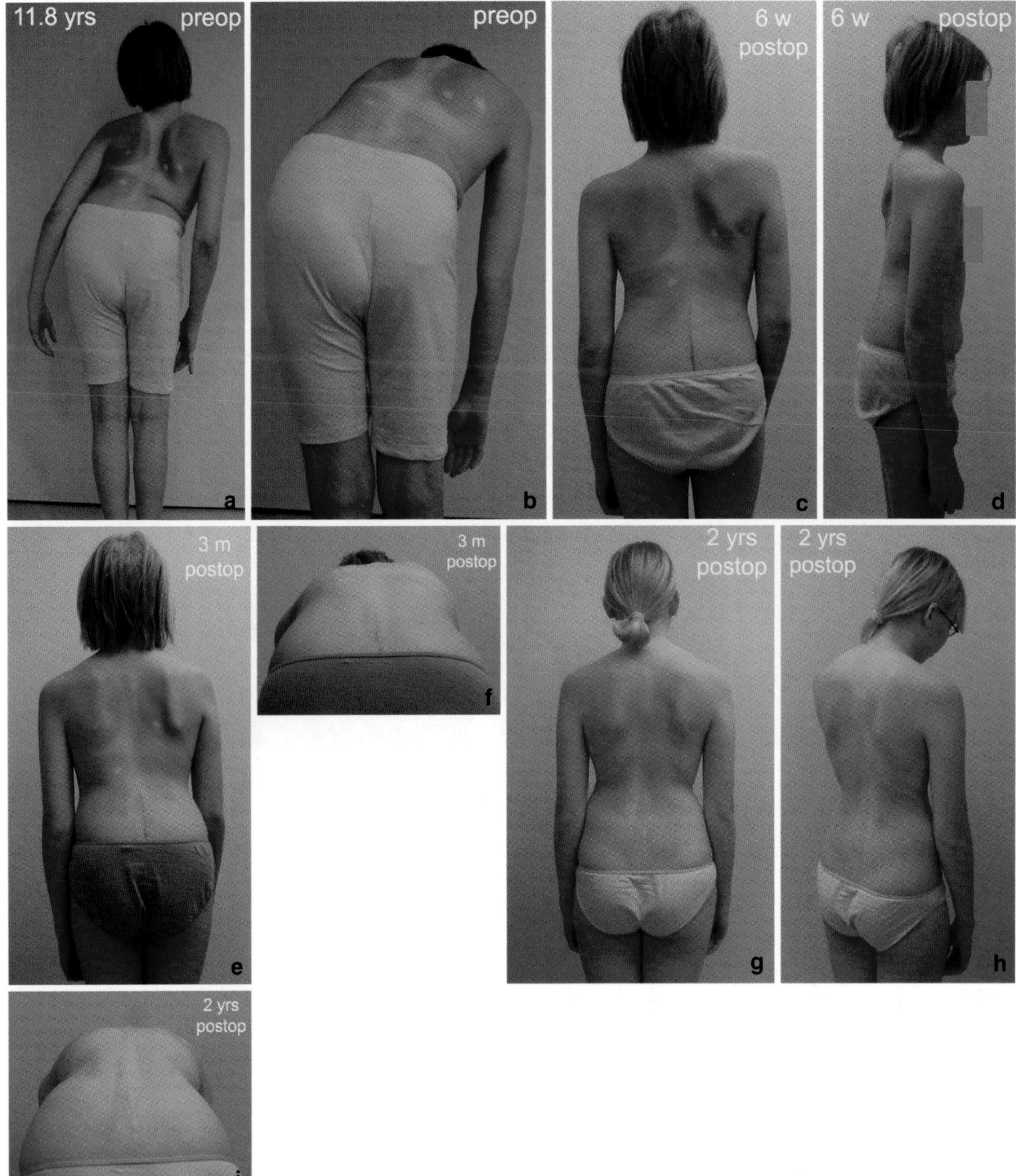

Fig. 25.13 An 11-year-old girl with a painful high-grade slip, severe balance problems, and a significant secondary scoliosis. (**a–i**) Clinical pictures, pre operative to 2 years post operative follow up

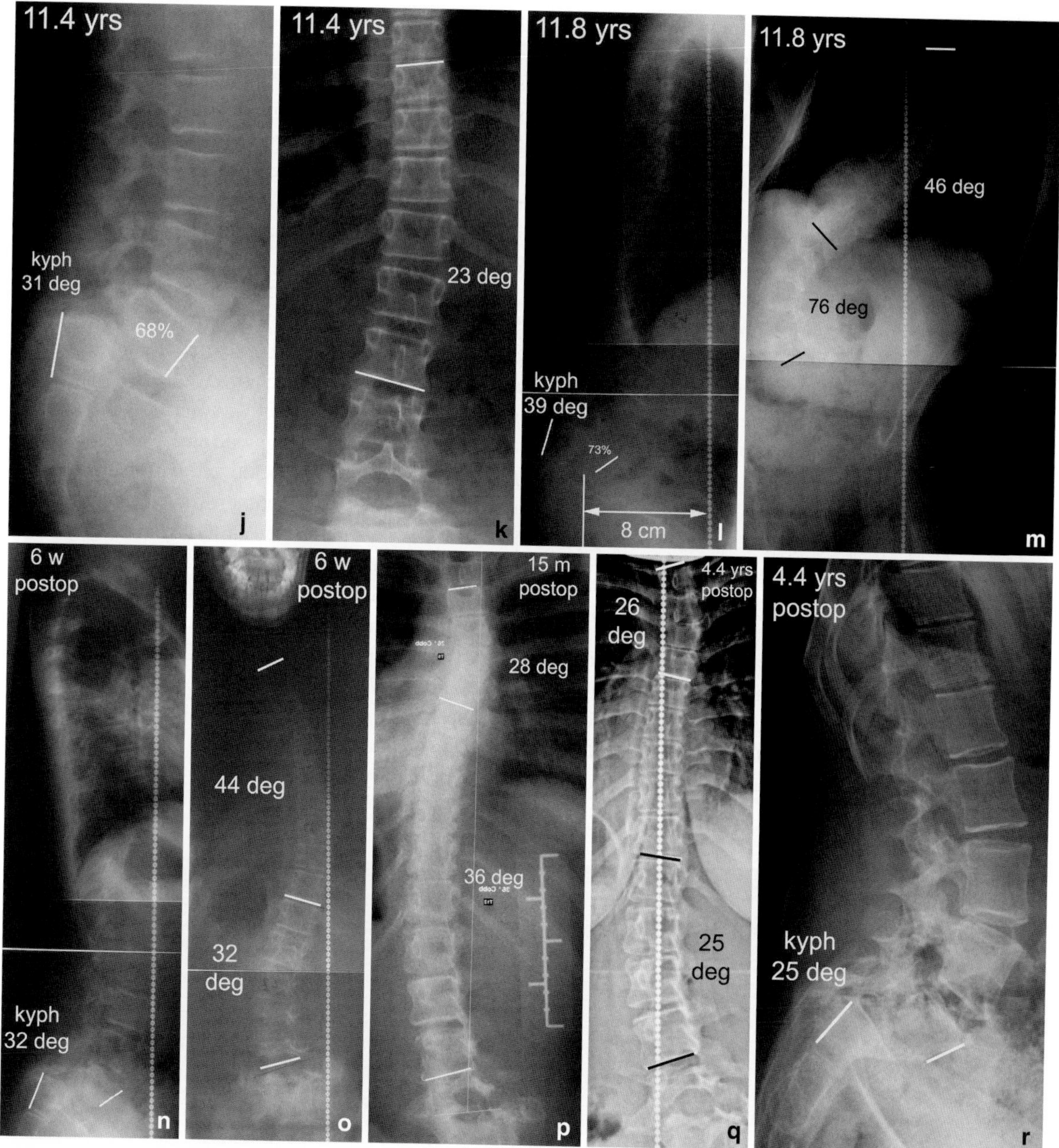

Fig. 25.13 (continued) (**j–r**) Plane radiographs, pre operative to 4.4 years post operative follow up. The patient was treated by uninstrumented combined in situ fusion without decompression. Note rapid preoperative deterioration within 4 months. Because of considerable residual scoliosis 6 weeks after surgery, a Boston brace was applied. The brace treatment was stopped after 13.5 months when overcorrection of the curve was observed (**p**). Very satisfactory clinical (**g–i**) and radiographic outcome (**q**, **r**)

capability of the growing spine. Lubicky [81], in his comment on this topic, stated: "Are we so stubborn and arrogant that we cannot accept the possibility that we feel has to be better on anatomic improvement is in fact not better when viewed from the patients' eyes? Or are we right and the outcomes instruments just cannot demonstrate it? Who knows?".

At this stage of knowledge, the author considers active instrumented slip reduction in children and adolescents only when the slip is not reducible in the supine-hyperextension radiograph sufficiently to allow for adequate anterior fusion. The aim of the (partial) reduction in those cases is to improve the position of the slipped vertebra to facilitate successful anterior interbody fusion. Reduction should then always be combined with decompression to allow visual control of the nerve roots during the maneuvre.

25.4.3.3 Spondyloptosis

Spondyloptosis is a very special and rare situation. It requires thorough investigation and serious consideration of individual solutions as there is not a single approach. There are different degrees of ptosis: The vertebra may be just "fallen off" the sacrum and is still very mobile. However, it may be also situated very caudally in front of S2 and appear almost unmovable. The clinical presentation is variable, too. It reaches from very mild symptoms to severe neurological impairment. A traction radiograph and a hyperextension radiograph in supine position should be taken to demonstrate the mobility of the slipped vertebra. MRI shows the configuration of the spinal canal, the cauda equina, and the exiting nerve roots.

If there is no neurological impairment, one can perform a posterolateral in situ fusion from L3 to S1 and add a transsacral strut graft according to Bohlman. This is effective if solid fusion is achieved. It does, however, not improve the cosmetic aspect very much. If the vertebra appears to be mobile enough one can reduce it by halo-femoral traction or intraoperatively with pedicle screw instrumentation depending on the severity. Decompression should be always performed in these cases. Combined fusion ensures a stable result (Fig. 25.14).

Another option is the resection of the slipped vertebra and instrumented fusion of L4 onto the sacrum as proposed for spondyloptosis by Gaines and Nichols [36] Gaines [37] and Lehmer et al. [75] This seems to be the *ultima ratio* if it is not possible to get the vertebra by means of reduction safely into a satisfactory position for fusion (Fig. 25.15). These complex

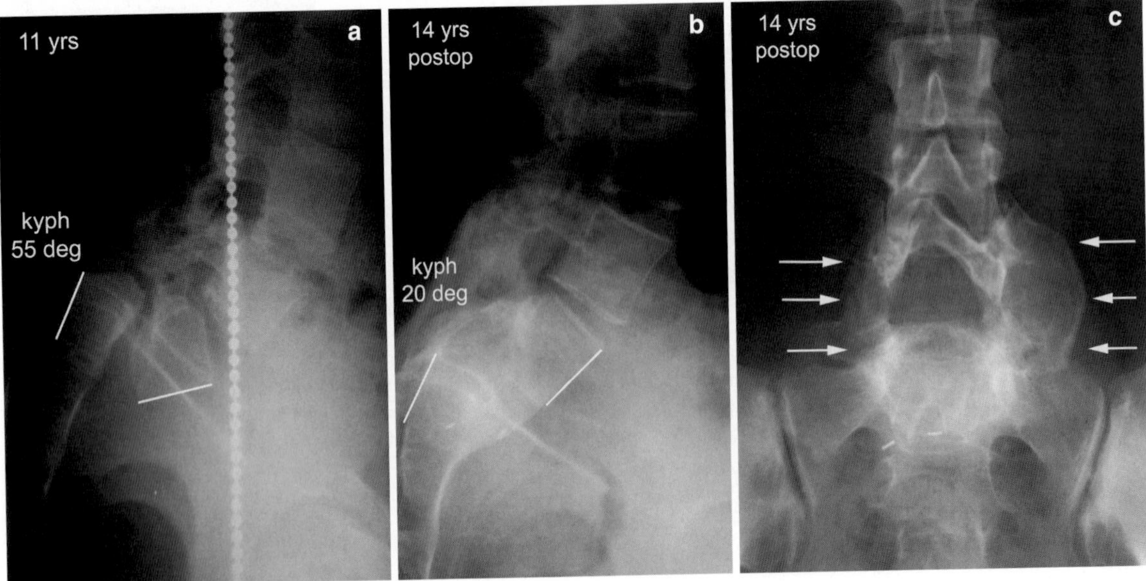

Fig. 25.14 (**a**) Standing lateral radiograph of an 11-year-old girl with L5 spondyloptosis, (**b**) Lateral radiograph 14 years after instrumented reduction, decompression, and combined fusion shows satisfactory alignment and healed anterior fusion, (**c**) Solid posterolateral fusion (*arrows*) is seen on the ap radiograph

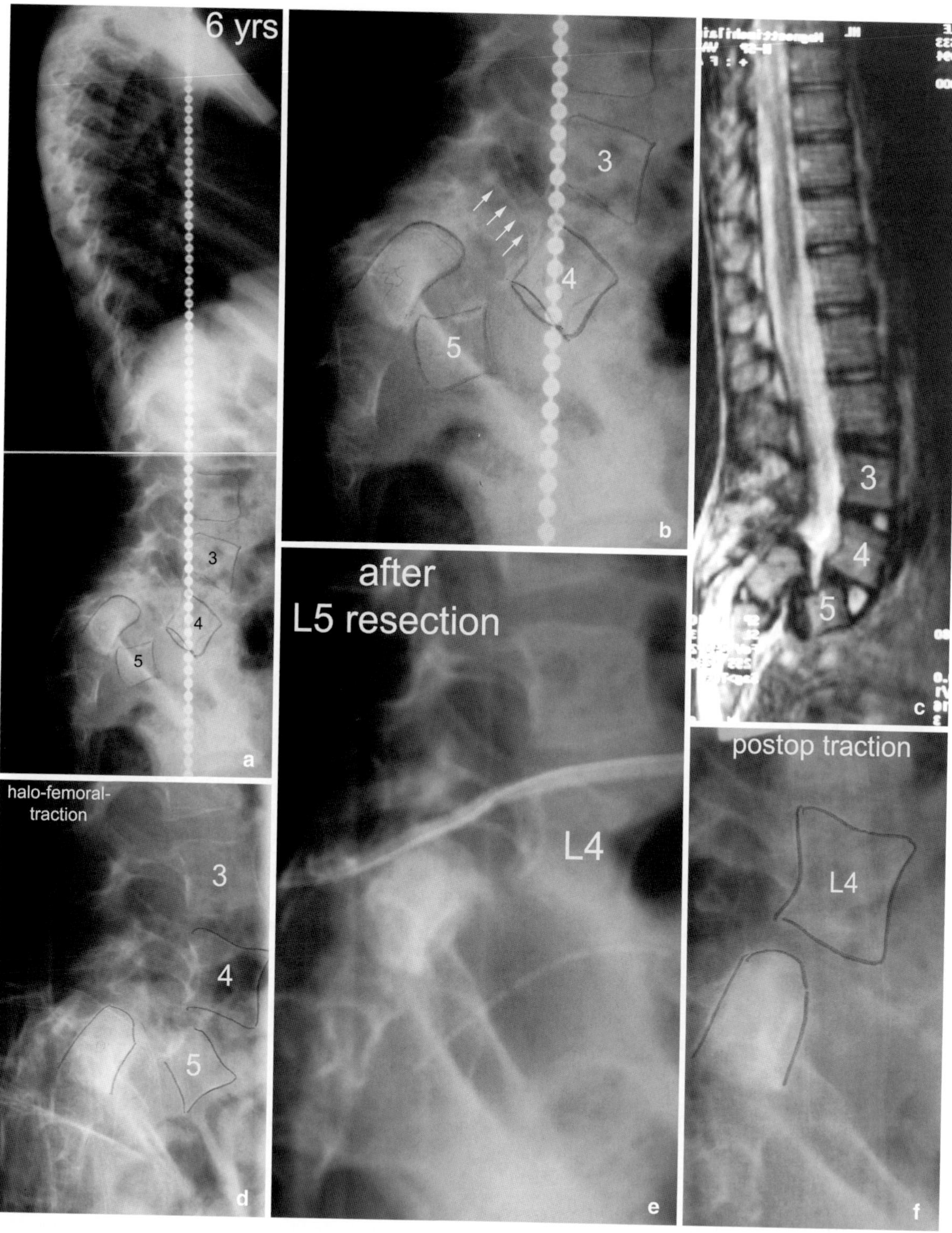

Fig. 25.15 Resection of L5 (Gaines' procedure) in a 6-year-old boy with osteogenesis imperfecta and spondyloptosis. (**a**) Preoperative lateral radiograph shows L5 spondyloptosis but acceptable sagittal balance. (**b**) Close-up of the preoperative lateral film, note elongated pedicles (*arrows*). (**c**) Preoperative MR image. (**d**) Partial reduction after halo-femoral traction. Traction had to be stopped because of developing bilateral peroneal weakness. (**e**) Radiograph after L5 resection. (**f**) Reduction of L4 on S1 after postoperative halo-femoral traction

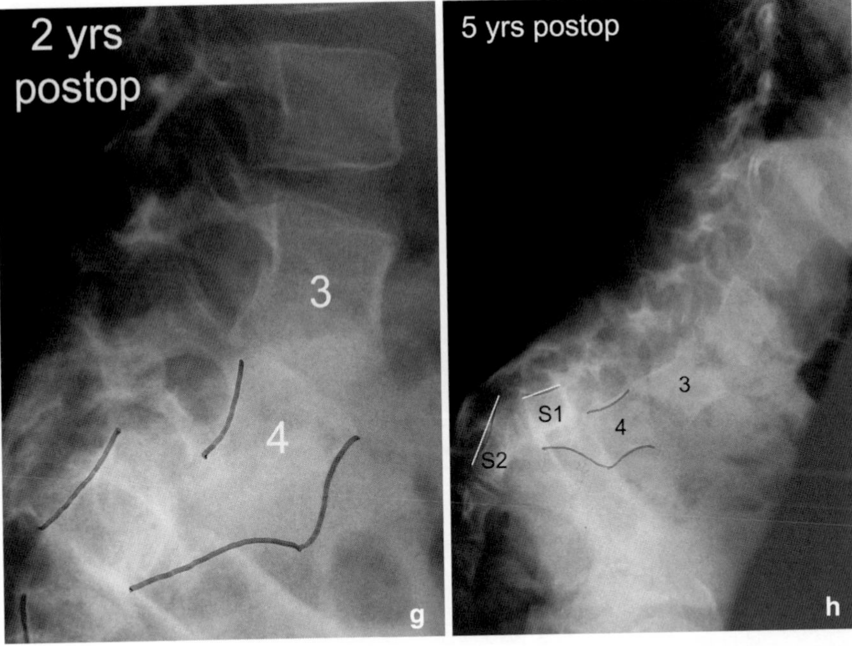

Fig. 25.15 (continued) (**g**) Solid fusion 2 years after anterior spondylodesis using an autologous fibular inlay-graft. (**h**) Five years after the operation, severe impairment of the sagittal profile due to bending of the sacrum at the level S1–S2. The patient is neurologically intact and free of pain

procedures, however, should be performed only by experienced spine surgeons familiar with the special pathoanatomical features of the deformity.

25.4.4 Spondylolisthesis in Very Young Children

As mentioned in the introduction, the literature on spondylolisthesis in children up to 12 years is sparse. Publications on children of preschool age (under 7 years) including a greater number of individuals are extremely rare. Several case reports are available.

King [61] analyzed lumbar radiographs of 500 (250 girls, 250 boys) normal first grade school children who were between 5 ½ and 6 ½ years old. Twenty two (4.4%) of them had spondylolisthesis, nine out of 250 girls and 13 out of 250 boys. In "several children", a slip up to 75% was present. There was no history of trauma. None of the children had any back symptoms. At re-examination after 6–10 years of follow-up, four additional cases were detected. All the children were still asymptomatic. Radiographs from some of the parents and siblings of the children with spondylolisthesis were obtained, too. The incidence in those was up to 69%. The author stressed that this finding supports the opinion that spondylolisthesis is hereditary. He also stated that in many children the slip occurs mainly before the age of 6. However, one has to note that the follow-up in this study was not long enough to exclude slip progression during the adolescent growth spurt in all children.

Zippel and Abesser [174] obtained ap- and lateral lumbar radiographs from 530 children of a pediatric orthopaedic outpatient clinic. All these children were free of any low-back symptoms. Their age ranged from 1–10 years. If the isthmus was not seen clearly in the primary radiograph, additional oblique films were taken. Low-grade spondylolisthesis was found in 3 out of 293 (1%) children in the age group 1–6 years and in 7 out of 237 (3%) in the age group 7–10 years. In the younger age group, all slips were at L5. One child in the elder age group had undergone operative treatment for myelomeningocele earlier. There is no follow-up data available of this series.

Pfeil [109] took lumbar radiographs from 500 normal children aged up to 6 years. Bilateral spondylolysis and low-grade spondylolisthesis were found in nine children (1.8%). The youngest child was a boy of 1 ½ year. There were further four boys of 3 years, one of 4 and two of 5 years. The only girl in this group was 6 years old. The mother of one of the 3 year old boys had spondyloptosis. None of the nine children had any subjective symptoms.

Beguiristáin and Diaz-de-Rada [7] presented a series of eight preschool children with a mean age of 3.5 years (range 9 months to 5 years) out of 188 spondylolisthesis patients younger than 20 years at diagnosis. All patients had slips at L5. There is some confusion in the publication concerning the classification of the cases. According to the text, four slips were isthmic, two dysplastic, one traumatic, and one iatrogenic. In Table 25.1 of the same paper, three cases are categorized as being isthmic, three dysplastic, one traumatic, and one iatrogenic. Two slips were high-grade, one dysplastic 87%, and one traumatic 57% slip. In the remaining four, the slip ranged from 18% to 48%. The two patients with the iatrogenic and the traumatic slip resp. had pain at admission. In the other six cases, the reason for investigation was scoliosis in four, kyphosis or skin alteration in one each. The mean follow-up was 11.5 (9–14) years. Three patients were treated operatively. A 4-year-old patient was operated at the time of diagnosis because of high-grade slip (87%). In situ arthrodesis was performed. The technique (levels? appoach?) is not described in detail. After 11 years of follow-up, the patient was asymptomatic, the slip measured 95%. The youngest patient a girl with a 15% slip was diagnosed at the age of 9 months due to a skin alteration. She was operated at the age of 11 years because of progression to 53%. Posterior fixation with hooks and rods from L3 to the sacrum was performed. The patient developed pseudarthrosis and was reoperated successfully 9 months later with pedicle screw fixation from L4 to S1. After 2-year follow-up, the patient was free of symptoms. No further progression of the slip occurred. The third surgically treated patient was a girl with a 25% slip at the age of 3 years. Progression of the slip to 50% was detected at the age of 11. Combined fusion L5 to S1 with pedicle screw instrumentation was performed. Three years after the operation, the patient was asymptomatic. The slip was 28%. Three non-surgically treated patients had slips from 18 to 47%. To one of them, a 3-year-old girl with 47% of slip, restriction of sports activities was recommended. The remaining two were allowed to live without any restrictions. No braces were used. After follow-up until maturity, no slip progression was seen in those three. The 5-year-old boy with the lumbosacral luxation-fracture (so-called traumatic spondylolisthesis, slip 57%) was treated by reduction under general anesthesia and plaster immobilization for 3 months. He had a complete unilateral motor deficit and impaired sensibility at L5 and a partial S1 motor deficit at admission. Neurological symptoms resolved. The patient was asymptomatic at 14-year follow-up with a slip of 15%. The patient with the iatrogenic slip of 25% had undergone tumor surgery at the age of 4 years. He was followed for 14 years. He remained symptomfree, and there was no progression of the slip.

Out of a clinical series of 63 patients aged 0–19 years, McKee et al. [91] found seven children in the age group up to 4 years, the youngest being 16 months old. Twenty-one children belonged to the group 5–9 years. The gender distribution was equal. Eighteen out of these 28 children under age 10 were symptomfree. The ten symptomatic children had lumbar pain, none had radiating pain. Three had spondylolysis without any slip, 24 had a low-grade slip, and one child had a high-grade slip. Out of the whole patient population (63 patients), only five patients were operated on. However, it is not known if any operated child belonged to the group under the age of 10 years as the ages of the operated patients are not presented in the paper. In their discussion, the authors stress that usually children under the age of 10 years do not have radiating pain, which seems to be present more in elder children and adolescents.

In the study by Seitsalo [137], out of the five children under the age of 7, four were asymptomatic at diagnosis. After postoperative mean follow-up of 14.5 years, no difference in outcome after fusion was detected if compared with children over 7 years.

The youngest patient in the literature was described by Borkow and Kleiger [13]. In this boy, a kyphotic deformity of the lumbosacral region was detected after birth. At the age of 15 weeks, a lateral radiograph of the lower lumbar spine and the sacrum revealed a kyphotic displacement of L4. The child developed normally, but its gait was described as "wide based shuffeling". The hip radiographs were normal. At the age of 11 years, a lax right patella was stated. One year later, recurrent dislocations of the patella started. Although no back problems were reported nor any slip progression occurred, posterolater fusion from L3 to the sacrum was performed at the age of 13 ½ years. Fusion was successful. And after short-term follow-up the patient was free of symptoms. Looking at the radiographs in the publication, one gets the impression that this was a congenital lumbosacral kyphosis due to an anterior failure of formation of the L5 vertebral body. In fact, the authors also discussed this possibility in their paper, but they preferred the explanation that a real slip had happened in utero (see Fig. 25.15).

A patient with a unilateral spondylolysis and 4 mm slip of L5 at the age of 10 months was reported primarily by Laurent and Einola [73]. When she was re-examined at age 10, the lysis and the slip were still visible. At final follow up, 25 years after the first presentation, the isthmus was healed and there was no slip anymore. The patient was free of any complaints and played volleyball actively.

Wild et al. [164], in a case report, described an 18-month-old boy with L5 spondyloptosis and spina bifida occulta L4 to S1. The condition was deemed congenital although there is no prove in the paper that the deformity has been present already at birth. The boy had episodes of recurrent falls and inability to stand and walk lasting no longer than 30 min. The history was otherwise uneventful. There were no objective neurological findings. At the age of 5 years, the child was hyperactive and demonstrated a waddling gait and lower limb muscle hypoplasia. There was L4/L5-weakness, a mild foot deformity and ileopsoas contacture which resolved after stretching. The degree of vertebral slip was unchanged. A three stage procedure (back-front-back) was performed: bilateral L5 laminectomy and root decompression, partial resection of the L5 vertebral body, reduction of L5, interbody fusion L5 to S1, and posterior fixation from L2 to the sacrum. Nine months later the instrumentation was removed and posterolateral fusion L5 to S1 was added. Nine years after the operation, the patient had a normal alignment of the lumbosacral spine and was practising sports actively.

Wertzberger and Peterson [162] published a case of a girl developing a spondylolysis and a low-grade slip at the age of 18 months during an observational period after repeated radiotherapy and chemotherapy for histiocytosis X. She was free of back symptoms. During a 2-year follow-up the radiographic picture did not change. Nor did the patient get symptoms from her spine. No treatment was applied.

Kleinberg [63] described a case of a 17-months-old girl which was admitted for treatment of a congenital dislocation of the hip. The back was clinically normal. The child had been walking for a few weeks. No trauma was known. On routine radiographs, a forward slip of L5 of more than 50% of its length was seen. A "gap or cleft" in the pedicle visible on the lateral radiograph was interpreted as being the inborn cause for the slip. Therefore, the case was claimed to represent a true congenital spondylolisthesis.

Finnegan and Chung [31] reported a case of a very special L5 spondyloptosis in a 3-year-old girl. The child was born small-for-age at gestation week 37 and developed erythroblastosis fetalis. The mother detected a lump in the back of the child when it started to walk at the age of 1 year. No trauma was reported. A doctor was consulted because of out-toeing at the age of 3. The child exhibited a "wide-based shuffling gait" with stiff knees. The muscle tonus was slightly increased in the lower extremities, as were the tendon reflexes. But there was no hamstring tightness. The skin sensation in the perineal area was decreased. The plain radiograph showed a spondyloptosis of L5 being situated in front of S1. At the same time, L5 was also displaced anteriorly in relation to L4, i.e., L 5 was slipped forward out of the vertebral row. Owing to that, the posterior inferior corner of the L4 vertebral body was riding on top of the dome-shaped sacrum. This is extraordinary because usually the whole upper vertebral column is moving forward with the slipping vertebra. Myelography demonstrated a filling defect at the slip level. Decompression was performed by unilateral laminectomy L3 to L5 and excision of the posterior part of the L5 vertebral body. A posterior and a posterolateral fusion from L3 to L5 was added. The outcome was favorable after 3 months of follow-up. Concerning the etiology, the authors of the papers did not believe that it was possible to determine the cause of the slip exactly. They questioned whether this was a usual spondylolytic slip and favored the explanation that this was possibly a "complete congenital spondylolisthesis".

The vast majority of very young children with a vertebral slip seem to be free of pain. An exceptional case of low-back pain symptoms in a very young patient with spondylolisthesis was published by Lucey and Gross [82]. They saw a girl of 2 years and 8 months who had an uneventful history until she started to complain about back pain at the age of 2 years. The pain was not related to activities nor was there any trauma. On physical examination, the spine looked normal. There was no tenderness but a pilonidal cyst at the lower back. Neurology and her gait were normal. The popliteal angle was 20° bilaterally. On the primary radiograph, there was a "unilateral (?) grade 1 spondylolisthesis" of L5. Two months later, the slip had progressed to 27%. MRI was normal. An antilordotic cast (later a brace) was applied. The girl became pain free. No healing of the pars defect was seen during a period of 8 months.

In conclusion, children of preschool age with spondylolisthesis may have low-back pain, but the majority seems to be pain free. Often, the lysis or the slip is diagnosed incidentally during investigations for other diseases. Some cases are detected because of posture anomalies, scoliosis, or gait problems. Slip progression does not appear to be a common phenomenon during this age period. Despite that, regular radiographic follow-up is advisable. If operation is deemed to be necessary uninstrumented posterolateral fusion is the method of choice.

25.4.5 Exotic Spondylolisthesis

The term exotic spondylolisthesis was coined by Lubicky [80] for unusual cases with vertebral slips due to bone or soft tissue anomalies often related to syndromes. This chapter is based to a large extend on Lubicky's recent review paper. There can be developmental disturbances in the facet joints or elongation of the pars interarticularis or the pedicles due to poor bone quality or spina bifida. Pathologic increased soft tissue laxity may also be a contributing factor.

Some cases of spondylolisthesis in *osteogenesis imperfecta* have been published in the literature [4, 6, 62, 80, 116]. Usually elongation of the pedicles is seen in those cases. Assessment and diagnosis is often difficult as a significant other spine deformity may be present. No specific recommendations for treatment are existing. In asymptomatic nonambulators, operative treatment is probably not indicated. In walking children with symptoms, it seems reasonable to stabilize the segment with combined fusion.

King and Bobechko [62] found four cases of spondylolisthesis due to elongated pedicles among 60 patients with osteogenesis imperfecta. Three of the four had also scoliosis. No treatment for spondylolisthesis was applied. The age of the patients was not mentioned.

The case published by Rask [116] was a 40-year-old man with a low-grade slip of L5 who had a back injury at the age of 4 years. Back pain persisted for many years following the injury. It is assumed that he had sustained a pars interarticularis fracture during that childhood injury. No treatment was necessary.

Barrack et al. [4] described a case of spondylolysis after prior posterior spinal fusion.

Basu et al. [6] reported on two cases. A 10-year-old girl had elongated pedicles of L4 and L5 causing a low-grade slip on both levels. A successful uninstrumented anterior L3 to S1 fusion was performed at age 11. Later, a posterior instrumentation and fusion from T1 to L1 was carried out for thoracic scoliosis. At 3-year follow-up she had no back problems. The second patient was an 11-year-old girl suffering from low-back and coccygeal pain since 1 year. She had elongated lumbar pedicles and a high-grade slip of L5. In addition, a lumbar hyperlordosis and thoracic scolisis were present. She was developing also leg pain. In situ fusion was planned.

At the author's institution, one case of spondyloptosis in a 6-year-old boy with osteogenesis imperfecta was treated by resection of L5 and fusion of L4 to the sacrum. Fusion was successful and the patient is still clinically free of symptoms. No neurological complications occurred. However, obviously due to the poor bone quality, the sacrum started to bend into kyphosis causing significant cosmetic impairment (see Fig. 25.15). This example shows that especially in young patients with systemic disease long follow-up is mandatory to ensure the lasting benefit of an operative procedure.

A few cases of spondylolisthesis in *neurofibromatosis* type I have been described in the literature [80]. As in osteogenesis imperfecta, they are often accompanied by other severe spinal deformity. Treatment should follow common rules. In operative treatment, the poor bone quality should be taken in consideration. Therefore, combined fusion is advisable if operative treatment is deemed to be necessary.

McCarroll [90] analyzed radiographs of 46 patients with neurofibromatosis. Four of them had spondylolisthesis. Two were accidental findings; the other two had low-back pain. The age of the patients is not reported. No details are given concerning follow-up or treatment.

Crawford [23] published a series of 82 patients with neurofibromatosis. Fifty of them had spinal deformities. One out of the 50 had a vertebral slip. The case was not described in detail. In a later publication including another 34 patients, no additional case of spondylolisthesis was found [24]. The authors conclude that spondylolisthesis is not as common in neurofibromatosis patients as compared with the general population.

Spondylolisthesis has been reported also in connection with *Marfan's syndrome* [65, 172].

Sponseller et al. [147] investigated two different groups of patients with Marfan's syndrome Among 82 skeletally mature patients, five (6%) had a low-grade slip, the mean slip being 30%. Out of 56 patients of all age groups with scoliosis of more than 10° and a radiologic follow-up of more than 2 years, three had spondylolisthesis, one low-grade and two high-grade (mean 60%). No information is provided on slip progression, symptoms, or treatment. The authors hypothesize that the frequency of spondylolisthesis in Marfan's may not be higher than in the general population. But the degree of slip is greater probably because of the altered ligament properties and shear resistance of the disc.

Winter [172] presented a report on two operated cases of spondyloptosis: a 13-year-old and a 16-year-old male. Both patients showed the typical posture of a high grade slip. Both had back pain and leg pain. Their hamstrings were tight. There were no neurological findings, nor bladder dysfunction. One was treated by decompression and uninstrumented posterolateral fusion from L3 to S1. At 4-year follow-up, the patient had no complaints and the fusion was sound. The other patient had preoperative halo-femoral traction for 2 weeks, bilateral laminectomy L4 and L5, posterolateral fusion L3 to S1, postoperative traction for 3 weeks more, and subsequent anterior fusion L5–S1. This was followed by 4 months of bed rest in a plastercast and after that a body cast with one leg included for further 3 months. At follow-up after 2 years, the patient was pain free and had normal neurology. The fusion was solid.

Taylor [153] published a case of an 11-year old girl with Marfan's and a high-grade L5 slip and a 70° c-shaped lordoscoliosis. She had pain in her left buttock, leg, and foot. Hamstrings were tight, and ankle jerks were absent. L5 laminectomy and posterolateral fusion from L4 to S1 was performed. She was mobilized in a plasterspika after 2 weeks. The fusion healed within 6 months. The patient was free of symptoms. Further follow-up of the spondylolisthesis was not presented. The scoliosis progressed and was operated on 14 months later.

Spondylolisthesis in *Ehlers-Danlos syndrome* was reported by Nematbakhsh and Crawford [101]. A 2-year-old girl was evaluated for transient paraparesis of the upper extremities. An unstable slip of C2 was found and treated by fusion from C1 to C3. Owing to subsequent instability of the adjacent segment the fusion had to be extended to C5. At the age of 4 years, she started having back pain, and at 7 years radiographs revealed a low-grade L5 spondylolisthesis with pars defects. At that time she was diagnosed having Ehlers-Danlos Type VI. The slip progressed during 4 years to 75%. A successful uninstrumented posterolateral fusion L4 to S1 was performed when she was 13 years old. No complications occurred. The long-term outcome was not reported. Lubicky [80] reported having treated at least one other patient with Ehlers-Danlos and spondylolisthesis. He underlines the risks related to poor bone quality and wound healing and recommends treating them in a similar way as Marfan patients.

In patients with *Myelomeningocele*, spondylolisthesis should be very common due to the developmental disturbance of posterior vertebral elements. The incidence reported ranges from 5.9 to 28.6% [58]. In the study of Mardjetko et al. [86], ambulatory patients with spina bifida had an incidence of spondylolisthesis twice as high as nonambulatory patients. All slips were low-grade. During 5 years of follow-up no progression was seen. There was no correlation between the level of the spina bifida and the degree of slip. According to Lubicky [80], two patients of that series had been operated on, one because of pain, the other for tethered cord release. Operative stabilization is advised for pain, progressive deformity, or neurological impairment.

Stanitski et al. [148] performed a radiographic evaluation of 305 patients aged 7–22 years with myelomeningocele. They found L5 spondylolisthesis in 18 (5.9%) patients. The majority (75%) of them were between 7 and 14 years old. All affected patients were walkers. The mean slip was 37%, ranging from 12 to 56%. Fourteen were low-grade and four high-grade slips. Patients with spondylolisthesis had a greater lumbar lordosis than patients without a slip. Furthermore, lumbar lordosis was positively related to the slip percentage. During a follow-up from 2 to 7 (mean 2.5) years, no slip progression was detected. None of the patients had symptoms from the spondylolisthesis. No comments concerning treatment are given in that paper.

Overall, spondylolisthesis in various syndromes represents a very mixed conglomerate of problems. As a general recommendation, the author agrees fully with Lubicky [80] who wrote that one "will need to use common sense and well-accepted general principles when encountering such clinical problems". Long-term follow-up is to be recommended in operated as well as in nonoperated patients to ensure a favorable final outcome.

References

1. Albanese M, Pizzutillo PD (1982) Family study of spondylolysis and spondylolisthesis. J Pediatr Orthop 2:496–499
2. Antoniades SB, Hammerberg KW, DeWald RL (2000) Sagittal plane configuration of the sacrum in spondylolisthesis. Spine 25:1085–1091
3. Baker DR, McHollick W (1956) Spondyloschisis and spondylolisthesis in children. J Bone Jt Surg Am 38:933–934
4. Barrack R, Whitecloud TS, Skinner HB (1984) Spondylolysis after spinal instrumentation in osteogenesis imperfecta. South Med J 11:1453–1454
5. Bartolozzi P, Sandri A, Cassini M et al (2003) One-stage posterior decompression-stabilization and trans-sacral interbody fusion after partial reduction for severe L5-S1 spondylolisthesis. Spine 28:1135–1141
6. Basu PA, Noordeen MHH, Elsebaie H (2001) Spondylolisthesis in osteogenesis imperfecta due to pedicle elongation. Report of two cases. Spine 26:E506–E509
7. Beguiristáin JL, Diaz-de-Rada P (2004) Spondylolisthesis in pre-school children. J Pediatr Orthop B 13:225–230
8. Belfi LM, Orlando Ortiz A, Katz DS (2006) Computed tomography evaluation of spondylolysis and spondylolisthesis in asymptomatic patients. Spine 31:E907–E910
9. Bell D, Ehrlich M, Zaleske D (1988) Brace treatment for symptomatic spondylolisthesis. Clin Orthop 236:192–198
10. Beutler WJ, Fredrickson BE, Murtland A et al (2003) The natural history of spondylolysis and spondylolisthesis. 45-year follow-up evaluation. Spine 28:1027–1035
11. Bodner RJ, Heyman S, Drummond DS et al (1988) The use of single photon emission computed tomography (SPECT) in the diagnosis of low-back pain in young patients. Spine 13:1155–1160
12. Boos N, Marchesi D, Zuber K et al (1993) Treatment of severe spondylolisthesis by reduction and pedicular fixation. Spine 18:1655–1661
13. Borkow SE, Kleiger B (1971) Spondylolisthesis is the newborn. A case report. Clin Orthop 81:73–76
14. Boxall D, Bradford DS, Winter R et al (1979) Management of severe spondylolisthesis in children and adolescents. J Bone Jt Surg Am 61:479–495
15. Bradford DS (1985) Spondylolysis and spondylolisthesis in children and adolescents. Current concepts in management. In: Bradford DS, Hensinger RM (eds) The pediatric spine.Thieme, New York, pp 403–423
16. Bradford DS, Iza J (1985) Repair of the defect in spondylolysis and minimal degrees of spondylolisthesis by segmental wire fixation and bone grafting. Spine 10:673–679
17. Bridwell KH (2006) Point of view. Spine 31:170
18. Buck JE (1970) Direct repair of the defect in spondylolisthesis. J Bone Jt Surg Br 52:432
19. Burkus JK, Lonstein JE, Winter RB et al (1992) Long-term evaluation of adolecents treated operatively for spondylolisthesis. J Bone Jt Surg Am 74:693–704
20. Carl RL, Noonan KJ, Nemeth BA (2007) Isthmic spondylolisthesis in a nonambulatory patient. Spine 32:E723–E724
21. Cavalier R, Herman MJ, Cheung EV et al (2006) Spondylolysis and spondylolisthesis in children and adolescents: I. Diagnosis, natural history, and nonsurgical management. J Am Acad Orthop Surg 14:417–424
22. Cheung EV, Herman MJ, Cavalier R, et al (2006) Spondylolysis and spondylolisthesis in children and adolescents: II. Surgical management. J Am Acad Orthop Surg 14: 488–498
23. Crawford AH (1981) Neurofibromatosis in childhood. In: Murray GD (ed) Instructional course lectures Vol XXX. C V Mosby, St. Louis, Toronto/London, pp 56–74
24. Crawford AH, Bagamery N (1986) Osseous manifestation of neurofibromatosis in childhood. J Ped Orthop 6:72–88
25. Cyron BM, Hutton WC (1979) Variations in the amount and distribution of cortical bone across the partes interarticulares of L5. A predisposing factor in spondylolysis. Spine 4:163–167
26. Cyron BM, Hutton WC, Troup JDG (1976) Spondylolytic fractures. J Bone Jt Surg [Br] 58-B:462–466
27. d'Hemecourt PA, Zurakowski D, Kriemler S et al (2002) Spondylolysis: returning the athlete to sports participation with brace treatment. Ortopedics 25:653–657
28. Dick WT, Schnebel B (1988) Severe Spondylolisthesis. Reduction and internal fusion. Clin Orthop 232:70–79
29. Fairbank JCT, Couper J, Davies JB et al (1980) The Oswestry low back pain disability questionnaire. Physiotherapy 53:271–273
30. Farfan HF, Osteria V, Lamy C (1976) The mechanical etiology of spondylolysis and spondylolisthesis. Clin Orthop 117:40–55
31. Finnegan WJ, Chung SMK (1975) Complete spondylolisthesis in an infant. Am J Dis Child 129:967–969
32. Fredrickson BE, Baker D, McHolick WJ et al (1984) The natural history of spondylolysis and spondylolisthesis. J Bone Jt Surg Am 66:699–707
33. Frennered K (1994) Isthmic spondylolisthesis among patients receiving disability pension under the diagnosis of chronic low back pain symdromes. Spine 19:2766–2769
34. Friberg S (1939) Studies on spondylolisthesis. Acta Chir Scand 55(Suppl):7–131
35. Fujii K, Katoh S, Sairyo K et al (2004) Union of defects in the pars interarticularis of the lumbar spine in children and adolescents. The radiological outcome after conservative treatment. J Bone Jt Surg [Br] 86-B:225–231
36. Gaines RW, Nichols WK (1985) Treatment of spondyloptosis by two stage L5 vertebrectomy and reduction of L4 onto S1. Spine 10:680–686
37. Gaines RW (2005) L5 vertebrectomy for the surgical treatment of spondyloptosis. Thirty cases in 25 years. Spine 30:S66–S70
38. Gillet P, Petit M (1999) Direct repair of spondylolysis without spondylolisthesis, using a rod-screw construct and bone grafting of the pars defect. Spine 24:1252–1256
39. Grobler LJ, Robertson PA, Novotny JE et al (1993) Etiology of spondylolisthesis. Spine 18:80–91
40. Grzegorzewski A, Kumar SJ (2000) In situ posterolateral spine arthrodesis for grades III, IV and V spondylolisthesis in children and adolescents. J Ped Orthop 20:506–511
41. Haher TR, Gorup JM, Shin TM et al (1999) Results of the scoliosis research society outcome instrument for evaluation of surgical outcome in adolescent idiopathic scoliosis. A multicenter study of 244 patients. Spine 24:1435–1440
42. Hanson DS, Bridwell KH, Rhee JM et al (2002) Dowel fibular strut grafts for high-grade dysplastic isthmic spondylolisthesis. Spine 27:1982–1988

43. Hanson DS, Bridwell KH, Rhee JM et al (2002) Correlation of pelvic incidence with low- and high-grade isthmic spondylolisthesis. Spine 27:2026–2029
44. Harvey CJ, Richenberg JL, Saifuddin A et al (1998) Pictorial review: the radiological investigation of lumbar spondylolysis. Clin Radiol 53:723–728
45. Hefti F, Seelig W, Morscher E (1992) Repair of lumbar spondylolysis with a hook-screw. Int Orthpedics 16:81–85
46. Hefti F, Brunazzi M, Morscher E (1994) Spontaverlauf bei Spondylolyse und Spondylolisthesis. Orthopäde 23:220–227
47. Helenius I, Lamberg T, Österman K et al (2005) Scoliosis research society outcome instrument in evaluation of long-term surgical results in spondylolysis and low-grade spondylolisthesis in young patients. Spine 30:336–341
48. Helenius I, Lamberg T, Österman K et al (2005) Posterolateral, anterior, or circumferential fusion in situ for high-grad spondylolisthesis in young patients: a long-term evaluation using the scoliosis research society questionnaire. Spine 31:190–196
49. Herman MJ, Pizzutillo PD (2005) Spondylolysis and spondylolisthesis in the child and adolescent. A new classification. Clin Orthop 434:46–54
50. Higashino K, Sairyo K, Sakamaki T et al (2007) Vertebral rounding deformity in pediatric spondylolisthesis occurs due to deficient of enchondral ossification of the growth plate. Spine 32:2839–2845
51. Huang RP, Bohlman HH, Thompson GH et al (2003) Predictive value of pelvic incindence in progression of spondylolisthesis. Spine 28:2381–2385
52. Ishikawa S, Kumar J, Torres BC (1994) Surgical treatment of dysplastic spondylolisthesis. Results after in situ fusion. Spine 19:1691–1696
53. Ivanic GM, Pink TP, Achatz W et al (2003) Direct stabilization of lumbar spondylolysis with a hook-screw. Spine 28:255–259
54. Jackson DW, Wiltse LL, Cirincione RJ (1976) Spondylolysis in the femal gymnast. Clin Orthop 117:68–79
55. Johnson GV, Thompson AG (1992) The Scott wiring technique for direct repair of lumbar spondylolysis. J Bone Jt Surg [Br] 74-B:426–430
56. Johnson JR, Kirwan EO'G (1983) The long-term results of fusion in situ for severe spondylolisthesis. J Bone Jt Surg [Br] 65-B:43–46
57. Kajiura K, Katoh S, Sairyo K et al (2001) Slippage mechanism of pediatric spondylolysis. Biomechanical study using immature calf spines. Spine 26:2208–2213
58. Karlin L, Citrone BA, Zimbler S (1990) The association of spondylolisthesis in myelomeningocele. Paper presented ant the Annual Meeting of the Pediatric Orthopaedic Soiciety of North America. San Francisco
59. Kilian HF (1853) De spondylolisthesi gravissimae pelvangustiae caussa nuper detecta. Commentatio anatomico-obstetricia. Litteris Caroli Georgii Bonn
60. Kimura M (1968) My method of filling the lesion with spongy bone in spondylolysis and spondylolisthesis. Orthop Surg 19:285–295
61. King AB (1966) Experiences with spondylolisthesis. Bull Johns Hopk Hosp 118:2–9
62. King JD, Bobechko WP (1971) Osteogenesis imperfecta. An orthopaedic description and surgical review. J Bone Jt Surg [Br] 53-B:72–89
63. Kleinberg S (1934) Spondylolisthesis in an infant. J Bone Jt Surg 16:441–444
64. Komatsubara S, Sairyo K, Katoh S et al (2006) High-grade slippage of the lumbar spine in a rat model of spondylolisthesis. Spine 31:E528–E534
65. Kumar SJ, Guille JT (2001) Marfan Syndrom. In: Weinstein SL (ed) The pediatric spine, Lippincott Williams and Wilkins, Philadelphia, PA
66. Labelle H, Roussouly P, Berthonnaud É et al (2005) The importance of spino-pelvic balance in L5-S1 developmental spondylolisthesis. Spine 30:S27–S34
67. Lamberg TS, Remes VM, Helenius IJ et al (2005) Long-term clinical, functional and radiological outcome 21 years after posterior or posterolateral fusion in childhood or adolescence isthmic spondylolisthesis. Eur Spine J 14:639–644
68. Lamberg T, Remes V, Helenius I et al (2007) Uninstrumented in situ fusion for high-grade childhood and adolescent isthmic spondylolisthesis: long-term outcome. J Bone Jt Surg Am 89:512–518
69. Lambl D (1881) Primitive Spondylolysis und deren Verhältnis zur Steatopyga an der hottentottischen Venus. Zbl Gynäkol 5:256–259
70. Lambl W (1858) Das Wesen und die Entstehung der Spondylolisthesis. Beitr Geburtsk u Gynäkol 3:1–79
71. Lance EM (1966) Treatment of severe spondylolisthesis with neural involvement. J Bone Jt Surg Am 48:883–891
72. Laurent LE (1958) Spondylolisthesis. A study of 53 cases treated by spine fusion and 32 cases treated by laminectomy. Acta Orthop Scand 35(Suppl):7–45
73. Laurent LE, Einola S (1961) Spondylolisthesis in children and adolescents. Acta Orthop Scand 31:45–64
74. Laurent LE, Österman K (1976) Operative treatment of spondylolisthesis in young patients. Clin Orthop 117:85–91
75. Lehmer SM, Steffee AD, Gaines RW (1994) Treament of L5-S1 spondyloptosis by staged resection with reduction and fusion of L4 onto S1 (Gaines procedure). Spine 19:1916–1925
76. Lenke LG, Bridwell KH, Bullis D et al (1992) Results of in situ fusion for isthmic spondylolisthesis. J Spinal Disord 5: 433–442
77. Lenke LG, Bridwell KH (2003) Evaluation and surgicat treatment of high-grade isthmic dysplastic spondylolisthesis. AAOS Intruct Course Lectures 52:525–532
78. Loder RT (2001) Profiles of the cervical, thoracic, and lumbosacral spine in children and adolescents with lumbosacral spodylolisthesis. J Spinal Disord 14:465–471
79. Louis R (1988) Reconstitution isthmique des spondylolyses par plaque et greffes sans athrodèse. A propos de 78 cas. Rev Chir Orthop 74:549–557
80. Lubicky JP (2005) Unusual spondylolisthesis. Spine 30:S82–S87
81. Lubicky JP (2006) Point of view. Spine 31:591–592
82. Lucey SD, Gross R (1995) Painful spondylolisthesis in an two-year-old girl. J Ped Orthop 15:199–201
83. Mac-Thiong J-M, Labelle H (2006) A proposal for a surgical classification of pediatric lumbosacral spondylolisthesis based on the current literature. Eur Spine J 15:1425–1435
84. Magora A (1976) Conservative treatment in spondylolisthesis. Clin Orthop 117:74–79
85. Marchetti PG, Bartolozzi P (1997) Classification of spondylolisthesis as a guideline for treatment. In: Bridwell KH,

DeWald RL (eds) The textbook of spinal surgery, 2nd edn. Lippincott-Raven Publishers, Philadelphia, PA

86. Mardjetko S, Knott P, Ellis P et al (2002) A longitudinal retrospective study to determine the incidence and the risk of progression of spondylolisthesis in children with spina bifida. Paper #10. 37th Annual Meeting of the Scoliosis Research Society, Sept 18–21, 2002, Seattle, Washington
87. Mardjetko S, Albert T, Andersson G et al (2005) Spine/SRS Spondylolisthesis summary statement. Spine 30:S3
88. Marty C, Boisaubert B, Descamps H et al (2002) The sagittal anatomy of the sacrum among young adults, infants, and spondylolisthesis patients. Eur Spine J 11:119–125
89. Matthiass HH, Heine J (1986) The surgical reduction of spondylolisthesis. Clin Orthop 203:34–44
90. McCarroll HR (1950) Clinical manifestations of congenital neurofibromatosis. J Bone Jt Surg Am 32:601–617
91. Mc Kee BW, Alexander WJ, Dunbar JS (1971) Spondylolisthesis and spondylolysis in children: A review. J L'Ass Canad Radiol 22:100–109
92. Miller SF, Congeni J, Swanson K (2004) Long-term functional and anatomical follow-up of early detected spondylolysis in young athletes. Am J Sport Med 32:928–933
93. Miyagi S (1971) Spondylolysis in Japan. Verhandl Dtsch Orthop Gesellsch Beilh Z Orthop 119–124
94. Moe JH, Winter RB, Bradford DS et al (1978.) Scoliosis and other spinal deformieties. WB Saunders, Philadelphia
95. Molinari RW, Bridwell KH, Lenke LG (1999) Complications in the surgical treatment of pediatric high-grade isthmic dysplastic spondylolisthesis. Spine 24:1701–1711
96. Moreton RD (1966) Spondylolysis. J Amer Med Ass 195: 671–674
97. Morscher E, Gerber B, Fasel J (1984) Surgical treatment of spondylolisthesis by bone grafting and direct stabilization of spondylolysis by means of a hook screw. Arch Orthop Trauma Surg 103:175–178
98. Muschik M, Hähnel H, Robinson P et al (1996) Competetive sports and the progression of spondylolisthesis. J Ped Orthop 16:364–369
99. Muschik M, Zippel H, Perka C (1997) Surgical management of severe spondylolisthesis in children and adolescents. Spine 22:2036–2043
100. Natarajan RN, Garretson RB, Biyani A et al (2003) Effects of slip severity and loading directions on the stability of isthmic spondylolisthesis: a finite element study. Spine 11: 1103–1112
101. Nematbakhsh A, Crawford AH (2004) Non-adjacent spondylolisthesis in Ehlers-Danlos syndrome. J Ped Ortop 13-B: 336–339
102. Newman PH (1963) The etiology of spondylolisthesis. J Bone Jt Surg 45-B:39–59
103. Nicol RO, Scott JHS (1986) Lytic spondylolysis. Repair by wiring. Spine 11:1027–1030
104. Nordström D, Santavirta S, Seitsalo S et al (1994) Symptomatic lumbar spondylolysis. Neuroimmunologic Studies. Spine 19:2752–2758
105. O'Brien JP, Mehdian H, Jaffrey D (1994) Reduction of severe lumbosacral spondylolisthesis. Clin Orthop 300:64–69
106. Österman K, Lindholm TS, Laurent LE (1976) Late results of removal of the loose posterior element (Gill's operation) in the treatment of lytic lumbar spondylolisthesis. Clin Orthop 117:121–128
107. Österman K, Österman H (1996) Experimental lumbar spondylolisthesis in growing rabbits. Clin Orthop 332: 274–280
108. Pease CN, Najat H (1967) Spondylolisthesis in children. Special reference to the lumbosacral joint and treatment by fusion. Clin Orthop 52:187–198
109. Pfeil E (1971) Spondylolysis und Spondylolisthesis bei Kindern. Z Orthop 109:17–33
110. Pfeil E (1971) Experimentelle Untersuchungen zur Frage der Entstehung der Spondylolyse. Z Orthop 109:231–238
111. Pfeil J, Niethard FU, Cotta H (1987) Die Pathogenese kindlicher Spondylolisthesen. Z Orthop 125:526–433
112. Phalen GS, Dickson JA (1961) Spondylolisthesis and tight hamstrings. J Bone Jt Surg Am 43:505–512
113. Poussa M, Tallroth K (1993) Disc herniation in lumbar spondylolisthesis. Acta Orthop Scand 64:13–16
114. Poussa M, Schlenzka D, Seitsalo S et al (1993) Surgical treatment of severe isthmic spondylolisthesis in adolescents. Reduction or fusion in situ. Spine 18:894–901
115. Poussa M, Remes V, Lamberg T et al (2006) Treatment of severe spondylolisthesis in adolecence with reduction or fusion in situ: long-term clinical, radiologic, and functional outcome. Spine 31:583–590
116. Rask MR (1979) Spondylolisthesis resulting from osteogenesis imperfecta. Clin Orthop 139:164–166
117. Remes VM, Lamberg TS, Tervahartiala PO et al (2005) No correlation between patient outcome and abnormal lumbar MRI findings 21 years after posterior or posterolateral fusion for isthmic spondylolisthesis in children and adolescents Eur Spine J 14:833–842
118. Remes V, Lamberg T, Tervahartiala P et al (2006) Long-term outcome after posterolateral, anterior, and circumferential fusion for high-grade isthmic spondylolisthesis in children and adolescents. Spine 31:2491–2499
119. Rosenberg NJ, Bargar WL, Friedman B (1981) The incidence of spondylolysis and spondylolisthesis in nonambulatory patients. Spine 6:35–38
120. Ruf M, Koch H, Melcher RP et al (2006) Anatomic reduction and monosegmental fusion in high-grade developmental spondylolisthesis. Spine 31:269–274
121. Ruiz-Cotorro A, Balius-Matas R, Estruch-Massana A et al (2006) Spondylolysis in young tennis players. Br J Sports Med 40:441–446
122. Sagi HC, Jarvis JG, Uthoff HK (1998) Histomorphic analysis of the development of the pars interarticularis and its association with isthmic spondylolysis. Spine 23:1635–1640
123. Sailhan F, Gollogly S, Roussouly P (2006) The radiographic results and neurologic complications of instrumented reduction and fusion of high-grade spondylolisthesis without decompression of the neural elements: a retrospective review of 44 patients. Spine 31:161–169
124. Sairyo K, Goel VK, Grobler LJ (1998) The pathomechanics of isthmic lumbar spondylolisthesis. A biomechanical study in immature calf spines. Spine 23:1442–1446
125. Sairyo K, Katoh S, Sakamaki T (2004) Vertebral forward slippage in immature lumbar spine occurs following epiphyseal separation and its occurence is unrelated to disc degeneration. Spine 29:524–527
126. Sairyo K, Goel VK, Masuda A et al (2006) Three dimensional finite element analysis of the pediatric lumbar spine. Part II: Biomechanical change as the initiating factor for

pediatric isthmic spondylolisthesis at the growth plate. Eur Spine J 15:930–935

127. Sakamaki T, Sairyo K, Katoh S et al (2003) The pathogenesis of slippage and deformity in the pediatric lumbar spine. Spine 28:645–651
128. Saraste H (1986) Symptoms in relation to the level of spondylolysis. Internat Orthop 10:183–185
129. Scaglietti O, Frontino G, Bartolozzi P (1976) Technique of anatomical reduction of lumbar spondylolisthesis and its surgical stabilization. Clin Orthop 117:164–175
130. Schlenzka D, Poussa M, Seitsalo S et al (1991) Intervertebral disc changes in adolescents with isthmic spondylolisthesis. J Spinal Disord 4:344–352
131. Schlenzka D, Seitsalo S, Poussa M et al (1993) Premature disc degeneration: source of pain in isthmic spondylolisthesis in adolescents? J Ped Orthop 1-B:153–157
132. Schlenzka D, Seitsalo S, Poussa M et al (1993) Operative treatment of symptomatic lumbar spondylolysis and mild isthmic spondylolisthesis in young patients: direct repair of the defect or segmental fusion? Eur Spine J 2:104–122
133. Schlenzka D, Remes V, Helenius I et al (2006) Direct repair for treatment of symptomatic spondylolysis or mild isthmic spondylolisthesis in young patients: no benefit in comparison to segmental fusion after a mean follow-up of 14.8 years. Eur Spine J 15:1437–1447
134. Schulitz KP, Niethard FU (1980) Strain on the interarticular stress distribution. Measurements regarding the development of spondylolysis. Arch Orthop Trauma Surg 96: 167–202
135. Seitsalo S, Österman K, Poussa M (1988) Scoliosis associated with lumbar spondylolisthesis. A clinical survey of 190 young patients. Spine 13:899–904
136. Seitsalo S, Österman K, Poussa M et al (1988) Spondylolisthesis in children under 12 years of age: long-term results of 56 patients treated conservatively or operatively. J Ped Orthop 8:516–521
137. Seitsalo S (1990) Operative and conservative treatment of moderate spondylolisthesis in young patients. J Bone Jt Surg 72-B:908–913
138. Seitsalo S, Österman K, Hyvärinen H et al (1990) Severe spondylolisthesis in children and adolescents. A long-term review of fusion in situ. J Bone Jt Surg 72-B:259–265
139. Seitsalo S, Österman K, Hyvärinen H et al (1991) Progression of spondylolisthesis in children and adolescents. A long-term follow-up in 272 patients. Spine 16:417–421
140. Seitsalo S, Schlenzka D, Poussa M (1992) Solid fusion vs. non-union in long-term follow-up of in situ fusion without internal fixation in symptomatic spondylolisthesis in young patients. Eur Spine J 1:163–166
141. Seitsalo S, Poussa M, Schlenzka D (1993) The occurrence of lumbar spondylolisthesis in relatives of patients with symptomatic spondylolisthesis. Finn J Orthop Traumatol 16:181–183
142. Seitsalo S, Antila H, Karrinaho T (1997) Spondylolysis in ballet dancers. J Dance Med Sci 1:51–54
143. Shelekov A, Haideri N, Roach J (1993) Residual gait abnormalities in surgically treated spondylolisthesis. Spine 18:2201–2205
144. Sherman FC, Rosenthal RK, Hall JE (1979) Spine fusion for spondylolysis and spondylolisthesis in children. Spine 4:59–67
145. Shuffleberger HL, Geck MJ (2005) High-grade isthmic dysplastic spondylolisthesis. Monosegmental surgical treatment. Spine 30:S42–S48
146. Smith JA, Deviren V, Berven S, et al (2001) Clinical outcome of trans-sacral interbody fusion after partial reduction for high-grade L5-S1 spondylolisthesis. Spine 26:2227–2234
147. Sponseller PD, Hobbs W, Riley LH et al (1995) The thoracolumbar spine in Marfan symdrome. J Bone Jt Surg Am 77:867–876
148. Stanitski CL, Stanitski DF, LaMont RL (1994) Spondylolisthesis in myelomeningocele. J Ped Orthop 14:586–591
149. Steiner ME, Micheli LJ (1985) Treatment of symptomatic spondylolysis and spondylolisthesis with a modified Boston brace. Spine 10:937–943
150. Steward TD (1953) The age incidence of neural arch defects in Alaska natives, considered from the standpoint of etiology. J Bone Jt Surg 35:937–950
151. Sys J, Michielsen J, Bracke P et al (2001) Nonoperative treatment of active spondylolysis in elite athletes with normal X-ray findings: literature review and results of conservative treatment. Eur Spine J 10:498–504
152. Taillard W (1954) Le spondylolisthesis chez l'enfant et l'adolescent. Etude de 50 cas. Acta Orthop Scand 24: 115–144
153. Taylor LJ (1987) Severe spondylolisthesis and scoliosis in Marfan's syndrome. Case report and review of the literature. Clin Orthop 221:207–211
154. Tiusanen H, Schlenzka D, Seitsalo S et al (1996) Results of anterior and combined lumbar fusion for treatment of severe isthmic spondylolisthesis in young patients. J Ped Orthop 5-B:190–194
155. Transfeld EE, Mehbod AA (2007) Evindence-based medicine analysis of ithmic spondylolisthesis treatment including reduction versus Fusion in situ for high-grade slips. Spine 32:S126–S129
156. van Ooij A, Weijers R, van Rhijn L (2003) Remodelling of the sacrum in high-grade spondylolisthesis: a report of two cases. Eur Spine J 12:332–338
157. Vialle R, Miladl L, Wicart P et al (2005) Le traitement chirurgical du spondylolisthésis lombo-sacré à grand déplacement de l'enfant et de l'adolescent. À propos d'une série continue de 20 patients au recul moyen de 5 ans. Rev Chir Orthop 91:5–14
158. Vialle R, Charosky S, Padovani J-P et al (2006) Surgical treatment of high-grade lumbosacral spondylolisthesis in childhood, adolescent and young adult by the "double-plate" technique: a past experience. Eur Spine J 15:1210–1218
159. Villiaumey J (1968) Spondylolisthésis lombaire chez des jumeaux. Rev du Rhum 35:130–133
160. Virta L (1991) Lumbar spondylolytic spondylolisthesis in adults. Turku University, Thesis
161. Ward CV, Latimer B (2005) Human evolution and the development of spondylolysis. Spine 30:1808–1840
162. Wertzberger KL, Peterson HA (1980) Acquired spondylolysis and spondylolisthesis in the young child. Spine 5:437–442
163. Whitesides TE, Horton WC, Hutton WC et al (2005) Spondylolytic spondylolisthesis. A study of pelvic and lumbosacral parameters of possible etiologic effect in two genetically and geographically distinct groups with high occurence. Spine 30:S12–S21

164. Wild A, Jäger M, Werner A et al (2001) Treatment of congenital spondyloptosis in an 18-month-old patient with a 10-year follow-up. Spine 26:E502–E505
165. Wiltse LL (1961) Spondylolisthesis in children. Clin Orthop 21:156–163
166. Wiltse LL, Widell EH, Jackson DW (1975) Fatigue fracture: the basic lesion in isthmic spondylolisthesis. J Bone Jt Surg Am 57:17–22
167. Wiltse LL, Jackson DW (1976) Treatment of spondylolisthesis and spondylolysis in children. Clin Orthop 117:92–100
168. Wiltse LL, Newman PH, Macnab I (1976) Classification of spondylolysis and spondylolisthesis. Clin Orthop 117:23–29
169. Wiltse LL (1977) Spondylolisthesis and its treatment. In: Ruge D, Wiltse LL, (eds). Spinal disorders. Lea and Febiger, Philadelphia
170. Wiltse LL, Spencer CW (1988) New uses and refinements of the paraspinal approach to the lumbar spine. Spine 13: 696–706
171. Wiltse LL, Rothman LG (1989) Spondylolisthesis: classification, diagnosis, and natural history. Semin Spine Surg 1: 78–94
172. Winter RB (1982) Severe spondylolisthesis in Marfan's syndrome: report of two cases. J Ped Orthop 2:51–55
173. Wynne-Davies R, Scott JHS (1979) Inheritance and spondylolisthesis. A radiographic family survey. J Bone Jt Surg 61-B:301–305
174. Zippel H, Abesser EW (1965) Zur Wirbelbogendysplasie und Spondylolisthesis im ersten Lebensdezennium. Arch Orthop Trauma Surg 58:242–259
175. Zippel H, Runge H (1976) Pathologische Anatomie und Pathogenese von Spondylolyse und Spondylolisthesis im Kindesalter. Z Orthop 114:189–191
176. Zippel H (1980) Wirbelgleiten im Lendenbereich. J.A.Barth Leipzig

Section IV

Management of Spinal Deformity in the Growing Child: Non-Surgical

Casting for Early Onset Scoliosis

26

James O. Sanders

Key Points

- Progressive infantile scoliosis is potentially fatal.
- Proper derotational casting does not appear to be associated with increasing rib or chest wall deformity.
- Serial derotational casting in younger, particularly nonsyndromic, children can result in a cure.
- Casting has an important role in older children in delaying the need for surgical intervention.

Infantile idiopathic scoliosis comes in two basic varieties, benign or resolving and progressive, which is potentially fatal. Mehta [5] was able to distinguish resolving from progressive scoliosis by using the rib vertebral angle difference (RVAD) on an early supine radiograph. The RVAD nearly follows the 80/20 rule – 80% of curves with an RVAD of 20 or more continue to progress while only 20% of those with lesser angles progress. She identified cases with rib phase with stage II, where the rib head of the convex apex overlaps the vertebra body, as always progressive. Her findings have been confirmed by others [2, 4, 8].

Early onset scoliosis is one of the few potentially fatal spinal anomalies if untreated. Unfortunately, treatment can also result in poor thoracic growth and thoracic insufficiency syndrome (TIS) as described by Campbell et al. [1]. Current treatments, primarily the VEPTR and growing rods [7], aim at delaying definitive fusion and almost never focus on a cure. Definitive fusion before the age 10 years is fraught with problems. Each of these methods has difficulties. Growing rods often fracture, pull loose, develop infections, and create a variant of the crankshaft phenomena with growth. The VEPTR has similar complications to growing rods with the additional problem of creating stiff, noncompliant chest walls.

Casting represents another alternative for scoliosis, which was quite common until the development of effective spinal instrumentation. Casting itself can create pressure sores, significant rib or mandibular deformities, and constrict the chest. "Cast syndrome" even denotes the historical term for superior mesenteric artery syndrome. However, many of these problems seem to be the result of indiscriminate casting of all types of scoliosis using improper techniques combined with a limited understanding of spinal and particularly of chest wall deformities. Scoliosis casting comes in several varieties. The most commonly used method in the United States is Risser casting [1], which uses a three-point bend for correction. Although it is possible to obtain significant curve correction with this technique, it does not sufficiently account for rotational abnormality, and, especially in younger children with flexible bones, can cause significant rib deformities and chest constriction. More recently, Mehta [6] described her results of casting in 136 patients with infantile scoliosis using the technique of Cotrel and Morel [3] with the philosophy that early rapid growth, if guided by the cast, would assist an initially curved spine to straighten. We have used serial casting in a select group of patients with success in curing the curve in younger patients with less severe curves and in delaying surgery in older children.

J.O. Sanders
Department of Orthopaedics and Rehabilitation,
University of Rochester, 601 Elmwood Avenue, Rochester,
NY 14642, USA
e-mail: James_Sanders@urmc.rochester.edu

B. A. Akbarnia et al. (eds.), *The Growing Spine*,
DOI: 10.1007/978-3-540-85207-0_26, © Springer-Verlag Berlin Heidelberg 2011

26.1 Influence of Age and Etiology

The age at treatment onset and etiology are crucial and significant factors in treatment success. Mehta found that casting would be much more likely to be successful if started below the age 2 years. Our results are nearly identical with the patients achieving nearly full correction starting at average age of 1.1 years and full correction rare in those started above the age of 18 months. Casting to resolution typically takes a year or more. Mehta identified four physiological patterns: a "sturdy phenotype" with good muscle mass and tone, a "slender phenotype" with more delicate features, ligamentous laxity, and more rapidly progressive curves, those with known syndromes, and those with unknown syndromes. In her series, all groups responded if treatment was initiated early with smaller curves. In older patients with larger curves, the prognosis worsened from the sturdy to the slender to named and unnamed syndromes. We have not found her classification of slender and sturdy reproducible in our hands and have divided the patients into the simple categories of idiopathic or syndromic. Older and syndromic patients usually have less correction. Our goal in these older and syndromic patients is to delay the need for surgery until the spine has achieved sufficient growth for good pulmonary function as an adult. This endpoint is not well defined, but the hope is to delay fusion until the adolescent growth spurt. Both the VEPTR and growing rods are alternatives in this group of patients, though we believe proper casting creates less spine or chest wall stiffness while still allowing spinal growth, though we lack comparison studies. Casting assumes and important role in delaying surgery for those patients with responding but not resolving curves.

26.2 Technique of Casting

Once the diagnosis of progressive scoliosis is made, based on either a progressive Cobb angle or a RVAD of more than 20° at presentation, casting is recommended. We have typically required an MRI of the spine before casting, but some centers initiate casting before the MRI. Mehta's program consists of cast changes under anesthesia in younger patients every 8–16 weeks until the curve was nearly resolved followed by an underarm brace, which may be weaned if the patient's curve correction continues. We base our cast changes on the child's growth rate with changes in every 2 months for those aged 2 years and below, 3 months for those aged 3 years, and 4 months for those aged 4 years and above. We aim for curves less than 10° supine out of the cast and then use a brace molded under anesthesia just like the cast. Children are occasionally braced during the summer months with resumption of casting in the fall.

A proper casting table is crucial. We have used both a Risser and a Cotrel frame, but found them quite large for small children. Mehta has designed a table marketed by AMIL, which leaves the head, arms, and legs supported but the body free. The Salt Lake City Shriners Hospital uses a custom table that performs a similar function of supporting the child in traction while leaving the body free for the cast application. Patients are intubated since thoracic pressure during the cast molding can make ventilation temporarily difficult. Older children might be successfully managed without anesthesia, but it is impractical in very young children. A silver impregnated shirt is used as the innermost layer. Head halter and pelvic traction assists in stabilizing the patient and in narrowing the body (Fig. 26.1). Even though traction can correct the curve while applied, the position cannot be retained in the cast once traction is released, and the body recoils unless the cast also supports the occiput or the mandible. For curves with an apex above T8, the shoulders are incorporated, and high thoracic curves may require a mandibular extension. A mirror slanted under the table is useful for visualizing the rib prominence, the posterior cast, and the molds. A thin layer of webril is applied with occasional felt on significant bony

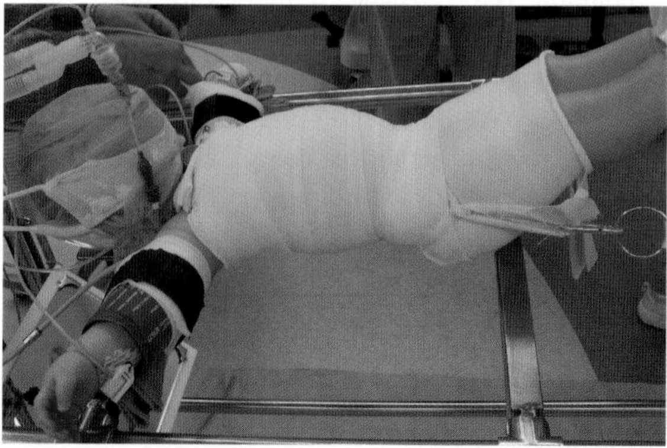

Fig. 26.1 Patient positioning on a casting frame with head halter and pelvic traction. The body is free while the patient remains well supported

prominences. Mehta uses crape paper that is removed after the casting leaving plaster on the skin except at pressure points protected by felt. If there is a lumbar curve, the hips are slightly flexed to decrease lumbar lordosis and facilitate curve correction.

Plaster, or, in smaller curves, typically less than 20°, fiberglass, is applied. The pelvis portion, as the foundation, is well molded. It is important that the cast not push the ribs toward the spine and consequently narrow the space available for the lung. Rather, the posteriorly rotated ribs are rotated anteriorly to create a more normal chest configuration with counter rotation is applied through the pelvic mold and upper torso (Fig. 26.2). While the Cotrel/Morel technique and Mehta's modifications use an over-the-shoulder cast, we have had excellent success staying below the shoulders since most infantile curves have low apices, typically at T10–11 with nearly identical results to Mehta's. An anterior window is made to relieve the chest and abdomen while preventing the lower ribs from rotating (Fig. 26.3). A posterior window is made on the concave side allowing the depressed concave ribs and spine to move posteriorly (Fig. 26.4). A proper cast corrects the curve and the rotation without deforming the ribs toward the spine (Fig. 26.5).

Initiation of casting at a younger age, moderate curve size (<60°), and an idiopathic diagnosis carry a better prognosis than an older age of initiation, curve >60°, and a nonidiopathic diagnosis. We have had no worsening of the space available for the lung (SAL) and no worsening rib deformities.

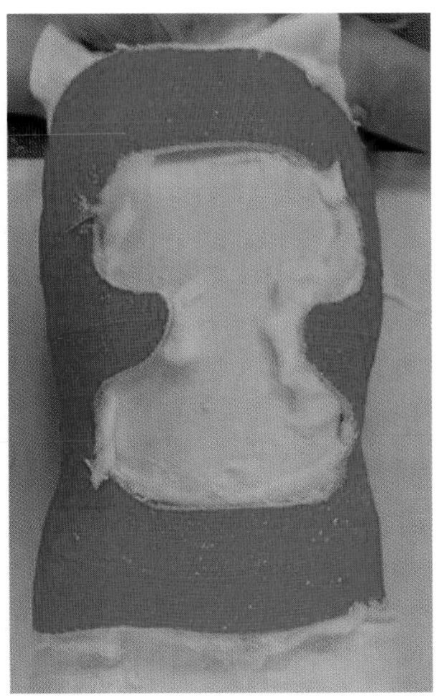

Fig. 26.3 Anterior window made to relieve chest and abdomen while keeping the inferior anterior ribs controlled

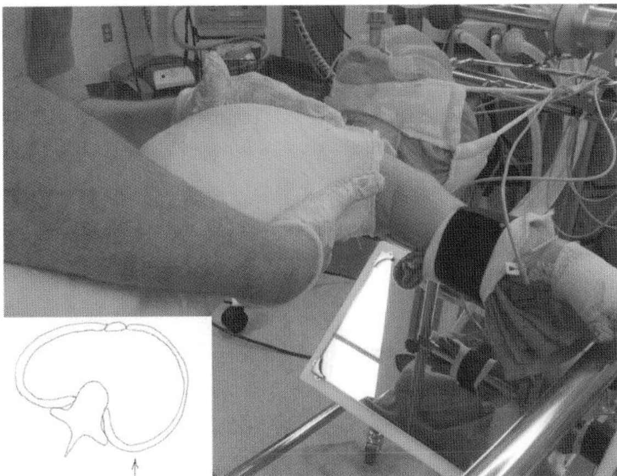

Fig. 26.2 Proper technique of molding with rotational correction applied from posteriorly rather than laterally. Counter rotation is applied through the pelvis and shoulders

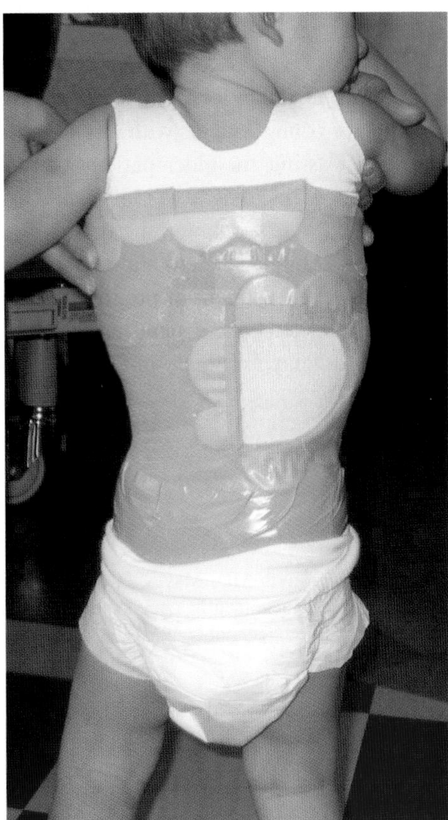

Fig. 26.4 Posterior window on the concavity coming to the midline, allowing the ribs to rotate posteriorly and the patient to escape the pressure on the convexity

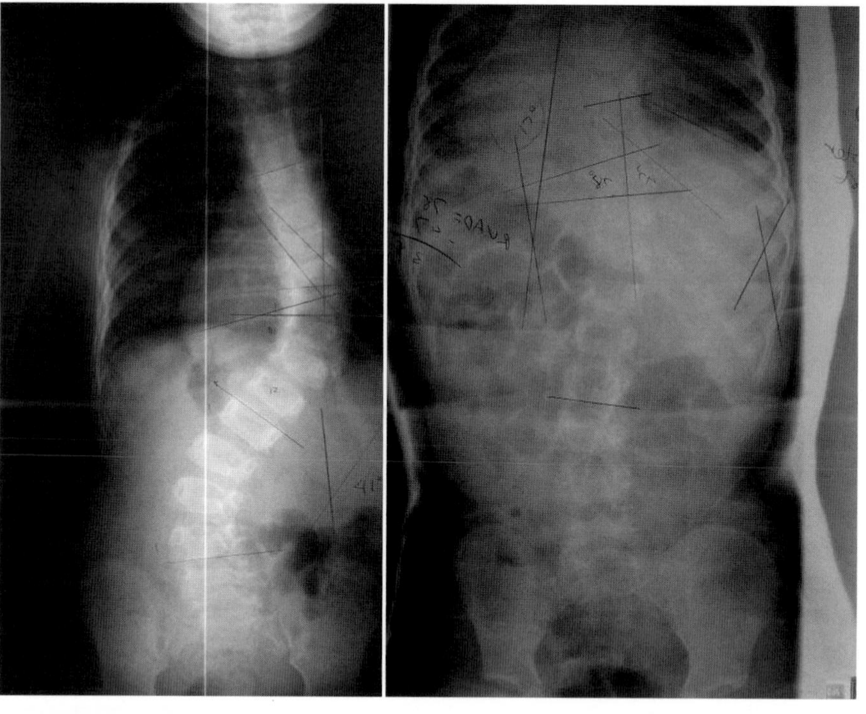

Fig. 26.5 Radiographs in the cast demonstrating derotation and lack of deformation of the convex ribs toward the spine

Serial casting for infantile scoliosis often results in full correction in young patients with idiopathic curves less than 60°. Casting for older patients with larger curves or nonidiopathic diagnosis still results in curve improvement and a long delay in the time before surgery. The Cotrel technique of derotation casting appears to play a role in the treatment of progressive infantile scoliosis with cures in young patients and reductions in curve size with a delay in surgery in older and syndromic patients.

References

1. Campbell RM Jr., Smith MD, Mayes TC et al (2003) The characteristics of thoracic insufficiency syndrome associated with fused ribs and congenital scoliosis. J Bone Joint Surg Am 85-A:399–408
2. Ceballos T, Ferrer-Torrelles M, Castillo F et al (1980) Prognosis in infantile idiopathic scoliosis. J Bone Joint Surg Am 62:863–875
3. Cotrel Y, Morel G (1964) The elongation-derotation-flexion technic in the correction of scoliosis. Rev Chir Orthop Reparatrice Appar Mot 50:59–75
4. Ferreira JH, Janeiro Rd, James JI (1972) Progressive and resolving infantile idiopathic scoliosis. The differential diagnosis. J Bone Joint Surg Br 54:648–655
5. Mehta MH (1972) The rib-vertebral angle in the early diagnosis between resolving and progressive infantile idiopathic scoliosis. J Bone Joint Surg Br Vol 54:230–242
6. Mehta MH (2005) Growth as a corrective force in the early treatment of progressive infantile scoliosis. J Bone Joint Surg Br 87:1237–1247
7. Thompson GH, Akbarnia BA, Campbell RM Jr (2007) Growing rod techniques in early-onset scoliosis. J Pediatr Orthop 27:354–361
8. Thompson SK, Bentley G (1980) Prognosis in infantile idiopathic scoliosis. J Bone Joint Surg Br 62-B:151–154

27 Orthotic Management for Infantile and Juvenile Scoliosis

John B. Emans

Key Points

- Orthotic treatment is a useful adjunct to cast treatment of infantile idiopathic scoliosis.
- Orthotic treatment is most successful in juvenile idiopathic scoliosis, particularly in single curves in the middle of the spine.
- Successful brace treatment of early onset scoliosis requires an effective brace, a committed multidisciplinary team, and an involved family.
- Bracing can cause irrevocable harm to the growing thorax if pressure is inappropriately applied or continued too long in spite of worsening thoracic deformity.

27.1 Introduction

This chapter attempts to discuss the contemporary role of orthotic treatment of idiopathic early onset spinal deformity. Orthotic treatment has limited efficacy in congenital scoliosis, and orthotic treatment of paralytic deformities, although useful, varies greatly by etiologic diagnosis, type of deformity, and goals of treatment. These latter uses of bracing are beyond the scope of this discussion.

Bracing has always occupied a prominent position in the treatment of early-onset idiopathic spinal deformity. Over the last 2 decades, orthotic treatment has come to be questioned as an effective treatment for adolescent idiopathic scoliosis for the lack of prospective, randomized evidence supporting the efficacy of orthotic treatment [9, 10, 15, 16], in spite of a preponderance of nonrandomized series suggesting efficacy [48]. Incontrovertible evidence for the efficacy of bracing in infantile and juvenile idiopathic scoliosis is similarly lacking. Retrospective series, experience, and expert opinion strongly suggest that bracing can be effective in juvenile, and to a lesser extent, in infantile idiopathic scoliosis. Brace treatment of juvenile idiopathic scoliosis is approached with enthusiasm in continental Europe, yet greeted with skepticism in much of the United States. This author approaches the subject with the impression that nonoperative treatments (casting or bracing) are the preferable treatment and can be effective in moderate idiopathic early onset deformity (Figs. 27.1 and 27.2).

Success or failure in bracing depends partly upon the goals chosen for treatment. Establishing realistic, specific, and transparent goals early in orthotic treatment of early onset deformity facilitates rational expectations by the practitioner and family. Is the goal complete correction, prevention of worsened deformity, or slowing of progressive deformity, acknowledging that surgery will eventually be needed? Complete, lasting correction with repetitive casting is a reasonable goal in early, selected infantile idiopathic scoliosis as demonstrated by Mehta [37], and is anecdotally occasionally also achieved in moderate juvenile idiopathic scoliosis treated by bracing alone (see Fig. 27.2). Complete correction is rarely achieved in progressive infantile idiopathic scoliosis by orthotic treatment alone and repetitive casting may be a better choice. Complete correction as a goal can help motivate families and patients assuming there is some

J.B. Emans
Department of Orthopaedic Surgery, Children's Hospital, Boston, MA 02115, USA
e-mail: John.Emans@childrens.harvard.edu

B. A. Akbarnia et al. (eds.), *The Growing Spine*,
DOI: 10.1007/978-3-540-85207-0_27, © Springer-Verlag Berlin Heidelberg 2011

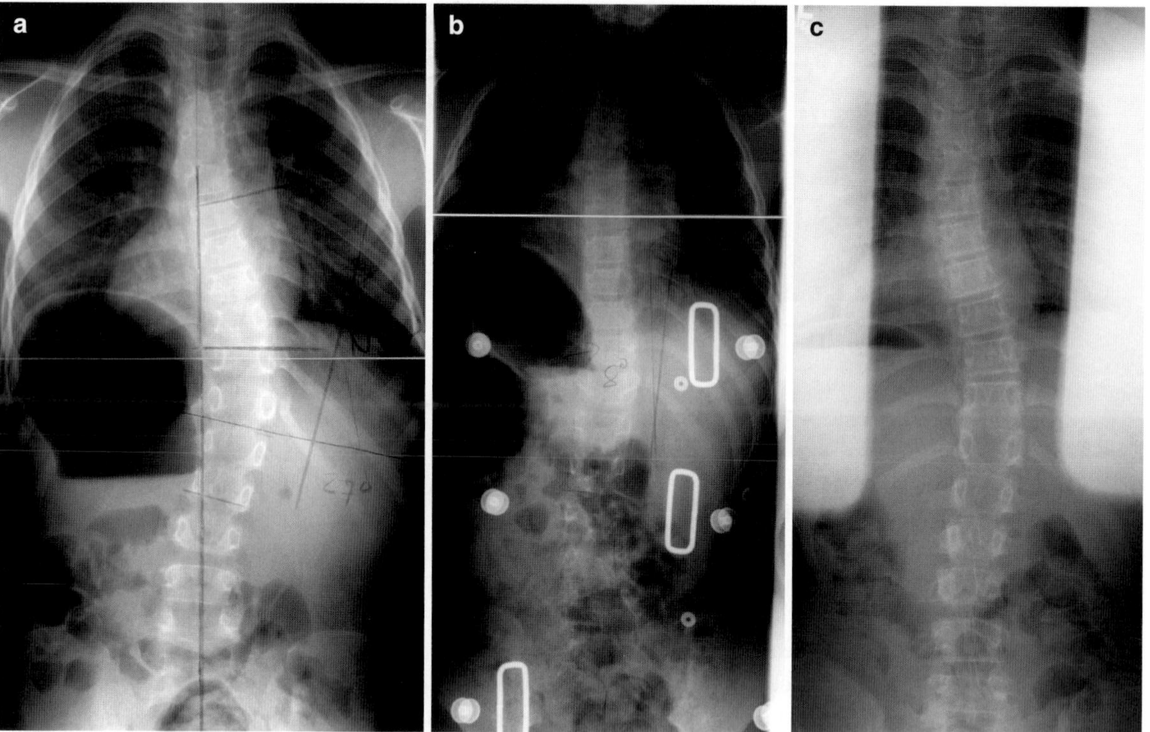

Fig. 27.1 Juvenile idiopathic scoliosis. Scoliosis was noted at the age of 6 years and progressed to 30° by the age of 7 years (**a**). Full-time brace treatment began at the age of 7 years (**b**) and continued through the age of 13 years, then parttime at the request of the patient. At follow-up at the age of 18 years after 1 year out of brace, there is a stable 25° curve (**c**)

chance of achieving that goal. In more severe early-onset scoliosis where complete correction is unlikely, orthotic treatment is sometimes viewed as a temporizing measure, stabilizing deformity for years, allowing for more growth before initiating surgical treatment, and allowing the child to remain free of the need for repetitive surgical intervention with growing rods (Fig. 27.3). Orthotic treatment to allow for more growth with eventual surgery anticipated can be successful in achieving the dual goals of a longer spine and fewer operations, but also may lead to inappropriate delay and worsened, irrevocable, thoracic deformity (Figs. 27.4 and 27.5). The availability of modern growth-oriented surgical treatments for spinal deformity such as expandable spinal rods or VEPTR should lower the threshold for discontinuance of bracing and initiation of surgery to a point *before* spine or chest deformity become too severe.

Effective brace treatment of early onset scoliosis demands appropriate indications, practical expectations, an effective brace, and committed care-givers. Creating an effective scoliosis orthosis requires some level of skill and experience, and although well-documented bracing systems of many types are available, it is difficult to be successful in early onset scoliosis without experience at some level. Not all techniques applicable to adolescents are transferable to early onset scoliosis. Fortunately, the appropriateness of the specific orthosis and its potential effectiveness is easily assessed by radiographs taken in the brace. Commitment to bracing at the level of the physician (and the rest of the medical team), orthotist, and family is critical for success. Absence of dedication by any of the team will subvert the efforts of the others. Patient compliance with requested brace usage is a major barrier to success in adolescents but much less problematic in younger children with early-onset deformity if families are committed to brace wear. Often, the most likely member of the team to lack commitment is the physician, who may imply "try this brace for a while, it probably won't work; come back and see me when you need an operation".

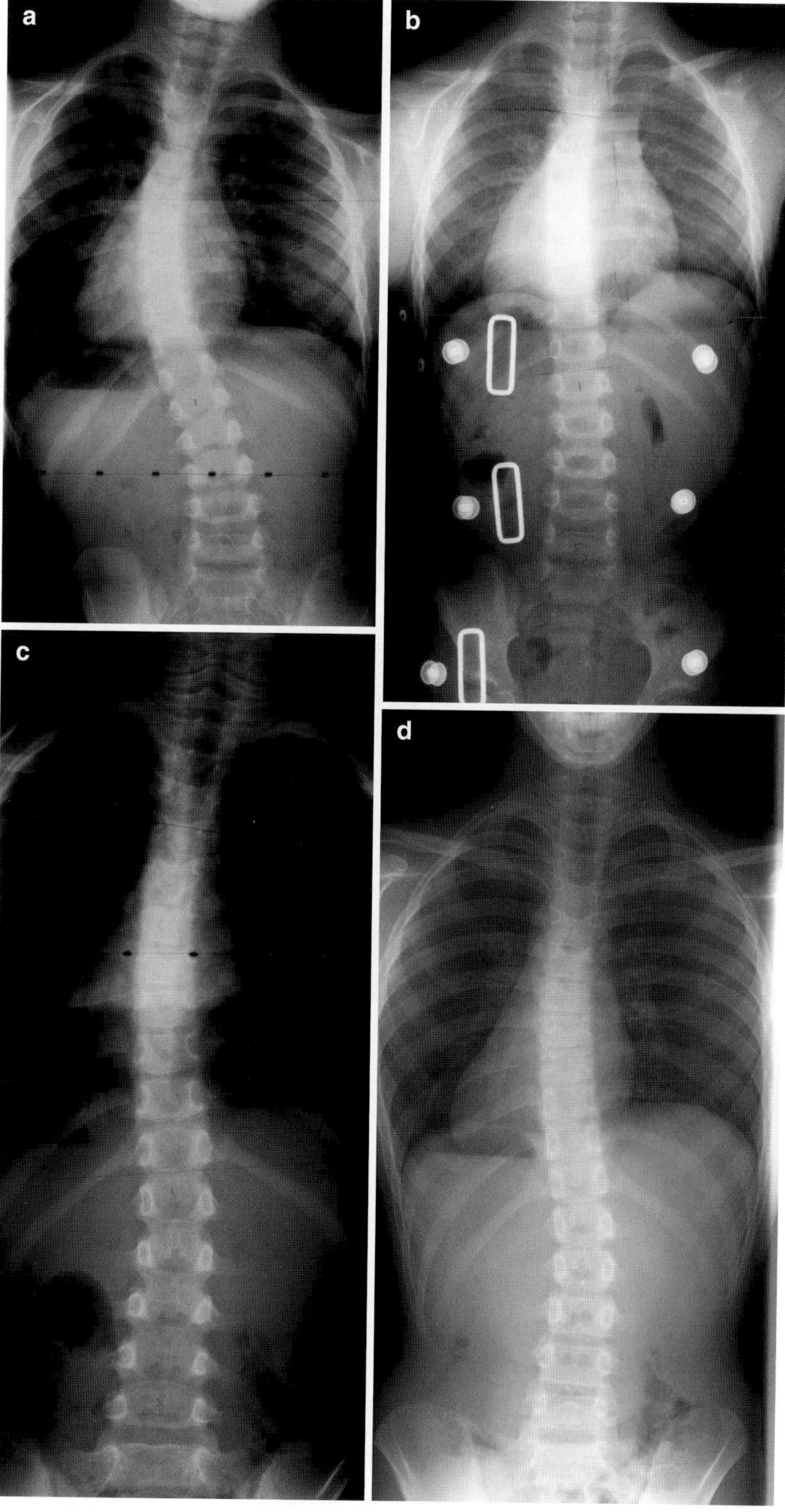

Fig. 27.2 Juvenile idiopathic scoliosis. Scoliosis noted at the age of 3 ½ years (**a**) and full-time bracing initiated with good in-brace correction (**b**). At the age of 6 years, correction was maintained (**c**). Part-time bracing and correction were maintained through adolescence (**d**)

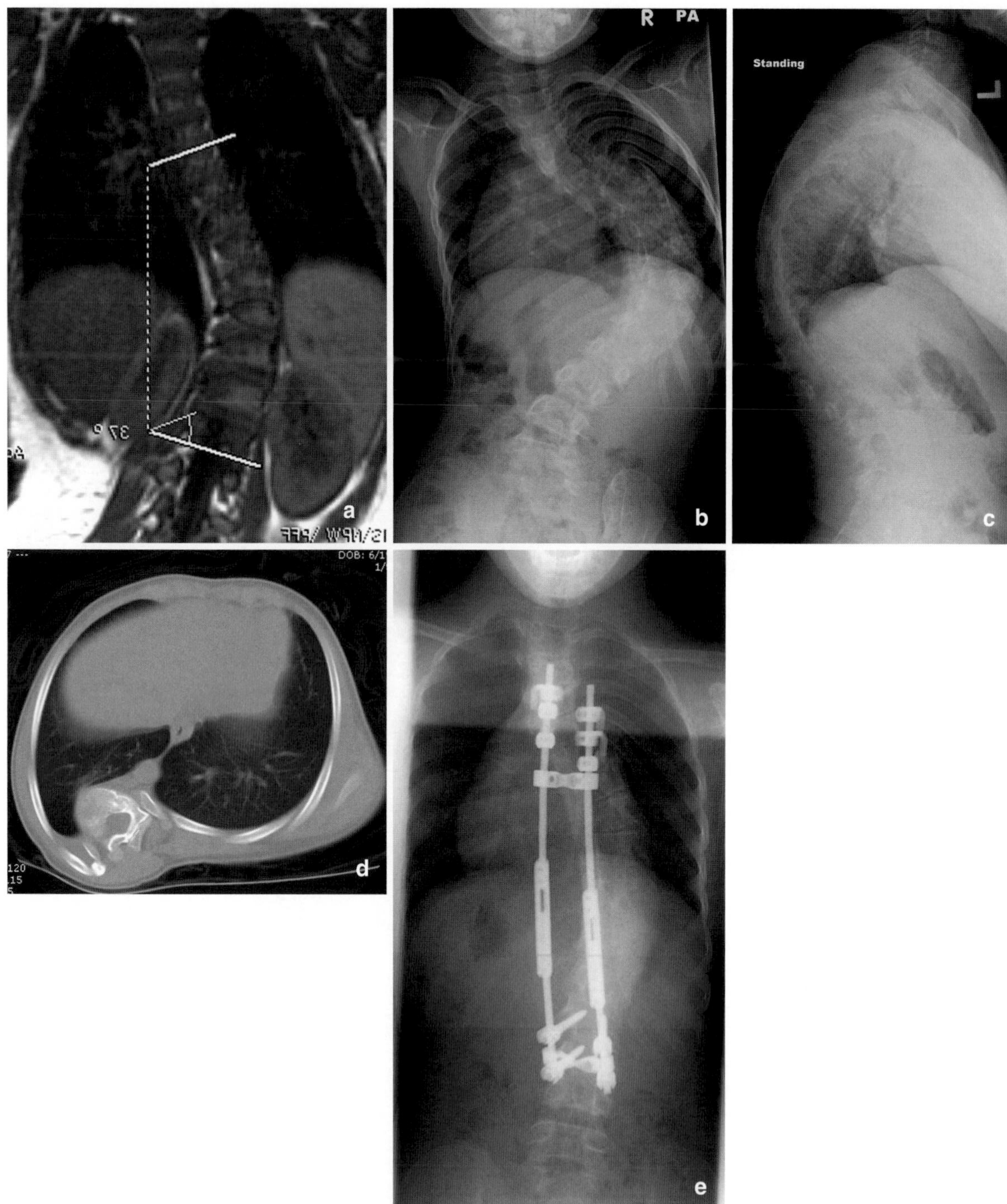

Fig. 27.3 Infantile idiopathic scoliosis. Treatment began at 18 months with full-time brace treatment (**a**). Referred for growing rods at the age of 7 years when rib prominence and thoracic deformity had worsened (**b–d**). Spine and thoracic deformity have been fairly well-controlled by dual growing rods from the age of 7 to 11 years (**e**). Growing rods had been suggested at the age of 2 years, but declined by the family. Earlier surgical intervention would have resulted in an easier initial surgical procedure, but the child was spared 5 years of surgical interventions and 10 surgical lengthening procedures by brace treatment from the age of 18 months until 7 years

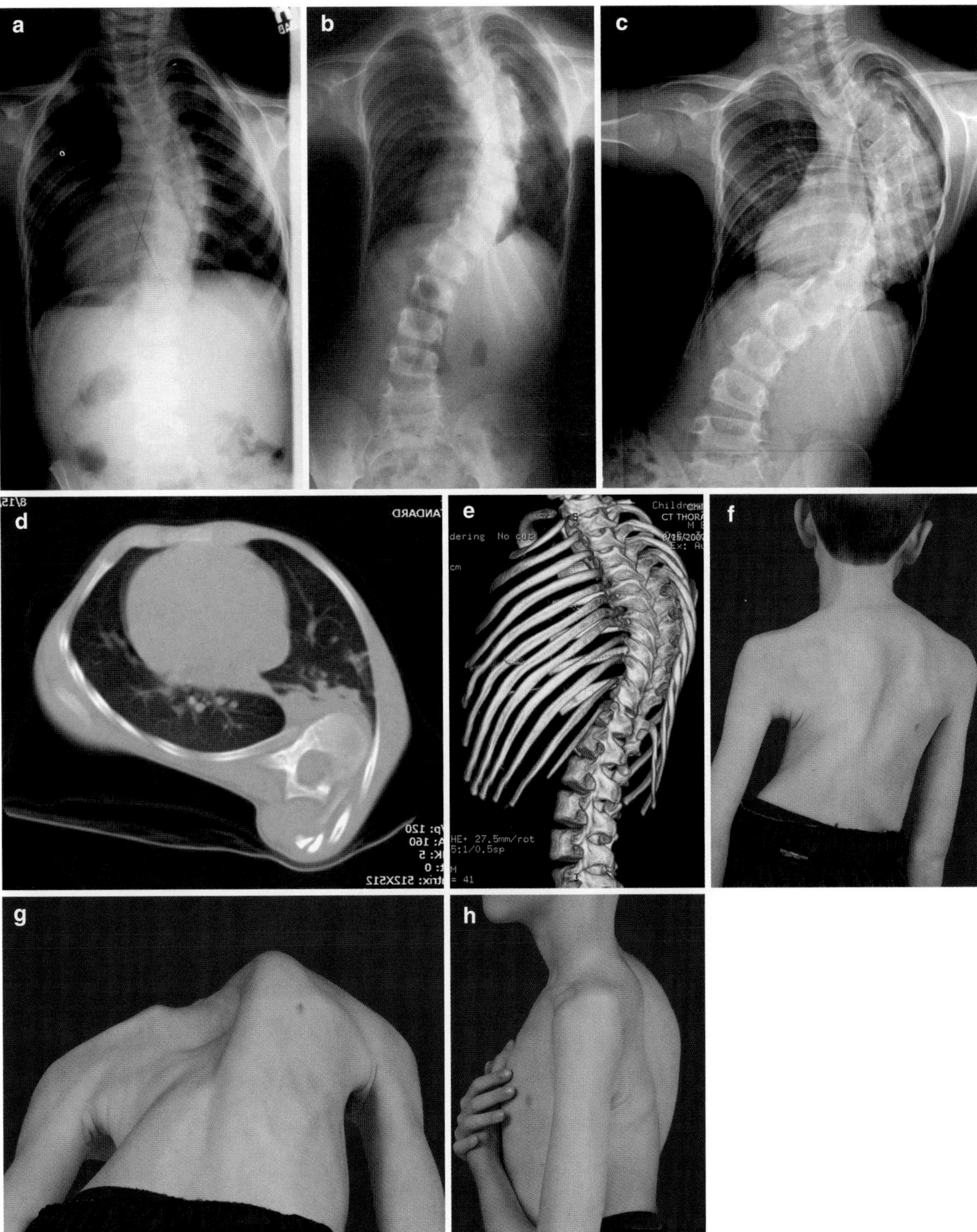

Fig. 27.4 Infantile idiopathic scoliosis treated with repetitive casting and bracing beginning at the age of 2 years. Initial thoracic deformity at the age of 3 years (**a**) was modest, worse at the age of 5 years (**b**), and severe at the age of 8 years (**c**), with pulmonary function tests approximately 50% of predicted and early restrictive lung disease. The convex thorax is collapsed, with the ribs assuming a vertical orientation or "collapsing parasol deformity" as described by Campbell. Thoracic deformity is demonstrated on CT (**d, e**). An area of the posterior convex thorax normally occupied by lung is occluded. Thoracic deformity is clinically apparent (**f–h**). Spinal deformity can be controlled surgically at this stage, but the chest deformity will not be completely improved by surgical means. Earlier intervention with a growth-oriented technique such as dual growing rods or VEPTR might have controlled both spine and chest deformity and led to a better result

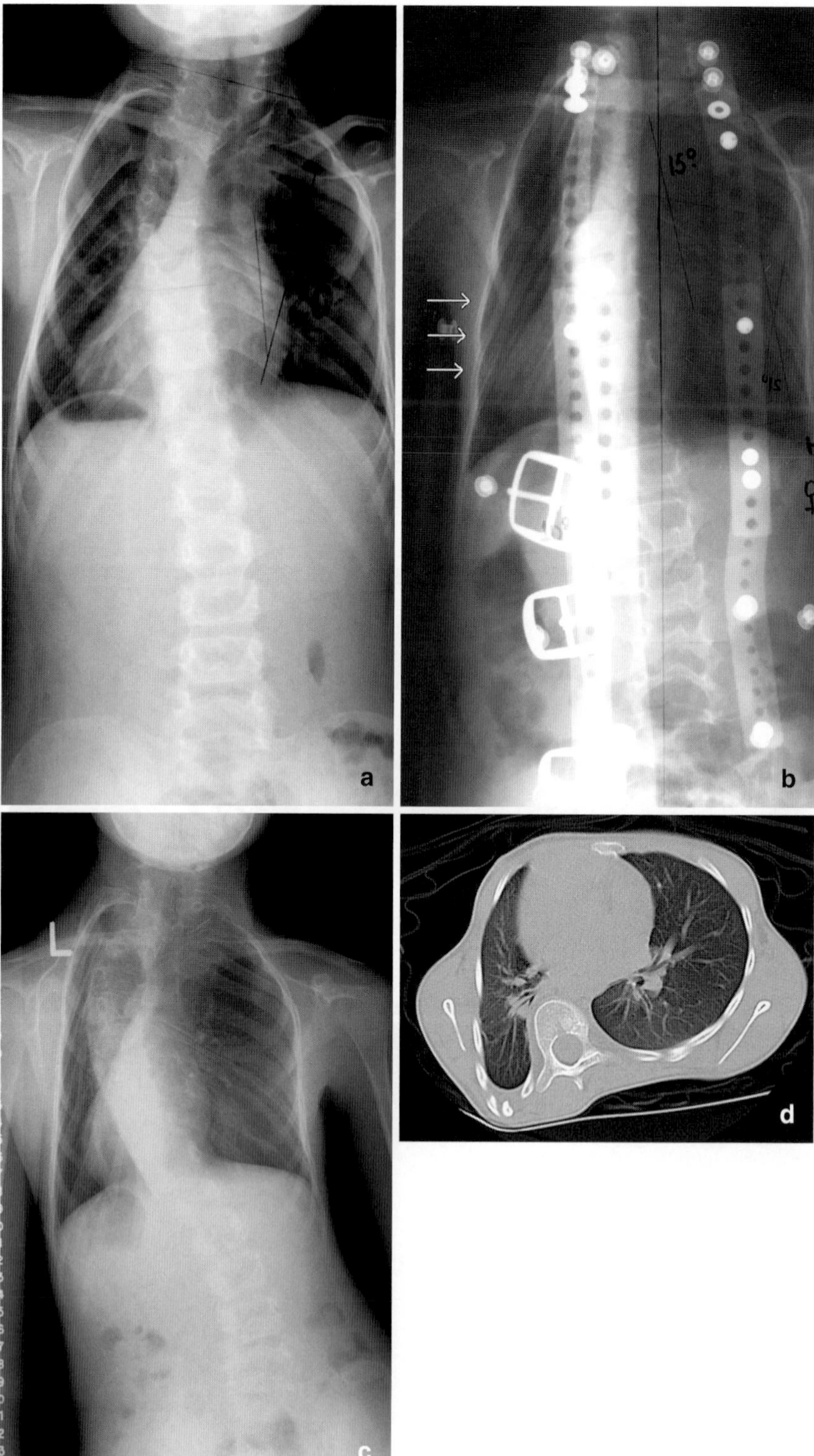

Fig. 27.5 Congenital scoliosis in the upper thoracic spine was treated with circumferential in situ fusion at the age of 2 years (**a**). The normally segmented curve below was then treated with a full-time Milwaukee brace with a pad pressure applied directly laterally over the convex chest wall (**b**). At the age of 9 years, the child was referred for surgical treatment because of curve progression (**c**) while still using the brace. Chest deformity with a severe collapse of the convex chest wall (**d**), however, has been evolving for years and is now irrevocable. Earlier growing rods would have been a better choice than persistent brace management

27.2 Evidence for Efficacy of Bracing in Early Onset Idiopathic Scoliosis

Mehta's [37] experience with casting for infantile idiopathic scoliosis is now well documented and shows remarkable, lasting correction of many patients in whom treatment was begun early and even some long-term improvement in many in whom referral was late. This experience clearly shows that the deformed growing spine can be guided through growth not just with stabilization of deformity but with actual long-term improvement in deformity, and that complete correction may be possible if the early infantile growth rate is harnessed to curve correction. The obvious advantage of casting includes full time use without the need for adherence to bracing regimens. Mehta's [37] series included patients up to 48 months in age and her experience is relevant to bracing of early onset curves as it shows convincingly that with growth and appropriate application of external pressure, the deformed growing spine can be changed for the better. Mehta [36] has also advocated the use of serial plaster casts in juvenile scoliosis, but this is less well documented. Experience with brace treatment alone for infantile idiopathic scoliosis is sparsely reported [8, 21–23, 29, 36]. McMaster and Macnicole [35] documented Milwaukee brace treatment in 27 children with infantile idiopathic scoliosis, of whom only five did not require surgery during adolescence.

Experience reported with brace treatment of juvenile idiopathic scoliosis is encouraging. With notable exceptions [13, 24, 30, 33, 34, 36, 46], this experience is blended into reports on success or failure with adolescent idiopathic scoliosis. Robinson and McMaster [46], in analyzing curve patterns in juvenile idiopathic scoliosis, reported 88 of 109 patients who were treated with a brace. Arthrodesis was needed in 67 of 84 thoracic curves, but in only 3 of 20 thoracolumbar or lumbar curves. Curve correction in brace was best below the age of 6 years and early in bracing. Noonan et al. [40] discouraging report of bracing in idiopathic scoliosis included patients as young as the age of 8 years, but juvenile patients are not distinguished from the rest, although the authors noted a higher failure rate in patients under the age of 12 years. Our experience with the Boston Brace system in 295 patients [12] included 34 juveniles in the age of 10 years or less. When compared with adolescents in the study, patients less than 10 years old at initiation of bracing had a higher rate of surgery, but also a higher mean correction at the end of bracing in those who did not need surgery. There were very few juveniles whose curves remained the same by the end of growth, probably reflective of the large amount of growth and opportunity for change in either direction during treatment. We felt that bracing as a whole for this group was successful. Mean curve correction at the end of bracing was 25% for juveniles. Of all patients between the age of 4 and 10 years at initiation of brace treatment, only 5 of 34 went on to surgery. Of those less than the age of 10 years starting bracing with curves between 30 and 49°, only 2 of 11 went on to surgery. Tolo and Gillespie [53] reported on 44 patients braced for juvenile scoliosis, among whom, 16 went on to surgery and felt that part-time brace use might be effective. Jarvis et al. [24] reported on 23 patients and also felt part-time bracing was effective. Kahanovitz et al. [25] reported on treatment of 15 juveniles with part-time bracing and noted success for patients who had curvatures less than 35° at the onset of part-time bracing and whose rib vertebrate angle difference remained less than 20°. All these studies suffer from being retrospective selective reviews without either cohort controls or prospective controls. With the exception of Noonan, however, all observed encouraging outcomes for juveniles treated with braces. The Scoliosis Research Society prospective study of bracing in idiopathic scoliosis by Nachemson et al. [39] demonstrated efficacy in bracing for adolescent idiopathic scoliosis, but does not include patients below the age of 10 years.

Long-term studies of outcome after bracing for adolescent idiopathic scoliosis [1, 7] indicate a favorable long-term result with regards to pain and function. All show a cohort of patients functioning well with no report of major psychological impairment and no impairment of bone density when bracing begins in adolescence. The less optimistic functional outcome for early onset scoliosis as a group is well documented by Goldberg et al. [17, 18], and Pehrsson et al. [42]. Masso et al. [34] reported no difference in child health questionnaire results in braced patients with juvenile idiopathic scoliosis when compared with those only observed. No other reports of long-term functional outcome after bracing in early onset deformity are found. We may probably safely conclude that juveniles with moderate curves at the end of growth have long-term outcomes similar to their adolescent counterparts, while those with more severe curves requiring early surgery are more likely to demonstrate respiratory insufficiency and functional deficits associated with a short, fused spine.

27.3 Decision-Making in Orthotic Treatment of Early Onset Idiopathic Scoliosis

Goal-oriented thinking is helpful in assessing patients with early onset spinal deformity. Broadly-stated goals for early onset deformity patients include achieving maximum spine growth and length, maximum spine flexibility, optimal respiratory function and lung growth, and a minimum of hospitalizations and procedures. Some goals are frequently at odds with others, but utilizing these goals to assess patient status will often help make the choice between observation, bracing, and surgery more rational. Families should understand these goals, and the care of early onset deformity, as a logical progression toward a final, functionally acceptable spine at the end of growth and treatment.

Indications for bracing are different in infantile and juvenile idiopathic scoliosis. In infantile scoliosis, casting should be considered as the preferred treatment and the decision to observe or treat based on the criteria advocated by Mehta. The first 2 years of growth can be viewed as an opportunity to maximally correct the spine deformity. Indications for bracing in infantile idiopathic scoliosis are probably restricted to bracing after serial cast treatment or infants who do not tolerate casting, or those with gastro-esophageal reflux, severe eczema, severe sleep apnea, or where casting is simply not available. Full-time brace treatment of progressive or persistent infantile scoliosis may then be appropriate. If bracing is undertaken in infancy, great care should be taken to not apply pressure over the thorax, except as a part of a derotation maneuver and to allow adequate room for expansion of the thorax (Fig. 27.6b, c). Braces should follow the same principles outlined by Mehta for casting. An improperly designed brace applied full time can quickly create a new thoracic deformity in the infant in excess of or equivalent to that created by an improperly applied cast.

Indications for orthotic treatment of juvenile idiopathic scoliosis are suggested by published results of brace treatment, likelihood of curve progression, and biomechanical curve simulations. This center has utilized a Cobb angle in excess of 20° as a lower threshold for orthotic treatment in juvenile idiopathic curves. We agree with Winter [56] and urge that curves over 20° should be considered for brace treatment in all juveniles, assuming that the curve has been persistent or progressive and is in a region of the spine accessible to bracing. Biomechanical models [19, 50, 51] of scoliosis suggest that at approximately 25° of curvature, the load required to deform the spine diminishes significantly and that conversely, if the curve can be diminished to well under 25°, then vertebrae may be loaded much more symmetrically. Stokes et al. demonstrated asymmetric growth of rat tail vertebrae in response to asymmetric loading [52]. The rationale for early bracing of moderate curves (those in excess of 20° in juveniles) is the assumption that by placing the growing spine under straighter mechanical load, there is some chance for spine remodeling toward symmetry, and progression is less likely during the preadolescent period of rapid growth. Sanders et al. [49] and many others have shown the early adolescent growth phase to be the period of greatest risk for progression of scoliosis, while Lonstein and Carlson [31] and Charles et al. [6] quantified the relationship between growth phase, curve magnitude, and the risk of progression. The goal of early bracing of moderate juvenile idiopathic scoliosis should be to enter the rapid preadolescent growth phase, when risk of progression is highest, with as little deformity as possible.

Early onset scoliosis associated with syringomyelia, Chiari malformation, or a tethered spinal cord should also be considered for brace treatment. Although surgical treatment of the Chiari malformation, syringomyelia, or tethered cord often results in improvement in the associated spinal deformity, the spinal deformity may continue to worsen if there is established deformity or persistent neuraxis abnormality [14]. Surgeons and families may falsely assume that by alleviating the presumed etiologic cause of the deformity, the deformity itself will probably resolve spontaneously as it frequently does if the deformity is mild. Many patients with established kyphotic

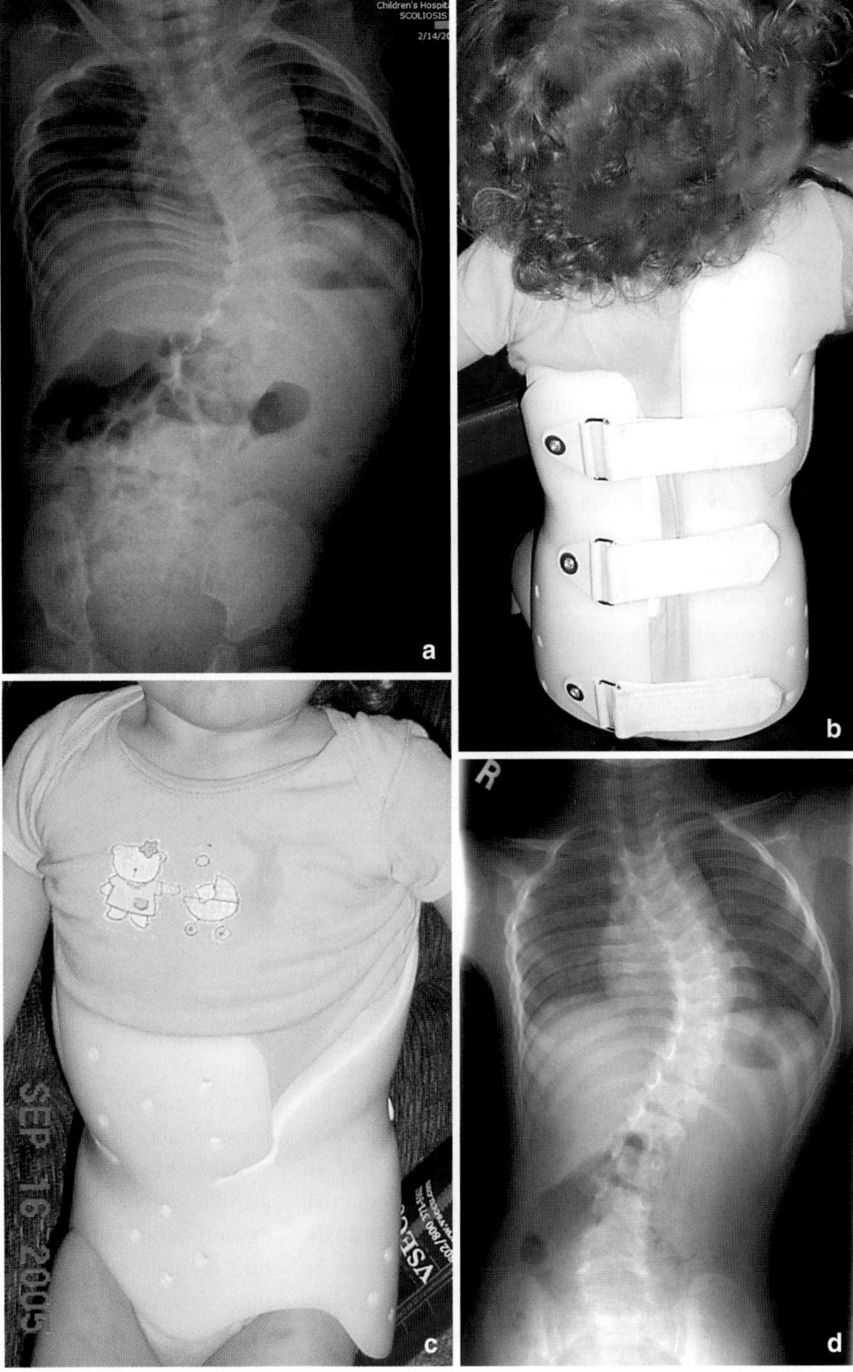

Fig. 27.6 Infantile scoliosis with tethered spinal cord. Scoliosis noted at the age of 6 months. No treatment was initiated and no MRI was done until the age of 2 years. In spite of detethering performed at the age of 2 years, scoliosis progressed at the age of 2 1/2 years (**a**) and bracing was initiated. Full-time custom- molded Boston brace is well-tolerated, asymmetric, and has large areas of relief opposite any area of pressure (**b**, **c**). At the age of 6 years, bracing continues with some progression of curve and mild thoracic deformity (**d**). Dual growing rods was planned, if worsening continued

deformity or scoliosis in excess of approximately 30° may develop progressive deformity during the rapid growth of preadolescence, even though the neuraxis abnormality has been treated. Although a trial of observation following decompression of the Chiari malformation or syringomyelia or tethered cord is appropriate, if the deformity persists as excessive kyphosis or greater than 20° of scoliosis, treatment as in idiopathic juvenile scoliosis should be instituted.

Contraindications to bracing include certain curve locations, very large curves, associated thoracic lordosis, advanced chest deformity, and some medical and psychological conditions. Multiple reports of brace treatment of adolescent idiopathic scoliosis note the poor results of bracing in upper thoracic curves, triple curves, and curves at the lumbo–sacral junction. Although the Milwaukee brace is felt to be the most appropriate brace for curves with apices above T6, reported results [32] are not encouraging, leading most practitioners to observe rather than treat the upper thoracic curves. Jarvis et al. [24], Lenke et al. [30], and McMaster and Macnicole [35], in their series of juvenile idiopathic scoliosis, did not specifically note curves with predominantly high thoracic apices, suggesting that this is an uncommon curve pattern in juvenile idiopathic scoliosis. Jarvis et al. [24] noted more success in juveniles with single thoracic and thoracolumbar curves than with double major curves, mirroring our experience with adolescent and juvenile idiopathic scoliosis. Most curves with high thoracic apices are accompanied by secondary, less structural lower curves of lesser magnitude, which may be successfully treated by bracing. Surgical correction of the high thoracic curve followed by brace treatment of the lower curve(s) is also an option when the upper thoracic curve is rapidly progressive.

Thoracic hypokyphosis or thoracic lordosis is a nearly universal accompaniment of idiopathic thoracic curves, and is often cited as a contraindication to brace treatment, yet Mannherz et al. [33] found thoracic hypokyphosis in only 20% of their series of juvenile idiopathic curves. Although frequently mentioned [12, 32–34, 39, 44], guidelines for the treatment of thoracic lordosis and hypokyphosis are not clear. Our practice has been to treat associated thoracic hypokyphosis with a brace modified to include posterior cephalad extensions of the brace intended to encourage thoracic kyphosis. For true thoracic lordosis (less than 0° of thoracic kyphosis), bracing may be counterproductive and produce more thoracic lordosis. Thoracic lordosis, in association with thoracic scoliosis, may however be the ideal indication for surgical guided-growth procedures such as anterior vertebral stapling [4].

Large curves (in excess of 60–90°) are rarely permanently stabilized by repetitive casting or bracing in juveniles. Although bracing may be used for large curves to allow more growth before a planned surgical intervention, many large curves are best dealt with by surgical intervention such as dual growing rods. Moderately large curves in the adolescent may be successfully treated with bracing as demonstrated by Wiley et al. [55] and Katz and Durrani [27] and also in some juveniles. In our Boston Brace series [12], none of the three juveniles, aged 4–10 years, with curves 40–49° at initiation of bracing needed surgery after bracing and follow-up. Our present practice is to attempt bracing in larger juvenile curves between 40° and 60°, provided that there is acceptable chest deformity, but will switch to dual growing rods if the chest deformity worsens significantly.

Significant chest deformity [5, 17] often accompanies more severe juvenile scoliotic curves and may be a contraindication to bracing. Continued brace treatment may worsen the chest deformity while seemingly stabilizing the spine deformity. The more advanced the chest deformity is, the more likely that the patient will be left at the end of surgical treatment with a functionally significant thoracic deformity and increased risk of respiratory insufficiency as an adult [17, 42]. In most severe juvenile idiopathic scoliosis, final instrumentation and fusion is generally successful in achieving a balanced, stable, minimally deformed spine at the end of treatment. However, surgical treatment is rarely successful in restoring normal chest shape and normal chest compliance when there has already been a severe chest deformity. Therefore, chest deformity should not be allowed to worsen beyond a point at which it is irrevocable. Surgical treatment such as dual growing rods should be instituted earlier.

Some associated medical conditions are also contra-indications to bracing. Severe gastro-esophageal reflux [28] may be exacerbated by abdominal pressure from a brace and may be a contraindication. Failure to thrive or anorexia nervosa may be aggravated by a constrictive brace or any orthosis. Patients with severe asthma may not tolerate bracing during periods of exacerbation. Patients with difficulties with temperature regulation will also be affected by bracing, and those in very warm climates may not tolerate full time orthotic use. Those with severe eczema or other skin conditions often will not tolerate the continued contact between skin and the brace. Adverse psychological reactions to bracing are commonplace in adolescents, less common in juvenile patients, but may still be a contraindication to bracing. Family ambivalence toward treatment or failure to be supportive of the braced child is a relative contraindication to brace treatment. Similarly, if the physician and team do not really believe that bracing is beneficial, or have limited experience or insufficient skill to be successful with bracing, it is probably preferable to observe or operate rather than treat with a brace.

When should we switch to surgical treatment from bracing? A common and difficult issue is when to switch from brace treatment to surgical treatment for deformity in the growing spine. We suggest that the decision to switch to surgical treatment should be based more on progression and severity of the thoracic deformity than the magnitude of spinal deformity. A large thoracic curve stabilized by bracing, with minimal chest deformity may continue to be managed by bracing in anticipation of eventual definitive fusion (Fig. 27.7). At final operation, the spinal deformity can be stabilized, and the thoracic deformity and function will be acceptable. In contrast, if a moderate thoracic curve is associated with a severe or progressive chest deformity, brace treatment should be abandoned in favor of growing rods, or if old enough, definitive fusion (see Fig. 27.3). This attitude is based on the observation that surgical treatment is generally successful in correcting and stabilizing spine curvature, but poor at correcting severe chest deformity and restoring normal thoracic compliance and respiratory function. Brace treatment should be stopped and surgical treatment should begin before chest deformity becomes irrevocable or severe.

Bracing should also be abandoned in favor of surgical treatment if continued brace treatment will cause a more extensive spinal fusion at a later stage. Persisting with brace treatment of some progressive thoracic curves may cause increasingly larger lumbar curves and the need to eventually include the lumbar curve in the final fusion. Switching to growing rods or fusion for control of the thoracic curve may save the lumbar curve from eventual fusion.

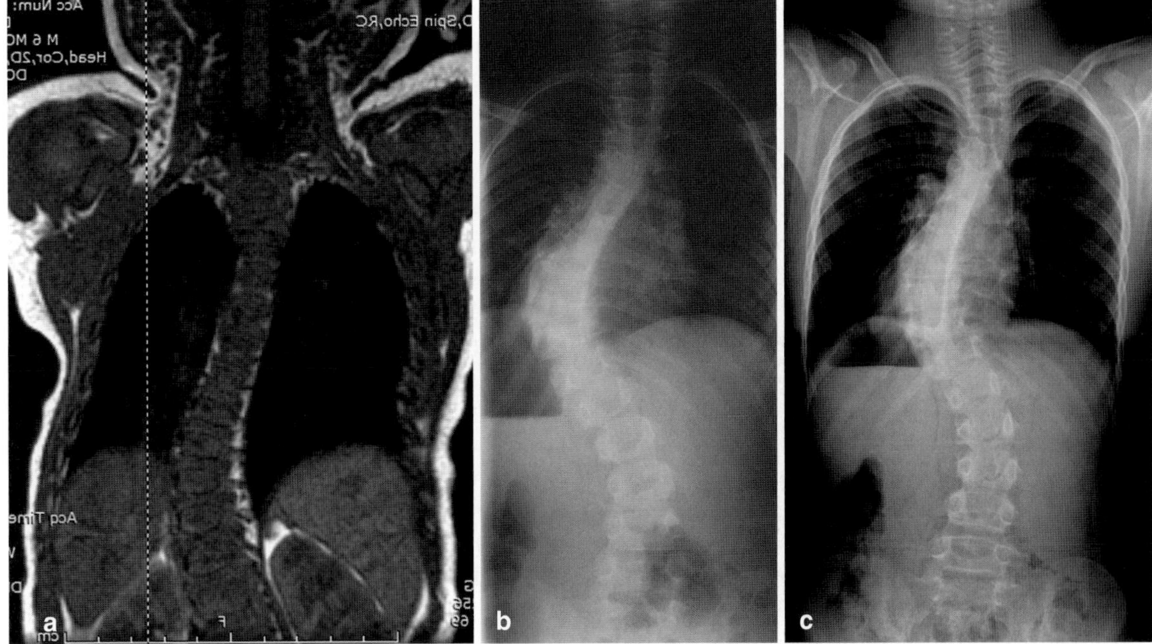

Fig. 27.7 Infantile idiopathic scoliosis. Bracing was begun at age 20 months with thoracic Cobb angle of 60° (MRI at 18 months of age (**a**)) and has been continued full-time in a TLSO, (age of 6 years seen on (**b**)), with an emphasis on allowing chest expansion opposite the pressure pads. By the age of 11 years, the curve has increased minimally to 70° (**c**) with minimal thoracic deformity. If a rapid increase in either chest deformity or curvature starts in the preadolescent growth phase, definitive fusion or growing rods can be accomplished. Otherwise, fusion and instrumentation can wait until later in growth

27.4 Bracing Techniques

Brace types available for orthotic treatment of early onset scoliosis vary greatly. Available rigid braces include traditional CTLSO braces such as the Milwaukee brace, TLSO braces such as the Boston Brace, Wilmington brace, Cheneau or Rigo-Cheneau brace, and night time only, "overcorrecting" braces such as the Charleston and Providence braces. Nonrigid braces such as the Kalabas and SpineCor systems are also available. Manuals and technical details for most North American bracing systems (Milwaukee, Boston, Charleston, Providence, and Charleston) are available online at the Scoliosis Research Society http://www.srs.org/professionals/bracing_manuals/. Most physicians will have experience with a limited number of bracing techniques, and it is probably preferable to use a familiar technique with which the team is skilled, than to attempt an unknown method for the first time.

Principles of correction are remarkably similar among brace types and probably never completely achieved. Braces should be constructed based on principles of the particular bracing system, but applied and modified as needed to the individual patient. The orthotist and physician must communicate about the orthosis to be constructed and the orthotist must have access to and base the brace upon radiographs in both coronal and sagittal planes, as well as an examination of the patient. Common principles espoused by all systems include the recognition that idiopathic scoliosis is a three-dimensional deformity and that correction should be sought in all three planes by forces applied in all three dimensions. Brace construction should be planned in all dimensions. Coronal deformity is corrected by lateral pressure, rotational deformity by rotational pressure on both the front and back of the brace, and sagittal malalignment may be improved or should not be made worse. Every system, in one form or another, provides an area of relief, void, or window in the brace opposite the applied force, to both enhance the asymmetry of the force and provide an area into which the spine may shift as it moves toward a corrected position. Wherever possible, derotation forces are coupled, so that, for example, derotation of a typical right thoracic curve will include posterior to anterior pressure on the right posterior rib hump and anterior to posterior pressure on the left anterior rib prominence. No unnecessary constriction should occur, particularly of the chest. Continued application of force to the growing chest can create an irreversible thoracic deformity of greater significance than the underlying spinal deformity [5] (see Fig. 27.5).

Physical therapy is prescribed on a variable basis in North America, but in the opinion of the author, specific, individualized physical therapy is an important adjunct to full-time bracing in the child, old enough to cooperate. The Milwaukee and Boston systems as well as the Rigo-Cheneau and other European systems place great emphasis on coordinated physical therapy. Purported benefits include reduction of associated lower extremity contractures, enhanced in-brace correction through active in-brace exercises, strengthening to counteract the inevitable weakening of trunk muscles by a full-time brace, and improvement of thoracic hypokyphosis or other sagittal malalignment. Contact with an informed and enthusiastic physical therapist on a regular basis further reinforces the team commitment to the individual patient. Physical therapy for night-time only bracing may be much less important, but some juveniles as well as adolescents may exhibit pelvic obliquity associated with infra-pelvic contractures, including the ilio-tibial band or tensor fascia femoris. Physical therapy alone has generally been considered in North America to be of little value in preventing progression or reducing scoliosis. However, there has been enthusiasm in Europe and increasing enthusiasm in North America for specific, individualized, intensive programs of physical therapy such as the Schroth technique [45] with some limited data to demonstrate its effectiveness in mild curves [54].

Assessment of patient progress during bracing should include postero-anterior (PA) and lateral radiographs both in and out of the brace. However, in early onset scoliosis, radiographic assessment will likely continue for many years, with the potential for many radiographs during a potentially sensitive period of growth. Based on a large cohort of women treated for scoliosis, Hoffman et al. [20] and Morin Doody et al. [38] suggested that frequent exposure to low-level diagnostic radiation during childhood or adolescence might increase the risk of breast cancer. Reporting on an expanded cohort [47], recently, there appeared only to be a borderline-significant radiation dose response, not related to stage of development at first exposure, but increased significantly by a family history of breast cancer. Limiting the lifetime radiation exposure is nonetheless desirable in early onset patients. We generally require PA and lateral views before bracing, and obtain PA and lateral views in the brace once the brace is maximally adjusted, to assess brace construction, pad placement, and in-brace correction. The in-brace radiograph as well as the brace on the patient are assessed to see that maximum correction has been achieved and that the original plan, as agreed upon by the orthotist and prescribing physician, has been followed and is effective. Most follow-up radiographs are taken out of brace at intervals that are as widely spaced as feasible, usually when the data from the follow-up radiograph is needed for a treatment decision.

In-brace correction as seen on radiographs has been noted by multiple studies [1, 12, 26, 27, 32, 34, 37, 46, 55] to be a meaningful prognostic sign for eventual success or failure in bracing. In-brace correction is presumably related to both the inherent flexibility of the individual curve, brace construction, and strap tension [3]. The physician cannot influence the first factor, but the latter two can be improved by increased skill in brace construction and patient/family diligence. When in-brace correction is less than anticipated, a careful reassessment of the brace and plan for brace construction should be undertaken. We use 50% correction in the brace as a goal, always expecting to see this in single thoracolumbar curves and most thoracic curves in juveniles (see Figs. 27.1, 27.2, 27.6, and Figs. 27.8, 27.9).

Full- vs. part-time bracing is often debated, with advocates for each. Definitions of "full-time" vary greatly; in our program, our "full-time" goal is 20h daily, with additional time-out of the brace allowed for organized sports. While traditional bracing programs (MWB, Wilmington, Boston) have included "full-time" bracing, success has also been noted with part-time bracing systems (Charleston, Providence). For adolescent idiopathic scoliosis, meta-analysis [48] suggests full-time use is more effective than part-time use. Katz et al. [26] showed that particularly for larger curves, full-time Boston Brace use was more effective than part-time Charleston bracing. Yet, they also demonstrated that for smaller single thoracolumbar or single lumbar curves, a part-time Charleston brace was as effective as a full-time orthosis. Two series of brace treatment of juvenile idiopathic scoliosis [24, 25] used part-time bracing and generally noted success. Tolo and Gillespie [53] began with patients with full-time, and then switched many patients to part-time when the curve was controlled, noting success with part-time use when RVAD fell toward zero or became negative with treatment. This has been similar to our practice; we encourage full-time use but if the curve as measured out of the brace is greatly reduced and below approximately 15°, part-time use will be instituted with close observation, particularly in the preadolescent growth phase. Many patients will need to shift back to full-time use during the preadolescent growth phase.

A team approach to management of bracing of all ages is sought at most pediatric deformity centers and is felt by the proponents of Milwaukee, Wilmington, and Boston bracing to be germane to successful bracing. Typically, the "team" is composed of physician, orthotist, physical therapist, and nurse or other coordinator. We also view the family and patient as part of the team. Decisions and assessment of progress are made openly where possible, and if at all feasible, all members see the patient at each visit, assessing the patient's progress and the fit of the brace, a practice that we think fosters better brace wear compliance by the patient and family. All members of the team understand brace construction principles, and are encouraged to assess and critique the individual orthosis. This model is possible at a medical center, but more difficult at individual office practices or satellite centers. Still, it is possible to promote team communication with orthotist, physical therapist, and coordinator, even though they may be physically separated. Each patient represents a unique deformity, with individual physical findings, contractures, and curve patterns as well as specific lifestyle, activity, and emotional needs. Each patient deserves the best effort of each of these team members.

27.5 Current and Future Developments

Developments in imaging technology, computer-assisted modeling (see Chap. 8), and genetics (see Chap. 50) may improve the quality and specificity of bracing for juvenile idiopathic spine deformity.

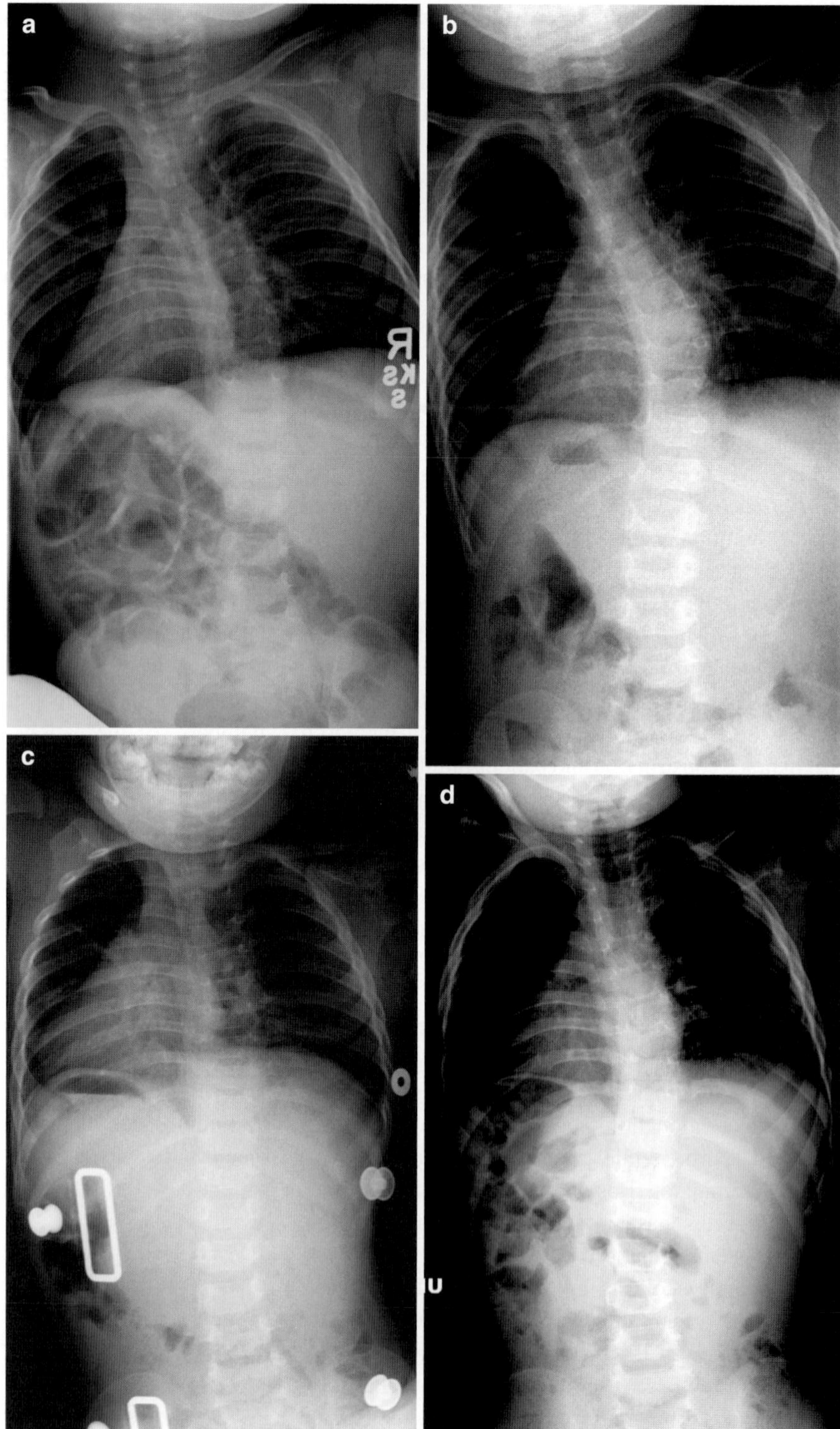

Fig. 27.8 Infantile idiopathic scoliosis. This 18-month-old child (**a**) with infantile idiopathic scoliosis did not tolerate an attempted cast treatment. By 24 months (**b**), the curve had increased further and a custom-molded TLSO was begun with substantial in-brace correction (**c**). Substantial in-brace correction should be expected and sought. At the age of 4 years, bracing has continued and some correction is maintained (**d**). Full-time bracing for infantile idiopathic scoliosis can be employed if casting is not tolerated, or vice-versa

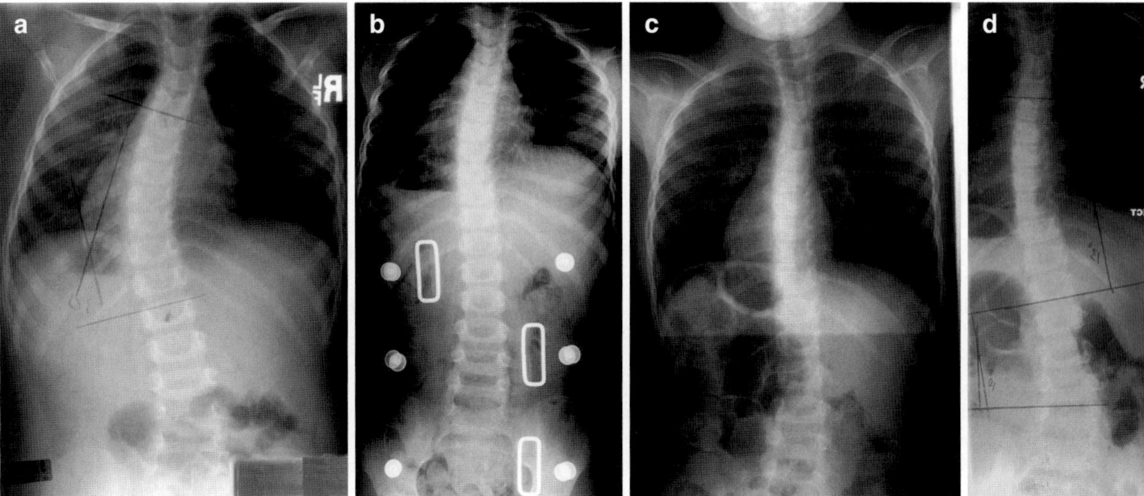

Fig. 27.9 Juvenile idiopathic scoliosis. This child began full-time brace treatment at the age of 3 years for a persistent curve noted for 6 months (**a**). Good in-brace correction was achieved (**b**). At the age of 7 years, curve is minimal out of the brace (**c**) and brace was discontinued. By the age of 9 years, there had been some reoccurrence of the curve and part-time bracing was initiated (**d**)

Dubousset et al. [11] and others have described the rapid low-dose acquisition of three-dimensional images. The availability of such images on a regular basis should help rationalize treatment decisions about early onset spinal deformity and permit brace construction based on three-dimensional data. Ogilvie et al. [41] have studied the genetic predisposition to idiopathic scoliosis in a limited population and suggested that it may be possible to predict progressive idiopathic scoliosis on the basis of genetic markers. The ability to identify patients at risk and initiate nonsurgical treatment early, in theory would facilitate earlier and more successful treatment of juvenile idiopathic scoliosis before curves have become too structural. Computer-aided acquisition of brace shapes from body contours [43, 57] has been reported to improve patient's acceptance and patient's fit of rigid TLSO braces. Aubin et al. [2] has been able to correlate real-time measurement of forces between pads and the patient with computer-generated models, and demonstrate improved brace correction with such designs. Effective braces presently require a maximum in orthotist skill and experience. Brace design and construction according to computer-generated guidelines offer the hope of more widely available, effective orthosis for the treatment of juvenile idiopathic scoliosis.

References

1. Andersen MO, Christensen SB, Thomsen K (2006) Outcome at 10 years after treatment for adolescent idiopathic scoliosis. Spine 31:350–354
2. Aubin CE, Labelle H, Cheriet F et al (2007) Tridimensional evaluation and optimization of the orthotic treatment of adolescent idiopathic scoliosis. Med Sci 23:904–909
3. Beausejour M, Petit Y, Grimard G et al (2002) Relationships between strap tension, interface pressures and spine correction in brace treatment of scoliosis. Stud Health Technol Inform 88:207–211
4. Betz RR, Kim J, D'Andrea LP et al (2003) An innovative technique of vertebral body stapling for the treatment of patients with adolescent idiopathic scoliosis: a feasibility, safety, and utility study. Spine 28:S255–S265
5. Campbell RM Jr, Smith MD (2007) Thoracic insufficiency syndrome and exotic scoliosis. J Bone Joint Surg Am 89(Suppl 1):108–122
6. Charles YP, Daures JP, de Rosa V et al (2006) Progression risk of idiopathic juvenile scoliosis during pubertal growth. Spine 31:1933–1942
7. Danielsson AJ, Nachemson AL (2003) Back pain and function 22 years after brace treatment for adolescent idiopathic scoliosis: a case-control study-part I. Spine 28:2078–2085; discussion 86
8. Dobbs MB, Weinstein SL (1999) Infantile and juvenile scoliosis. Orthop Clin North Am 30:331–341; vii
9. Dolan LA, Weinstein SL (2007) Surgical rates after observation and bracing for adolescent idiopathic scoliosis: an evidence-based review. Spine 32:S91–S100

10. Dolan LA, Donnelly MJ, Spratt KF et al (2007) Professional opinion concerning the effectiveness of bracing relative to observation in adolescent idiopathic scoliosis. J Pediatr Orthop 27:270–276
11. Dubousset J, Charpak G, Dorion I et al (2005) A new 2D and 3D imaging approach to musculoskeletal physiology and pathology with low-dose radiation and the standing position: the EOS system. Bull Acad Natl Med 189:287–297; discussion 97–300
12. Emans JB, Kaelin A, Bancel P et al (1986) The Boston bracing system for idiopathic scoliosis. Follow-up results in 295 patients. Spine 11:792–801
13. Figueiredo UM, James JI (1981) Juvenile idiopathic scoliosis. J Bone Joint Surg Br 63-B:61–66
14. Flynn JM, Sodha S, Lou JE et al (2004) Predictors of progression of scoliosis after decompression of an Arnold Chiari I malformation. Spine 29:286–292
15. Goldberg CJ, Dowling FE, Hall JE et al (1993) A statistical comparison between natural history of idiopathic scoliosis and brace treatment in skeletally immature adolescent girls. Spine 18:902–908
16. Goldberg CJ, Dowling FE, Fogarty EE et al (1995) School scoliosis screening and the United States preventive services task force. An examination of long-term results. Spine 20: 1368–1374
17. Goldberg CJ, Moore DP, Fogarty EE et al (2002) The natural history of early onset scoliosis. Stud Health Technol Inform 91:68–70
18. Goldberg CJ, Gillic I, Connaughton O et al (2003) Respiratory function and cosmesis at maturity in infantile-onset scoliosis. Spine 28:2397–23406
19. Haderspeck K, Schultz A (1981) Progression of idiopathic scoliosis: an analysis of muscle actions and body weight influences. Spine 6:447–455
20. Hoffman DA, Lonstein JE, Morin MM et al (1989) Breast cancer in women with scoliosis exposed to multiple diagnostic x rays. J Natl Cancer Inst 81:1307–1312
21. Hopper WC Jr, Lovell WW (1977) Progressive infantile idiopathic scoliosis. Clin Orthop Relat Res (126):26–32
22. James JI (1971) Infantile idiopathic scoliosis. Clin Orthop Relat Res 77:57–72
23. James JI (1975) The management of infants with scoliosis. J Bone Joint Surg Br 57:422–429
24. Jarvis J, Garbedian S, Swamy G (2008) Juvenile idiopathic scoliosis: the effectiveness of part-time bracing. Spine 33:1074–1078
25. Kahanovitz N, Levine DB, Lardone J (1982) The part-time Milwaukee brace treatment of juvenile idiopathic scoliosis. Long-term follow-up. Clin Orthop Relat Res (167): 145–151
26. Katz DE, Richards BS, Browne RH et al (1997) A comparison between the Boston brace and the Charleston bending brace in adolescent idiopathic scoliosis. Spine 22:1302–1312
27. Katz DE, Durrani AA (2001) Factors that influence outcome in bracing large curves in patients with adolescent idiopathic scoliosis. Spine 26:2354–2361
28. Kling TF Jr, Drennan JC, Gryboski JD (1981) Esophagitis complicating scoliosis management with the Boston thoracolumbosacral orthosis. Clin Orthop Relat Res (159): 208–210
29. Koop SE (1988) Infantile and juvenile idiopathic scoliosis. Orthop Clin North Am 19:331–337
30. Lenke LG, Dobbs MB (2007) Management of juvenile idiopathic scoliosis. J Bone Joint Surg Am 89(Suppl 1):55–63
31. Lonstein JE, Carlson JM (1984) The prediction of curve progression in untreated idiopathic scoliosis during growth. J Bone Joint Surg Am 66:1061–1071
32. Lonstein JE, Winter RB (1994) The Milwaukee brace for the treatment of adolescent idiopathic scoliosis. A review of one thousand and twenty patients. J Bone Joint Surg Am 76:1207–1221
33. Mannherz RE, Betz RR, Clancy M et al (1988) Juvenile idiopathic scoliosis followed to skeletal maturity. Spine 13:1087–1090
34. Masso PD, Meeropol E, Lennon E (2002) Juvenile-onset scoliosis followed up to adulthood: orthopaedic and functional outcomes. J Pediatr Orthop 22:279–284
35. McMaster MJ, Macnicol MF (1979) The management of progressive infantile idiopathic scoliosis. J Bone Joint Surg Br 61:36–42
36. Mehta MH (1992) The conservative management of Juvenile Idiopathic Scoliosis. Acta Orthop Belg 58(Suppl 1):91–97
37. Mehta MH (2005) Growth as a corrective force in the early treatment of progressive infantile scoliosis. J Bone Joint Surg Br 87:1237–1247
38. Morin Doody M, Lonstein JE, Stovall M et al (2000) Breast cancer mortality after diagnostic radiography: findings from the U.S. scoliosis cohort study. Spine 25:2052–2063
39. Nachemson AL, Peterson LE (1995) Effectiveness of treatment with a brace in girls who have adolescent idiopathic scoliosis. A prospective, controlled study based on data from the brace study of the scoliosis research society. J Bone Joint Surg Am 77:815–822
40. Noonan KJ, Weinstein SL, Jacobson WC et al (1996) Use of the Milwaukee brace for progressive idiopathic scoliosis. J Bone Joint Surg Am 78:557–567
41. Ogilvie JW, Braun J, Argyle V et al (2006) The search for idiopathic scoliosis genes. Spine 31:679–681
42. Pehrsson K, Larsson S, Oden A et al (1992) Long-term follow-up of patients with untreated scoliosis. A study of mortality, causes of death, and symptoms. Spine 17:1091–1096
43. Perie D, Aubin CE, Lacroix M et al (2002) Personalized biomechanical modeling of Boston brace treatment in idiopathic scoliosis. Stud Health Technol Inform 91:393–396
44. Raso VJ, Russell GG, Hill DL et al (1991) Thoracic lordosis in idiopathic scoliosis. J Pediatr Orthop 11:599–602
45. Rigo M, Quera-Salva G, Villagrasa M et al (2008) Scoliosis intensive out-patient rehabilitation based on Schroth method. Stud Health Technol Inform 135:208–227
46. Robinson CM, McMaster MJ (1996) Juvenile idiopathic scoliosis. Curve patterns and prognosis in one hundred and nine patients. J Bone Joint Surg Am 78:1140–1148
47. Ronckers CM, Doody MM, Lonstein JE et al (2008) Multiple diagnostic X-rays for spine deformities and risk of breast cancer. Cancer Epidemiol Biomarkers Prev 17: 605–613
48. Rowe DE, Bernstein SM, Riddick MF et al (1997) A meta-analysis of the efficacy of non-operative treatments for idiopathic scoliosis. J Bone Joint Surg Am 79:664–674

49. Sanders JO, Browne RH, Cooney TE et al (2006) Correlates of the peak height velocity in girls with idiopathic scoliosis. Spine 31:2289–2295
50. Schultz AB, Hirsch C (1974) Mechanical analysis of techniques for improved correction of idiopathic scoliosis. Clin Orthop Relat Res 66–73
51. Schultz AB (1984) Biomechanical factors in the progression of idiopathic scoliosis. Ann Biomed Eng 12:621–630
52. Stokes IA, Spence H, Aronsson DD et al (1996) Mechanical modulation of vertebral body growth. Implications for scoliosis progression. Spine 21:1162–1167
53. Tolo VT, Gillespie R (1978) The characteristics of juvenile idiopathic scoliosis and results of its treatment. J Bone Joint Surg Br 60-B:181–188
54. Weiss HR, Klein R (2006) Improving excellence in scoliosis rehabilitation: a controlled study of matched pairs. Pediatr Rehabil 9:190–200
55. Wiley JW, Thomson JD, Mitchell TM et al (2000) Effectiveness of the boston brace in treatment of large curves in adolescent idiopathic scoliosis. Spine 25: 2326–2332
56. Winter RB (2000) Expert editorial: bracing for idiopathic scoliosis: where do we go now? J Prosthet Orthot 12:2–4
57. Wong MS, Cheng JC, Lo KH (2005) A comparison of treatment effectiveness between the CAD/CAM method and the manual method for managing adolescent idiopathic scoliosis. Prosthet Orthot Int 29:105–111

28 Halo-Gravity Traction

Charles E. Johnston II

Key Points

- A safe, effective method to obtain complex/exotic deformity correction non-operatively
- Upright patient positioning and halo anchorage avoids morbidity from supine positioning and head halters
- Advantages/indications:

  Rigid deformity, especially kyphosis, wherein acute correction carries increased neurological risk

  Osteopenia, which compromises effective acute instrumented correction

  Pre-existing respiratory compromise/thoracic insufficiency syndrome sufficient to compromise anesthesia or other external means of deformity treatment

  Contraindications:

  Pre-existing neurological deficit

  Intra-canal mass lesion (extradural, intramedullary) or significant canal stenosis

28.1 Introduction

Traction is a traditional orthopaedic technique to produce, among other things, correction of a deformity. As applied to early onset spine deformity, it can be used as an effective method to obtain correction prior to spinal fusion, or as a delaying tactic to produce correction so that another non-operative or fusionless method can be applied more effectively. In the past, traction has been applied by the use of various neck and head halters combined with pelvic or leg harnesses or with skeletal traction. Most of these methods require the patient to remain supine in bed with longitudinal traction being applied via attachments to the bed frame, thus immobilizing the patient in a non-upright and non-movable position. Not surprisingly, the duration of such traction is limited by the physical, psychological and medical complications, which can befall a bedridden patient.

Because the traction is applied via a halo device, discomfort or intolerance from the head attachment portion of the traction is avoided – as opposed to halter methods, which are notorious for producing chin and facial discomfort and irritation, thus limiting the effectiveness of the method. Because gravity is the method of force application to the lower body, the legs remain unrestrained, and the patient is mobile. Many young patients seem totally unaware of the presence of the halo on the skull once they recover from the immediate pain of pin application to the skull – a process which often takes no more than 24 h following application. From that point on, the morbidity from halo-gravity traction is so minimal that it can be continued for several months if necessary to produce maximum deformity correction as well as improve respiratory status in anticipation of further surgical or non-operative treatment.

28.2 Indications

Patients with early onset spinal deformity often present with co-morbidities and physical characteristics, which can significantly challenge and compromise *any*

C.E. Johnston II
Texas Scottish Rite Hospital, 2222 Welborn Street, Dallas, TX 75219–3924, USA
e-mail: charles.johnston@tsrh.org

B. A. Akbarnia et al. (eds.), *The Growing Spine*,
DOI: 10.1007/978-3-540-85207-0_28, © Springer-Verlag Berlin Heidelberg 2011

surgical treatment plan. Specifically, those with syndromic or "exotic" diagnoses possess diminutive osteopenic bony elements, which severely curtail the possibility of acute deformity correction due to weakness of the bone-implant interface. Frequently, their deformity is rigid and/or kyphotic, in which case posterior distractive methods of correction (rod systems, VEPTR's) are compromised by the need for extreme contouring of the expandable device, leading to ineffective distraction and proximal anchor failure by posterior cut-out, if not immediately peri-operatively, then later by fatigue "plowing" or fracture due to the unfavorable biomechanical forces – especially in kyphosis (Fig. 28.1a-c). Neurological risk from acute correction is always a concern in such patients, especially if severe deformity requires canal manipulation by osteotomy or vertebral resection to achieve it. Relative canal stenosis, from previous fusion for example, is another cause for neurological concern with acute correction, especially if the previous fusion might produce cord compression at a junctional segment due to fusion mass overgrowth or a juxta-fusion hypermobile segment [4]. Patients with severe thoracic deformity, especially as a sequela of neglect or ineffective previous treatment, may present with respiratory failure or thoracic insufficiency syndrome, in which case traction is indicated as a preliminary step to improve respiratory mechanics and make them a more suitable surgical candidate. Such respiratory compromise, as well as hypotonia and weakness, chest wall defects, skin intolerance or anesthesia, and mental retardation may eliminate external means of deformity control, such as bracing or casting, from consideration.

Patients with severe deformity are also not candidates for bracing or casting purely from biomechanical considerations related to curve magnitude. Curves exceeding approximately 53° are corrected more effectively by longitudinal distraction forces than by the laterally-directed (transverse) forces [14], such as would be realized with a cast or brace. Large, stiff curves thus may not benefit from use of the latter, being poorly tolerated due to excess skin pressure associated with inefficient transverse loads, as well as rib and chest wall deformation caused by the lateral rib pressure. In these instances, halo-gravity traction has been an invaluable method to achieve deformity correction, and indirectly, improve respiratory mechanics [11, 12]. We have noted up to 10% increase in predicted vital capacity *acutely* in several patients who benefit from the elongation of the chest wall associated with

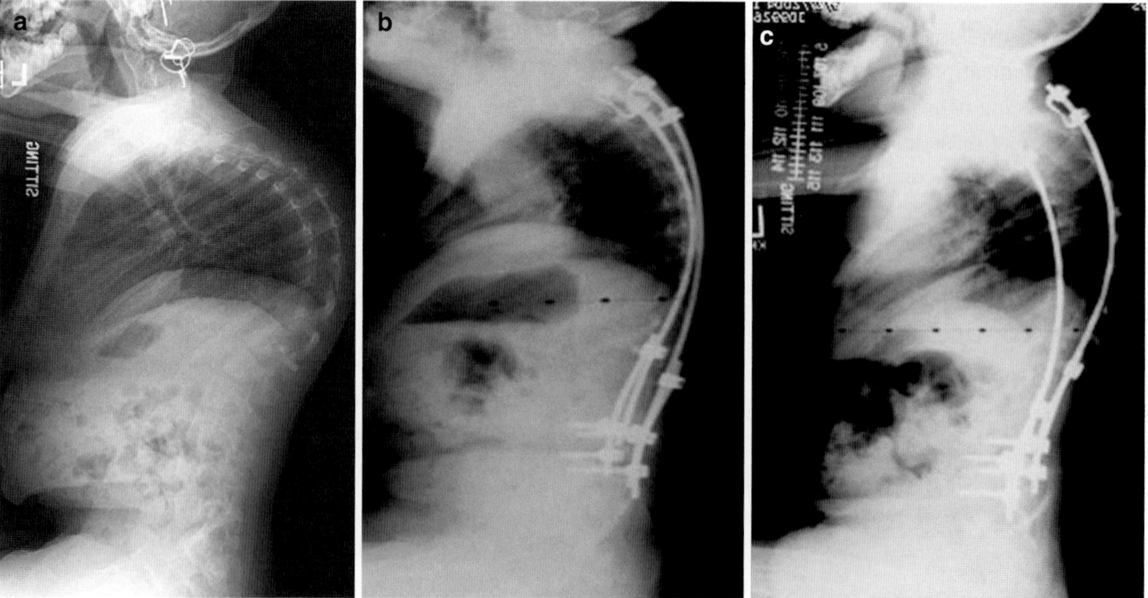

Fig. 28.1 (**a**) Preoperative lateral radiograph of a non-ambulatory child with collapsing kyphoscoliosis due to spastic quadriparesis. (**b**) Immediate postoperative radiograph following bilateral rib-to-pelvis growing rod instrumentation. (**c**) Two months postoperative. One of the bilateral hook claws has pulled through the upper rib attachments with loss of fixation and correction

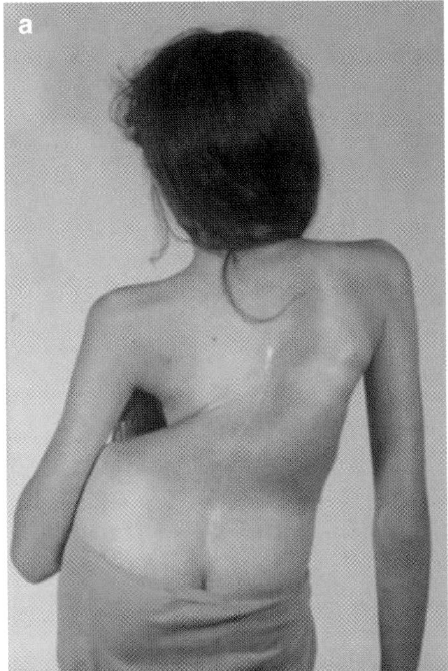

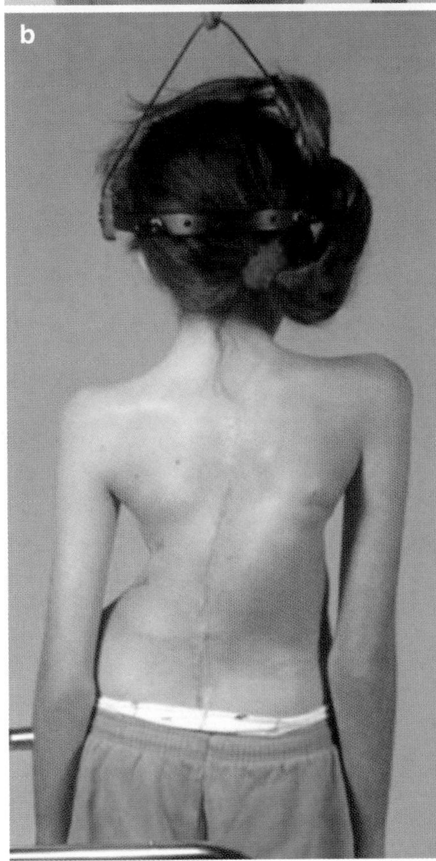

Fig. 28.2 (**a, b**) Elongation of the thorax in a patient undergoing osteotomies of a previous fusion mass and halo-gravity traction

the spinal elongation/correction (Figs. 28.2a, b and 28.3a–d). Improving the restrictive component of the deformity probably results from more efficient diaphragmatic excursion in the elongated abdomen as well as from rib separation on the concavity, providing more effective inspiration and consequently respiration. This appears to be the physiologic explanation for this acute vital capacity increase during traction.

Halo-gravity traction has been found to be almost uniformly safe [11, 12]. The only absolute *contraindications* to its use would be bone stock in the skull insufficient to gain halo purchase due to underlying diagnoses such as osteogenesis imperfecta or fibrous dysplasia (Fig. 28.4a, b); pre-existing neurological deficit (paraparesis) due to an intra- or extramedullary lesion (tumor, syrinx), or severe canal distortion with stenosis [4] (Fig. 28.5a-c). Otherwise, any patient with severe rigid deformity with or without kyphosis, potential or actual thoracic insufficiency syndrome, osteopenia, and increased potential neurological risk from acute instrumented correction is a candidate for halo-gravity traction as a preliminary step before other operative treatment, to reduce the occurrence of instrumentation or neurological complications and to improve respiratory function and suitability for general anesthesia.

28.3 Technique

Halo-gravity traction is not a new method of treatment of spinal deformity, having been developed soon after the halo apparatus was first described in the 1960s at Rancho Los Amigos hopsital [10] Stagnara [13] (1971) popularized the gravity-traction method, which was introduced at our institution after it was demonstrated to this author by Zielke in 1984 during a visit to the latter's clinic in Germany. The indications for which these early authors used halo-gravity traction were essentially the same as its use for us today – neuromuscular "collapsing" deformity in the Rancho experience and as an adjunct to neglected deformity in older patients with respiratory insufficiency, as well as in the young patient with syndromic or exotic spinal deformity.

Halo application requires general anesthesia for children of this age group, using the maximum number of pins possible [9, 12] (Fig. 28.6a–e). Experience has shown that the use of numerous pins actually decreases

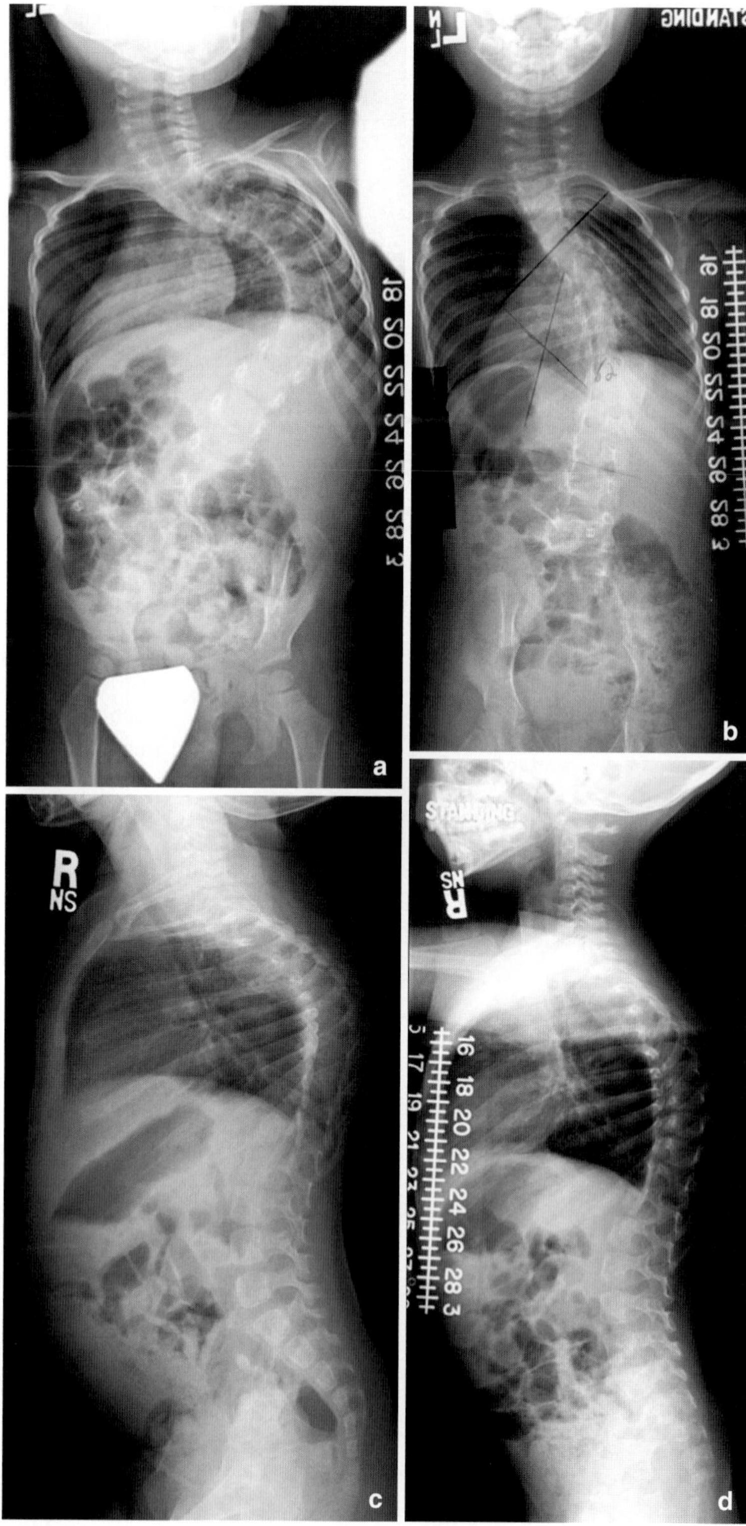

Fig. 28.3 (**a**) A Standing radiograph of an 18 month old girl with a 107° infantile idiopathic scoliosis. Note the "jamming" of the concave ribs and the severe penetration of the spine into the convex thorax. (**b**) Improvement in traction after 2 months. Space between concave ribs is now obvious, and the convex lung field appears expanded due to apical spine translation to the concavity occurring with distraction. The curve is reduced to 62° in traction. (**c, d**) Improvement of thoracic hyperkyphosis while in traction

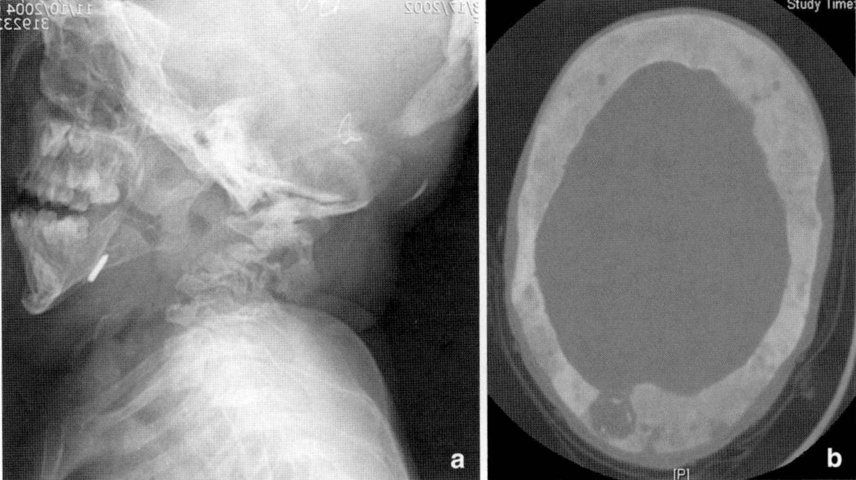

Fig. 28.4 (**a**) Absence of occipital bone in a patient with Loeys-Dietz syndrome. This patient is unsuitable for halo placement. (**b**) Skull in severe fibrous dysplasia, which is also unsuitable for halo placement

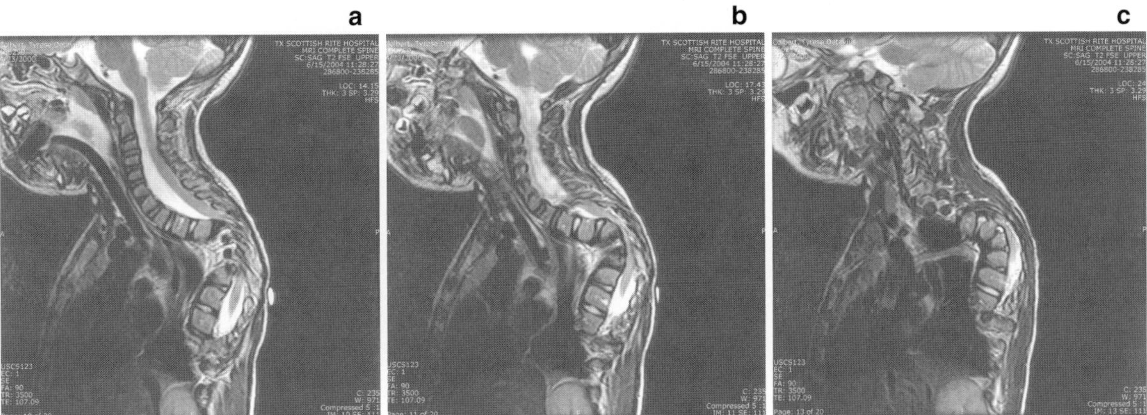

Fig. 28.5 (**a–c**) MRI images of spinal cord compression in a patient with paraplegia and kyphoscoliosis due to Pierre Robin syndrome. This patient is *not* a candidate for HGT

the incidence of pin infection or loosening of any *single* pin, as well as pin direction being as perpendicular to the skull as possible [1, 3]. Pins are tightened to a torque approximately equaling the age of the child – e.g. a 4-year-old patient's pins are tightened to four inch-pounds of torque, using a calibrated torque wrench. Because of variation in skull thickness and location of sutures, computed tomography (CT) scanning of the skull has been recommended to control pin placement [7, 15], but in practice such thickness determination has not altered intended pin location when multiple pins are used and the penetration is controlled by torque determination. Frontal and occipital areas are commonly adequate for safe, secure placement. Upright overhead traction via a traction bale attached to a wheelchair or standing frame, using a spring-loaded fish scale or other dynamic traction device (see Fig. 28.6b–d), is begun the following day, initially with 5–10 pounds of traction. The amount of time and weight is increased to tolerance under careful neurological surveillance. All patients should have cranial nerve testing once a shift while upright in traction, as well as motor and sensory testing of upper and lower extremities, especially during the phase of increasing traction. Eventually traction force exceeding 50% of body weight may be achieved, with cervical pain being the usual limiting factor. The goal of just lifting the patient's buttocks off the wheelchair seat while sitting,

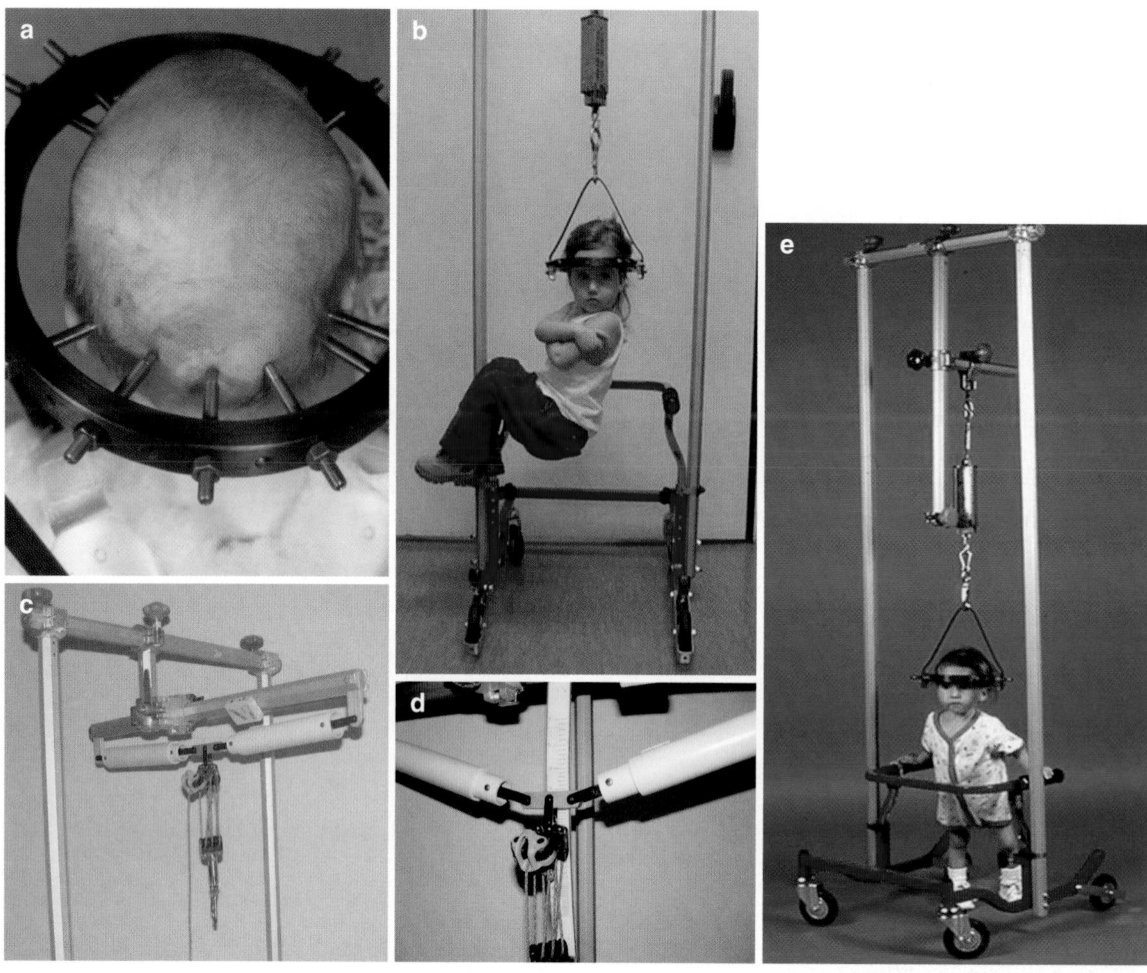

Fig. 28.6 (**a**) Ten halo pins in the skull of a 9-month-old infant. (**b**) Patient suspended by fish scale traction device. Although dynamic, this dangling activity is not encouraged. (**c**) Currently-used dynamic spring loaded traction apparatus with windlass pulleys. (**d**) Fifteen pounds traction in dynamic spring apparatus. (**e**) Obligatory walking on tiptoes while in overhead walker. If the patient is able to achieve flatfoot position, this is the maximum necessary traction amount

or being on tiptoes in the standing frame can usually be attained within 2 weeks (see Fig. 28.6e). The use of nighttime traction, making the treatment program more or less continuous, can be added by providing a cervical traction frame to the patient's bed, usually a gatched bed with the head portion elevated to act as countertraction [2]. Out-patient (home) traction can be attempted if caregivers are appropriately trained and vigilant. Radiographs are obtained in traction once every 3–4 weeks until a plateau of correction is reached. Remaining in traction without complication and with gradual deformity improvement over a period of 6 months is *not* unusual.

28.4 Complications

Complications of traction include pin site infections, which are relatively common (up to 20% incidence) [8] but also usually controlled with oral antibiotics and pin care. As mentioned earlier, placement of extra pins at the time of halo application usually decreases the incidence of individual pin sepsis by presumably making the halo-cranial interface more stable. Intra-cranial abscess from septic pin penetration of the dura has previously been emphasized as an uncommon but serious halo complication [5, 6], although this complication is now rarely reported in more recent series and has never occurred at our institution.

Pin pain in the absence of pin tract infection suggests loosening, another relatively common occurrence, and mandates that the pin torque be checked by tightening the pin(s), under sedation if necessary. Cervical pain (axial) without radicular symptoms is also common, and probably indicates the limit of tolerable traction [2]. In older patients (>10 years), the pain associated with continual traction is a more frequent complaint, and while it may limit the amount of weight that can be eventually applied, it rarely produces symptoms which negate the efficacy of the method. Obviously any patient with a severe or unrelenting neck pain must be evaluated radiographically for cervical pathology (Fig. 28.7), which in our series has occurred but once in >100 cases.

True neurological complications are rare and mainly depend on the rapidity of adding weight. Reversible cranial nerve lesions have been reported [2, 8], which responded to decreasing the amount of traction. Similarly, nausea and dizziness with nystagmus have been reported and are reversible with temporary traction relief [11]. On the other hand, motor paresis can occur rapidly at the onset of traction application, but is associated with pre-existing abnormalities of the cord or a stenotic spinal canal [4], and may not necessarily resolve with immediate discontinuance of traction. Thus *any* pre-existing cord or canal abnormality automatically constitutes a contraindication to halo-gravity traction – indeed, *any* form of traction – especially if there is a pre-existing paraparesis, which can be decompressed.

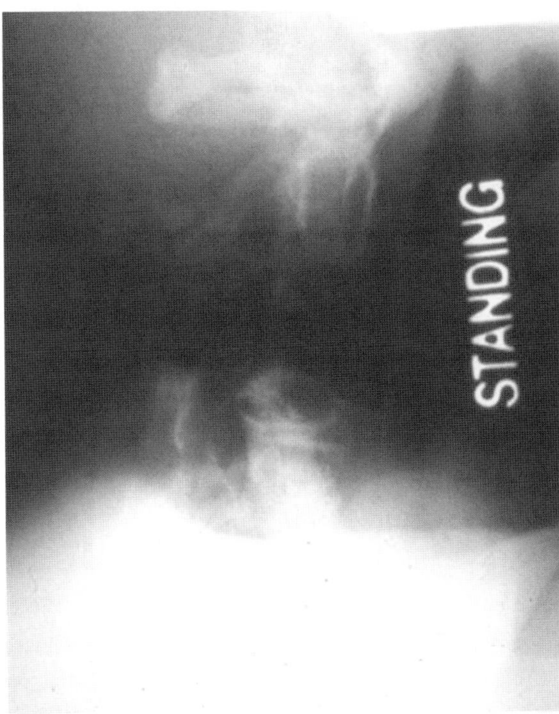

Fig. 28.7 A patient with known Klippel-Feil anomalies of the cervical spine was undergoing halo-gravity correction when there was a sudden increase in neck pain and facial numbness and dysesthesias. This separation at C2–3 occurred at the first non-fused segment cephalad to a long congenitally-fused segment from C3 to the upper thoracic spine. The traction was immediately discontinued, with resolution of the neurological symptoms

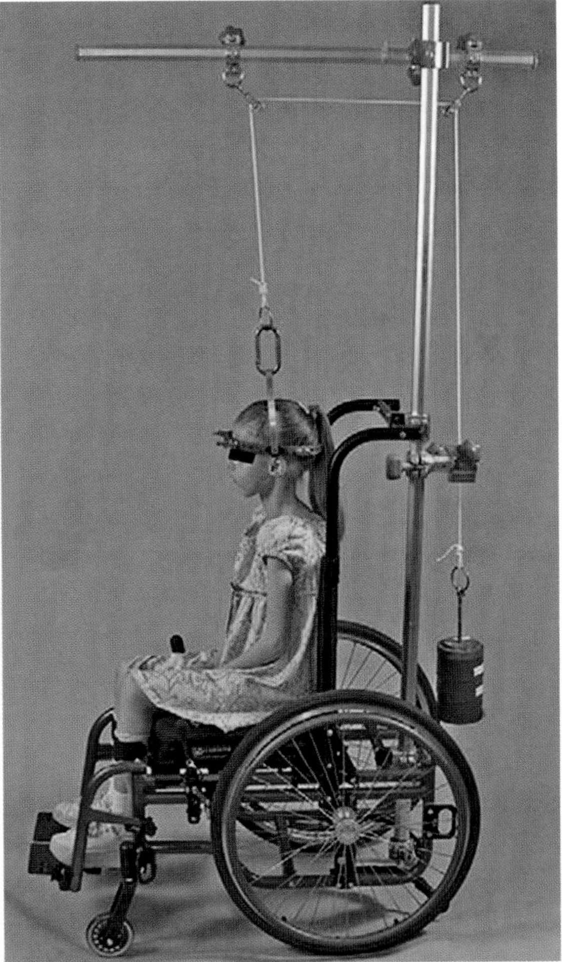

Fig. 28.8 Wheelchair traction using classic orthopaedic traction pulleys and fixed weights. Note the absence of arms on the wheelchair (not recommended). The patient cannot auto-relieve the amount of weight by raising herself up off the seat, as the weight amount is fixed (as opposed to a spring device), and the lack of chair arms makes auto-relief even more difficult

The *safety* of the method may rely on the ability of the patient to auto-relieve the traction stretch by pushing up on the wheelchair arms or walker hand rails as necessary if uncomfortable and the "stretch" is excessive. Such safety is secured by using a spring-loaded traction appliance such as a common fish-scale or other device where spring tension provides the "weight", and shortening the spring decreases the weight amount (see Fig. 28.6a–e). Although classic orthopaedic traction pulleys with weights are commonly used, these provide less flexible traction, and as the amount of weight is constant, the patient cannot auto-relieve the excessive weight by pushing up on wheelchair arms or tip-toeing (Fig. 28.8). If a series of pulleys in different directions are required, thus adding additional friction in the system, the patient may not be able to "bounce" in the traction, losing the dynamic feature, and again preventing auto-relief and safety. For this reason, spring-type devices are recommended whenever possible (see Fig. 28.6a–e).

28.5 Current Results

Radiographic improvement in spinal deformity is usually seen within 1–2 weeks of instituting traction, but as suggested earlier, longer cycles of treatment are normally utilized to produce more correction until a "plateau" is reached wherein no further improvement seems to occur (see Fig. 28.3a–d). Thirty percent to 40% correction of coronal and sagittal plane Cobb deformity typically occur over periods of 2–21 weeks of traction, whether for definitive correction and fusion [11, 12] or as a preliminary treatment for use of Veptr or growing rods [4] (Fig. 28.9a–c). Equally important is the improvement in trunk length (5–6 cm average) and trunk shift [11, 12] (see Fig. 28.2a, b).

In addition to the radiographic improvement, other positive changes that are not always easy to quantify have been observed. Although many patients do not have an *objective* improvement in pulmonary function tests (PFT's) while in traction, there is often a sense of

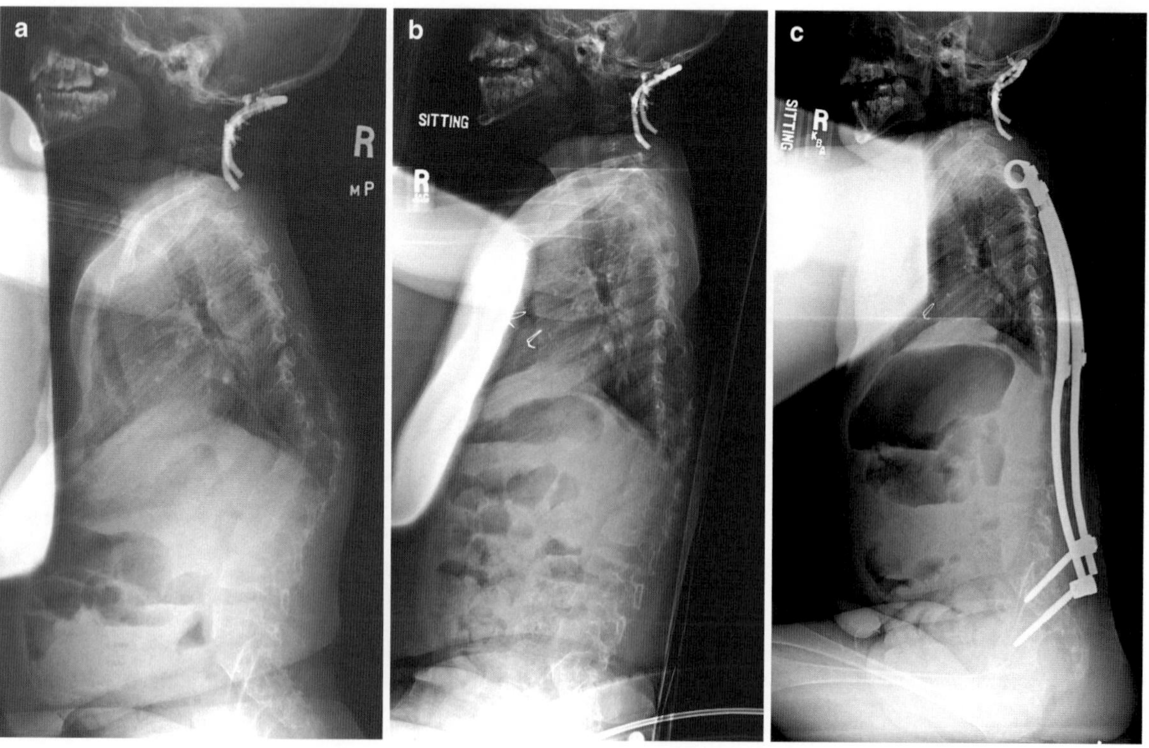

Fig. 28.9 (**a**) Preoperative paralytic kyphosis in a 3 year boy with cervical myopathy due to basilar invagination associated with skeletal dysplasia. He was unable to tolerate any external bracing or casting due to skin discomfort and gastro-esophageal reflux. (**b**) Lateral radiograph after 3 months in traction during which his nutrition improved and there was a 5 kg weight gain. (**c**) Immediate postoperatively following insertion of bilateral rib-to-pelvis expandable devices

improved well-being and respiratory "reserve" during the time in traction, which translates into postoperative ICU mechanical ventilation becoming unnecessary, even though it may have been predicted as part of the preoperative evaluation and one of the indications to proceed with traction. The surgical stabilization following traction also tends to be less technically difficult, since as much as 75–85% of the eventual deformity correction has already been achieved by the time instrumented correction is attempted [4], and the instrumentation can be implanted with less contouring and much less stress on the anchors, especially if there is preexisting kyphosis, which has been improved by the traction. Finally, if there are any nutritional or metabolic issues preoperatively, which might jeopardize wound healing, these can easily be dealt with during the weeks in preparatory traction (see Fig. 28. 9a–c).

References

1. Copley LA, Pepe MD, Tan V, Sheth N, Dormans JP (1999) A comparison of various angles of halo pin insertion in an immature skull model. Spine 24:1777–1780
2. D'Astous JL, Sanders JO (2007) Casting and traction treatment methods for scoliosis. Orthop Clin N America 38: 477–484
3. Dormans JP, Criscitiello AA, Drummond DS, Davidson RS (1995) Complications in children managed with immobilization in a halo vest. J Bone Joint Surg [Am] 77:1370–1373
4. Emans JB, Johnston CE II, Smith JT (2007) Preliminary halo-gravity traction facilitates insertion of growing rods or VEPTR devices in severe early onset spinal deformity. Presented at the 42nd Scoliosis Research Society. Edinburgh, Scotland, pp 5–8
5. Garfin SR, Botte MJ, Waters RL, Nickels VL (1986) Complications in the use of halo fixation device. J Bone Joint Surg [Am] 68:320–325
6. Garfin SR, Botte MJ, Nickel VL (1987) Complications in the use of the halo fixation device (letter). J Bone Joint Surg [Am] 69A:954
7. Letts M, Kaylor D, Gouw G (1988) A biomechanical analysis of halo fixation in children. J Bone Joint Surg [Br] 70: 277–279
8. Limpaphayom N, Skaggs DL, McComb G, et al (2007) Complications of halo use in children. Presented at the 42nd Scoliosis Research Society. Edinburgh, Scotland, pp 5–8
9. Mubarak SJ, Camp JF, Vuletich W, Wenger DR, Garfin SR (1989) Halo application in the infant. J Pediatr Orthop 9:612–614
10. Nickel VL, Perry J, Garrett A, Heppenstall M (1968) The halo. A spinal skeletal traction fixation device. J Bone Joint Surg [Am] 50:1400–1409
11. Rinella A, Lenke L, Whitaker C, Kim Y, Park SS, Peele M, Edwards CII, Bridwell K (2005) Perioperative halo-gravity traction in the treatment of severe scoliosis and kyphosis. Spine 30:475–482
12. Sink EL, Karol LA, Sanders J, Birch JG, Johnston CE, Herring JE (2001) Efficacy of perioperative halo-gravity traction in the treatment of severe scoliosis in children. J Pediatr Orthop 21:519–524
13. Stagnara P (1971) Cranial traction using the "halo" of Rancho Los Amigos. Rev Chir Orthop Reparatif Appar Mat 57:287–300
14. White AA III, Punjabi MM (1976) The clinical biomechanics of scoliosis. Clin Orthop Rel Res 118:100–112
15. Wong WB, Haynes RJ (1994) Osteology of the pediatric skull. Considerations for halo pin placement. Spine 19: 1451–1454

Crankshaft Phenomena Following Spinal Fusion in the Growing Child

29

Nobumasa Suzuki and Kota Watanabe

Key Points

> Posterior spinal fusion in patients less than 10 years of age and Risser stage 0, may result in "crankshaft phenomenon."

> Other factors associated with "crankshaft phenomena" include rotational changes, increased lateral trunk shift, apical rib-vertebral angle, and changes in rib deformity.

> "Crankshaft phenomena" can be prevented by an intervertebral anterior spinal fusion in selected cases.

29.1 Introduction

In situ posterior spinal fusion (PSF) was initially performed for the primary treatment for congenital scoliosis. Later, in conjunction with PSF, segmental spinal instrumentation became the treatment of choice for idiopathic and congenital scoliosis. This was due to the emergence of Harrington rod instrumentation to correct the deformity and reduce the incidence of pseudoarthrosis. However, because of problems of halting the posterior longitudinal spinal growth of the fused area and continued spinal deformity caused by crankshaft phenomenon, PSF with instrumentation has been avoided for patients with infantile and juvenile idiopathic scoliosis. As a result, until the emergence of fusionless or growing rod techniques, the preferable management of infantile and juvenile idiopathic scoliosis was conservative treatment until the child reached 10 years of age or older [15].

N. Suzuki (✉)
Saiseikai Central Hospital, Scoliosis Center,
1-4-17 Mita, Minato-ku, Tokyo,108-0073,
Japan
e-mail: nobumasa@po.jah.ne.jp

29.2 The Problems of Corrective Fusion with Instrumentation in Idiopathic Scoliosis

29.2.1 Halting of Further Longitudinal Spinal Growth

When considering PSF, the amount of remaining longitudinal spinal growth had been one of the most important concerns. Whether the fusion mass can grow longitudinally has also been controversial. Hallock et al. [5] reported that based on a review of 15 patients who had undergone a PSF in early childhood for tuberculosis that the fusion mass could elongate due to biological plasticity. The entire fusion area grew 37% less anteriorly and 45% less posteriorly than normal vertebrae, and the fused normal vertebrae grew 23% less anteriorly and 36% less posteriorly than adjacent normal unfused vertebrae. Risser et al. [19] in a review of 100 cases of PSF performed in children between 2 and 12 years of age that the fusion mass elongated by the stress of continued growth of the unfused anterior vertebra. However, it became widely accepted that the posterior fusion mass prevented further longitudinal growth in the fused area, leading to production of a relative shortening of the spine by skeletal maturity. Johnson and Southwick [9] reported that when a fusion mass was unquestionably solid and fairly massive, there was little increase in length of the fused area. They concluded that a small increase in length could

B. A. Akbarnia et al. (eds.), *The Growing Spine*,
DOI: 10.1007/978-3-540-85207-0_29, © Springer-Verlag Berlin Heidelberg 2011

be accounted for by magnification and technical factors. However, it was impossible to rule out a small amount of growth. Moe et al. [17] reviewed 42 patients fused between 1 and 10 years of age and followed for a mean of 49 months. They found no change in the length of the fusion mass in 20 patients, a length increase of 1–2 mm in 10 patients, a length decrease of 1–2 mm in 5 patients, and an increase of 3–5 mm in 7 patients. Winter [28] reported that in 75 patients with a spinal fusion performed at 10 years of age or younger, the mean lengthening was 1 mm after a mean of 9.5 years postoperatively. Furthermore, Winter [29] produced a formula from standard growth tables, which yields an approximate potential shortening of a spine caused by spinal fusion: centimeters of shortening = 0.07 × number of vertebrae fused × number of years of remaining growth. After the emergence of spinal instrumentations, most surgeons believed that the longitudinal growth in the fused area ceased. Letts and Bobechko [13] reported on 57 patients treated by spinal fusion at 7 years of age or younger, including 19 patients with Harrington rod instrumentation, that a PSF halted further longitudinal growth in the fused area. Hefti and McMaster [7] reported that in 24 children with infantile or juvenile idiopathic scoliosis treated by PSF with Harrington rod instrumentation before the age of 11 years, all longitudinal growth in the posterior elements ceased during a mean of 4.5 years of follow-up.

29.2.2 Loss of Correction

Hallock et al. [5] first reported the loss of correction after PSF in 1957. They speculated that the fusion acted as a posterior tether that aggravates the primary curve in the growing spine. Roaf [20] reported that a PSF alone would not control a progressive spinal deformity when there was marked imbalance of growth potential. McMaster and Macnicol [15] in a review of 12 infantile idiopathic scoliosis treated by PSF prior to 10 years of age found that a loss of correction of 17° occurred after a mean of 7 years of postoperative follow-up. Nearly all of the loss of correction occurred during the adolescent growth spurt. Even after the emergence of Harrington rod instrumentation, the loss of correction was a problem in infantile and juvenile scoliosis. Hefti and McMaster [7] reviewed 24 patients with infantile or juvenile idiopathic scoliosis who had a PSF and Harrington rod instrumentation before 11 years of age. They recognized that anterior growth was accommodated by narrowing of intervertebral disc spaces initially, but finally the vertebral bodies bulged laterally toward the convexity and pivoted on the posterior fusion, resulting in loss of correction, increasing vertebral rotation, and recurrence of the rib hump. Dubousset et al. [3] applied the term "crankshaft phenomenon" to the progression of a deformity after a solid posterior spinal fusion. They reviewed 40 children with idiopathic and neuromuscular scoliosis treated by posterior spinal fusion and Harrington or Luque rod instrumentation prior to Risser stage one. Thirty-nine patients had curve progression over the postoperative follow-up period. They noted that progression was an inevitable consequence of asymmetry of remaining growth between the anterior and posterior columns and that it was proportional to the number of vertebrae fused and the number of years of growth remaining. Later, other authors also reported the progression after PSF in immature patients with idiopathic scoliosis [11, 12, 18, 21, 24].

Quantification of the crankshaft phenomenon is difficult clinically and radiographically, since the changes in curve measurement do not entirely represent the emergence of crankshaft phenomenon. Lee and Nachemson [12] reported on 63 consecutive patients with idiopathic scoliosis who were all in Risser sign 0 at the time of surgery. Eight patients showed rotational progression with no increases in curve measurement. Five patients demonstrated curve progression but no rotational progression. These findings were also supported by Dubousset et al. [3]. Consequently, the evaluation of the crankshaft phenomenon should include not only the curve measurement but also rotational changes, increased lateral trunk shift, changes in apical rib–vertebral angle, translation of the apical vertebra toward the chest wall, and changes of rib deformity.

29.2.3 Prediction and Prevention of Crankshaft Phenomenon

Since the crankshaft phenomenon is related to the remaining asymmetric anterior growth potential, maturity signs such as the Risser sign [12], the Tanner stage [21], the presence of open triradiate cartilage [6, 11, 21, 24], the peak height velocity [24], and chronologic age [12] must be evaluated in the prediction of crankshaft phenomenon. Sanders et al. [24] reviewed 43 idiopathic scoliosis patients who had undergone a PSF at a Risser grade 0 at a mean age of 12.4 years. Open triradiate cartilages were observed in 23 patients and closed triradiate cartilages in 20 patients. After a mean of 4 years of follow-up, the crankshaft phenomenon was seen in one patient who had a closed triradiate cartilage and in 10 patients who had the open triradiate cartilages. There was a mean curve increase of 22° in these patients. However, Hamil et al. [6] reported, based on 33 patients (14 idiopathic, 11 congenital, 5 dysplastic, and 3 neuromuscular) who were Risser 0 preoperatively, that an open triradiate cartilage was not an absolute prognostic predictor for the occurrence of crankshaft phenomenon. Besides preoperative curve magnitude, rotational magnitude, apical rib–vertebral angle, residual curve magnitude, and thoracic versus lumbar curve location, further evaluations were assumed to be predictive factors [18, 23, 24, 26]. Lee and Nachemson [12] reported a model using three factors: chronologic age, skeletal age, and apical rib–vertebral angle difference (RVAD) for prediction of postoperative curve progression. Using this three-factor model, 81% of all patients were classified correctly as progressive or nonprogressive with a false-positive rate of 10%.

Thus far, the only method to prevent the crankshaft phenomenon is an anterior intervertebral fusion. Dubousset et al. [3] discussed that younger patients might require a combined anterior and posterior fusion to achieve stable correction. However, the precise indications for an anterior fusion are still controversial. A patient with Risser sign 0 is not a sufficient candidate for combined anterior and posterior fusion. The iliac crest apophysis ossification first appears at a mean of 8 months after menarche [8, 25]. Furthermore, menarche also was not predictive for the progression of deformity since menarche occurred about 2 years after the onset of the pubertal growth spurt, and there was a less than a 3% increase in height after menarche [1, 2, 22]. An open triradiate radiographical cartilage or observed radiographically is believed to be useful in determining the candidate for anterior fusion in patients with Risser sign 0 [11, 21, 24]. Lapinsky and Richards [11] concluded that in skeletally immature children (open triradiate cartilage and Risser sign 0) with idiopathic scoliosis, the addition of anterior spinal fusion with a posterior spinal fusion and segmental spinal instrumentation was helpful in preventing the crankshaft phenomenon. Roberto et al. [21] reported that anterior and posterior spinal fusion should be considered in prepubertal (Tanner I) patients with open triradiate cartilages.

29.3 Spinal Fusion with or Without Instrumentation in Congenital Scoliosis

Spinal fusion without instrumentation is commonly performed for congenital scoliosis. Spinal instrumentation is becoming more widely used for congenital scoliosis since it allows earlier postoperative ambulatory treatment, better intraoperative correction, and may reduce the incidence of pseudoarthrosis. Hall et al. [4] reviewed 31 patients who underwent a PSF for congenital scoliosis and compared those with Harrington rod instrumentation to those who had no instrumentation. They concluded that fusion without instrumentation was sufficient if a curve was of lesser magnitude that did not need correction (less than 40°, with no trunk imbalance). However, Harrington rod instrumentation could obtain and maintain better correction more consistently than was possible using a corrective postoperative cast without instrumentation. Winter et al. [31] reviewed 323 cases of congenital scoliosis who underwent PSF with or without Harrington rod instrumentation. Two hundred and ninety cases were operated between the ages of 5 and 19 years and were followed for 2 years or more with a mean follow-up of 6 years. He divided the patient into two groups: instrumented and non-instrumented. The instrumented group was older (mean age, 12.8 years when compared with 9.8 years) and had a slightly more severe curve (mean, 58° compared with 53°). Though the demographics of the groups were slightly different, the correction rate was better in the instrumented group (36% when compared with 28%). The mean loss of correction was same (6°) in both groups, and the pseudoarthrosis rates were almost same (6.2% in the instrumented group with 7.4% in the non-instrumented group when compared). The numbers of patients with significant curve progression were also similar (13% in the instrumented group with 14% in the non-instrumented group). However, infection and paralysis were seen only in the instrumented group. The two patients with paraplegia were treated without wake-up test or intraoperative spinal cord monitoring. They concluded that Harrington rod instrumentation allowed slightly better correction but was associated with the only cases of paraplegia and infection in his series. However, larger curves in older children appear to be appropriate for instrumentation, since the curve correction and maintenance of the correction was more difficult by a plaster cast alone.

29.4 Crankshaft Phenomenon in Congenital Scoliosis

The crankshaft phenomenon has been documented in children with congenital scoliosis who have had early PSF [10, 14, 27, 30, 31]. Previous reports by Winter et al. [30, 31] showed that 14% of patients had recognized curve progression of more than 10°. The concept of crankshaft phenomenon was not established at that time. Terek et al. [27] reviewed 23 patients who were operated on before 10 years of age. Operative procedures consisted of various kinds of posterior spinal fusions as well as anterior and posterior hemiepiphysiodeses. Seven of the 23 patients had curves that progressed more than 10°, and 6 of these demonstrated a crankshaft phenomenon. Kesling et al. [10] reviewed 54 patients with congenital scoliosis treated with a PSF. The patients were all classified as Risser 0 and with open triradiate cartilages. They were followed until the end of growth (mean follow-up period of 12 years). The crankshaft phenomenon, measured as a curve increase of more than 10°, was seen in 15% of the patients.

The crankshaft phenomenon can be prevented by an anterior spinal fusion [10, 16, 27]. However, prediction of crankshaft is more difficult than in idiopathic scoliosis because of complicated asymmetric anterior growth caused by vertebral anomalies. Terek et al. [27] reported that the only statistically predictive factor in their study was the length of follow-up. Kesling et al. [10] reported that an earlier surgery and a larger (>50°) curve at the time of surgery were the predictive factors for the crankshaft phenomenon. Lopez-Sosa et al. [14] reported a review of 84 patients with single curves. Sixty-five patients eventually underwent spinal fusion and 19 were treated nonoperatively with bracing or observation. The incidence of crankshaft phenomenon and curve progression varied with the complexity of vertebral deformities. Thus, they concluded that because of the uncertainty of remaining growth potential in congenitally dysplastic vertebrae, future growth in the spine should be considered before undertaking operative procedures.

References

1. Anderson M, Hwang SC, Green WT (1965) Growth of the normal trunk in boys and girls during the second decade of life; related to age, maturity, and ossification of the iliac epiphyses. J Bone Joint Surg Am 47:1554–1564
2. Calvo IJ (1957) Observations on the growth of the female adolescent spine and its relation to scoliosis. Clin Orthop 10:40–47
3. Dubousset J, Herring JA, Shufflebarger H (1989) The crankshaft phenomenon. J Pediatr Orthop 9:541–550
4. Hall JE, Herndon WA, Levine CR (1981) Surgical treatment of congenital scoliosis with or without Harrington instrumentation. J Bone Joint Surg Am 63:608–619
5. Hallock H, Francis KC, Jones JB (1957) Spine fusion in young children; a long-term end-result study with particular reference to growth effects. J Bone Joint Surg Am 39-A: 481–491
6. Hamill CL, Bridwell KH, Lenke LG et al (1997) Posterior arthrodesis in the skeletally immature patient. Assessing the risk for crankshaft: is an open triradiate cartilage the answer? Spine 22:1343–1351
7. Hefti FL, McMaster MJ (1983) The effect of the adolescent growth spurt on early posterior spinal fusion in infantile and juvenile idiopathic scoliosis. J Bone Joint Surg Br 65: 247–254
8. Izumi Y (1995) The accuracy of Risser staging. Spine 20:1868–1871
9. Johnson JTH, Southwick WO (1960) Bone growth after spine fusion: a clinical survey. J Bone Joint Surg Am 42:1396–1412
10. Kesling KL, Lonstein JE, Denis F et al (2003) The crankshaft phenomenon after posterior spinal arthrodesis for congenital scoliosis: a review of 54 patients. Spine 28:267–271
11. Lapinksy AS, Richards BS (1995) Preventing the crankshaft phenomenon by combining anterior fusion with posterior instrumentation. Does it work? Spine 20:1392–1398
12. Lee CS, Nachemson AL (1997) The crankshaft phenomenon after posterior Harrington fusion in skeletally immature patients with thoracic or thoracolumbar idiopathic scoliosis followed to maturity. Spine 22:58–67
13. Letts RM, Bobecbko WP (1974) Fusion of the scoliotic spine in young children. Clin Orthop 101:136–145
14. Lopez-Sosa F, Guille JT, Bowen JR (1995) Rotation of the spine in congenital scoliosis. J Pediatr Orthop 15:528–534
15. McMaster MJ, Macnicol MF (1979) The management of progressive infantile idiopathic scoliosis. J Bone Joint Surg Br 61:36–42

16. McMaster MJ, Ohtsuka K (1982) The natural history of congenital scoliosis. A study of hundred and fifty-one patients. J Bone Joint Surg Am 64:1128–1147
17. Moe JH, Sundberg B, Gustilo R (1964) A clinical study of spine fusion in the growing child. J Bone Joint Surg Br 46:784–785
18. Mullaji AB, Upadhyay SS, Luk KD et al (1994) Vertebral growth after posterior spinal fusion for idiopathic scoliosis in skeletally immature adolescents. The effect of growth on spinal deformity. J Bone Joint Surg Br 76:870–876
19. Risser JC, Norquist DM, Cockrell BR Jr et al (1966) The effect of posterior spine fusion on the growing spine. Clin Orthop Relat Res 46:127–139
20. Roaf R (1960) Vertebral growth and its mechanical control. J Bone Joint Surg Br 42:40–59
21. Roberto RF, Lonstein JE, Winter RB et al (1997) Curve progression in Risser stage 0 or 1 patients after posterior spinal fusion for idiopathic scoliosis. J Pediatr Orthop 17: 718–725
22. Root AW (1973) Endocrinology of puberty. I. Normal sexual maturation. J Pediatr 83:1–19
23. Sanders JO, Evert M, Stanley EA et al (1992) Mechanisms of curve progression following sublaminar (Luque) spinal instrumentation. Spine 17:781–789
24. Sanders JO, Herring JA, Browne RH (1995) Posterior arthrodesis and instrumentation in the immature (Risser-grade-0) spine in idiopathic scoliosis. J Bone Joint Surg Am 77: 39–45
25. Scoles PV, Salvagno R, Villalba K et al (1988) Relationship of iliac crest maturation to skeletal and chronologic age. J Pediatr Orthop 8:639–644
26. Shufflebarger HL, Clark CE (1991) Prevention of the crankshaft phenomenon. Spine 16:S409–S411
27. Terek RM, Wehner J, Lubicky JP (1991) Crankshaft phenomenon in congenital scoliosis: a preliminary report. J Pediatr Orthop 11:527–532
28. Winter RB (1971) The effects of early fusion on spine growth. In: Zorab PA (ed) Scoliosis and growth. Churchill Livingstone, Edinburgh, London, pp 98–104
29. Winter RB (1977) Scoliosis and spinal growth. Orthop Rev 6:17–20
30. Winter RB, Moe JH (1982) The results of spinal arthrodesis for congenital spinal deformity in patients younger than five years old. J Bone Joint Surg Am 64:419–432
31. Winter RB, Moe JH, Lonstein JE (1984) Posterior spinal arthrodesis for congenital scoliosis. An analysis of the cases of two hundred and ninety patients, five to nineteen years old. J Bone Joint Surg Am 66:1188–1197

30 Convex Growth Arrest for Congenital Scoliosis

Muharrem Yazici and Ozgur Dede

Key Points

- Convex growth arrest (CGA) has been used in patients with congenital spinal deformity, enabling the progression to cease or even reverse the deformity with subsequent growth of the spinal column.
- Growth control of the convex side, which is relatively longer along the length of the vertebral column than the concave side, not only stops progression but also leads to spontaneous correction given that the concave side has growth potential.
- CGA is accepted as a safe procedure that generally does not result in serious complications. More significant problems include unpredictability of the curve behavior after the procedure, and incapability to control the spinal balance.

30.1 Background

The physes (growth plates) are the cartilage zones between the metaphysis and epiphysis of bones that are responsible for the major part of longitudinal growth of long bones. Owing to the imbalances in the growth of the physeal plates, a variety of deformities arise on the extremities, such as limb length discrepancies and angular deformities. Modulation of growth on one or both sides of a growth plate is therefore a potential treatment alternative for the growing skeletons. Thus, limb length discrepancy and deformity correction that interferes with the development at the growth plates has long been tried and practiced since the early 1930s [17, 19, 27, 8].

Congenital spinal deformities result from anomalous vertebrae that in the end produce deformities in the coronal and sagittal planes due to the longitudinal growth imbalances. Typically, there are hemivertebrae or bars that cause an imbalanced growth of the vertebral column, causing convexity and concavity occurring simultaneously on opposite sides. Modulation of vertebral growth on either the convex or concave side of the curve (growth arrest or growth enhancement, respectively) theoretically seems to be an early and effective treatment alternative for the growing spine. Early attempts at arresting growth of the convex side have been reported, notably that of stapling performed by Smith et al. [23]. Then, in 1963 Roaf [21] reported his surgical technique and corresponding patient outcome in utilizing unilateral growth arrest for congenital scoliosis. Convex anterior and posterior growth arrest has been used in patients with congenital spinal deformity, enabling the progression to cease or even reverse the deformity with subsequent growth of the spinal column [1, 3, 6, 10, 11, 24, 26, 29, 30]. Theoretically, growth control of the convex side, which is relatively longer along the length of the vertebral column than the concave side, not only stops progression but also leads to spontaneous correction given that the concave side has growth potential. The convex growth arrest (CGA) procedure based on this concept has been popularized due to its safety, efficacy, and simplicity when compared with other surgical alternatives [1, 3, 6, 10, 11, 24, 26, 29, 30, 32].

M. Yazici (✉)
Department of Orthopaedics and Traumatology,
Hacettepe University, Faculty of Medicine,
06100 Sihhiye, Ankara, Turkey
e-mail: yazioglu@hacettepe.edu.tr

B. A. Akbarnia et al. (eds.), *The Growing Spine*,
DOI: 10.1007/978-3-540-85207-0_30, © Springer-Verlag Berlin Heidelberg 2011

30.2 Classical Indications and Contraindications

CGA is not suitable for every congenital spinal deformity. Several criteria have been defined in the literature. These commonly accepted criteria dictate a purely scoliotic curve composed of less than five segments with a magnitude of less than 70° in a patient not over 5 years of age. Sagittal plane deformity, cervical involvement, intraspinal anomalies, posterior arch defects (e.g. myelomeningocele), and unilateral bars are considered to be contraindications for this procedure.

30.3 Techniques

The original technique described by Winter [30] and Andrew et al. [1] consists of anterior and posterior interventions to the spinal column. Separate anterior and posterior exposures are performed; these surgeries can be done either during the same session or with a week in between. Initially, the cartilaginous end plates and the intervening discs are partially excised whereby the gap is filled with bone grafts using an anterior approach to the spinal column. Then, using a posterior approach, the zygoepiphyseal facet joints are removed and filled with bone grafts to produce a fusion effect. A protective cast is applied 4–7 days after the operation. It is then removed at 4–6 months when the fusion is evident on radiographs.

30.4 Results

One of the earliest studies by Smith et al. [23] did not report any improvement with their stapling method, which was argued to be due to the anatomy and the bony structure of the vertebrae. It was further argued that the growth rate of the vertebrae is much less than those of the long bones, as well as the soft cancellous bone not causing enough compression on the endplates. Roaf [21] reported his results of using anterior epiphysiodesis and posterior intra-articular fusion on 188 patients. There were no cases of complete correction, only those with limited improvement. These results were argued by Andrew et al. [1] to be partly due to the extra pleural approach that only provided a limited exposure and resection of the posterior ends of several ribs on the convex side.

Marks et al. [14] reported results for the use of anterior and posterior convex hemiepiphysiodesis for congenital scoliosis with a mean follow-up period of 8.8 years on 57 patients. Furthermore, the rate of change of the Cobb angle was decreased but not reversed when deformity was due to an unsegmented bar. For the complex anomalies, they reported an increase in the final Cobb angle from a mean of 61° to 70°. The rate of progression reversed or decreased in 97% of the hemivertebra patients, with a change in the mean Cobb angle from 41° pre-operatively to 35° post-operatively. Lumbar anomalies and the younger patient age resulted in better corrections. Additionally, Uzumcugil et al. [25] reported their results on 32 patients utilizing anterior and posterior approaches. Forty-one percent of the patients had true epiphysiodesis effect, 47% of the patients had fusion, and only 12% of the patients showed an increase in the curvature in an average follow-up of 40 months.

The classically defined indications of the procedure have been commonly stretched by a number of authors. There are conflicting reports in the literature when the variables that are commonly accepted to affect the outcome of the convex hemiepiphysiodesis surgery are considered. A recent paper by Uzumcugil et al. [25] scrutinized these variables in a series of 32 patients and also provided an extensive review of the series in the literature. The fusion, epiphysiodesis effects, and progression rates were calculated collectively among the studies. Anomalies consisting of hemivertebrae instead of unsegmented bars have repeatedly been reported to yield a more favorable outcome [1, 6, 10, 12, 24, 30]. This may be originating from the fact that in the presence of an unsegmented bar it is believed to be impossible for the concavity to grow. On the other hand, it has also been shown that fusion of the one upper and one lower segment of the bar may result in an improvement of the deformity. From natural history studies, it is known that more severe and progressive deformities occur either in the thoracolumbar region [16, 22] or the thoracic spine [31]. However, Thompson et al. [24] reported that hemivertebra in the lumbar spine had the best prognosis when treated with CGA. Walhout et al.

reported that complex deformities in the thoracolumbar and upper thoracic regions were more favorable than those in the lower thoracic region when CGA was the treatment modality [26]. These mixed results show that there is no preference between the upper and lower spine for CGA. For a successful CGA, the preoperative curve magnitude was reported to be less than 50–60° [16] whereas there are other studies showing that curves less than 70° also have favorable results [10, 11, 30]. The number of vertebrae included in the curve was also reported to have an effect on the outcome of the surgery. Best results were reported with curves that affect five consecutive segments or less [10, 11, 30]. On the other hand, longer curves have been successfully treated with CGA (25). Presence of an intraspinal anomaly, either treated or not, does not seem to have a negative effect on the progression of congenital curves [9, 15, 18, 28]. However, Reigel et al. [20] reported that the technique of release of tethering for lumbar and sacral scoliosis produces a stabilized or improved scoliosis, whereas it does not stop the progression of scoliosis in the thoracic level. The upper age limit set for an effective CGA was reported to be 5 years [1] since most of the vertebral growth occurs before this age. However, it should be noted that other work has suggested that the procedure is effective in children older than 5 years without signs of advanced skeletal maturity [10, 25]. Although the existence of a sagittal plane abnormality (i.e., kyphosis or lordosis) is accepted as a contraindication for CGA, this issue has not been discussed in detail [1, 10, 24, 26, 30]. Comprehensive analysis of the literature reveals two possible effects of a sagittal plane abnormality on the outcome of CGA: progression of sagittal plane deformity despite well-stabilized scoliosis [8], or unsatisfactory control of the deformity in all three planes [1, 10, 26, 27]. Dubousset et al. [6] and Kieffer and Dubousset [11] reported that CGA could be used even in patients with kyphoscoliosis or lordoscoliosis. Their findings appeared to contradict with the assumption that the presence of a sagittal plane deformity negatively affects the outcome of the CGA procedure as mentioned above (Fig. 30.1).

As can be seen overall, none of the variables including age, type of the anomaly, presence of sagittal deformity or intraspinal anomaly, and the length of the curve were found to significantly affect the outcome of the procedure.

30.5 Problems

CGA is accepted as a safe procedure that generally does not result in serious complications except for infections (wound or chest) and traction neuropraxias of either the intercostals or thigh cutaneous nerves, which are related to anterior surgery [1, 3, 6, 10, 11, 21, 24, 26, 29, 30]. More significant problems include unpredictability of the curve behavior after the procedure, and incapability to control the spinal balance.

30.6 Proposed Solutions and Modifications

For each of the drawbacks mentioned previously, potential solutions were proposed by a number of authors. Keller et al. [10] and King et al. [12] reported an alternative method, which avoids the anterior surgery and thus the risks related to it. This method consists of a posterior approach utilizing transpedicular curettage of the endplates anteriorly. Posterior hemiepiphysiodesis is done as in the original technique. Transpedicular approach has potential advantages over the standard two-staged operation in that it decreases the neurovascular complications by avoiding the anterior approach. On the other hand, a potential disadvantage is the chance for an incomplete hemiepiphysiodesis of the anterior endplates, which in turn might cause rotational deformities.

Bandi et al. [2] reported a modified technique that spares the segmental vessels during the anterior epiphysiodesis surgery in order to decrease the neurological complications. It was argued that as the level of segmental vessel ligation increased, there was a corresponding increase in the risk of spinal cord damage; therefore, it was suggested that caution should be taken when several segmental arteries are to be ligated in the clinical setting.

Anterior and posterior hemiepiphysiodesis using a transpedicular approach with short segment instrumentation follow-up was reported by Ginsburg et al. [7]. Their series, however, consisted of ten patients with an average follow-up time of 29.7 months. They reported either no improvement or a decrease in the curves of seven of their patients. Conclusions were drawn that CGA with a transpedicular approach is an

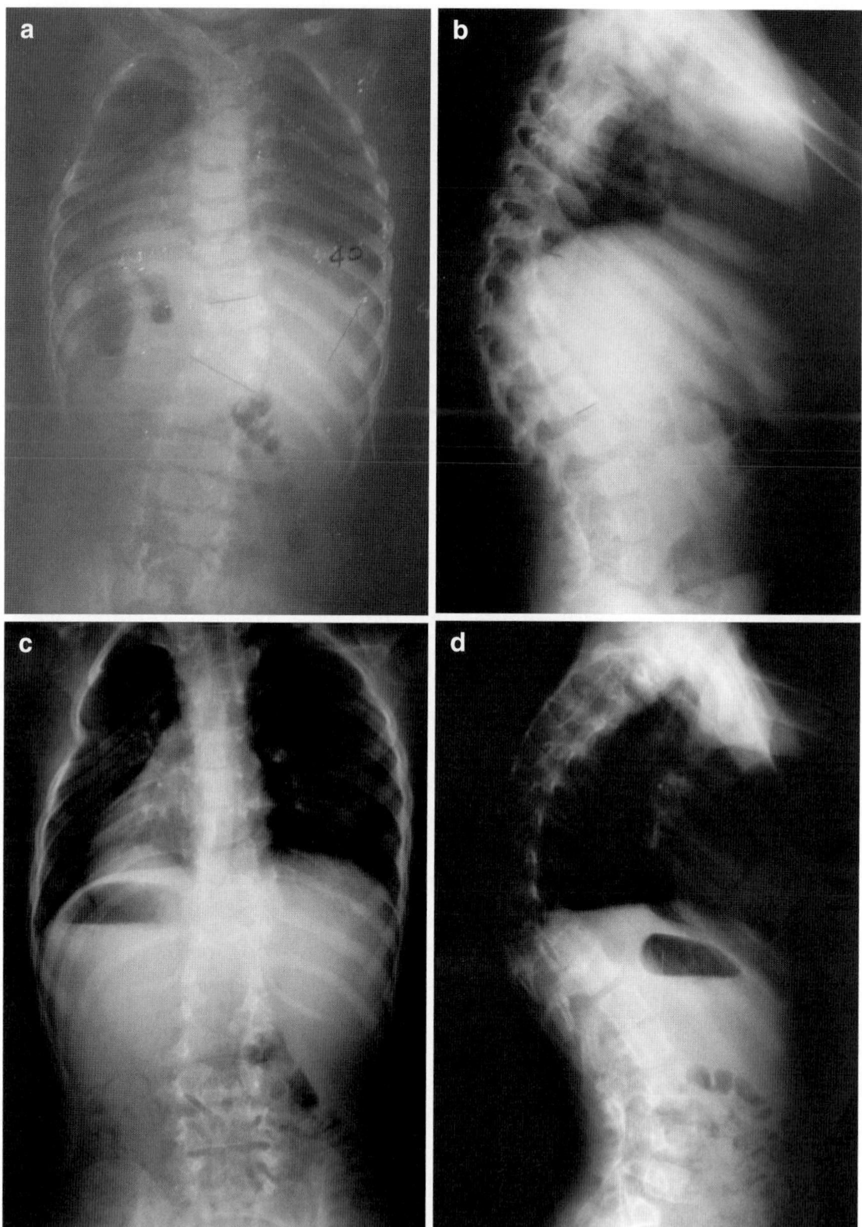

Fig. 30.1 (**a**) Thoracolumbar scoliosis and (**b**) a concurrent sagittal plane deformity in a 4-year-old patient. Fourth-year follow-up radiographs showing almost total correction of (**c**) spinal deformity with (**d**) slight improvement in the sagittal deformity

effective method for congenital scoliosis, especially when done earlier in premenarche patients and patients with open triradiate cartilages.

Cheung et al. [4] reported their results using convex hemiepiphysiodesis with concave distraction. They suggested that this procedure could be recommended for children with severe deformities and decompensation in the lower thoracic spine. The concave distraction produces immediate improvement in the coronal balance such that there is no need to wait for uncertain growth-mediated correction in patients who undergo convex fusion only.

Another modification that has been proposed by the Hacettepe group is the addition of posterior instrumentation with transpedicular screws [33]. Specifically, transpedicular screws were shown to control growth of the vertebral column in both longitudinal [13] and transverse planes [5] in animal studies. Transpedicular screws were placed in all the vertebrae that were fused to eliminate the need for an anterior surgery and acute

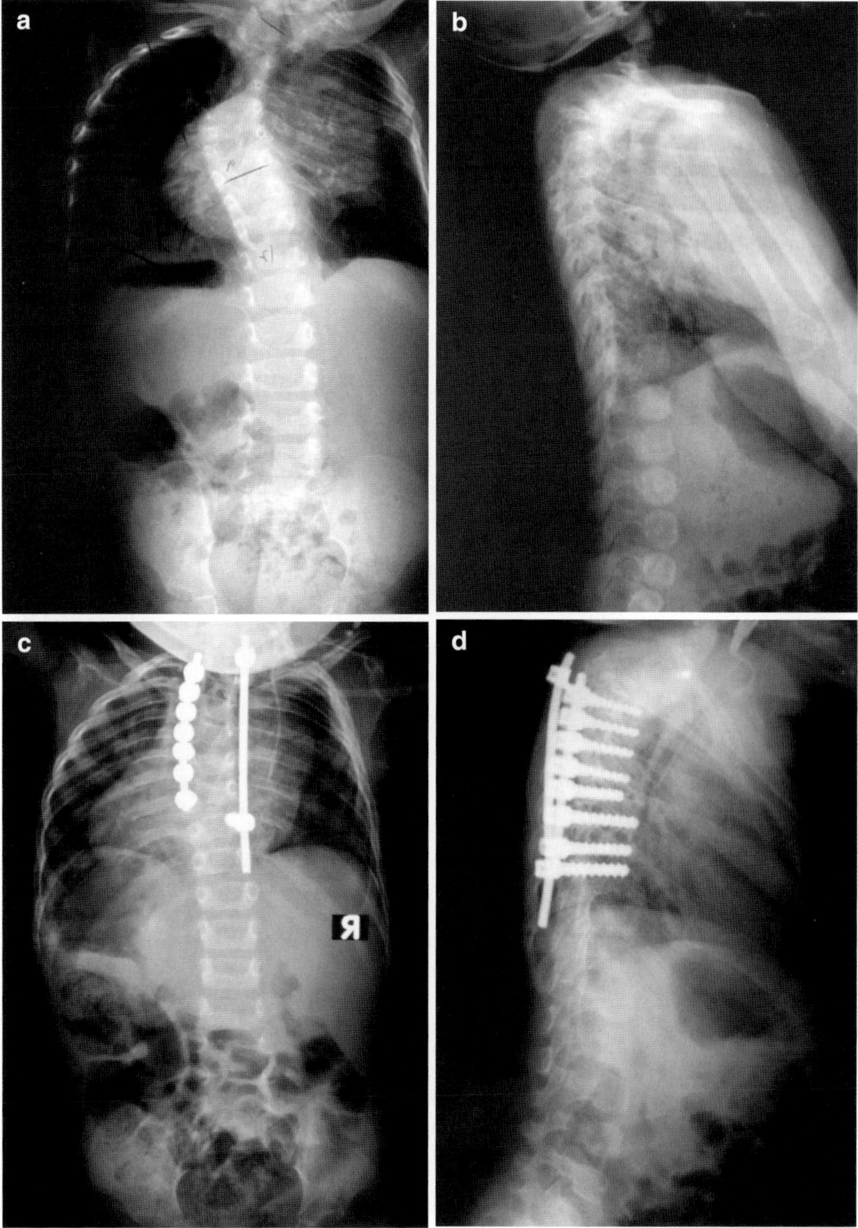

Fig. 30.2 Young female patient (1.5 years of age) with a *left* thoracic scoliosis shown from (**a**) anteroposterior and (**b**) mediolateral views prior to treatment. Patient after convex hemiepiphysiodesis and concave distraction that provided (**c**) accurate correction of the deformity while (**d**) the concave distraction reduced trunk imbalance

compression-rotation maneuvers were employed to correct the deformity in ten patients. Added posterior instrumentation provided an initial correction, thereby decreasing the unpredictability of the curve. This procedure controls the progression of the curve and provides a correction of the deformity although trunk balance is not achieved in every case. Therefore, recently concave distraction without fusion has been added to convex compression and fusion as it might better achieve trunk balance in patients (Fig. 30.2).

30.7 Conclusion

CGA appears to be an effective procedure to halt the progression of the curve with an expected correction over time in scoliosis patients without signs of advanced skeletal maturity. Overall, the main problem seems to be the unpredictability of the results. To alleviate this problem, there have been several proposed solutions, but it is still quite early to make conclusions, since there are no long-term studies on such modifications.

In younger children, for cosmetically acceptable curves, CGA is still a very valid alternative. For more severe and imbalanced curves, hemivertebrectomy or apical vertebral resection and addition of instrumentation can generally be the treatment of choice. However, when major reconstructive surgeries are considered too risky because of the age of the child, CGA can be considered a way to stabilize the deformity until the child grows. In this way, further reconstruction is not precluded.

References

1. Andrew T, Piggott H (1985) Growth arrest for progressive scoliosis: combined anterior and posterior fusion of the convexity. J Bone Joint Surg [Br] 67:193–197
2. Bandi S, Davis BJ, Ahmed el-NB (2007) Segmental vessel sparing during convex growth arrest surgery–a modified technique. Spine J 7(3):349–352
3. Bradford DS (1982) Partial epiphyseal arrest and supplemental fixation for progressive correction of congenital spinal deformity. J Bone Joint Surg [Am] 64:610–614
4. Cheung KM, Zhang JG, Lu DS et al (2002) Ten-year follow-up study of lower thoracic hemivertebrae treated by convex fusion and concave distraction. Spine 27(7):748–753
5. Cil A, Yazici M, Daglioglu K et al (2005) The effect of pedicle screw placement with or without application of compression across the neurocentral cartilage on the morphology of the spinal canal and pedicle in immature pigs. Spine 30(11): 1287–1293
6. Dubousset J, Katti E, Seringe R (1993) Epiphysiodesis of the spine in young children for congenital spinal deformities. J Pediatr Orthop 1:123–130
7. Ginsburg G, Mulconrey DS, Browdy J (2007) Transpedicular hemiepiphysiodesis and posterior instrumentation as a treatment for congenital scoliosis. J Pediatr Orthop 27(4):387–391
8. Green WT, Anderson M (1947) Experiences with epiphyseal arrest in correcting discrepancies in length of the lower extremities in infantile paralysis; a method of predicting the effect. J Bone Joint Surg 29:659
9. Keim HA, Greene AF (1973) Diastematomyelia and scoliosis. J Bone Joint Surg [Am] 55:1425–1435
10. Keller PM, Lindseth RE, DeRosa GP (1994) Progressive congenital scoliosis treatment using a transpedicular anterior and posterior convex hemiepiphysiodesis and hemiarthrodesis. Spine 19:1933–1939
11. Kieffer J, Dubousset J (1994) Combined anterior and posterior convex epiphysiodesis for progressive congenital scoliosis in children aged less or equal 5 years. Eur Spine J 3:120–125
12. King AG, MacEwen GD, Bose WJ (1992) Transpedicular convex anterior hemiepiphysiodesis and posterior arthrodesis for progressive congenital scoliosis. Spine 17:S291–S294
13. Kioschos HC, Asher MA, Lark RG et al (1996) Overpowering the crankshaft mechanism. The effect of posterior spinal fusion with and without stiff transpedicular fixation on anterior spinal column growth in immature canines. Spine 21(10):1168–1173
14. Marks DS, Sayampanathan SR, Thompson AG et al (1995) Long-term results of convex epiphysiodesis for congenital scoliosis. Eur Spine J 4(5):296–301
15. McMaster MJ, Ohtsuka K (1982) The natural history of congenital scoliosis: a study of two hundred and fifty-one patients. J Bone Joint Surg [Am] 64:1128–1147
16. McMaster MJ (1984) Occult intraspinal anomalies and congenital scoliosis. J Bone Joint Surg [Am] 66:588–601
17. Métaizeau JP, Wong-Chung J, Bertrand H et al (1998) Percutaneous epiphysiodesis using transphyseal screws (PETS). J Pediatr Orthop 18:363
18. Miller A, Guille JT, Bowen JR (1993) Evaluation and treatment of diastematomyelia. J Bone Joint Surg [Am] 75:1308–1317
19. Phemister DB (1993) Operative arrestment of longitudinal growth of bones in the treatment of deformities. J Bone Joint Surg 15:1
20. Reigel DH, Tchernouka K, Bazmi B et al (1994) Change in spinal curvature following release of tethered spinal cord associated with spina bifida. Pediatr Neurosurg 10:30–42
21. Roaf R (1963) The treatment of progressive scoliosis by unilateral growth-arrest. J Bone Joint Surg [Br] 45:637–651
22. Shahcheraghi GH, Hobbi MH (1999) Patterns and progression in congenital scoliosis. J Pediatr Orthop 19:766–775
23. Smith A, De F, von Lackum WH, Wylie R (1954) An operation for stapling vertebral bodies in congenital scoliosis. J Bone Joint Surg [Am] 36-A:342–348
24. Thompson AG, Marks DS, Sayampanathan SR et al (1995) Long-term results of combined anterior and posterior convex epiphysiodesis for congenital scoliosis due to hemivertebrae. Spine 20(12):1380–1385
25. Uzumcugil A, Cil A, Yazici M et al (2004) Convex growth arrest in the treatment of congenital spinal deformities, revisited. J Pediatr Orthop 24(6):658–666
26. Walhout RJ, van Rhijn LW, Pruijs JEH (2002) Hemi-epiphysiodesis for unclassified congenital scoliosis: immediate results and mid-term follow-up. Eur Spine J 11: 543–549
27. White JW, Stubbins SG (1944) Growth arrest for equalizing leg lengths. JAMA 126:1146
28. Winter RB, Moe JH, Eilers VE (1968) Congenital scoliosis. A study of 234 patients treated and untreated. Part I-II. J Bone Joint Surg [Am] 50:1–47
29. Winter RB, Haven JJ, Moe JH et al (1974) Diastematomyelia and congenital spinal deformities. J Bone Joint Surg [Am] 56:27–39
30. Winter RB (1981) Convex anterior and posterior hemiarthrodesis and hemiepiphysiodesis in young children with progressive congenital scoliosis. J Pediatr Orthop 1:361–366
31. Winter RB, Lonstein JE, Denis F et al (1988) Convex growth arrest for progressive congenital scoliosis due to hemivertebra. J Pediatr Orthop 8:633–638
32. Winter RB, Lonstein JE, Boachei-Adjei O (1996) Congenital spinal deformity. J Bone Joint Surg [Am] 78:300–311
33. Yazici M, Demirkiran HG, Ahmadi H et al (2007) Instrumented convex hemiepiphysiodesis in treatment of congenital scoliosis. J Child Orthop I:255–276

31 Kyphectomy in Myelomeningocele

John F. Sarwark, Ritesh R. Shah, and Neel Jain

Key Points

- Kyphectomy in myelomeningocoele requires careful preoperative evaluation and postoperative care
- Kyphectomy is a technically demanding procedure
- Kyphectomy is safe and efficacious when techniques are used that reduce perioperative morbidity

31.1 Background

Intervention to restore sagittal balance has been well accepted in patients with severe kyphotic deformities to improve postural stability and sitting balance. Kyphectomy-type reconstructive surgery can be a useful treatment modality, specifically in patients with myelomeningocele, to achieve this goal. With significant sagittal plane spinal deformities, kyphectomy and instrumentation allows for satisfactory long-term correction.

The indications and surgical technique have been well described in the literature. With recent advances in operative techniques, the procedure has demonstrated safety and efficacy as an effective surgical management for the child with severe sagittal plane deformity and for the orthopaedic surgeon.

Myelomeningocele is defined as a defect of the neural tube during embryonal development. With failure of closure of the caudad end of the neural tube, there is a resulting sac that may contain spinal cord, nerve roots, and meninges [7]. Commonly, the level of the defect correlates with the patient's neurological deficits. Congenital vertebral anomalies, some producing scoliosis and kyphosis, have been associated with myelomeningocele secondary to the malformations that occur. Kyphotic deformities in myelomeningocele, although not as common as scoliosis, are commonly associated with high motor level deficit involving thoracic or upper lumbar levels [3, 9, 17].

The kyphotic deformity in myelomeningocele patients is progressive and as a result, one must consider early intervention (see also Chaps. 20 and 34). Kyphosis progression can approximate 8° annually in most children, and patients may already have a significant deformity present at birth [17]. The underlying progressive nature of the curve has been attributed to the lack of muscular stabilization. The erector spinae musculature are displaced anterior to the axis of the spine and, with a hypertrophied psoas and the tenodesis effect of the crus of the diaphragm, create a strong flexor moment on the spine. Additionally, once patients become upright with sitting, the flexion moment arm is compounded by gravity and a progressive kyphotic deformity results. Ultimately, the deformity becomes fixed and structural and the vertebral bodies become wedge-shaped [2, 3].

31.2 Medical/Neurosurgical Issues

Prior to early neurosurgical intervention, the mortality rate of patients with myelomeningocele was as high as 90–100% [16]. With early intervention including sac closure and ventriculoperitoneal shunt placement,

J.F. Sarwark (✉)
Department of Orthopaedic Surgery, The Children's Memorial Hospital, 2300 Children's Plaza, Chicago, IL 60614, USA
e-mail: jsarwark@childrensmemorial.org

B. A. Akbarnia et al. (eds.), *The Growing Spine*,
DOI: 10.1007/978-3-540-85207-0_31, © Springer-Verlag Berlin Heidelberg 2011

the survival rates have significantly improved. There is a very high incidence of associated hydrocephalus necessitating shunt placement. Additionally, owing to an associated abnormal development of the cephalad portion of the neural tube, there is an association with Arnold-Chiari II malformation. Surgical repair of the Chiari II malformation is indicated in up to 15–35% of patients. The procedures include an occipital craniotomy and upper cervical laminectomy for decompression [7].

Another commonly associated neurosurgical condition is tethered spinal cord syndrome. Symptomatic tethering of the spinal cord may occur in 25–30% of patients with myelomeningocele. Given that most patients undergo sac closure, dural scarring is inevitable and almost always seen on magnetic resonance imaging. Therefore, tethered spinal cord syndrome is a clinical diagnosis with radiographic confirmation. Signs and symptoms include back and leg pain, motor and strength deterioration, urodynamic changes, rapid progression of scoliosis or kyphosis, and spasticity/contracture. This condition is treated with tethered cord release (TSCR)-neurosurgical exploration of the scarred dural sac with mobilization of the tight nerve roots and filum terminale. Patients may ultimately not recover their baseline motor or sensory function. Without appropriate recognition and early TSCR an orthopaedic surgeon may not adequately treat a kyphotic deformity if there is an underlying tethered cord syndrome [16, 18].

Associated medical issues with regard to kyphotic deformity in these patients include both urological and gastrointestinal. Patients may have neurogenic bladder dysfunction depending on the level of the spinal cord lesion. This may ultimately lead to urinary incontinence and impaired bladder emptying. Ultimate management may entail prevention of infections and monitoring of renal function. Patients may also have an abnormal anal sphincter tone and anorectal sensation leading to problems with bowel incontinence and constipation [7].

Non-surgical management of the kyphotic deformity usually proves futile. With the abnormal posture that results from the kyphotic deformity, patients often rely on the upper extremities for sitting stability and support. A patient may experience severe loss of independence as there is a dependence on use of the hands for sitting. Conservative, non-surgical treatment including bracing has proven to be ineffective and ultimately does not prevent progression. Additionally, there may be associated skin breakdown at the level of the spinal deformity and this can lead to a vicious cycle of pressure sores. The ulceration over bony prominences combined with thin, scarred, and insensate skin leads to a difficult problem [2, 3].

31.3 Perioperative Management

Patients require an extensive preoperative evaluation involving a multidisciplinary approach. The neurosurgeon should be actively involved and the ventriculoperitoneal shunt should be tested [3]. Additionally, it can be worthwhile to determine the anatomic course of the abdominal aorta. It has been shown that the abdominal aorta is at little risk during kyphectomy correction surgical techniques as the aorta does not follow the path of the kyphosis, rather spanning it anteriorly [3, 17]. Also, given the potential for chronic wound issues, it might be necessary to consult a plastic surgeon preoperatively to optimize the wound healing potential. It may be necessary to admit the patient preoperatively for wound care, including prone nursing care up to 2 weeks [14]. Postoperatively, the combined involvement of physical and occupational therapy is necessary to aid in the patient's recovery. Additionally, an orthotist may also be utilized to fabricate a thoracolumbosacral orthosis.

31.4 Surgical Strategies: General

The objectives of a kyphectomy procedure are complete restoration of sagittal alignment, balance, and stability while simultaneously allowing the child to grow and achieve appropriate truncal height. Surgical correction for congenital kyphosis is performed for the clinical manifestations of the kyphotic deformity rather than absolute radiological measurements. The primary indications for operative intervention include increasing spinal deformity, the need for primary skin closure over the spinal dysraphic defect and protuberant bone; recurrent decubitus skin ulceration over the kyphotic apex causing chronic debilitation; inability of placement in an upright sitting or standing position without the use of both upper extremities for support; reduction in the anterior abdominal wall available surface area prohibiting necessary gastroenterology or urology procedures and fitting of appliances; significant compression of abdominal contents during upright posture creates upward pressure on the diaphragm and respiratory compromise. Costal margin impingement on the pelvis may cause pain and discomfort [1]. The major contraindications to surgical intervention are associated medical condition prohibiting a surgery of this magnitude [16].

Currently, the most well-studied surgical procedure for kyphectomy is vertebral resection with modified Luque fixation (resection kyphectomy). As shown by Lindseth and Stelzer [8] in 1979, in addition to vertebral resection of the apex of the kyphotic deformity, resection of 1.5–2.5 vertebral bodies cephalad to the apical vertebra must also be performed to best correct the lumbar kyphosis and distal rigid compensatory thoracic lordosis. The extent of resection must extend to the lordotic segment. One of the often cited limitations of this procedure includes the potential inability to allow for complete preservation of the dural sac and subsequent potential life-threatening postoperative complications that may occur, specifically acute hydrocephalus [15]. Additionally, this procedure leads to vertebral shortening and an indirect reduction of tension on the spinal cord [17].

A second, more recent, kyphectomy surgical technique is subtraction (decancellation) vertebrectomy. Conceptually, the decancellation kyphectomy technique is a lordosing intravertebral apical osteotomy over multiple lumbar levels. This procedure obviates the need to perform a cordectomy and the resulting associated morbidities of cerebrospinal fluid flow problems such as meningitis and acute hydrocephalus [17]. Additionally, this method is not a complete resection of a significant portion of the spinal column, allowing for preservation of spinal height. The lordosing kyphectomy is tethered along the length of the anterior longitudinal ligament, thus avoiding tension on neurovascular structures. The advantages of this newer procedure when compared with the prior vertebral resection include a satisfactory sagittal correction, preservation of the dural sac leading to fewer shunt complications, less blood loss, and decreased operative time [15]. The preferred age for surgery seems to be between 2 and 5 years, when the anteroposterior diameter reaches a 25 mm minimum [17].

With either the resection kyphectomy or decancellation kyphectomy, stable instrumentation is required to stabilize the osteotomies and sagittal correction, prevent recurrence, and allow for seating stability. The sacropelvis should be included distally – in most instances – to prevent lumbosacral sagittal plane deformity. Additionally, the instrumentation must correct the developmental thoracic lordosis by including the thoracic spine to the level of T4–T6. A wide range of long-term results has been generated when performing a resection kyphectomy using different instrumentation techniques. However, the current consensus is that segmental posterior spinal instrumentation with inclusion of the sacropelvis is necessary to attain and maintain sagittal correction [10].

31.5 Surgical Technique Specific

31.5.1 Vertebral Resection Kyphectomy Technique

The procedure is performed with the patient under general anesthesia, prone positioning, a radiolucent operating table, and a frame or chest rolls. A posterior midline longitudinal incision is used and developed through the area of previous closure. If a tissue expansion procedure has been completed, the tissue expanders are removed at the conclusion and closure of the case. The thoracic paraspinal muscles are subperiosteally dissected from the thoracic posterior spinal elements. At the lumbosacral junction, the dural sac is dissected, and the proximal stump is oversewn. Evidence of a functioning shunt must be determined preoperatively. Of note, the visualization of cerebrospinal fluid during this portion of the procedure precludes closure of the neural plaque in fear of precipitating acute hydrocephalus [10]. Then, the dural sac is retracted proximal to the osteotomy site.

Dissection is performed laterally and anteriorly around the kyphosis in order to access the sinus of the kyphosis. The kyphectomy is then performed via vertebral excision of the proximal aspect of the apical vertebra and one to two vertebral bodies cephalad to the kyphotic apex [8].

Modified segmental instrumentation using the Luque technique as outlined by McCall [10] may be utilized to correct and stabilize the kyphectomy. Contoured Luque rods are brought through the S1 foramen bilaterally, with the distal ends lying on the anterior aspect of the sacrum. The distal ends of the Luque rods are bent in accordance with the patient's sacral inclination, approximately 20–40°. A cross-link is placed distally near the sacral foramen to prevent rod migration and rotation. The rods are placed just medial to the lateral masses at the level of the osteotomy site and subsequently wired to the higher level thoracic lamina sequentially starting at T4, progressively reducing the osteotomy site and creating more rigid fixation. The osteotomy site is augmented with bone from the vertebrectomy to perform a local arthrodesis.

31.5.2 Subtraction (Decancellation) Kyphectomy Technique

The operation is performed with the patient under general anesthesia and prone positioning using a radiolucent operating table and frame or chest rolls. The procedure is performed through a posterior midline incision. The laminar bars are subperiosteally exposed laterally and medially. The dorsal laminar bar overlying each respective neuroforamen is resected for isolation of each pedicle needed for decancellation. The thecal sac and nerve roots are mobilized medially in the subperiosteal plane. The pedicle is entered with a curette from one side, and the cancellous bone is progressively evacuated from the vertebral body to the midline. Subsequently, this canal is packed and the procedure is repeated on the contralateral side, resulting in a cortical shell of vertebral body. A fine curette is used to etch a line in the anterior cortex of the vertebral body from pedicle to pedicle. The osteotomy will close or hinge on this line. This decancellation procedure is then repeated over contiguous levels from caudad to cephalad, usually beginning at L4 and progressing to L1. A correction of 45° per vertebral level can be expected with restitution of lumbar lordosis, thoracic kyphosis, and sagittal balance [17].

Stable instrumentation is required to stabilize the multilevel osteotomies and correction, prevent recurrence, and allow for seating stability and long-term stability. Again, the sacropelvis must be included distally to prevent lumbosacral sagittal plane deformity. Additionally, the instrumentation must correct the rigid developmental thoracic lordosis by including the thoracic spine to the level of T4–T6. Instrumentation techniques include posterior stabilization with neutral or sagittally contoured, paired rods; segmental thoracic hooks or sublaminar wires; lumbosacral pedicle screw fixation with intrasacral distal rod insertion (Roger Jackson Technique) [6]; and limited arthrodesis at the lumbosacral fixation points allowing growth proximally [15]. Furthermore, a growing construct can be attempted by extraperiosteal dissection for thoracic lamina exposure, limited lumbosacral arthrodesis, preservation of cartilaginous endplates at the decancellated levels, and utilization of segmental thoracic hooks, sublaminar wires, or cables [17].

31.5.3 Results

The results from the resection kyphectomy have varied dependences on the form of instrumentation. However, from these prior studies, it has been agreed that segmental spinal instrumentation with sacral fixation is important to obtain and maintain kyphectomy correction and stability.

Heydemann and Gillespie [4] published the first study reviewing resection kyphectomy and segmental spinal instrumentation, using sublaminar wiring at the osteotomy site supplemented with Luque rods placed anterior to the sacrum distally with average postoperative kyphosis measuring 32.8°. McCarthy et al. [11] in 1989 concluded that long posterior spinal fusion with Luque rod instrumentation achieved the best outcomes; and the Dunn-McCarthy modification involved placement of Luque rods into the sacral ala. In the longest follow-up evaluation of any kyphectomy technique to date, Litner and Lindseth [9] demonstrated that resection kyphectomy resulted in an average correction to 40° kyphosis postoperatively and 62° at follow-up. Huang and Lubicky [5] illustrated that resection kyphectomy and posterior spinal instrumentation using Luque rods resulted in an average correction of 21° postoperatively and 23.7° at follow-up. McCall [10] in 1998 showed an average correction of 15° kyphosis postoperatively and 20° of kyphosis at follow-up assessment with an average postoperative correction of 91°. Overall, these studies and others have demonstrated average postoperative corrections of 84–94% and average final 5 year retained corrections of 81–93% performing resection kyphectomies with rigid segmented fixation with Luque rods [4, 5, 9, 10, 11,12].

On the other hand, the decancellation kyphectomy results as shown by Nolden, et al. [15] Sarwark et al. in 2002 from the author's institution, also demonstrated a substantial improvement in sagittal correction. In this study, the average correction attained immediately

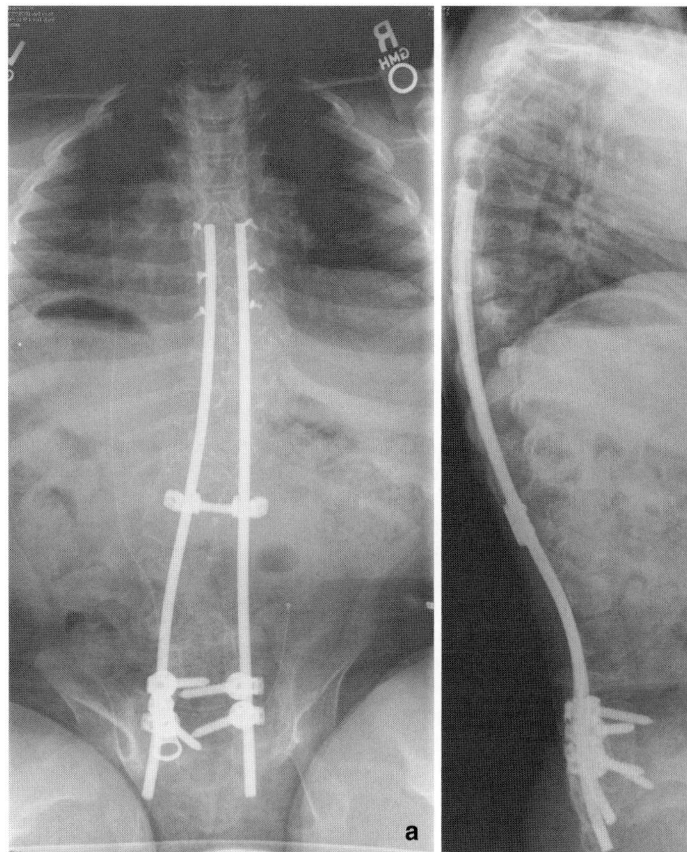

Fig. 31.1 (**a**) Postoperative AP image of subtraction kyphectomy and instrumentation. A growth construct is placed proximally to allow for column growth with arthrodesis only in the Lumbosacral region. (**b**) Postoperative lateral image of subtraction kyphectomy and instrumentation. Lumbosacral fixation includes L5 and S1 pedicle screw fixation and intra alar rod insertion. Rod countour is normal sagittal profile

postoperatively was 3° of lordosis, and at latest follow-up the correction was stabilized at 20° kyphosis. These findings represent an average postoperative correction of 91° and an average final correction of 66°. When performing a decancellation kyphectomy, an average immediate postoperative correction of 96% is attained and an average final 2 year correction of 87% is retained [14] (Fig. 31.1a, b). Furthermore, it has been stated that when compared with the resection kyphectomy, the decancellation kyphectomy resulted in diminished overall morbidity including substantially decreased intraoperative blood loss, decreased acute VP shunt malfunctions, and decreased mortality [15].

Although decancellation kyphectomy appears to have similar results in sagittal corrections as the resection kyphectomy with significantly decreased morbidity, it is important to note that long-term studies of decancellation kyphectomy are still pending. However, the decancellation kyphectomy procedure seems to be an efficacious option with decreased morbidity when compared with the resection kyphectomy.

31.6 Summary

Congenital kyphosis in children with myelomenigocele precludes significant functional and social development. It is associated with high rates of impairment including multiple shunt revisions, loss of ambulation, self-esteem issues, diminished skin integrity, and urologic problems [13]. Surgical intervention has been shown to be beneficial to the developing child. Both vertebral resection kyphectomy and subtraction (decancellation) kyphectomy procedures have been described and utilized with successful results. Whether performing a resection kyphectomy or decancellation kyphectomy, it seems that the benefits of improved sagittal correction, better sitting balance, enhanced pulmonary, gastroenterologic, and urologic function, improved skin integrity, and overall superior function outweigh the risks. The surgical techniques for correction of the kyphotic deformity have historically been associated with high morbidity and mortality. Although long-term studies are still pending, the author's experience demonstrates that the decancellation vertebrectomy is a safe and efficacious procedure for correction and stabilization of myelomeningocele kyphosis in young patients. The cautious surgeon is well advised to seek assistance in performing either procedure during their learning phase. Additionally, with either surgical technique, it is important to have long-term follow-up to verify longitudinal growth after spinal instrumentation [17].

References

1. Eckstein HB, Vora RM (1972) Spinal osteotomy for severe kyphosis in children with myelomeningocele. J Bone Joint Surg 54(2):328–333
2. Furderer S, Hopf C, Schwarz M et al (1999) Orthopedic and neurosurgical treatment of severe kyphosis in myelomeningocele. Neurosurg Rev 22(1):45–49
3. Guille JT, Sarwark JF, Sherk HH et al (2006) Congenital and developmental deformities of the spine in children with myelomeningocele. J Am Acad Orthop Surg 14(5): 294–302
4. Heydemann JS, Gillespie R (1987) Management of myelomeningocele kyphosis in the older child by kyphectomy and segmental spinal instrumentation. Spine 12(1):37–41
5. Huang TJ, Lubicky JP (1994) Kyphectomy and segmental spinal instrumentation in young children with myelomeningocele kyphosis. J Formos Med Assoc 93(6):503–508
6. Jackson RP, Hamilton AC. CD screws with oblique canals for improved sacral fixation: A prospective clinical study of the first fifty patients. Seventh Proceeding of the International Congress on Cotrel-Dubousset Instrumentation. Montpellier, France: Sauramps Medical, 1990:75–86
7. Kolaski K (2006) Myelomeningocele. Emedicine.com
8. Lindseth RE, Stelzer L Jr (1979) Vertebral excision for kyphosis in children with myelomeningocele. J Bone Joint Surg 61(5):699–704
9. Lintner SA, Lindseth RE (1994) Kyphotic deformity in patients who have a myelomeningocele. Operative treatment and long-term follow-up. J Bone Joint Surg 76(9):1301–1307
10. McCall RE (1998) Modified luque instrumentation after myelomeningocele kyphectomy. Spine 23(12):1406–1411
11. McCarthy RE, Dunn H, McCullough FL (1989) Luque fixation to the sacral ala using the Dunn-McCarthy modification. Spine 14(3):281–283
12. McMaster MJ (1998) The long-term results of kyphectomy and spinal stabilization in children with myelomeningocele. Spine 13(4):417–424
13. Mintz LJ, Sarwark JF, Dias LS et al (1991) The natural history of congenital kyphosis in myelomeningocele. A review of 51 children. Spine 16(Suppl 8):S348–S350
14. Niall DM, Dowling FE, Fogarty EE et al (2004) Kyphectomy in children with myelomeningocele: a long-term outcome study. J Pediatr Orthop 24(1):37–44
15. Nolden MT, Sarwark JF, Vora A et al (2002) A kyphectomy technique with reduced perioperative morbidity for myelomeningocele kyphosis. Spine 27(16):1807–1813
16. Sarwark JF (1996) Spina bifida. Pediatr Clin N Am 43(5):1151–1158
17. Sarwark JF (1999) Kyphosis deformity in myelomeningocele. Orthop Clin N Am 30(3):451–455; viii–ix
18. Sarwark JF, Weber DT, Gabrieli AP et al (1996) Tethered cord syndrome in low motor level children with myelomeningocele. Pediatr Neurosurg 25(6):295–301

Hemivertebrectomy

32

Gérard Bollini, Pierre-Louis Docquier, Yann Glard, Franck Launay, Elke Viehweger, and Jean-Luc Jouve

Key Points

- Resection is now a routinely used technique to treat a progressive spinal deformity due to a hemivertebra.
- The goal of resection is to correct the deformity in both coronal and sagittal planes and to avoid any further deterioration.
- The choice between a posterior only procedure or anterior and posterior combined approach to remove the hemivertebra is still debated.

32.1 Background

The natural history of congenital scoliosis has been well documented. The degree of scoliosis produced by a hemivertebra (HV) depends on its type, site, the number of HV, and patient age. When the HV is fully segmented or semi-segmented, progression of deformity is usually unavoidable.

Depending on the HV location, evolution of deformities is different. Thoracolumbar and lumbosacral junctions represent transitional areas between the mobile lumbar spine and a less or nonmobile segment (thoracic spine or sacrum). The HV located in these two transitional areas evolves to trunk shift. Moreover, in the thoracolumbar location, HV leads rapidly to torsional deformity so that an anatomical posterior convex compression can transform into a concave mechanical compression. In the thoracolumbar and lumbar location, sagittal alignment is important with risk of significative kyphosis. On the contrary, lumbosacral location does not present risk of kyphotic deformity. Single, fully segmented HV located at the thoracolumbar junction can deteriorate at a rate of 2–3.5° per year, in the lumbar area (between L2 to L4) deterioration of 1.7° per year in case of fully segmented HV and 1° in case of semi-segmented HV can be expected and fully segmented HV located at the lumbar sacral junction can deteriorate at a rate of 1.5° per year.

For the surgical management of congenital scoliosis, hemivertebral excision has a potential advantage over convex epiphyseodesis by addressing the deformity directly thus allowing immediate correction of both the frontal and the sagittal plane.

Royle [35] in 1928 was the first who performed a hemivertebra resection. Von Lackum and Smith [44] also reported on five cases in 1933.

He initially performed his surgery in one stage but later reported on a two-stage procedure consisting of vertebral body excision first followed later by posterior excision and fusion. In 1932, Compere [17] performed a thoracolumbar hemivertebra excision followed by turnbuckle cast correction in two patients. Wiles [45] in 1951 reported good correction of scoliosis after thoracic hemivertebrectomies in two patients but severe kyphosis developed in both patients and paraplegia developed in one. Goldstein [20] in 1964 reported on one case of lumbosacral hemivertebra resection. Hodgson [23] in 1965 reported safe results using an anterior approach to remove hemivertebra. A case of paraplegia following hemi vertebra resection was published by Winter [46] in 1976. Carcassone et al. [13] in 1977 and Onimus and Michel [33] in 1978 reported on two cases each of hemivertebral resection by an anterior and posterior approaches in two stages to treat congenital scoliosis. In 1981, Bergoin et al. [3–5] reported in the French literature his technique to remove safely the hemivertebra using two separated approaches during the same operative session.

G. Bollini (✉)
Hôpital Timone Enfants, 264 Rue Saint Pierre, 13385 Marseille Cedex 5, France
e-mail: gerard.bollini@ap-hm.fr

B. A. Akbarnia et al. (eds.), *The Growing Spine*,
DOI: 10.1007/978-3-540-85207-0_32, © Springer-Verlag Berlin Heidelberg 2011

32.2 Hemivertebra Resection Concept

A hemivertebra is located laterally in the frontal plane (responsible for a scoliosis) and in the sagittal plane more or less posteriorly (responsible for a certain amount of kyphosis). These two components, scoliosis and kyphosis, can progress with growth in terms of Cobb angles and moreover in terms of numbers of vertebrae included in the main curves (frontal and sagittal).

That is the reason why it is mandatory, as soon as there is proof of progression, to perform HV excision before more than the two vertebrae adjacent to the HV become involved in the scoliosis process (i.e. torsional deformity). In our opinion this is before 3 years of age.

There are controversies today as to whether it is better to perform HV using a single posterior approach or an anterior and posterior approach in the same operative session. There are also controversies concerning the use of hooks or pedicle screws together with a rod system to stabilize the spine after such a resection.

32.2.1 Biological Concept

For a better understanding, we have to consider the HV resection in two parts.

32.2.1.1 First Part is the Resection of the Posterior Aspects of the HV

Whatever the technique used, this session is the same. Often the hemilamina is fused with the lamina above or below. In such a case, to determine which part of the lamina belongs to the hemivertebra, we evaluate using fluoroscopy, the location of the pedicle of the hemivertebra. It is afterwards easy to answer that question. Once the hemilamina belonging to the hemivertebra is identified, the resection starts by removing the hemispinous process, then the hemilamina. The facets of the HV can be missing or aplastic. When present, these facets must be removed as well as the transverse process of the HV. It is then easy to circumscribe the pedicle of the hemivertebra. This pedicle is then removed using a subperiosteal approach. The periosteum protects, the nerve roots above and below the pedicle.

32.2.1.2 Second Part is the Resection of the Anterior Aspects of the HV

Several options exist regarding this session:

First option is to remove only the osseous part of the HV (Fig. 32.1a-d)

Whether the approach is a single posterior or an anterior and posterior approach and whether we use hooks or pedicle screws, a correction effect is applied through compression forces on the convexity. At the end of the procedure, the surrounding growth structure of the HV are still active. Thus, the empty space will be filled with spontaneous new bone formation. The positive consequence is that we regain stability of the vertebral column in its anterior aspect, but the negative consequence is that we may observe "recurrence" at least partial of the HV. That explains the observed new bone mass at the site of the HV [38]. This option is the one used in

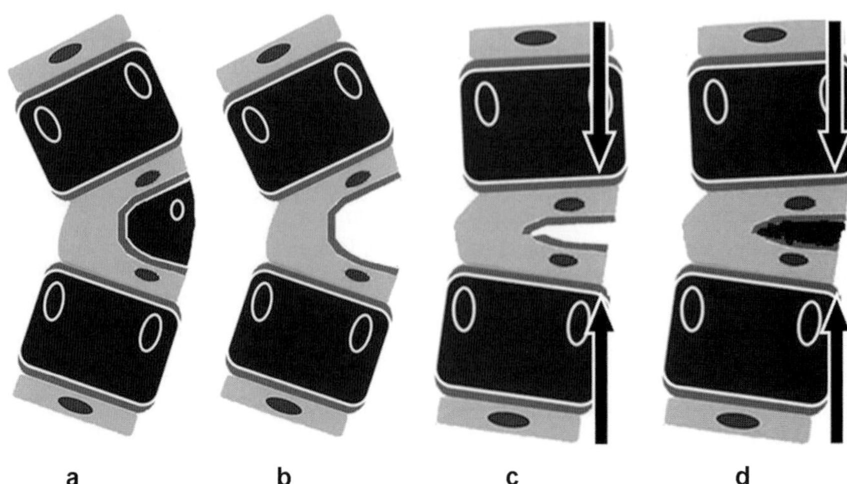

Fig. 32.1 *Black*: osseous part of the vertebrae. *Dark gray*: growing structures. *Light gray*: disc structures. (**a**) The HV to be removed. (**b**) The surrounding growing structures of the HV remain. (**c**) A compression force is applied. (**d**) The gap is spontaneously filled by new bone formation

the so-called “egg shell procedure” and is done usually by a posterior approach [31].

The second option (Fig. 32.2a-d) is to remove both the osseous hemivertebral body and the surrounding growth structure of the HV

At the end of this procedure, the growth structure of the adjacent vertebrae are still active. The negative consequence of this procedure is that the gap created is filled with a fibrous scar whose mechanical stability is doubtful. The relative positive consequence is this you may observe growth coming for the resting end plates of the vertebrae adjacent to the HV. We used the term “relative” because such a growth is correlated with distraction forces on the anterior aspect of the spinal column.

It is absolutely obvious that it is impossible to get an anterior arthrodesis between the two vertebrae adjacent to the HV and in the meantime to observe further growth coming from these same two vertebrae.

The third option (Fig. 32.3a-d) is to remove both the whole HV (osseous hemivertebral body + surrounding growth structure) and the end plates of the adjacent vertebrae on the convex side of the scoliosis

It is the only option that allows obtaining a convex epiphyseodesis under the condition that we add a bone

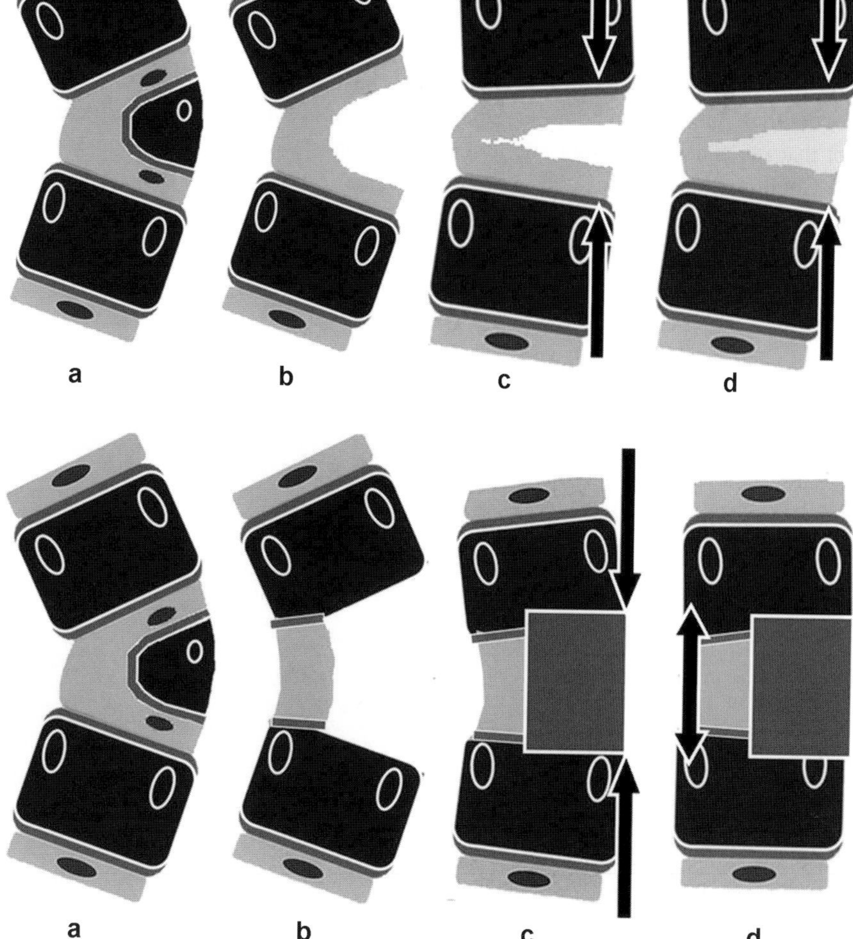

Fig. 32.2 *Black*: osseous part of the vertebrae. *Dark gray*: growing structures. *Light gray*: disc structures. (**a**) The HV to be removed. (**b**) The surrounding growing structures of the HV are removed. (**c**) A compression force is applied. (**d**) The gap is spontaneously filled by a fibrous scare

Fig. 32.3 *Black*: osseous part of the vertebrae. *Dark gray*: growing structures. *Light gray*: disc structures. (**a**) The HV to be removed. (**b**) The surrounding growing structures of the HV are removed as well as the disc and the convex growing structures of the adjacent vertebrae. (**c**) A compression force is applied. (**d**) The gap is filled by a bone graft

graft between the two adjacent vertebral bodies. The main point to understand is that at the end of such a procedure and after having applied the compression force on the posterior aspect of the vertebral column, there is still a large gap between the two adjacent vertebral bodies to fill, otherwise one may expect a secondary kyphotic deformity and/or a pseudoarthrosis.

In our opinion, it is the main reason to perform both a posterior and anterior approach, adding an anterior bone graft (usually a fibular segment), to correct the kyphotic component of the deformation as well as to prevent further kyphotic deformity. With this third option, you can expect an additional correction of the Cobb angle you obtain at the end of the procedure by further growth coming from the concave side of the deformity where growing structures are still active.

The fourth option (Fig. 32.4a-c) is to remove the whole structures between the two vertebral bodies of the vertebrae adjacent to the HV

This allows to correct the deformation and then to perform a total arthrodesis between these two vertebrae. This fourth option will be chosen whenever we have to treat an older child for whom the remaining growth is not that much and for whom additional correction of the Cobb angle by further concave growth cannot be expected. For these older children, anterior stability is of paramount importance.

32.2.2 Stability Concept

32.2.2.1 Primary Stability

Removal of a hemivertebra leaves an empty space posteriorly and anteriorly. To close the gap posteriorly and to ensure immediate posterior stability, one has to use compression hardware on the convex posterior aspect in the young children and on both sides older children. In our experience, we never encounter any breakage of the laminae using hooks. Except in case of HV located very posteriorly and as soon as the whole convex element are removed with the HV (option three), closing the posterior gap freed by the HV resection leaves an anterior gap open. This anterior gap decreases about 50% after posterior compression. Therefore, to obtain an anterior stability, one must add an anterior graft or a cage.

32.2.2.2 Secondary Stability

If the mechanical construct is responsible for immediate stability, late stability is devoted to anterior and posterior bone grafting.

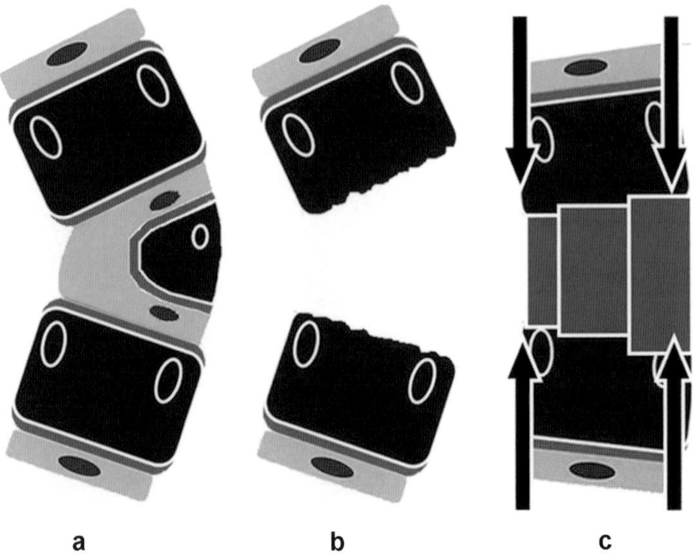

Fig. 32.4 *Black*: osseous part of the vertebrae. *Dark gray*: growing structures. *Light gray*: disc structures. (**a**) The HV to be removed. (**b**) The whole space between the two adjacent vertebral bodies is freed from all the structures. (**c**) A compression force is applied and the gap is filled with bone grafts

32.3 Our Personal Technique

32.3.1 Preoperative Evaluation

Radiologic imaging includes standing posteroanterior (PA) and lateral radiograph of the full spine. Magnetic resonance imaging (MRI) of the spine is performed to assess the neuroanatomy (exclude intrathecal abnormalities) and to study the segmentation of the HV and the growth plate. Renal ultrasound has to be done preoperatively to assess associated congenital renal system abnormalities.

32.3.2 Technique

Our philosophy is to perform posterior and anterior approach under the same anesthesia but in two different positions. This makes the surgery as safe as possible. (A lateral position is not the best one to perform the resection of the posterior elements of the HV.) For the posterior approach, the patient is in a prone position with the operative area accessibly for fluoroscopy. The pedicle of the HV is identified and the skin is marked, and a vertical midline incision is performed. In young children, only the convex aspect of the spine is freed from its soft tissue. The posterior approach has been previously described (see 32.1.1). Further insertion sites for laminar hooks in the adjacent proximal and distal laminae are prepared.

In case of significant kyphotic condition for a hemivertebra at the thoraco-lumbar junction, the convex posterior arthrodesis can extend two levels above the hemivertebra to be resected. At the end of this first posterior approach, the skin is temporarily closed with sutures and the patient is turned in a lateral position for a convex anterior approach. The anterior approach depends on the level of the hemivertbra; thoracophrenolombotomy for the thoracolumbar HV, lombotomy with retroperitoneal approach for the lumbar or lumbo – sacral HV. When the anterior spine is exposed, the posterior approach is reopened. The body of the HV lies very laterally and is easily found. Resection of the whole hemivertebral body plus the surrounding growth structures is performed as well as resection of the disc and growing structures of the adjacent vertebral bodies. This resection stops at the midline of the vertebral column avoiding damage in the young child on the concave side. During this time, anterior bleeding can be easily controlled using a light posterior compression of the intercostal vessels.

Then, two hooks, one above the upper adjacent convex lamina and one below the lower adjacent convex lamina are inserted in the already prepared site. A rod is introduced and a posterior compression is applied allowing reduction of the posterior gap freed by the HV resection. The anterior gap is only tightened by about 50%. Baby-CD in the past and now Legacy 3.5. instrumentation were used in children until 5 years of age. In case of weakness of S1 lamina after removal of a lumbosacral hemivertebra, an S1 pedicle screw can be used or the patient can wear a pantaloon cast. Hosalkar et al. [25] designed a new device for fixation at the lumbosacral junction. Autogenous anterior fibular grafting is done. The harvested fibular graft is presented anterolaterally during the posterior compression to control the kyphotic component of the deformity. Autogenous posterior convex grafting is realized as well using part of a rib if a thoracophrenolombotomy has been done or fibular grafting. The two approaches are then closed. Postoperatively, the patient wears a previously moulded brace for 6 months. A cell saver is used during the procedure and the recycled blood (if enough) is given to the child at the end of operation. Somatosensory cortical evoked potential spinal cord monitoring is used during the whole procedure.

32.3.3 Results

In our institution, from February 1987 to December 2003, 34 thoracolumbar, 26 lumbar, and 17 lumbosacral HV were excised. These 77 hemivertebrae were responsible for scoliosis or kyphoscoliosis with evidence of curve progression. Our experiences were reported in several publications [6–10]. Results of these procedures were reported using radiographic assessment of the deformity described in Fig. 32.5.

32.4 Discussion

Numerous authors have reported a series of HV resection using successive or simultaneous anterior and posterior operative approaches [11, 12, 18, 22, 24,

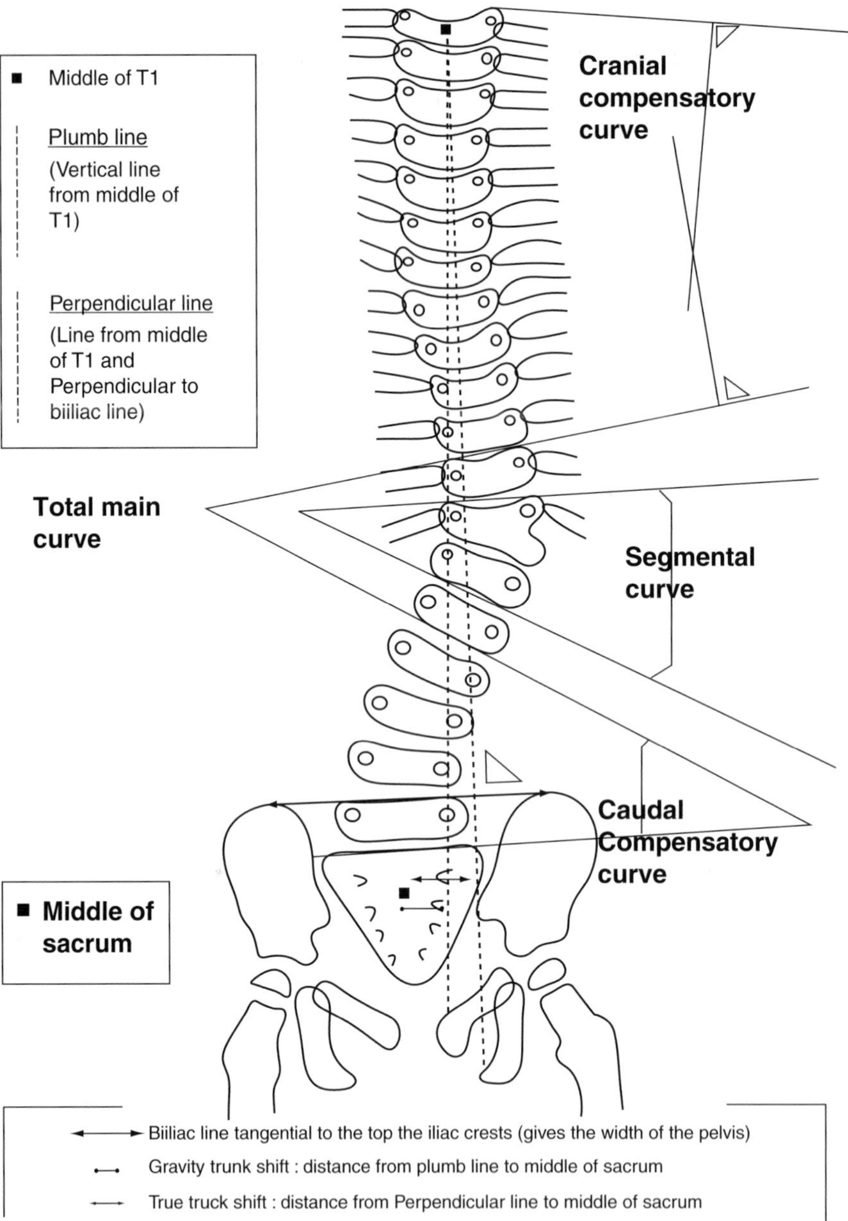

Fig. 32.5 Radiographic assessment of the deformity

26–30, 42, 43], posterior approach alone [32, 36–41], or anterior approach alone (18 for two cases [21]). No previous so large homogeneous series of HV excision than the present study exists in the literature.

This technique permits one to obtain immediate important correction of scoliosis and the result was stable over the time. However, in thoracolumbar HV location, there is a high rate of associated osseous malformations that could interfere with curve progression. It is difficult measuring angles to analyze the single result of HV excision, as it is influenced by other malformations. This can explain the number of additional surgeries due to curve progression in thoracolumbar hemivertebrae.

In our opinion, HV resection is indicated in thoracolumbar (Fig. 32.6a-e), lumbar (Figs. 32.7a-d, 32.8a-d, 32.9a-d), and lumbo-sacral (Fig.32.10a-c) areas when there is evidence of curve progression. However, indication in other localizations such as thoracic or cervicothoracic (Fig. 32.11a-d) is to be decided depending on the deformity, the rate of progression, and the type of hemivertebra. It is necessary to perform instrumentation

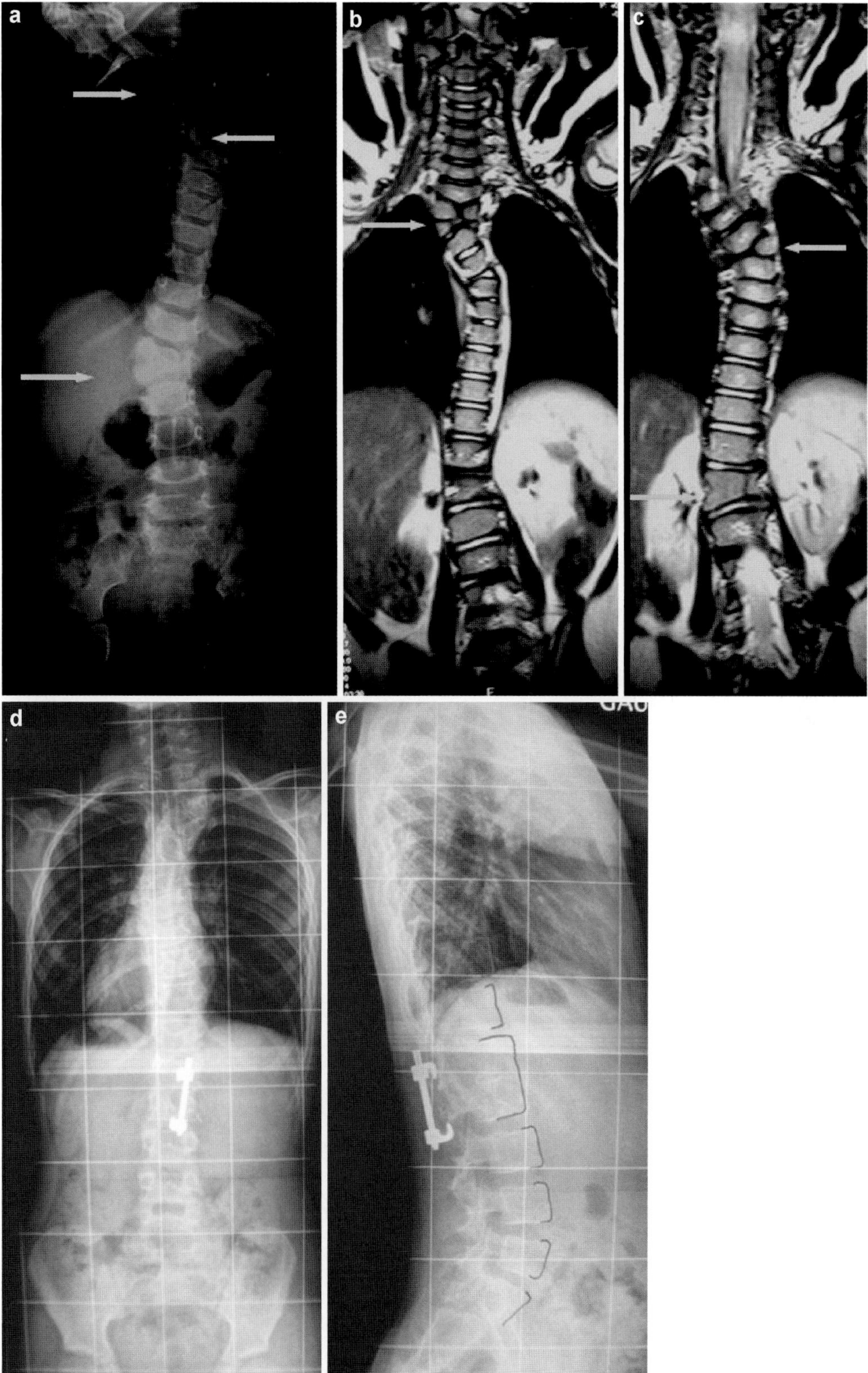

Fig. 32.6 Preoperative radiographs of a patient with thoracolumbar HV at 18 months of age before having resection procedure (**a**-**c**). Follow up radiographs 8 years 10 months after HV resection (**d**, **e**)

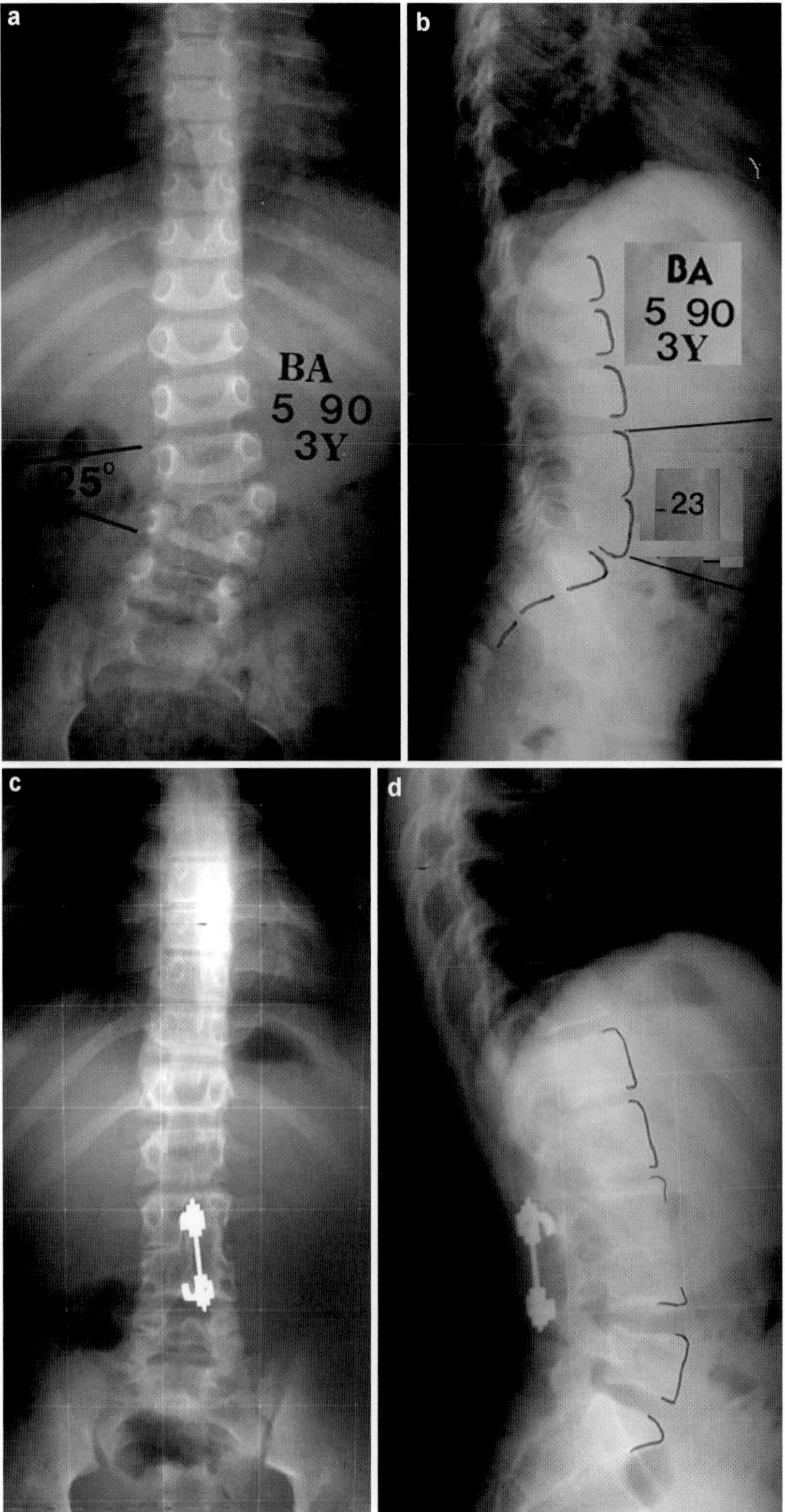

Fig. 32.7 Preoperative radiographs of a 3 year old child with lumbar HV before having resection procedure (**a**, **b**). Follow up radiographs at 15 years 10 months of age (**c**, **d**)

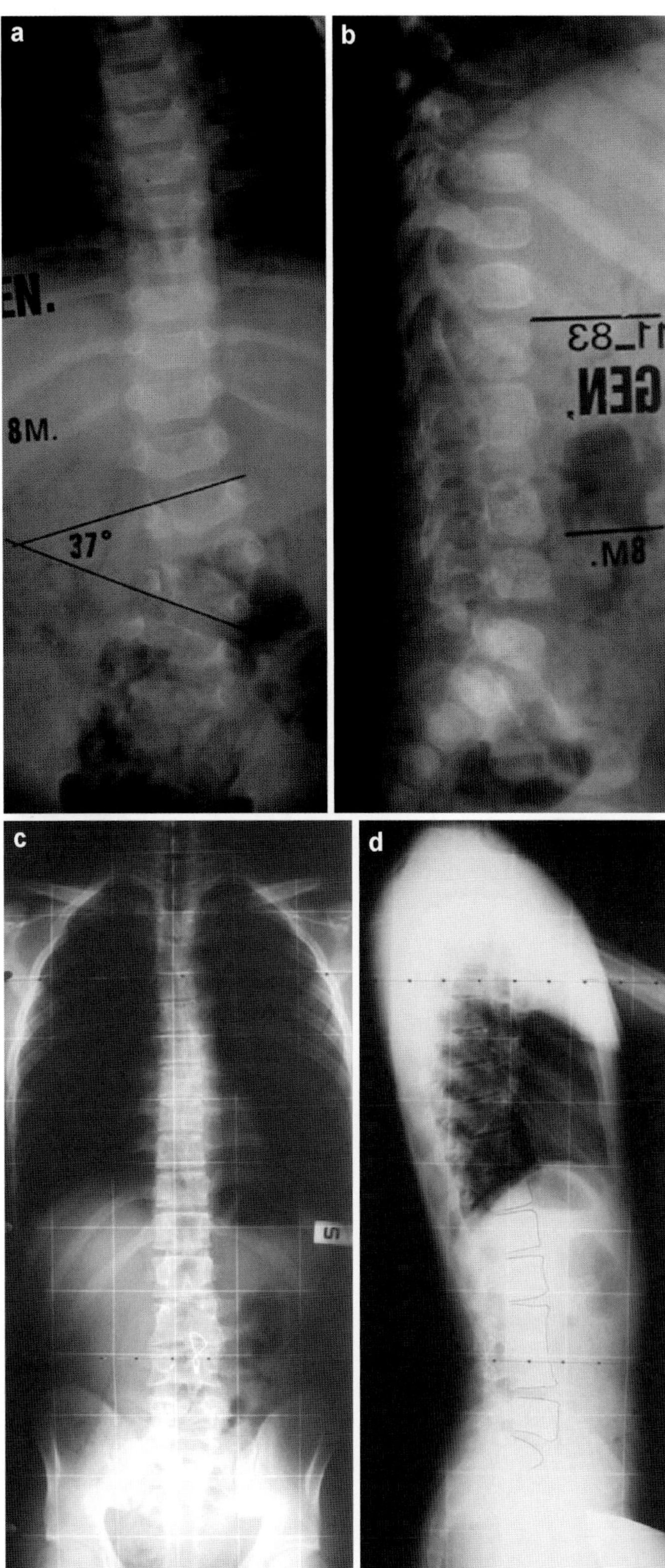

Fig. 32.8 Preoperative radiographs of a patient with lumbar HV at 1 year of age before having resection procedure (**a**, **b**). Follow up radiographs at 18 years 5 months of age (**c**, **d**)

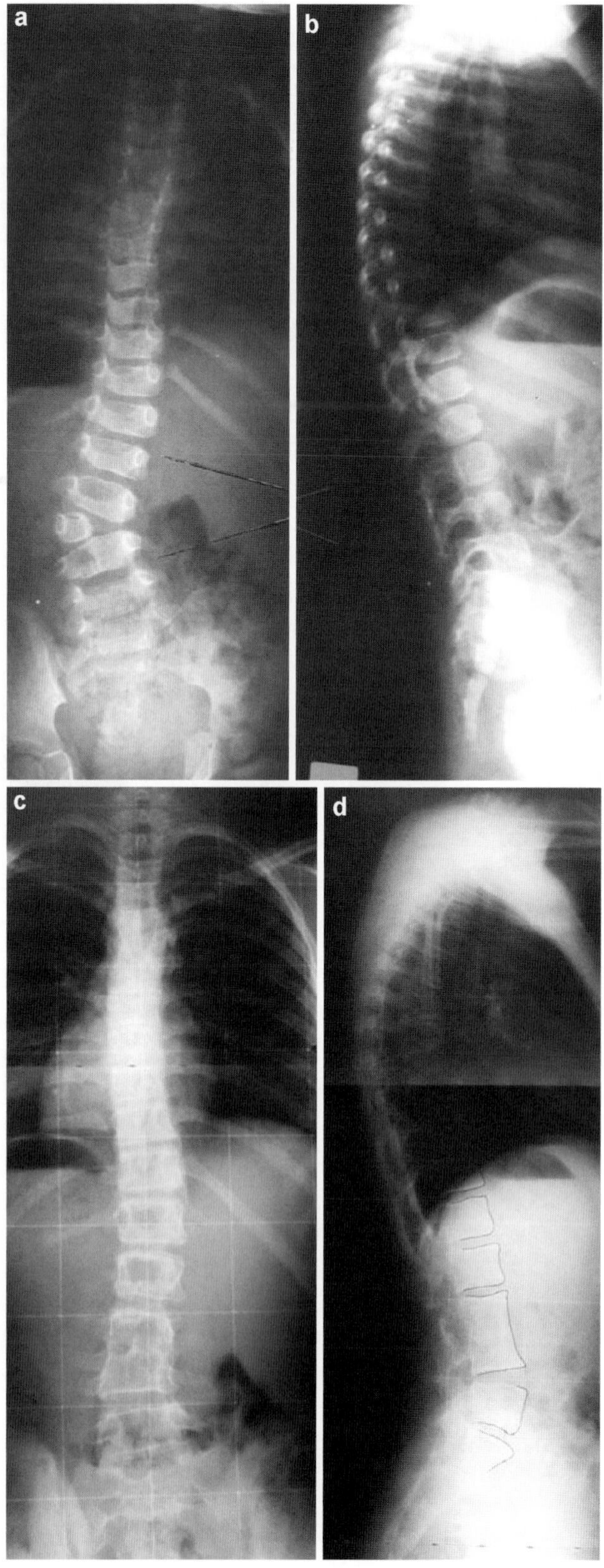

Fig. 32.9 Preoperative radiographs of a patient with lumbar HV at 1 year of age before having resection procedure (**a**, **b**). Follow up radiographs at 13 years 5 months of age (**c**, **d**)

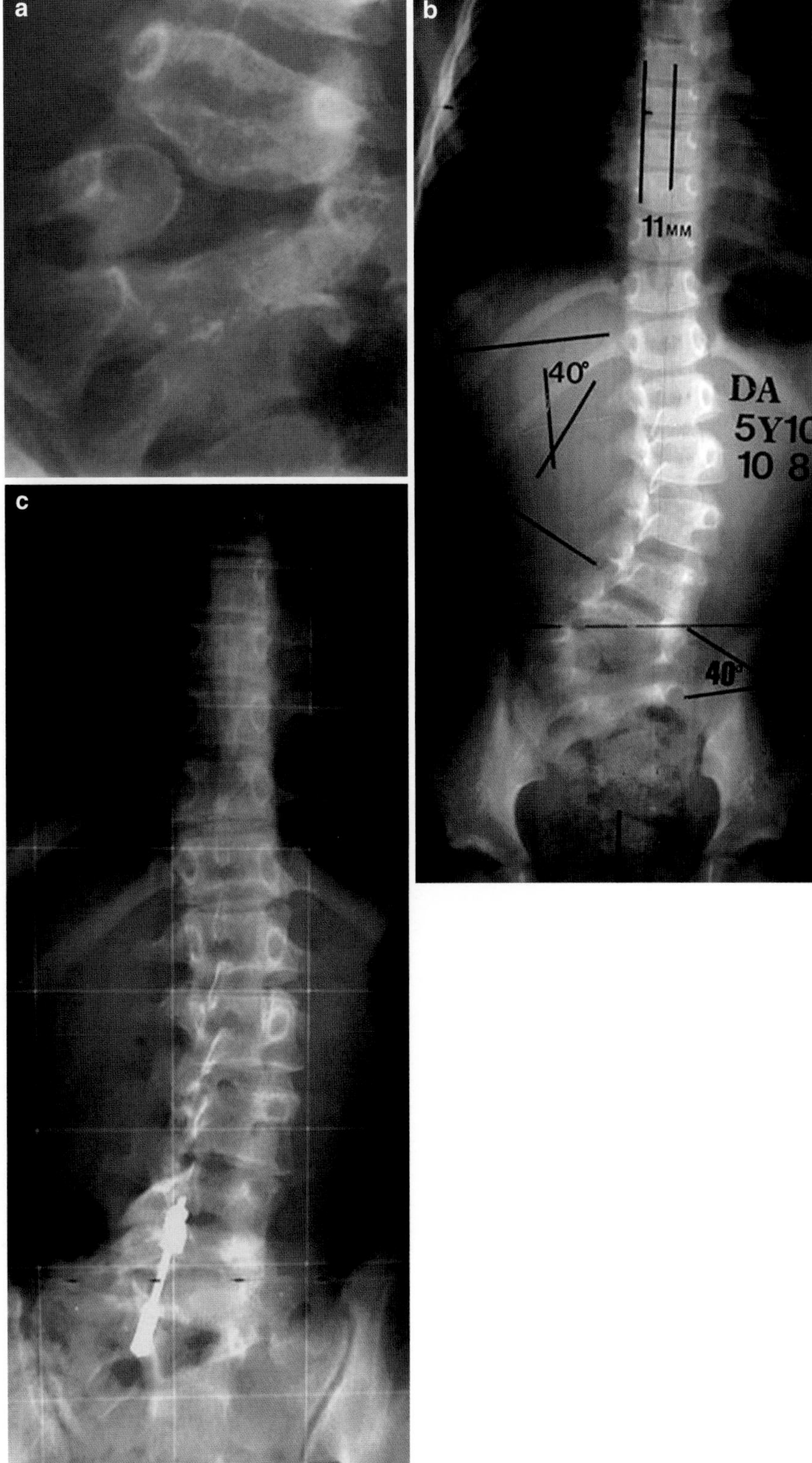

Fig. 32.10 Preoperative radiographs of a patient with lumbosacral HV at 5 years 10 months of age before having resection procedure (**a**, **b**). Follow up radiographs at 16 years 4 months of age (**c**)

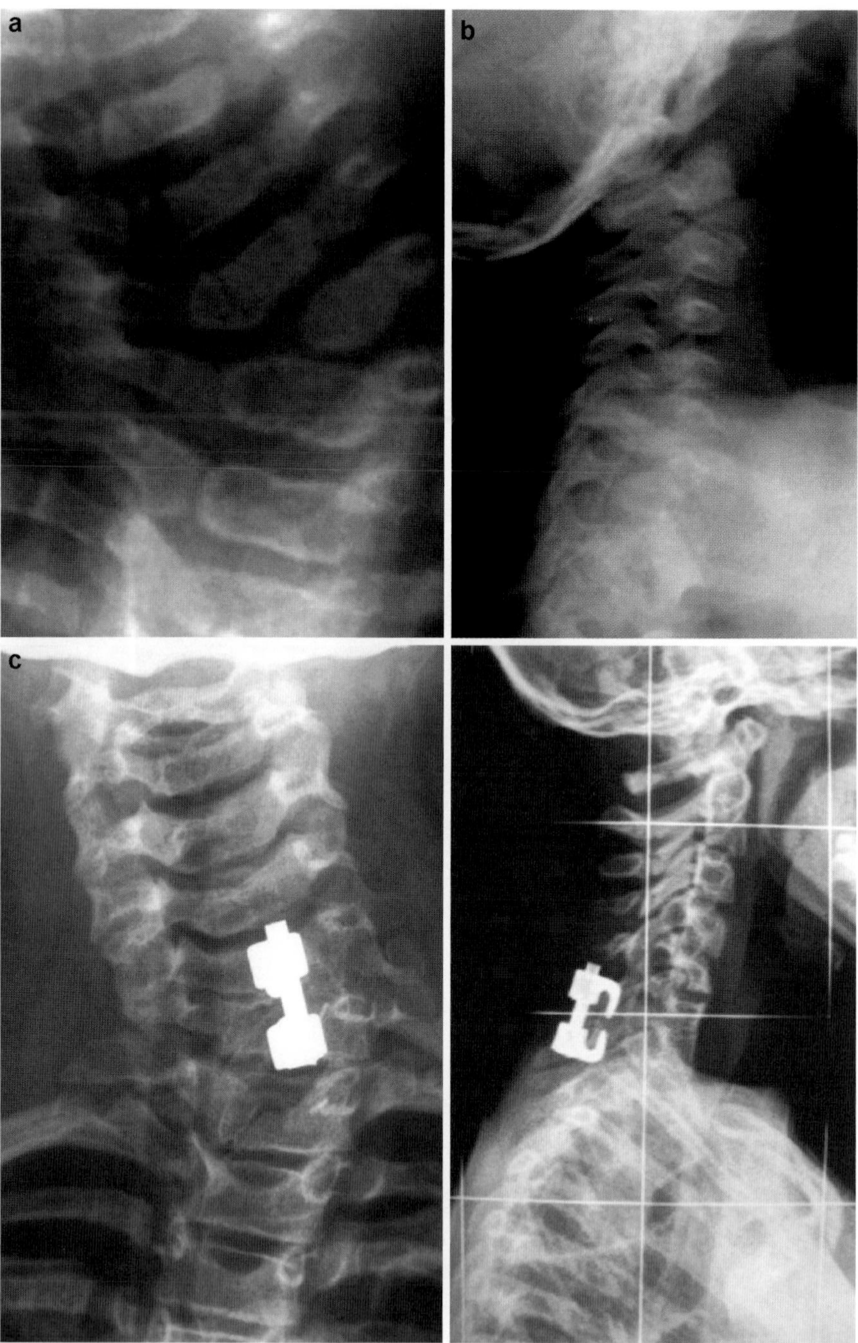

Fig. 32.11 Preoperative radiographs of a patient with cervicothoracic HV at 2 years of age before having resection procedure (**a**, **b**). Follow up radiographs at 11 years of age (**c**, **d**)

of the convexity after HV's resection because the HV excision creates instability. The material used for this instrumentation was the Baby-CD designed by the senior author with a trend to shift to the Legacy 3.5 in the more recent cases. This posterior instrumentation allows a convex compression by the mean of two hooks and a rod. It is convenient for moderate angulations in the thoraco-lumbar area and for lumbar and lumbosacral hemivertebrae. In case of important Cobb angulation with severe torsional deformity in the thoraco-lumbar area, the use of such instrumentation is not recommended because hooks are very close to the spinous processes (due to small laminae width) and can be in the concavity of the torsional process due to the amount of the vertebral torsion. In such cases, it is better to use pedicle screws or anterior instrumentation using screws in the vertebral bodies (Fig. 32.12a, b).

To discuss other options for resection of hemivertebrae, one has to understand that after such a removal the posterior compression permits one to close the posterior gap freed by the HV resection, whereas the anterior gap is only tightened by about 50%. That means that it is essential in our opinion to put a bone graft in front strong enough to maintain a primary stability against the spontaneous kyphotic effect. That is the reason why we use a fibular bone graft in front.

Ruf and Harms [36] argued that removal of a hemivertebra by a single posterior approach followed by convex and concave compression using pedicle screws and rods is the ideal procedure for correction in young children. They found no adverse effects putting pedicle screws in the very young. They showed at the SRS meeting in Edinburg (2007) two very astonishing data: first was that the pedicles screws inserted had a tendency to have their tips diverging during further growth and second is that on fluoroscopy mobility still exists at the level of the hemivertebra excision.

In our opinion, the only explanation for such data is that the removal concerns mainly the osseous part of the hemivertebra while the growing structure remains (at least partially) intact leading to some kind of fibrous pseudoarthrosis in front. We believe that such a pseudoarthrosis could lead to implant failure and further kyphotic deformity.

We believe that a single posterior approach could be a good indication for some kind of hemivertebra located very posteriorly but on a regular basis we think that a double approach in a single procedure is safer, has greater correction capabilities including a perfect control of the sagittal plane, decrease the likelihood of pseudoarthrosis, and prevent the development of crankshaft phenomenon. Except at S1 level, we never observed breakage of a lamina using laminar hooks, which means that it appears, except in specific cases (see above), not necessary to use pedicle screws. Figures 32.13a, b shows use of hooks even in the cervico-thoracic area.

The last point to be underlined is that it is not completely clear up to now whether using a pedicular screw, which crosses the neuro-central cartilage, in a 2 years old baby, should have any further consequences on the diameter of the spinal canal.

Ruf and Harms [37, 39] believed that "the benefit of pedicle screws exceeds their potential risk by far" while other authors [2, 14–16, 19, 34] demonstrated on animal models that the use of pedicle screws crossing the neuro-central cartilage reduces the diameter of the spinal canal.

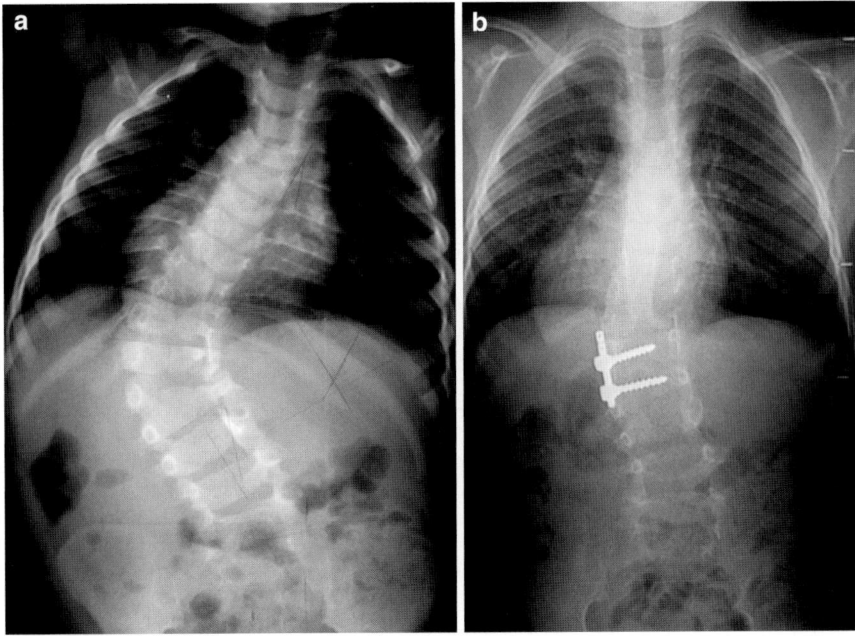

Fig. 32.12 Preoperative radiograph of a patient with thoracolumbar HV at 1 year 9 months of age before having resection procedure (**a**). Segmental instrumentation was done using screws after HV resection. Follow up radiographs at 7 years of age (**b**)

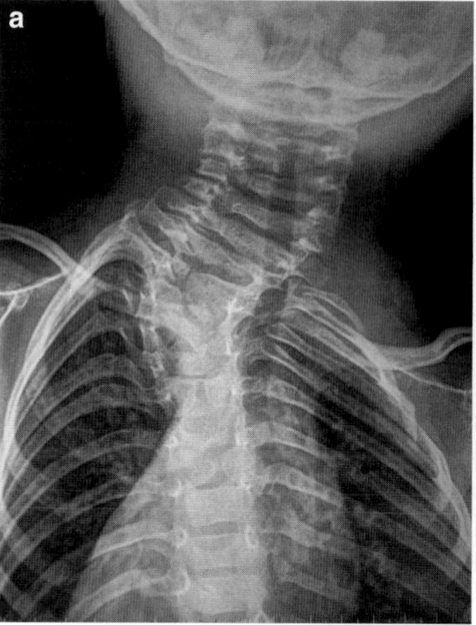

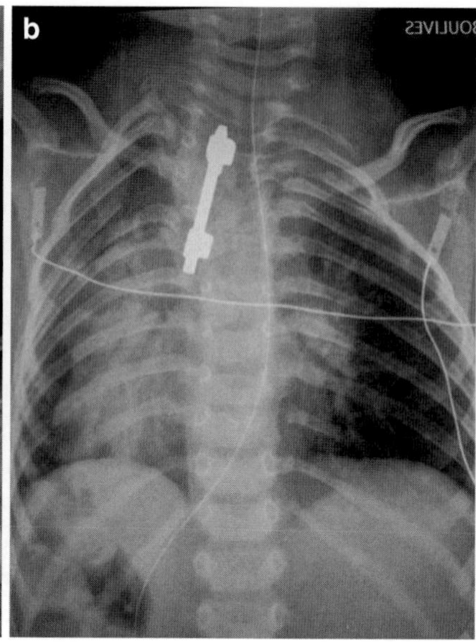

Fig. 32.13 Preoperative radiographs of a patient with cervicothoracic HV at 2 years of age before having resection procedure (**a**). Segmental instrumentation was done using hooks after HV resection (**b**)

To conclude, hemivertebra resection is now a routine technique widely used to treat a progressive spinal deformity due to a hemivertebra. The goal of such resection is to reduce the Cobb angle and to avoid any further deterioration. The choice between a posterior egg shell procedure and an anterior and posterior approach to remove the hemivertebra is still debated [1].

The surgeon who is in charge of the treatment needs to know any kind of treatment to choose the best one for each individual type and location of HV.

References

1. Banagan KE, Sponseller PD (2007) Surgical treatment of congenital scoliosis. Curr Opin Orthop 18:248–252
2. Beguiristain JL, De Salis J, Oriaifo A, et al (1980) Experimental scoliosis by epiphyseodesis in pigs. Int Orthop 4:317–321
3. Bergoin M, Carcassonne M, Choux M (1981) Technique sûre d'exérèse chirurgicale des hémi-vertèbres. Rev Chir Orthop 67:485–493
4. Bergoin M, Bollini G, Taibi L et al (1986) Excision of hemivertebrae in children with congenital scoliosis. Ital J Orthop Traumatol 12:179–184
5. Bergoin M, Bollini G, Gennari JM (1993) One-stage hemivertebral excision and arthrodesis on congenital oblique takeoff in children aged less than five years. J Pediatr Orthop B 1 108–112
6. Bollini G, Bergoin M, Labriet C et al (1993) Hemivertebrae excision and fusion in children aged less than five years. J Pediatr Orthop B 1:95–101
7. Bollini G, Docquier PL, Launay F et al (2005) Résultats à maturité osseuse après resection d'hémiverèbres par double abord. Rev Chir Orthop 91:709–718
8. Bollini G, Docquier PL, Viehweger E et al (2006) Lumbar hemivertebra resection. J Bone Joint Surg 88A:1043–1052
9. Bollini G, Docquier PL, Viehweger E et al (2006) Lumbosacral hemivertebrae resection by combined approach. Spine 11:1232–1239
10. Bollini G, Docquier PL, Viehweger E et al (2006) Thoracolumbar hemivertebrae resection by double approach in a single procedure. Spine 15:1745–1757
11. Bradford DS, Boachie-Adjei O (1990) One stage anterior and posterior hemivertebral resection and arthrodesis for congenital scoliosis. J Bone Joint Surg 72A(4):536–540
12. Callahan BC, Georgopoulos G, Eilert RE (1997) Hemivertebral excision for congenital scoliosis. J Pediatr Orthop 1:96–99
13. Carcassonne M, Gregoire A, Hornung H (1977) L'ablation de l'hémi-vertèbre "libre": traitement préventif de la scoliose congénitale. Chirurgie 103:110–115
14. Cil A, Yazici M, Daglioglu K et al (2003) The effect of pedicle scew placement with or without compression on the morphology of the spinal canal and pedicle in immature pigs. Eur Spine J 12 (Suppl 1):S30–S31
15. Cil A, Yazici M, Alanay A, et al (2004) Letters to the Editor. Spine 14:1593–1594
16. Coillard C, Rhalmi S, Rivard CH (1999) Experimental scoliosis in the minipig: study of vertebral deformations. Ann Chir 8:773–780
17. Compere EL (1932) Excision of hemivertebra for correction of congenital scoliosis. J Bone Joint Surg 14A:555–562
18. Deviren V, Berven S, Emami A et al (2001) Excision of hemivertebrae in the management of congenital scoliosis involving the thoracic and thoracolumbar spine. J Bone Joint Surg 83B:496–500
19. Dimiglio A (1992) Early spinal growth. J Pediatr Orthop 2:102–107

20. Goldstein LA (1964) The surgical management of scoliosis. Clin Orthop 35:95–115
21. Gregoire A, Hornung H, Yaffi D et al (1977) Intérêt de la résection précoce des hémivertèbres dans les scolioses congénitales. Ann Chir Inf 6:419–424
22. Hedequist D, Emans J (2007) Congenital Scoliosis. J Pediatr Orthop 1:106–116
23. Hodgson AR (1965) Correction of fixed spinal curves. J Bone Joint Surg 47A:1221–1227
24. Holte DC, Winter RB, Lonstein JE, et al (1995) Excision of hemivertebrae and wedge resection in the treatment of congenital scoliosis. J Bone Joint Surg 77A:159–171
25. Hosalkar HS, Luedtke LM, Drummond DS (2004) New technique in congenital scoliosis involving fixation to the pelvis after hemivertebra excision. Spine 22:2581–2587
26. King JD, Lowery GL (1990) Results of lumbar hemivertebral excision for congenital scoliosis. Spine 7:778–781
27. Klemme WR, Polly D, Orchowski JR (2001) Hemivertebral excision for congenital scoliosis in very young children. J Pediatr Orthop 6:761–764
28. Lazar RD, Hall JE (1999) Simultaneous anterior and posterior hemivertebra excision. Clin Orthop 364:76–84
29. Leatherman KD, Dickson RA (1979) Two stages corrective surgery for congenital deformities of the spine. J Bone Joint Surg 61B(3):324–328
30. Leong JCY, Day GA, Luk KDK et al (1993) Nine year mean follow up of one-stage anteroposterior excision of hemivertebrae in the lumbosacral spine. Spine 14:2069–2074
31. Mikles MR, Graziano GP, Hensinger RN (2001) Transpedicular eggshell osteotomies for congenital scoliosis using frameless stereotactic guidance. Spine 20:2289–2296
32. Nakamura H, Matsuda H, Konishi S et al (2002) Single-stage excision of hemivertebrae via the posterior approach alone for congenital spine deformity. Spine 1:110–115
33. Onimus M, Michel CR (1978) Problèmes posés par la résection des hémi vertèbres lombo-sacrées. Chir Pediatr 19: 119–121
34. Papp T, Porter RW, Aspden RM (1994) The growth of the lumbar vertebral canal. Spine 19:2770–2773
35. Royle ND (1928) The operative removal of an accessory vertebrae. Med J Aust 1:467–468
36. Ruf M, Harms J (2002) Hemivertebra resection by a posterior approach. Spine 10:1116–1123
37. Ruf M, Harms J (2002) Pedicle screws in 1 and 2 year old children: technique, complications, and effect on further growth. Spine 27:E460–E466
38. Ruf M, Harms J (2003) Posterior hemivertebra resection with transpedicular instrumentation: early correction in children aged 1 to 6 years. Spine 18:2132–2138
39. Ruf M, Harms J (2004) Answer to a letter. Spine 14: 1594–1596
40. Ruf M, Jensen R, Harms J (2005) Hemivertebra resection in the cervical spine. Spine 4:380–385
41. Shono Y, Abumi K, Kaneda K (2001) One-stage posterior hemivertebra resection and correction using segmental posterior instrumentation. Spine 7:752–757
42. Slabaugh PB, Winter RB, Lonstein JE et al (1980) Lumbosacral hemivertebrae. Spine 3:234–244
43. Ulrich EV, Moushkin AY (1993) Surgical treatment of scoliosis and kyphoscoliosis caused by hemivertebrae in infants. J Pediatr Orthop B 1:113–115
44. Von Lackum HL, Smith A (1933) Removal of vertebral bodies in the treatment of scoliosis. Surg Gynecol Obstet 57: 250–256
45. Wiles P (1951) Resection of dorsal vertebrae in congenital scoliosis. J Bone Joint Surg 33A:151–153
46. Winter RB (1976) Congenital kyphoscoliosis with paralysis following hemivertebra excision. Clin Orthop 119:116–125

33 Vertebral Osteotomy

Francisco Sànchez Pérez-Grueso

Key Points

- Techniques for correcting fixed spinal deformity, rarely used in the past, has become more popular in recent years.
- Indicated mostly in congenital deformities and in cases previously fused.
- There is an increased risk of neurological complications.
- Single osteotomy should involve three columns of the spine and should be located at the apex of the deformity.
- Multiple osteotomies normally occur in the posterior elements, creating several points of instability.
- The use of transpedicular implants adapted to children's size improves correction and stability.
- Rib osteotomies are rarely indicated in the pediatric age, because the rib cage is still not completely developed and has some flexibility.

33.1 Introduction

Vertebral osteotomy is a surgical technique used to treat fixed deformities in both coronal and sagittal planes by mobilizing and correcting vertebral malalignments. Vertebral osteotomy has always been considered to have a high risk of neurological injury [8]; therefore, its use in pediatric spine surgery has been relatively limited. Nonetheless, in recent years, this technique has become more widely used, in part because of the advances made in intraoperative monitoring of the nerve structures and the attainment of more extensive experience.

Vertebral osteotomy is indicated in rigid spinal deformities, caused by congenital defects or after vertebral fusions. When the procedure is contemplated for children, it is very important to take into consideration the potential for growth in this group of patients.

In single vertebral osteotomy, correction is achieved at only one level. The procedure should comprise the anterior and posterior portions of the vertebral body, as well as the posterior vertebral elements, including the pedicles, to be effective. Multiple vertebral osteotomies are performed mainly on the posterior vertebral elements and include several segments. The corrective force is distributed all along the multiple osteotomized levels.

The most important factor to consider when planning the correction is protection of the nerve structures. Application of corrective forces in distraction and lateral displacement of the vertebral segments have higher risk of paralysis. Forces in compression are safer and generally much better tolerated.

33.2 Single Osteotomy

A single osteotomy should involve the anterior, middle, and posterior portions of the spine; if not, the intact portion will impede correction (unless it is an intervertebral disc). Basically, the procedure consists of

F.S. Pérez-Grueso
Hospital La Paz, Pedro Rico,
131 8 G 28029, Madrid, Spain
e-mail: pérezgrueso@terro.es

B. A. Akbarnia et al. (eds.), *The Growing Spine*,
DOI: 10.1007/978-3-540-85207-0_33, © Springer-Verlag Berlin Heidelberg 2011

excision of a wedge of bone with the base corresponding to the convex side of the deformity at the apex, regardless of whether the deformity involves the frontal or sagittal plane [3] (Fig. 33.1a–d). The approach can be through the anterior and posterior portion of the spine, or only through the posterior part; the latter approach is currently more common, particularly for deformities in angular kyphosis (also see Chap. 34).

Correction is achieved by closing the excised wedge; hence, compression is the main corrective force that comes into play. In some cases, particularly in kyphosis, it is necessary to apply distraction at the same time as compression at the apex of the wedge (concavity) to avoid excessive buckling of the spinal cord (Fig. 33.2a–d). While performing the correction maneuvers, it is of utmost importance to avoid any

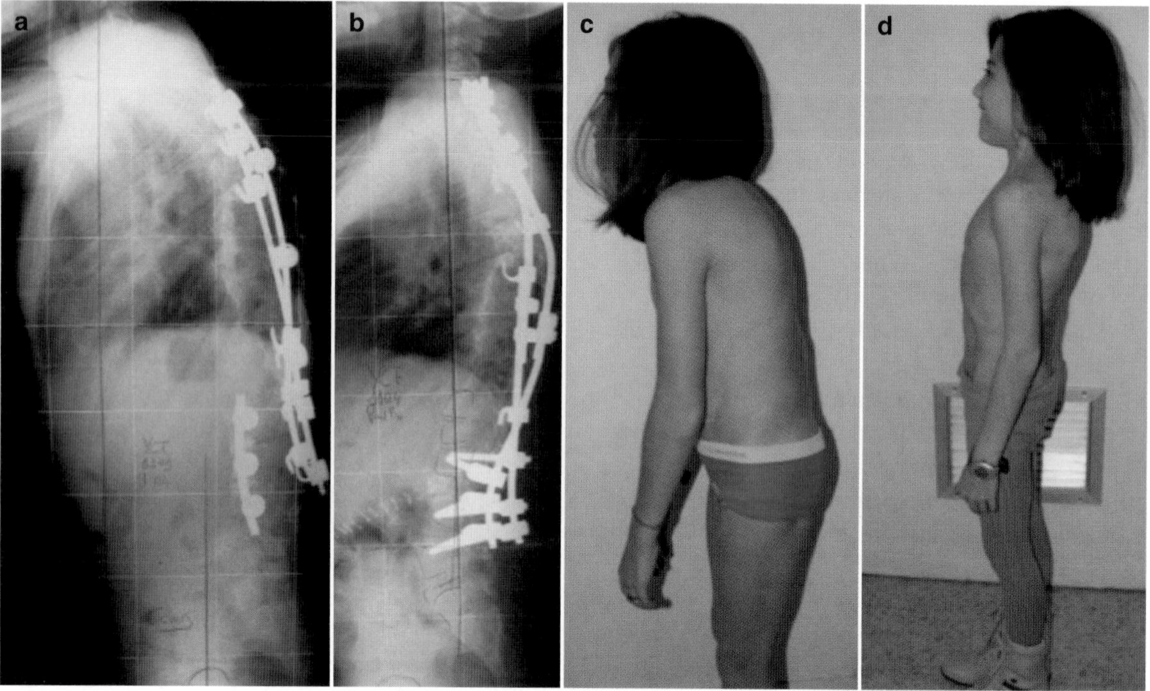

Fig. 33.1 (**a-d**) Correction of sagittal plane deformity by single level anterior and posterior osteotomy

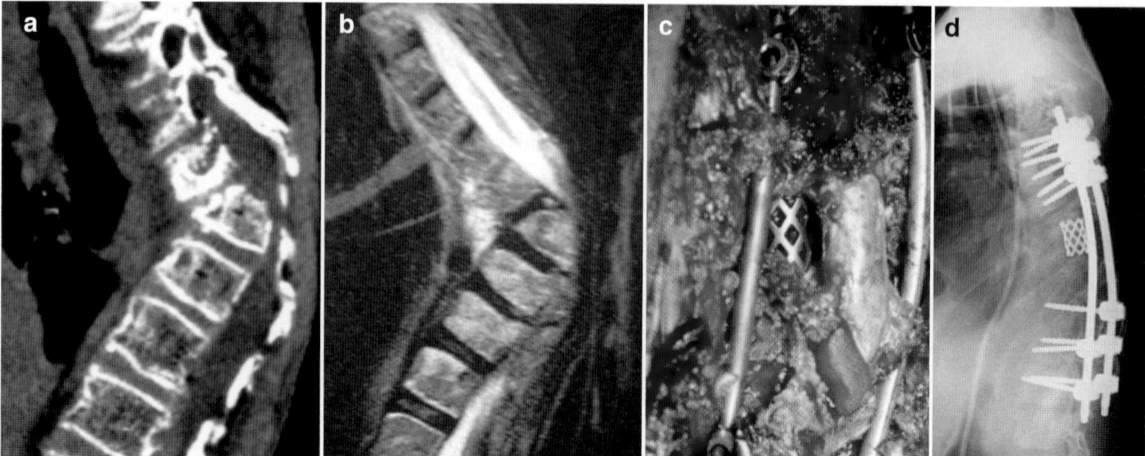

Fig. 33.2 (**a-d**) Preoperative and postoperative imaging of a child with Gorham syndrome who had single posterior closing anterior opening osteotomy for acute kyphosis. Note a titanium cage anteriorly

translational displacement of the free vertebral segments, which can easily result in an irreversible neurological deficit.

33.3 Multiple Osteotomies

Multiple osteotomies are usually performed on the posterior vertebral arches, unless there is a previous anterior interbody fusion (Fig. 33.3a–h). The objective is to obtain correction by creating several points of mobility along the deformity, it is essential that there is flexibility in the anterior portion of the spine.

One of the main advantages of multiple osteotomies is the fact that deformities encompassing both the frontal and sagittal planes can be corrected simultaneously. The corrective forces are distributed along the deformity, and the osteoligamentous continuity of the spinal column is maintained, thereby avoiding sudden translations in any plane.

Each osteotomy site should be centered over the foramen; osteotomy at the level of the pedicle will impede closure of the osteotomy (Fig. 33.4). The width of each osteotomy line should not exceed 10 mm to assure closure when the correction forces are applied and to avoid empty spaces that could lead to pseudoarthrosis.

The principal disadvantage of multiple osteotomies is that uniform correction distributed over each resected level often cannot be achieved: the greatest part of correction is achieved at a few levels, whereas the others remain partially open. The main indications for this surgical technique are the long deformities affecting several segments and deformities involving both the frontal and sagittal planes.

33.4 Use of Spinal Instrumentation

Among the main benefits of transpedicular implants with a size adapted to children are the considerable correction that can be obtained and the immediate stability provided by posterior as well as anterior instrumentation. Ruff [5,6] have reported the effectiveness and safety of these implants for the treatment of vertebral deformities in the pediatric population and the absence of long-term unfavorable repercussions on the size of the spinal canal.

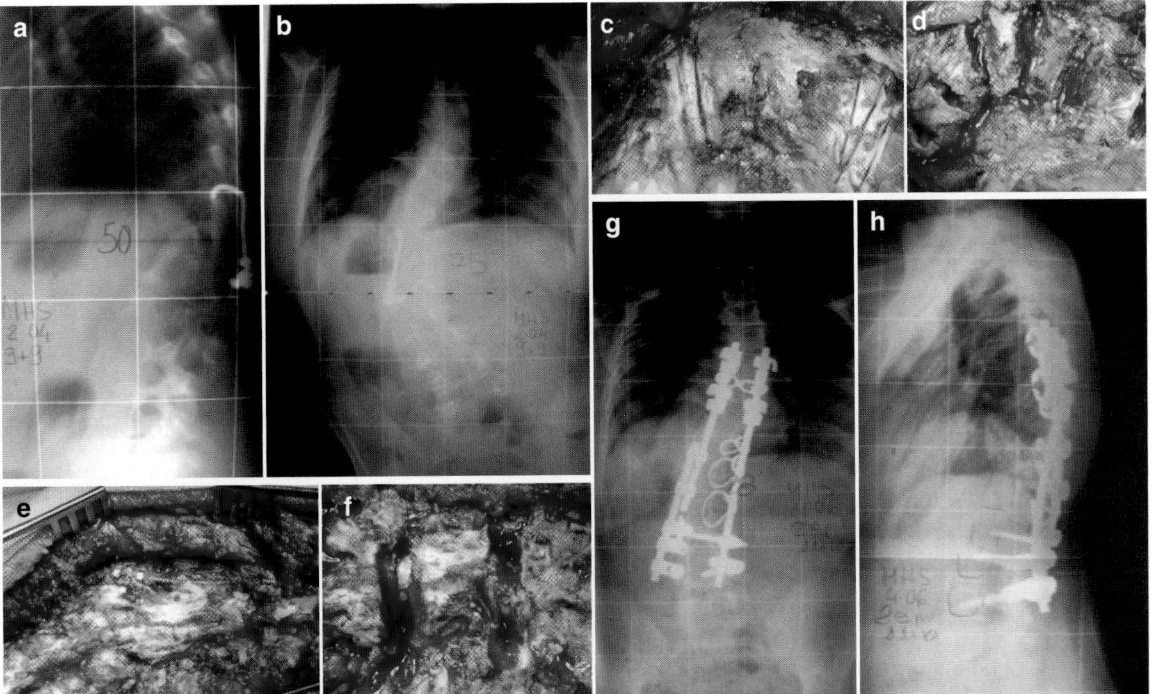

Fig. 33.3 (**a-h**) Reconstruction of complex and fixed congenital deformity by multiple anterior and posterior osteotomies

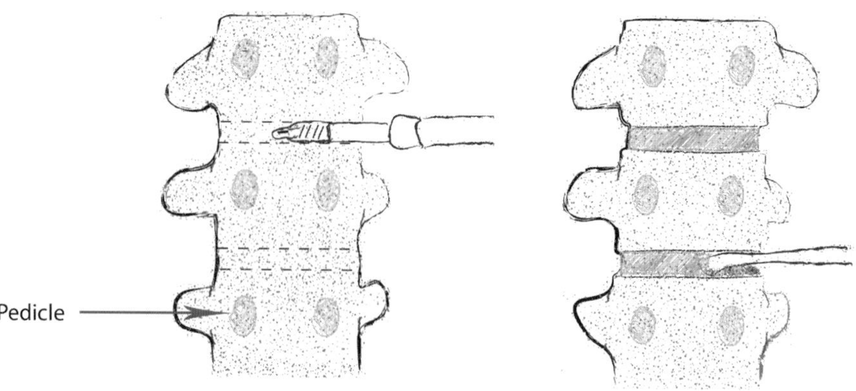

Fig. 33.4 Osteotomy through a previous fusion mass. Pedicle and foramen as a guidance to the osteotomy line. (Redrawn from [7]. Raven Press)

Lastly, it is important to emphasize the improvements in quality of life obtained with these implants, as long period of bed rest and rigid plaster cast are avoided.

33.5 Rib Osteotomies

The rib cage deformity can be seen either in the convexity, where the ribs are displaced and rotated posteriorly, or in the concavity, with the ribs turned anteriorly. Rib osteotomies are rarely indicated in the pediatric age group because the rib cage is still not completely developed and the repercussions on its growth can be highly unfavorable.

In patients with more mature bone status, rib osteotomies can be very useful for correction of the spinal deformity and to improve the cosmetic appearance. The greatest drawback of the technique is the possible negative effect on pulmonary function.

33.5.1 Rib Osteotomies at the Concavity

This procedure is only indicated in cases of rigid thoracic curves and significant cosmetic alteration produced by flattening of the hemithorax at the concavity of the curve. The objectives are to provide greater capacity for translation and correction of the spine by avoiding the theoretical barrier produced by the ribs and to improve the appearance of the back by decreasing the existing flattening of the thorax in the concavity of the deformity [1].

33.5.2 Osteotomies of the Ribs at the Convexity

This is a common technique, frequently used in adolescents and young adults [2]. By removing a small segment of rib near the spine, the deformed costal arch can be lowered, thereby significantly improving the typical rib hump seen in thoracic scoliosis. A slight decrease in respiratory function has been described following thoracoplasty at the convexity, but this deficit recovers over time [4].

References

1. Asher M, Lai SM, Burton D, Manna BRN (2004) Maintenance of trunk deformity correction following posterior instrumentation and arthrodesis for idiopathic scoliosis. Spine 29(16):1782–1788
2. Betz RR, Steel HH (1997) Thoracoplasty for rib deformity. In: Bradford DS (ed) Master techniques in orthopaedic surgery. Lippincott-Raven, Philadelphia, PA, pp 209–227
3. Chewning SJ, Heinig CF (1994) Osteotomy. In: Weinstein SL (ed) The pediatric spine: principles and practice. Raven Press, New York, pp 1443–1458
4. Lenke LG, Bridwell KH, Blanke K et al (1995) Analysis of pulmonary function and chest cage dimension changes after thoracoplasty in idiopathic scoliosis. Spine 20:1343–1350
5. Ruf M, Harms J (1996) Spinal growth after transpedicular instrumentation in one and two year old children. A ten year follow up. SRS 41st annual meeting. Monterey. Ca. Paper # 28
6. Ruf M, Harms J (2002) Pedicle screws in 1- and 2-year-old children: technique, complications, and effect on further growth. Spine 27(21):E460–E466
7. Weinstein S (1994) The pediatric spine. Principles and practice. Raven Press, New York, pp 1457
8. Winter RB (1983) Congenital deformities of the Spine. Thieme Straton, New York

34 Vertebral Resection

Dezsö Jeszenszky and Tamás Fülöp Fekete

Key Points

- Severe, early onset spinal deformities are likely to progress and can become life-threatening.
- Correction of such deformities is recommended as soon and as completely as possible to prevent the formation of secondary structural changes and to ensure balanced spinal growth.
- In the case of severe primary deformity of a short section of the spine (angular deformity), vertebral resection, a surgical procedure involving removal of at least one vertebra with the adjoining two intervertebral discs, is recommended.
- Vertebral resection allows substantial correction while keeping the length of instrumentation/fusion as short as possible.

34.1 Introduction

High-grade spinal deformities in the early years of life involve abnormalities in all planes, such that the use of a simple term such as scoliosis or kyphosis to describe them is usually inaccurate. Furthermore, the emphasis is on the young age of the patient and hence the potential for growth.

Severe early onset scoliosis (EOS), wherein conventional surgical treatment methods are not applicable, are relatively rare. However, since such severe deformities can be life-threatening in young children, surgical intervention is unavoidable and should be carried out as soon as possible. A deformed section of the spine not only affects the development of the remaining healthy spine regions, but also influences the development of the chest wall, and hence the lungs, and the extremities too. Chest wall deformity in the early years of life results in a decreased development of alveoli and thus an irreversible decrease of lung-function [4, 7, 16]. As development in early childhood is very dynamic and rapid [5], even a small delay in correction of a major spinal deformity leads to significant secondary damage to healthy structures and functions (breathing, gait, etc.) (Fig. 34.1a–d). A radical and swift spinal correction is needed in this setting, and this can be provided by vertebral resection (VR).

Vertebral resection (also known as vertebral column resection, columnotomy or vertebrectomy) is a radical surgical intervention in terms of the associated risks of neurological damage and the long-term effects on the growing spine, trunk, and ultimately the whole body. We use the term vertebral resection only to describe a circumferential resection of at least one vertebra of the spinal column along with the adjoining intervertebral discs.

Although VR has been used for several decades, the minimal literature that exists on the procedure is limited to its application in adolescents and adults [1–3, 10, 15]. There is minimal data concerning vertebral resection in the growing spine [13]. Hence, a sound synthesis of the general rules in spinal surgery and pediatric surgery is needed to appropriately apply VR in EOS. In our opinion, vertebral resection can be even more effective in the growing spine than in adolescents

D. Jeszenszky (✉)
Spine Unit, Schulthess Clinic, Lengghalde 2,
8008 Zürich, Switzerland
e-mail: dezsoe.jeszenszky@kws.ch
www.schulthess-clinic.ch

B. A. Akbarnia et al. (eds.), *The Growing Spine*,
DOI: 10.1007/978-3-540-85207-0_34, © Springer-Verlag Berlin Heidelberg 2011

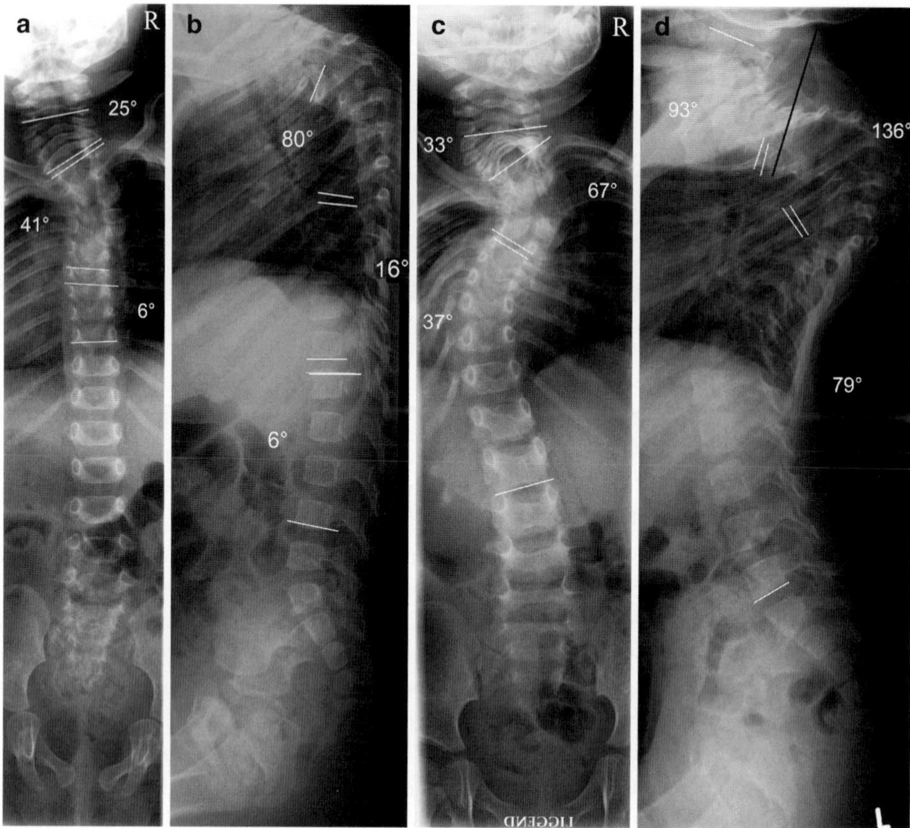

Fig. 34.1 EOS caused by an unknown syndrome (**a**, **b**). Sitting lateral and posteroanterior (PA) radiographs of a girl 9 months of age show a high thoracic kyphoscoliotic curve pattern. The Cobb angles were as follows: *left* cervical scoliosis, 25° (C4–T1); *right* thoracic scoliosis, 41° (T2–T6); *left* thoracic scoliosis, 6° (T7–T10); cervical lordosis, not measurable on the first radiographs; thoracic kyphosis, 80° (T2–T6); thoracic lordosis, 16° (T7–T12); lumbar kyphosis, 6° (L1–L4) (**c**, **d**). The follow-up shows a rapid deterioration in 15 months time. The supine radiographs demonstrate a thoracic kyphosis of 136° (T2–T7) and a *right* thoracic scoliosis of 67° (T2–T6). Note how rapidly the thorax collapses along with the spine. This results in a worsening of lung function. At admission at 2 years of age, the patient suffered from resting dyspnea, and had to lean on something to support her upper body and expand her chest to be able to breathe. Note the positions of the pedicles at the upper thoracic area. The *black line* in the lateral view indicates the trajectory of a planned pedicle screw. In this severe deformity, pedicle screws at this region cannot be inserted because of spatial limitations of the skull

and adults. It not only rapidly corrects deformity but also guides further development.

34.2 Evaluation

The undertaking of a thorough history and physical examination is important. Often, the children affected are so young that they have not yet achieved the ability to stand or even sit. Hence, it does not make sense to evaluate sitting or upright imbalance. Also, they usually do not complain of any pain. The main reason the children's guardians seek medical attention is usually the rapid progression of visible spinal deformity (trunk asymmetry).

Identification and treatment of any concomitant medical problems is necessary prior to consideration of surgical intervention. This is not always straightforward as some EOS are accompanied by extremely rare or even unknown syndromes.

The respiratory status of the patients should be thoroughly evaluated, which is often difficult in very young patients. If pulmonary function testing is compromised, it should be optimized preoperatively, possibly with Halo-traction.

The physical examination focuses on flexibility of the deformity as well as on evaluation of coronal and sagittal plane decompensation. It is important to evaluate the locomotor function as a whole with a focus on the ability to sit or stand, whenever possible. Further, the search for any accompanying pathologies of the extremities, such as contractures or instabilities of major joints, is important. A thorough neurological examination will reveal any signs of abnormality, after which further electrophysiological examinations might be justified.

Radiological evaluation includes standing (sitting in non-ambulatory patients) full-spine radiographs in posteroanterior and lateral views. The magnitude of curves is determined in both the coronal and sagittal planes using the standard Cobb method. In some severe deformities it may be impossible to measure the Cobb angles correctly. Trunk balance is determined by measuring the deviation from the midline at the sacrum of a plumb line dropped from the spinous process of C7 on the posterior anterior view and from the body of C7 on the lateral view. Special radiographs are necessary for evaluating the flexibility of the deformity. Anteroposterior radiographs are taken in a supine position with manually forced right and left bending with the pelvis fixed. Manual axial traction full-spine radiographs in posteroanterior (PA) and lateral views are necessary. These are all possible in standing, sitting or supine positions. All candidates for VR should be evaluated by magnetic resonance imaging (MRI). Computed tomography (CT) and/or CT-myelography are used to evaluate spinal anatomy. 3D reconstruction of the CT scans helps to better understand the pathoanatomy and the structural changes of the spine. If any intraspinal pathology such as syringomyelia, diastematomyelia, tumor, or tethering is discovered, its management has to be considered prior to correction of the deformity.

34.3 Management

Generally, the indications for surgical intervention are similar to those for any spinal deformities (progression, pain, imbalance, neurological deficit or deterioration of pulmonary function). However, the most important surgical indication for VR in EOS patients is a rigid, severe and angular curvature on a short section of the spine. This type of deformity usually progresses rapidly. VR is a salvage procedure; it is indicated if other surgical techniques would not be sufficient to achieve an acceptable correction and balance of the spine (Table 34.1). VR is applicable for severe deformity of any origin such as congenital, neuromuscular disease, developmental anomaly, tumor, etc.

The ultimate goal of surgery is to halt progression and to achieve radical correction of the deformity to balance growth and improve pulmonary function. This should be achieved with a rigid internal fixation and fusion of the spine over the shortest possible section. A biomechanically appropriate, stable internal fixation obviates the need for any postoperative orthosis. The short arthrodesis allows for motion preservation of the primarily unaffected areas of the spine.

If the planned instrumentation and correction cannot be carried out because of the existing configuration of the curve and/or insufficient lung-function, a preoperative reduction of the curve is necessary (see Fig. 34.1b and Fig. 34.2a, b). For this purpose, halo-gravity traction is suitable. To provide an acceptable means of continuous traction for several weeks or months, halo-gravitational-traction devices are used for each of the major body positions (halo-wheelchair, halo-bed and ambulatory halo-frame). For further details, see Chap. 28 – Halo-gravity traction.

It is of paramount importance to have experienced pediatric anesthesia and critical care teams to assist with the management of EOS patients. Preoperative evaluation by the anesthesia team several weeks prior to surgery is

Table 34.1 Comparison of different surgical techniques for severe early onset spinal deformities (authors' experience)

	In situ fusion	Stapling	Growing rods	Shilla	VR	VEPTR
Applicability in severe deformities	+	+	++	++	+++	++
Correction, rate/speed	+	+	++	++	+++	+
Grade of immediate correction	0	0/+	++	++	+++	++
Ability to prevent secondary structural changes	+	+	++	++	+++	+
Surgical risks/Complication rate	+	++	++	++	+++	+++
Immediate effect on thorax size after surgery	0	0	++	++	+++	++
Long-term effect on thorax function	0	+	++	++	++	+
Technically demanding	+	++	++	++	+++	+

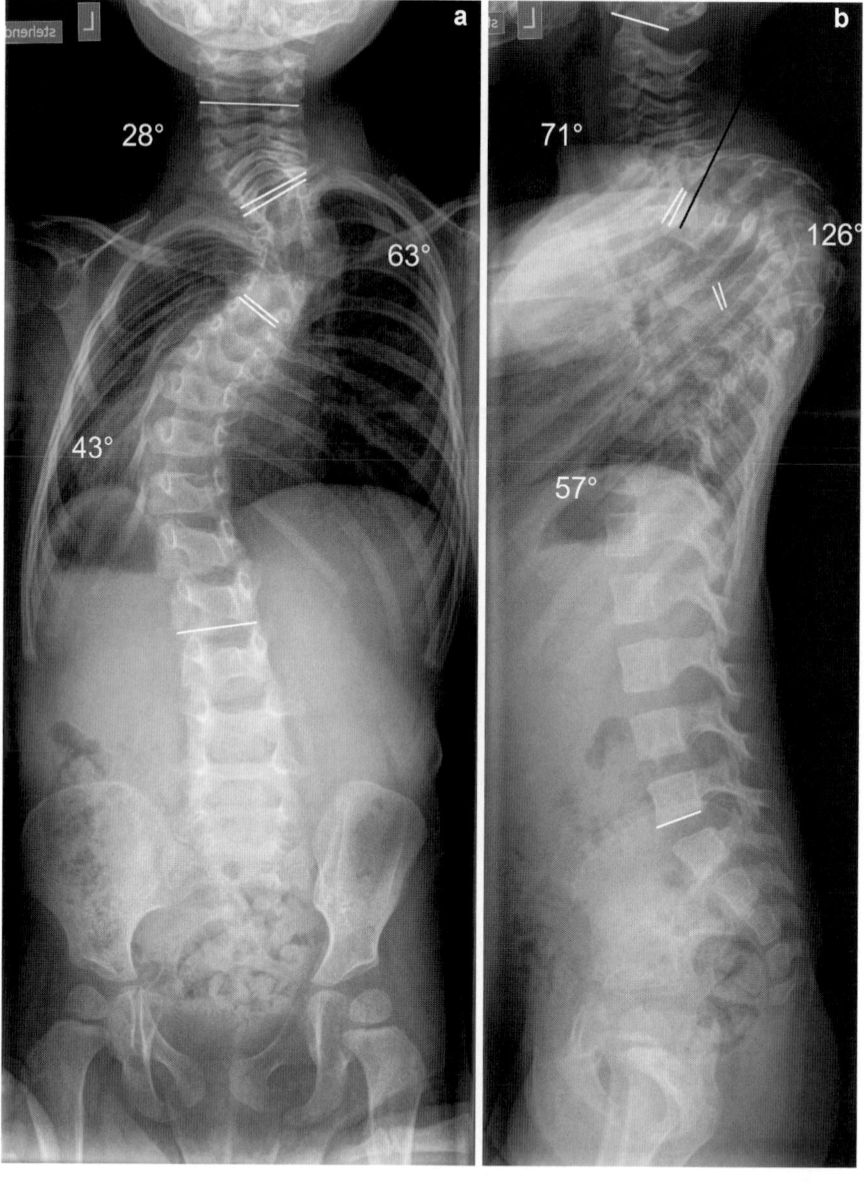

Fig. 34.2 Same patient as in Fig. 34.1.(**a**, **b**) Notable correction in terms of spinal alignment and chest configuration is achieved after 2 months of halo traction. There were three consequences of halo-gravity traction: first, lung function improved considerably and the activity level of the child increased; second, the cervical lordosis decreased from 93 to 71°, so the instrumentation with pedicle screws in the upper thoracic area became feasible (the *black line* again indicates the planned trajectory of the T2 pedicle screw); third, it became obvious which part of the curvature was rigid and through the improvement of the deformity the surgery was made less demanding

useful and is encouraged since many patients have multi-organ disorders as part of a syndrome. Blood loss is often substantial and pulmonary function requires careful monitoring and support during the immediate postoperative period. Use of a cell saver is recommended.

Radical correction is considered to be associated with a high-risk of neurological injury. The use of multimodal intraoperative monitoring (MIOM) reduces the risk of intraoperative neurological injury [6]. MIOM is a very helpful tool for safe and relaxed surgical work; it obviates the need for any form of wake-up tests. A good collaboration between anesthetist and monitoring neurologist is important. Hypotensive anesthesia helps to reduce intraoperative blood loss, but it can complicate the interpretation of MIOM.

34.4 Surgical Procedure

The more traditional techniques for correction of EOS, including posterior in situ fusion and instrumented fusion, convex growth arrest, kyphectomy, hemivertebrectomy, insertion of growing rods, thoracic expansion, vertebral osteotomy, non-fusion and motion preservation techniques, have been described elsewhere in this book.

In the case of severe angular spinal deformity, even a pedicle subtraction osteotomy or a series of osteotomies might not be sufficient to achieve acceptable correction and, instead, VR is needed. Careful preoperative planning is required to determine the number of vertebrae to be removed during surgery. However, we recommend a certain amount of flexibility in terms of the extent of resection. The preoperative plan can be modified according to the intraoperative findings. It is sometimes necessary to remove two or even three apical vertebrae, but the number of vertebrae to be removed should be kept as low as possible. It is therefore advisable to begin with resection of a single vertebra. Further resection can be performed in a stepwise fashion, if necessary. In some cases, additional spinal osteotomies might even be required.

34.4.1 Surgical Technique

Posterior spinal surgery is recommended, as this has more advantages compared with combined approaches [15]. There is no thoracotomy, and no postoperative thorax wall scarring. The posterior approach allows all the necessary steps for safe VR and correction. It provides continuous visual control of the neural structures during resection and correction. A costotransversectomy on one or on both sides in the thoracic area or removal of the transverse processes in the lumbar area is performed for good visualization and a capacious working area. This approach also allows for safe circumferential preparation around the vertebral body and control of the segmental vessels. One drawback is the difficulty in controlling the major vessels in the prevertebral area. In some cases, a combined anterior-posterior or posterior-anterior-posterior approach cannot be avoided [3, 8, 9].

Technically there is no major difference to VR described elsewhere [3, 15]. In contrast to the usual subperiosteal preparation, preservation of the periosteal layer is attempted to avoid unnecessary spontaneous fusion and allow for unaltered or minimally altered growth. This is followed by verification of the correct levels using fluoroscopy, usually in an anteroposterior view. The next step is to identify the entry points of all planned transpedicular screws by using anatomical landmarks. Ordinary 22 Gauge needles or other guides are then inserted into the pedicles. Fluoroscopy control in anteroposterior and lateral views is recommended. The next step is to preparation of pedicles for insertion of screws using a 1.5 mm drill, insertion of pre-bent K-wires into each hole, and once again performing fluoroscopy inspection in two views. Depending on what is revealed in the images acquired, fine adjustments can be made at the next step, where a 2.0 or 2.5 mm drill or pedicle probe is used for final preparation of the pedicle, 2.7, 4.0, 4.75 or 5.0mm diameter screws can be used instead. Screws are preferable to hooks or wires because of their greater anchoring capacity and thus better potential to achieve and maintain the correction (primary stability) [11, 14]. The placement of pedicle screws at strategically important sites prior to vertebral resection is of extreme importance, since it allows the control of spinal alignment and hence protection of the neural structures in an otherwise extremely unstable intraoperative situation.

It is useful to mark the exiting nerve roots using a simple rubber band. A single nerve root may be sacrificed in the thoracic area between T3 and T9. This helps to perform a more secure resection.

In the correction of coronal and sagittal deformities, all correction maneuvers can be used. During correction, the dura has to be continuously checked visually; dural pulsation is a good sign, but it is certainly not a reliable indicator of neural function. Even with the use of MIOM, correction still needs to be carried out slowly and carefully.

Anterior support is important; this is either achieved by bone-on-bone contact or, in the case of a longer defect, anterior reconstruction (e.g. with cage). To facilitate bony fusion, morsalized autologous bone (e.g., removed rib and vertebra) is recommended. In the authors' experience, rib resection (thoracoplasty) on the convex side and osteotomy on the concave side should be avoided. These structures are usually flexible enough in EOS patients. On the basis of intraoperative findings, careful consideration of additional osteotomies and further resection might be necessary.

Unfortunately, intraoperative radiographs often fail to indicate whether the spine is correctly aligned with respect to the plumb line; the balance of the spine can only be evaluated accurately in an upright position (standing or sitting). If the postoperative films demonstrate residual imbalance in the sagittal or coronal plane, further correction should be undertaken as soon as possible.

34.4.2 Postoperative Management

Pedicle screw instrumentation provides enough stability to mobilize patients without any external orthosis; therefore, children can ambulate immediately after surgery. They do not need to be encouraged to get up and mobilize themselves, as this usually happens as soon as wound pain subsides. Physiotherapy for improvement of lung function is recommended.

Radiographic and clinical follow-ups should be performed at regular intervals: 8 weeks, 6 months, 1 year after surgery at least until fusion is consolidated and mature. Depending on the rate of growth, further follow-ups are carried out at 6-month or 1-year intervals. Lung function tests might also be important.

34.4.3 Documentation

We recommend thorough documentation of deformities with radiographs and photographs (Fig. 34.3). The photographs should be taken in a standardized fashion preoperatively and postoperatively. Videos might also be useful to document dynamics. Such documentation, repeated also at the regular follow-ups, allows for analysis of the development and change of deformity

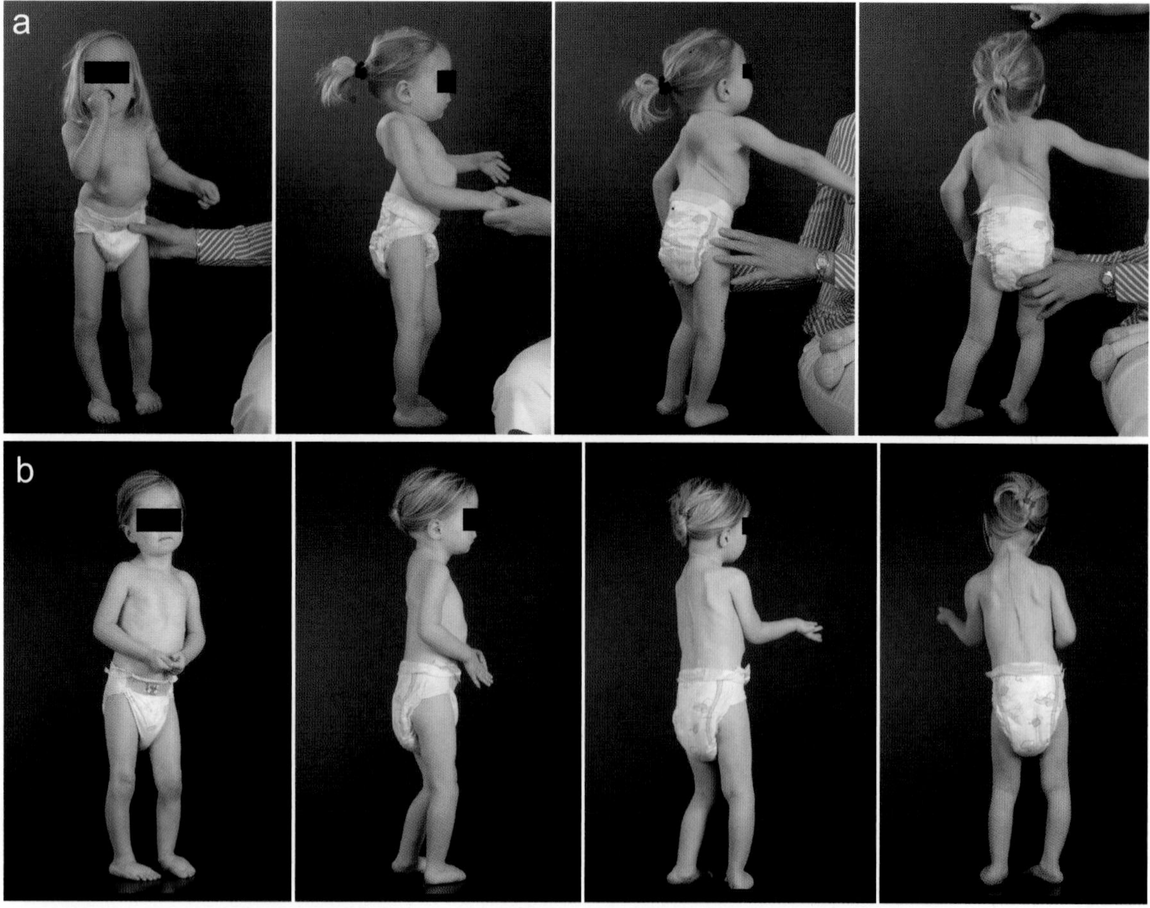

Fig. 34.3 Same patient as in Fig. 34.2. Comparison of the preoperative (**a**) and immediately postoperative (**b**) images demonstrates the marked change of the whole body caused by the radical spinal correction through vertebral resection – and all achieved as a direct and immediate result of the surgery itself. In addition, the patient is able to stand independently through the improved balance of the spine. The time factor is very important. The sooner the correction is achieved, the less secondary changes can occur through the deformity-related, abnormally guided development

of the whole body. This is not only helpful for scientific or professional purposes, but it also helps to show the results to the patients and their parents.

34.5 Discussion

There are many etiologies of EOSs, which include congenital, neuromuscular, and idiopathic forms, and they can present as part of various syndromes.

Ideally one should not let a spinal deformity progress to a severe stage. If severe curves develop because of the delay in treatment for any reason, severe chest deformity can develop, resulting in cardiopulmonary problems. In extremely severe cases, children can present with dyspnea at rest, because of their being at the limit of their respiratory compensatory mechanisms. Some surgeons advocate only incomplete correction, which is considered to reduce the risk of the surgery [4]. However, the best long-term results are obtained with total correction of the deformity. Complete restoration of physiological curvatures should be aimed for in young children. The abnormality is in many aspects obvious, but the management of children with progressive, severe EOS has proven difficult. Attempting any type of conservative treatment in this setting is hazardous and highly questionable.

Most of the well established treatment methods for EOS (e.g., posterior growing rod procedures, hemi-epiphysiodesis, VEPTR, Shilla, etc.) can only be applied in the case of mild, moderate or moderately-severe deformities. They cannot be used for extremely severe deformities, either due to technical difficulties or because of their slow effect (Table 34.1).

For the treatment of a severe EOS, a VR can be applied. This radical surgical technique is often used in adolescents and adults. However, its application in young children is not yet established; there is a lack of treatment standards, and there are no recommendations in the literature. This results in uncertainty and perplexity for the treating physicians. Desperate parents often present their child after being recommended different (and often contradictory) treatment methods, while they witness the progression of deformity. VEPTR is often recommended but only after a hesitant wait, which is often too long, such that VEPTR can no longer be applied due to curve progression. Furthermore, if thorax deformity is secondary to spinal deformity, it is advisable to treat the spine first rather than to treat the spine indirectly through the primarily intact chest.

If there is a severe and rigid primary deformity on a short segment, vertebral resection should be considered. After the decision for VR has been made, further delay is unacceptable. Prevention of secondary changes is paramount. However, this does not mean that the process should be initiated in a hurry, before all relevant issues have been carefully considered.

First, these young children already have a short spine and hence a short trunk due to their spinal deformity. Performing a vertebral resection and thereby further shortening the spine might sound contradictory. Some surgeons consider that such a shortening will be associated with a further decrease of pulmonary function [13]. This point is debatable, since the length of the spine is not the most important factor in determining lung function and development. A more important factor is the curvature of the spine and consequently the volume, configuration, and function of the chest. As such, we have to aim for as short a resection as possible while achieving maximal correction of the spine (and hence the chest) in as short a time as possible. Spinal resection with correction of the deformity (Fig. 34.4 a, b) stops unbalanced growth of the spine, which in turn will result in an overall lengthening of the trunk in the long run. The surgery itself shortens the spine, which is better tolerated by the spinal cord. The situation is analogous to another spine shortening procedure, the resection of a hemivertebra. The latter is a less radical procedure, performed in less severe deformities, but it used to be regarded as a difficult and demanding procedure; in the meantime, it has become a standard treatment method [12].

Second, in contrast to adolescent and adult deformities, balance of the spine is not the most important factor to consider. More important are the severity of deformity and the rate of progression. In most cases, these young patients have not yet developed any upright posture and therefore the term spinal balance is not applicable. In the case that the young patient is already able to sit or stand, the balance of the spine can be determined. If imbalance is present, it can reinforce the surgical indication. However, values describing imbalance in the adult spine are not transferable to children in the first 5 years of life because of their principally different body proportions.

For surgical indications in adolescent and adult deformity surgery, there are relatively clear-cut values to indicate the degree of deformity and the point at which one should intervene. Such limits cannot be applied to a severe early onset curvature. Instead, it

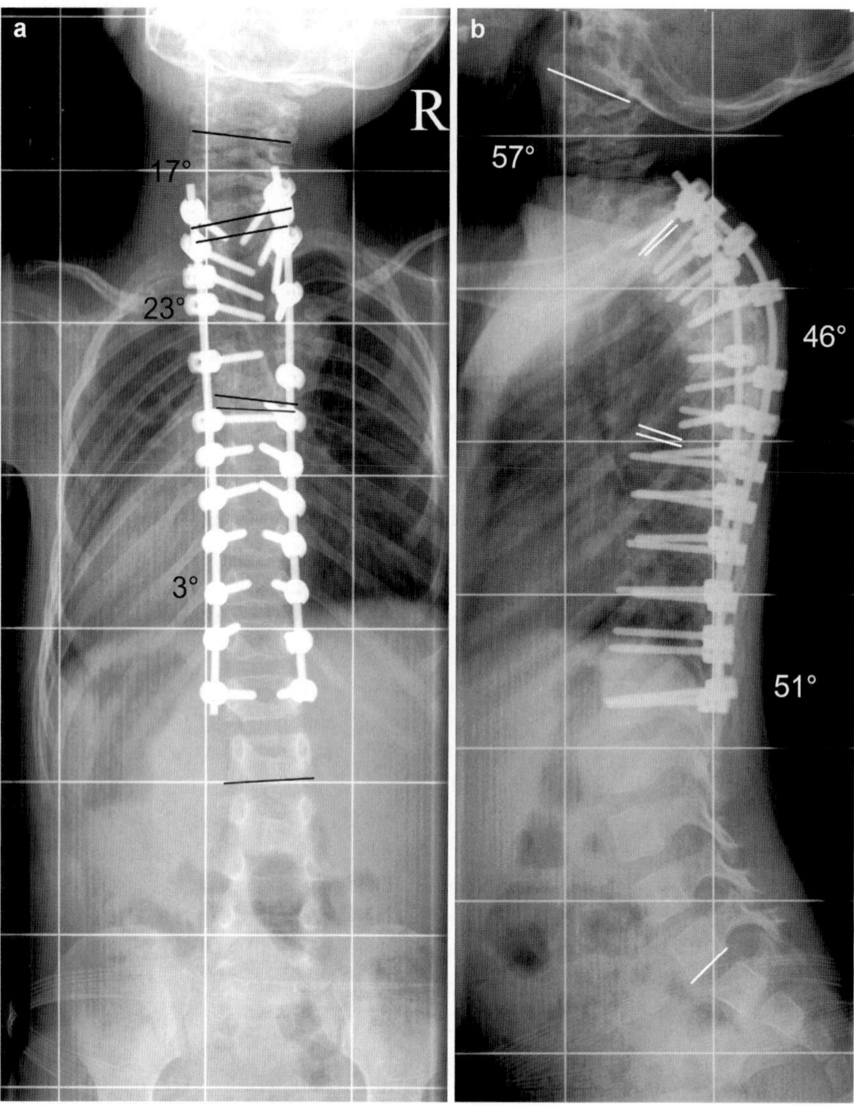

Fig. 34.4 Same patient as in Fig. 34.2. (**a**, **b**) Subperiosteal preparation was used during the surgical procedure to avoid spontaneous fusion. Polyaxial pedicle screws with a diameter of 3.5 mm were inserted between T1 and L1 on both sides, and were connected with 3 mm rods on either side. Such a long instrumentation was required to correct the secondary hyperlordosis in the thoracic area. A bone-on-bone fusion was only performed between T4 and T6. The autologous bone material gained by the resection of the T5 vertebra was used to enhance fusion. Resection of the T5 vertebra was performed with costotransversectomy T5 and T6 on the *right side* and T5 on the *left side* through a posterior approach. The thoracic kyphosis thus decreased to 46° and the *right thoracic* scoliosis decreased to 23° between T2 and T6. Note the near physiological sagittal and coronal alignment of the spine and the marked change of the chest wall immediately after surgery. The almost complete correction of the deformity resulted in correct alignment at the non-instrumented area. This allowed for an undisturbed development of the spine, preventing secondary structural changes at the previously healthy spine segments. A partial implant removal is subsequently worth considering to free up the non-fused segments T1–T2 and the segments between T7 and L1. If some residual deformity still exists, a change to a dual growing-rod or Shilla technique is possible

always has to be evaluated individually, in view of progression. Although it is a salvage procedure, it should be considered a prophylactic intervention in relation to the rest of the spine.

As mentioned earlier, halo-gravity traction for several weeks or months preoperatively is necessary in certain cases for various reasons. It causes stretching of abnormally shortened soft-tissues (including vessels, muscles, ligaments, etc.) and the spinal curvature decreases such that instrumentation becomes possible. It also alters the chest volume, improving pulmonary function. In children with initial respiratory insufficiency, a marked improvement in the performance of daily activities can be observed.

Vertebral resection is a complete circumferential resection, or disconnection of the spine, which allows realignment in any direction. The realignment is limited by the neural structures, mainly the spinal cord itself. During realignment, the pivot point is in the spinal cord area. Although, with regards to the spine, this is a shortening procedure, from the point of view of the spinal cord, it is effectively a neutral or minimally shortening procedure. It therefore allows a large amount of freedom to realign the spine with a high, but acceptable risk of neurological injury.

Reliable, strong but also short anchoring is necessary to achieve and maintain correction, for which the pedicle screw–rod system seems to be the most appropriate.

Owing to continued growth of the spine following a vertebral resection procedure, a change to the growing rod instrumentation might become necessary if correction is incomplete.

The experience with VR in EOS is currently limited but the initial results are encouraging. The improved pulmonary function and more optimal spinal balance result in an increased ability to perform daily activities and an improved quality of life, making it a worthwhile treatment for certain severe early onset spinal deformities.

34.6 Summary

The most important aim of treatment in early onset spinal deformities is to correct the deformity as soon and as completely as possible. This ensures a balanced growth of healthy regions of the spine. It also prevents the development of secondary structural changes. Ideally, the treatment focus should not extend beyond the site of primary deformity; the surgical correction should be kept as short as possible.

Severe EOS is usually due to either rapid progression or unnecessary hesitation in introducing a corrective treatment. If the deformity is on a relatively short segment (angulated deformity), a vertebral resection is indicated, i.e., a surgical procedure involving removal of at least one vertebra with the adjoining two intervertebral discs. Such a removal of the severely deformed section of the spine allows for a short fusion whilst providing the fastest and greatest correction of the deformity. It therefore ensures balanced growth of the rest of the spine. If a complete correction cannot be achieved, vertebral resection provides the option to reduce severe deformity such that more established forms of treatment for a less pronounced deformity can then be used.

It is the most radical surgical treatment option. Currently, it is only used if other treatment modalities are considered likely to fail. However, as more and more experience is gained with the procedure, a widening of the indication spectrum is foreseeable, to also include less-pronounced deformities. In this case, it would be regarded as preventive surgery where rapid progression is otherwise expected.

The most important factor in the treatment of EOS is the early onset of treatment.

References

1. Boachie-Adjei O, Bradford DS (1991) Vertebral column resection and arthrodesis for complex spinal deformities. J Spinal Disord 4:193–202
2. Bradford DS, Tribus CB (1994) Current concepts and management of patients with fixed decompensated spinal deformity. Clin Orthop Relat Res:64–72
3. Bradford DS, Tribus CB (1997) Vertebral column resection for the treatment of rigid coronal decompensation. Spine 22:1590–1599
4. Dickson RA (2001) Early-onset idiopathic scoliosis. In: Weinstein SL (ed) The pediatric spine: principles and practice. Lippincott Williams and Wilkins, Philadelphia, pp 321–328
5. Dimeglio A (2001) Growth in pediatric orthopaedics. J Pediatr Orthop 21:549–555
6. Eggspuehler A, Sutter MA, Grob D et al (2007) Multimodal intraoperative monitoring during surgery of spinal deformities in 217 patients. Eur Spine J 16(Suppl 2):S188–S196
7. Emery JL, Mithal A (1960) The number of alveoli in the terminal respiratory unit of man during late intrauterine life and childhood. Arch Dis Child 35:544–547
8. Floman Y, Micheli LJ, Penny JN et al (1982) Combined anterior and posterior fusion in seventy-three spinally deformed patients: indications, results and complications. Clin Orthop Relat Res 164:110–122
9. Kostuik JP, Maurais GR, Richardson WJ et al (1988) Combined single stage anterior and posterior osteotomy for correction of iatrogenic lumbar kyphosis. Spine 13: 257–266
10. Leatherman KD (1973) The management of rigid spinal curves. Clin Orthop Relat Res (93):215–224.

11. Liljenqvist U, Hackenberg L, Link T et al (2001) Pullout strength of pedicle screws versus pedicle and laminar hooks in the thoracic spine. Acta Orthop Belg 67:157–163
12. Ruf M, Jensen R, Jeszenszky D et al (2006) Hemivertebra resection in congenital scoliosis – early correction in young children. Z Orthop Ihre Grenzgeb 144:74–79
13. Sponseller PD, Yazici M, Demetracopoulos C et al (2007) Evidence basis for management of spine and chest wall deformities in children. Spine 32:S81–S90
14. Suk SI, Lee CK, Kim WJ et al (1995) Segmental pedicle screw fixation in the treatment of thoracic idiopathic scoliosis. Spine 20:1399–1405
15. Suk SI, Chung ER, Kim JH et al (2005) Posterior vertebral column resection for severe rigid scoliosis. Spine 30:1682–1687
16. Thurlbeck WM (1982) Postnatal human lung growth. Thorax 37:564–571

35 Single Growing Rods

George H. Thompson and Jochen P. Son-Hing

Key Points

- Single growing rods are beneficial in the treatment of early onset scoliosis.
- The complication rate with single growing rods is moderately high, with rod breakage being the most common.
- Cosmesis is less than ideal with "crankshaft" phenomena being a major problem.

35.1 Introduction

Progressive early onset scoliosis (EOS) poses unique challenges to those involved in management. The objective in such cases is to minimize or prevent curve progression while allowing for spinal growth and therefore increased thoracic cage volume and lung growth and development. Serial Risser casts and orthotics can be used initially [2, 12], but can be hampered by difficulties with compliance, expense, and sub-optimal mechanical control of the deformity, particularly as the child gets older. At the other extreme, definitive surgical treatment using anterior spinal fusion (ASF) or posterior spinal fusion (PSF) and segmental spinal instrumentation (SSI) can stabilize curve progression, even preventing crankshaft [8, 11, 20], but in such cases, this may result in a disproportionately short trunk that can further adversely affect thoracic cage and lung development.

To bridge these options, growing rods have been developed as a means to both control the spinal deformity and allow spinal, thoracic cage and lung growth and development. Growth modulation techniques have been attempted but with limited success. Growing rods can either be single or dual rods. These rods require periodic lengthening in an attempt to maintain alignment of the spine during growth. Earlier attempts to facilitate this usually incorporated a single Harrington rod [5–7, 13, 14, 21, 24] or employed Luque rods or "Luque Trolleys" [10, 17–19]. Later, Morin [15] introduced the concept of proximal and distal "claw" foundations for fixation of the growing rods. The growing rod technique with which we have had the most experience is a single growing rod with proximal and distal "claw" foundations.

35.2 Surgical Technique for Single Growing RODS

35.2.1 *Intraoperative*

Our single growing rod construct consists of a proximal "claw" with hooks and a distal construct of either hooks or pedicle screws. The technique is similar to other spine procedures. (Fig. 35.1a–d) After induction of general anesthesia, the patient is positioned prone on either the Hall-Relton four poster frame or a Jackson table. Typically, a long, mid-line incision is made over that portion of the spine that is to be instrumented. The exact length is based on preoperative planning. The subcutaneous tissues are divided and the fascia exposed. One spinous process proximally and distally delineating the

G.H. Thompson (✉)
Division of Pediatric Orthopaedic Surgery, Rainbow Babies and Children's Hospital, University Hospitals Case Medical Center, 11100 Euclid Avenue, Cleveland, Ohio 44106, USA
e-mail: ght@po.cwru.edu

B. A. Akbarnia et al. (eds.), *The Growing Spine*,
DOI: 10.1007/978-3-540-85207-0_35,

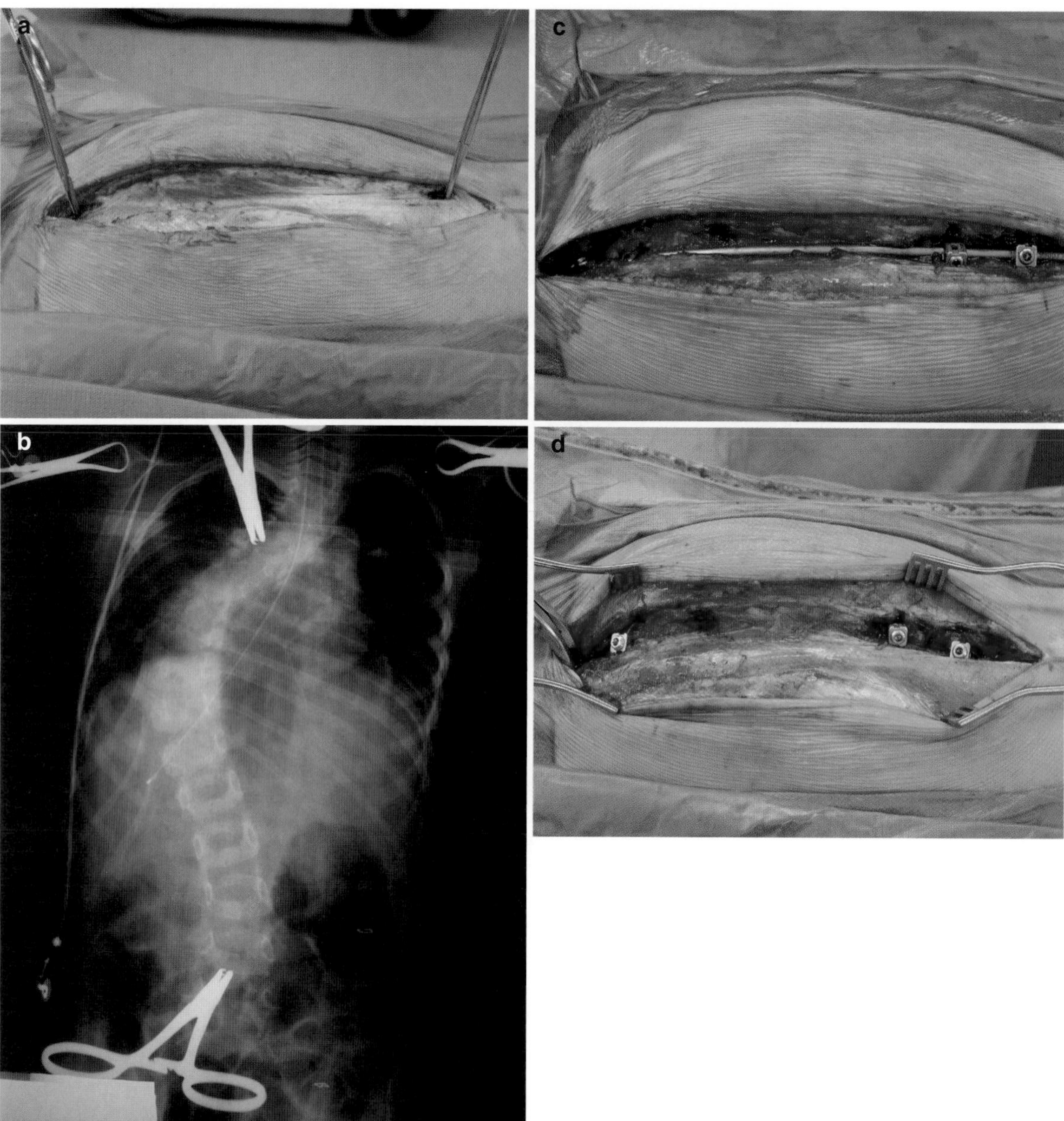

Fig. 35.1 (**a**) Intraoperative photograph demonstrating the incision and the exposure for the upper and lower foundations. The spinous processes at the planned levels are identified and marked. A radiograph is obtained to confirm the preplanned levels. (**b**) Intraoperative antero-posterior (AP) radiograph demonstrating identification of the foundation sites. (**c**) Hooks are typically used for the upper foundation and hooks and/or screws for the lower foundation. Hooks spanning two vertebral segments for the proximal and distal foundation were used in this patient. The muscle has been separated to allow the rod to lie as close to the bone as possible. However, the laminae, facets and spinous processes are not exposed except at the foundation sites, which are fused. (**d**) Following rod insertion a long segment of rod is *left* extending below the lower foundation. This is used to expand the rod and maintain spinal length. The fascia is closed over the instrumentation

foundation sites is exposed and marked with a clamp. Intraoperative radiographs are obtained to identify the preplanned foundation sites. Once this has been accomplished, then the two or three adjacent vertebrae are exposed subperiosteoally. The fascia between the foundation sites is also divided and the muscle thinned so that the rod will lie close to the spine. However, the laminae are not exposed or visualized. The distal foundation is usually constructed first. In the beginning, we used a claw construct with an over-the-top laminar hook proximally and a sublaminar hook distally. This allowed compression between the hooks. However, in the last 5 years, we have used a pedicle screw construct for the distal foundation. The proximal foundation consists of an over-the-top laminar hook proximally and a sublaminar hook in the next distal vertebrae. Occasionally, this may extend one additional level distally. This also allows for a compression once the rod has been inserted. The size of the rod is based on the size of the patient. In most small children, a 5.5 mm rod is used, while in older children, a 6.35 mm rod is used. The interval between the foundations is measured with a silk suture and the rod measured. Typically, an additional 5 or 6 cm is added to this measurement to compensate for the initial distraction and to have enough extra length to allow it to be expanded at subsequent surgeries. The rod is appropriately contoured and inserted. When hooks are utilized for the distal foundation, they occasionally need to be open hooks to allow for the rod to be appropriately seated. Once the rod is inserted, it is grasped with rod holders and rotated to allow for a relatively normal sagittal plane alignment. The upper foundation is typically tightened first. The rod is distracted distally. This is always done under intraoperative neuromuscular monitoring. There are 4 or 5 cm of rod extending below the lower hook or screw. This is used for subsequent lengthenings. The wound is closed in layers. The fascia is closed over the entire construct. Typically, a drain is placed over the top of the fascia. The subcutaneous tissues and skin are closed in a standard manner. The latter is typically a subcuticular closure.

35.2.2 Postoperative Management

The rods are lengthened periodically, usually every 6 months. As long as there is enough rod available proximally or distally from the foundation for lengthening, this area alone can be exposed (Fig. 35.2). For example, in the case in which rod length is available caudal to the distal foundation, a rod holder is placed cephalad to the distal foundation, a distracter is placed between the rod holder and the foundation, the set screws in the foundation are loosened, and the distracter is used to lengthen the rod. This maneuver increased the rod length now present between the proximal and distal foundations, at the expense of the available rod length caudal to the distal foundation. One must ensure to finish by using a compressor on the distal foundation to re-tension this claw or pedicle screw segment, before tightening the set screws again.

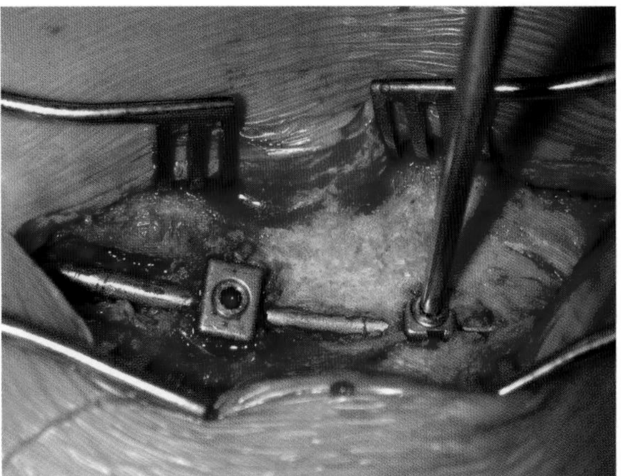

Fig. 35.2 Rod lengthening is performed through the lower foundation. The set screws loosened and rod elongated between the foundations. The corner foundation is then retightened. When the rod has been fully expanded additional lengthenings can be accomplished by dividing the rod at the thoracolumbar junction and applying a tandem connector

In the situation in which there is no longer enough rod available above or below the terminal foundations, two options are available. The first option is to cut the rod in the thoracolumbar region and place a tandem connector over the cut ends. The construct can then be lengthened even further through this connector. The thoracolumbar region is selected because of its lack of significant kyphosis or lordosis, allowing ease of placement of the connector. The second option is to remove the rod and insert a new, longer one. It is possible in such a circumstance to minimize the surgical dissection by exposing only the terminal foundations, and using the submuscular tunnel to introduce the new rod; however, it is essential in such instances to do this in a very controlled manner, since the rod can be directed into the thoracic cage if significant care is not used [7].

35.2.3 Definitive Fusion

Definitive fusion is performed once the patient reaches sufficient age (approximately 10 years for girls and 12 years for boys), size and maturity (Fig. 35.3a–e) Usually, this involves conversion from

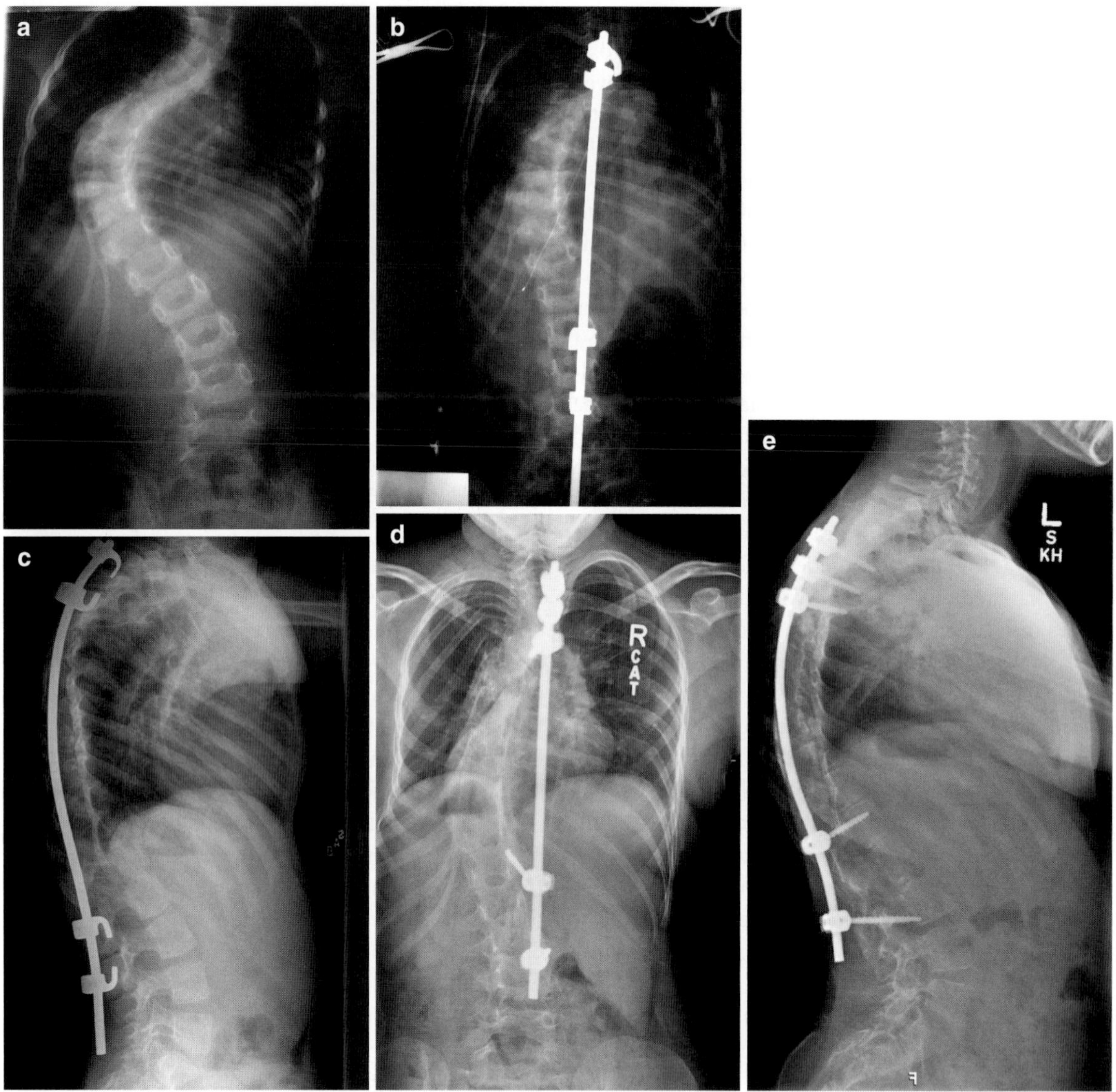

Fig. 35.3 (**a**) Preoperative postero-anterior (PA) radiograph of the patient in Fig. 35.1. She is a 4-year, 2-month old female with infantile idiopathic scoliosis. She has an 85° *left* thoracic curve between T6 and L2. (**b**) Postoperative PA radiograph showing that her curve has been reduced to 35°. Note the long length of rod below the lower foundation from which the rod will be lengthened in the future. (**c**) Postoperative lateral radiograph showing her sagittal plane alignment. She has a moderate increase in thoracic kyphosis and lumbar lordosis. (**d**) Antero-posterior radiograph 7 years postoperative at 11 years of age showing her final fusion and correction. Her major curve measures 46°. She has undergone one major revision to all pedicle screw construct. Because of the extensive fusions proximally and distally, a dual rod system was not inserted. (**e**) Lateral radiographs showing maintenance of sagittal plane alignment. She has maintained her moderate increase in the thoracic kyphosis (72°) and lumbar lordosis (52°)

the single growing rod to a standard dual rod construct for a PSF and SSI with or without an ASF. We have found that conversion to a dual rod construct allows better correction than simply performing facetectomies, repeat lengthening of the single rod, and bone grafting.

35.3 Current Results

In 2001, our first published report on this technique was a retrospective review of 29 patients who underwent submuscular rod placement for the treatment of severe, progressive early onset scoliosis or kyphoscoliosis [1].

Of these, 11 patients also had a short anterior and posterior apical fusion to aid with correcting and stabilizing the deformity. In this study, the mean age at surgery was 6.7 years (range, 1–11 years). The mean preoperative major curve was 66° (range, 42–112°), the immediate mean postoperative curve was 38° (range, 16–70°), and the mean curve at last follow-up was 47° (range, 28–79°). The preoperative mean thoracic kyphosis was 35° (range, 5–72°) and postoperative mean kyphosis was 42° (range, 25–72°). The preoperative mean lumbar lordosis was 38° (range, 12–60°) and postoperative mean lordosis was 31° (range, 5–52°). No significant junctional kyphotic deformities were observed proximal or distal to the instrumentation. Lengthenings were performed when the curves had progressed 15–20°. The mean number of lengthenings per patient was two (range, 0–5 lengthenings). At the time of the study's publication, nine patients had reached a suitable age and been converted to a definitive PSF and SSI. Nine complications occurred in seven patients (24%). The best correction was obtained after initial insertion of the submuscular rod, and although initial correction was sometimes maintained, it was never improved. Curve control, nonetheless, was generally felt to be satisfactory.

In 2005, we combined with the San Diego Center for Spinal Deformities in a retrospective review examined 28 patients treated either with single or dual growing rods who had completed their submuscular rod lengthenings, had been converted to a definitive PSF and SSI, and had a minimum follow-up of 2 years [22]. Five patients had a single submuscular rod with a short apical fusion, 16 patients had a single growing rod alone, and seven patients had dual growing rods. In this study, patients who had received a short apical fusion had the worst results, with eight complications in four patients (80%) and less than optimal spinal growth. In contrast, the single growing rod group who did not have an apical fusion had the lowest complication rate, with five complications in three patients (19%), and the best frontal and sagittal plane balance. The initial correction, maintenance of correction, amount of growth per year, and the percentage of expected T_1–S_1 growth was best with dual rods. This group had two complications in seven patients (29%). The sagittal plane alignment was not seen to be a problem in any of the groups, and both the single and dual rod groups had good initial correction of the spinal deformity while enabling continued spinal growth.

Finally, in 2007, the review of Thompson et al. [23] on the three systems, presently used for the surgical treatment of early-onset scoliosis, was published. In addition to single and dual growing rods, this review examined the Vertically Expandable Prosthetic Titanium Rib (VEPTR) implant. It concluded that all three techniques have the ability to be effective in providing the surgical control of progressive EOS. Most importantly, all these systems allowed spinal growth and lung development, despite a moderate complication rate.

35.4 Controversies

A number of the controversies with respect to single growing rods center around the high complication rate associated with their use. Two of the more concerning issues during the period over which lengthenings occur are rod breakage and hook displacement, while the incidence of wound infections, neurological injury, and other complications has been substantially less. Other studies aside from the ones previously discussed have reported a significant incidence of complications. Klemme et al. reported 33 implant-related problems in 25 of their 67 patients (37%), and these included 21 hook dislocations and 12 rod breakages [7]. They also reported on one case of death occurring intraoperatively, related to deflection of a rod into the retroperitoneum and thoracic cage during exchange of the rod through the submuscular tunnel.

Rod breakage and hook displacement are complications that can be addressed at the time of detection. Our philosophy has been to treat rod breakage as an opportunity for an unscheduled lengthening. Furthermore, rod breakage implies some degree of repetitive loading and therefore is an excellent indicator that an autofusion has not yet occurred. Hook dislodgement can be particularly problematic at the site of an upper thoracic kyphosis, and careful consideration of the patient's sagittal profile must be considered prior to placement of the upper claw construct. The increasing use of pedicle screws may prove to be an excellent adjustment in such situations, since they provide three-column fixation and have been shown to be placed safely in the upper thoracic spine [3, 9].

Mineiro and Weinstein [13] have expressed concerns about the utility of growing rods for another reason: spinal growth. Although they conceded satisfactory results in 11 patients treated with a subcutaneous Harrington rod prior to definitive fusion, they questioned whether an appropriate amount of spinal growth had been achieved and the relative merit of the number of procedures required to produce these results. They noted mean spinal growth of only 2.0 cm (range, 0.5–4.5 cm). In the Klemme et al. [7] study no patients received an apical fusion, and curve progression was arrested or improved in 44 children, whereas 23 had continued progression. Spinal growth here was noted to be 0.08 cm/vertebral segment per year (range, 0–0.23 cm/segment/year), with slightly better absolute mean spinal growth of 3.1 cm (range, 0–10.2 cm). Therefore, it has been proposed that patients may benefit more from a single anterior and posterior spinal fusion and segmental spinal instrumentation at a young age.

However, we have observed that the spine does continue to grow, as documented by continued curve progression after initial instrumentation with the growing rod. The additional spinal length that occurs from each rod lengthening should be reflective of spinal length that would not have been achieved if a formal fusion had been performed. For this reason, we analyzed the T1–S1 length, which is an indication of spinal growth and truncal height [23]. Our results indicated that with lengthenings at 6-month intervals regardless of the amount of curve progression, there is an adequate percentage of expected T1–S1 growth in single growing rod patients. This study does agree that a concomitant short apical fusion is not advisable, since this procedure may stiffen the spine and thereby decrease the amount of spinal growth. Despite this, it should also be noted that the amount of spinal growth achieved even in the apical fusion group in this study was better than in previous studies using Harrington rod instrumentation without fusion [7, 13]. In addition, the alternative option of doing a single anterior and posterior spinal fusion and segmental spinal instrumentation at a young age is not without its own potential complications. Much of Newton et al. [16] developmental work regarding video-assisted thoracoscopic surgery for anterior spinal release and fusion was centered on its utility in reducing the chest wall morbidity associated with open thoracotomy. Dobbs et al. [4] has taken this a step further and advocates posterior-only surgery to obviate any compromise of pulmonary function engendered by entering the thoracic cavity.

Implicit in the concern over stunted spinal growth is the belief that insertion of a growing rod will cause premature spinal fusion. In our experience, the aim is to obtain localized areas of spinal fusion at the superior and inferior claw constructs. The intermediate areas often appear to be fused, but further observation intraoperatively reveals that this consists of facet joint ossification that, once debrided, does not interfere with obtaining further spinal deformity correction during definitive fusion. Interestingly, this concern may be mitigated by the use of single rather than dual rod constructs, the latter of which offer a stiffer construct during the lengthening phase of treatment.

35.5 Conclusions

The current results indicate that the use of a single growing rod can be considered a useful adjunct in the surgical management of severe progressive spinal deformities in early-onset scoliosis. This technique can help minimize curve progression while allowing continued spinal growth. Complication rates are moderate, but often manageable even in an elective setting. Short anterior and posterior apical fusions should be avoided because of adverse effects on long-term spinal growth and deformity correction and an increased incidence of complications. We strongly recommend postoperative bracing for all patients. This technique has been well tolerated and accepted by our children and their families.

References

1. Blakemore LC, Scoles PV, Thompson GH et al (2001) Submuscular Isola rods with or without limited apical fusion in the management of severe spinal deformities in young children: preliminary report. Spine 26:2044–2048
2. D'Astous JL, Sanders JO (2007) Casting and traction treatment methods for scoliosis. Orthop Clin North Am 38:477–484
3. Daubs MD, Kim YJ, Lenke LG (2007) Pedicle screw fixation (T1, T2, and T3). Instr Course Lect 56:247–255
4. Dobbs MB, Lenke LG, Kim YJ, et al (2006) Anterior/posterior spinal instrumentation versus posterior instrumentation alone for the treatment of adolescent idiopathic scoliotic curves more than 90 degrees. Spine 31:2386–2391
5. Gillespie R, O'Brien J (1981) Harrington instrumentation without fusion. J Bone Joint Surg Br 63:461
6. Harrington P (1962) Treatment of scoliosis: correction and internal fixation by spine instrumentation. J Bone Joint Surg Am 44:591–610

7. Klemme WR, Denis F, Winter RB et al (1997) Spinal instrumentation without fusion for progressive scoliosis in young children. J Pediatr Orthop 17:734–742
8. Lapinksy AS, Richards BS (1995) Preventing the crankshaft phenomenon by combining anterior fusion with posterior instrumentation. Does it work? Spine 20:1392–1398
9. Lehman RA Jr, Lenke LG, Keeler KA et al (2007) Computed tomography evaluation of pedicle screws placed in the pediatric deformed spine over an 8-year period. Spine 32:2679–2684
10. Luque ER (1982) Paralytic scoliosis in growing children. Clin Orthop 163:202–209
11. Marks DS, Iqbal MJ, Thompson AG et al (1996) Convex spinal epiphysiodesis in the management of progressive infantile idiopathic scoliosis. Spine 21:1884–1888
12. Mehta MH (2005) Growth as a corrective force in the early treatment of progressive infantile scoliosis. J Bone Joint Surg Br 87:1237–1247
13. Mineiro J, Weinstein SL (2002) Subcutaneous rodding for progressive spinal curvatures: Early results. J Pediatr Orthop 22:290–295
14. Moe JH, Kharrat K, Winter RB et al (1984) Harrington instrumentation without fusion plus external orthotic support for the treatment of difficult curvature problems in young children. Clin Orthop Relat Res 185:35–45
15. Morin C (1991) Pediatric Cotrel-Dubousset instrumentation system. In: Bridwell KH, Dewald RL (eds) The textbook of spinal deformity. JB Lippincott, Philadelphia, pp 212–217
16. Newton PO, Marks M, Faro F et al (2003) Use of video-assisted thoracoscopic surgery to reduce perioperative morbidity in scoliosis surgery. Spine 28:S249–S254
17. Patterson JF, Webb JK, Burwell RG (1990) The operative treatment of progressive early onset scoliosis: a preliminary report. Spine 15:809–815
18. Pratt RK, Webb JK, Burwell RG et al (1999) Luque trolley and convex epiphysiodesis in the management of infantile and juvenile idiopathic scoliosis. Spine 24:1538–1547
19. Rinsky LA, Gamble JG, Bleck EE (1985) Segmental instrumentation without fusion in children with progressive scoliosis. J Pediatr Orthop 5:687–690
20. Roberto RF, Lonstein JE, Winter RB et al (1997) Curve progression in Risser stage 0 or 1 patients after posterior spinal fusion for idiopathic scoliosis. J Pediatr Orthop 17: 718–725
21. Tello CA (1994) Harrington instrumentation without arthrodesis and consecutive distraction program for young children with severe spinal deformities: experience and technical details. Orthop Clin North Am 25:333–351
22. Thompson GH, Akbarnia BA, Kostial P et al (2005) Comparison of single and dual growing rod techniques followed through definitive surgery: a preliminary study. Spine 30: 2039–2044
23. Thompson GH, Akbarnia BA, Campbell RM Jr (2007) Growing rod techniques in early-onset scoliosis. J Pediatr Orthop 27:354–361
24. Vanlommel E, Fabry G, Urlus M et al (1992) Harrington instrumentation without fusion for the treatment of scoliosis in young children. J Pediatr Orthop B 1:116–118

Dual Growing Rods

36

Behrooz A. Akbarnia, Gregory M. Mundis Jr., and Pooria Salari

Key Points

- Growing rod technique has evolved throughout the last 50 years.
- Dual growing rod is a valuable technique to correct and maintain deformity correction and allow the growth of the spine and thorax.
- This treatment technique requires a long-term commitment by the surgeon and the family.
- Adherence to the technique detail is imperative.
- Complications are frequent, but manageable when treated by an experienced spine or pediatric orthopaedic surgeon.

36.1 Introduction

Surgical treatment of early onset scoliosis (EOS) is one of the most difficult challenges in modern pediatric spine surgery. This arises from the fact that young children with progressive spine deformity can have life-threatening cardiopulmonary complications and face severe consequences if left untreated. Ideal timing and type of intervention remains debatable. However, our understanding of the natural history and treatment options for this condition is steadily increasing and new techniques are being developed. It is understood that the development of scoliosis at an early age will have a more significant impact on spinal growth, thoracic volume, and cardiopulmonary development. Appropriate treatment of the spinal deformity in these children in a timely manner is necessary to avoid these consequences.

Growth friendly techniques for the treatment of EOS usually fit into three categories: distraction-based, compression-based, and growth-guided procedures [24]. The last two options have been described in separate chapters. The common procedures in the first group are chest wall distraction techniques such as rib devices and growing rods used primarily for the spine. In this chapter, we will discuss indications, current surgical techniques, and complications of dual growing rod technique in EOS.

From the time Harrington [9] introduced instrumentation without fusion in 1962, the growing rod techniques have evolved from one rod and two hooks placed subcutaneously [18] to the current dual rod technique [1]. Historical background will be discussed in more detail for better understanding of the principles behind dual growing rod surgery.

36.2 Background

The indications and goals of surgery have changed significantly over the years. Currently the recommendation for surgery among children with infantile or juvenile scoliosis is Cobb 45° or greater and documented progression. The trend to operate is a reflection of our improved understanding of the natural history of this disease and significant advances in surgical technology [16].

Historically, the goal was to achieve a straight but shortened spine by early spine fusion when the curves

B.A. Akbarnia (✉)
Department of Orthopaedics, University of California, San Diego and San Diego Center for Spinal Disorders, 4130 La Jolla Village Drive, Suite 300, La Jolla, CA 92037, USA
e-mail: akbarnia@ucsd.edu

B. A. Akbarnia et al. (eds.), *The Growing Spine*,
DOI: 10.1007/978-3-540-85207-0_36, © Springer-Verlag Berlin Heidelberg 2011

could not be controlled. These goals quickly changed after Dubousset [8] described the crankshaft phenomenon. This phenomenon is seen in skeletally immature patients following posterior spinal fusion. The posterior fusion mass acts as a tether to the growth of the anterior column, resulting in increase of rotational deformity. Sanders et al. [22] identified patients with Risser 0 and open triradiate cartilage as the population at maximum risk for crankshaft after posterior arthrodesis. To avoid this phenomenon, anterior spinal fusion was recommended in addition to posterior fusion. It was later discovered that limiting the growth of the immature spine with an anterior/posterior fusion had significant untoward effects on pulmonary development, chest growth, and height. Spine growth has been described by Dimeglio [7] who outlined two peaks in spinal growth: 0–5 and 9–15 years. Using his data, one can predict the expected height loss from an anterior/posterior arthrodesis. Winter [30] similarly described a formula to calculate the expected height loss: multiply 0.07 × number of segments fused × number of years of growth remaining. Being able to predict this is a valuable tool in educating family and being aware of the potential ramifications of fusion at an early age. The negative consequences of early fusion on pulmonary and thoracic development have been a strong motivating factor in the development of surgical techniques aimed at reducing morbidity and early mortality.

Advances in surgical treatment have been accompanied by a paradigm shift in the goals of surgical management of infantile idiopathic scoliosis (IIS) and juvenile idiopathic scoliosis (JIS). No longer is a short but straight spine acceptable. Some spine deformity is acceptable if spine and chest growth can be maintained, allowing for more normal pulmonary development.

Harrington [9] was the first to describe internal fixation without fusion among 27 post-polio and idiopathic patients; however, his article did not describe the long-term follow-up among this subset of patients. His surgical technique included a subperiosteal dissection placing a single distraction rod on the concavity of the curve attached to hooks at both ends. The idea was to maintain spinal growth without fusion, correct deformity, and control residual deformity. He ultimately concluded that children under the age of 10 years were candidates for fusionless surgery and those older than 10 years needed definitive arthrodesis.

Moe et al. [18] modified the technique described by Harrington and limited the subperiosteal dissection to the site of hook placement and passed the rod subcutaneously. The rod was also modified to have a smooth, thicker central portion to prevent scar formation to the threads and allow for sagittal contouring. Lengthenings were performed when there was a loss of correction (Cobb 10° or more). Both the children treated for idiopathic scoliosis showed a considerable decrease in curve magnitude. They reported a 50% complication rate including rod breakage and hook dislodgement from the rod or lamina.

Marchetti and Faldini [14] described their "end fusion technique" in 1977. The initial surgery included fusion of two vertebrae at each end of the curve. Six months later, these foundations were used as strong anchor points for hook placement. A rod was then placed connecting the two ends after subperiosteal dissection. Lengthening was then performed periodically. A Milwaukee brace was used as external support. The first patient treated by Marchetti and Faldini with this method was a 11-year-old girl with a thoracolumbar curve of 148°; the patient had a curve of 69° at the end of treatment 4 years later.

In 1977, Luque and Cardoso [11] described their technique of fusion-less surgery with segmental spinal instrumentation. Luque [12] modified this technique by adding sublaminar wires and replacing the Harrington rod with an L-shaped rod. This technique was later coined as the Luque trolley technique. The initial series included 47 paralytic patients who grew an average of 4.6 cm over the instrumented segment and an initial curve correction of 78%. Although early results were promising, the system grew out of favor due to the extensive subperiosteal exposure and reports of early fusion. Sublaminar wire passage also created scar tissue and weakened the lamina resulting in more difficult definitive fusion surgery.

Pratt et al. [20] later performed a retrospective review of 26 patients treated with Luque trolley instrumentation with and without convex epiphysiodesis. Of the 8 patients treated with Luque trolley alone all showed significant curve deterioration. Of those treated with epiphysiodesis, 7 of 13 worsened, 4 remained unchanged, and 2 improved. Growth was 49% as predicted in the Luque trolley alone group and 32% among those undergoing combined surgery.

Mardjetko et al. [15] in 1991 performed a retrospective review of 9 patients who underwent Luque instrumentation without fusion. Average preoperative curve is 51°. All the 9 patients had at least one revision. All

Table 36.1 Review and comparison of selected published literature

Authors	Number of patients	Average initial elongation pre- to postinitial (cm)	Average growth of instrumented area (cm) during treatment	Average total length increase of the spine (cm)	T1-S1 increase (cm/year)	Space available for lung (SAL) ratio (pre/final)	Number of complications per patient
Moe et al. [19]	20	Not reported	2.9	Not reported	Not reported	Not reported	1.1
Luque et al. [11]	43	Not reported	2.6	Not reported	Not reported	Not reported	0.3
Klemme et al. [10]	67	Not reported	3.1	Not reported	Not reported	Not reported	0.81
Blakemore et al. [6]	29	Not reported	Not reported	Not reported	Not reported	Not reported	0.3
Akbarnia et al. [1]	23	5.0	4.67	9.64	1.21	0.87/1	0.57
Akbarnia et al. [2]	13	5	5.7	10.7	1.46	Not reported	0.46

revisions were technically demanding due to extensive fibrosis and weakened laminar bone. Follow-up curves averaged 51° with an average gain in spinal height of 5.8 cm. Only a small portion of this growth was derived from the instrumented levels. Spontaneous fusion was documented in all the 9 patients.

In 1997, Klemme et al. [10] reported their 20 year follow-up of the Minnesota experience. Sixty seven children were treated with various diagnoses. Curve magnitude improved from 67° at initial internal fixation to 47° at definitive fusion. They felt that the amount of correction obtained declined with consecutive lengthenings (average 6.1 procedures per patient). Curve progression was arrested or improved in 44 of 67 patients with an average curve reduction of 30%. Of the remaining 23 patients, 12 were neuromuscular and the curves progressed 33% on an average.

Blakemore et al. [6] reported on 29 patients with progressive kyphoscoliosis treated with a single submuscular Isola rod with or without apical fusion or convex hemiepiphysiodesis. Apical fusion was performed on curves >70° and on those curves that were stiff on bending radiographs. All wore a Milwaukee brace postoperatively. Mean Cobb improved from 66 to 38° immediately postoperative and 47° at latest follow-up. Overall complication rate was 24% and included hook dislodgement (5), rod breakage (3), and superficial wound infection (1).

In 2005, Akbarnia et al. [1] building on the experience of McCarthy and Asher, described the dual growing rod technique for EOS. The original series included 23 patients treated with dual growing rods using Pediatric Isola instrumentation and specially made tandem connectors. All the patients had curve progression over 10° and unsuccessful treatment with bracing or casting. They reported on 189 procedures of which 151 were lengthenings. Mean preoperative curve improved from 82 to 38° after initial surgery, and correction was maintained to 36° at last follow-up or postspinal fusion. Average growth from T1-S1 was 1.21 cm/year excluding the initial correction. Space available for lung (SAL) ratio in patients with thoracic curves improved from 0.87 to a normal ratio of 1.0. Complications occurred in 48% (11/23) of patients during the course of treatment. These included hook dislodgment, rod breakage, and superficial wound infections. They found this to be both a safe and effective technique for treating EOS [2]. See Table 36.1 for summary of the literature.

36.3 Indications

Principles governing the treatment of EOS are adhered to when applying the dual growing rod technique. There is a trend in recent years to employ a more aggressive treatment strategy. In IIS curve progression greater than 10°, Cobb angle greater than 35°, and RVAD greater than 20° should prompt active treatment. When curve magnitude reaches 45° and the progression is documented surgical management is usually recommended. Patients with JIS follow principles similar to those with adolescent idiopathic scoliosis. Documented curve progression, and curve magnitude greater than 45° are indications for surgical intervention. Cobb angle alone should not be the main indication for surgical treatment. Deterioration of pulmonary function and other associated conditions leading to the impairment of quality of life may also be main indications for surgical intervention (Table 36.2).

Table 36.2 Surgical indications

Indications for operative vs. Nonoperative treatment in early onset scoliosis	
Nonoperative	Cobb angle <20°[1]
	RVAD<20°[1]
	Phase 1 rib head[1]
Operative	Cobb angle >25°[1]
	RVAD<20°[1]
	Phase 2 rib head[1]
	Failure of brace/casting treatment
	Documented progression of curve

[1]Idiopathic infantile scoliosis only

Once the decision is made to treat the child surgically, the question should be asked as to which method will most consistently give good results with the least or most manageable complications for that particular child. The growing rod technique has the best indication in patients with idiopathic, neuromuscular, or syndromic scoliosis and absence of congenital anomalies. The dual growing rod has been found superior in clinical outcome to single rod technique. A recent comparison of dual vs. single rod constructs by Thompson et al. [28] highlights this debate. The results quite convincingly favor the dual growing rod technique. Although the overall complication rate was slightly higher (3/16 vs. 2/7), the amount of initial correction obtained and final correction sustained, as well as improved growth rate and T1-S1 length, make this a more effective treatment. The presence of a second rod allows some leeway for revision when one rod breaks or undergoes plastic deformation. In the single rod construct, a broken rod or implant complication is usually something that cannot wait until the next scheduled lengthening (Table 36.3).

Bess et al. [5] further highlighted these differences in his Growing Spine Study Group (GSSG) data base review of 910 growing rod surgeries. He found that the need for reoperation was lower in the dual vs. single group for complications. Also, the rate of implant-related complications was higher in the single rod group. Superficial wound problems were greater in the dual rod group due to the bulkiness of implants, but did not lead to a need for additional surgeries. The construct of the dual rod is also biomechanically favorable with improved initial curve correction and maintenance of correction.

Table 36.3 Comparison of single and dual rod techniques [28]

	Single rod	Dual rod
Unplanned trips to OR	Increased risk	–
Implant-related complications	Increased risk	–
Infection	No difference	No difference
Growth (mm/year)	6.8	11.3
Initial corrections (Cobb) (%)	38	47
Maintenance of correction (%)	14	40

Although the dual growing rod system may be somewhat more prominent than single rods, it certainly is lower profile than the current available rib devices such as VEPTR. Furthermore, dual growing rods more specifically address the pathology it treats compared to VEPTR. When comparing this technique to VEPTR, the main distinction that should be made is in the very indication. If a patient has thoracic insufficiency syndrome (TIS) with multiple congenital anomalies and stiff thorax, then the VEPTR may provide a better treatment modality. However, in children with scoliosis without chest wall anomalies and TIS, it could be argued that the growing rod constructs is lower profile and more directly addresses the spinal deformity. With its anchor points on the cephalad and caudal ends of the spine, it avoids attachment to the ribs and the associated complications thereof. As the goal of this technique is growth modulation, it can be argued that placing anchors on a mobile segment away from the spine (on ribs) will result in a lower transmission of force on the spine, and consequently stimulate less growth. For this reason, when growth modulation is the goal, dual growing rods are the most reliable way to accomplish this. No information of T1-S1 length is available following VEPTR procedures to date (Tables 36.4 and 36.5).

The dual growing rod technique remains an investigational device that is not yet FDA approved for this indication and like most of the devices for this age group is being used off label in the United States. For this reason, there are no absolute indications or contraindications. Dual growing rods have been used for the treatment of scoliosis with the diagnoses of such conditions as: IIS and JIS, neuromuscular, and congenital scoliosis, neurofibromatosis, Ehlers Danlos, cerebral palsy, myelodysplasia, Marfan syndrome, Sotos syndrome, Beals syndrome, chromosomal abnormalities, Ulrich syndrome, Prader–Willi syndrome, thoracogenic-neuroblastoma, multiple pterygium syndrome, and Proteus syndrome.

The dual growing rod may not be an effective procedure when there is no further growth potential or in

Table 36.4 Indications for distraction-based devices

	Indications	Contraindications
Chest wall distraction (VEPTR[1])	Thoracic insufficiency syndrome[2]	Skeletal maturity
	Skeletally immature[2]	Poor rib bone stock
	Congenital Scoliosis/fused ribs	Absence of proximal ribs
	Chest wall deficiency	
Spine distraction (growing rods)	IIS	Skeletal Maturity
	JIS	
	Neuromuscular scoliosis	
	Scoliosis associated with syndromes	

IIS infantile idiopathic scoliosis; *JIS* juvenile idiopathic scoliosis
[1]Vertically Expandable Prosthetic Titanium Rib (Synthes Inc.)
[2]FDA indications

Table 36.5 Predictable complications of two distraction based non fusion techniques

Growing Rod	Chest Wall Distraction
Multiple surgeries, infection	Multiple surgeries, infection
Rod breakage	Drift of device attachments, brachial plexus injury
Spine stiffness or fusion	Chest wall stiffness

patients with TIS and chest wall problems. One also has to be careful in the presence of kyphosis to take precautions to avoid complications due to kyphosis, as discussed later in this chapter.

36.4 Technique

36.4.1 Initial Dual Rod Procedure

Patient is brought to the operating room and general anesthesia is induced. Prophylactic antibiotics are administered. Patient is placed on the table in prone position over chest roles for small children and over a frame or Jackson table for larger patients. The entire back is prepped and draped in usual fashion.

The procedure includes preparation of cephalad and caudal foundations for anchor placement and performing a limited fusion, rod contouring, rod passage, and application of connectors. The index procedure can usually be performed through one or two midline incisions [2].

36.4.2 Technique of Preparing Foundations

A foundation is defined as an assembly of at least two anchors and one or two rods that are stable and strong enough to accept corrective loads and to resist deforming loads without dislodgement of the anchors or plastic deformation of the rod [31]. In a typical dual rod technique, we have used four anchors (hooks or screws) for each foundation for maximum stability (Fig. 36.1a–d). The exposures at the foundations are the only locations where the exposures are subperiosteal. Meticulous technique is employed to avoid a broad exposure and risking the occurrence of spontaneous fusion.

Selection of foundation sites is based on the type and location of the curve as well as the patient's age and diagnosis. Patients with neuromuscular scoliosis for example, may require longer instrumentation compared to those with IIS or JIS. The upper foundation anchors are generally placed at the T2–T4 levels in a claw fashion. If hooks are used at the upper foundation, the author's preference is a supralaminar location for superior hooks. The inferior hooks are placed sublaminar under the lamina (facet), similar to the technique used with original Harrington hooks, in a "claw" construct (Fig. 36.2a, b) The superior hooks can be staggered over two or three levels to avoid crowding the spinal canal if this is a concern. Staggering hook levels, however, may interfere with the use of a transverse connector at the foundation level. In that case, the connector is attached just below the lower hooks. It is utmost crucial to achieve the best foundation stability at the initial surgery to reduce the possibility of failure, even at the expense of exposing three instead of two levels. A study by Mahar et al. [13] demonstrated the increased stability of a screw construct over hooks alone or hooks with cross-connectors showing the significance of adding a cross link if all hook construct is used. We utilize both hooks and screws for foundations. It is our preference to use pedicle screws whenever possible; however, if anatomical considerations make this difficult, then hooks are another excellent option (Fig. 36.3a–c).

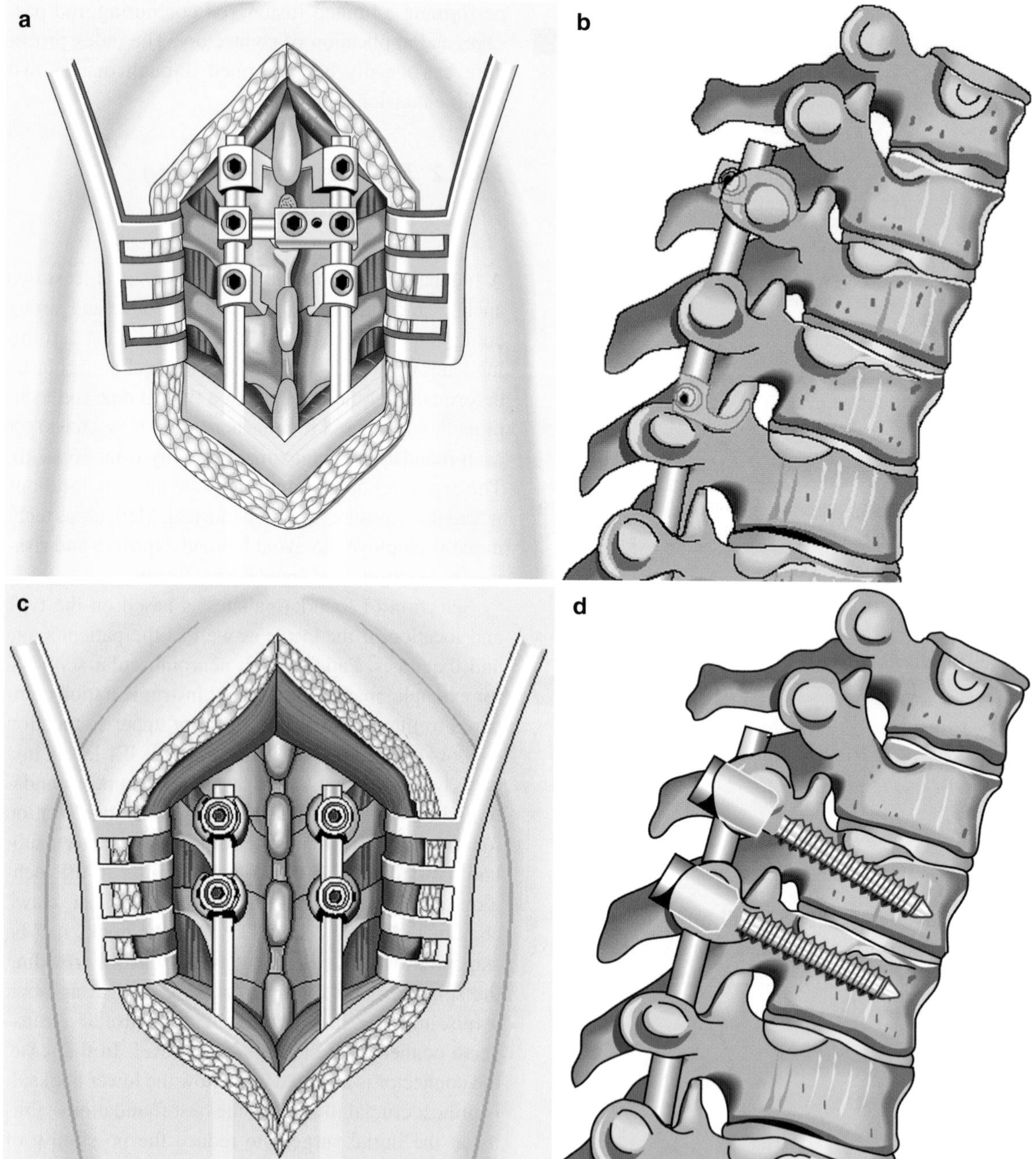

Fig. 36.1 Anteroposterior and lateral view of upper foundations using four hooks and a cross connector (**a**, **b**) or four screws (**c**, **d**)

The caudal foundation is generally instrumented with four pedicle screws. The foundation levels are typically three levels below the lower end vertebra of the major curve. In the presence of pelvic obliquity, such as neuromuscular scoliosis, the distal foundation may be extended to the sacrum or ilium using intrailiac fixations. It is extremely important that the foundations be stable and as strong as the bone quality permits. Bone graft or bone graft substitutes is used to augment bony fusion across at the foundation sites including a facet fusion and secure foundation anchors.

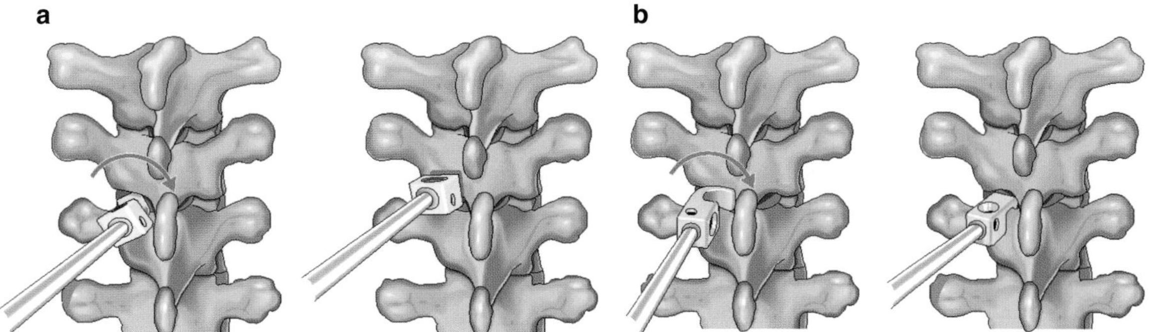

Fig. 36.2 Hook insertion maneuvers. Infralaminar hooks are inserted applying lateral to medial rotary motion (**a**) supralaminar hooks can be placed by medial to lateral rotation of hook holder (**b**)

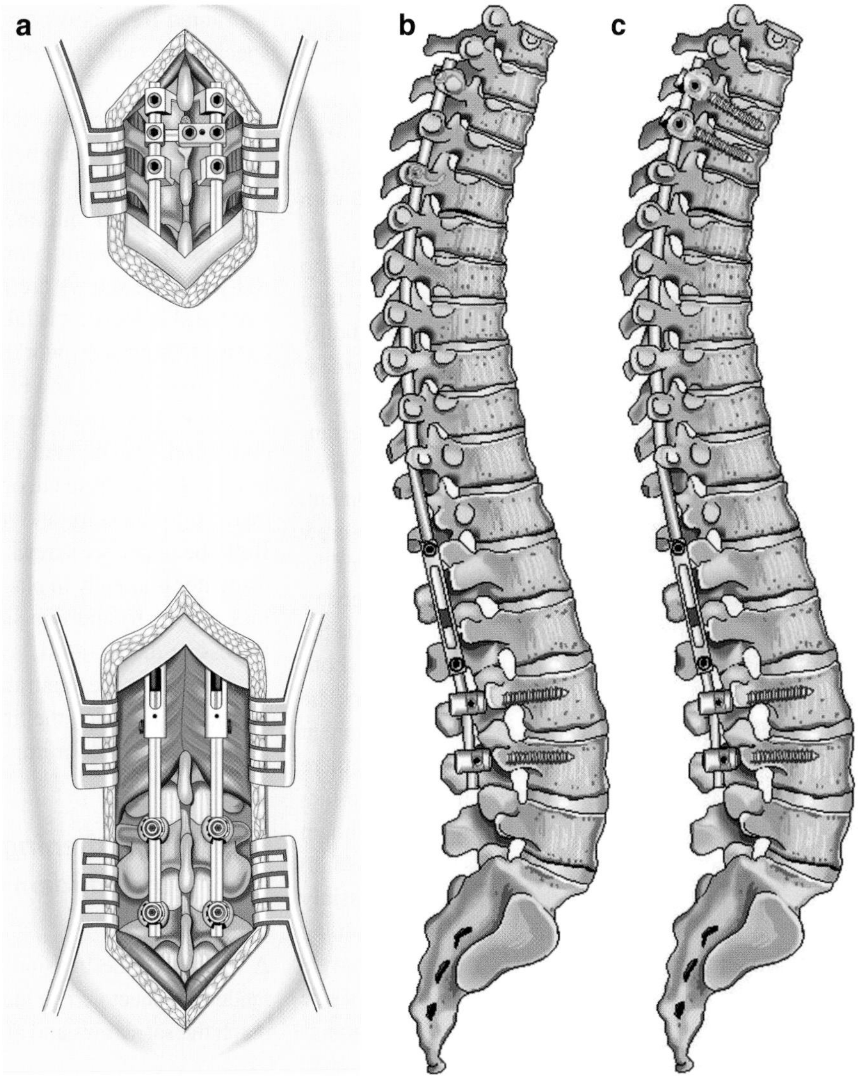

Fig. 36.3 Considering patient's age, anatomical provision and bone quality screws and hooks can be used as upper and lower anchors to provide strong foundations (**a–c**)

36.4.3 Insertion of Dual Rods and Anchors

A low profile pediatric implant system, with appropriate dimensions, such as 4.5 mm diameter stainless steel or titanium rods, is usually used. The rods are measured and cut into four segments, two for each side, and contoured for sagittal alignment. When tandem connectors are used, the rods should be cut in the region where the rod ends meet mostly at the thoracolumbar junction as this will be the best site for the tandem connectors. Appropriate contouring may help to correct the kyphosis using a cantilever maneuver when the deformity is flexible. One has to avoid extreme sagittal correction in one session to avoid anchor failure. The individual rods are passed subfascially as the tip of the rod is felt at all times through the skin until it appears at the site of the upper foundation. They will then be secured to their respective anchors and a cross link can be added if necessary. Mahar et al. did not show any benefit of cross-connecting if four pedicle screws are used for fixation, but did find significantly more strength associated with a cross-link and hook foundation. The lower foundation is then prepared and contour rods are connected to the caudal anchors. The tandem connectors are then placed at the thoracolumbar junction by first sliding them cephalad and then caudal. The thoracolumbar region is chosen for tandem connectors, as this is an area of the spine that is anatomically straight. The tandem connectors are rigid and do not bend; therefore, this location has the least effect on sagittal alignment. Lengthenings are done mostly by loosening the screw for the upper rod; therefore, only a short segment of the lower rod should be attached to the tandem connector leaving room for more of the upper rods to be inside the connector. This segment of the rod should not be contoured to allow entry into the straight connector. The tandem connectors are placed in their least prominent position to achieve the lowest profile possible. If there are set screws with connectors, they can be placed facing either medially or laterally. Turning the tandem connectors medially (set screw heads facing medial) makes the reach easier for the screws and possibly allows minimally invasive access during lengthening procedures. The lateral placement however may have a lower profile. Another option for rod connection is side to side connection. When side to side connection is used, the location of the connectors may vary and the rods in those segments can remain contoured for appropriate sagittal alignment.

At this point, an initial correction and lengthening is performed; however, extreme care is taken to avoid overdistraction and immediate implant or neurological complication.

36.5 Lengthenings

Currently, we perform lengthening of the growing rods every 6 months [1]. In otherwise healthy children, this procedure can be performed on an outpatient basis at a hospital or ambulatory surgery center. In children with significant comorbidities, an inpatient stay may be warranted for recovery and a children's hospital with specialized care is preferred. Spinal cord monitoring should be considered during lengthening procedures.

Fluoroscopy can be used to identify the location of the connector, the gap between the rods within the tandem connector, and identify the site of the *proximal* set-screws. A small midline incision is made, centered between the tandem connectors and at the site of the rod-gap if all screws are medial or posterior. It is vital that the skin incision is taken to the depth of the tandem connectors prior to working laterally so that only one skin flap is created and to save good skin thickness and coverage. The gap on the side of the spine needing more correction (usually the concave side) is exposed and freed of fibrous tissue in order to fit the special distractor inside the connector and into the gap between the rods. Both the upper set-screws are loosened (ensure that the distractor is already in place for lengthening to avoid any loss of length) and one side is lengthened (Fig. 36.4a) Excessive distraction is avoided. The set-screw is then tightened. On the contralateral side, the distraction is performed to match the first side unless differential distraction is desired for improved coronal balance.

36.5.1 Lengthening Outside the Tandem Connector

A small midline incision is made just cephalad to the tandem connector. The incision must be long enough to reach the set screws and accommodate a rod holder. The

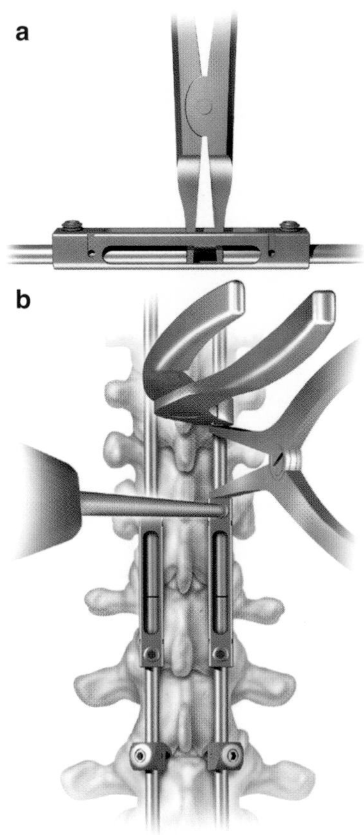

Fig. 36.4 Distraction can be done with special tandem connector distractor (**a**) or using a rod holder and a distractor outside the tandem connector (**b**)

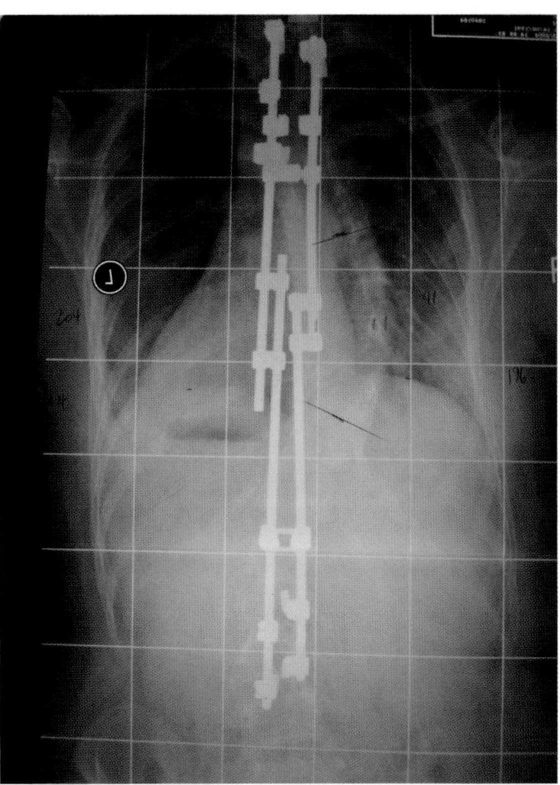

Fig. 36.5 When the side to side connector is used, the rods can be lengthened by tightening the appropriate set screws of each connector and distracting the connectors to achieve distraction or compression. (Courtesy of Mr. David Marks)

same meticulous exposure is performed to approach the rods. The exposure is completed on both sides prior to lengthening. A rod holder is then placed cephalad to the tandem connector, with enough room to place a distractor between the rod holder and the connector (Fig. 36.4b). Both the set screws are released and sequential lengthening as described above is performed. The indications to employ this technique is when the rods are too close to each other within the connector and the distractor will not fit. If the rods are too far away from each other within the connector then small pieces of rod can be placed within the connector to avoid a larger skin incision.

Excessive distraction force *must* be avoided especially at the first lengthening, to avoid implant complications. The timing of lengthening is universally at 6-month intervals. As the number of lengthenings increase and growth potential decrease, the interval can be longer. They are stopped when no further distraction is achieved and therefore are ready for final fusion. When the side to side connector is used, the rods can be lengthened by tightening the appropriate set screws of each connector and distracting between the connectors to distract the rods (Fig. 36.5). Based on which of the two screws are tightened, distraction or compression can be achieved using only distraction between two connectors.

36.6 Final Fusion

Final fusion usually necessitates the removal of growing rod system, complete exposure of the spine, identifying any possible fusion areas, correction of residual deformity and reinstrumentation with arthrodesis. It may require multiple osteotomies to achieve correction. The levels of fusion are usually the same as the levels spanned in the growing rod construct (Fig. 36.6a–h).

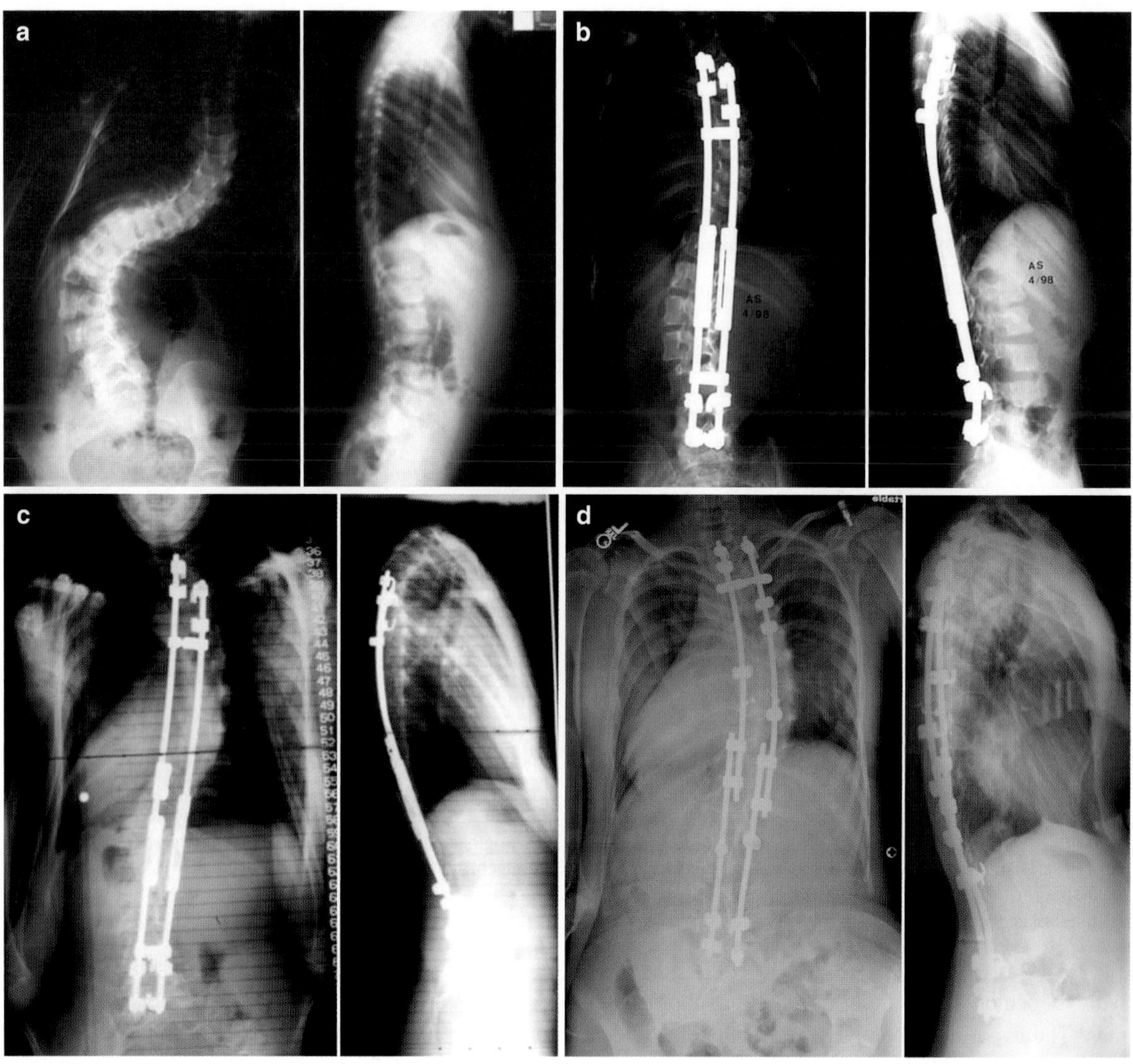

Fig. 36.6 A 4-year-old girl with Marfans syndrome (**a**). Patient underwent dual growing rod insertion for treatment of severe progressive scoliosis (**b**). Same patient after 7 years active treatment with frequent lengthening, before final fusion (**c**) and after final fusion (**d**)

Exceptions to this include patients who have progressive curves above or below the foundations, an example being neuromuscular patients with pelvic obliquity. For more details regarding reduction maneuvers and instrumented fusion and different osteotomy techniques, please see respective Chaps. 29 and 33.

36.6.1 Spinal Cord Monitoring

Although neurological risks are unlikely during growing rods surgery, neuromonitoring is commonly used in initial surgeries and often in lengthening/exchange procedures. Sankar et al. [23] reported a temporary neurological event among 782 growing rod surgeries (incidence rate = 0.1%). This was caused by pedicle screw misplacement and resolved after 3 months. In their report, the incidence of intraoperative neuromonitoring changes were 0.9, 0.9, and 0.5% in initial surgery, revision surgery, and lengthening respectively. Recently, a case of delayed neurological deficit was reported by Akbarnia et al. [4], who had delayed neurological deficit after rod exchange procedure despite normal intraoperative somatosensory evoked potential (SSEPs), Hoffmann reflexes (H-reflexes), and EMGs the patient had

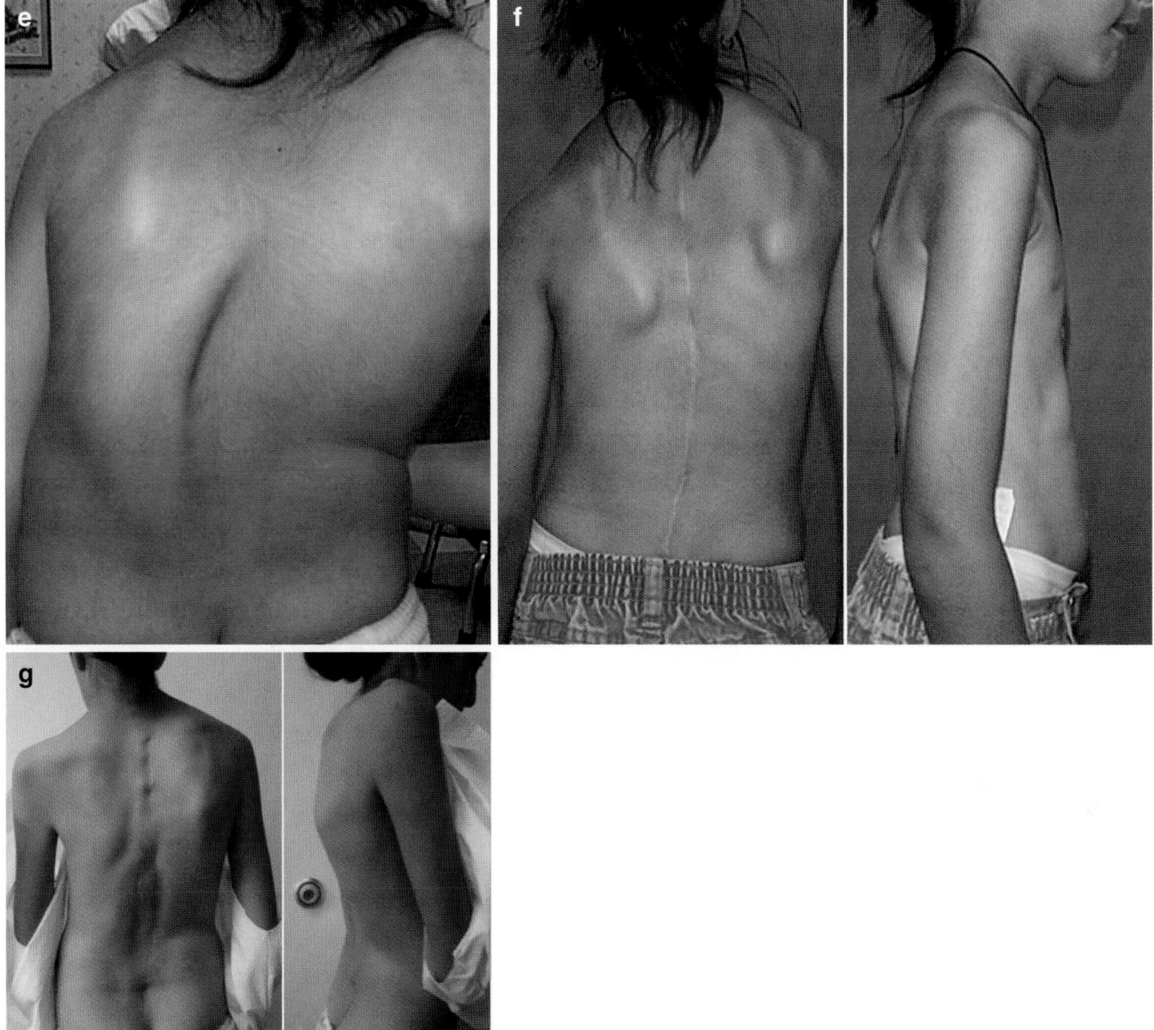

Fig. 36.6 (continued) Clinical images showing the same patient, pre-initial surgery **(e)**, post-initial surgery **(f)**, and post-final spinal fusion **(g)**

full recovery after rod shortening. This highlights the need for more sensitive neuromonitoring techniques.

Despite the early historical success of SSEP monitoring, reliance on this one modality is no longer adequate for the patients who present for surgical correction of complex deformities. Hence multimodality neurophysiologic monitoring of the spinal cord including highly sensitive-specific transcranial electric motor-evoked potentials (tceMEPs) has a definite place in the context of growing rod placement and lengthening/adjustment procedures. For more details on neuromonitoring please see Chap. 40.

36.7 Complications (Fig. 36.7a–g)

Complications following growing rod techniques have been a problem since its first description by Harrington [9]. In his series, the complication rate was 48% (32/67) for the duration of the treatment. Mineiro et al. [17] reported on their experience using subcutaneous rodding with consecutive distraction procedures. Of the 53 surgical procedures performed in 11 patients, 17 complications were reported for overall complication rate of 32%. Their conclusion was that single subcutaneous rods had acceptable results; however, one has to weigh the potential benefits gained against the risks to achieve these modest gains.

The development of dual growing rods was prompted by this high complication rate. Akbarnia et al. [1] were the first to report on the dual growing rod technique. They reported complications in 11 of 23 patients (48%). Four of the 23 patients required unplanned trips to the operating room (17%). Complications included 2 patients with deep wound infections requiring a total of six unplanned surgical procedures. Both the patients were treated by debridement and primary wound closure with one patient requiring removal of one of the rods which was eventually replaced. Four patients had four superficial wound problems, 2 of which required unplanned surgeries to treat a draining fistula and an incision granuloma. Implant-related complications

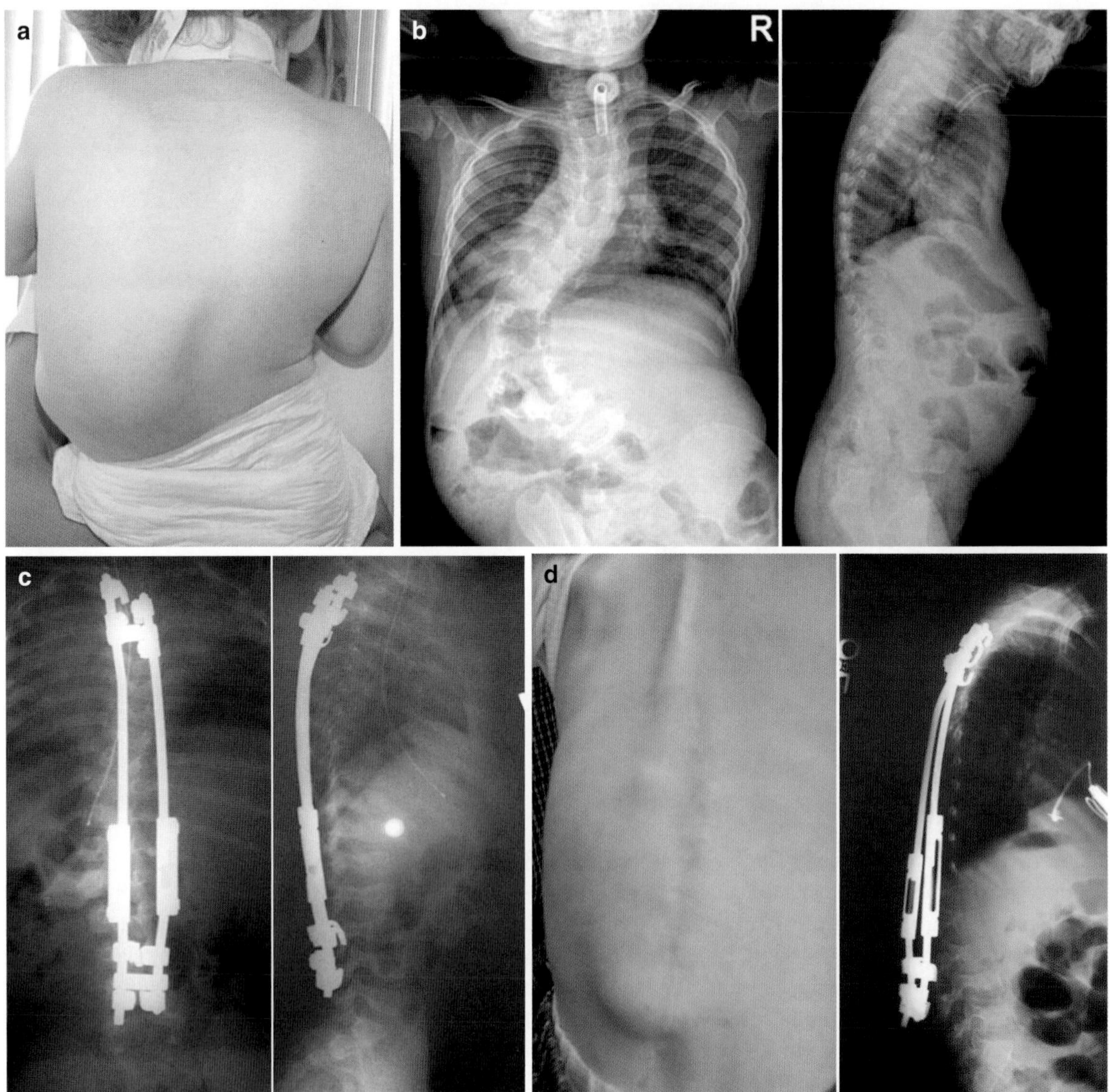

Fig. 36.7 (**a–g**) A 30-month-old boy with idiopathic scoliosis (**a**). Anteroposterior and lateral preinitial surgery radiographs (**b**). The patient underwent dual growing rod insertion from T3 to L4. Hooks were used at upper foundation (T3–T4) and lower foundation (L3–L4) (**c**). During 7 years active treatment, patient had multiple complications, treated through planned/unplanned surgeries. Hooks pull-out at lower foundation; hooks were replaced by pedicle screws (**d**)

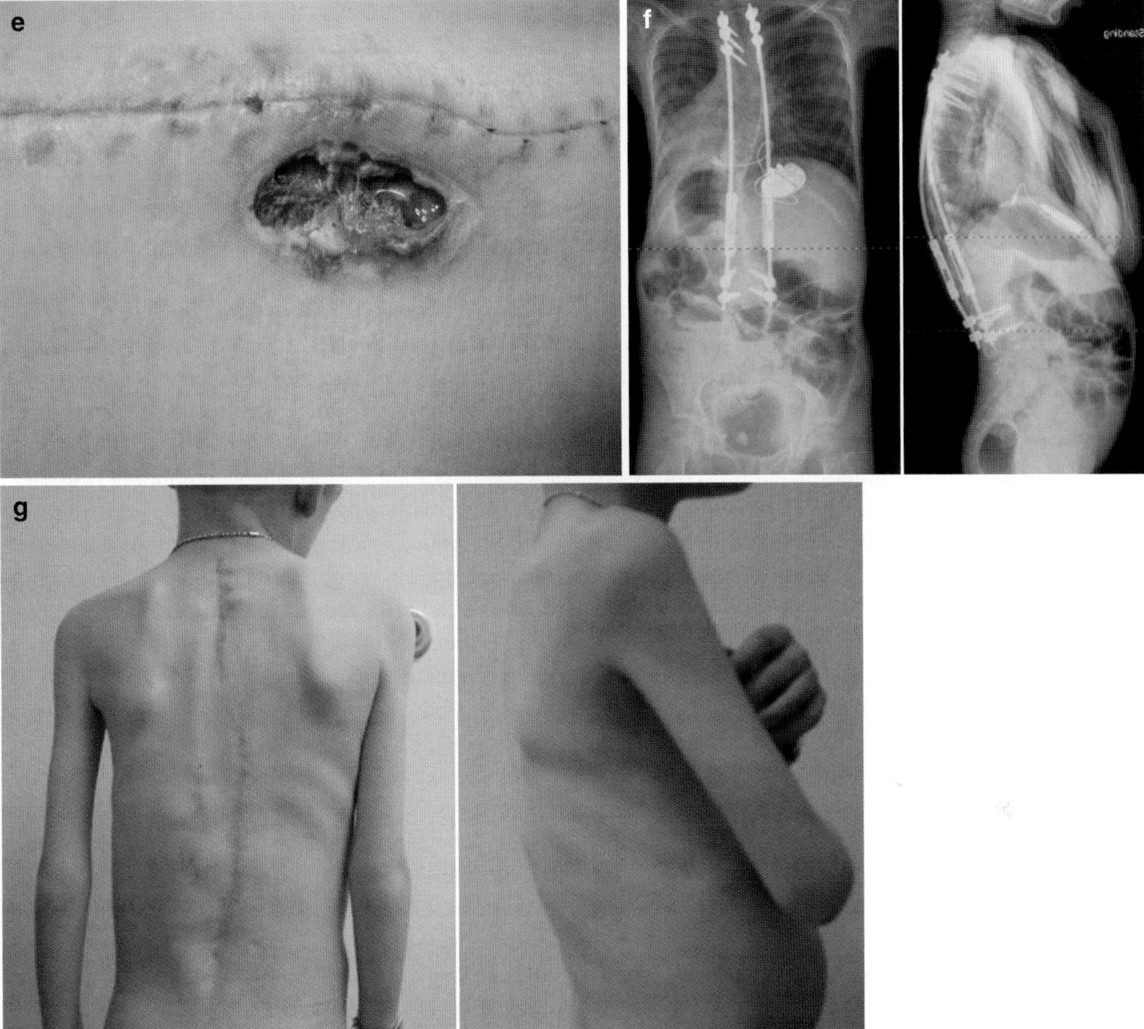

Fig. 36.7 (continued) Infection and skin loss in the same patient happened between two lengthenings, treated in an unplanned surgery with irrigation, debridement, and secondary closure (**e**). Latest follow-up radiographs at the age of 10 years; all the hooks were replaced with screws throughout the treatment period (**f**). Clinical photos at the age of 10 and after 7.5 years of active treatment (**g**)

included two rod breakages, two hook dislodgment, and one screw pullout in 5 patients. All implant-related complications were addressed during planned lengthening procedures. Two alignment-related complications occurred in 2 patients including one crankshaft phenomenon and one junctional kyphosis requiring extension of the construct during a planned lengthening. Unplanned procedures accounted for 4% of the total surgical interventions (8/189).

Thompson et al. [28] compared single vs. dual growing rods among 28 consecutive patients. He divided the study into three groups: Group 1, single submuscular rod with apical fusion, group 2, single growing rod alone, group 3, dual growing rods. Group 1 included four of 5 (80%) patients who sustained eight complications including three rod breakages and 5 hook displacements. Three of 16 patients (19%) sustained five complications in group 2. These included three rod breakages, one hook displacement, and one superficial wound infection. Two of the 7 patients (29%) in group 3 had sustained two complications. These included one broken rod and one superficial infection. When rod breakages and hook displacements were analyzed separately no difference was found between the three groups.

Akbarnia et al. [2] in 2008 reported on the dual growing rod techniques followed for 3–11 years until final fusion. They found that 6 of 13 patients (46%) experienced 13 complications during the treatment period. Eight occurred after final fusion. Four patients had multiple complications. Eight complications occurred during the treatment phase and five after final arthrodesis. No neurological deficit, junctional kyphosis, or crankshaft phenomenon was noted. Complications included three implant-related complications in 3 patients. Two patients had two rod breakages both of which were noted just before treatment completion and therefore were addressed at final fusion. Upper hooks pulled out in a third patient requiring unplanned surgery to replace the upper anchors. The same patient underwent two additional surgeries to address a deep wound infection. Another patient developed a wound granuloma requiring unplanned surgery for primary wound closure and debridement. One other patient with Pterygium syndrome experienced three general complications including a chylothorax after anterior annulotomy, superior mesenteric artery syndrome leading to a DVT in a major vessel, and an implant-related complication requiring rod exchange at the time of final fusion. Eight unplanned surgeries were performed during the treatment period accounting for 8% (8/102) of the total surgical interventions.

Bess et al. [5] have recently reported the GSSG data on 897 growing rod procedures (single and dual growing rods) among 143 patients. Complication rate per procedure was 19% (177/910). Eighty-one of 143 patients (57%) had a minimum of one complication. Nineteen of 94 (20%) patients with single rods had unplanned procedures due to implant complications compared to 7 of 83 patients with dual rods (8.4%). Thirteen of 52 (13%) patients with subcutaneous rods had wound complications compared to 9/90 (10%) patients with submuscular rods ($p<0.05$).

They were also able to demonstrate an increased risk for complications with increasing number of procedures. Complication risk increased 13% with each successive procedure. More importantly, however, they demonstrated that not all complications require a separate surgical procedure. Furthermore, they identified factors under the control of treating surgeons to reduce complications and unplanned surgery. These factors include: age at initial implantation, number of procedures performed during the treatment period, use of dual growing rods, and submuscular rod placement. Younger children are at higher risk for complications during the treatment period for several reasons: They have less soft tissue coverage, smaller bone, less physiologic reserves than older children, and younger age at initial instrumentation implies a longer treatment course and increased number of operations needed until final fusion.

Dual growing rods reduced implant-associated complications and unplanned surgery for two possible reasons. Dual rods reduce the mechanical stress on a rod compared to the single rod construct. This becomes a very important factor when combining fusionless technology with instrumentation as the construct will incur continued loading and micromotion. This leaves the implants susceptible to fatigue and mechanical failure. Another benefit of the dual growing rod construct is seen when one of the rods fail. In this instance, one rod remains, maintaining correction and stability, possibly delaying revision until the next planned lengthening procedure.

Another way to avoid further complication is by placing the rod submuscular rather than in the subcutaneous tissues. Subcutaneous rods were placed initially to reduce the risk of spontaneous spine fusion, due to subperiosteal exposure of the spine. It has been demonstrated however that there were more total and wound complications with subcutaneous rod placement. Bess et al. [5] also demonstrated that subcutaneous rods had more implant prominence as well as implant-related unplanned procedures compared to the submuscular dual growing rods. Furthermore, the subcutaneous group had the highest rate of overall wound complications (11/35). Unplanned surgery was reduced to the greatest extent in patients with submuscular dual growing rods where the planned to unplanned surgery ratio was 20:1. Patients with single growing rods placed subcutaneously had the worst planned to unplanned surgery ratio of 7.4:1.

In summary, the complication rate remains high, despite advances in technology and an improved understanding of the natural history of early-onset scoliosis. Though complications remain a problem, we have found ways to avoid unplanned surgery. Having the knowledge of the various complications and their incidence will allow us to communicate more effectively with family and caregivers and allow for a more informed consent.

36.7.1 How to Avoid Complications

Indications: Proper patient selection is the key for improved outcomes. Consider the diagnosis, age, and clinical presentation especially the pulmonary condition. The younger the patient and more surgical procedures, the more the possibility of complications. If feasible, surgery can be delayed using nonoperative treatment such as casting, bracing, and sometimes traction.

Technique: When exposing for the placement of foundation, avoid subperiosteal dissection except in foundation sites. Proper selection of foundation levels, proper position of connectors, and delicate handling of skin coverage are of utmost importance. Frequent lengthening assures maximum growth achievement. If the patient has a rigid curve and/or kyphosis consider preoperative traction or annulotomy to improve flexibility. It is wise not to try to correct all the sagittal deformity in one sitting. Since the patient is brought to the operating room often for lengthening, the deformity can be corrected by gradual rod contouring to more normal alignment (Fig. 36.8a, b) (Table 36.6).

Complications should be diagnosed and treated early to avoid major catastrophes. Some complications are unavoidable and relates to the natural growth of the child. For example, if a small screw is placed in a very young child, it will be necessary to revise the foundation at some point in the future and should not be considered as complications and should be anticipated and planned. In case of rod breakage, replacement may be a better strategy than connecting two broken rods. If a rod breaks, one can wait until the time of scheduled lengthening and exchange the rods. We recommend changing both the rods if one breaks since the incidence of second rod breakage is significantly higher.

Skin problems and infections should be addressed aggressively to avoid long-term problems by debridment, antibiotics and healthy skin coverage. Implant exchange is usually not necessary but long-term antibiotics are given until the laboratory work becomes normal.

36.8 Results

In 1984, Moe et al. [19] reported on his outcomes after Harrington instrumentation. Cobb angle improved from 70° preoperatively to 38° at the time of last surgery. They also reported on T1-S1 growth and found an average growth of 2.9 cm across the instrumented area for all patients and an overall growth of 3.8 cm. The gain achieved during initial curve correction was not counted. Klemme et al. [10] reported on 67 children with progressive scoliosis using a single rod distraction-based technique. Curve magnitude improved from 67° at initial instrumentation to 47° (30%) at definitive fusion. Growth across the unfused spinal segments averaged 1 cm/year (0.08 cm/segment/year). Average number of spinal segments instrumented was 13.7.

Tello [27] described his experience with 44 children treated with Harrington instrumentation without fusion. He reported on 12 patients who went on to final fusion with an average curvature correction of 32%.

Akbarnia et al. [1] in 2005 were the first to report the clinical outcomes following dual growing rod surgery. Their early results included data collected with a minimum of 2 years follow-up after initial surgery. Follow-up averaged 4.02 years with an average of 6.6 lengthenings per patient at an interval of 7.4 months. Average Cobb improved from 82 to 38° after initial surgery and 36° at last follow-up or postfinal fusion. T1-S1 increased by 1.21 cm/year. The SAL ratio among thoracic curves improved from 0.87 to 1.0. Complication rates were reported as 48%.

In 2008, Akbarnia et al. [2] reported on the results of 13 patients with no previous surgery and noncongenital curves who underwent dual growing rod therapy and were followed to final fusion. Average age was 6.6 years at initial growing rod surgery and 11 years at final fusion. Patients underwent an average of 7.8 surgeries including initial growing rods and final fusion. Cobb angle improved from average 81° preinitial to 36° postoperatively and 28° after final fusion. The patients underwent on an average 5.2 lengthenings at an interval of 9.4 months. Average growth was 1.46 cm/year for a total of 5.7 ± 2.9 cm over 4.37 ± 2.4 years. When analyzing a cohort of children with more frequent lengthenings (≤6 months), he found a statistical improvement in growth rate (1.8 cm vs. 1 cm/year) and Cobb correction (79 vs. 48%) (Fig. 36.9).

Sponseller et al. [26] recently reported the outcome of growing rods fixed to the pelvis. He included 36 patients of which 30 were dual growing rods. A cross-link was used in the dual iliac fixation group to provide improved construct stability. Overall, there was significant improvement in coronal and sagittal balance. Among the 6 patients with final fusion, mean gain in

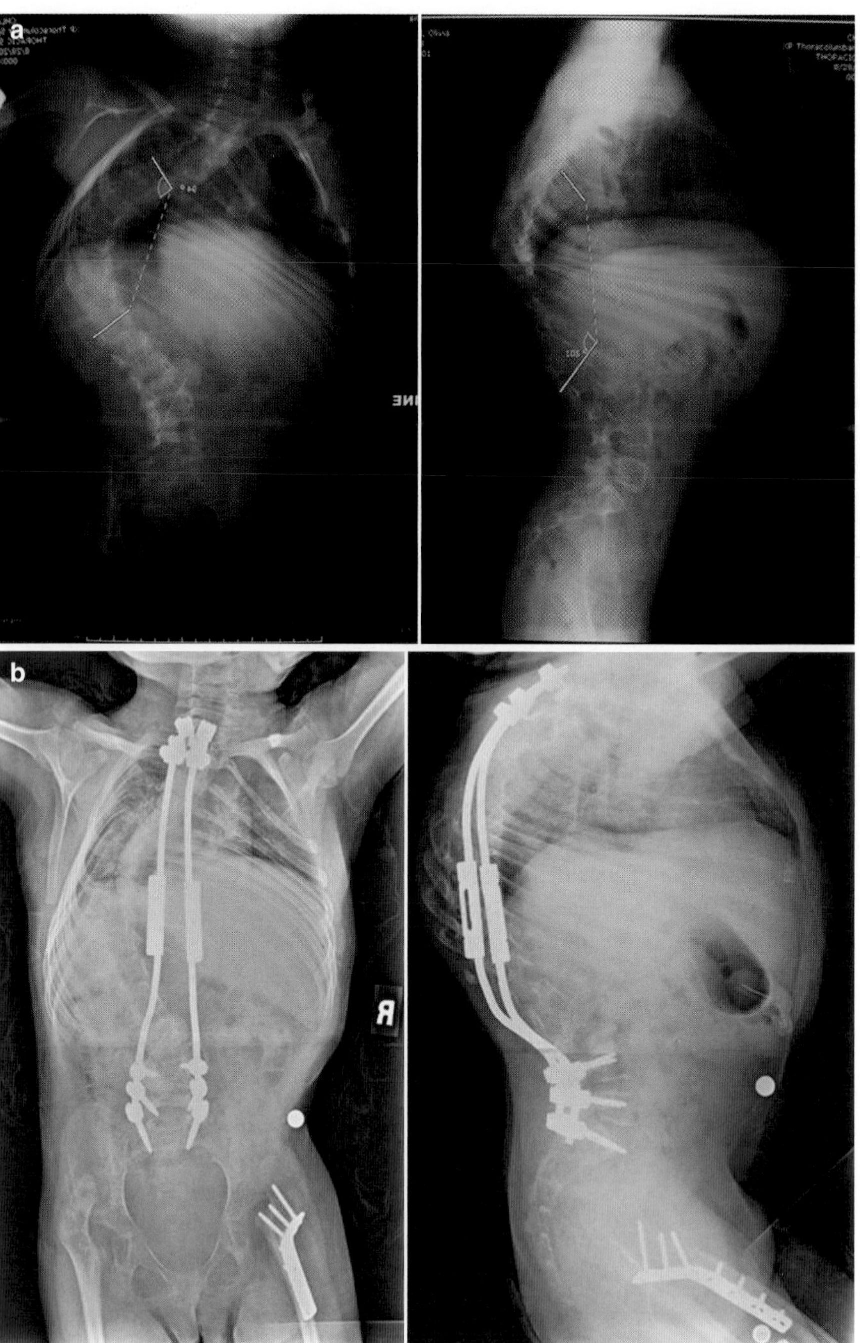

Fig. 36.8 Dual growing rods in a patient with severe kyphoscoliosis. (**a**) Postoperative radiographs show considerable correction after surgery (**b**)

T1-S1 was 8.6 cm of which 4 cm occurred during the lengthening period. The dual iliac fixation group has a statistical advantage over single rod fixation regarding correction of deformity (47 vs. 25%) and pelvic obliquity (67 vs. 44%). Iliac screws also showed overall superiority compared to sacral fixation with regard to correction of major Cobb, and pelvic obliquity. Pelvic fixation, regardless of the technique, resulted in greater percentage improvement in pelvic obliquity than in correction of major curve. All the 12 patients who

Table 36.6 Recommendations for minimizing complications

Growing rod pitfalls and avoidance	
Pitfall	**Avoidance**
Proximal junctional kyphosis	Bend the proximal rods into appropriate kyphosis Preserve interspinal ligaments Proximal construct should be around T2 or T3, DO NOT end construct in kyphotic segment Add more support in addition to foundations such as wires or tape
Tandem connector problems	Place at thoracolumbar junction (T10-L2, a normally straight area of the spine) if possible and smaller size connectors if used in other spinal segments
Primary surgery failures	When in doubt instrument longer Construct usually ends at L3-L5 Use pedicle screw instrumentation at caudal foundation Cephelad foundation use either pedicle screws or hooks with a crosslink In rigid curves consider preoperative traction and or anulotomy With pelvic obliquity consider instrumentation to pelvis
Growth not occurring as expected	Ensure lengthening every six months but consider limitation
Premature fusion	Meticulous surgical technique Avoid overexposing the spine Apply less invasive techniques Frequent lengthenings
Wound problems	Avoid mishandling tissue Careful layered closure Avoid use of electrocaudery near skin Use low profile implants If tissue coverage cannot be obtained involve plastic surgery for coverage

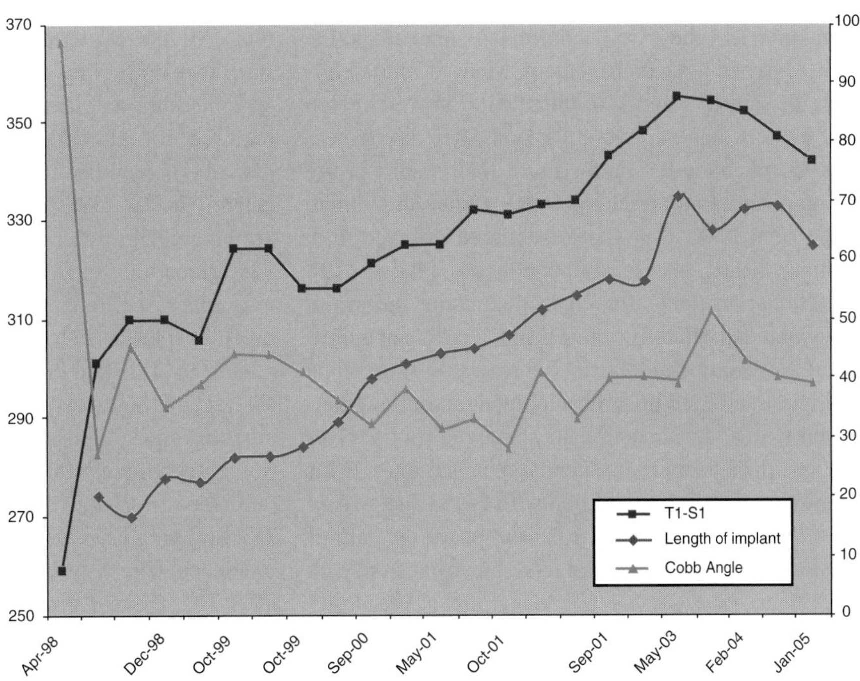

Fig. 36.9 T1S1 and Cobb angle changes in a 4-year-old patient with Marfans syndrome treated with dual growing rods (7 years follow-up)

were expected to ambulate given their neurological status were able to do so after surgery.

There are several points worth reiterating regarding improved outcome in patients who undergo dual growing rod surgery. The initial surgical treatment of scoliosis is by far the most important procedure to predict long-term success. This includes choosing which growing rod construct to use, and levels to be included. In general, the upper thoracic spine is used as the proximal foundation, and caudally, the levels are chosen based on curve pattern, but in general, span the thoracolumbar junction (L2 or below). More frequent lengthenings (≤6 months) do seem to lead to more correction and improved radiographic outcomes, but with a higher number of complications. Complication rates remain high; however, dual growing rods lead to fewer unplanned surgeries, with most complications addressed at routine lengthening. Pelvic fixation can be safely applied to a growing rod in cases where distal fixation is appropriate. Dual iliac screws with a caudal crosslink have the best outcome.

36.9 Discussion

EOS represents one of the most complex conditions challenging the pediatric spine surgeons. These patients have a variety of underlying etiologies in addition to their spine and chest wall abnormalities that add to the complexity of their management. Many of these children die in their infancy if untreated. It is well known that even if they survive childhood, their life expectancy is much shorter. Furthermore, their quality of life is significantly impaired and some studies show them to be even lower than that of children afflicted with asthma, heart disease, or childhood cancer [29]. Traditional methods for correcting spine deformity have included spinal fusion. This method is not appropriate for young children since it results in short spine and chest and lung underdevelopment and often associated with an increase in their spinal deformity. Over the past decade, there has been a renewed interest for improving the care of children with EOS. The goal of these new treatment options is to improve the care of these children. There are obstacles, however, from lack of evidence-based research, and significant variability of treatment methods once the indication for treatment is established.

There has been increasing interest in the development of new technique and devices for surgical treatment of patients with EOS. Furthermore, there has been favorable legislature passed by US congress such as "The Pediatric Medical Device Safety and Improvement Act of 2007" which has improved the regulatory process; however, most of the new techniques for the treatment of patients with EOS involves off label use of pediatric devices. There are also obstacles for proving the effectiveness of methods since it requires evidence-based studies that cannot be easily done in this population.

Recent attempts have led to the establishment of Growing Spine Committee of Scoliosis Research Society and Study Groups conducting multicenter studies. One such study group is GSSG established in 2002.

36.10 Growing Spine Study Group

GSSG www.growingspine.org is an international study group which was founded in 2002. This study group is supported by the Growing Spine Foundation and Orthopaedic Research and Education Foundation to independently perform research and education, and focuses mainly on research on EOS. Currently, 18 centers from United States and other countries are actively involved in GSSG prospective data collection. All the activities are performed under Health Insurance Portability and Accountability Act (HIPPA), and Institutional Review Board (IRB) approval is required for all data submissions. A total of 470 patients (November 2009 report) with EOS have been entered in the GSSG data base and this number is growing. Diagnostic subgroups include 98 congenital, 124 idiopathic (84 Infantile, 40 Juvenile), 123 neuromuscular (24 cerebral palsy, 36 muscular disease, 34 myelodysplasia, 29 others), 113 syndromic, and 12 others. In 2007 and 2008, the GSSG has presented 12 abstracts at Scoliosis Research Society (SRS) annual meeting and/or International Meeting on Advanced Spine Techniques (IMAST). Many articles have been published from the GSSG data base [1, 2, 23, 25, 26, 28]. Studying EOS has been a challenge due to its rare incidence. The contribution of many surgeons to the GSSG has created an unique opportunity to study EOS in a growing number of patients using a multicenter data base.

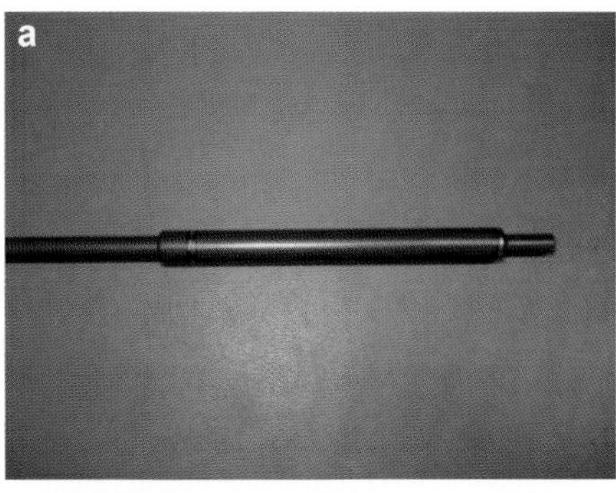

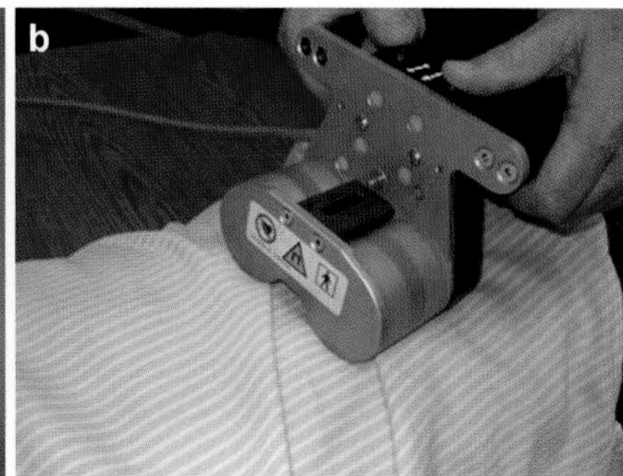

Fig. 36.10 Multiple attempts have been made to utilize technology for less invasive treatment of scoliosis in young children. MAGEC is an example of devices that has been made and is currently in experimental phase. It comprises two major elements, an implantable distraction rod (**a**) and an external adjustment device (**b**). The Initial animal studies have been encouraging [3]. Clinical studies are underway

36.11 Future Direction

There has been significant progress in recent years in our understanding of the natural history and outcomes of treatment in children with EOS. However, there exists a great deal of variation in indications as well as treatment methods [21]. This is partially due to a lack of standardized methods of categorizing the heterogeneous EOS population and difficulties in evaluating outcomes. The study groups using multicenter clinical studies should help standardizing the data collection and management and conduct quality research.

The recent enthusiasm in developing new technology and devices such as remotely controlled distraction-based mechanisms [3] will lead to less invasive procedures and minimize the complications associated with the current techniques (Fig. 36.10).

Finally, to assess the effect of the treatment methods on the natural history of EOS requires long-term follow-up of these patients with the collection of meaningful clinical and other important data. We have come a long way in 50 years, but certainly much more to learn in the next 50 years.

References

1. Akbarnia BA, Marks DS, Boachie-Adjei O et al (2005) Dual growing rod technique for the treatment of progressive early-onset scoliosis: a multicenter study. Spine 30(17 suppl): S46–S57
2. Akbarnia BA, Breakwell LM, Marks DS et al (2008) dual growing rod technique followed for three to eleven years until final fusion;the effect of frequency of lengthening. Spine 33(9):984–990
3. Akbarnia BA, Mundis G, Salari P et al (2009) Innovation in Growing Rod technique; Study of safety and efficacy of Remotely Expandable Rod in animal model. J Child Orthop 3(6):503–533
4. Akbarnia BA, Oliveira D, Salari P et al (2009) Neurological complication after growing rod implants exchange: a case report. J Child Orthop 3:145–168
5. Bess S, Akbarnia BA, Thompson GH et al (2010) Complications in growing rod treatment for early onset scoliosis: Analysis of 897 surgeries. J Bone Joint Surg Am: In Press
6. Blakemore LC, Scoles PV, Poe-Kochert C et al (2001) Submuscular Isola rod with or without limited apical fusion in the management of severe spinal deformities in young children: preliminary report. Spine 26(18):2044–2048
7. Dimeglio A (1993) Growth of the spine before age 5 years. J Pediatr Orthop 1-B:102–107
8. Dubousset J, Herring JA, Shufflebarger H (1989) The crankshaft phenomenon. J Pediatr Orthop 9(5):541–550
9. Harrington PR (1962) Treatment of scoliosis. Correction and internal fixation by spine instrumentation. J Bone Joint Surg Am 44-A:591–610
10. Klemme WR, Denis F, Winter RB et al (1997) Spinal instrumentation without fusion for progressive scoliosis in young children. J Pediatr Orthop 17(6):734–742
11. Luque E, Cardosa A (1977) Segmental spinal instrumentation in growing children. Orthop Trans 1:37
12. Luque ER (1982) Paralytic scoliosis in growing children. Clin Orthop (163):202–209
13. Mahar A, Bagheri R et al (2007) Biomechanical comparison of different anchors (foundations) for the pediatric dual growing rod technique. Spine J 8(6):933–939
14. Marchetti PG, Faldini A (1978) "End fusions" in the treatment of some progressive scoliosis in childhood or early adolescence. Orthop Trans 2:271

15. Mardjetko SM, Hammerberg KW, Lubicky JP et al (1992) The Luque trolley revisited. Review of nine cases requiring revision. Spine 17(5):582–589
16. Mehta MH (1972) The rib-vertebra angle in the early diagnosis between resolving and progressive infantile scoliosis. J Bone Joint Surg Br 54(2):230–243
17. Mineiro J, Weinstein SL (2002) Subcutaneous rodding for progressive spinal curvatures: early results. J Pediatr Orthop 22(3):290–295
18. Moe J, Cummine J, Winter R et al (1978) Harrington instrumentation without fusion combined with the milwaukee brace for difficult scoliosis problems in young children. Scoliosis Research Society, Cambridge, MA
19. Moe JH, Kharrat K, Winter RB et al (1984) Harrington instrumentation without fusion plus external orthotic support for the treatment of difficult curvature problems in young children. Clin Orthop (185):35–45
20. Pratt RK, Webb JK, Burwell RG et al (1999) Luque trolley and convex epiphysiodesis in the management of infantile and juvenile idiopathic scoliosis. Spine 24(15):1538–1547
21. Salari P, Oliveira D, Akbarnia BA et al (2009) Infantile idiopathic scoliosis; variations in preferred treatment options. In: The 16th International Meeting on Advanced Spine Techniques (IMAST) Vienna, Austria
22. Sanders JO, Herring JA, Browne RH (1995) Posterior arthrodesis and instrumentation in the immature (Risser-grade-0) spine in idiopathic scoliosis. J Bone Joint Surg Am 77(1):39–45
23. Sankar WN, Skaggs DL, Emans JB et al (2009) Neurologic risk in growing rod spine surgery in early onset scoliosis: is neuromonitoring necessary for all cases. Spine 34(18):1952–1955
24. Skaggs DL (2008) Terminology for early onset scoliosis and chest wall deformities.In: The Second International Congress on Early Onset Scoliosis & Growing Spine (ICEOS), Montreal, Quebec
25. Sponseller PD, Thompson GH, Akbarnia BA et al (2009) Growing rods for infantile scoliosis in Marfan syndrome. Spine 34(16):1711–1715
26. Sponseller PD, Yang JS, Thompson GH et al (2009) Pelvic fixation of growing rods; comparison of constructs. Spine 34(16):1706–1710
27. Tello C (1994) Harrington instrumentation without arthrodesis and consecutive distraction program for young children with severe spinal deformities. Experience and technical details. Orthop Clin North Am 25(2):333–351
28. Thompson GH, Akbarnia BA, Kostial P et al (2005) Comparison of single and dual growing rod techniques followed through definitive surgery: a preliminary study. Spine 30(18):2039–2044
29. Vitale MG, Matsumoto H et al (2008) Health-related quality of life in children with thoracic insufficiency syndrome. J Pediatr Orthop 28(2):239–243
30. Winter R (1997) Scoliosis and spinal growth. Orthop Rev 6:17–20
31. Yazici M, Asher M et al (2000) The safety and efficacy of Isola-Galveston instrumentation and arthrodesis in the treatment of neuromuscular spinal deformities. J Bone Joint Surg Am 82(4):524–543

37 VEPTR Expansion Thoracoplasty

Robert M. Campbell

Key Points

- VEPTR expansion thoracoplasty procedures treat volume depletion deformities of the thorax which cause thoracic insufficiency syndrome.
- Thoracic insufficiency syndrome is the inability of the thorax to support normal respiration or lung growth.
- Conditions such as congenital scoliosis and fused ribs, early onset scoliosis and infantile scoliosis, myelomeningocele, and congenital deficiencies of the chest wall can be addressed by VEPTR expansion thoracoplasty without inhibiting the growth of the spine.
- Advances in imaging techniques such as dynamic magnetic resonance imaging (MRI) of the lungs will enable a better understanding of the biomechanical deficits of the thorax in thoracic insufficiency syndrome.

37.1 Introduction

37.1.1 *Thoracic Insufficiency Syndrome: Anatomic Basis*

Thoracic insufficiency syndrome (TIS), a new characterized disease [4], is the inability of the thorax to support normal respiration or lung growth. It is the prime indication for the treatment by VEPTR (vertical expandable prosthetic titanium rib) expansion thoracoplasty. The natural history of thoracic insufficiency syndrome can easily be lethal in cases of untreated early-onset spine and chest wall deformity, but overall TIS is not well understood and is just beginning to be characterized in the literature [9].

The thorax is a complex, dynamic chamber of respiration that both supports and rhythmically expands the lungs during breathing. Structurally, the thorax consists of the spine, as its posterior pillar, the rib cage [18], the sternum, and the diaphragm. As the respiratory pump [4], it must provide normal, stable volume for the underlying lung through rigidity of the chest wall, as well as the ability to change that volume. These are termed the two thoracic characteristics of breathing [4].

Abnormalities of the thorax, including congenital structural problems of the thoracic spine, the rib cage, and the diaphragm, result in *primary* thoracic insufficiency syndrome. These, unfortunately, are not the only problems degrading thoracic function. Abnormalities of the lumbar spine may also critically affect thoracic performance in an indirect fashion. The diaphragm may also be compromised unilaterally or bilaterally in *secondary* thoracic insufficiency syndrome [3] either when there is a collapse of the torso inferiorly through lumbar kyphosis in myelomeningocele or when there is pelvic obliquity due to thoracolumbar scoliosis, both causing a relative obstruction to excursion of the diaphragm. Clinically, these children have a Marionette's sign with the patient's head bobbing synchronously with respiration with the diaphragm, in effect, doing a push up against body weight [3].

The only practical aspect of TIS that is currently treatable is the volume reduction of the thorax. VEPTR expansion thoracoplasty can enlarge a constricted thorax, either unilaterally or bilaterally, with the assumption that

R. M. Campbell
Division of Orthopaedics, The Children's Hospital of Philadelphia, Division of Orthopaedics, 2nd Floor, Wood Center, 34th Street and Civic Center Blvd, Philadelphia, PA 19104, USA
e-mail: campbellrm@email.chop.edu

B. A. Akbarnia et al. (eds.), *The Growing Spine*,
DOI: 10.1007/978-3-540-85207-0_37, © Springer-Verlag Berlin Heidelberg 2011

the underlying diaphragm can make use of the new volume of lung that goes on to fill the expanded thoracic volume, but such an approach cannot restore chest wall motion, and it is not known whether such procedures enhance diaphragmatic function. These aspects of TIS await future developments to better address them. The first step in VEPTR treatment is to classify the thoracic volume depletion deformity so that the proper VEPTR surgical strategy is chosen.

37.1.2 Volume Depletion Deformities of the Thorax

Three-dimensional thoracic deformity is defined in the three anatomic planes: coronal, sagittal, and transverse. These were recently defined as volume depletion deformities (*VDD*) of the thorax [9] (Table 37.1, Fig 37.1a–d): Type I is a volume depletion deformity due to absent ribs and exotic scoliosis. This is a physiologic unilateral thoracic hypoplasia in which the underlying anatomic defect is prolapse of the lung into the chest with effective volume loss. Examples of this include the VATER association as well as absent ribs and congenital scoliosis (see Fig. 37.1a). The next volume depletion deformity of the coronal anatomic plane is fused ribs and scoliosis, called a Type II deformity. This is also a unilateral thoracic hypoplasia, but due to constriction of the lung secondary to fused ribs that longitudinally constrict the hemithorax. Examples include VATER association, fused ribs and congenital scoliosis, and thoracogenic scoliosis from prior thoracotomy (see Fig. 37.1b). There are two types of global volume depletion deformity of the thorax: Type IIIA is a foreshortened thorax with bilateral longitudinal constriction of the lungs from loss of thoracic height; this is commonly seen in Jarcho-Levin Syndrome (see Fig. 37.1c), and a Type IIIB deformity when there is a transverse constriction of the thorax with secondary lateral constriction of the lungs from rib deformity; this is found in Jenue's Asphyxiating Thoracic Dystrophy (see Fig. 37.1d). Type III-B deformity is also found in wind-swept deformity of the thorax [4] owing to thoracic spine rotation and lordosis in scoliosis without primary rib abnormality. The VEPTR expansion thoracoplasty strategy for each volume depletion deformity of the thorax is different. In mixed types of volume depletion deformity, VEPTR surgical treatment should address each individual segment of thoracic deformity with either appropriate longitudinal or lateral expansion of the constricted thorax.

37.1.3 FDA Indications for VEPTR Expansion Thoracoplasty

- *Presence of Thoracic Insufficiency Syndrome*
- *Skeletally Immature patient*

Anatomic Diagnosis

- *Absent ribs*
- *Constrictive chest wall syndrome, including fused ribs and scoliosis*
- *Hypoplastic Thorax*
- *Scoliosis of congenital or neurogenic origin without rib anomaly*

Table 37.1 Thoracic volume depletion deformities

Type of volume depletion deformity	Thoracic deficit	Mechanism of lung volume loss	Examples
I. Absent ribs and exotic scoliosis	Unilateral thoracic hypoplasia	Lung prolapses into the chest with volume loss	VATER, absent ribs and congenital scoliosis
II. Fused ribs and exotic scoliosis	Unilateral thoracic hypoplasia	Constriction of lung due to fused ribs shortening hemithorax	VATER, fused ribs and congenital scoliosis, thoracogenic scoliosis from prior thoracotomy
IIIa. Foreshortened thorax	Global thoracic hypoplasia	Bilateral longitudinal constriction of lungs from loss of thoracic height	Jarcho-Levin syndrome
IIIb. Transverse constricted thorax	Global thoracic hypoplasia	Lateral constriction of lungs from rib deformity	Jeune's asphyxiating thoracic Dystrophy, windswept deformity of the thorax in scoliosis

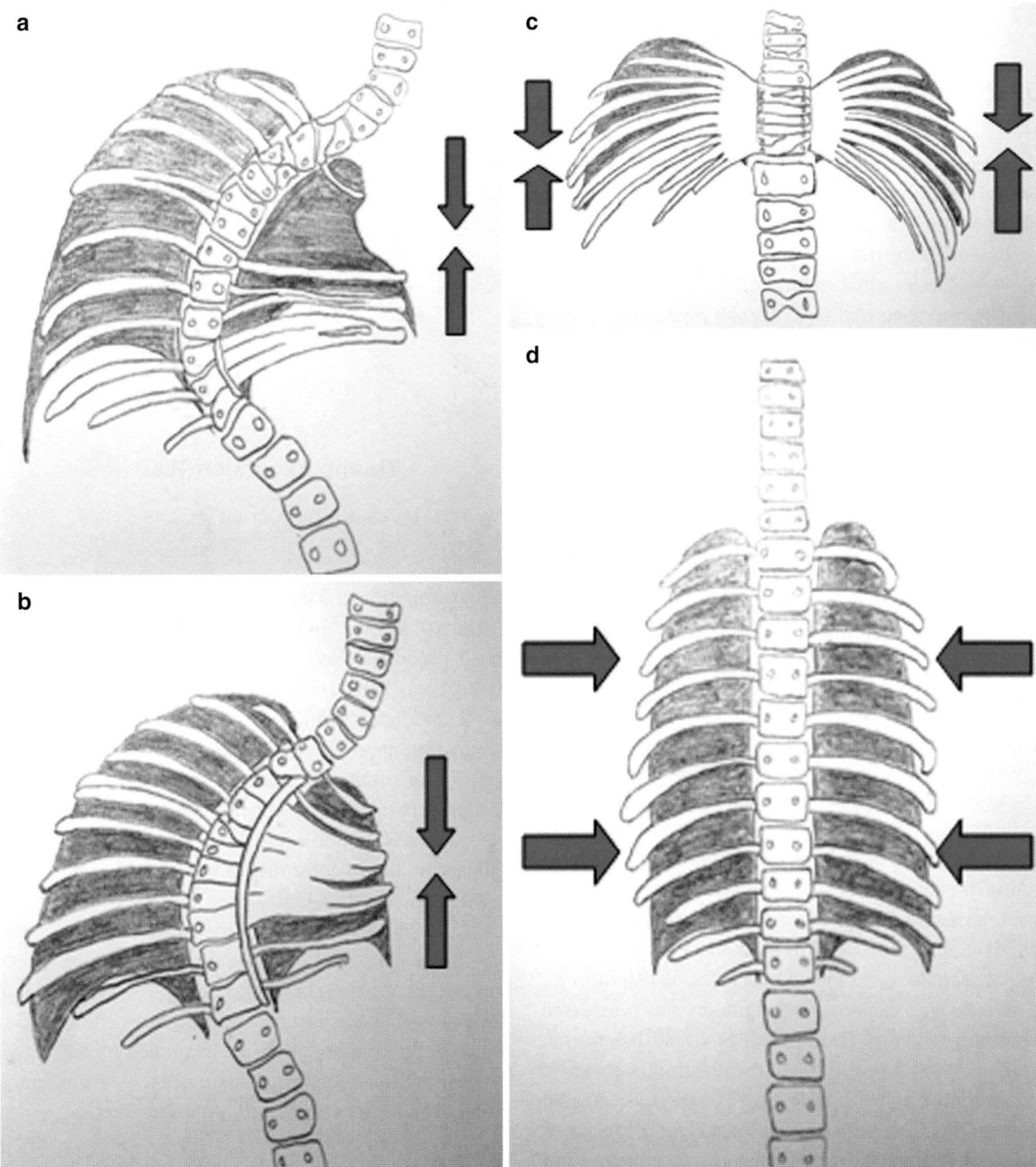

Fig. 37.1 (**a**) Type I thoracic volume depletion deformity: Absent ribs and scoliosis. (**b**) Type II thoracic volume depletion deformity: Fused ribs and scoliosis. (**c**) Type IIIa volume depletion deformity of the thorax: Spondylothoracic dysplasia (Jarcho-Levin syndrome). (**d**) Type IIIb volume depetion deformity of the thorax: Jeune's asphyxiating thoracic dystrophy

37.2 VEPTR Preoperative Assessment

37.2.1 Clinical Examination

It is important to obtain a detailed history in children with thoracic insufficiency syndrome: When was the onset of clinical deformity? What were past surgical treatments? Are there associated morbidities such as renal, gastrointestinal, central nervous system and cardiac system abnormalities? A good respiratory history should be taken to note past episodes of pneumonia, bronchitis, asthma attacks or needs for respiratory support during illness. If the patient is on oxygen, or dependent on more invasive respiratory support, the degree of respiratory insufficiency should be defined by the assisted ventilator ratings (AVR) [2, 9].

AVR Ratings:

+0: no assistance, on room air;
+1: supplemental oxygen required;
+2: night time ventilation/CPAP
+3: part time ventilation/CPAP;
+4: full time ventilation.

An increase in AVR suggests progressive clinical respiratory insufficiency, and this is a strong indication for treatment. Pulmonary function tests are practical in children aged 5 years or older [16]; so past testing, if available, would be helpful in determining any deterioration of vital capacity as determined by decreasing percent normal vital capacity. Clinical history, noting the child's ability to respond to pulmonary challenge such as play activities and running, can also be helpful.

On physical examination respiratory rate is assessed. Normal respiratory rate at birth is 40–80 breaths/min and, up to age 5 years, 20–40 breaths/min, with 15–25 breaths/min being normal from age 6–12 years and adult values, 15–20 breaths/min, are reached after 15 years of age [16]. Respiratory rate at rest above these values suggest occult respiratory insufficiency [4]. The chest is assessed for clinical deformity and the circumference measured at the nipple line and compared with normal values for age to discern percentile normal [21].

The thumb excursion test [4] is performed to clinically measure the ability of each side of the chest to contribute to respiration by rib cage expansion. In this test, the examiner's hands are placed around the base of the thorax with the thumbs posteriorly pointing upward at equal distances from the spine (Fig. 37.2).

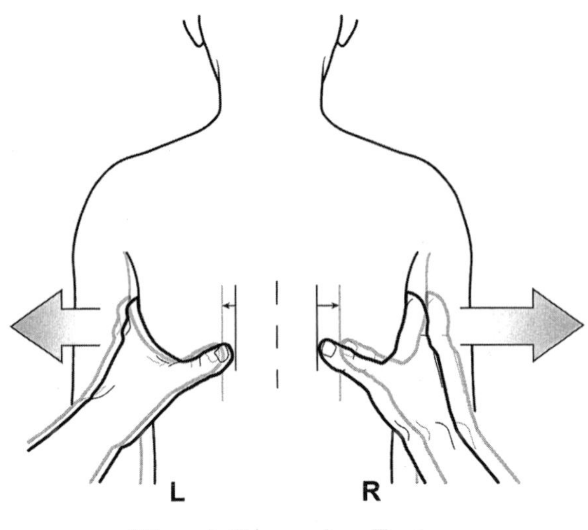

Fig. 37.2 The thumb excursion test

With respiration, the thumbs move away from the spine symmetrically because of the anterior lateral motion of the chest wall. Greater than 1 cm excursion of each thumb away from the spine during inspiration is graded as +3, and this is normal, 0.5–1 cm excursion is graded +2, motion up to 0.5 cm is graded as +1, and complete absence of motion is graded +0. Each hemithorax is graded separately. The concave fused rib hemithorax often has a +0 thumb excursion test, and if there is significant rib hump deformity of the convex hemithorax, it will also be stiff and also have a +0 TET.

"Collapsing torso" deformities, resulting in secondary thoracic insufficiency syndrome may raise pressure on the diaphragm by proximity to the pelvis and are assessed by the presence of the Marionette sign [3]. Both the lips and fingertips are examined for any signs of cyanosis and fingertips for evidence of clubbing, suggesting long term clinical hypoxia.

37.2.2 Imaging Studies

The patients with thoracic insufficiency syndrome should have a weight bearing anterior–posterior (PA) lateral radiographs of the entire spine, including the chest and pelvis, on the same radiograph. The radiograph is analyzed for Cobb angle, interpedicular line ratio [3], the height of the thoracic spine in centimeters, and the space available for lung [4]. The height of the thorax is determined by the radiographic height of the patient's thoracic spine, and this distance is divided by the normal thoracic spinal height for age [12], deriving a percentage normal. The lateral radiograph defines a loss of sagittal depth of the thorax either due to pectus excavatum or thoracic spinal lordosis. The AP and lateral radiographs enable identification of the volume depletion deformities of the thorax [9] in the coronal and sagittal planes of the thorax.

Computed tomography (CT) scans of the entire chest and lumbar spine are performed at 5 mm intervals, unenhanced [1] with the scanner set for pediatric dosage to minimize radiation exposure [13, 19]. Usually Type I, Type II, and Type III volume depletion deformities have a diminished thoracic volume on CT scan in the coronal plane reconstructions. In Type I and Type II volume depletion deformities, wind swept deformity of the chest is also common with severe reduction in transverse volume of the convex hemithorax. Its severity can be defined by measurements of spinal rotation, the posterior hemithorax symmetry ration, and the thoracic rotation of the CT scan cut at the level of maximum deformity [4]. CT lung scan volumes can be computed [14, 15]. Full chest CT scans may be taken at yearly follow up if percent normal lung volumes are being followed to detect progressive thoracic volume loss. A more limited CT scan, localized at the level of maximum deformity, may also be followed yearly if CT lung volumes are not felt to be necessary. Both ventilation perfusion lung scans and 3 mm cut CT scans with airway reconstruction can define airway compression deformity, if necessary. All patients should also undergo MRI studies of the entire spinal cord to rule out spinal cord abnormalities. Either ultrasound or fluoroscopy of the diaphragm can be performed to document diaphragmatic function, but dynamic MRI study of the lungs (Fig. 37.3a, b) will show great detail of diaphragm and chest wall function [10].

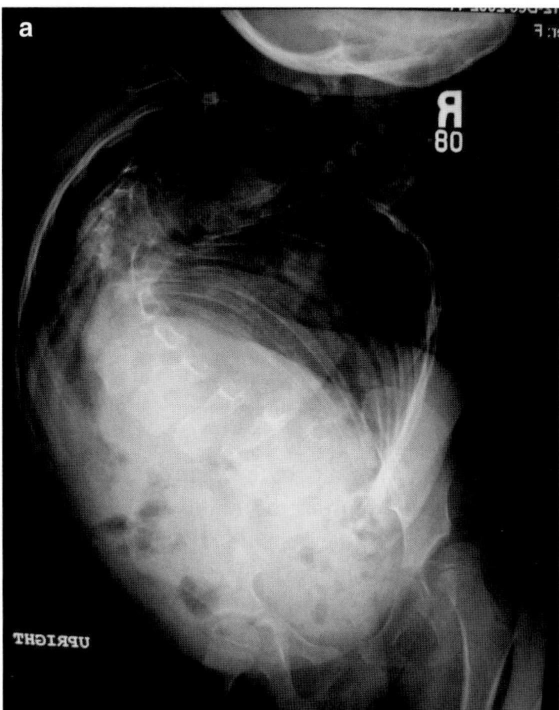

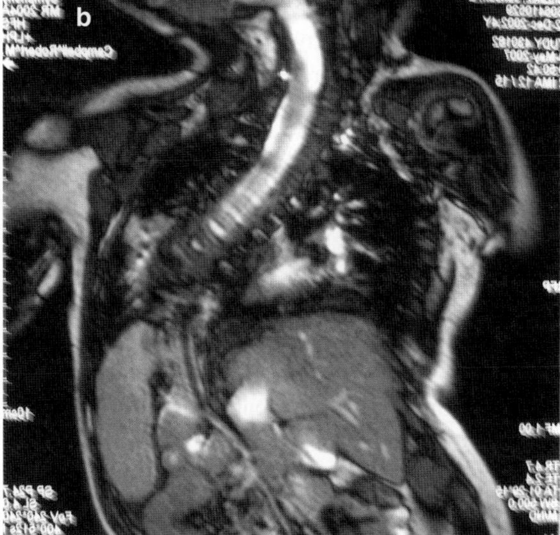

Fig. 37.3 (**a**) Severe scoliosis. (**b**) PA dynamic lung MRI of the thorax. Note intrusion of the liver into the chest from the iliac crest malposition, obstructing diaphragmatic motion

37.2.3 Specific Cardiopulmonary Studies

Routine spirometry pulmonary function studies are feasible for children aged 5 years or older, and infant pulmonary function tests can be performed in younger patients, if available. When there is spinal deformity present, the overall height of the patient is usually decreased, and care must be taken to use arm span instead of height for normalization of pulmonary function test results. Pulse oximetry studies are useful to detect significant amount of hypoxia. When there is a question of early cor pulmonale, echocardiograms are performed to detect tricuspid valve regurgitation.

37.3 VEPTR Expansion Thoracoplasty Treatment Strategies

VEPTR expansion thoracoplasty is a general category of surgical procedures that can expand the volume-constricted thorax when there is three-dimensional deformity of the thorax due to spine deformity, as well as primary rib cage deformity. The VEPTR device is made by Synthes Spine Company of West Chester, PA and is available under FDA Humanitarian Device Exemption with Institutional Review Board approval required for the use of the device at each institution. Multiple types of expansion thoracoplasties address each type of volume depletion deformity of the thorax. All the procedures have in common the ability to enlarge the constricted area of the hemithorax with the goals of restoring thoracic volume, stability, and symmetry, with correction of spinal deformity without fusion, to allow growth of the thorax afterwards. In contrast to classic spine fusion, in which the instrumentation "drives" the deformity correction, in VEPTR surgery the thorax first undergoes acute surgical reconstruction to increase volume and correct deformity, then the VEPTR devices are added to stabilize the reconstruction. VEPTR procedures may be used in patients as early as 6 months and up to skeletal maturity.

Contraindications for VEPTR treatment include a bone age of skeletal maturity, when lung growth has certainly been completed, so that there is little chance of a thoracic enlargement triggering pulmonary growth. One possible exception is chest wall instability, which may benefit from VEPTR treatment regardless of age, but FDA compassionate exemption may be needed for this use in the US. Another contraindication is poor rib bone stock or proximal absence of ribs for VEPTR attachment. Biphosphinates may strengthen ribs enough to allow VEPTR use. In proximal rib absence, rib autografts and the use of a longitudinally osteotomized clavicle as a vascularized pedicle graft may provide a bony "first rib" for VEPTR attachment. Severe comorbidities that make repetitive surgeries impractical are also a relative contra-indication, especially when cardiac or pulmonary disease are the primary reason for the patient's respiratory disability and the thorax is not the major problem. Soft tissue coverage is critical for VEPTR success, but commonly children with respiratory insufficiency have a calorie deficit from the work of tachypnea and may have percent normal body weight of less than 5%. Diet supplements, or even G tube therapy, may be necessary to increase the soft tissue coverage for VEPTR implantation, and a minimum percent normal body weight of 25% is recommended before proceeding to surgery. Poor lung function of itself is not a contraindication for VEPTR treatment.

37.4 Surgical Technique

37.4.1 The General VEPTR Implantation Surgical Approach

The patient is placed in a lateral decubitus position with the primary thoracic deformity on the upward side (Fig. 37.4a–c). The prone position may also be used if exposure does not extend too far anteriorly, but the decubitus positon helps correct deformity in cases of severe scoliosis. Spinal cord and upper extremity status are monitored by both somatosensory evoked potentials and motor evoked potentials. A central arterial line is placed. Prophylactic IV antibiotics are given and maintained for 5 days or until are drains are out. A modified curvi-linear thoracotomy incision is used, extending anteriorly between the ninth and tenth rib. Once the chest wall flap is elevated, the common insertion of the middle and posterior scalene muscles are identified to determine the location of the nerovascular bundle just anterior to it. After complete exposure of the rib cage, the paraspinal muscles are next reflected by cautery medially up to the tips of the transverse processes of the spine. Care must be taken not to expose the spine to prevent inadvertent fusion. The underlying chest wall deformity is then assessed for the degree of instability, constriction of underlying lung by rib fusion, anomalous insertion of the ribs into the spine, and sites for device placement (see Fig. 37.4b). Surgical strategy depends on the specific type of volume depletion deformity to be addressed, with complex deformity involving more than one type requiring combined techniques. In general, unilateral constriction of the thorax is addressed by an expansion thoracoplasty, termed an opening wedge thoracostomy. The lengthened hemithorax is then stabilized by a hybrid VEPTR device from proximal ribs to lumbar spine [5], sized so that the rib sleeve does not extend below the inferior end plate of T12. Hybrid devices are always inserted in a proximal

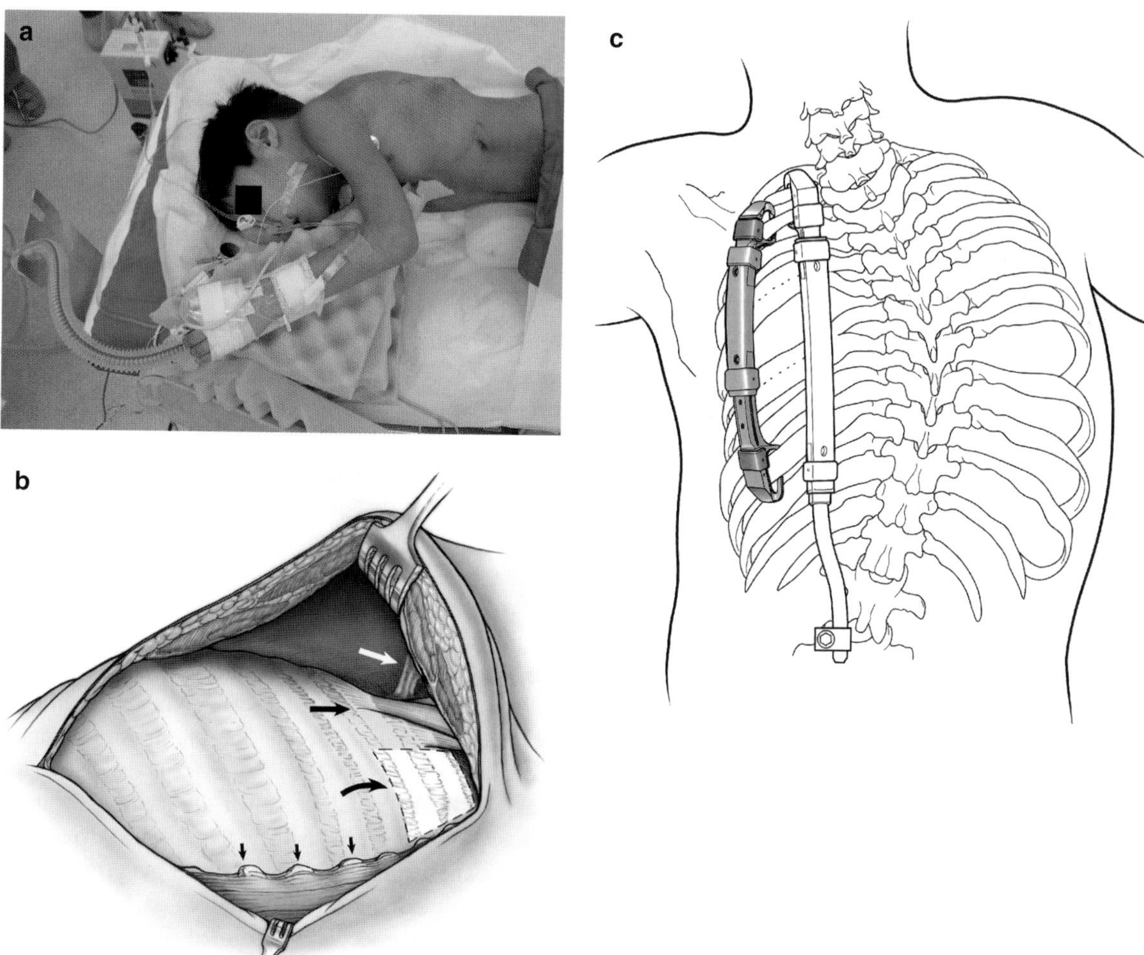

Fig. 37.4 (**a**) General patient positioning for VEPTR thoracoplasty. (**b**) VEPTR exposure: white arrow notes neurovascular bundle, hatched area is the safe zone for superior cradle attachment, small arrows show tips of the transverse processes. (**c**) Standard VEPTR construct

to distal direction to avoid penetrating the chest and causing cardiopulmonary injury. In patients younger than 18 months, hybrid devices are impractical because of inadequate spinal canal width for a spinal hook, so a single rib-to-rib VEPTR is used instead. When such a child reaches 2 or 3 years of age, the rib-to-rib device can be easily converted to a hybrid device which controls scoliosis better than the rib-to-rib devices. If space permits, a second device, rib-to-rib, is added laterally in the posterior axillary line to load share (see Fig. 37.4c). If there are areas of chest wall instability more anteriorly, additional longitudinal rib-to-rib VEPTR devices are implanted as needed with care to place them well below the neurovascular bundle. Once the thoracic reconstruction has been completed and VEPTR devices are in place, then the combined muscle and skin flapped are stretched to provide increased soft tissue coverage for the expanded hemithorax. The goal of all types of VEPTR expansion thoracoplasties is to correct the thoracic deformity with maximum expansion longitudinally and laterally of the constricted hemithorax in unilateral disease, or to increase thoracic volume and symmetry in bilateral disease in a staged fashion. The thorax should be equilibrated as much as possible in all planes, increasing space available for lung [4] on the concave side to 100%, with symmetrical hemithorax width on radiograph, and symmetrical hemithorax volumes in the transverse plane on the CT scan.

For closure, the scapula is first brought distally to the approximate anatomic position, and the pulse oximeter reading on the upper arm and somatosensory and motor evoked potentials are checked for signs of acute thoracic outlet syndrome. Patients with very anomalous proximal ribs, distracted into the area of the brachial plexus by VEPTR expansion thoracoplasty, are at the risk of getting this syndrome and early signs are decrease in ulnar nerve tracings and diminished pulse. Usually relaxation of the position of the scapula, allowing a more proximal position, resolves this problem. If continued alterations in pulse oximeter or spinal cord monitoring are encountered, even with relaxation of the closure, it may be necessary to resect the anterior-lateral portion of the first and second rib, lateral to the devices, to provide clearance for the brachial plexus in the reconstructed thorax.

Two subcutaneous Jackson Pratt drains are used. In patients when there is substantial defect in the pleura greater than 4 cm, it is repaired with Surgisis® by Cook Medical [20] with an addition of a chest tube. Patients are usually left intubated 24–72 h. VEPTR thoracic reconstruction acutely alters pulmonary function mechanics to a much greater extent than a standard thoracotomy, so immediate extubation is often not well tolerated. The hematocrit is checked daily for 3 days. Although blood loss usually averages 50 mL [3], continual oozing underneath the large flaps results in a 50% risk of postoperative transfusion. Generally, a hematocrit of 30% or greater is optimal for oxygen carrying capacity for these patients. Fluid management should be on the restrictive side to prevent acute pulmonary edema.

Once weaned off the ventilator, the patient can be transferred to the surgical ward. Jackson Pratt drains are removed when their individual drainage decreases to 20 cc or less over a 24 h period. Chest tubes are removed once their drainage equals 1 cc/kg of patient weight or less over 24 h.

If the patient goes into respiratory distress after drains and chest tubes are removed, consider checking for acute reaccumilation of the pleural effusion with compression of the lung. Temporary chest tube drainage can address this through placement of an anterior "pig-tail" chest tube.

Vigorous pulmonary toilet, including percussion, is needed postoperatively. The patients are mobilized as soon as possible. No bracing is used because of the potential constrictive effects. Specific postoperative care is detailed in other reports [5, 7].

37.5 VEPTR Expansion Procedures

Twice a year, the devices are expanded under general anesthesia to accommodate growth of the patient [5]. We do not use spinal cord monitoring for expansion procedures unless the primary implantation procedure was associated with monitoring/neurological changes, but some surgeons monitor all VEPTR procedures. Prophylactic IV antibiotics are given and maintained for 2 days. Each individual device is accessed by a 3 cm incision, with care taken to preserve a thick muscle flap over the devices by meticulous soft tissue technique to minimize the risk of skin slough. If the distraction lock is exposed through the thoracotomy incision, a freer elevator is inserted proximally along the top of the device and used to elevate the overlying muscle. Cautery is inserted into the soft tissue tunnel created by the freer elevator, and is used to release the muscle deeply on each side of the device so that a thick muscle flap is mobilized with the free edge at the skin incision. The same approach is used distally. When the skin incision parallels the device, the muscle incision is made by cautery *along the side of the device* at the distraction lock site of the rib sleeve, then the cautery is turned sideways to release the muscle flap off the device. The full thickness muscle flap is reflected by a freer elevator, the distraction locks of the device are removed, and the expansion procedure performed (Fig. 37.5). When there is a medial device, usually a hybrid, extending from proximal ribs down to lumbar spine, it is first expanded until the reactive force increases substantially and then the device is locked with a new distraction

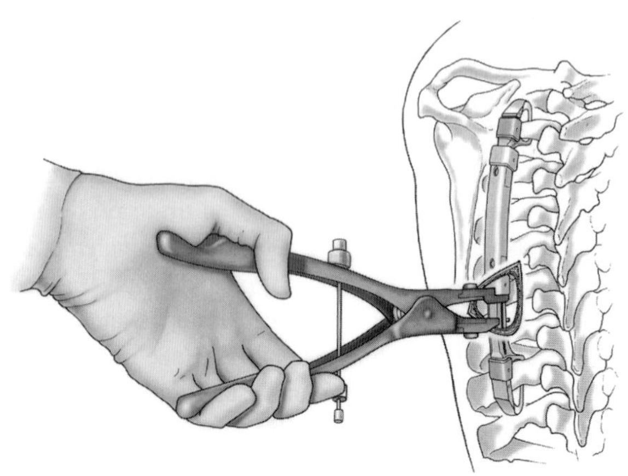

Fig. 37.5 VEPTR expansion

lock at its new length. The adjacent devices are then expanded approximately half that distance, the distraction lock replaced and locked into its new length. When there are bilateral devices to expand, first the concave hemithorax are expanded and locked, then the devices on the convex side are expanded and locked. The mobilized muscle flaps are closed without tension over the locks when device expansion is complete.

37.6 VEPTR Replacement Procedures

The VEPTR device expansion is somewhat limited in the very small sizes of 4 and 5 cm, but it progressively increases with longer devices. Once completely expanded, change out of the central rib sleeve portion and the inferior cradle is needed. This is usually accomplished through a limited access, central incision at the distraction point, a small incision over the superior cradle, and then a third incision over the lumbar hook or the inferior cradle [5] (Fig. 37.6). Prophylactic IV antibiotics are given and maintained for 3 days, or until any drains are out. The device is unlocked from the spinal hook and the superior cradle, removed, and then replaced with a longer device. The new device is locked into place, and then tensioned, much as is done during an expansion procedure. We use spinal cord monitoring for VEPTR replacement procedures.

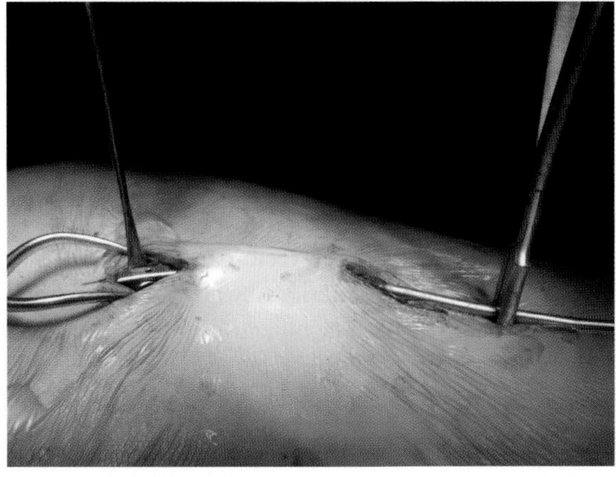

Fig. 37.6 VEPTR replacement through "skip" incisions

37.7 Specific VEPTR Surgical Strategies

37.7.1 Type I Volume Depletion Deformity: Rib Absence and Scoliosis

The stabilization VEPTR expansion thoracoplasty for a Type I VDD is performed through the usual thoracotomy incision with the goal of lateral and longitudinal expansion of the underlying collapsed hemithorax with stabilization of flail segment [2]. The thoracostomy is performed in the usual fashion. Care must be taken not to damage the lung when the skin incision is over the chest wall defect, and generally there is a large spine defect in the area of the chest wall defect, so care must be taken not to violate dura in the exposure.

The initial VEPTR device is commonly placed adjacent to the spine. The first step is implantation of the superior rib cradle. Commonly it is attached to the proximal ribs above the chest wall defect, either on the bottom rib of the rib cluster, or on a more proximal rib. In the latter case, a 1 cm incision is made by cautery in the intercostal muscle, immediately beneath the rib of attachment. Next a Freer elevator is then inserted, pushing through the intercostal muscle to the lower edge of the rib, stripping the combined pleura/periosteum layer off from the rib anteriorly. A second portal is the placed by cautery above the rib of attachment. A second Freer is inserted in this portal, pointing distally to strip off the periosteum of the rib anteriorly, and the two Freers should touch in the "chopstick" maneuver [3], to confirm that a continuous soft tissue tunnel has been made. The VEPTR trial instrument is then inserted into the portals to enlarge them superiorly and inferiorly. At least 1 cm of bone should be encircled by the superior rib cradle. If the rib chosen is too slender, then two ribs are encircled with an extended cradle cap added to the construct to encircle it. The rib cradle cap is inserted by forceps into the superior portal, facing laterally, to avoid the great vessels and the esophagus, then turned distally. Next, the superior rib cradle is then inserted into the inferior portal, mated with the cradle cap and attached with a cradle cap lock. The superior cradle is gently distracted by forceps superiorly to test for instability. If unstable, the superior cradle can be moved another level distally to a stronger rib for attachment. Superior cradle insertion is similar when the attachment rib has fibrous adhesions instead of intercostal muscles linking it to the ribs above and below. However, when the superior cradle needs to be placed within a mass of fused ribs, the inferior portal for the superior cradle is created by a bone burr, creating a slot 5 by 1.5 mm, and a 5 mm superior portal is cut by burr for placement of the cradle cap.

An opening wedge thoracostomy is then performed through the flail segment of the chest, usually requiring release of the fibrosed pleura, then the proximal ribs are distracted upward so that they become horizontal in orientation. With the Synthes rib distractors holding the opening wedge thoracostomy open to the corrected position, a correct length VEPTR rib sleeve and inferior cradle is then attached to the previously placed rib cradle and extended down to a stable rib near the inferior margin of the thorax, commonly the ninth or tenth rib.

When there is significant scoliosis, a hybrid VEPTR from rib to spine is often needed. With the Synthes rib spreader left in place to continue to lengthen the constricted chest wall through the thoracostomy, a separate paraspinous skin incision, 5 cm long, is then made 1 cm lateral to the midline at the level of the proximal lumbar spine. A flap is elevated medially to expose the midline of the spine. Cautery is used to longitudinally section the apophysis of the two posterior spinous processes at the correct interspace and a Cobb elevator used to strip the spine laterally. The ligamentum flavum is then resected and the laminar hook inserted. Gelfoam is placed over the exposed dura. A bone block of autograft, usually from rib resection, is then placed from the superior lamina to the top of the hook, anchoring it with a single level fusion. To hold the hook in place until the bone block fuses, a #1 prolene suture is wrapped around the shank of the hook and underneath the posterior spinous process at that level. Next, the size of hybrid lumbar extension rib sleeve needed is determined by measuring from the bottom of the rib of attachment encircled by the superior rib cradle down to the endplate of T12. This can usually be estimated by palpating the 12th rib clinically. The distance in centimeters should correspond to the number inscribed on the rib sleeve and the hybrid lumbar extension. The hybrid device is assembled and locked with a distraction lock. To estimate the proper length, the device is then placed into the field with the rib sleeve engaged into the implanted superior cradle proximally and the spinal rod marked by a skin marker approximately 1.5 cm below the bottom of the spinal hook. The hybrid is removed from the field and the rod cut smoothly by a rod cutter. Avoid using a bolt cutter because the resulting sharp edges may cut through the overlying soft tissues. The end of the rod is bent into slight lordosis and valgus by a French bender so that the rod will line up with the axis of the spine after implantation and conform to the lordosis of the lumbar spine.

Next a subfascial canal is created for safe passage of the sized lumbar hybrid extension. A long Kelley clamp is threaded from the proximal incision, through the paraspinal muscles, into the distal incision, with care taken not to violate the chest wall and the pericardium. A #20 chest tube is then attached to the clamp, and the tube pulled upward into the proximal incision. The end of the rod of the hybrid is then placed into the chest tube, and the device carefully guided through the muscle by the chest tube into the distal incision. The tube is removed, and the rod threaded into the hook, and then upward into the superior cradle. A distraction lock engages the superior cradle to the rib sleeve.

To perform the initial tensioning of the device, a Synthes C-ring is attached to the rod just above the hook, and a VEPTR distractor used to distract the device from the hook through the C ring. The hook is then tightened. The Synthes rib distractor is then removed from the thoracostomy. If there is adequate distraction from the hybrid device, then the proximal ribs should remain horizontal, and the combined corrected opening wedge thoracostomy and rib defect interval should be maintained. Additional VEPTR devices are then placed at a 3–4 cm intervals anteriorly, much like a "picket fence", to provide expansion for the thorax and stability for the underlying lung (Fig. 37.7a, b). Proximally, these additional devices should be placed well below the neurovascular bundle to avoid compression. To provide extra stability for the chest wall, a segment of distal ribs may be osteotomized apart inferiorly then rotated upward, than tied by nonabsorbable suture to the VEPTRs.

If there is scoliosis extending into the lumbar spine, or if there is considerable pelvic obliquity, then the hybrid can extend down to the iliac crest with attachment by an S-hook. This is termed an "Eiffel Tower" construct because the force vectors from iliac crests to proximal ribs have an inferior upward and central orientation. The S hook attachment to mid iliac crest is termed "iliac crest pedestal" fixation. This construct is also a powerful means to address pelvic obliquity [11] (see Figs. 37.7a, b).

Mal-insertion of the hemidiaphragm, usually attached too far proximally, is treated by circumferential release,

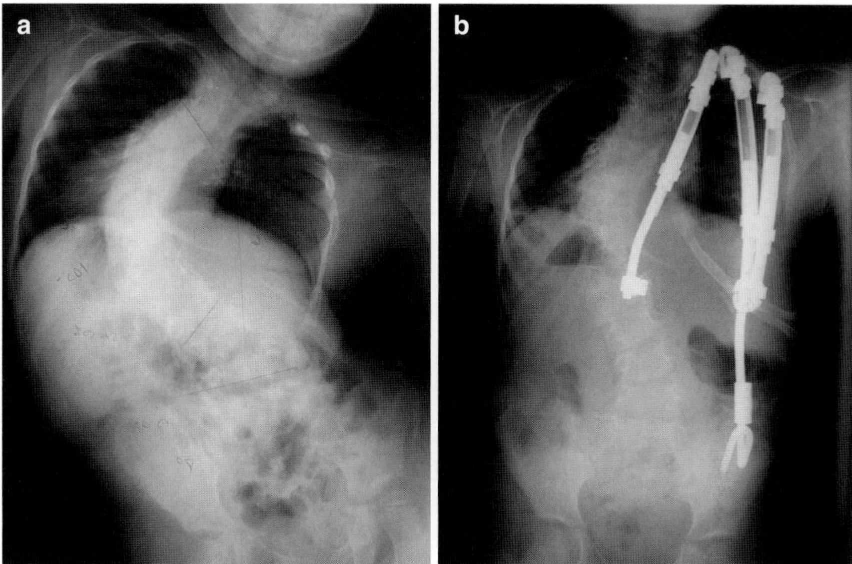

Fig. 37.7 (**a**) Preoperative radiographs of a rib absence patient. (**b**) Postoperative radiographs VEPTR procedure for rib absence

with transposition distally to the most inferior circumference of the reconstructed thorax to provide both additional volume and also a better biomechanical dome shape.

37.7.2 Type II Volume Depletion Deformity: Fused Ribs and Scoliosis

The VEPTR expansion thoracoplasty for this volume depletion deformity is an opening wedge thoracostomy [3, 5, 7]. The approach is very similar to that for absent ribs, but the volume depletion deformity of fused ribs commonly requires a transverse osteotomy at the apex of the constricted hemithorax from the transverse processes of the spine to the rib costochonral junction. A superior cradle anchor for the VEPTR device is first placed in an appropriate stable rib in the proximal segment of the constricted hemithorax, just lateral to the tip of the transverse process. The most proximal placement possible is the second rib; more proximal rib cradle location endangers the brachial plexus. Two ribs may be encircled by the cradle for enhanced stability. The opening wedge thoracostomy is then performed. If there is a large bone plate of fused ribs, the section is cut apart transversely from anterior to posterior by a Kerrisan ronguer. A number four Penfield elevator is threaded underneath the line of bone resection to protect the lung. Sometimes an adjacent line of fibrosis between ribs just above or below the middle of the bone plate is identified and this can also be used as the cleavage point for the opening wedge thoracostomy. If there is solid bone extending medially from the tip of the transverse process down to the spine at the posterior point of the thoracostomy, then it is resected with ronguer under direct vision, carefully pulling free the final fragment of bone away from the spine with a curved curette to avoid canal violation.

AO bone spreaders are then inserted into the thoracostomy interval and used to widen it, and then the Synthes rib spreaders are next inserted to hold the hemithorax out to corrected length. The pleura are carefully stripped proximally and distally by a Kidner, often with only minimal tearing. When the proximal fused ribs are oriented in the horizontal orientation, then correction is felt to be adequate. Next, a rib-to-rib device is inserted in a younger patient, or, in an older patient, a hybrid device is placed down to lumbar spine [5]. Detailed operative technique is available in prior reports [5, 7]. An additional rib-to-rib device may be added in the posterior axillary line, parallel to the more medial device, to share load and provide stability to the area of opening wedge thoracostomy (Fig. 37.8a, b). If there is flail chest present after the thoracostomy, then it is possible to perform a centralization transport of inferior fused ribs by osteotomizing them from the lower segment of the chest, and then displacing them upwards into the defect to increase stability of the

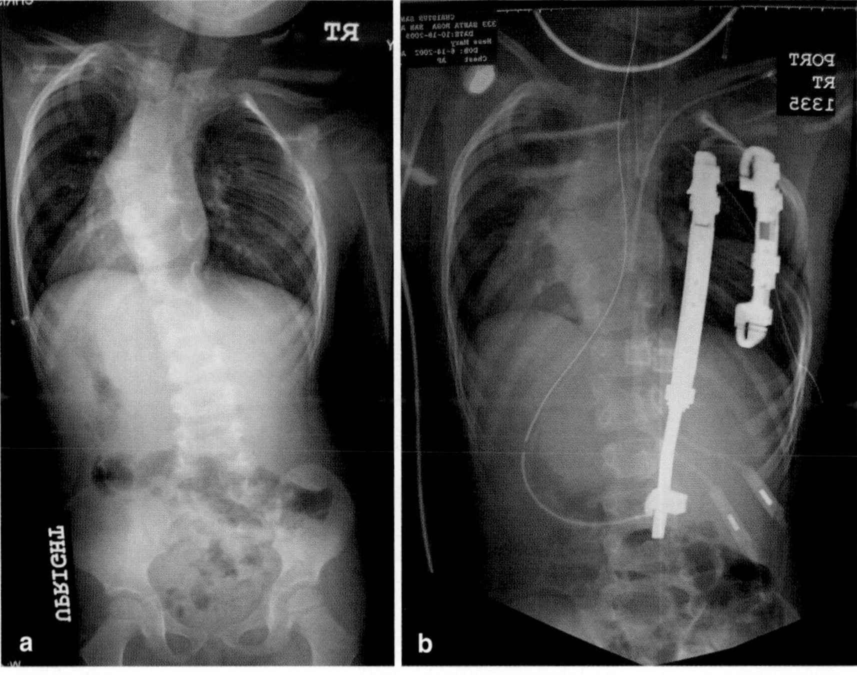

Fig. 37.8 (**a**) Preoperative radiographs of a rib fusion and congenital scoliosis patient. (**b**) Postoperative radiographs of a rib fusion VEPTR procedure

construct, attaching them by non absorbable suture to the device. Closure is in the usual fashion.

Results of 27 children treated with this volume depletion deformity by VEPTR opening wedge thoracoplasty, with average of 5.7 year follow up, noted average correction of 25°, with space available for lung increasing from 63 to 80% at follow up [3] with evidence of growth in length of the unilateral and unsegmented bars on the concave side of rigid congenital curves [1]. The most common complications noted were asymptomatic migration of the hybrid devices superiorly through the ribs of attachment at an average follow-up of 3 years, requiring reinsertion into either a reformed rib or a rib more proximal or distal. Infection rate was 1.9% per procedure, skin slough was present in 15% of patients and were treated by debridement and local flap rotation. Two patients, early in the series, had brachial plexopathy, which is treated by repositioning of devices and one patient had acute respiratory distress syndrome. One patient died of post operative pneumonia. Those patients operated on under age 2 years, when lung growth by alveolar cell multiplication is most rapid, had an average vital capacity of 58% normal at last follow up; those patients older than age 2 years at time of surgery had average 44% vital capacity percent normal, while three patients with history of spinal fusion early in life had a vital capacity of 36% predicted at time of follow up [3]. VEPTR treatment of congenital scoliosis and fused ribs also improves trunkal decompensation, head shift, and neck tilt [8].

37.7.3 Type II Volume Depletion Deformity: Myelomeningocele

One difference between VDD VEPTR treatment for fused ribs and scoliosis and myelomeningocele patients is the absence of posterior elements for hybrid VEPTR attachment in the myelomeningocele patients, as well as the presence of poor skin centrally from the myelomeningocele closure compromising central exposure. The former can be addressed by attachment of the hybrid VEPTR to the iliac crest, bypassing the deficit in posterior elements, and the latter by slightly skewing the incision laterally to avoid the poor skin.

Patients with myelomeningocele needing VEPTR treatment generally have progressive congenital scoliosis with fused ribs of the concave hemithorax, causing *primary* thoracic insufficiency syndrome, but these children also may have *secondary* thoracic insufficiency syndrome, when there is significant lumbar kyphosis placing the torso too close to the pelvis, blocking effective diaphragmatic excursion. Another cause of secondary thoracic insufficiency syndrome is thoraco-lumbar scoliosis,

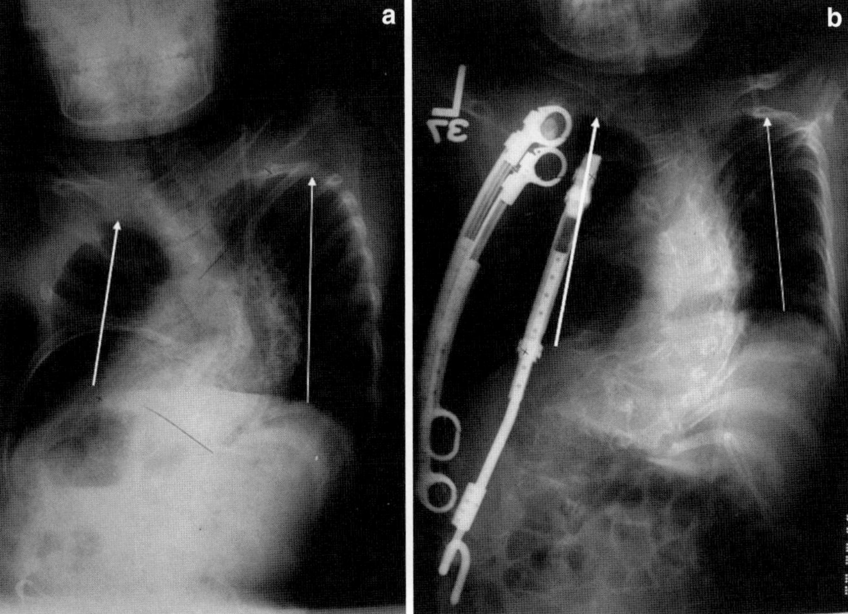

Fig. 37.9 (**a**) Myelomeningocele. (**b**) Postoperative VEPTR treatment of myelomeningocele

which causes the concave side iliac crest to intrude into the chest with blockage of unilateral diaphragmatic excursion. Both concerns require VEPTR treatment to reverse the proximity problem of the diaphragm to the pelvis. Secondary thoracic insufficiency syndrome in myelomeningocele from flexible lumbar kyphosis can be addressed by bilateral VEPTRs extending from the proximal ribs to the iliac crests, an "Eiffel Tower construct".

In a study of ten patients with myelomeningocele, treated by VEPTR with an average of 5.75 years follow-up, the average scoliosis was 73°, and, at follow-up after VEPTR treatment, was an average of 46°. Six of these patients had flexible lumbar kyphosis, averaging 43°, with a positive marionette sign, indicating secondary thoracic insufficiency, but, with VEPTR treatment, the decrease of lumbar kyphosis was an average of 26° with resolution of their marionette signs [11]. The SAL improved from 66 to 83% at follow-up, and the thoracic spine height increased 5.8 mm/year (Fig. 37.9a, b).

37.7.4 Type IIIb/ II Volume Depletion Deformity: Early Onset Scoliosis

VEPTR opening wedge thoracostomy, used to treat extensive thoracic congenital scoliosis and fused ribs of the concave hemithorax, can also address early onset scoliosis with a similar opening wedge thoracostomy approach, using intercostal muscle lysis rather than transverse rib osteotomy of the concave hemi-thorax. The type IIb volume depletion deformity is from the transverse constriction of the chest due to the wind swept deformity from spine rotation into the convex hemithorax. The type II VDDD hemithorax constriction is identified by the area of multiple persistent intercostal space narrowing of the concave hemithorax in the AP bending films. The apex of the curve is often distal to this area of rib cage constriction. The superior distraction point, where the superior cradle is attached, should be at the proximal end of the curve. Care must be taken to not place it in the compensatory curve above the structural curve since the distraction force will just increase the compensatory curve without correction of the true curve. The soft tissue approach is identical to that for fused ribs and congenital scoliosis.

The superior cradle is placed in the usual fashion. Once the area of intercostal muscle narrowing is identified, then the central narrow interval is released by cautery, with a right angle clamp under the muscle to protect the underlying pleura. The pleura is mobilized by a Kidner, two to three ribs above and below the interval. Another opening wedge thoracostomy can be made two ribs above or below the initial release, if the area of constriction is widespread. The ribs are distracted apart by the Synthes rib spreader to lengthen the constricted

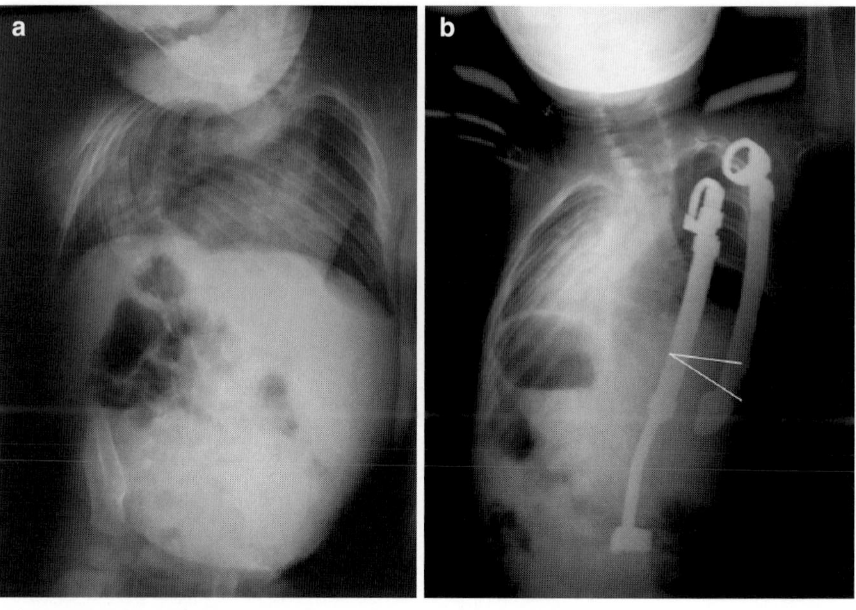

Fig. 37.10 (**a**) Early onset scoliosis. (**b**) Postoperative VEPTR treatment of early onset scoliosis

hemithorax. An unilateral rib to spine VEPTR hybrid is then placed. A second rib-to-rib VEPTR device is often added to load share (Fig. 37.10a, b). Other constructs that can be used are bilateral rib to spine VEPTR hybrids, a unilateral rib to pelvis via Dunn-McCarthy hook VEPTR hybrids, or bilateral rib to pelvis via Dunn-McCarthy hook VEPTR hybrids.

VEPTR expansion thoracoplasty treatment of early onset scoliosis remains controversial. Some argue that the presence of a VEPTR on the chest wall will eventually stiffen the chest, adversely affecting respiration, but since the chest wall is already irreversibly stiff preoperatively, it seems unlikely that the VEPTR will affect chest wall stiffness one way or the other. It is assumed that growing rods do not stiffen the chest wall because of their central placement, but often the rods extend over the ribs on the concave side of the curve.

The ideal nonfusion surgical system to treat early onset scoliosis currently does not exist. VEPTR surgery does increase the size of the constricted thorax, so that the diaphragm can take advantage of the increased lung volume, but no known treatment, including VEPTR, can restore active motion to a chest wall stiffened by the distortion of spine deformity. This component of TIS will have to be addressed by future forms of instrumentation and most likely will need to be corrected early when the chest wall distortion is mild and the biomechanical deficit reversible. In addition, an accurate, standardized laboratory means of measuring unilateral chest wall excursion is needed to assess chest wall stiffness in spinal deformity and to define the effect of surgical treatment on active chest wall expansion.

37.7.5 Type IIIa Volume Depletion Deformity: Jarcho-Levin Syndrome

This bilateral hemithorax constriction is treated with bilateral opening wedge thoracostomies in a staged fashion [6]. For Jarcho-Levin Syndrome due to spondylocostal dysostosis, the technique is very similar to that for the Type II volume depletion deformity of fused ribs and congenital scoliosis. The concave hemithorax is addressed first with opening wedge thoracostomy, then the other side is expanded 3–4 months later if there is significant longitudinal constriction. For patients with Jarcho-Levin Syndrome due to spondylothoracic dysplasia with minimal, if any, scoliosis and crab-shaped fused chest wall, staged opening wedge thoracostomies are performed, through a "V" shaped osteotomy of the densely fused hemithorax with the apex adjacent to the tip of the transverse process in the mid portion of the spine (Fig. 37.11a, b). A VEPTR is placed 2–3 cm lateral to the transverse process of the spine to provide maximum expansion of the hemithorax. The same procedure is performed on the contralateral side approximately 3 months after the first surgery (see Fig. 37.11b).

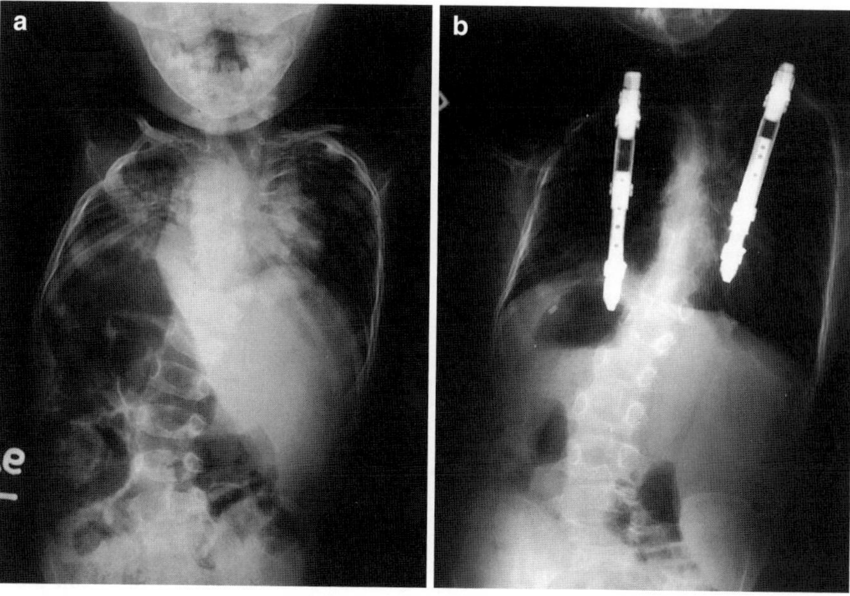

Fig. 37.11 (**a**) Jarcho-Levin Syndrome. (**b**) Treatment of Jarcho-Levin by bilateral VEPTRs after wedge osteotomies of the fused chest wall

37.8 Minimizing Complications

37.8.1 Overall Complication Rates

Campbell and Smith [9] reported complications of 1412 procedures in 201 patients between 1989 and 2004.

VEPTR surgeries have the tendency for complications inherent to all repetitive surgery approaches, with growing rod technique being the most equivalent (Table 37.2). Each surgical incision, whether for the primary implantation, expansion, or replacement of a VEPTR, is a new opportunity for skin slough, infection, or other operative complication. The long duration of VEPTR treatment also increases risk of migration of devices. The most common VEPTR complication is an asymptomatic upward migration of the superior cradle of the device into the rib of attachment over time. It is not due to breakage of the rib or erosion, but rather a remodeling process of the rib reacting from the stress of the distraction forces of the device. Within a few months of implantation, the rib of attachment begins to thicken, extending bone beneath the rib cradle, strengthening the interface between the device and the rib. As the years go by, the device appears to gradually "move" upward to lie centrally in the middle of the thickened rib. This is probably due to remodeling of the rib from constant upward pressure of the rib cradle, much like the way braces induce gradual movement of teeth through the bone of the jaw over time. Eventually, the device begins to emerge through the upper edge of the rib, and may completely dislodge, but often either clinical prominence or radiograph appearance will identify the problem early, and allow reattachment during a scheduled VEPTR expansion surgery. Even if there is complete dislodgement, there are often minimal symptoms, because the device is covered by the thick muscle of the trapezius. As a rule, the longer a patient has an implanted device, the higher the likelihood of migration. To factor in the time component of VEPTR migration, a migration index, representing the risk per year of complete migration per patient, was derived which is based on the number of complete migrations per patient divided by years since implantation.

Infection in VEPTR patients is often associated with skin slough. Many of these patients have comorbidities, such as myelomeningocele or syndromes, that probably make them prone to surgical infection. VEPTR breakage is rare, with most incidents occurring with earlier design devices.

37.8.2 VEPTR Device Complications

VEPTR patients have complex, rare spine and chest wall deformities, with a significant incidence of spinal cord abnormalities, and a high rate of neurological injury should be expected from the large corrections in spinal deformity from VEPTR techniques, but neurological injury from VEPTR surgery is rare, usually transient, and, unlike spinal surgery, is unique in that upper extremities are more involved than the lower

Table 37.2 Complications of VEPTR and two reported single growing rod series

	San Antonio [9]	Klemme et al. [17]	Tello [22]
(proc/pt)	201 pts (7.02)	67 pts (6.1)	44 pts (3.4)
f/u	6 years	3.1 years	4.75 years
• Infect rate/ proc	3.3%	1.5%	5.3%
• Skin slough	8.5%	4.5%	13.6%
• Migration	0.09 mig/year	0.1 mig/year	0.029 mig/year
– % pts	27%	31%	14%
– Time	3.2 years	?	?
• Device breakage	6%	18%	27%

extremities. Upper brachial plexopathy has been seen in five early San Antonio VEPTR patients, all resolving spontaneously except one patient who has small residual dyesthesias. The probable basis for brachioplexopathy in VEPTR patients is the compression of the brachial plexus by expansion thoracoplasty elevation of malformed, fused ribs, documented in one patient on MRI [8]. Improved monitoring of procedures has decreased the incidence of this complication.

There have been three lower extremity neurological injuries in our experience. One was a monoplegia after a dural tear from a spinal canal violation with a ronguer. This almost completely resolved a year after surgery. Another was a delayed paraplegia in a patient with sharp, angular congenital kyphosis. There was normal SSEP's and wake-up test during surgery, but delayed paraplegia was evident when the patient awoke from respiratory support sedation several days post implantation. Removal of the device did not improve neurological status and the paraplegia is permanent. The third "injury" was a poorly communicative patient with a VP shunt who presented several days post VEPTR expansion procedure with refusal to walk. Neurological examination was equivocal. Shunt malfunction was present, and during revision the VEPTR was shortened. The patient began to walk again post op, but it is unclear whether the shunt malfunction or VEPTR surgery was the basis for the change in ambulatory status.

In summary, most VEPTR complications are treatable, and the frequency can be tolerated in view of the probable long term pulmonary benefit.

37.8.3 Prevention of Complications

To prevent neurological injury during VEPTR implantation, the preoperative CT scan should be checked carefully for areas of dysraphic spine within the area of approach. In these areas, dissection should be cautious, with medial exposure only above and below the areas of dysraphism. Particularly dangerous is an area of mid-thoracic spine dysraphism where the medial edge of the scapula lies within the spinal canal on the concave side of the curve. The usual thoracotomy approach in this anatomic variant, cutting through the rhomboid muscles with cautery, would result in direct spinal cord injury. To avoid this, the scapula should be retracted posteriorly with a rake to pull it out of the spinal canal, and the rhomboid muscles sectioned directly off the bone of the scapula, away from the area of dysraphism. There is also risk of lumbar spine dysraphism of the posterior spinal elements in patients with extensive congenital scoliosis. Use a large Cobb elevator in stripping the paraspinal muscles to minimize the risk of violating the canal during exposure.

To avoid premature device migration, use an extraperiosteal soft tissue sparing technique when performing cradle insertion or opening wedge thoracostomies, avoiding the stripping of rib periosteum, because of the subsequent risk of devascularization. To avoid distal migration of a rib-to-rib device, be sure the device is well aligned to the osseous ribs of attachment. Usually the standard superior rib cradle and the inferior rib cradle of the rib-to-rib VEPTR are in neutral position, but if the inferior osseous rib of attachment is oriented differently from the superior rib, then the VEPTR may not fit well around the inferior rib. A 30° angled right handed or left handed inferior VEPTR cradle may be used to better fit the inferior cradle around the rib in such a situation.

In placement of lumbar hooks, it is important not to violate the cortex of the lamina of attachment because this weakens its ability to withstand the distraction forces. If the interspace is too small for the hook, then a superior laminotomy of the inter-space is performed. It is important to place the hybrid lumbar extension in the lumbar spine below any areas of junctional kyphosis seen on the lateral weight bearing radiograph. The VEPTR hook should be placed at least two levels below any junctional kyphosis to prevent accentuating the kyphosis.

37.8.4 Treatment of Complications

Superior migration of a rib cradle is treated by accessing the cradle, usually at time of expansion surgery, through a limited incision of the proximal portion of the thoracotomy incision, and reimplanting it into the rib of attachment which is usually reformed, or a more distal rib. Curved curettes are extremely useful for shaving the hypertrophied rib down to acceptable size for reimplantation of the rib cradle. Inferior cradle migration is treated in a similar fashion.

For infection, debridement without removal of devices is generally performed and with irrigation by a dilute betadine solution. The skin edges are then loosely approximated with Prolene sutures, leaving a 5 mm gap in the wound, allowing it to close by secondary intention. The patient is maintained on 4–6 weeks of IV antibiotics with culture results determining the specific antibiotic. Sometimes it is helpful to add a wound Vac® overlying the device to help it with healing.

Recurrent infections require removal of the rib sleeve and the lumbar hybrid extension or the inferior rib cradle, and the patient is maintained on 6 weeks of antibiotics. When sedimentation rate/C-reactive protein has normalized, and the wound is healed, then reinsertion of the device can be considered.

Skin slough is treated by debridement and mobilization of flaps. Primary closure is possible, but loose approximation with proline suture is preferred. In patients with long standing VEPTR devices, dense soft tissue scarring sometimes occurs over devices and recurrent skin slough becomes a problem. For these patients soft tissue expanders are placed laterally to mobilize skin, the scar resected, and then the new skin is transferred posteriorly over the devices with the assistance of a plastic surgeon.

Acknowledgment This chapter is to acknowledge Dr. Melvin D. Smith (1941–2008), a tireless contributor to the understanding and treatment of thoracic insufficiency syndrome.

References

1. Campbell RM, Hell-Vocke AK (2003) Growth of the thoracic spine in congenital scoliosis after expansion thoracoplasty, J Bone Joint Surg Am 85:409–420
2. Campbell RM, Smith MD (2003) Reconstruction of the thorax in patients with absent ribs and flail chest physiology using vertical expandable prosthetic titanium ribs (VEPTR). Poster Presentation, American Association of Pediatric Surgeons Annual Meeting
3. Campbell RM Jr, Smith MD, Mayes TC et al (2003) The effect of opening wedge thoracostomy on thoracic insufficiency syndrome associated with fused ribs and congenital scoliosis. J Bone Joint Surg Am 85-A:1615–1624
4. Campbell RM Jr, Smith MD, Mayes TC et al (2003) The characteristics of thoracic insufficiency syndrome associated with fused ribs and scoliosis. J Bone Joint Surg Am 85-A:399–408
5. Campbell RM Jr, Smith MD, Hell-Vocke AK (2004) Expansion thoracoplasty: the surgical technique of opening-wedge thoracostomy. Surgical technique. J Bone Joint Surg Am 86(Suppl 1):51–64
6. Campbell RM, Smith MD, Taichi et al (2004) The treatment of thoracic insufficiency syndrome associated with spondylocostal dysotosis and spodylothoracic dyplasia. Presented at the Scoliosis Research Society Meeting, Buenos Aires
7. Campbell RM (2005) Operative strategies for thoracic insufficiency syndrome by vertical expandable prosthetic titanium rib expansion thoracoplasty. Operative Tech Orthopaed 15:315–325
8. Campbell RM, Adcox B, Smith MD et al (2007) The Effect of mid-thoracic VEPTR opening wedge thoracostomy on cervical -thoracic congenital scoliosis. Spine 32:2171–2177
9. Campbell RM Jr, Smith MD (2007) Thoracic insufficiency syndrome and exotic scoliosis. J Bone Joint Surg 89-A(Suppl 1):108–122
10. Campbell RM Jr, Aubrey A, Smith MD et al (2008) The characterization of the thoracic biomechanics of respiration in thoracic insufficiency syndrome by dynamic lung MRI: a preliminary report. Presented at the International Congress of Early Onset Scoliosis, Montreal, Canada
11. Campbell RM, Smith MD, Simmons III JW et al (2008) The treatment of secondary thoracic insufficiency syndrome of myelominingocele by a hybrid VEPTR "Eiffel Tower" construct with S-Hook Iliac Crest pedestal fixation. Presented at IMAST, 2007, Bahamas, and Poster Exhibit. AAOS, San Francisco
12. DiMeglio A, Bonnel F (1990) Le rachis en croissance. Springer, Paris
13. Donnelley LF, Emery KH, Brody AS et al (2001) Minimizing radiation dose for pediatric body applications of single-detector helical CT: strategies at a large children's hospital. AJR Am J Roentgenol 176:303–306
14. Gollogly S, Smith JT, Campbell RM (2004) Determining lung volume with three dimensional reconstructions of CT scan data: a pilot study to evaluate the effects of expansion thoracoplasty on children with severe spinal deformities. J Pediatr Orthop 24(3):323–328
15. Gollogly S, Smith JT, White SK et al (2004) The volume of lung parenchyma as a function of age: a review of 1050 normal CT scans of the chest with three-dimensional volumetric reconstruction of the pulmonary system. Spine 29(18): 2061–2066
16. Hoekelman RA (1987) In: Hoelkelman RA, Blatman S, Friedman SB, Nelson NM, Seidel HM (eds). Primary pediatric care. Mosby. St. Louis
17. Klemme W, Denis D, Winter R et al (1997) Spinal Instrumentation without Fusion. J Pediatr Orthop 17: 734–742
18. Openshaw P, Edwards S, Helms P (1984) Changes in rib cage geometry during childhood. Thorax 39:624–627

19. Paterson A, Frush DP, Donnelly LF (2001) Helical CT of the body: are setting adjusted for pediatric patients? AJR Am Roentgenol 176:297–301
20. Smith MD, Campbell Jr (2006) RM Use of a bioabsorbable patch for reconstruction of large thoracic cage defects in growing children. J Pediatr Surg 41:46–49
21. Smith's Hereditary Malformations (1988) Jones KL (ed) W.B Saunders, Philadelphia, pp 694
22. Tello J (1994) Subcutaneous rods and scoliosis. Ortho Clin N Am 167:87–95

Revision Spine Surgery in the Growing Child

38

Oheneba Boachie-Adjei and Matthew E. Cunningham

Key Points

- Revision spine surgery in the growing child occurs infrequently, other than when performed for predetermined controlled growth of the spine.
- Revision surgery poses a significant technical challenge, which requires a comprehensive and multidisciplinary team approach.
- Surgeon must have a complete understanding of the primary deformity and reason for index surgery failure, of how this affects the revision surgery plan, and must comprehend the residual growth potential of the spine.
- The treating surgeon must be familiar with the various surgical techniques to achieve optimal balance correction while allowing maximum growth, preserving motion segments and reducing complications.

38.1 Overview

The need for spinal surgery in pediatric patients is uncommon and estimated at approximately 1–10/100,000 of all children, with surgical indications ranging from intra- or extra-dural neoplasms requiring laminectomies and excision, to spinal deformity requiring correction and stabilization in adolescent idiopathic scoliosis [9, 30, 44, 51]. Intermediate and long term (greater than 5 years) rates of problems following index procedures are reported to be as high as 25–50% [19, 29, 38], while results at shorter follow-up have much lower rates of issues such as junctional degeneration, junctional kyphosis, and instrumentation failure. Problems leading to repeat surgery for adolescent idiopathic scoliosis patients over a 15 year period have been reported from two institutions, and show that 4.6–12.9% of patients had one or more surgeries after their index procedure, most commonly for infection, symptomatic implants and pseudarthrosis [22, 40]. This estimate is considerably lower than the reported 26–46% rate of junctional kyphosis [19, 20, 22], and higher than the 1.3–1.5% rate of pseudarthrosis reported for the group [3, 22], indicating that decision for surgical revision is made on a case by case basis. Owing to good short term surgical results, requirement for revision spine surgery while children are still in their growing phase is uncommon, if interval surgeries for "growing rod" lengthenings are not considered.

Patient diagnoses at the time of index spinal surgery include congenital deformity, neuromuscular conditions (e.g., cerebral palsy or muscular dystrophy), connective tissue disorders (e.g., Marfan's syndrome or Ehlers Danlos), idiopathic deformity, Scheuermann's kyphosis, and neoplastic etiologies requiring laminectomy for intradural excisions (e.g., neuroblastoma, astrocytoma or meningioma). The available English language literature does not definitively detail the relative rates of surgical intervention for these diagnoses, nor are there large studies for each of the diagnoses with sufficient follow-up to document the relative rates for required revision surgery. Smaller studies have reported rates for postsurgical problems and revisions for many of the common deformity diagnoses. In a series of 17 patients treated for Scheuermann's kyphosis with posterior

O. Boachie-Adjei (✉)
The Scoliosis Service, Hospital for Special Surgery, New York, NY 10021, USA
e-mail: boachie@hss.edu

B. A. Akbarnia et al. (eds.), *The Growing Spine*,
DOI: 10.1007/978-3-540-85207-0_38, © Springer-Verlag Berlin Heidelberg 2011

fusion with multiple posterior element osteotomies, one case of each proximal and distal junctional kyphosis were reported that did not require revision surgery at minimum of 2 year follow-up [15]. Two similar studies of Scheuermann's patients (n = 23 and 39) reported instrumentation problems requiring revision in 10–13% of patients [26, 27]. Children with congenital spinal deformities had requirement for repeat surgery in 6.3–33% of cases [17, 34, 35, 42, 47], with rates of pseudarthrosis [17, 34] and instrumentation problems [17, 42] that were approximately 10%. Revision rates for skeletally immature patients with cerebral palsy range from 5.8 to 18%, with indications including crankshaft phenomenon, deformity progression, and instrumentation problems [11, 13]. Perhaps the highest rates of surgical revision are in the myelomeningocele population where revisions for deformity progression average 10%, but wound problems requiring removal of instrumentation range from 10 to 75% [28, 37]. Overall, independent of diagnosis, pediatric spine deformity revision rates occur at about 10% of the index case rates.

This chapter summarizes the approach to revision spine surgery in the growing child, and reviews the senior author's experience in this regard for the 5-year period from 1995 to 2000. Clinical presentation prior to revision, required patient evaluation, revision surgery goals and indications, and a brief overview of revision surgery techniques are reviewed. We also describe illustrative cases for pediatric spine revision surgery.

38.2 Clinical Presentation, Evaluation and Diagnosis

Children in need of revision spine surgery present with a limited number of symptoms. Namely, these presentations are for pain, obvious deformity progression, and loss of clinical function [11, 13, 22, 40, 45]. Pain can be the result of pseudarthrosis with or without consequent implant fatigue failure, prominent implants either as sub-optimally placed at the index procedure or after dislodgement [13, 17, 40, 46], or due to muscle fatigue in the setting of pain or decompensation after index procedures. Deformity progression can be in the setting of very young patients fused from posterior only approach that have anterior element overgrowth and crankshaft phenomenon [41, 43], patients who have "adding on" of levels proximally or distally after being fused over too short of a spinal segment [49, 50], or those patients who have degeneration above or below a fusion that leads to instability and junctional kyphosis or complex junctional deformity [20, 29, 32, 38, 45]. Functional losses, such as loss of walking tolerance in the setting of junctional stenosis below a fusion, may not only be easily articulated by the patient but also be more subtle as in the requirement for increased oxygen by nasal cannula in a patient who already has cardiopulmonary compromise in the setting of slowly progressive spinal deformity.

The evaluation should begin with a thorough history and physical examination, with emphasis placed on defining the timing and character of symptoms. While conducting the history with young patients, be attentive to subtle information that is available in the examination room. For example, in the young or non-verbal child, observation of the patient in undisturbed activity or while they interact with their parent may demonstrate valuable information about asymmetry in extremity movements, gait or balance problems, and behaviors that indicate the location of the problem (rubbing the skin over a painful implant, or demonstrating dyspnea or tachypnea due to compromised pulmonary status). Obtain as detailed an account of the index procedure as possible, including preoperative radiographs, operative notes, and a thorough description of the postoperative course, along with serial radiographs. This information will document and quantify deformity progression if present, and will demonstrate the chronology and potential associations of pertinent radiographic findings to the symptoms reported. A detailed account of what happened to the patient prior to presentation for revision will provide the physician with the best means to diagnose why the index procedure failed and what revision surgery can be offered to remedy the clinical situation.

Symptoms that occur acutely, either in the first few weeks after the index procedure or abruptly after a long symptom free interval from the index surgery, suggest implant related problems [11, 40]. Point tenderness over a prominent portion of the instrumentation may suggest irritation of superficial soft tissue. Radiographs will help to define the implant responsible, and examining serial radiographs from the index procedure and up to presentation will help define if this is a newly dislodged instrumentation, or a new inflammatory process in the overlying skin of chronically prominent implants. An injection of local anesthetic and a corticosteroid can be considered for further diagnosis and potential therapeutic intervention, but will likely be poorly tolerated in younger patients. Definitive management involves implant removal, but this should be delayed until definitive fusion is confirmed, unless overlying skin is tented and threatens breakdown. Patients and their families should be warned that deformity may progress after removal of instrumentation [39]. A febrile patient, or a patient with a diffusely tender wound, with or without signs of local infection, should be considered to have a deep wound infection and must be evaluated accordingly [16]. Complete blood count with differential, and serology for inflammatory markers such as erythrocyte sedimentation rate and C-reactive protein should be obtained in addition to radiographs of the instrumented segment in two planes to evaluate lucency around the implants that often is associated with infected instrumentation. If the white blood cell count and inflammatory markers are not sufficiently supportive of the diagnosis of infection, peripheral blood cultures can be obtained, the instrumentation can be cultured by image-guided or open biopsy, or a gallium scan can be obtained to support a diagnosis of deep infection of the implants [1, 18, 31]. If infection is diagnosed in the setting of an unfused spine or immature fusion, irrigation and debridement will be needed followed by suppressive antibiotics; maturely fused spines with deep infections involving the instrumentation require implant removal, and proper management with surgical and chemotherapeutic modalities to clear the infection. Consultation with a pediatric infectious disease specialist is recommended.

Pain symptoms with a more gradual onset, or those that have a gradual onset that acutely worsen, could represent pseudarthrosis. On examination, the patient may have increased and painful motion through the region of the fusion, and tenderness to palpation in specific locations of the spine. Pain symptoms may be the result of inflammation and painful motion at the site of a single or multiple pseudarthroses, or may be associated with the instrumentation (increased strain at a nearby bone-instrumentation interface or fractured implants). Radiographs should be obtained in orthogonal planes to assess the entire length of the instrumented fusion, with coned down and oblique views obtained in areas where there is suspicion for non-healing of the fusion [4, 23, 24]. If radiographs do not demonstrate lucencies in the fusion mass or broken implants, then computerized tomography (CT) of the fusion or bone scan should be considered. Another etiology for gradual onset of lower back pain complaints is muscular deconditioning of the lumbar extensors. This is suggested on physical examination by tenderness within and spasm of the paraspinals below the fusion segment, and tenderness symptoms elicited with patients returning from a bent-forward position. It is an uncommon finding in children, due to their expected high activity levels, but typically is found in conjunction with other pain generators that limit general activity levels and predispose to muscular deconditioning. Addressing the primary pain generator, and restoring general activity typically leads to spontaneous strengthening and conditioning of the musculature, and resolution of symptoms.

Apart from pain, a common presentation for revision deformity surgery evaluation is continued deformity progression [11, 40]. This may take the from of shoulder asymmetry, enlarging thoracic rib hump or lumbar prominence, decompensation in the coronal or sagittal plane, or diagnosis based on follow-up radiographs from the index procedure without clinical complaints. Perhaps the most feared complication in spinal surgery of the growing child is that of crankshaft phenomenon. This is typically seen in skeletally immature children who are fused at a very early age (possibly with open triradiate cartilages, and Risser 0 or 1) by a posterior approach alone [41, 43]. Continued growth of the vertebral bodies within the length of the posterior fusion leads to progressive deformity, which is typically seen in the coronal and axial planes due to residual scoliosis after the index procedure. Deformity progression can be recognized as progression of Cobb measurement by 10° or more within the length of the index fusion as assessed through serial radiographs, or by progressive clinical rotational deformity documented by photographs or quantified by increasing angle of trunk rotation measured by scoliometer. Loss of shoulder, coronal or sagittal balance may be indicative of crankshaft phenomenon, but these are also encountered when post-operative deformity is due to "adding on" of segments outside of the index fusion, and with degeneration of segments flanking the index fusion. Treatment of crankshaft phenomenon typically requires anterior spinal fusion (epiphysiodesis) to arrest the anterior spinal growth driving the deformity progression, along with posterior osteotomies and revision fusion to correct and stabilize the spine.

"Adding on" of segments proximal or distal to a fusion typically occurs in the setting of an index fusion that was not sufficiently long to correct and control the spinal deformity present [49, 50]. Deformity left untreated by the index procedure then progresses in the expected manner, worsening in until the completion of skeletal growth. The diagnosis is suspected when obvious deformity progression is seen by any of a multitude of clinical parameters, and is confirmed with serial radiographs documenting progression of the Cobb measurements. Junctional kyphosis, or more broadly junctional degeneration, is a different pathological process, involving accelerated degeneration and instability at segments proximal or distal to an index fusion [19, 20, 25, 32]. This is a diagnosis that is not commonly encountered in the growing child, but is seen frequently in the older adolescent population and in the young adult population after spinal fusion. Clinical suspicion for junctional kyphosis should be raised when patients have a feeling of "falling forward" of either their head and shoulders or their trunk. Failure of the degenerating segment forward in the sagittal plane is thought to be more common due to the kyphogenic mechanics of posterior placement of the spine in the body; however, decompensation of the spine can also occur in the coronal plane with loss of balance laterally. Junctional degeneration is evaluated with orthogonal radiographs scrutinized for gross evidence of degeneration (arthrosis, disk height loss) and excessive angulation at the segment in question (Cobb measurement greater than 10°) [20, 32]. Typical management of added on segments or mild junctional degeneration involves extension of the posterior fusion to include the involved segments. For advanced junctional degeneration associated with central or neuroforaminal stenosis at the effected level, decompression and fusion of the level is required.

Functional losses may be the most difficult symptoms for the physician and patient to quantify and identify as symptoms of deformity progression or failure of an index spinal deformity surgery. Complaints may include increasing leg tiredness with walking associated with degeneration and stenosis below an index fusion, or can be as subtle as an increased percent inspired fraction of oxygen (FiO_2) requirement in a young patient with baseline pulmonary compromise that is being worsened by crankshaft phenomenon. Maintaining vigilance to the complaints reported by the patient, and correlating these with observations made on imaging studies will often lead to expedient diagnosis of the pathology. A low threshold should be maintained for obtaining multidisciplinary consultations to further evaluate vague clinical functional losses including pulmonology, cardiology, gastroenterology, and physiatry/physical therapy.

Complete evaluation of the patient requires a thorough history and physical examination characterizing the complaint and its chronology as described earlier, and supplemental testing including imaging, routine laboratory work up, and possibly specialized testing. Orthogonal radiograph views of the entire spine are a requirement, and can be supplemented with oblique views, coned down views of specific areas of concern, and special views (e.g., Fergusen's view of the lumbosacral junction). Stress views may be added to assess for motion within a suspected area of pseudarthorsis, or to assess the flexibility of a segment being evaluated for revision posterior fusion in the setting of "adding on." If further delineation of bony architecture is required, a CT scan of the area of interest is the study of choice. To evaluate the neural canal and foramina outside of the index fusion, magnetic resonance imaging (MRI) is the study of choice, but due to interference of the magnetic field from instrumentation, evaluation of the neural canal within the instrumented segment is best done with a CT-myelogram. Evaluations for spinal infection can include tagged white blood cell scans, but increased sensitivity and specificity are obtained for spine infection with the combination of gallium and bone scans [31]. Routine blood work should be checked, and additional tests should be considered in the setting of very thin patients (pre-albumin, transferrin, and total lymphocyte count), patients with potential metabolic bone problems (vitamin D level , NTX-1, osteocalcin, and bone specific alkaline phosphatase), and if infection is suspected (erythrocyte sedimentation rate, c-reactive protein, and surveillance peripheral blood cultures). If a thoracic fusion is needed, and particularly if entry into the chest is required, pulmonary function testing should be performed, along with obtaining a pediatric pulmonology consultation. Additional pediatric multidisciplinary consultations should also be obtained as indicated.

Ultimate diagnosis for the index surgery failure may be obvious from the initial evaluation, or may be only evident after review of the clinical data including operative notes, serial radiographs, and notes documenting the postoperative clinical course. A critical appraisal of the diagnosis should be completed to be certain that the clinical complaints, testing and other data are explained by the proposed etiology in their entirety. If symptoms or observations are not explained by the diagnosis, then alternate etiologies or combinations of problems should be considered. An example could be a patient with obvious crankshaft phenomenon who is also experiencing significant pain symptoms, or who has a fever, who may have a concurrent pseudarthrosis or deep infection. Suspicion for complete and accurate diagnosis should be maintained to optimize preparedness for the operating room, and to minimize "surprises" that may adversely affect the level of care delivered.

38.3 Goals for Treatment and Surgical Considerations

Goals for revision deformity surgery vary slightly depending upon the specifics of the revision surgery required. All revision surgeries will have the goals of stable reconstructions that lead to solid fusions, physiological coronal and sagittal balance postoperatively, and minimization of risks for curve progression, transfusion, neurological injury, infection, pulmonary problems, and future surgical requirements. In the setting of patients presenting with pain symptoms, an obvious goal is for relief of discomfort; this is predictable in the setting of pseudarthrosis or symptomatic instrumentation, but is less predictable when the pain generator is not obvious, such as in the patient with pain in the setting of "adding on" of deformity below or above an index fusion. Patients and family members should be counseled about the reasonable expectation for achieving postoperative goals in language that they are able to understand, to avoid dissatisfaction with surgical results in the postoperative period.

Surgical considerations are different from case to case, and are dictated by both the nature of the index procedure, and etiology of the surgical failure. Strategies for revision fusions with correction include extension of posterior fusion, revision of index fusion with or without posterior osteotomies, and revision anterior/posterior spinal fusion. Posterior osteotomies through the posterior fusion mass for minor corrections (Smith-Petersen osteotomy) [48], resection of a posterior wedge of bone through all three spinal columns for major corrections (pedicle subtraction osteotomy) [7, 36], and resection of segments of the entire vertebral column from a posterior only approach for debridement and decompression in addition to major deformity correction (posterior vertebral column resection) [5, 33]. Anterior/posterior procedures are indicated for anterior spine growth arrest in the setting of crankshaft phenomenon, when prior anterior fusion was used but residual deformity is not acceptable, and when mobilization of a stiff spine is required for optimal correction [2, 6, 14, 21].

38.3.1 Smith-Petersen Osteotomy

Smith-Petersen osteotomies (SPOs) are performed by completing resections of the posterior fusion mass, sparing the lamina at the level of the transverse processes and pedicles [48]. Revision fixation can then be obtained with hooks, wires or pedicle screws into desired segments. Deformity correction is accomplished through relative translation, derotation and compression/distraction of the vertebrae with reference to one another. Average correction expected from a single SPO is approximately 10°, and is dependent upon the amount of bone resected from the prior fusion and the amount of mobility present in the intervertebral disk at the level being corrected [10]. Patients who have had prior anterior fusion at a particular spinal segment are not candidates for SPOs for deformity correction of that level at revision, but can have SPOs performed proximal or distal to an anterior fusion mass if SPOs will help to level the lowest instrumented vertebra or otherwise provide spinal balance.

38.3.2 Pedicle Substraction Osteotomy

Pedicle subtraction osteotomies (PSOs) are performed through a posterior only approach, and compromise a complete transection of the bony spinal column through the vertebral level chosen [7, 8, 36]. They are designed to remove a wedge of bone that will result in correction of the spine in one or multiple planes after apposition of the osteotomy site [8]. Ideally, the anterior cortex of the vertebral body involved in the osteotomy is left intact, and acts as a hinge for the closing wedge resection. Laminotomies are performed proximally and distally to the osteotomized level, to allow the dura and contents adequate room to reposition after the osteotomy is closed. Rigid fixation during and after the osteotomy is essential to prevent spinal translation and neural injury. The osteotomy gets its name from the typical planes that are used in the bony posterior resection wedge, just above and below the level of the pedicles, which results in resection of the pedicles. Single level PSOs result in corrections of approximately 30°, but can be modified to provide more or less correction by the size of the posterior wedge of bone removed [10]. Ultimate limitation of correction is limited by the posterior height of the vertebral body, and the desire to preserve the disk integrity above and below the osteotomized level. Corrections in sagittal, coronal or complex planes can be accomplished through asymmetric bone removal from side to side, effectively rotating the closing wedge from the anteroposterior plane toward one side or the other. PSOs are three column osteotomies, with posterior or posterolateral shortening, and therefore do not depend upon the mobility of the intervertebral disks for the correction obtained.

38.3.3 Vertebral Column Resection

Posterior vertebral column resection (VCR) is similar to the pedicle subtraction osteotomy in that there is a complete resection of the spinal column, but differs in the exposure required, and extent of bone resected [5, 33]. The concept of VCR is to complete a total vertebrectomy through a costotransversectomy approach (for the thoracic spine), allowing deformity correction and anterior decompression or debridement of the level(s) resected. It requires rigid fixation of the vertebral column during the resection and afterward, and the anterior spine requires reconstitution with a titanium mesh cage, or the equivalent, packed with bone graft [5, 12]. VCR is a very powerful technique for focal correction of deformity, and renders the spine reducible in coronal, sagittal and axial planes.

Appropriate clinical use of these techniques requires the surgeon to critically assess the revision surgical problem, and the structural changes required in the spine to obtain optimal results. For example, in a patient with crankshaft phenomenon, a PSO or VCR could result in correction of deformity, but neither of these addresses the anterior vertebral overgrowth driving the deformity; a better option is multilevel anterior/posterior revision surgery. For the patient with short-segment (focal) deformity, multiple level SPOs can be attempted to provide global correction of balance, with lower expectation of correction of the focal deformity. Intraoperatively, if further correction of the focal deformity is desired, then a PSO can be added to the procedure with the posterior closing wedge osteotomy providing the focal deformity correction. Similarly, if the PSO is not able to obtain the amount of correction desired, then the osteotomy can be converted to a VCR to maximally mobilize the spine for deformity correction. Use of the posterior osteotomies in a stepwise manner allows a "trial" of the less complex techniques to be attempted prior to exposing them to the increased potential for morbidity associated with the complex osteotomy procedures.

38.4 Author's Experience

In the period between 1995 and 2000, the senior author (OBA) treated 28 pediatric patients requiring revision spine deformity surgery. There were nine boys and 18 girls with average age at revision surgery of 13 years (range 4–18 years). Twelve patients had diagnosis of congenital scoliosis, eight with adolescent idiopathic scoliosis, two each with Marfan's syndrome and post-laminectomy kyphosis (tumor resections), and four patients with neuromuscular scoliosis (two with muscular dystrophy and one with cerebral palsy). Index operations were instrumented posterior fusions in 17, instrumented anterior/posterior fusions in three, instrumented anterior fusion in one, non-instrumented anterior/posterior fusions in four, and posterior laminectomy in three. Each patient had an average of three surgeries prior to the revision deformity surgery (range 1–12 prior surgeries). All patients had increasing spinal deformity, and ten patients had instrumentation related problems, including three with broken rods. Spinal deformity encountered included crankshaft phenomenon in eleven patients, progressive kyphosis in six, and pseudarthrosis in three. Pain was a major determinant of surgical indication in seven patients.

The type of revision surgical intervention was determined on a case by case basis, with 25 patients receiving anterior/posterior fusions, and three being treated with posterior spinal fusions. Instrumentation was used in all cases. Surgical revision for the 11 crankshaft phenomenon patients was anterior/posterior fusion, as dictated by their disease. The pseudarthrosis patients were also managed with anterior spinal fusion to best guarantee solid arthrodesis across the segment, and posterior instrumented fusion for correction and compression across the segment. Additional anterior procedures were indicated for osteotomy of unacceptable residual deformity, and to mobilize the spine for improved correction. Stand alone posterior spinal fusions were performed as a simple extension in one patient, and were combined with posterior osteotomies in two patients. Post operative correction in the coronal plane was from 67° (range 32–115) preoperatively to 36° (20–60) postoperatively, for an average correction of 43% (range 17–66%). Sagittal measurements in the thoracic spine averaged 57° (range 20–107) of kyphosis preoperatively and 51° (range 20–95) of kyphosis postoperatively, and in the lumbar spine were 66° (range 40–106) of lordosis preoperatively and 60° (range 40–88) of lordosis postoperatively.

Major complications occurred in three patients, and included one superficial wound dehiscence, one pleural effusion/pneumothorax, one junctional kyphosis, and one proximal hook implant dislodgement. Each of these required invasive intervention, and each patient eventually fully recovered. No events of neurological deficit, deep infection, or death occurred. No patients required placement of tracheostomy, despite nine patients having preoperative forced vital capacity averaging 30% of predicted (range 20–40%). None of the 28 patients have required further spine surgery.

The first illustrative case is a 17 year old girl who had underwent posterior selective thoracic spinal fusion for adolescent idiopathic scoliosis 6 years prior to presentation. (Fig. 38.1a, b) She was indicated for the index procedure after failing brace management of the deformity, and was fused instrumented with CD implants from T4 to T11. In the period after the index surgery, she experienced progressive spinal deformity and pain symptoms throughout the spine and into the lower extremities that interfered with her ability to sit, stand or walk for more than a few minutes. She was neurologically intact, and otherwise very healthy. Radiographs obtained preoperative to the revision demonstrated apex right thoracic curve of 60°, apex left lumbar curve of 50°, and 36° of global kyphosis in the thoracic segment (see Fig. 38.1a). Diagnosis of "adding on" below the

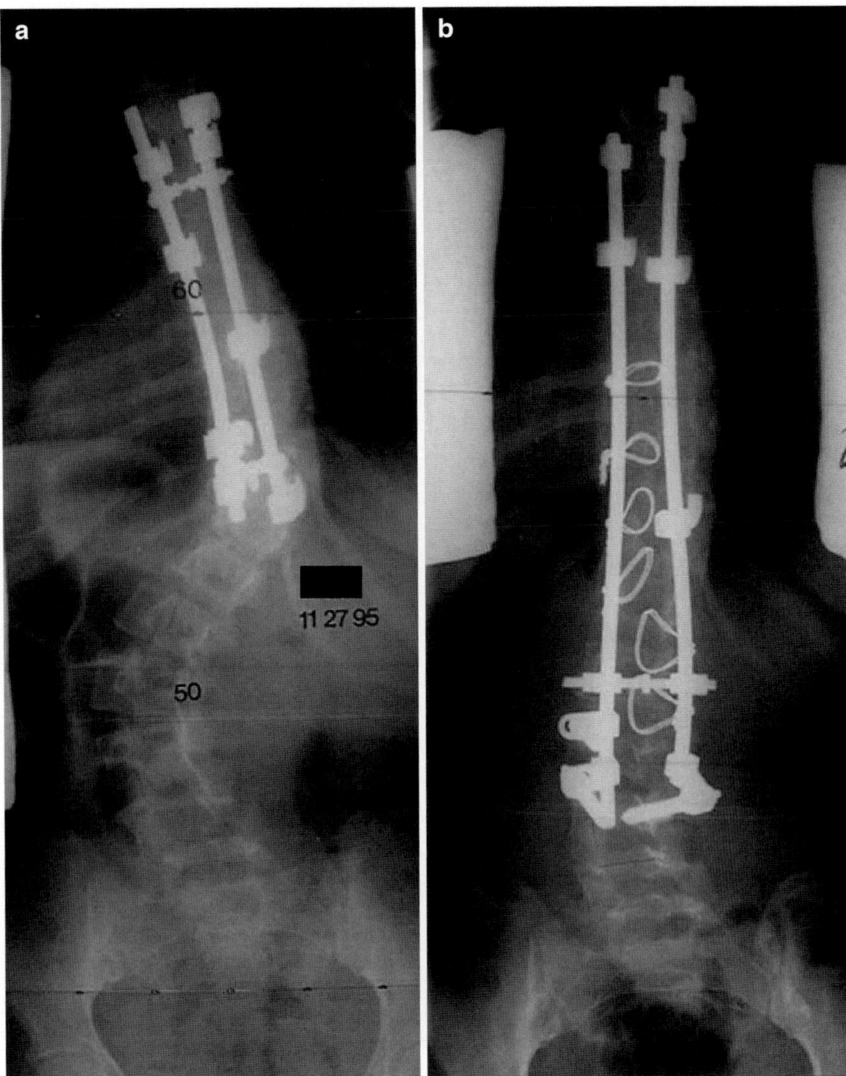

Fig. 38.1 Illustrative case: 17 year old girl with "adding on" below prior posterior spinal fusion. (**a**) Is an image of the anteroposterior radiograph taken prior to the revision deformity surgery demonstrating apex right thoracic curve of 60°, and apex *left* lumbar curve of 50°. (**b**) Is an image of a 6 month postoperative anteroposterior radiograph showing revision instrumentation and deformity correction to 25° in the thoracic and 20° in the lumbar spines

prior fusion was made, and the patient was indicated for revision surgery for removal of instrumentation, posterior osteotomies (Smith-Petersen osteotomies distally) to allow correction, and distal extension of posterior instrumented fusion to L4. The patient underwent the planned procedure with use of an ISOLA hybrid construct and distal pedicle screws, along with right sided thoracoplasties and iliac crest bone graft harvest. By 2 months after the revision surgery she required no pain medicine, and preoperative symptoms had resolved. At 6 months after the revision she had normal balance, apparently solid arthrodesis, and residual curve magnitudes of 25° thoracic and 20° lumbar, with 40° thoracic kyphosis and 65° lumbar lordosis (see Fig. 38.1b). She remains symptom free in long term follow-up, and is managed by a physician located closer to her home.

The second case is a 7 year old girl with Marfan's syndrome who had scoliosis diagnosed prior to 3 years of age (Fig. 38.2a, b). She had managed her spine deformity with bracing, then subcutaneous growing rods with interval lengthenings, and finally a definitive anterior and posterior spinal fusion with posterior instrumentation performed 4 months prior to presentation. Radiographs were available throughout the treatment course, and demonstrated that the proximal instrumentation from the definitive fusion procedure dislodged proximally, and that the spine developed increasing rotation and angular deformity. Operative management was slightly delayed due to her emaciated state, and need for nutritional optimization by gastroenterology consultation, along with placement of a gastrostomy tube and enteral supplementation. Her deformity at presentation was an apex left T5–T12 curve of 128° that measured 108° after application of axial traction, and fractional T12–L5 curve of 35° below (see Fig. 38.2a). She had global kyphosis of 60°, was Risser 0, and had three-dimensional imaging demonstrative of dural ectasia. She was indicated for revision anterior and posterior fusion with posterior instrumentation, and underwent anterior osteotomies

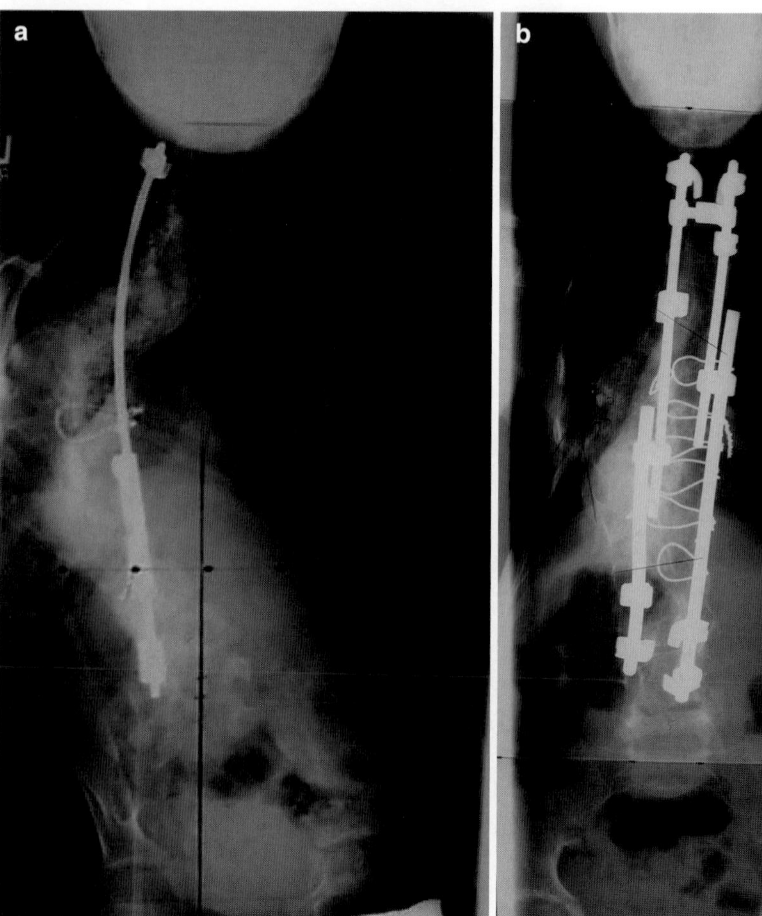

Fig. 38.2 Illustrative case: 7 year old girl with crankshaft phenomenon after definitive fusion. (**a**) Is an image of the anteroposterior radiograph taken prior to the revision deformity surgery showing loss of proximal fixation, main thoracic apex *left* curve from T5–T12 measuring 128° and fractional curve from T12–L5 measuring 35°. (**b**) Is an image of the anteroposterior radiograph taken postoperatively showing the revision instrumentation and correction of deformity with residual thoracic scoliosis of 40°

from T5–T12 and a staged posterior procedure. During the second stage posterior procedure, multiple Smith-Petersen osteotomies were performed, and an ISOLA four-rod construct was used to instrument from T2–L4 with claw and wire fixation. At most recent follow-up 7 years after the revision surgery, she had gained eight in. in height and 24 pounds in weight, was pain free and neurologically intact with a residual thoracic 40° scoliosis and 50° kyphosis (see Fig. 38.2b).

The final case illustration is a 14 year old girl who had diagnosis of VATER/VACTERL syndrome, and had three prior spine procedures for progressive kyphosis at the thoracolumbar junction (Fig. 38.3a, b). Prior spine procedures included a spinal cord detethering done at 8 years of age, a posterior fusion at age 9 that was noted to have deformity progression postoperatively, and was revised with combined anterior (T10–L5) and posterior (T4–L5) fusion at age 10. She had a subsequent proximal extension of the fusion 2 months following the anterior/posterior fusion to T3. In the interval since the most recent revision, the patient noted that her kyphosis was progressing, and reported mild pain over the kyphus, easy fatigability, and poor self image that prompted her to be home schooled. She was followed medically for hypertension, chronic renal insufficiency, and chronic urinary tract infections. She was neurologically intact distally, had obvious gibbus deformity and 1.5 cm left shoulder elevation. Radiographs showed single rod instrumentation T3–L5, apex right scoliosis T10–L4 21°, T8–L4 kyphosis 87°, and sagittal plumb line 17.7 cm anterior to the posterior border of S1 (see Fig. 38.3a). She had a multidisciplinary evaluation for preoperative clearances, and was indicated for posterior vertebral column resection T12–L2, revision instrumentation (second rod placement), correction and fusion. No extension of fusion was required, and reduction of the spine was completed using a four rod cantelever maneuver after placement of bone-graft filled titanium mesh cage in the T12–L2 vertebral body void. Immediately postoperatively she experienced anterior thigh decreased sensation, which gradually returned during the following 24 months. At 2 year follow-up she had physiological balance, markedly improved sagittal countour with residual kyphosis measured at 50°, normal neurological exam, no pain, and had returned to school (see Fig. 38.3b).

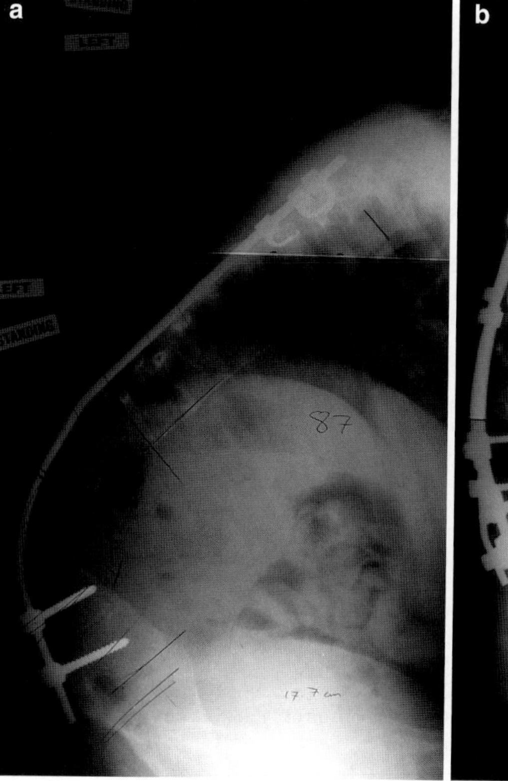

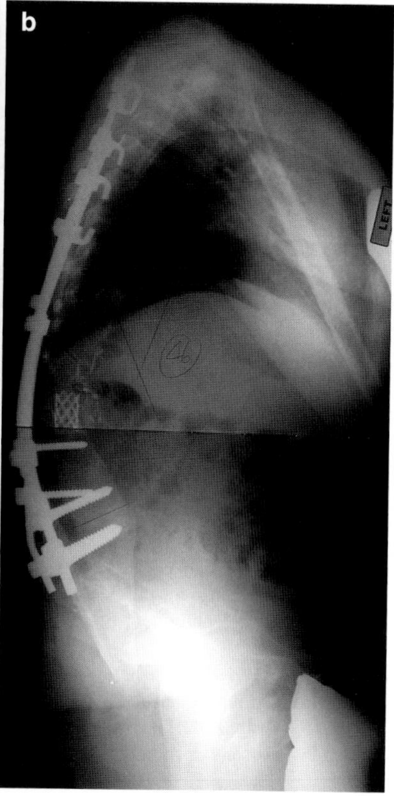

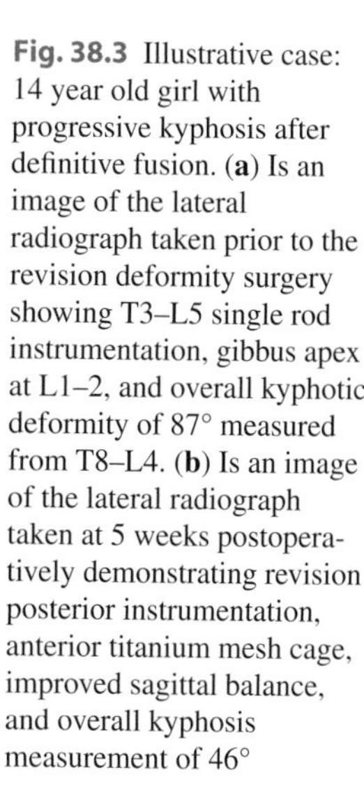

Fig. 38.3 Illustrative case: 14 year old girl with progressive kyphosis after definitive fusion. (**a**) Is an image of the lateral radiograph taken prior to the revision deformity surgery showing T3–L5 single rod instrumentation, gibbus apex at L1–2, and overall kyphotic deformity of 87° measured from T8–L4. (**b**) Is an image of the lateral radiograph taken at 5 weeks postoperatively demonstrating revision posterior instrumentation, anterior titanium mesh cage, improved sagittal balance, and overall kyphosis measurement of 46°

38.5 Summary

Revision spine surgery in the growing child is technically challenging and not encountered frequently. In approaching this complex problem the surgeon must have a complete understanding of the primary deformity and reason for index surgery failure, comprehend the residual growth potential of the spine and how this affects the revision surgery plan, and have a realistic appreciation of technical ability required to perform the procedures safely. Remember: first do no harm, and if in doubt do not hesitate to refer the patient to a more experienced surgeon or to ask for help. Indications and goals for revision surgery need to be agreed upon by the surgeon and the family of the child to assure that postoperative satisfaction is maximal, and preoperative planning must include a multidisciplinary evaluation to optimize both care delivered and surgical outcome.

References

1. Auh JS, Binns HJ, Katz BZ (2004) Retrospective assessment of subacute or chronic osteomyelitis in children and young adults. Clin Pediatr (Phila) 43:549–555
2. Berven SH, Deviren V, Smith JA et al (2003) Management of fixed sagittal plane deformity: outcome of combined anterior and posterior surgery. Spine 28:1710–1715; discussion 6
3. Betz RR, Petrizzo AM, Kerner PJ et al (2006) Allograft versus no graft with a posterior multisegmented hook system for the treatment of idiopathic scoliosis. Spine 31:121–127
4. Blumenthal SL, Gill K (1993) Can lumbar spine radiographs accurately determine fusion in postoperative patients? Correlation of routine radiographs with a second surgical look at lumbar fusions. Spine 18:1186–1189
5. Boachie-Adjei O, Ferguson JA, Pigeon RG et al (2006) Transpedicular lumbar wedge resection osteotomy for fixed sagittal imbalance: surgical technique and early results. Spine 31:485–492
6. Bradford DS, Tribus CB (1994) Current concepts and management of patients with fixed decompensated spinal deformity. Clin Orthop Relat Res 306:64–72
7. Bridwell KH, Lewis SJ, Lenke LG et al (2003) Pedicle subtraction osteotomy for the treatment of fixed sagittal imbalance. J Bone Joint Surg Am 85-A:454–463
8. Bridwell KH, Lewis SJ, Rinella A et al (2004) Pedicle subtraction osteotomy for the treatment of fixed sagittal imbalance. Surgical technique. J Bone Joint Surg Am 86-A(Suppl 1):44–50
9. Bunnell WP (1988) The natural history of idiopathic scoliosis. Clin Orthop Relat Res 229:20–25
10. Cho KJ, Bridwell KH, Lenke LG et al (2005) Comparison of Smith-Petersen versus pedicle subtraction osteotomy for the correction of fixed sagittal imbalance. Spine 30:2030–2037; discussion 8
11. Comstock CP, Leach J, Wenger DR (1998) Scoliosis in total-body-involvement cerebral palsy. Analysis of surgical treatment and patient and caregiver satisfaction. Spine 23:1412–1424; discussion 24–25
12. Cunningham ME, Charles G, Boachie-Adjei O (2006) Posterior vertebral column resection for VATER/VACTERL associated spinal deformity: A case report. HSS J 3:71–76
13. Dias RC, Miller F, Dabney K et al (1997) Revision spine surgery in children with cerebral palsy. J Spinal Disord 10: 132–144
14. Floman Y, Penny JN, Micheli LJ et al (1982) Osteotomy of the fusion mass in scoliosis. J Bone Joint Surg Am 64:1307–1316
15. Geck MJ, Macagno A, Ponte A et al (2007) The Ponte procedure: posterior only treatment of Scheuermann's kyphosis using segmental posterior shortening and pedicle screw instrumentation. J Spinal Disord Tech 20:586–593
16. Hahn F, Zbinden R, Min K (2005) Late implant infections caused by Propionibacterium acnes in scoliosis surgery. Eur Spine J 14:783–788
17. Hedequist DJ, Hall JE, Emans JB (2004) The safety and efficacy of spinal instrumentation in children with congenital spine deformities. Spine 29:2081–2086; discussion 7
18. Hoffer FA, Strand RD, Gebhardt MC (1988) Percutaneous biopsy of pyogenic infection of the spine in children. J Pediatr Orthop 8:442–444
19. Kim YJ, Bridwell KH, Lenke LG et al (2005) Proximal junctional kyphosis in adolescent idiopathic scoliosis following segmental posterior spinal instrumentation and fusion: minimum 5-year follow-up. Spine 30:2045–2050
20. Kim YJ, Lenke LG, Bridwell KH et al (2007) Proximal junctional kyphosis in adolescent idiopathic scoliosis after 3 different types of posterior segmental spinal instrumentation and fusions: incidence and risk factor analysis of 410 cases. Spine 32:2731–2738
21. Kostuik JP, Maurais GR, Richardson WJ et al (1988) Combined single stage anterior and posterior osteotomy for correction of iatrogenic lumbar kyphosis. Spine 13:257–266
22. Kuklo TR, Potter BK, Lenke LG et al (2007) Surgical revision rates of hooks versus hybrid versus screws versus combined anteroposterior spinal fusion for adolescent idiopathic scoliosis. Spine 32:2258–2264
23. Lauerman WC, Bradford DS, Transfeldt EE et al (1991) Management of pseudarthrosis after arthrodesis of the spine for idiopathic scoliosis. J Bone Joint Surg Am 73:222–236
24. Lauerman WC, Bradford DS, Ogilvie JW et al (1992) Results of lumbar pseudarthrosis repair. J Spinal Disord 5:149–157
25. Lee GA, Betz RR, Clements DH 3rd et al (1999) Proximal kyphosis after posterior spinal fusion in patients with idiopathic scoliosis. Spine 24:795–799
26. Lee SS, Lenke LG, Kuklo TR et al (2006) Comparison of Scheuermann kyphosis correction by posterior-only thoracic pedicle screw fixation versus combined anterior/posterior fusion. Spine 31:2316–2321
27. Lim M, Green DW, Billinghurst JE et al (2004) Scheuermann kyphosis: safe and effective surgical treatment using multisegmental instrumentation. Spine 29:1789–1794
28. Lintner SA, Lindseth RE (1994) Kyphotic deformity in patients who have a myelomeningocele. Operative treatment

and long-term follow-up. J Bone Joint Surg Am 76: 1301–1307
29. Lonstein JE (1977) Post-laminectomy kyphosis. Clin Orthop Relat Res 128:93–100
30. Lonstein JE (2006) Scoliosis: surgical versus nonsurgical treatment. Clin Orthop Relat Res 443:248–259
31. Love C, Patel M, Lonner BS et al (2000) Diagnosing spinal osteomyelitis: a comparison of bone and Ga-67 scintigraphy and magnetic resonance imaging. Clin Nucl Med 25:963–977
32. Lowe TG, Lenke L, Betz R et al (2006) Distal junctional kyphosis of adolescent idiopathic thoracic curves following anterior or posterior instrumented fusion: incidence, risk factors, and prevention. Spine 31:299–302
33. Magerl F, Coscia MF (1988) Total posterior vertebrectomy of the thoracic or lumbar spine. Clin Orthop Relat Res 232:62–69
34. McMaster MJ, Singh H (2001) The surgical management of congenital kyphosis and kyphoscoliosis. Spine 26:2146–2154; discussion 55
35. Montgomery SP, Hall JE (1982) Congenital kyphosis. Spine 7:360–364
36. Murrey DB, Brigham CD, Kiebzak GM et al (2002) Transpedicular decompression and pedicle subtraction osteotomy (eggshell procedure): a retrospective review of 59 patients. Spine 27:2338–2345
37. Niall DM, Dowling FE, Fogarty EE et al (2004) Kyphectomy in children with myelomeningocele: a long-term outcome study. J Pediatr Orthop 24:37–44
38. Papagelopoulos PJ, Peterson HA, Ebersold MJ et al (1997) Spinal column deformity and instability after lumbar or thoracolumbar laminectomy for intraspinal tumors in children and young adults. Spine 22:442–451
39. Rathjen K, Wood M, McClung A et al (2007) Clinical and radiographic results after implant removal in idiopathic scoliosis. Spine 32:2184–2188
40. Richards BS, Hasley BP, Casey VF (2006) Repeat surgical interventions following "definitive" instrumentation and fusion for idiopathic scoliosis. Spine 31:3018–3026
41. Roberto RF, Lonstein JE, Winter RB et al (2006) Curve progression in Risser stage 0 or 1 patients after posterior spinal fusion for idiopathic scoliosis. J Pediatr Orthop 1997;17: 718–725
42. Ruf M, Harms J (2003) Posterior hemivertebra resection with transpedicular instrumentation: early correction in children aged 1 to 6 years. Spine 28:2132–2138
43. Sanders JO, Little DG, Richards BS (1997) Prediction of the crankshaft phenomenon by peak height velocity. Spine 22:1352–1356; discussion 6–7
44. Schellinger KA, Propp JM, Villano JL et al (2008) Descriptive epidemiology of primary spinal cord tumors. J Neurooncol 87:173–179
45. Sciubba DM, Noggle JC, Marupudi NI et al (2007) Spinal stenosis surgery in pediatric patients with achondroplasia. J Neurosurg 106:372–378
46. Sink EL, Newton PO, Mubarak SJ et al (2003) Maintenance of sagittal plane alignment after surgical correction of spinal deformity in patients with cerebral palsy. Spine 28: 1396–1403
47. Smith JT, Gollogly S, Dunn HK (2005) Simultaneous anterior-posterior approach through a costotransversectomy for the treatment of congenital kyphosis and acquired kyphoscoliotic deformities. J Bone Joint Surg Am 87:2281–2289
48. Smith-Petersen MN, Larson CB, Aufranc OE (1945) Osteotomy of the spine for correction of flexion deformity in rheumatoid arthritis. J Bone Joint Surg Am 27-A:1–11
49. Suk SI, Lee SM, Chung ER et al (2003) Determination of distal fusion level with segmental pedicle screw fixation in single thoracic idiopathic scoliosis. Spine 28:484–491
50. Vaughan JJ, Winter RB, Lonstein JE (1996) Comparison of the use of supine bending and traction radiographs in the selection of the fusion area in adolescent idiopathic scoliosis. Spine 21:2469–2473
51. Wilson PE, Oleszek JL, Clayton GH (2007) Pediatric spinal cord tumors and masses. J Spinal Cord Med 30(Suppl 1): S15–S20

Anesthesia and Postoperative Management of Spinal Deformity Surgery in Growing Children

39

Ivan Florentino-Pineda

Key Points

- Because scoliosis surgery is multidisciplinary, several teams must work together to assure the best outcome.
- Early onset scoliosis may be associated with progressive restrictive lung disease, which increases the risks of pulmonary complications following surgical correction.
- The increased prevalence of malnutrition in patients with neuromuscular scoliosis is a significant concern and one that needs to be evaluated preoperatively.
- Mean blood loss per vertebral level correlates with the number of vertebral levels fused and has been reported to be as high as 500mL.
- In view of the ischemic nature of spinal cord injury, it is now suggested that mean arterial pressure (MAP) should be maintained in the low normal range.

39.1 Introduction

The number of pediatric scoliosis surgeries is increasing each year due to recent advances in spinal instrumentation, surgical techniques, and improved perioperative monitoring. A clear understanding of the disease processes with their associated changes in cardiovascular and respiratory function, the preservation of spinal cord blood flow, and techniques in monitoring spinal cord integrity are essential for a good outcome.

Anesthesia during correction of scoliosis in children must address surgical requirements for positioning and monitoring in addition to taking into consideration the associated comorbidities, age-related pathophysiology, and the potential for blood loss and vascular injury of the spinal cord. Children undergoing correction of spinal deformities present a significant challenge to the pediatric anesthesiologist due to not only wide spectrum of underlying pathology, but also the variable range of age and size.

Awareness of the risk of spinal cord injury (SCI) that will affect the function is critical. Expertise in the management of the patients in various positions; prevention of hypothermia secondary to exposure of a large surgical field for a prolong period of time; and severe hemorrhage, which can sometimes exceed the patient's total blood volume, are required. In the case of correction of spinal deformities, all of those situations may converge, demanding attentive intraoperative monitoring, particularly of spinal function, and an anesthesia plan tailored to maintain appropriate spinal cord perfusion, minimize blood loss, and allow for early awakening and extubation.

This chapter reviews spinal blood flow and autoregulation, preoperative assessment, anesthesia care, including one lung ventilation and blood preservation techniques, and postoperative management.

39.2 Spinal Cord Blood Flow and Regulation

The spinal cord vascular anatomy comprises separate anterior and posterior circulations that arise from the vertebral arteries and are supplemented by intercostals

I. Florentino-Pineda
Department of Anesthesiology, Children's Medical Center, 1446 Harper Street, BT-2651, Augusta, GA 30912-2700, USA
e-mail: iflorentino@mail.mcg.edu

B. A. Akbarnia et al. (eds.), *The Growing Spine*,
DOI: 10.1007/978-3-540-85207-0_39, © Springer-Verlag Berlin Heidelberg 2011

and lumbar vessels from the descending aorta. A single anterior spinal artery supplies the ventral two-thirds of the spinal cord, which includes the corticospinal tracts and motor neurons. Paired posterior spinal arteries form a plexus-like arrangement on the surface of the cord and supply the dorsal one-third of spinal cord parenchyma, which transmits proprioception and light touch. There is essentially no collateral flow between the anterior and posterior circulations [57].

The anterior spinal artery, which supplies motor neurons and tracts, is of uneven caliber and is not functionally continuous. The blood flow to the anterior spinal cord is supplemented by collateral flow through radicular arteries arising from the aorta. Only 6–8 of the 62 radicular vessels that present during development persist into adult life. The large distance between these radicular arteries leaves watershed areas at the upper thoracic and lumbar levels, making the spinal cord particularly vulnerable to ischemia. The great radicular artery of Adamkiewicz arises from the aorta between T8 and L3 nerve roots and supplements the blood flow to the anterior portion of the distal thoracic spinal cord and lumbar enlargement [1]. It provides up to 50% of the entire spinal cord blood flow and may be injured during aortic or spinal surgery or after spinal trauma [52].

The venous outflow of the spinal cord is divided into two systems, called the vertebral and venous plexuses. These internal and external plexuses communicate with each other and with the segmental systemic veins.

Animal data suggest that the spinal cord blood flow is controlled by the same factors and the same general physiological principles as the cerebral blood flow (CBF) [25]. Spinal cord blood flow is lower than CBF, because absolute spinal cord metabolism is lower than that of the brain. Blood flow to the spinal gray matter is about half that to the cerebral cortex, and the flow to the white matter is about one-third of that to spinal gray matter.

Spinal cord perfusion pressure (SCPP) is equal to MAP minus extrinsic pressure on the spinal cord. Pressures exerted by local extrinsic mechanical compression, such as tumor, hematoma, spinal venous congestion, and increased intraspinal fluid pressure can be important determinants of the SCPP. Spinal blood flow is maintained constant by vasodilatation or vasoconstriction of the cord's vasculature to accommodate for changes in MAP.

Limits of spinal cord blood flow autoregulation are 45–180 mmHg. Conditions that affect this autoregulatory mechanism include severe hypoxia, hypercapnia, and trauma [25, 51]. The spinal cord vasculature and cerebral vasculature react to changes in oxygen and carbon dioxide concentrations in a similar fashion.

39.3 Anesthesia Management

39.3.1 Preoperative Evaluation

Patients presenting for correction of spinal deformities present as two distinct groups: those with adolescent idiopathic scoliosis, who are usually well with good cardiorespiratory reserve, and those with secondary scoliosis, who may have very limited reserve and for whom the risks of surgery and anesthesia are greater. The preoperative anesthesia begins with a detailed assessment to identify patients at risk with the aim of decreasing morbidity and mortality related to surgical correction of deformities. The initial step is a thorough history and physical examination. Because of the known association of spinal column deformity with potentially serious alterations of the cardiovascular and respiratory systems, the preoperative anesthesia evaluation is directed primarily to these systems in order to exclude any preoperative factor that could make the surgical intervention too dangerous unless corrected (e.g. cardiac failure, severe pulmonary hypertension, clotting abnormalities, respiratory insufficiency, etc.). When such factors have been ruled out, the preoperative evaluation progresses to detect other factors that, although perhaps not life-threatening, could cause significant morbidity (e.g. malnutrition, muscle weakness, abnormal cough reflex, chronic aspiration secondary to gastroesophageal reflux). The outcome of these patients depends, to a significant degree, on their physiologic reserves to endure the high demands that spinal surgery entails. During their preoperative evaluation, it will be important to identify any physiologic abnormality and assess the degree of severity. Patients must be in optimal medical condition before planned surgery if uncomplicated intraoperative and postoperative courses are to be realized.

Because scoliosis surgery is multidisciplinary, several teams must work together to assure the best outcome. Patients with comorbidities will require an evaluation by pulmonary, cardiology, pediatric, and anesthesia services. Neurology should be involved in patients with significant underlying neurological conditions, and gastroenterology needs to be involved for patients with poor nutritional status or suspicion of a previously undiagnosed gastrointestinal disorder. In the physical examination during the preoperative evaluation of the patient with spinal scoliosis, special attention needs to be given to the airway anatomy, which can be severely deformed by abnormalities of the thoracic and cervical spine and may require fiberoptic assistance at the time of surgery.

Most cases of idiopathic scoliosis occur in otherwise healthy adolescent females, with only mild abnormalities that do not affect their intraoperative management. Preoperative assessment in these patients includes hemoglobin and coagulation function testing and a type-and-crossmatch. Autologous blood or directed-donor blood donation is highly recommended. Preoperative pulmonary function tests (PFTs) are only indicated for curves 60 to 80° or greater, if there is a history of reactive airway disease or if anteroposterior fusion is being performed.

39.3.2 Cardiopulmonary Involvement

Scoliosis may be associated with progressive restrictive lung disease, which increases the risks of pulmonary complications following surgical correction. Patients with preexisting respiratory disease have an increased risk of developing postoperative complications [18,33]. The spinal deformity significantly affects the respiratory mechanics, gas exchange, pulmonary vasculature, and chemical regulation of ventilation. As the curvature worsens, the severity of pulmonary and cardiovascular involvement increases, often resulting in respiratory failure, pulmonary hypertension, and cor pulmonale. Several factors are thought to play a role in the changes of lung volumes and decrease respiratory compliance. These include the abnormal development of the thoracic cage with a direct effect on the elastic properties of the respiratory system. In addition, the deformity will also affect the development of inspiratory and expiratory muscle forces [8, 49]. These changes occur earlier and are more pronounced in patients with congenital scoliosis than in those with adolescent scoliosis, which make age of onset a significant factor for treatment, because curves that demonstrate a major thoracic deformity before a child is 5 years of age are more likely to be associated with significant cardiopulmonary morbidity in addition to other growth abnormalities. Long-term cardiopulmonary complications of untreated scoliosis can include hypoxemia, hypercapnia, cor pulmonale, and pulmonary hypertension.

The goal of surgical treatment of scoliosis is to stop progression of the curve while allowing maximum growth of the spine, lungs, and thoracic cage, preventing the chronic hypoxemia and pulmonary hypertension that presents as the curve is left untreated. The literature supports surgical treatment of spinal deformities in pediatric patients in order to prevent cardiopulmonary morbidity; surgical treatment of infantile idiopathic scoliosis is recommended for progressive curves of 45° or greater in an immature child, indicating the current trend toward less tolerance of curve progression prior to operative intervention.

The effect of surgery on lung function depends on the surgical approach and type of surgery. Thoracic surgery decreases lung volumes, expiratory flow rates, and oxygenation after surgery as a result of the surgery itself, anesthesia, pain, and immobilization [63]. In adult studies, thoracic and upper abdominal surgery may reduce lung volumes and flow rates to 50–75% from their preoperative baseline values.

Because of developmental immaturity of the respiratory system and possibly decreased ability to cooperate with respiratory care, the decrements in children may be even worse [43]. This can lead to serious pulmonary complications, including pneumonia, respiratory failure requiring prolonged mechanical ventilation, bronchospasm, atelectasis, and exacerbation of the underlying chronic disease. Pulmonary function decreases immediately following scoliosis surgery, and the extent of this decrease has been documented in children. Yuan et al. [68] evaluated the immediate change in PFTs values in 24 children following scoliosis surgery and showed that PFT values fell by 60% after surgery. The PFT nadir was at 3 days. PFT values remained significantly decreased at 1 week, with values half of preoperative baseline. Most PFT values were near the preoperative baseline by 1–2 months postoperatively. No statistical significance was found between the degrees of decline in PFT with etiology of scoliosis. Based on their findings, the authors concluded that patients are still at risk for postoperative complications as long as 1 week after surgery. Neuromuscular scoliosis (NS) includes a wide variety of disorders, including muscular dystrophies, spinal muscular atrophies, and cerebral palsy. When taken as a group, patients with NS have increased postoperative complications [2, 37].

Although the role of preoperative PFT in patients with idiopathic scoliosis is controversial, PFT should be routinely performed in NS patients to assess the need for prolonged postoperative mechanical ventilation, as accurately as possible. In a study evaluating risk factors for prolonged ventilatory support in 125 patients with idiopathic and nonidiopathic scoliosis on whom PFTs were obtained in the preoperative visit, patients with neuromuscular disease were more likely to require prolonged mechanical ventilation than other diagnosis groups ($P < 0.0001$). After removal of the neuromuscular patients, no significant difference was observed in the risk of prolonged ventilation among other diagnosis groups ($P = 0.631$). The combination of age >13 years, neuromuscular disease, and FEV1 <40% almost undoubtedly predicted the need for prolonged mechanical ventilation in this study [69].

In addition to the restrictive lung deficit caused by the spinal deformity, children with neuromuscular disease have impaired pulmonary function from progressive muscle weakness and recurrent chest infections, as a consequence of poor cough and impaired airway protective reflexes. Of these conditions, Duchenne's muscular dystrophy (DMD) is the most common disorder, with an incidence of 1 in 3,300 male births. It is inherited as an X-linked disorder, which presents as weakness during the fourth to eighth years of life. The genetic defect results in a deficiency of the protein dystrophin in the skeletal, cardiac, and smooth muscle. As these patients enter their second decade of life, the myocardium is progressively affected; patients develop dystrophy cardiomyopathy and may present with arrhythmia, ventricular dilatation, and heart failure. Preoperative assessment in patients with muscular dystrophies should routinely include a 12-lead electrocardiogram and an echocardiogram.

The increased prevalence of malnutrition in patients with NS is a significant concern and one that needs to be evaluated preoperatively. Systemic implications of a sub-optimal nutritional status include poor wound healing and immunological depression; their presence makes these patients highly susceptible to postoperative complications [26].

Poor intake of vitamin K will cause depletion of vitamin K-dependent coagulation factors, resulting in preoperative coagulation dysfunction. Preoperative screening of coagulation function is required to detect any abnormality that may require optimization previous to surgery.

39.3.3 Conduct of Anesthesia

It is important during the planning of the anesthesia technique to take into consideration all the potential problems associated with spinal reconstruction. Aside from consideration of the cardiorespiratory risk, other important challenges during the administration of anesthesia for this operation in children and adolescents include management of a patient in the prone or lateral positions, prevention of hypothermia secondary to a long procedure with an extensive exposed area, potential for severe blood loss, the provision of one-lung ventilation when required for surgical access, and the preservation of adequate spinal cord perfusion.

Premedication should be guided by the patient's physical examination status. Midazolam administered orally or intravascularly in patients with intravenous access provides adequate anxiolysis, facilitating the transition to the operating room. For patients with abnormal airway anatomy on whom fiberoptic-assisted endotracheal intubation is planned, an anticholinergic agent such as glycopyrrolate will dry secretions and facilitate visualization. Following premedication, patients are transported to the operating room, where placement of ASA standard monitors is followed by induction of general anesthesia. The choice of induction of general anesthesia will be guided by the age of the patient, clinical status, and patient's preference. Inhalation induction with sevoflurane and combined nitrous oxide/oxygen mixture is the preferred method at our institution. In children and adolescents with intravenous access and appropriate cardiac reserve, propofol is the agent of choice; in those without optimal cardiac function, ketamine is a good option. After completion of induction and establishment of vascular access, muscle relaxation is normally achieved with a nondepolarizing muscle-blocking agent (NMBA). A single dose of the NMBA, administered during the induction of general anesthesia, provides optimal conditions for endotracheal intubation and will allow return of neuromuscular function to obtain baseline motor-evoked potentials (MEP) before surgery begins. Monitoring muscle relaxation with a nerve stimulator is the standard of care in any patient in whom muscle relaxation is used as part of the anesthesia technique; in patients with muscular disorders, the duration of action of these agents may be prolonged. Succinylcholine is contraindicated in Duchenne's muscular dystrophy, along with other dystrophic myopathies, because of increased risk of malignant hyperthermia; in patients with neuropathies, the potential for rhabdomyolisis, hyperkalemia, and cardiac arrest also precludes its use.

Immediately after the endotracheal tube is secured, venous access needs to be obtained in all children. Because of the potential of severe hemorrhage during spinal reconstruction, a minimum of two large peripheral intravenous lines will provide for adequate and prompt intravascular volume resuscitation in case of severe bleeding, and will also allow for the infusion of medications. Patients with poor intravenous access and those with significant comorbidities that could prolong hospital stay require central venous cannulation for appropriate intravascular access.

Monitoring during spinal surgery should routinely include ECG, pulse oximetry, capnography and anesthetic agent monitoring, temperature (core and peripheral), neuromuscular block, continuous neuromonitoring by somatosensory-evoked potential, and blood pressure. Owing to the probability that hemodynamic instability could occur during the course of the surgery, intravascular monitoring of blood pressure is required. Hemodynamic instability could be caused by either a reduction in preload, an increase in afterload, impaired contractility, or any combination of the above. The prone position alone can reduce the cardiac output from decreased venous return and increased intrathoracic pressure [60]. Major blood loss is a significant factor for reduction in preload, and in patients with impaired contractility, may not be well tolerated; inotropic support may be required, particularly in boys with DMD, to maintain appropriate hemodynamic parameters. Invasive intravascular monitoring is routinely obtained in most cases of pediatric spinal surgery by placement of an arterial canula allowing for continuous monitoring of blood pressure and frequent evaluations of acid–base status, blood gases, hemoglobin, hematocrit, and coagulation function. Monitoring for air embolism is also recommended in patients undergoing scoliosis repair. Measurement of unconsciousness by bispectral index (BIS™) allows titration of medication for the maintenance of anesthesia. A BIS value of <60 reflects depression of the brain function adequate to ensure unconsciousness during surgery [20, 27]. Titration of anesthesia agents using the BIS monitor to maintain an appropriate level of unconsciousness results in decreased drug utilization and more rapid recovery [19, 55]. In this regard, BIS monitoring serves as a useful intraoperative monitor for guiding drug administration during correction of spinal scoliosis.

When appropriate vascular access and monitoring have been established, and before positioning the patient on the operating table, children with idiopathic scoliosis are turned in a lateral position for an intrathecal administration of 5–10 μg/kg preservative-free morphine via a 24-gauge pencil point spinal needle. The addition of intrathecal morphine decreases MAP, blood loss, and anesthetic agent requirements, without affecting somatosensory-evoked potentials; in addition, it provides for up to 18 h of postoperative analgesia in children undergoing posterior spinal fusion [14, 21]. The final position of the patient on the operating table depends on the specific type of surgery but is generally prone or lateral. In the prone position, the patient in placed face down with supports placed beneath the upper chest, shoulders, and iliac crest, allowing freedom of abdominal movement to facilitate ventilation by preventing restriction of diaphragmatic movement.

The surgeon and the anesthesiologist must coordinate patient position, whether this involves a specific positioning frame (e.g. Hall-Relton) or type of headrest. Placement of the patient and appropriate padding of pressure points should be performed by the surgeon with the assistance of both nursing and anesthesia staff (Fig. 39.1).

The patient's arms should be placed in a well-padded position of no more than 90° of combined abduction and forward flexion, and care should be taken to avoid pressure in the axilla. The elbows should remain free of compression, with particular attention paid to the ulnar nerve. In the female patients, the breasts should be

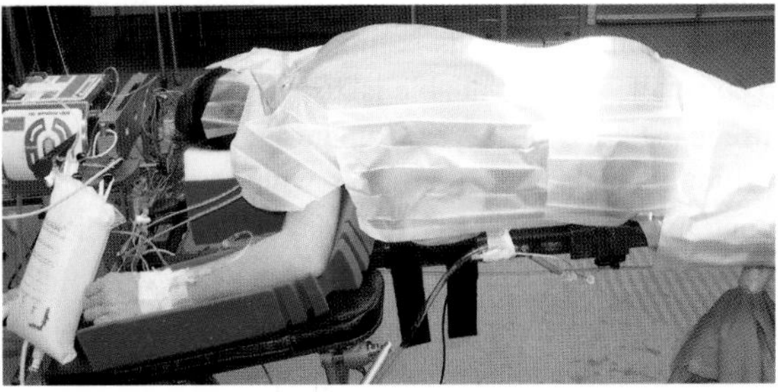

Fig. 39.1 Prone position with a Jackson table. The arms are extended less than 90° whenever possible. Pressure points are padded, and the chest and pelvis are supported to preserve pulmonary compliance and minimize intra-abdominal pressure

moved toward the midline, and generous padding should be placed over the anterior superior iliac spine in all patients to decrease the risk of injury to the lateral femoral cutaneous nerve. The knees should be flexed and the feet be supported, but the toes should be allowed to hang freely.

The most important factor that influences the choice of anesthesia agents is the use of evoked potentials to assess spinal cord integrity. Only small concentrations of inhalation agents are used. Maintenance of general anesthesia usually consists of continuous infusions of propofol and remifentanil. In patients with intrathecal morphine, the addition of remifentanil is not necessary.

39.3.4 One-Lung Ventilation (OLV)

Pediatric scoliosis surgery may require single-lung ventilation for surgical access. Current methods of lung isolation are inadequate for some or all of these children. Spinal access in pediatric scoliosis correction surgery may require lung collapse for several hours and is traditionally achieved in larger children with a double lumen tube (DLT) or with specially designed selective endobronchial blockers that are placed with the assistance of a fiberoptic bronchoscope like the Univent endotracheal tube (Fuji Systems, Tokyo, Japan) and the Arndt endobronchial blocker (Cook Critical Care, Birmingham, IN). Other alternatives to providing bronchial blockade, such as a Fogarty embolectomy catheter or main bronchus intubation with a conventional endotracheal tube, are limited by nonspecific design [12]. They can result in inadequate isolation that requires direct lung compression, which is potentially traumatic for lung tissues. Although DLT is the standard technique for lung isolation in thoracic surgery, its use in scoliosis patients is limited for several reasons. The smallest size available is 26 Fr, which prevents its use in patients <8–10 years of age and in those who are difficult to intubate. In patients with abnormal airway anatomy, placement of a DLT may not be possible and may be contraindicated due to the potential traumatic injury to the airway.

For younger patients and those in whom the DLT or the Univent endotracheal tube is not indicated, the Arndt endobronchial blocker (Cook Critical Care, Birmingham, IN) is an alternative for providing lung isolation. There are three commercially available sizes of this device: 5, 7, and 9 Fr. Its application and successful use in small patients undergoing scoliosis surgery has been reported [4].

In small children, use of the smallest blocker is limited by its external diameter and can be placed only via an endotracheal tube with an internal diameter of 4.5 mm or larger, requiring a thin pediatric bronchoscope.

Dexterity in fiberoptic bronchoscopy and familiarity with these devices are essential for their successful use. Although single-lung isolation provides the optimal surgical access, it is not without risk of potential serious complications due to migration and tracheal occlusion by endobronchial balloons, resulting in inadequate ventilation. Constant vigilance is required, including uninterrupted auscultation of breath sounds on the nonisolated lung and monitoring of airway resistance, in order to identify this problem promptly and avoid serious complications.

As ventilation into one-lung ventilation is blocked, active vasoconstriction of the pulmonary artery supplying the hypoxic lung occurs, leading to the diversion of blood to the better ventilated, nonhypoxic lung segments. This protective mechanism decreases the amount of shunt and improves the arterial oxygenation in the presence of regional lung hypoxia. This phenomenon is known as hypoxic pulmonary vasoconstriction (HPV); an understanding of this physiologic response is critical during the anesthesia management of patients with OLV, as inhalation anesthesia agents and other medications that produce vasodilatation (sodium nitroprusside, nitroglycerin, albuterol, nicardipine, verapamil) can interfere with HPV, causing systemic hypoxia.

Isoflurane and sevoflurane directly inhibit HPV to a similar degree in a dose-related manner. In vitro, intravenous anesthesia agents do not directly inhibit HPV. Propofol infusions in the range of 100–200 μg/kg/min do not inhibit HPV [28].

During OLV, adequate oxygenation can be a concern, especially in the supine position and in patients with poor pre-existing lung function. Therefore, it is important for anesthesiologists to be aware of all the variables that can influence oxygenation. Arterial oxygenation (Pa_{02}) is determined by pulmonary capillary oxygenation (Pc_{02}), mixed venous oxygenation (Pv_{02}), and shunt. Pc_{02} depends on alveolar oxygenation (PA_{02}), and therefore, on inspired oxygen and ventilation. Pv_{02} depends on tissue oxygen delivery, and therefore, on cardiac output (Qt) and oxygen consumption. Shunt blood flow through the atelectatic lung during

OLV depends principally on HPV rather than on the mechanical effects of lung collapse [37]. HPV is a function of both Pa_{02} and Pv_{02} [35]. General anesthetic agents can affect Pa_{02} by two possible mechanisms: they can alter Pv_{02} by altering Qt, and they can alter shunt flow directly by inhibition of HPV and indirectly by altering HPV through a change in Pv_{02}.

Anesthesia in patients with OLV is maintained with a combination of small inspiratory fractions of inhalation agents, supplemented with intravenous infusion drugs like remifentanil and propofol. Ventilation is maintained with tidal volumes of 8–10 mL/kg; the rate is adjusted to maintain normocarbia. Hypocarbia is avoided as it may interfere with HPV. If adequate oxygenation cannot be maintained with 100% oxygen to the nonoperative side, continuous positive airway pressure (CPAP) of 4–5 cmH_2O can be applied to the operative side. Although this could improve oxygenation, it may also distend the lung in the operative area. If CPAP fails, another option is to apply positive end-expiratory pressure (PEEP) to the nonoperative side. If both maneuvers fail to improve oxygenation, intermittent periods of double-lung ventilation will be required in order to provide adequate oxygenation.

39.4 Neurological Risk and Spinal Cord Monitoring

Paraplegia resulting from the operative treatment of scoliosis is the complication most feared by surgeons, anesthesiologists, and patients [3, 32]. Neurological injury is most often due to ischemic injury caused by spinal cord distraction or direct spinal cord compression by a hook or wire. The areas of the cord most vulnerable to ischemic injury are the motor pathways supplied by the anterior spinal artery. Rapid interventions, such as adjustment or removal of the hardware, can reverse neurological deficits and prevent permanent injury. Prevention of Spinal Cord Injury (SCI) begins with maintaining spinal cord perfusion with reasonable MAP and agreed transfusion thresholds [40].

Recognition of the high-risk case is essential. Congenital kyphosis, neurofibromatosis, skeletal dysplasias, and postinfectious scoliosis carry higher neurologic risk [31]. Congenital scoliosis also increases risk due to a higher incidence of occult spinal cord anomalies [7, 36]. Neurologic deficit prior to the onset of treatment indicates an increased possibility of additional injury [32].

Intraoperative spinal cord monitoring is an integral part of almost all surgeries for scoliosis in pediatric patients. While of limited value in patients with spinal deformity and minimal lower-extremity function associated with myelomeningocele or spinal cord injury, spinal cord monitoring is of great importance in most other patients. Somatosensory evoked potential monitoring (SSEP) was popularized in North America by Nash and Brown [41, 42] in the late 1970s and is used most commonly today. Studies have shown that reliable SSEP data can be obtained in up to 98% of those without preexisting neurologic disorders and in 75% of those with neuromuscular scoliosis (i.e., cerebral palsy) [45]. SSEP data may be influenced by multiple factors, including inhalation anesthesia agents; hence, the use of low-dose inhalational agents in conjunction with total intravenous anesthesia agents (propofol/remifentanil) so as to minimize the effect of the inhalation agents on the SSEP signals is recommended. Finally, patient core temperatures must be maintained at close to a normal range, as low body temperature may cause difficulty with reliable SSEP monitoring.

Motor-evoked potentials (MEPs) have been used less frequently than SSEPs; however, with technical advances, they are becoming more reliable and more widely available. MEPs can be elicited via cortical stimulation or direct stimulation of the spinal cord itself. MEPs are highly influenced by anesthesia technique, and again coordination between surgeon and anesthesiologist is necessary to maximize maintenance of reliable signals. Recently, reports have reviewed patients undergoing spinal surgery utilizing both SSEP and MEP monitoring. Padberg et al. [46, 47] found no false-negative results in 500 patients and concluded that combined SSEP and MEP monitoring eliminated the need for intraoperative wake-up tests in idiopathic scoliosis.

Finally, surgeon, anesthesiologist, and nursing staff must communicate regarding the use of the Stagnara wake-up test, if it is to be used effectively [11, 62]. Described by Vauzelle et al. [62] in 1973, this intraoperative determination of motor function is still the most widely used method and is considered by most to remain the gold standard. It is important to discuss the test with the patient prior to induction of anesthesia, because such discussion appears to improve the performance and accuracy of the test.

39.4.1 *Intraoperative Management of Neurological Insult*

If SCI is suspected, immediate confirmation and appropriate action are necessary to reduce the likelihood of permanent damage. The anesthesiologist should be informed and the patient's blood pressure, hematocrit, and oxygenations should be optimized [10]. In general, the following events should occur in a timely and coordinated fashion:

1. Wake-up test. The Stagnara wake-up test remains the gold standard to determine the presence or absence of injury to the anterior (motor) portion of the spinal cord. It requires two important elements: an anesthesiologist familiar with the procedure and a patient who can understand and follow directions. If the patient cannot follow directions due to mental retardation, significant preoperative weakness, or profound hearing loss, the surgeon will not be able to evaluate any abnormal result. Because the patient may struggle during this test, there is a risk of self-extubation [30]. Therefore, a gurney should be available in the room to turn the patient quickly into the supine position so that reintubation can be performed without delay.
2. Loading dose of steroids and the administration of maintenance-dose steroids. Methylprednisolone is currently the only medication recommended for the treatment of acute traumatic SCI, although other medications have been evaluated [29]. In addition to reducing inflammation and edema, pharmacologic doses of methylprednisolone are thought to act by membrane stabilization and reduction in free radical-induced lipid oxidation. The recommended protocol is methylprednisolone of 30 mg/kg as a loading dose, then 5.4 mg/kg every hour for the next 23 h [5, 6]. Use of steroids in situations of possible intraoperative SCI is not well documented in literature, but we think that the potential benefits of this protocol outweigh the possible risk.

Once the anesthesiologist has been asked to begin a wake-up test, it may take 15–20 min for the patient to become alert enough to comply with the test. If the surgeon is convinced that SCI has occurred, the loading dose of methylprednisolone may be given during this time, as there is evidence that early administration improves recovery in traumatic SCI. If there is doubt of an injury, the wake-up test is completed within a half-hour and the loading dose can be held until confirmation of SCI.

39.5 Anesthesia Techniques in Blood Conservation

Perioperative blood loss remains a significant concern for orthopaedic surgeons performing spinal fusion and instrumentation. Mean blood loss per vertebral level correlates with the number of vertebral levels fused and has been reported to be as high as 503 mL per segment [24]. Many factors affect blood loss in patients undergoing spinal fusion and instrumentation; the surgical technique employed, duration of surgery, number of vertebrae fused, site of autologous bone graft harvest, MAP, the pressure in the inferior vena cava, and patient position affect the total blood loss. In addition, there may be others factor influencing blood loss during scoliosis surgery that are not affected by current techniques to decrease intraoperative bleeding. Yarom et al. [66] described abnormal platelet in vitro function and ultrastructure in patients with idiopathic scoliosis, and Udén et al. [61] noted both an increased bleeding time and decreased ability of collagen to aggregate platelets in patients with scoliosis when compared with nonscoliotic controls. These factors are exacerbated in scoliosis patients with an underlying neuromuscular disorder. In one study comparing neuromuscular scoliosis patients with idiopathic scoliosis patients, the former were found to have a nearly sevenfold risk of losing over 50% of their estimated blood volume during scoliosis surgery, after adjusting for age, weight, number of levels fused, and coagulation profile [16]. Mean estimated blood loss associated with surgical procedures for neuromuscular scoliosis has been reported to range from 1,000 mL for anterior procedures to 2,000–3,000 mL for posterior approaches [54]. Disseminated intravascular coagulation has also been described in patients undergoing surgery for scoliosis, suggesting that extensive decortication may stimulate the intrinsic system of the coagulation cascade, promoting the production of kalikrein, bradykinin, and plasmin, thereby increasing fibrinolytic activity, which may ultimately lead to a consumptive coagulopathy and increase perioperative blood loss.

There is considerable evidence that transfusion of allogenic blood products is associated with serious complications, including transfusion reactions, transmission of infectious diseases, graft-vs. -host disease, acute lung injury, and immunosuppression.

Because major blood loss is to be expected, proper positioning, optimal ventilatory pressures, autologous blood donation, intraoperative hemodilution, the use of a cell saver, induced hypotension, and the use of antifibrinolytic agents should be considered. Transfusion decisions should be based on clinical judgment rather than reliance on a predetermined hemoglobin concentration as a "transfusion trigger."

39.5.1 Positioning and Ventilation

Proper positioning plays an important role in blood conservation in patients in the prone position. Placing the patient with support below the pelvis and shoulder leaves the abdomen free. It has been shown that, by preventing pressure on the abdominal wall, the pressure on the vena cava is minimized, thus reducing blood flow through collateral vertebral venous plexuses, known as Baston's plexus [50]. During mechanical ventilation, airway pressure increases, resulting in an increase in mean intrathoracic pressure. Because venous return to the thorax is dependent on the difference between peripheral venous pressure and intrathoracic pressure, venous return is, consequently, impeded during the inspiratory cycle of mechanical ventilation [64].

There is evidence that elevation in intrathoracic pressures during mechanical ventilation raises the peripheral vascular pressure to adequate level to affect blood loss. Spontaneous ventilation, on the other hand, assists venous return because of reduced mean intrathoracic pressure with inspiration. Therefore, the hemodynamic differences between spontaneous and mechanical ventilation can reduce intraoperative blood loss.

Another aspect of ventilation affecting venous return is expiratory and inspiratory resistance. Maintaining expiratory resistance as low as possible assists venous return by reducing intrathoracic pressure [65]. Appropriate management of reactive airway disease, appropriate setting of the inspiratory-to-expiratory ratio, allowance of adequate expiration time, and maintenance of unobstructed expiratory flows (e.g. avoidance of kinks or buildup of secretions in the endotracheal tube) may be beneficial in reducing blood loss.

39.5.2 Preoperative Autologous Blood Donation and Acute Normovolemic Hemodilution

Although preoperative donation of autologous blood was first suggested by Fantus in 1937, when he founded the first blood bank in the United States, the technique did not became popular until the 1980s. Advantages of this technique include reduced exposure to allogenic blood, the availability of blood for patients with rare phenotypes, reduction of blood shortages, avoidance of transfusion-induced immunosuppression, and the availability of blood to some patients who refuse transfusions based on religious beliefs. There are no limitations in regard to a patient's weight or age. Patients who weigh 50 kg or more can donate a standard unit of blood (450 mL), while those who weigh less than 50 kg can donate proportionately smaller volumes. The hematocrit (Hct) should be ≥33% prior to each donation. Red blood cell production can be augmented by iron supplementation and the administration of erythropoietin. Donations may be made every 3 days, but the usual practice is to donate one unit per week. The last unit should be donated at least 5–7 days before surgery to allow plasma proteins to normalize and to restore intravascular volume. Autologous blood donation in pediatric patients undergoing spinal fusion is an efficient blood-saving technique, especially in idiopathic scoliosis. In some centers, almost 80% of children and adolescents undergoing spinal fusion participate in the autologous blood predonation program; almost 90% of the participants avoid receiving allogenic blood. Patients with neurological causes of scoliosis less often participate in the predonation program and usually need transfusion of allogenic blood.

Acute normovolemic hemodilution (ANH) involves removing and temporarily storing two to four units of a patient's blood just before major elective surgery in which major blood loss is anticipated. The blood that has been withdrawn is then reinfused into the patient during or after surgery. Simultaneous infusions of crystalloids (3 mL of crystalloids per 1 mL of blood withdrawn) have been recommended. The rationale for the use of hemodilution is that, if intraoperative blood loss is relatively constant with or without preoperative normovolemic hemodilution, then it is better to lose blood at a lower rather than at a higher level of Hct.

This procedure lowers the patient's preoperative Hct to 28%. If the perioperative Hct level falls to 24%, the ANH blood units are reinfused in reverse order of their collection (i.e. last unit collected is the first unit transfused). The first unit of blood collected, and therefore the last unit reinfused, has the highest Hct, contains the most platelets, and has the highest concentration of clotting factors [39].

Clinical observations show that ANH reduces allogeneic blood use in 20–90% of patients with no difference in postoperative outcomes [22, 56]. Furthermore, ANH is substantially more cost-effective than transfusion. ANH has been shown to decrease perioperative transfusion requirements of adolescents undergoing extensive spinal surgery. By allowing patients to arrive at surgery with a higher preoperative hemoglobin and Hct levels and by decreasing the quantity of predonated autologous blood collected and therefore used, the hemodilution method may indirectly decrease the quantity of postoperative autologous transfusion in this population.

39.5.3 Controlled Hypotension

Controlled hypotension involves the use of pharmacological agents to lower the MAP to 50–65 mmHg. This method significantly decreases both intraoperative blood loss and blood requirement. Blood loss during controlled hypotension is at least in part dependent on venous pressure [38, 58].

The potential contribution of venous pressure to blood loss can be further understood from studies using epidural anesthesia. Modig et al. [38] demonstrated that both intraoperative and postoperative blood loss are significantly lower during epidural anesthesia when compared with general anesthesia in patients undergoing total hip replacement.

In view of the ischemic nature of spinal cord injury, it is now suggested that MAP should be maintained in the low normal range, and hypotension should be quickly corrected if there is a loss of MAP [40]. It has been shown that the spinal cord is more sensitive to distraction and/or compression during controlled hypotension than at normotension as measured by reduction in somatosensory-evoked potentials [23, 67].

Several different agents and methods are used in spinal surgery to provide controlled hypotension, including direct-acting vasolidators (sodium nitroprusside, nitroglycerine), calcium channel blockers, and intrathecal opioids.

Sodium nitroprusside produces a reliable decrease in blood pressure and at least initially increases spinal cord blood flow; however, it may be associated with tachyphylaxis, rebound hypertension, and toxicity. Nitroglycerin, which has been used successfully for controlled hypotension in adults, may be ineffective in children. Nicardipine is the first calcium channel-blocking agent for intravenous administration. It was introduced to prevent and treat spasm of cerebral arteries in patients with subarachnoid hemorrhage, but it has also been employed in adults to control perioperative hypertension. It does have some intrinsic negative chronotropic effects, which may limit the rebound tachycardia. Like other direct-acting vasodilators, nicardipine and other calcium channel antagonists may increase intracranial pressure. Studies comparing SNP with nicardipine have demonstrated several potential advantages of nicardipine, including fewer episodes of excessive hypotension, less rebound tachycardia, less activation of the rennin-angiotensin and sympathetic nervous systems, and in some studies, decreased blood loss. One disadvantage of nicardipine is that its effect is somewhat prolonged (20–30 min) following discontinuation of the infusion.

Administration of opioids is another approach to lowering intraoperative blood pressure and decreasing blood loss. With 20 µg/kg morphine mixed with 50 µg of sufentanil and 2 mL of preservative-free saline, administered at the level of T3–T4 in children anesthetized with 0.5% isoflurane in oxygen, hypotension to a MAP of 50–55 mmHg was achieved, without any additional pharmacological intervention [21]. Intraoperative blood loss was related to the MAP, and it was significantly lower in children anesthetized with intrathecal morphine than in the control group, which was anesthetized with intravenous sufentanil and 0.5–1% isoflurane. No effect of intrathecal opioids on somatosensory-evoked potentials was observed, while changes in amplitude and latency were observed in the control group. The mechanism of the hypotensive effect of intrathecal opioids may be the direct sympatholytic effect of intrathecal opioids at the spinal cord level [9].

The potential for an additive effect of spinal cord distraction and controlled hypotension emphasizes the importance of intraoperative evoked-potential monitoring when using controlled hypotension during these surgical procedures.

39.5.4 Hemostatic Drugs

Desmopressin acetate (DDAVP) is a synthetic analog of vasopressin with decreased vasopressor activity. DDAVP therapy causes a 20-fold increase in plasma levels of factor VIII and stimulates vascular endothelium to release von Willebrand factor (vWF). Factor VIII is a plasma glycoprotein that speeds up activation of factor X by factor IXa in the presence of a phospholipid surface and calcium ions. vWF mediates platelet adherence to vascular subendothelium by functioning as a protein bridge between glycoprotein Ib receptors on platelets and subendothelial vascular basement membrane proteins.

Intravenous DDAVP has been shown to reduce blood loss during scoliosis surgery in some patients. In patients with neuromuscular diseases undergoing spinal fusion, the overall blood loss was reduced in the treatment group when compared with placebo group, but the results were not statistically significant [59].

39.5.5 Antifibrinolytics

Epsilon-aminocaproic acid (EACA) and tranexamic acid (TA) are omega aminocarboxylic acid analogs of lysine. The antifibrinolytic effect of these drugs is due to the formation of a reversible complex with plasminogen, which prevents the fibrinolysis that would normally occur with activation of plasminogen to plasmin. As a result of this inhibition, fibrin is not lysed, which allows for the formation of a more stable clot. EACA is administered at an intravenous loading dose of 100–150 mg/kg, followed by infusion of 10–15 mg/kg/h. Ninety percent is excreted in the urine within 4–6 h of administration. TA is 6–10 times more potent than EACA and may be used at lower doses (loading dose of 10 mg/kg followed by an infusion of 1 mg/kg/h). Ninety percent is present in the urine after approximately 24 h. Adverse effects of EACA or TA may be related to the effect on coagulation function and the route of excretion. As these agents are cleared by the kidneys, their administration in the presence of renal or ureteral bleeding is not recommended because ureteral clot formation and possible obstruction may result. In 2001, Florentino-Pineda et al. [17] administered EACA or placebo (100 mg/kg followed by 10 mg/kg/h) to 28 adolescents undergoing posterior spinal fusion. Patients who received EACA had decreased intraoperative blood loss (988 ± 411 mL vs. 1,405 ± 670 mL, P = 0.024) and decreased transfusion requirements (1.2 + 1.1 U vs. 2.2 ± 1.3 U, P = 0.003). TA has been found to be similarly effective in decreasing blood loss in spinal fusion [53].

Aprotinin is a serine protease inhibitor derived from bovine lung. Among the proteases it can inhibit are trypsin, chymotrypsin, plasmin, tissue plasminogen activator (tPA), serum urokinase plasminogen activator, and both tissue and plasma kallilreins [15]. By inhibiting plasmin, aprotinin is able to inhibit fibrinolysis. In addition, by inhibiting kallikrein, activation of the intrinsic pathway of coagulation is inhibited or attenuated. Although aprotinin has also been shown to reduce blood loss and transfusion requirements during posterior spinal fusion in children [13], its potential side effects including anaphylactic reactions and renal failure, and recent reports of increased morbidity and mortality in adult patients undergoing cardiac revascularization who received aprotinin have made the utilization of this drug during spinal reconstruction no longer an option [34].

39.6 Postoperative Care

Children returning from surgery directly to the intensive care unit have a number of unique concerns. It is incumbent upon the care team to systematically address the needs of the patient and provide support during this critical phase.

39.6.1 Central Nervous System

Scoliosis patients should be monitored closely after surgery; the patient needs to be placed in an intensive care unit or a "step-down" unit for approximately 24 h. Postoperative monitoring should include close assessment of MAP and overall hemodynamic status. Anecdotal reports have hypothesized that the late-onset neurological changes within the immediate postoperative period may be the result of spinal cord ischemia in patients due to relative hypotension [48]. Postoperative analgesia must not overly sedate the patient or in any way mask the timely discovery of delayed or evolving neurological dysfunction. Family presence is often vital to assess children's level of activity and cognition, especially in the preverbal years or in the special-needs population.

Pain Control: Pain after spinal surgery usually requires the use of an opioid-based technique. In younger children, this may be by using a morphine infusion or a nurse-controlled analgesia. Children >7 years of age may be able to use patient-controlled analgesia. Infiltration of the wound at the end of surgery with local anesthetic will improve pain relief in the immediate postoperative period. Opioids should be supplemented with acetaminophen of 15 mg/kg/dose given every 4 h around the clock for the first 48 h. Muscle spasms present a unique challenge after posterior spinal fusion. Diazepam (0.05–0.2 mg/kg/dose Q 2–4 h, Max dose 0.6 mg/kg within an 8-h period) administered intravenously may prove a useful adjunct in the first 48 h as the musculature of the rib cage and back adjust to the new contour afforded after corrective surgery. Scoliosis surgery pain could also be managed with the use of an epidural infusion of opioids–local anesthetic combination with the catheter inserted by the surgeon at the end of the procedure [44]. Intrathecal morphine administered as part of intraoperative anesthesia management will provide for up to 18 h of postoperative analgesia in children undergoing posterior spinal fusion [14].

Respiratory: Many of these patients have restricted lung disease secondary to rib cage distortion that has led to decreased maximum voluntary ventilation over time. The goal is to extubate the children in the operating room or at least in the first 24 h. This goal is met with ease if the child had good pre-surgical respiratory function as demonstrated through pulmonary function testing. Often children are successfully extubated and require only face shield oxygen immediately, with non-invasive positive pressure ventilation reserved for the children who are unable to effectively ventilate despite optimal positioning and low sedation requirement. Over the years, there has been a wide increase in the devices available to the practitioner to aid in airway clearance. Some of the most frequently used include the following:

- *The FLUTTER® mucous clearance device and Acapella™* device are small handheld devices that provide positive expiratory pressure (PEP). Exhaling through the device creates oscillations or "flutters" in pressures in the airway, resulting in loosening of mucous. It also allows inhalation and exhalation without removing it from the mouth. It can support virtually any patient's lung capacity. This can be used with a mask or nebulizer as well for medication delivery.
- *Mechanical Insufflator–Exsufflator (CoughAssist)* is a portable electric device which utilizes a blower and a valve to alternately apply a positive and then a negative pressure to a patient's airway, in order to assist the patient in clearing retained bronchopulmonary secretions. Air is delivered to and from the patient via a breathing circuit incorporating a flexible tube, a bacterial filter, and either a facemask, a mouthpiece, or an adapter to a tracheostomy or endotracheal tube.
- *Intrapulmonary Percussive Ventilator (IPV)* is a type of mechanized chest physical therapy. Instead of a caretaker clapping or cupping the patient's chest wall, the IPV device delivers high-flow jets of air to the airways by a pneumatic flow interrupter at a rate of 100–300 cycles/min via a mouthpiece. The patient controls variables such as inspiratory time, peak pressure, and delivery rates.
- *Intermittent positive pressure breathing (IPPB)* devices use pressure to passively fill the lungs when a breath is initiated. An incorporated manometer and mechanical valves serve to terminate the flow of inspired air when a predetermined pressure is reached on inhalation. IPPB breathing circuits are designed for nebulizer-inhaled medication.
- *Vest® Airway Clearance System* generates increased airflow velocities that create cough-like shear forces and decreases secretion viscosity, thus assisting patients in mobilization of secretions from smaller to larger airways where they can more easily be removed by coughing. Patients often receive this therapy every 4–6 h while awake for 20-min sessions.

Cardiovascular: Blood pressure lability is frequently seen in the first 24 h after surgery, and thus, arterial line monitoring of blood pressure is recommended. Shock may develop secondary to hypovolemia from severe fluid losses during prolonged surgeries. Inotropic support may be required if contractility seems impaired, to ensure adequate perfusion in the patients.

Fluids/Electrolytes: Fluid losses during a prolonged surgery require appropriate volume replacement. It is not unusual for a child to receive up to 100 mL/kg of fluid during surgery. Excellent hand-off communication must occur between the anesthesia staff and intensive care team to ensure adequate understanding of the fluid-balance concerns for each patient. Children are often managed with Dextrose 5% + Normal Saline and Potassium Chloride 20 meq/L at maintenance rate.

Gastrointestinal: Enteral nutrition is often not started for the first 48–72 h, but should be engaged as soon as possible. Adequate nutrition promotes healing and will aid in the total recovery of the child. While under NPO, it is prudent for the child to begin taking prophylactic Zantac of 2 mg/kg/dose, given every 8 h intravenously, to prevent stress ulcer development.

Hematologic: Because blood loss may be profound, it is important to obtain a baseline hemoglobin and coagulation panel when the child returns from the OR. Monitoring of these parameters every 6 h for the first 24 h is not unreasonable, as many patients require packed red blood cell transfusion (over time, the threshold for transfusion has lowered, but many would agree that a hemoglobin <7 with a symptomatic patient is worthy of transfusion). Care should be taken to note the presence of a Jackson Pratt drain and the amount of drainage per hour. Drainage that exceeds 3–5 mL/kg/h is excessive, and these children will often require transfusion or correction of coagulation factors.

Infectious: After instrumentation, these children routinely receive broad-spectrum antibiotic coverage (Ancef 25 mg/kg/dose given intravenously every 8 h) for 72 h. Hyperthermia may be a clue to atelectasis and not herald an infection. However, removal of all invasive devices, i.e., Foley catheter, arterial line, and additional peripheral IVs, in a timely fashion will reduce the potential for hospital-acquired infections.

39.7 Summary

Care for children with spinal deformities starts well before their admission for surgery.

The anesthesiologist must address surgical requirements for positioning and monitoring, in addition to taking into consideration the associated comorbidities, age-related pathophysiology, the potential for blood loss, and vascular injury of the spinal cord. Care for these patients requires a number of pediatric subspecialists, and close communication and dedication are essential to providing these children the best opportunity for a safe operation and recovery.

References

1. Alleyne CH Jr, Cawley CM, Shengelaia GG et al (1998) Microsurgical anatomy of the artery of Adamkiewicz and its segmental artery. Neurosurgery 89:791–795
2. Anderson PR, Puno MR, Lovell SL et al (1985) Posoperative respiratory complications in non-idiopathic scoliosis. Acta Anaesthesiol Scand 29:186–192
3. Ben-David B, Taylor PD, Haller GS (1987) Posterior spinal fusion complicated by posterior column injury. A case report of a false negative wake-up test. Spine 12:540–543
4. Bird GT et al (2007) Effectiveness of Arndt Endobronchial Blockers in Pediatric Scoliosis Surgery: a case series Pediatric Anesthesia 17:289–294
5. Bracken MB, Shepard MJ, Collins WF et al (1990) A randomized, controlled trial of methylprednisolone or naloxone in the treatment of acute spinal-cord injury. Results of the second national acute spinal cord injury study. N Engl J Med 322:1405–1411
6. Bracken MB, Shepard MJ, Holford TR et al (1997) Administration of methylprednisolone for 24 or 48 hours or tirilazad mesylate for 48 hours in the treatment of acute spinal cord injury. Results of the Third National Acute Spinal Cord Injury Randomized Controlled Trial. National Acute Spinal Cord Injury Study. JAMA 277:1597–1604
7. Bradford DS, Heithoff KB, Cohen M (1991) Intraspinal abnormalities and congenital spinal deformities: a radiographic and MRI study. J Pediatr Orthop 11:36–41
8. Branthwaite MA (1986) Cardiorespiratory consequences of unfused idiopathic scoliosis. Br J Dis Chest 80:360–369
9. Breslow MJ, Jordan DA, Christopherson R (1989) Epidural morphine decreases postoperative hypertension by attenuating sympathetic nervous system hyperactivity. JAMA 261: 3577–3581
10. Bridwell KH, Lenke LG, Baldus C et al (1998) Major Intraoperative neurologic deficits in pediatric and adult spinal deformity patients. Incidence and etiology at one institution. Spine 23:324–331
11. Brustowicz RM, Hall JE (1988) In defense of the wake-up test. Anest Analg 67:1019
12. Campos JH (2002) Current techniques for perioperative lung isolation in adults. Anesthesiology 97:1295–1301
13. Cole JW, Murray DJ, Snider RJ et al (2003) Aprotini reduces blood loss during spinal surgery in children. Spine 28: 2482–2485
14. Dalens B, Tanguy A (1988) Intrathecal Morphine for Spinal Fusion in Children. Spine 13:494–498
15. Davis R, Whittington R (1995) Aprotinin: a review of its pharmacology and therapeutic efficacy in reducing blood loss associated with cardiac surgery. Drugs 49:954–983
16. Edler A, Murray DJ, Forbes RB (2003) Blood loss during posterior spinal fusion in patients with neuromuscular disease: is there an increase risk? Pediatr Anesth 13: 818–822

17. Florentino-Pineda I, Blakemore LC, Thompson GH et al (2001) The effect of epsilon aminocaproic acid on perioperative blood loss in patients with idiopathic scoliosis undergoing posterior spinal fusion. Spine 26:1147–1151
18. Froese AB (1979) Preoperative evaluation of pulmonary function. Pediatr Clin North Am 26:645–659
19. Gan TJ, Glass PS, Windsor A et al (1997) Bispectral index monitoring allows faster recovery from propofol, alfentanil, and nitrous oxide anesthesia. Anesthesiology 87:808–815
20. Glass PS, Bloom M, Kearse L et al (1997) Bispectral analysis measures sedation and memory effects of propofol, Midazolam, isoflurane, and alfentanil in healthy volunteers. Anesthesiology 86:836–847
21. Goodarzi M (1998) The advantages of intratechal opiods for spinal fusion in children. Pediatr Anesth 8(2):131–134
22. Goodnough LT, Shander A, Brecher ME (2003) Transfusion medicine: looking toward the future. Lancet 361:161–169
23. Grundy BL, Nash CL Jr, Brown RH (1982) Deliberate hypotension for spinal fusion: prospective randomized study with evoked potential monitoring. Can Anaesth Soc J 29(5): 452–462
24. Guay J et al (1994) Predicting blood loss in surgery for idiopathic scoliosis. Can J Anaesth 41:775–781
25. Holtz A, Nystrom B, Gerdin B (1988) Regulation of spinal cord blood flow in the rat as measured by quantitative autoradiography. Acta Physiol Scand 133:485–493
26. Jevsevar DS, Karlin LI (1993) The relationship between preoperative nutritional status and complications after an operation for scoliosis in patients who have cerebral palsy. J Bone Joint Surg 75-A(6):880–884
27. Kearse L, Rosow C, Zaslavsky A et al (1998) Biespectral análysis of the electroencephalogram predicts conciousness processing of nformation during propofol sedation and hypnosis. Anesthesiology 88:25–34
28. Keer LV et al (1989) Propofol does not inhibit hypoxic pulmonary vasoconstriction in humans. J Clin Anesth 1:284–288
29. Klemme WR, Burkhalter W, Polly DW Jr et al (1999) Reversible ischemic myelopathy during scoliosis surgery: a possible role for intravenous lidocaine. J Pediatr Orthop 19: 763–765
30. Koscielniak-Nielsen ZJ, Stens-Pedersen HL, Hesselbjerg L (1998) Midazolam-flumazenil versus propofol anesthesia for scoliosis surgery with wake-up tests. Acta Anesthesiol Scand 42:111–116
31. Lonstein JE, Winter RB, Moe JH et al (1980) Neurologic deficits secondary to spinal deformity. A review of the literature and report of 43 cases Spine 5:331–355
32. MacEwen GD, Bunnell WP, Sriram K (1975) Acute neurologic complications in the treatment of scoliosis. J Bone Joint Surg [Am] 57:404–408
33. Malmberg R, Dottori O, Berglund E (1965) Preoperative spirometry in thoracic surgery. Acta Anesthesiol Scand 9:57–62
34. Mangano DT, Tudor IC, Dietzel C et al (2006) The risk associated with aprotinin in cardiac surgery. N Engl J Med 354:353–365
35. Marshall C, Marshall BE (1983) Site and sensitivity for stimulation of hypoxic pulmonary vasoconstriction. J Appl Physiol 55:711–716
36. McMaster MJ (1984) Occult intraspinal anomalies and congenital scoliosis. J Bone Joint Surg [Am] 66:588–601
37. Miller FL, Chen L, Malmkvist G et al (1989) Mechanical factors do not influence blood flow distribution in atelectasis. Anesthesiology 70:481–488
38. Modig J, Karlstrom G (1987) Intra-and post-operative blood loss and haemodynamics in total hip replacement when performed under lumbar epidural versus general anaesthesia. Eur J Anaesthesiolo 4(5):345–355
39. Monk TG, Goodnough LT, Birkmeyer JD et al (1995) Acute normovolemic hemodilution is a cost-effective alternative to preoperative autologous blood donation by patients undergoing radical retropubic prostatectomy. Transfusion 35:559–565
40. Mooney J, Bernstein R, Hennrikus W et al (2002) Neurologic risk management in scoliosis surgery. J Pediatr Orthoped 22:683–689
41. Nash CL, Brown RH (1989) Current concepts review: spinal cord monitoring. J Bone Joint Surg [Am] 71:627–630
42. Nash CL, Long RA, Schatzingey LA et al (1977) Spinal monitoring during operative treatment of the spine. Clin Orthop 126:100–105
43. Newth CJL (1979) Recognition and management of respiratory failure. Pediatr Clin North Am 26:617–643
44. O'Hara JF Jr, Cywinski JB, Tetzalff JE et al (2004) The effect of epidural vs. intravenous analegesia for posterior spinal fusion surgery. Paeiatr Anaesth 14:1009–1015
45. Owen JA (1999) The application of Intraoperative monitoring during surgery for spinal deformity. Spine 24:2649–2662
46. Padberg AM, Komanetsky RE, Bridwell KH et al (1997) Neurogenic motor evoked potentials: a prospective comparison of stimulation methods. J Spinal Dis 11:21–24
47. Padberg AM, Wilson-Holden TJ, Lenke LG et al (1998) Somatosensory motor-evoked potential monitoring without a wakeup test during idiopathic scoliosis surgery. An accepted standard of care. Spine 23:1392–1400
48. Paonessa KJ, Hutchings F (1998) Delayed postoperative neurologic deficits following spinal deformity surgery. Paper presented at the Scoliosis Research Society Annual Meeting, New York, (Sept 16–20)
49. Pehrsson K, Larsson S, Oden A, Nachemson A (1992) Long-term follow-up of patients with untreated scoliosis. A study of mortality, causes of death, and symptoms. Spine 17:1091–1096
50. Relton JE, Hall JE (1967) An operation frame for spinal fusion. A new apparatus designed to reduce haemorrhage during operation. J Bone Joint Surg Br 49(2):327–332
51. Rubinstein A, Arbit E (1990) Spinal cord blood flow in the rat under normal physiological conditions. Neurosurgery 27: 82–86
52. Servais LJ, Rivelli SK, Dachy BA et al (2001) Anterior spinal artery syndrome after aortic surgery in a child. Pediatr Neurolo 24:310–312
53. Sethna N, Zurakowski D, Brustowicz RM et al (2005) Tranexamic acid reduces intraoperative blood loss in patients undergoing scoliosis surgery. Anesthesiology 102:727–732
54. Shapiro F, Sethna N (2004) Blood loss in pediatric spine surgery. Eur Spine J 13(Suppl 1):S6–S16
55. Song D, Joshi G, White PF (1997) Titration of volatile anesthesia using bispectral index facilitates recovery after ambulatory anesthesia. Anesthesiology 87:842–848
56. Spence RK, Cernaiau AC, Carson J et al (1993) Transfusion and surgery. Curr Probl Surg 30:1103–1180
57. Standring S (2004) Gray's anatomy: the anatomical basis of medicine and surgery. 39th ed. Churchill-Livingston, Edinburgh

58. Tate DE Jr, Friedman RJ (1992) Blood conservation in spinal surgery. Review of current techniques. Spine 17(12): 1450–1456
59. Theroux MC, Corddry DH, Tietz AE et al (1997) A study of desmopressin and blood loss during spinal fusion for neuromuscular scoliosis: a randomized, controlled, double-blinded study. Anesthesiology 87:260–267
60. Toyota S, Amaki J (1998) Hemodynamic evaluation of the prone position by transesophageal echocardiography. J Clin Anesth 10:32–35
61. Udén A, Nilsson IM, Willner S (1980) Collagen-induced platelet aggregation and bleeding time in adolescent idiopathic scoliosis. Acta Orthop Scand 51:773–777
62. Vauzelle C, Stagnara P, Jouviroux P (1973) Functional monitoring of spinal activity during spinal surgery. Clin Orthop 93:173–178
63. Vollmar B, Olinger A, Hildebrandt U et al (1999) Cardiopulmonary dysfunction during minimally invasive thoracolumboendoscopic spine surgery. Anesth Analg 88:1244–1251
64. West J (1982) Pulmonary pathophysiology – the essentials, 2nd edn. William and Wilkins, Baltimore, pp 187–201
65. Wildsmieth JA, Sinclair CJ, Thorn J et al (1983) Haemodynamic effects of induced hypotension with nitroprusside-trimetaphan mixture. Br J Anaesth 55(5):381–389
66. Yarom R, Muhlrad A, Hodges S et al (1980) Platelet pathology in patients with idiopathic scoliosis. Lab Invest 1980;159:490–492
67. Yeoman PM, Gibson MJ, Hutchinson A et al (1989) Influence of induced hypotension and spinal distraction on feline spinal somatosensory evoked potentials. Br J Anaesth 63(3): 315–320
68. Yuan N, Fraire JA, Margetis MM et al (2005) The effect of scoliosis surgery on lung function in immediate postoperative period. Spine 30(19):2182–2185
69. Yuan N, Skaggs Dl, Dorey F et al (2005) Preoperative predictors of prolonged postoperative mechanical ventilation in children following scoliosis repair. Pediatr Pulmonol 40: 414–419

Intraoperative Neurophysiological Monitoring During Corrective Spine Surgery in the Growing Child

40

Daniel M. Schwartz, Anthony K. Sestokas, and John P. Dormans

Key Points

- Multimodality neurophysiologic monitoring of spinal cord and brachial plexus function has a definite place in the context of growing rod and vertical expandable prosthetic titanium rib (VEPTR) placement and lengthening/adjustment procedures.
- Transcranial electric motor evoked potential (tceMEP) recording is the only viable method for monitoring the corticospinal tracts.
- Monitoring brachial plexus function with tceMEP and ulnar nerve SSEP recordings should be considered routine during VEPTR placement and adjustment.
- Total intravenous anesthesia and absence of neuromuscular relaxation optimize neurophysiological signal amplitude and reduce interpretation ambiguity.

40.1 Introduction

Operative management of scoliosis has undergone dynamic evolution over the course of the previous half century, particularly in the immediate past decade. Advances in multisegmental instrumentation and improved surgical technique have facilitated treatment of complex deformities, even in young children with progressive early onset scoliosis who are unresponsive to nonoperative treatment. These developments in spinal instrumentation and surgical management have been complemented by dramatic improvements in anesthesia care and intraoperative neurophysiological monitoring (IONM) of spinal cord and spinal nerve root function. Both these latter clinical specialties have played vital roles in making scoliosis surgery safe and effective across a broad range of patient populations.

This chapter discusses the role of intraoperative neurophysiological monitoring during surgical treatment of rapidly progressing spinal and/or thoracic cage deformity in young children, using temporary internal bracing.

40.2 What Neural Structures and Pathways Are at Risk?

In contrast to formal instrumented fusion of the spine involving placement of permanent fixation devices and application of multidimensional corrective forces, the insertion/adjustment of growing rods and other internal braces would seem to pose fewer risks of iatrogenic neurological injury. Although the neurological risks are likely to be diminished during these latter, less-extensive surgical procedures, they cannot be discounted completely. Assessment of risk to underlying neural structures follows from systematic analysis of the patient's pre-existing pathology in the context of the proposed surgical intervention. For example, treatment of early onset scoliosis with growing rods requires anchoring of the rods to the spine, commonly with pedicle screws. Medial misdirection of pedicle screws in the lumbar spine poses risk of contusive injury to the

D. M. Schwartz (✉)
Surgical Monitoring Associates, 900 Old Marple Road, Springfield, PA 19064, USA
e-mail: dan@surgmon.com

B. A. Akbarnia et al. (eds.), *The Growing Spine*,
DOI: 10.1007/978-3-540-85207-0_40, © Springer-Verlag Berlin Heidelberg 2011

spinal nerve roots, whereas in the thoracic spine, there is a risk of injury both to the roots and the spinal cord. Similarly, lengthening of growing rods, particularly in the presence of abnormal vasculature, spinal cord lesions, or hypotension may compromise normal blood supply to the spinal cord and predispose it to hypoxic injury. Other techniques, such as those that use internal bracing to expand the chest wall, can inadvertently stretch the brachial plexus [30]. Consequently, lessons learned from monitoring the spinal cord, spinal nerve roots, and brachial plexus during traditional surgical correction of spinal deformity appear to have direct application during surgical treatment of deformities in the growing child.

Neurological injury to the spinal cord usually has a mechanical or vascular etiology. Mechanical insults in the form of direct contusion or distortion of a neural element by a surgical instrument or spinal implant, such as a sublaminar hook, tend to manifest globally, producing alteration of both anterior motor and posterior sensory column function. By comparison, vascular insults due to stretch of critical vessels following lengthening or distractive maneuvers can present either as focal compromise to the motor tracts alone or more globally to include the sensory tracts. As a result, spinal cord monitoring *must* be a multimodality technique to allow for neurophysiologic surveillance of both pathways [28].

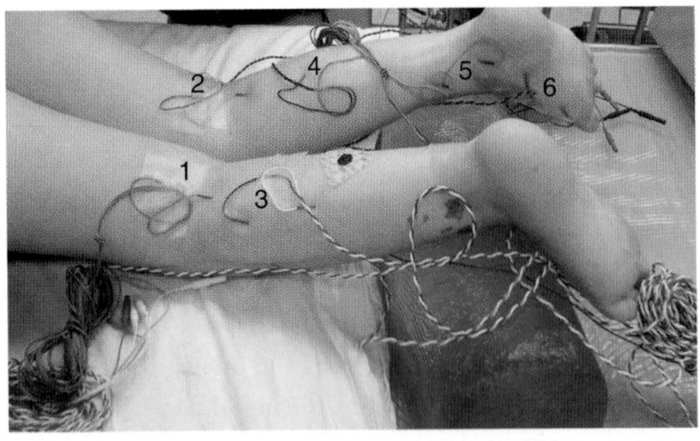

Fig. 40.1 Electrode positions for posterior tibial nerve SSEP, H-Reflex and Train-of-Four (TOF). (TOF is monitored to ensure clearance of the neuromuscular junction for optimal tceMEP recordings.) (**1**) *Left*: Popliteal Fossa (H-Reflex Stimulation Site); (**2**) *Right*: Popliteal Fossa (H-Reflex Stimulation Site); (**3**) *Left*: Gastrocnemius Muscle (H-Reflex and tceMEP Recording Site); (**4**) *Right*: Gastrocnemius Muscle (H-Reflex and tceMEP Recording Site) (**5**) *Right*: Posterior Tibial Nerve (TOF and SSEP Stimulation Site) (**6**) *Right*: Abductor Hallucis Muscle (TOF and tceMEP Recording Site). The *Left* posterior tibial nerve stimulation electrodes are not shown

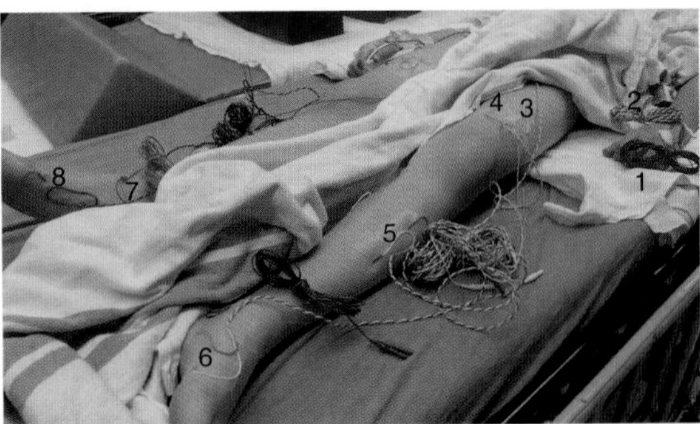

Fig. 40.2 Electrode position for eliciting upper and lower extremity tceMEPs. (**1–2**) *Left*: First Dorsal Interosseous Muscle; (**3–4**) *Left*: Quadriceps Muscle; (**5**) *Left*: Tibialis Anterior Muscle; (**6**) *Left*: Abductor Hallucis Muscle (also used for TOF recording); (**7**) *Right*: Posterior Tibial Nerve SSEP and TOF stimulating site; (**8**) *Right*: Abductor Hallucis Muscle (also used for TOF recording)

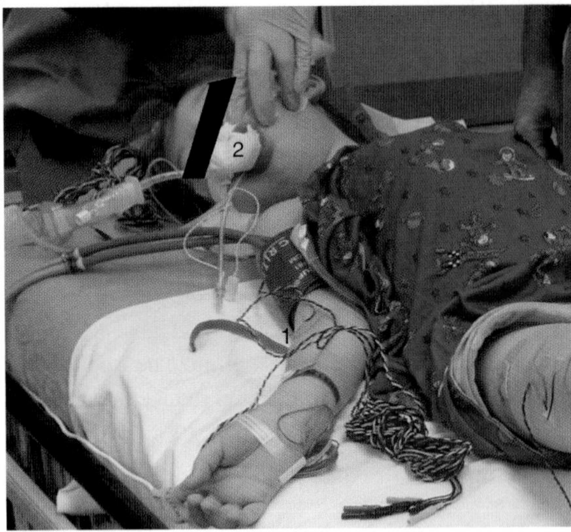

Fig. 40.3 (**1**) Recording electrode over the *right* Deltoid and Biceps muscles for upper extremity tceMEP recordings during VEPTR. (**2**) Position of the bite Block for tongue bite protection

Figs. 40.1–40.3 show a typical intraoperative setup for multimodality monitoring of neurological function during vertical expandable prosthetic titanium rib (VEPTR) and growing rod surgery. These electrode composites provide neurophysiologic monitoring coverage of the spinal cord sensory and motor pathways, brachial plexus, neuromuscular junction, and adequacy of anesthesia. The specific recording electrodes for cortical and subcortical somatosensory-evoked potentials (SSEP) and EEG, as well as the stimulating electrodes for transcranial electrical motor-evoked potential activation are not shown.

40.3 Neuromonitoring Modalities

Despite the early historical success of SSEP monitoring during surgical correction of scoliosis, reliance on this modality is no longer adequate for the growing population of patients who present for surgical correction of increasingly complex deformities. As the SSEP is mediated by the posterior sensory columns and reflects integrity of spinal cord white matter, it provides no direct information about the condition of the descending motor tracts or spinal cord gray matter structures which are particularly susceptible to vascular insult. Hence, when used alone to monitor spinal cord function, SSEPs carry a definite risk of false-negative findings, even among patients with adolescent idiopathic scoliosis [12, 14, 30]. Because of the distractive or lengthening maneuvers needed for deformity correction both with traditional fusion and contemporary nonfusion techniques, there is increased opportunity for excessive vascular stretch and ischemic spinal cord injury. This may not manifest in the SSEP, either at all, or within the critical period necessary to initiate timely intervention for injury reversal.

In response to the limitations of SSEP monitoring, other techniques have been introduced to assess the descending spinal cord motor tracts and anterior column function. These include transcranial electric motor evoked potentials (tceMEPs) and the Hoffmann reflex (H-reflex). The highly debated and often misunderstood neurogenic "motor" evoked potential (NMEP) is discussed separately in this chapter because of several seminal studies that point to its sensory origin.

40.3.1 *Transcranial Electric Motor Evoked Potentials*

tceMEPs are neuroelectric events elicited from descending motor pathway structures including the corticospinal tract (CST), spinal cord interneurons, anterior horn cells, peripheral nerves, and skeletal muscles. These potentials are triggered by delivering electrical pulse trains to the brain through subdermal scalp electrodes over the motor cortex, as illustrated in Fig. 40.4. Following depolarization of the cortical motor neurons, efferent neural signals course through the internal capsule to the caudal medulla where CST fibers decussate and descend into the spinal cord motor tracts. CST

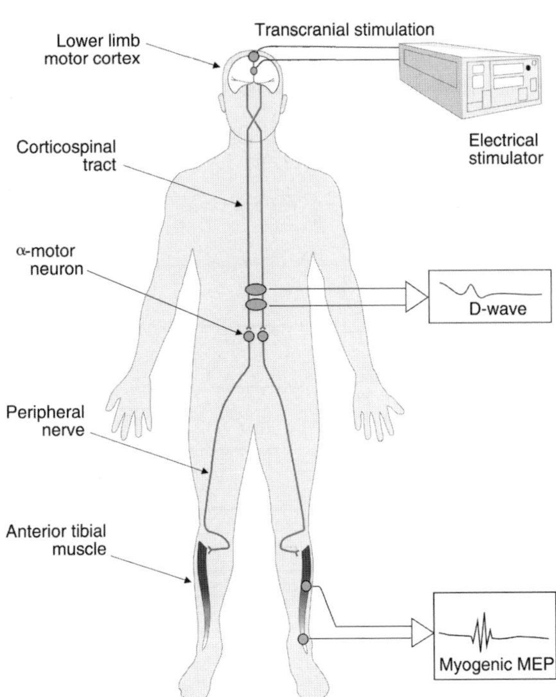

Fig. 40.4 Schematic of tceMEP stimulation and recording

axons enter the spinal cord gray matter, interact with the spinal interneurons, and go on to synapse with alpha motor neurons that innervate the peripheral muscle.

Compound muscle action potentials representing motor-evoked potentials can thus be recorded from upper and lower extremity peripheral muscle with subdermal needle electrodes at the end of this neural chain. Because of the high sensitivity–specificity of tceMEPs for the identification of spinal cord and spinal nerve root injury [1, 10, 12, 14, 19], they should now be considered as the gold standard for monitoring spinal cord motor function during complex spine surgery.

The sensitivity of tceMEPs to motor pathway insult is illustrated in Fig. 40.5 which shows the time course of tceMEP monitoring in a 9-year-old female undergoing revision of growing rod for the treatment of neuromuscular scoliosis. This child presented preoperatively with bilateral upper and lower extremity weakness, though she was weight-bearing and capable of taking several steps with support. Reference to Fig. 40.5 shows that soon after placement of pedicle screws at T2–3, there was acute tceMEP amplitude diminution at left tibialis anterior (TA) and right abductor hallucis (AH) recording sites, and complete loss of the right tibialis anterior response. Moments later, the patient became hypotensive

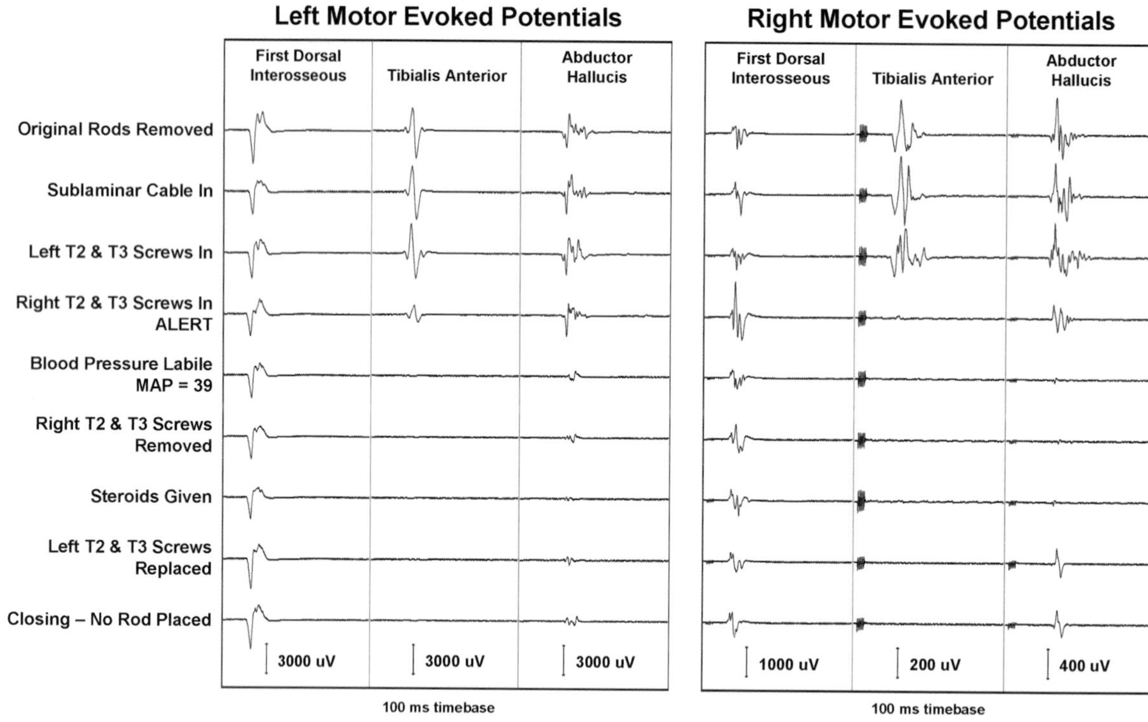

Fig. 40.5 Time course showing acute tceMEP loss following pedicle screw placement at T2–3 in a 9-year-old female undergoing revision of growing rod for treatment of neuromuscular scoliosis

with a mean arterial pressure (39 mmHg) well below the threshold level for spinal cord ischemia (see Chap. 39 for further discussion). At this time, there was bilateral loss of lower extremity tceMEPs, with the exception of a barely observable response (10% of baseline amplitude) over the left AH. Note, however, that control responses from the left and right upper extremities (first dorsal interosseous muscle) remained unchanged.

Despite all attempts to raise the blood pressure, replace screws, and begin a spinal cord injury course of methylprednisolone, the tceMEP amplitudes never improved. Predictably, the child emerged from anesthesia exhibiting further deterioration of lower extremity motor function.

40.3.2 The Hoffman Reflex

The H-reflex, recorded from gastrocnemius muscle following stimulation of the tibial nerve at the popliteal fossa, is a neurophysiologic correlate of the ankle stretch reflex influenced by upper motor neurons and other supra-segmental structures of the spinal cord and brain. The H-reflex reflects the functional integrity of complex motor control subsystems in the highly integrated ascending, descending, and interneuronal pathways of the spinal cord. It is thought that severe, acute spinal cord injury results in suppression of the H-reflex, which is observable within moments of insult. When amplitude suppression has exceeded 90%, and has persisted for the rest of the surgery, patients have awakened with profound postoperative neurological deficit consistent with spinal shock [16].

Because of its neurophysiological underpinnings, and the fact that the anesthesia requirements for recording an H-reflex are not as restrictive as those for tceMEP monitoring, a minority of clinical neurophysiologists has proposed H-reflex monitoring as an equivalent substitute for tceMEPs [37]. Hicks [11] compared the results of H-reflex monitoring to the postanesthesia ankle clonus test in a diverse population of 292 spine surgery patients. The H-reflex predicted the outcome of the ankle clonus test in 80% of the cases, leading Hicks [11] to conclude that the H-reflex was a reliable predictor of spinal cord injury during spine surgery. Of the three patients in the series who exhibited loss of the H-reflex intraoperatively, all had subsequent recovery to baseline prior to closure. There were no patients with permanent loss of the H-reflex and none with postoperative deficits, making comparison of results with known sensitivity of tceMEPs to spinal cord injury difficult at best.

Our experience with the H-reflex has not been as positive as that reported by others, particularly in very young children. All too often, the responses are either variable or there is significant inter-leg amplitude asymmetry for recorded H-waves. Moreover, we have observed dissociations between H-reflex responses and tceMEPs on several occasions, suggesting that the former may be less sensitive than the latter to predisposing factors for spinal cord injury.

An example of such dissociation is illustrated in Fig. 40.6. This figure shows intraoperative transcranial electrical motor-evoked potentials and H-reflex responses recorded from a 42-month-old female during a third lengthening of growing rod to treat 68° kyphotic deformity of the thoracic spine. The patient's history is significant for the resection of thoracic teratoma at 1 month of age, initial placement of growing rod at 10 months with removal at 15 months, and subsequent biopsy of spinal cord lesion with reinsertion of growing rod at 23 months of age.

Following lengthening of the growing rod, tceMEPs disappeared from multiple lower extremity myotomes, including bilateral tibialis anterior, gastrocnemius, and abductor hallucis muscles. There were no concomitant changes in the H-waves recorded from bilateral gastrocnemius muscles during this period. Upon decrease in distraction and elevation of mean arterial blood pressure, motor-evoked potential amplitudes returned to baseline range. There were no new postoperative

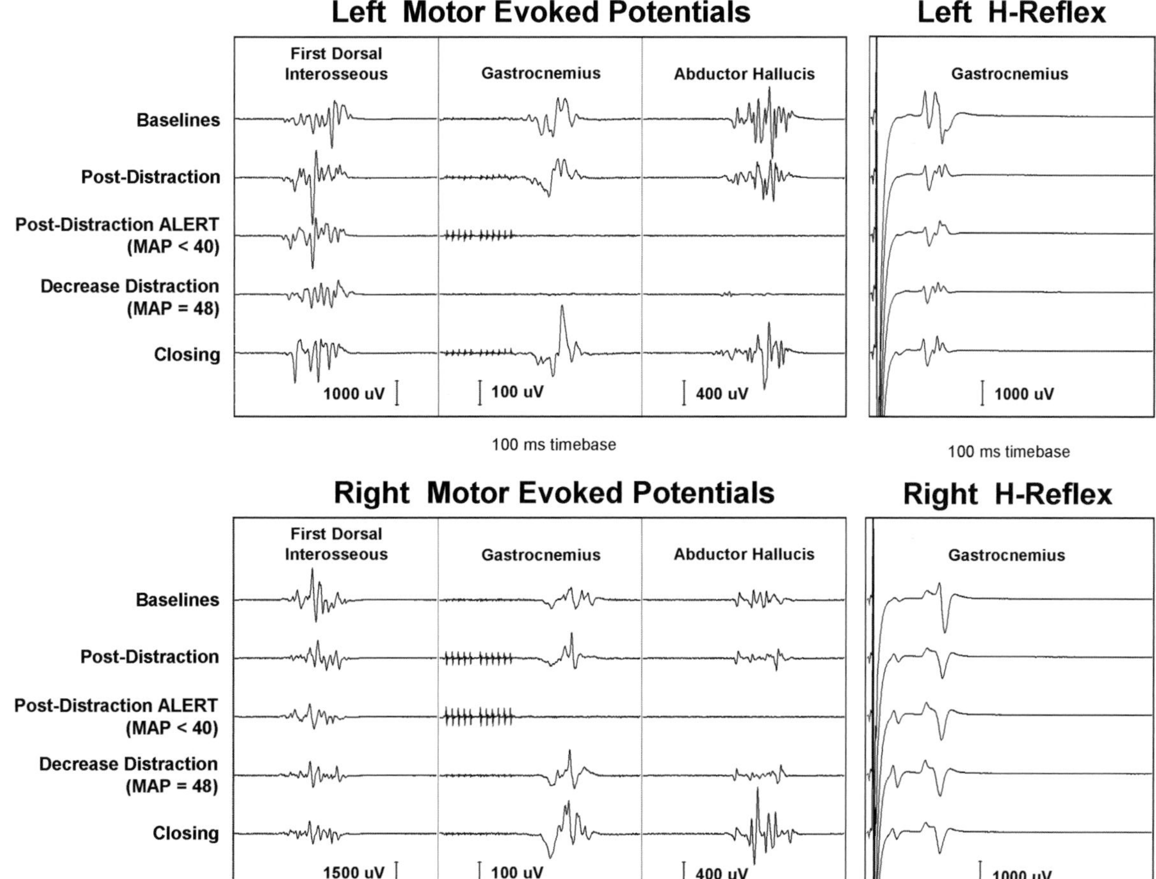

Fig. 40.6 Example of the dissociation between transcranial electrical motor-evoked potentials and H-responses recorded from a 42-month-old female during a third lengthening of growing rod. Note the loss of tceMEPs with no significant change in H-responses

neurological sequelae. In light of such examples, where H-reflex responses have been insensitive to surgical and physiological conditions known to be risk factors for postoperative deficit, we have come to view its role in neuromonitoring somewhat differently from that described by Hicks [11] or Toleikis et al [37].

Unlike tceMEPs which are both highly sensitive and specific for evolving spinal cord injury, the H-reflex appears to be more specific than being sensitive. That is, while presence of the H-wave cannot be equated to a prediction of no neurological injury, acute loss of the response could point to spinal shock. For that reason, we would caution not to view the H-reflex as a substitute for tceMEP monitoring, but rather as an adjunct. Moreover, in the presence of discrepancy between the results of the two monitoring modalities, greater interpretive weight should be given to tceMEP findings. To be sure, it is not a "new standard" as posited by Toleikis and Toleikis [37].

40.3.3 Neurogenic-Evoked Potentials Are Sensory Not Motor

There is considerable evidence dating back to 1992 that NMEP predominantly reflects the functional integrity of posterior column sensory tracts rather than anterior column motor pathways [5, 6, 17, 18, 21, 23, 33, 35]. The general conclusion drawn from these studies is that the NMEP is triggered by antidromic activation of posterior column sensory fibers that communicate with alpha motor neurons via collateral branches at a segmental level. Thus, NMEPs are insensitive to a wide variety of surgical and vascular insults to the motor tracts of the spinal cord by virtue of the sensory pathways that mediate them. As such, it may be more appropriate to label these responses NSEPs (neurogenic sensory-evoked potentials) or DASEPs (descending antidromic sensory-evoked potentials).

Despite the body of evidence pointing to a sensory origin for the NMEP, it continues to have its proponents as a viable technique for monitoring the spinal cord [3, 34]. While there is a general consensus in the surgical neurophysiology community that its use in place of the tceMEP provides a false sense of protection for spinal cord motor tract function, the ultimate decision to continue monitoring with NMEPs lies with the neurophysiological monitoring personnel and surgeons at each hospital facility [7].

In our experience, neurogenic-evoked potentials have played a limited role as an adjunctive modality for monitoring spinal cord sensory function, since we began the routine use of tceMEPs to monitor the motor tracts over 15 years ago. The contribution of neurogenic-evoked potentials is further limited by observations that they can disappear in the presence of rigid spinal instrumentation due to current shunting [25]. This creates interpretative ambiguity for the neuromonitoring professional and can result in a false-positive result just at the time of deformity correction, leading to unnecessary intervention.

40.3.4 Monitoring Spinal Nerve Roots

To the extent that growing rods are anchored to the spine with pedicle screws, individual spinal nerve roots may be at risk of injury from medial pedicle breaches and should be monitored using spontaneous and electrically-stimulated electromyography, as well as tceMEPs [19]. The principles and techniques for testing pedicle screw placement with electrical stimulation, which have been described in detail for the mature spine in numerous publications, are equally applicable to the growing spine. Note that stimulation threshold criteria for detection of medial pedicle breaches may have to be adjusted downwards from those reported for adults to account for smaller pedicles in children.

40.3.5 Monitoring the Brachial Plexus

There has been recent interest in the evaluation of patients who have a congenital spinal deformity together with chest-wall abnormalities leading to thoracic insufficiency syndrome. The VEPTR has been effectively utilized for the treatment of these challenging patients by expanding the chest during the growing years to allow for maximum lung development, while also treating the spinal deformity. As is common with a new technique, there is a debate on the value of intraoperative neuromonitoring during VEPTR surgery.

The most commonly reported neurological complication during VEPTR procedures is brachial plexus injury [2, 9, 31]. In a multicenter investigation on the use of neuromonitoring, Skaggs et al. [31] reported that 8 of 299 (2.3%) children presented with new onset postoperative neurologic sequelae. Of these, 6 patients showed deficits limited to the upper extremities, which resolved within 12 months for 5 patients and were incompletely resolved after four years for the sixth. They emphasized two potential underlying causes. First, the brachial plexus often drapes over the first rib and may be subject to compression or entrapment during VEPTR expansion; therefore, they recommended that the device not be placed at this level. Second, while lifting the scapula, pressure may be applied inadvertently to the brachial plexus, particularly in patients with a hypoplastic chest, requiring adjustment of retractive forces when alerted by neuromonitoring changes.

Risk to the brachial plexus and other upper extremity peripheral nerves is not limited to VEPTR procedures. Fig. 40.7 shows one example of unilateral tceMEP and upper extremity SSEP loss in a 5-year-old female undergoing growing rod lengthening. Her status was post Chiari decompression and repair of myelomeningocele.

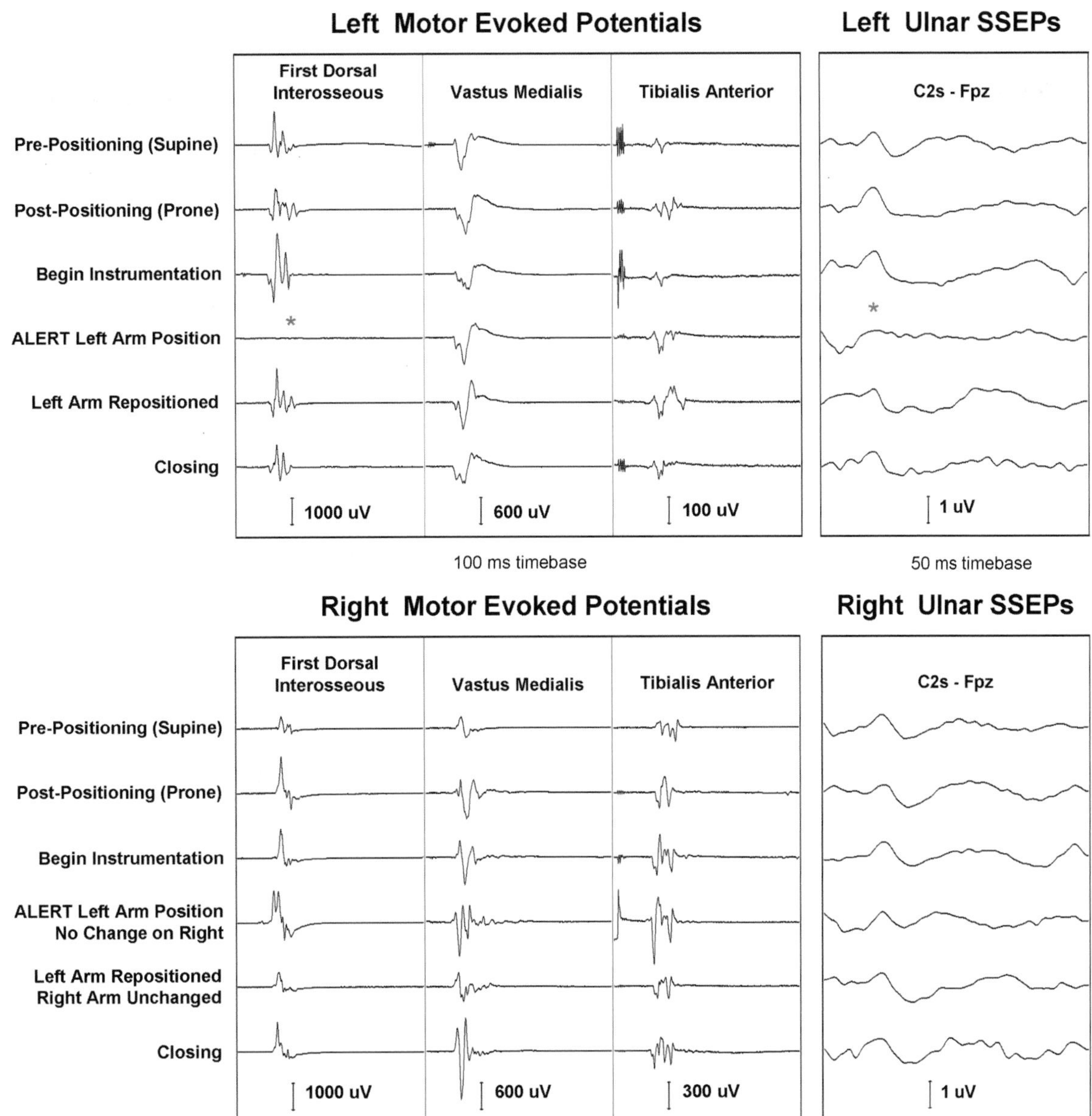

Fig. 40.7 Example of unilateral tceMEP and upper extremity SSEP loss in a 5-year-old female undergoing growing rod lengthening indicative of emerging brachial plexopathy

During hook placement, there was an acute tceMEP amplitude decrease followed by complete loss over the left first dorsal interosseous muscle (FDI) recording site, accompanied by a > 60% drop of the left ulnar nerve SSEP. Unchanged tceMEPs from both legs and the right hand pointed to the left upper extremity as the site of emerging injury. Upon repositioning the left arm, both the tceMEP and SSEP responses returned to baseline.

In our experience, one of the tangential benefits of intraoperative neuromonitoring is the detection of impending brachial plexopathy or other peripheral neuropathies [27, 30]. As in the case of the spinal cord, monitoring sensitivity for peripheral nerve injury is improved by using both sensory- and motor-evoked potential modalities [29].

40.3.6 Anesthesia Considerations

The role of anesthesia for optimized delivery of IONM care has been both underestimated and misunderstood by many. IONM personnel all too often have an inadequate understanding of the goals of anesthesia and the pharmacodynamics of different anesthetic agents, as well as how each agent interferes with the generation of neurophysiologic signals. Likewise, it is not uncommon for the anesthesiologist or nurse anesthetist to have an equally poor appreciation of the influence of such agents and their aggregate effect on the neurophysiologic signals.

All general anesthetic agents depress synaptic function in the brain and spinal cord gray matter, resulting in amplitude suppression of neurophysiologic signals that cross those synapses. The goal, then, is to meet the conventional anesthetic requirements of amnesia, hypnosis, analgesia, and akinesis without compromising neurophysiological signals to the point where they are too small or variable for meaningful interpretation.

Inhaled volatile agents such as isoflurane, desflurane, sevoflurane, as well as nitrous oxide, present the greatest challenges of synaptic suppression and consequent depression of cortical SSEP and tceMEP amplitudes [4, 8, 13, 15, 20, 24, 26, 32]. While some claim to be able to record neurophysiological signals in the presence of these potent anesthetics, they do so under suboptimal conditions, even when the agents are present at low levels of concentration. In these situations, there is maximal opportunity for interpretive ambiguity or overall inability to monitor, owing to the fact that the signal amplitudes are either near the physiologic noise floor or completely absent [36]. Schwartz et al. [26] have stated that the use of these potent anesthetic agents (and nitrous-oxide) is perhaps the biggest reason why many surgeons and neuromonitoring personnel complain of an inability to record stable and acceptably large-amplitude tceMEPs.

To circumvent the amplitude-suppressive effects of these inhalational agents and nitrous oxide, we transitioned to a propofol-narcotic total intravenous anesthetic technique soon after Diprivan (propofol) was introduced some 25 years ago, initially, to optimize cortical SSEPs, and later, transcranial electric motor-evoked potentials. Using constant infusion delivery, average propofol concentrations of 150 μg/kg/min, in combination with remifentanil (0.2–0.5 μg/kg/min) and intermittent dosing of midazolam (0.1–0.2 mg/kg) provide adequate amnesia, hypnosis, and analgesia for the majority of spine patients, both pediatric and adult, without compromising tceMEP and cortical SSEP amplitudes. (Caveat: propofol infusion rates that cause burst suppression on EEG will have significant depressive effects both on cortical SSEP and tceMEP amplitudes, similar to inhalational anesthetics; therefore, it is best to maintain a range between 125 and 175 μg/kg/min.)

Drugs which act at the neuromuscular junction have profound effects on tceMEP and EMG monitoring, both of which depend on nerve root depolarization and innervated muscle contraction. Any use of neuromuscular blockade either will diminish tceMEP amplitude significantly or abolish the response completely. In keeping with the theory of maximizing neurophysiological response amplitudes to optimize interpretation of signal change, no muscle relaxants should be used except to facilitate intubation.

Recently, dexmedetomidine, an α-2 agonist, has been suggested as an anesthetic adjuvant during spine surgery because of its sedative, analgesic, and neuroprotective properties [22]. Adding dexmedetomidine also enables reduction of propofol requirements, which helps facilitate more rapid emergence at the conclusion of surgery. We have been evaluating the effects of dexmedetomidine on tceMEP and cortical SSEP amplitudes over the last few years. In general, a marked dose-dependent suppression of tceMEP amplitudes without concomitant changes in cortical

SSEP amplitudes has been observed when holding propofol steady at 100 μg/kg/min and varying the dexmedetomidine infusion rate between 0.2 and 0.7 μg/kg/hr [22]. Until the effects of dexmedetomidine on tceMEP amplitudes are better understood, it is best to titrate infusion rates for each individual patient by establishing the threshold at which tceMEP amplitudes begin to decrease.

40.3.7 Hemodynamic Considerations

Nonanesthetic factors that can influence the size of neurophysiologic signals include spinal cord perfusion pressure, mean arterial blood pressure, hematocrit, and blood volume. Although regulation of spinal cord perfusion is not as well understood as its cerebral perfusion counterpart, similar principals seem to apply (for further discussion see Chap. 39). Hence, decreases in mean arterial blood pressure below the autoregulation threshold for adequate spinal cord perfusion will result in a significant decrease in tceMEP amplitudes. We believe that if spinal cord blood flow and the associated delivery of oxygen and nutrients to neural tissue are reduced around the same time when spinal corrective maneuvers (i.e. growing rod lengthening) are applied, there may be increased risk of spinal cord injury.

All too often, we have noticed that children undergoing surgery for scoliosis correction are volume-depleted both prior to and during surgery. This challenges maintenance of a recommended mean arterial blood pressure, preferably 65 mmHg or more, to ensure adequate spinal cord perfusion pressure during deformity correction. Treatment of the ensuing hypotension with an alpha-agonist such as phenylephrine usually offers only temporary relief by elevating blood pressure transiently and thus increasing tceMEP amplitudes. What follows, however, is a picket-fence phenomenon, where the mean pressure drops again, as do tceMEP amplitudes, until pharmacologic intervention is reinitiated. It is usually more productive to address issues related to volume depletion, blood loss, and hematocrit proactively rather than reactively. Given the sensitivity of the spinal cord to ischemic injury, avoidance of prolonged controlled hypotension as a strategy for minimizing intraoperative blood loss is highly recommended.

40.4 Conclusions

The use of intraoperative neuromonitoring during growing rod and VEPTR procedures is still debatable. Our experience has been that neuromonitoring serves a valuable purpose and is well-justified for routine use both during initial implant placement and subsequent adjustment. The sensitivity of tceMEPs to emerging spinal cord injury has been well established; however, the value of neuromonitoring for the detection of brachial plexus and other positionally related peripheral nerve injuries during these procedures should not be underestimated.

References

1. Bose, B, Sestokas AK, Schwartz DM (2007) Neurophysiological detection of iatrogenic C5 nerve injury during anterior cervical spine surgery. J Neurosurg 6:381–385
2. Campbell RM Jr, Smith MD, Mayes TC et al (2004) The effects of opening wedge thoracostomy on thoracic insufficiency syndrome associated with fused ribs and congenital scoliosis. J Bone Joint Surg Am 86-A(8):1659–1674
3. Cheh G, Lenke LG, Padberg AM et al (2008) Loss of spinal cord monitoring signals in children during thoracic kyphosis correction with spinal osteotomy: why does it occur and what should you do? Spine 33:1093–1099
4. Chen Z (2004) The effects of isoflurane and propofol on intraoperative neurophysiological monitoring during spinal surgery. J Clin Monit Comp 18:303–308
5. Deletis V (1993) Intraoperative monitoring of the functional integrity of the motor pathways. In: Devinski O, Berie A, Dogali M (eds) Electrical and magnetic stimulation of the brain and spinal cord. Advances in neurology, vol 63. Raven, New York, pp 201–214
6. Deletis V (2001) The "motor" inaccuracy in neurogenic motor evoked potentials. [Editorial]. Clin Neurophys 112:1365–1366
7. Devlin VJ, Schwartz DM (2007) Intraoperative neurophysiologic monitoring during spinal surgery. J Am Acad Orthop Surg 15:549–560
8. DiCindio S, Schwartz DM (2005) Anesthetic management for pediatric spinal fusion: implications of advances in spinal cord monitoring. Anesthesiol Clin N Am 23:765–787
9. Emans JB, Caubet, Francois J et al (2005) The treatment of spine and chest wall deformities with fused ribs by expansion thoracostomy and insertion of vertical expandable prosthetic titanium rib: growth of thoracic spine and improvement of lung volumes. Spine 30:S58–S68
10. Fan D, Schwartz D, Vaccaro A et al (2002) Intraoperative neurophysiologic detection of iatrogenic C5 nerve root injury during laminectomy for cervical compression myelopathy. Spine 27(22):2499–2502

11. Hicks G (2006) The intraoperative gastrocnemius H-reflex predicts post-anesthetic clonus in patients during surgeries of the spine. J Clin Monit Comp 20:59(A)
12. Hilibrand A, Schwartz D, Sethuraman V et al (2004) Comparison of transcranial electric motor and somatosensory evoked potential monitoring during cervical spine surgery. J Bone Joint Surg Am 86:1248–1253
13. Kalkman CJ, Traast H, Zuurmond WW et al (1991) Differential effects of propofol and nitrous-oxide on posterior tibial nerve cortical somatosensory evoked potentials during alfentanil anesthesia. Br J Anaesth 66:483–489
14. Kelleher MO, Tan G, Sarjeant R et al (2008) Predictive value of intraoperative neurophysiological monitoring during cervical spine surgery: a prospective analysis of 1055 consecutive patients. J Neurosurg: Spine 8:215–221
15. Kincaid MS, Souter MJ, Bryan PD et al (2007) Somatosensory and motor evoked potentials during sevoflurane and propofol anesthesia. Paper Presented at the Annual Meeting of the American Society of Anesthesiologists. San Francisco
16. Leppanen R, Maguire J, Wallace S et al (1995) Intraoperative lower extremity muscle activity as an adjunct to conventional somatosensory evoked potentials and descending neurogenic monitoring in idiopathic scoliosis. Spine 20:1872–1877
17. Leppanen R, Madigan R, Sears C et al (1999) Intraoperative collision studies demonstrate descending spinal cord stimulated evoked potentials are mediated through common pathways. J Cin Neurphysiol 16:170
18. Leppanen R (2004) From the electrodiagnostic lab … Where we see that spinal cord stimulated descending neurogenic evoked potentials(DNEPs) are mediated by antidromic sensory rather than motor systems. Spine J 4(6):712–715
19. Lieberman JA, Lyon R, Feiner J et al (2008) The efficacy of motor evoked potentials in fixed sagital imbalance deformity correction surgery. Spine 33:414–424
20. Liu FHC, Wong HK, Chia CP et al (2005) Effects of isoflurane and propofol on cortical somatosensory evoked potentials during comparable depth of anaesthesia as guided by bispectral index. Brit J Anaesth 94:193–197
21. MacDonald DB (2006) Intraoperative motor evoked potential monitoring: update and overview. J Clin Monit Comput 20:348
22. Mahmoud M, Senthikumar S, Sestokas AK et al (2007) Loss of transcrabnial motor evoked potentials during pediatric spine surgery with dexmedetomidine. Anesthesiology 106:393–396
23. Minahan RE, Sepkuty JP, Lesser RP et al (2001) Anterior spinal cord injury with preserved neurogenic 'motor' evoked potentials. Clin Neurophysiol 112:1442–1450
24. Scheufler K-M, Zentner J (2002) Total intravenous anesthesia for intraoperative monitoring of motor pathways: an integral view combining clinical and experimental data. J Neurosurg 96:571–579
25. Schwartz DM, Drummond D, Ecker M (1996) Influence of rigid spinal instrumentation on the neurogenic motor evoked potential. J Spine Dis 9:439–445
26. Schwartz DM, Schwartz JA, Pratt RE et al (1997) Influence of nitrous-oxide on posterior tibial nerve cortical somatosensory evoked potentials. J Spin Disord 10:80–86
27. Schwartz D, Drummond D, Hahn M et al (2000) Prevention of positional brachial plexopathy during surgical correction of scoliosis. J Spinal Dis 13(2):178–182
28. Schwartz D, Sestokas A (2002) A systems-based algorithmic approach to intraoperative neurophysiological monitoring during spinal surgery. Sem Spine Surg 14(2):36–145
29. Schwartz D, Albert T, Sestokas et al (2006) Neurophysiological identification of position-induced neurologic injury during anterior cervical spine surgery. J Clin Mont Comput 20(6):437–444
30. Schwartz DM, Auerbach JD, Dormans JP et al (2007) Neurophysiologic detection of impending spinal cord injury during surgery for adolescent idiopathic scoliosis: a comparison of transcranial electric motor and somatosensory evoked potential monitoring. J Bone Joint Surg 89: 2440–2449
31. Skaggs DL, Choi PD, Rice C, Emans J, Song KM, Smith JT, Campbell RM (2009) Efficacy of intraoperative neurologic monitoring in surgery involving a vertical expandable prosthetic titanium rib for early-onset spinal deformity. J Bone Joint Surg Am 91:1657–1663
32. Sloan TB, Heyer EJ (2002) Anesthesia for intraoperative physiologic monitoring of the spinal cord. J Clin Neurophys 19:430–443
33. Su CF, Hahhighi SS, Oro JJ et al (1992) "Backfiring" in spinal cord monitoring. High thoracic spinal cord stimulation evoked sciatic response by antidromic sensory pathway conduction, not motor tract conduction. Spine 17: 504–508
34. Succato DJ (2008) In response to Devlin VJ, Schwartz DM: Inraoperative monitoring during spinal surgery. Letter to the Editor. J Am Acad Orthop Surg 16:61–62
35. Toleikis J, Skelly J, Carlvin A et al (2000) Spinally elicited peripheral nerve responses are sensory rather than motor. Clin Neurophysiol 111:736–742
36. Toleikis JR, Toleikis SC, Braverman B (2006) Monitoring motor evoked potentials: is TIVA really necessary. J Clin Monit Comp 20(A):64–65
37. Toleikis JR, Toleikis SC (2007) Intraoperative monitoring of spinal cord function with H-reflex responses: The new standard. Paper presented at the Annual Meeting of the American Society of Anesthesiologists. pp 13–17

41 Nursing Care

Patricia Kostial, Connie Poe-Kochert, and Phyllis D'Ambra

Key Points

- Patient and family education by the nurse or similar health care professional is critical to improve the quality of care.
- To become a valuable member of the team, nurses caring for children with complex early onset scoliosis should attempt to learn as much as possible using all available resources.
- Well informed nurses can help surgeons to provide early detection of potential complications.
- Treatment of early onset scoliosis is a long-term commitment by the family and the medical team and nursing support is essential.

41.1 Overview

Early onset scoliosis (EOS) is a less common but often progressive scoliosis subtype. The etiology of EOS can vary, and diagnoses include infantile idiopathic scoliosis (IIS – diagnosed through 3 years of age), juvenile idiopathic scoliosis (JIS – diagnosed between 4 and 10 years of age), neuromuscular, congenital, neurofibromatosis (NF), thoracogenic, and syndromic scoliosis (Marfan, etc.).

Progressive scoliosis in early childhood can lead to serious health problems that comprise pulmonary, including Thoracic Insufficiency Syndrome [4] and severe spinal deformity. As a result of these potential problems, early treatment is important. Nonoperative care may be ineffective and may increase pulmonary risks in some groups. Traditional operative treatment has included spinal fusion, which itself can cause problems including growth arrest of the spine, restriction of the thorax and lung development, as well as potential crankshaft of the spine (asymmetrical growth of the anterior spinal column in the presence of a posterior spinal fusion which creates a tethering of the posterior column). Growing rods and VEPTR (vertical expandable titanium rib prosthesis) for the treatment of EOS have been studied, and early results have documented scoliotic curve improvement and maintenance as well as spinal, thorax, and lung growth [1, 3, 8].

The care for children with EOS is demanding not only on the child, but the parents and family members who must deal with the long-term aspects of not only the treatment, but in many cases, the other medical problems stemming from their disease process. The role of the nurse is critical in assessing, evaluating, and providing appropriate care at the appropriate time.

41.2 Family Education

Often, families of children with progressive EOS have obtained multiple surgical opinions for their child's care. It is not uncommon for these surgical opinions to vary, thus leading to frustration on the parents' part due to the lack of evidence-based information available to them. Fortunately, the number of scientific presentations and publications has started to grow over the past few years, increasing the knowledge of the results, albeit short-term, of the current treatment methods available. Families should strongly consider going to a center that is actively involved in the treatment of EOS, including participation in the research needed to answer

P. Kostial (✉)
San Diego Center for Spinal Disorders, 4130 La Jolla Village Drive, Suite 300, La Jolla, CA 92037, USA
e-mail: pkostial@sandiego-spine.com

B. A. Akbarnia et al. (eds.), *The Growing Spine*,
DOI: 10.1007/978-3-540-85207-0_41,

the complex questions stemming from this medical problem. Once the family has been evaluated by a surgeon at such a center, family education can then be initiated both by the surgeon and his or her educational liaison.

Regardless of the recommended treatment (nonoperative vs. operative), the family must remember that EOS treatment is a long-term commitment on the part of the child and the family. Whether the treatment involves serial cast applications, bracing, surgical placement and lengthening of Growing Rods or VEPTR device, etc., the care of the child must be consistent until the end of the treatment period. This can be quite daunting to the family, especially if treatment is recommended at a very young age. In addition, the child's family must be fully aware of the treatment options, the benefits and risks (potential complications) of each option, and the anticipated treatment period (in years). Willingness to commit to long-term care must be expressed by the parents in order to move forward with any treatment program.

Many of the EOS centers are now study sites of the Growing Spine Study Group (GSSG), a group of spine surgeons located around the world, who are committed to learning the most effective and safe ways to treat EOS and other early onset spinal deformities. As a result, part of the educational process will be to ask the family to consent to having their child participate in prospective studies (involving an ongoing review of the child's medical records and diagnostic studies). These centers emphasize that participation in the GSSG's studies will in no way change the care offered to their child, but allows the group to collect observational data on many children over time to better study various current and future treatments, especially by subgroups such as diagnosis, age, etc.

Education for the family must always consider the child first and then the spinal problem. Growth and development milestones are critical at very young ages. Treatment and the education about treatment should keep growth and development in mind, especially in the cognitively normal and ambulatory patient populations. As many of the treatments can be either repetitively invasive or impose upon body image (long-term casting or bracing), keeping the family focused on its child's developmental milestones as well as attempting to maintain balance in the family is important. Other siblings may feel that they are not getting attention due to their "sick" brother or sister. Parents should be reminded to keep the family in focus to avoid this pitfall. Also, many children with EOS may be quite active physically and cognitively, and every effort should be made to allow the child to engage in age-appropriate activities. This will help reduce the child's image of being "sick" or appearing "sick" to others. For example, a child having growing rods inserted may need to wear a special TLSO brace for the first 6 months to allow the bone anchors attached to the spine to heal. After that, the child is weaned out of the brace for the duration of the treatment, which may be many years, and is allowed to do most physical activities. This will help improve the child's self esteem and self image. Parents are reminded that potential risks of this relatively unrestricted activity could result in a problem such as a rod fracture, which is anticipated as a possible treatment outcome and is often treated at the time of the next scheduled lengthening to avoid unnecessary surgery.

Each surgeon and his or her team must establish a rapport with the patient and family for the best long-term success. Families who are well informed about commitment and potential risks are far more cooperative than those who have not been allowed to have an active role along with the treatment-planning team.

It is also important to note that families will likely to go through financial, social, and emotional stress at any time when they deal with a long-term health problem of a family member. The treatment of EOS is no different. Families may find themselves reaching their maximum insurance coverage and having to seek state aid to continue receiving care. The doctor and EOS team need to be very tuned into the family's needs and concerns, and be ready to assist. Counseling may be necessary for those requiring financial, social, or other assistance.

41.3 Nonoperative Care

41.3.1 Bracing

A brace or orthosis is named for the part of the body in which it supports. A thoracic, lumbar, sacral orthosis (TLSO) may be prescribed as a nonoperative treatment for scoliosis. One such brace that may be used in young children is the Kalibus brace (see Chap. 27). The purpose of the brace is to stop the curve from progressing.

To clean, condition, and prevent skin breakdown, rubbing alcohol and cornstarch is applied before each brace application. Rubbing alcohol is applied at the waistline and where the edges of the brace touch the skin, and it dries quickly. Cornstarch is applied to the same areas where the rubbing alcohol was applied to help absorb skin moisture. Do not use creams, lotions, or Band-Aids under the brace because they may cause a rash or skin breakdown. The skin should be observed for areas of redness, irritation, discoloration, or puffiness. This may indicate a need for the brace to be adjusted.

Children can wear any clothes in which they are comfortable. Pants or shorts may need to be one to two sizes larger in order to fit. Jogging suits, bib overalls, and wrap around outfits are comfortable and easy to put on. In general, clothing with elastic waistbands or drawstrings are easier to fit. Looser fitting clothing will usually not reveal the outline of the brace. If a Milwaukee brace is prescribed, turtle necks or scarves can help to cover the neck ring and throat mold. This may also help prevent hair from being caught in the screws on the neck ring.

Physical activity and playing are important for children. All activities are encouraged if the brace is being used as a nonoperative treatment. However, the brace should be removed before swimming, showering, and tub bathing.

41.3.2 Casting

Body casts, such as Risser casts, are another form of nonoperative treatment. The purpose is to stop the curve from progressing. Sometimes, the curve may improve with casting [5, 7].

Parents are usually pleasantly surprised on how well a child adapts to wearing the body cast once the initial adjustment is completed. Parents have commented that the cast is not only more comfortable for their child; it is better tolerated than wearing a brace.

If the cast is utilized as a nonoperative treatment, there are very few restrictions. Most pertain to water: tub baths, showers, or swimming with the cast, are not permitted as the cotton web roll or padding would absorb the water and act as a sponge. Playing around sand is not advised as the sand can easily lodge under the cast and become abrasive. Other restrictions may be disorder-specific.

Stockinet, layers of cotton web roll, and plaster or fiberglass are applied to make a well-molded body cast. Extending the stockinet and web roll over the edges secured to the outside of the cast with staples helps to keep the edges of the cast well padded. This also eliminates the time and need for pedaling the cast with adhesive tape.

Creating an adequate opening in the abdominal area of the cast makes a difference in comfort, tolerance, respirations, digestion, and keeping the skin clean. As children are predominately "abdominal breathers," having an opening in this area is important. It is not uncommon for the abdomen to protrude from the cast, especially after eating.

A common concern of parents is keeping their child clean and preventing the cast from smelling and itching. Although keeping the cast clean and dry can be a challenge for parents of those children who are not toilet-trained, it is possible. Each concern can be addressed by teaching proper skin care.

Moisten a long, narrow cloth with rubbing alcohol. Alcohol is used instead of soap because it cleans, toughens the skin, dries quickly, and does not leave a residue on the skin. Thread the cloth under the cast from the top to the abdominal opening and from the abdominal opening to the bottom of the cast. Move the cloth back and forth over the skin. If the child lies on their abdomen, it creates extra space to clean the skin on the back. Itching under the casts is caused by dead, flaking skin and moisture. Cleaning the skin on a regular basis with rubbing alcohol can prevent itching, as it removes the dead skin. Lotions are not applied because they tend to soften the skin. Loose powders are avoided as they can cake and cause a rash under the cast.

One of the most important aspects of cast care is preventing the cast from becoming wet. The inside of the cast has layers of cotton web roll for padding. If the cotton becomes wet, it is difficult to dry; the child's skin can break down, develop a rash, or become macerated.

Padding the bottom of the cast with chuxs along with tucking the diaper inside the cast goes a long way to prevent wetting and soiling of the cast. Changing the diaper frequently and placing a sanitary pad in the diaper to absorb the urine also is helpful.

The skin around the cast is observed for redness, irritation, discoloration, and puffiness, which indicates the need for cast adjustment. Unusual odor, burning, or discomfort needs to be investigated. If the cast becomes wet, dry the inside using a hair dryer set on low or cool. If the cast has a strong odor, rub the outside of the cast with deodorant powder, baking soda, or Fabreze to help absorb the odor.

There are several ways to shampoo the child's hair:

- Place the child on the kitchen counter, with their head over the sink.
- The child may lean over the bathtub and use a spray hose.
- The child may lie across a bed with the head hanging over the side of the bed.

Arrange a large sheet of plastic (a trash bag cut open) under the head to form a trough for the water to run into a tall wastepaper basket next to the bed. Cover the cast with plastic to prevent it from becoming wet while washing the child's hair.

Clothing tips are the same as for brace use. It is important to note that the child should always wear a T-shirt over the cast to cover the opening at the top of the cast. This will help prevent food or toys from falling inside the cast by accident.

41.4 Operative Care

Traditional spinal fusion can pose problems when performed on the growing spine (and indirectly, the thorax). Fusions limited to a posterior approach only may correct the curve, but growth of the anterior spine in the presence of a posterior fusion (tether) may cause the spine to crankshaft, thus causing increased spinal deformity. Knowing this, a 360° fusion is often considered the treatment of choice, thus arresting the growth of the spine both posteriorly and anteriorly. This method is more effective in controlling the scoliotic deformity, but in very young children, it will also retard spinal, thorax, and lung growth. In some, serious pulmonary disease may result.

The concept of growing rods is not a new one. Harrington [2], the developer of Harrington Rod Instrumentation (HRI) for the treatment of scoliosis caused by the Polio epidemic, recognized the risks inherent in fusing the young pediatric spine. Early attempts of using spinal rods without fusion proved difficult, demonstrating a high rate of complication.

With the evolution of better spinal implants with anchor designs which are more capable to maintaining spinal fixation than their predecessors, growing rod spinal constructs are being used around the globe.

Originally developed as a single rod system, growing rods are most commonly being used as a two (dual) rod system now in the U.S. A recent publication [8] sited the advantages of dual rod over single rod systems, including better maintenance of the curve and better spinal growth. For this reason, the dual growing rod technique is described in this chapter.

Chest-wall deformities can also cause scoliosis and Thoracic Insufficiency Syndrome. For rib distraction-based procedures, VEPTR will be described as the representative technique for treatments directed specifically to chest-wall-related deformities.

The operative techniques for both growing rods and VEPTR are beyond the scope of this chapter (see Chaps. 35, 36 and 37) (Table 41.1).

41.5 Complications

The treatment of EOS, both nonoperative and operative, carries risks. While casting or bracing may seem to be an innocuous form of treatment, skin breakdown can be problematic to the point of discontinuing care in severe cases. Also, thorax growth must always be considered with this treatment to prevent restricting the thorax during critical growth.

Likewise, surgical treatments such as growing rods, VEPTR, and other growth friendly treatments that are intended to control the deformity while allowing growth can also have surgical or medical complications. It is possible for one child to have multiple problems during the treatment period over many years. Implant problems can be minor or major, wound problems, such as deep wound infection may require long-term antibiotic treatment to avoid removal of the implants. Well informed nurses can help surgeons to provide early detection of potential complications.

41.6 Preoperative Teaching

41.6.1 Growing Rods

The surgeon and his/her liaison should attempt to initiate education regarding treatment options with the family well before preoperative planning, if possible. This will help build trust between the surgical and patient/family team members. A close rapport between the medical team and the family is the goal. This will

Table 41.1 Information on patient care with respect to nonfusion techniques

	Placement of growing rod	Lengthening	Placement of VEPTR	VEPTR lengthening
Length of stay	4–5 days	ASU* <23 h	5–7 days	ASU* <23 h
Length of surgery	5 h	30–60 min	4–5 h	30–60 min
Pre op labs	CBC, basic chemistry	None	CBC, basic chemistry	None
	Type and screen; T and C for directed donation		Type and screen; T and C for directed donation	
	U.A. for neuromuscular patients		U.A. for neuromuscular patients	
Pre op tests	PA and Lat spine	PA and Lat spine	PA and Lat spine	PA and Lat spine
	Side bending; traction		Side bending; traction	
	CT of the thorax		CT of the thorax	
	MRI		MRI	
	PFT, EKG		PFT, EKG	
Tubes placed	2 IV's, foley catheter, E.T. Tube	1 IV	2 IV's, foley catheter, E.T. Tube	1 IV
	Central or arterial line, if needed	E.T. Tube	Central or arterial line, if needed	E.T. Tube
	Hemovac		Hemovac	
	MSO4, ativan	Marcaine in surgery; tylenol #3	Morphine IV, OnQ, to PCA for the older child	Marcaine in surgery; tylenol # 3
Pain meds	Tylenol #3	Zofran for nausea		Zofran for nausea
Return to school	2–3 weeks	3–5 days	2–4 weeks	5–7 days

*Ambulatory Surgical Unit

be helpful to all over time as care progresses and especially if a complication should develop.

Education should be ongoing throughout the treatment plan, but is critical prior to the first surgery. Written material, if available, should be provided to the family as well to assist in the retention of the complex information provided.

The goals of treatment need to be emphasized throughout the treatment plan. For the growing rod treatment, curve control and allowance of spinal growth over time are the main objectives. Details of the initial surgery including the implant components, what they are, their function initially and over time, the need for temporary external immobilization (surgeon's choice), what to expect before, during and after the surgery, the length of the surgery (approximately 5 h for the initial surgery and 30–60 min for a lengthening), the length of the hospital stay (4–5 days for the initial surgery and up to 23 h for a lengthening), home care instructions, benefits, risks, and anticipated outcomes of the initial and all treatment procedures need to be communicated at this time. Attention to any unique patient/family needs should also be addressed and the family assured that its needs are being considered. Any necessary medical clearance requirements from other specialists should be obtained and discussed with the family as well. If the family requires any other special services, financial or otherwise, it is best to set this up prior to the first surgery.

Discussion regarding ongoing care is equally important, including the need for frequent lengthening until the child is no longer benefiting from the treatment, or otherwise must be stopped for medical reasons. If a final fusion is likely needed at the end of the treatment period, this must also be included in the preoperative education with the family. Knowledge of the complete treatment plan is critical for trust between the surgeon and the family. Complication risks, especially those that are anticipated such as rod fracture, need to be explained to the family, and depending on the circumstances, will be addressed during a planned or unplanned surgery. The surgeon needs to communicate that it is likely for a complication to occur at some point during the treatment and rapid communication from the family to the surgeon followed by complete evaluation and explanation of the problem and the anticipated treatment from the surgeon to the family is very important.

If the patient/family is being asked to participate in a clinical study, this is the time to present the details of the study to the family, including all required HIPAA and IRB consent documents, so the family will feel at ease about the nature of the study and does not feel they are being pressured to participate. All educational and study consents provided to the family for signature should be given to the family, in copy form, to keep as part of their educational records.

Lastly, having one person on the team as the liaison between the surgeon and family is very important in promoting trust, rapport, and communication as the child's treatment progresses over time.

41.6.2 VEPTR

Campbell and Smith, developed the VEPTR program. This program was designed to treat children with congenital disease that includes congenital scoliosis with or without vertebral anomalies and/or fused or absent ribs. The chest-wall deformity due to anomalies of ribs causes thoracic insufficiency which leads to lung failure. There are a variety of disorders that cause thoracic insufficiency including Jeune's, Vater, and more. Surgery includes treating the congenital scoliosis and addressing the chest-wall deformity.

The population of children that this procedure is designed for is usually very ill. Some children are ventilator-dependent and may have a tracheostomy as well as have feeding problems. The procedure, which includes cutting the ribs and placing rods for future expansion, is difficult and requires specialized training by the physician. Children undergoing VEPTR will have multiple hospitalizations.

Presented with the potential complexity of the orthopaedic intervention in the treatment of these children, the nurse becomes acutely aware of the importance of her first-line observations. Management of the patient at any phase of treatment demands knowledge and skills so that complications are reduced and therapeutic effect can be achieved.

From the moment of introduction to the family regarding hospitalization, the nursing approach determines the degree of patient and family participation, understanding, and cooperation.

Reduction of fear through a well-thought out orientation can ease the patient and family through what otherwise could be a very traumatic experience. Physiologic responses have a direct relationship to compliance. Stressful experiences do not elicit patient or family compliance.

A surgical plan of care that introduces sophisticated mechanical devices and equipment requires a nursing practitioner, or similar liaison, who is skilled in the intricacies of observation, maintenance of equipment and problem-solving. Corrective action must be superseded by correct application of principles. Problems should be solved by appropriate and timely intervention.

Nursing must emerge as a body of knowledge that supplements assessment, develops a standard of care outlining the individuals needs with the task at hand, and continually seeks to reassess the consumers responses and anticipate outcomes.

The VEPTR patient population will have repeated procedures over the course of their lifetime. Planned actions need to be established, assuring that the surgical corrections and hospitalization are both seen by the patient and family as growth experiences. The treatment will span years. Sacrifice and cooperation will be needed by all members of the family unit. The nurse becomes the pivotal part of the team by helping the family and patient bridge the gap between knowledge and inexperience.

The preoperative evaluation and conference becomes the vehicle to bridge the knowledge deficit and secure trust in the team and anticipate outcomes in relationship to understanding, acceptance, and follow-up.

41.7 Preoperative Planning (All Techniques)

41.7.1 Preoperative Testing: Initial Surgery

Thorough preoperative planning, teaching, and testing are important for surgery, recovery, and to reduce the risk of complications. Preoperative testing can be completed 1–3 weeks before surgery, in most cases.

Preoperative testing usually includes lab work: Complete blood count (CBC) and Type and Screen (T and S). Other labs including basic chemistry, coagulation, and nutritional panel is usually driven by the patient's disease process and need.

Radiological examinations include: Posterior–anterior (PA) and lateral views of the entire spine (sitting if the patient is unable to stand), supine right and left maximum bending views, and a traction film before or after the patient is anesthetized. Magnetic resonance imaging (MRI) of the entire spine should be obtained (if it was not completed prior) to rule out intra-spinal abnormalities such as tethered cord, congenital components, Arnold Chiari malformation, or syrinx [6]. The MRI may need to be obtained under sedation or general anesthesia as many of the patients are very young and/or unable to cooperate or hold still for extended period of time. Computed tomography (CT) scan of the thorax assists in assessing for thoracic insufficiency [4].

Consultations and tests from other medical services such as cardiology or pulmonary may be necessary depending on the child's co-morbidities. Surgery may need to be postponed if the patient is not medically cleared for surgery until the cause is determined and treated.

41.7.2 Preoperative Testing: Lengthening Procedures

Most cases are usually considered outpatient, therefore no lab work or other testing may be necessary, however this will be up to individual surgeon's discretion based on comorbidity issues.

41.8 Perioperative Care

41.8.1 Growing Rods: Initial and Complex Revision Surgery

Once the child is asleep, an endotracheal tube, two large bore intravenous lines, arterial and/or central line, and a Foley catheter are placed. After the surgery is completed, a Hemovac or Jackson Pratt drainage tube is placed.

Patients are positioned prone using the Jackson Frame. If the child is too small for the frame, chest rolls are utilized using two to three surgical towel rolls. The length of the rolls should be from the axilla to the iliac crest. Place the two rolls on top of the folded blankets to make a platform to make room for the endotracheal tube and allow the abdomen to be free of pressure. A folded blanket with a gel pad under thighs keeps the knees free. Two to three blankets with a gel pad are placed under lower legs to keep toes free and knees flexed. Arms are abducted and elbow is flexed 90°. Padding or a folded blanket placed under each arm protects the elbows and arms.

After the initial placement of the growing rods, the orthotist can mold the patient for a TLSO in the operating room while the child is under anesthesia. This allows time for the brace to be completed by the time the patient is ready for discharge.

The nursing care before and after the initial insertion of growing rod(s) is very similar to the nursing care after a posterior spinal fusion. The patient may recover in the Pediatric Intensive Care Unit (PICU) or on a patient division, depending on the co-morbidity of the patient or at the discretion of the surgeon.

41.8.2 VEPTR: Initial and Complex Revision Surgery

The patient is kept in the prone position in the operating room. A Foley catheter is placed. An arterial line will be used and depending on the pulmonary function, the patient may be placed on a ventilator. The procedure can require 3–4 h for the initial implants.

The patient is placed in the lateral decubitus position with the thoracic area prepped and draped free. This exposure allows for the monitoring of the patient and access to the chest wall.

41.8.3 Growing Rods: Lengthening Procedures

Growing-rod lengthening is completed approximately every 6 months. The perioperative care is simpler than the initial placement of the rod(s). As the procedure is short and there is usually very little blood loss and preoperative lab work or other special tests are usually not necessary. Only one IV is required along with an endotracheal tube. A Foley catheter is not needed. Positioning in the operating room is the same as with the placement of the growing rod. Injection of ¼–½% Marcaine in the surgical incision after closure makes a significant difference with pain management. Occasionally, one dose of Morphine may be needed in the PACU. Tylenol #3 is started at home the evening of surgery.

Patients are usually discharged home from the Post Anesthesia Care Unit (PACU). Patients who have tracheostomies and ventilators are observed in the PACU for respiratory issues immediately following surgery.

If none has been developed, they are also discharged from the PACU. If extensive revision of the implants is needed, observation (23 h admit) would be indicated for pain management. Another reason a patient might need to stay overnight or be observed would be related to nausea and vomiting. Administering Zofran during surgery often prevents this. Delaying clear liquids for a few hours after surgery also helps.

41.8.4 VEPTR: Lengthening Procedures

When the patient is admitted for lengthening, it is a 1-day procedure. The patient will have an IV started for pre-op antibiotics. Child Life Therapist will meet the child and family during every admission. Patient is taken to OR and the incision is made for the lengthening. Post-op, the patient goes to Recovery Room with a small dressing at the incision site. Parents will meet patient in the recovery room. The patient will be released home the same day if no problems arise.

41.9 Postoperative Care

41.9.1 Growing Rods: Initial Surgery

Postoperatively, the patient participates in a routine every 2 h which consists of log rolling from side to back to side, isometric exercises, and incentive spirometer or similar respiratory care appropriate for the child's age and ability. Sitting is added on the first or second postoperative day; walking on the second to third day. Ambulating up and down the stairs is permitted. The brace is donned while out of bed and allowed off when showering or lying in bed.

The patient may be NPO for up to 3 days, as it takes 3 days for the GI system to resume normal activity. Once the patient passes flatus, clear liquids are started and the diet is advanced as tolerated. IV fluids should continue until adequate fluid intake by mouth is achieved. If a patient is at nutritional risk, hyper alimentation is advised. It is common for patients to have less appetite for a week after discharge. As a result, temporary weight loss often occurs. Small frequent meals can help encourage adequate nutritional intake. Dulcolax suppositories are given on the second to third postoperative day until the patient has a bowel movement. The Foley catheter is usually removed on the second or third postoperative day.

IV antibiotics are administered for 24–48 h. Standard pain management for patients having posterior spine surgery would be indicated for patients having initial placement of the growing rods including Spinal Duramorph, Morphine IV push, or PCA (for the older child). Supplemental IV Ativan is beneficial to relieve muscular tension or spasms caused by straightening the spine. PO pain meds consisting of Tylenol # 3 or Percocet are initiated once the patient tolerates clear liquids.

Prior to discharge, the patient can take a shower. Tub bathing is usually permitted 7–10 days after discharge, or when the skin incision is healed. Increasing activity with the brace on is encouraged. Ambulating up and down stairs is permitted. Patients often return to school at 2 weeks post discharge. Parents are instructed to call if there is swelling, redness, drainage, or open areas along their child's incision, increase in back pain, fever, or other symptoms that were not present previously. Questions are always encouraged.

A brace or cast may be prescribed after growing rods are first inserted. Skin care and clothing tips are the same whether the brace/cast is utilized, nonoperatively or after surgery. Body contact sports or activities in which one can be pushed, bumped, or jarred should be avoided.

41.9.2 VEPTR: Initial Surgery

The post-op care of the patient with a VEPTR procedure is similar to that of patient with associated co-morbidities who has had growing rods. Post-op, the patient will be in the ICU and placed on a ventilator depending on their pulmonary function. The precaution with these children relates to their level of illness prior to surgery including their limited pulmonary function and feeding disorders. Owing to their preoperative level of health, these children particularly require close observation.

The patient will be NPO until passing flatus. They will require an IV until fluid intake is adequate. They will be allowed to start on clear liquids and progress to solids in 3–4 days. The patient will be placed on a bowel regimen using Miralax, Dulcolax, or suppository until a bowel movement is achieved. The Foley catheter is used for 2–3 days post-op.

The patient will be given antibiotics for 24–48 h post-op. The pain management team is involved with post op medication ranging from morphine IV, OnQ, to PCA for the older child.

Depending on the patient's preoperative ability to ambulate, the patient will be sitting up 1 day after surgery and ambulating with the assistance of P.T. 2–3 days post-op. The patient may have a brace for ambulation that can usually be removed at night when sleeping.

Patients are allowed to shower 7–10 days post-op and have a tub bath 10 days post-op. The patient may ambulate up and down stairs. They may sleep in their regular bed when they go home. Children under the age of 5 years may have a difficult time with pulmonary toilet post-op. It is especially difficult using an incentive spirometer. Having the child blow bubbles has the same effect and the child will embrace this treatment.

Patients usually are discharged in 5–7 days depending on their pulmonary status and pain control. Patients will have a 1-week follow-up appointment with the doctor. They will have access to staff for questions and concerns regarding their home care. Taking a post-op VEPTR patient home can be a frightening experience for a parent, and parents need to know that they have access to medical staff at all times.

Discharge instructions include when to call:

- Fever over 101
- Drainage from wound
- Shoulder asymmetry
- Bump over surgical area
- Uncontrolled pain

41.9.3 Growing Rods: Post Lengthening Care

Patients may ambulate (or if nonambulatory, be up in a wheelchair) at home the first post-op night. Progression to normal activity is encouraged. Many patients return to school within 2–5 days after rod lengthening. Physical education class is permitted except for body contact sports. The back dressing is removed 2 days after surgery. Some patients' skin is sensitive to certain tape. Alternative tapes can be utilized or web roll can be wrapped around the patient to keep the back dressing in place instead of tape. Showering is permitted approximately 4 days after surgery; tub bath approximately 1 week later, or, when incision is healed.

41.9.4 VEPTR: Post Lengthening Care

Patients are instructed to keep incision dry and may resume all activities in 5–7 days. The patient may take a shower 7 days post-op or when suture is cut at incision line. Family is instructed to observe for possible wound infection, implant failure and/or retractable pain. Parents are instructed to look for change in height, shoulder level, and whether implant is prominent. Families have access to their nurse daily and can call with any concerns regarding post-op recovery.

41.9.5 Growing Rods: Post Final Fusion Care

The nursing care post final fusion is the same as posterior spinal fusion and similar in experience to the patient's initial surgery for rod implantation.

Caring for patients and parents having growing rod treatment can be challenging, yet rewarding. Nurses can make a significant difference in the patients' treatment, attitude, and team's problem-solving. As the treatment continues for a long time, the nurse becomes close to the patient and family sharing its struggles and successes.

41.10 Future Treatment: Evolution from Knowledge

With improved techniques including less invasive means of allowing for controlled growth and curve maintenance, such as growth guided techniques or magnetic devices which allow growth without repeated, frequent surgeries, it is believed that children with EOS may be treated earlier than before (40–50° curves at start of treatment vs. 80–90° curves). A question with regard to earlier treatment is will a final fusion be necessary at the end of treatment? It is hypothesized that if early brace treatment for AIS can potentially prevent spinal fusion surgery, early growth friendly procedures might also prevent the need for definitive spinal fusion for those EOS patients in the idiopathic scoliosis population or possibly, all diagnosis groups.

So far, only retrospective study data points to effective curve maintenance and spinal growth over time. Only prospective, long-term analysis will determine if certain children treated with the growing-rod technique and similar techniques may not require final fusion.

The GSSG, acknowledging that more needs to be learned about the care of children with EOS, hopes to address this and many other questions in the future.

References

1. Akbarnia BA, Marks DS, Boachie-Adjei O (2005) Dual growing rod technique for the treatment of progressive early-onset scoliosis: a multicenter study. Spine 30(17 suppl):S46–S57
2. Akbarnia BA (2008) Growing rod technique for the treatment of progressive early-onset scoliosis in fusionless surgery for spine deformity. In: Kim DH, Betz, RR, Huhnsh, Newton Po (eds) Surgery of the pediatric spine, Thieme, New York, pp 810–818
3. Campbell RM, Hell-Vocke A (2003) Growth of the thoracic spine in congenital scoliosis after expansion thoracoplasty. J Bone Joint Surg 85-A(3):409–420
4. Campbell RM, Smith MD, Mayes RC, et al (2003) The characteristics of thoracic insufficiency syndrome associated with fused ribs and congenital scoliosis. J Bone Joint Surg Am 85:399–408
5. Dimeglio A (1993) Growth of the spine before age 5 years. J Pediatr Orthop 1:102–107
6. Gupta P, Lenke LG, Bridwell KH (1998) Incidence of Neural axis abnormalities in infantile and juvenile patients with spinal deformity. Is magnetic resonance image screening necessary? Spine 23:206–210
7. Mehta M (1984) Infantile idiopathic scoliosis. In: Dickson RA, Bradford DS (eds) Management of spinal deformities. Butterworth, London, pp 101–120
8. Thompson GH, Akbarnia BA, Kostial P et al (2005) Comparison of single and dual growing rod techniques followed through definitive surgery: a preliminary study. Spine 30(18):2039–2044

42 Long-Term Effects of Instrumented Fusion in Growing Children

Lawrence G. Lenke

Key Points

- There are rare indications for fusion in patients with early onset (Infantile and very young juvenile) idiopathic scoliosis, except for considering periapical fusions, along with some form of growing instrumentation for those with >90–100° of scoliosis.
- Congenital spine deformities that are amenable to short resection and realignment procedures can often be best treated with concomitant short-segment instrumentation and fusion.
- Patients with actual/impending spinal cord neurological deficit should undergo appropriate spinal decompression along with instrumentation and fusion, regardless of their age.
- Although the goal should always be to obviate/minimize spinal fusion in the skeletally immature patient, there are still many patients/conditions where either a short or more extensive fusion procedure may be in the best interest of the patient's overall health and development. Individual assessment and treatment will always be essential in this patient population.

42.1 Introduction

The control of progressive spinal and chest-wall deformity in young children is an extremely difficult problem. Intuitively, gaining control of a spinal deformity and limiting progression while maximizing the ultimate growth potential of the entire spinal column and ribcage would be beneficial. Thus, much effort has been expended in the last decade to apply various growth modulation techniques in order to avoid spinal fusion in young and highly skeletally immature children. However, there certainly are circumstances where fusion may be the best option for these patients, and these limited but extremely important indications will be highlighted in this chapter. In addition, potential long-term consequences of spinal fusion in the young child will be discussed.

42.2 Patient Characteristics

The chronologic separation of idiopathic scoliosis falls into two categories: **infantile** from birth to 2 years and 11 months, and **juvenile** from the age of 3–9 years and 11 months. There is also an early and late onset scoliosis category which lists the age of 6 years as the distinction between these two groups [5]. As we know that spinal fusion limits the axial spinal column growth and ultimate height, the younger the patient, the more detrimental the spinal fusion. In addition, as retarded spine growth also limits trunk and ribcage growth, fusion also has a potentially significant detrimental effect on pulmonary development, chest volume, and function. We know that alveolar growth is rapid and continues until the age of 8 years; however, ultimate

L. G. Lenke
Washington University School of Medicine,
660 South Euclid Avenue, Campus Box 8233, St. Louis,
MO 63110, USA
e-mail: lenkel@wudosis.wustl.edu

B. A. Akbarnia et al. (eds.), *The Growing Spine*,
DOI: 10.1007/978-3-540-85207-0_42, © Springer-Verlag Berlin Heidelberg 2011

pulmonary function increases until the age of 18 years primarily due to the increased thoracic cavity volume [2]. Thus, every effort should be made to maximize the spinal growth in the thoracic region, ultimate spinal column height, and chest wall and ribcage alignment in the very young child. In later juvenile years, this becomes especially important for males versus females, as males tend to develop later and their spine growth often continues until the late teenage years.

Besides chronologic age issues, patient diagnosis becomes extremely important as well. Although infantile idiopathic scoliosis (IIS), as well as juvenile idiopathic scoliosis (JIS) are the prototype diagnostic categories for the young child with a spinal deformity, there are also quite a number of other diagnoses seen in children with progressive spinal deformity. These include congenital spine and/or rib deformities, various types of genetic syndromes such as neurofibromatosis, connective tissue disorders such as Marfan and Ehlers-Danlos syndromes, bone dysplasias such as Hurler's syndrome, neuromuscular disorders such as cerebral palsy and myelodysplasia, and those that fall under the "exotic" category of unusual spinal abnormalities and rare diagnostic categories such as prune-belly syndrome.

42.2.1 Infantile Idiopathic Scoliosis

In those patients who present with a spinal deformity under the age of 3 years, there are very few indications to consider fusion in these very young patients with otherwise idiopathic curves [1]. Although there is a tendency to avoid any type of apical fusion in patients with rather severe IIS deformities, in the past, this was a viable option and may still be so today [9]. However, this would be reserved for patients with curves over 90–100°, and in very selective and individualized circumstances (Fig. 42.1a–h). If surgery is contemplated in an IIS patient with a severe deformity, we strongly recommend a period of halo-gravity traction prior to any surgical intervention for maximal spinal correction in this patient group that have very small vertebrae and relative osteoporosis due to their small stature. Following several weeks of halo-gravity traction, a circumferential apical fusion of 3–5 levels may be performed with the posterior application of some type of growing rod construct covering the full extent of the scoliosis deformity. The goal of treatment would be continued growth of the areas cephalad and caudad to the apex following consolidation of the apical fusion. It is important to minimize the number of thoracic levels fused for reasons mentioned earlier, especially with reference to the pulmonary system and development. One can argue that a posterior-only growing rod or a chest-wall growing system would be a better option for these patients. However, in patients having a severe deformity such that the rotated apex nearly touches the lateral ribcage, the risk of crankshaft phenomenon with posterior-only application of instrumentation is still extremely high. Another alternative would be a limited convex hemiepiphysiodesis anteriorly and a hemiarthrodesis posteriorly. However, in a severely rotated deformity, it is extremely difficult to know where the true "convexity" of the disc is at the apex because of the severe deformity. Thus, proceeding to a full growth arrest via a circumferential fusion may be the best option.

42.2.2 Juvenile Idiopathic Scoliosis

As the chronologic age of the patient increases, the indications for spinal fusion with progressive deformity increase as well. Although a juvenile becomes an adolescent at 10 years of age, performing a spinal fusion for progressive scoliosis in a 9-year-old female would seem very reasonable for many surgeons. One definite concern with the procedure is whether a circumferential approach is needed to resist the crankshaft phenomenon in these skeletally immature patients [3]. This concern has lead to three surgical techniques: a traditional anterior as well as posterior fusion with posterior instrumentation, an anterior instrumented fusion if feasible, and more recently, a posterior fusion utilizing segmental pedicle screw fixation. Although there are no good long-term studies demonstrating the efficacy of this last approach, it is being performed in many centers by many surgeons throughout the world, who utilize pedicle screw constructs routinely. For an older juvenile patient with a very severe deformity, it is probably best to consider a circumferential fusion to control the progressive deformity prior to the growth spurt, than to attempt to control the deformity during the rapid growth phase of the adolescent growth spurt [4, 6]. Ideally, this should be performed after 8 years of age as alveolar development is finished, with less detrimental effect on the pulmonary system in the long term.

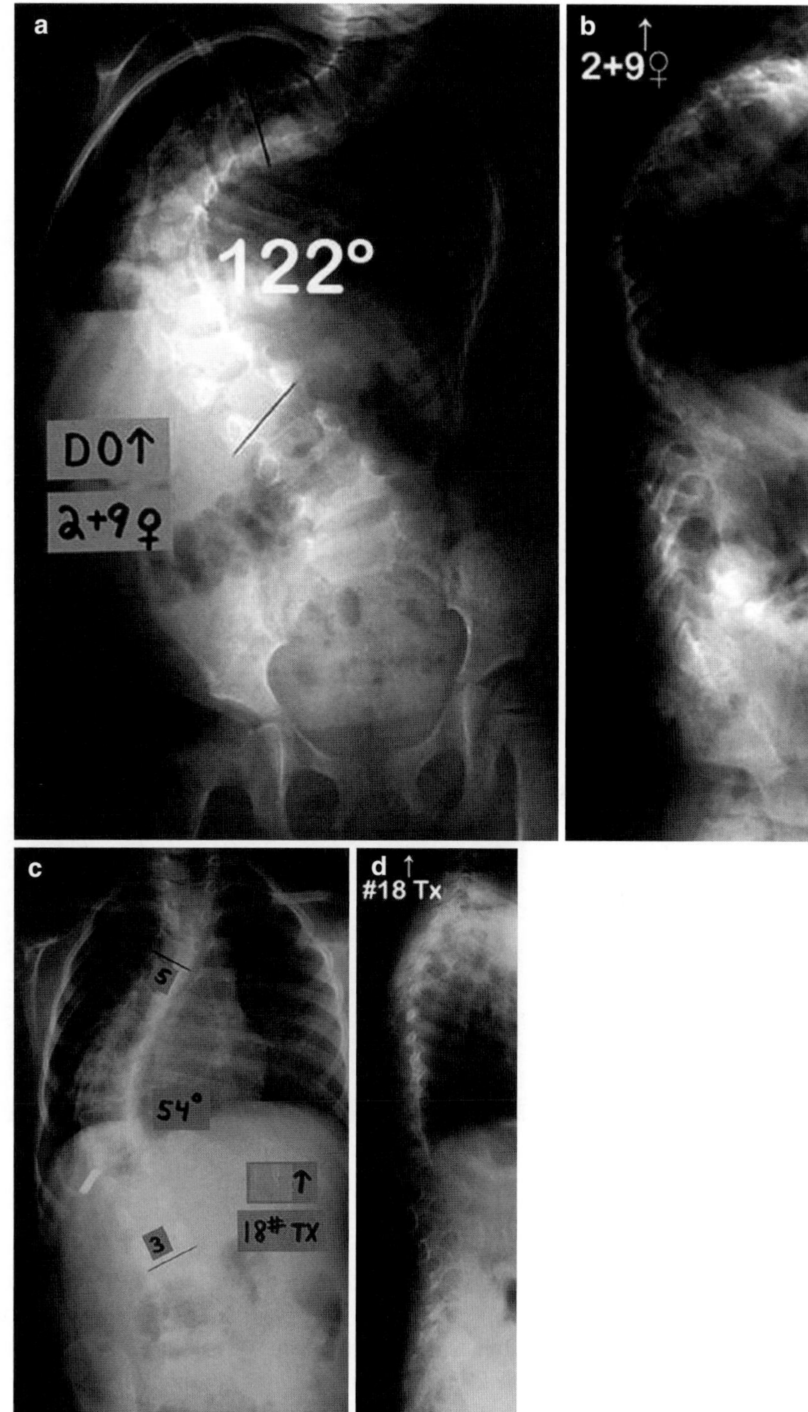

Fig. 42.1 Patient is a 2 + 9-year-old female with infantile idiopathic scoliosis. She had a normal spine MRI and a negative genetics evaluation. (**a, b**) Posterior-anterior (PA) and lateral radiographs showing a 122° scoliosis deformity. (**c, d**) She was placed in preoperative halo-gravity traction, and underwent a five-level anterior apical release and fusion. Following, she had further traction reducing her scoliosis to 54°

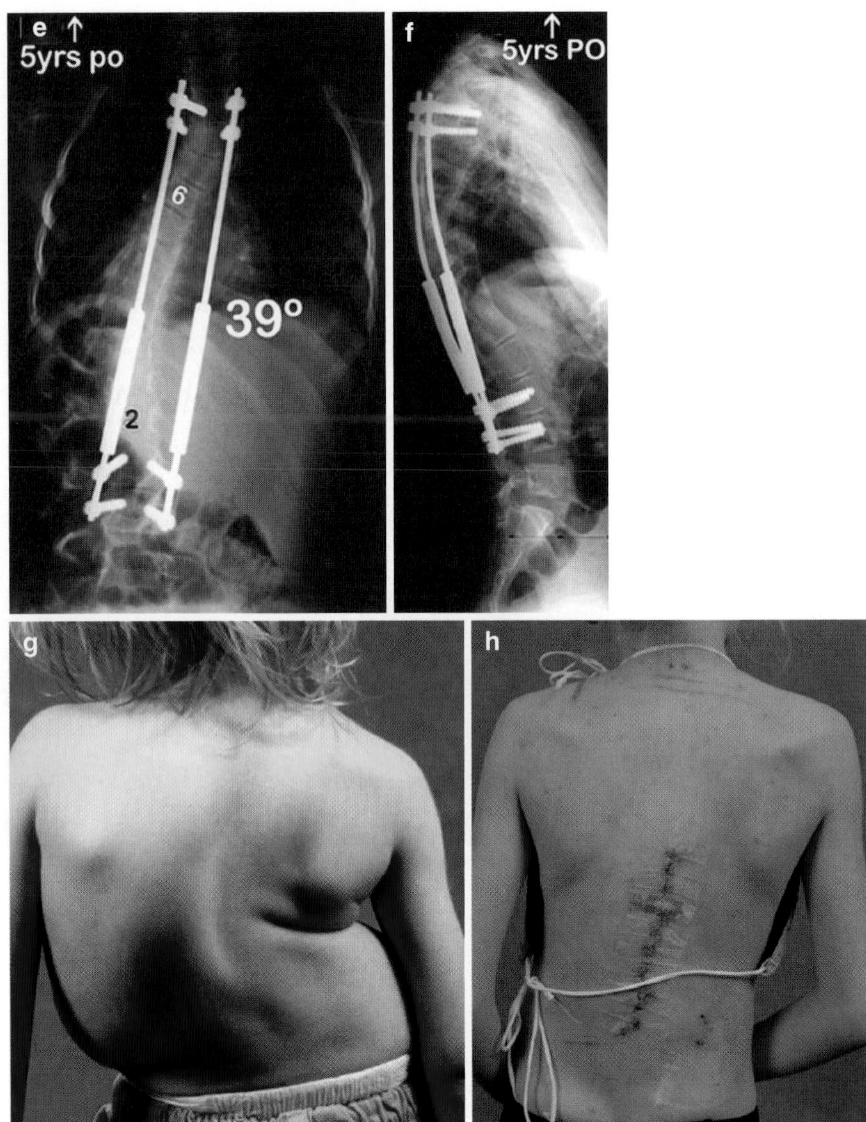

Fig. 42.1 (continued) (**e**, **f**) She then underwent posterior growing rod placement from T3 to L4. At 5 years postoperative, her coronal curve is maintained at 39°. (**g**, **h**) Her preoperative and postoperative (growth-rod lengthening) coronal photographs show the marked improvement in her clinical alignment as well as the growth of her trunk over time

42.2.3 Congenital Spinal Deformities

For patients with isolated congenital deformities, a unilateral, fully segmented nonincarcerated, hemivertebra resection with a short spinal fusion has become a preferred method of treatment. Often a near-complete correction of the congenital deformity can be obtained from a single operation, often performed from a posterior-only approach. The indications for a longer spinal fusion in congenital deformities are more controversial. However, a congenital dislocation of the spine (CDS), with or without neurological deficit, has been a nearly universal indication for spinal fusion as soon as the patient is old enough to tolerate the operation, usually in the first to second year of life. The spinal column is extremely unstable and there is a high risk of spontaneous and/or progressive neurological deficit including full paralysis, which can occur if left untreated. Traditional methods of treatment have included circumferential fusion with casting followed by brace immobilization. However, we have seen a very high pseudarthrosis rate with that method, and now prefer to add posterior instrumentation, if at all possible, to stabilize the spinal column during the fusion process. Similar to the above-mentioned CDS patient with a severe deformity, those with a severe congenital deformity may be best treated with a posterior-only or circumferential spinal fusion as a better alternative, than allowing the deformity to progress into the adolescent years.

42.2.4 Genetic Syndromes

Unfortunately, many genetic syndromes have musculoskeletal conditions involving progressive spinal deformity. Some of the more common are those involving the connective tissues, such as Marfan disease and Ehlers-Danlos syndrome. This becomes a detrimental combination involving a large deformity, very lax connective tissues, and a young patient. Growth modulation techniques should be utilized in the highly immature patient, but again, once patients are near the late juvenile years, consideration for an apical if not complete spinal fusion of the deformity should be entertained. These patients may ultimately develop severe, life-threatening deformities if left untreated because of their poor connective tissues; hence, surgical intervention can produce a secure and stable spinal column which is certainly advantageous.

42.2.5 Neuromuscular Disorders

There is a spectrum of diagnoses involved in neuromuscular spinal deformity. Unfortunately, most patients do not benefit from a prophylactic orthosis, especially when their deformity reaches severe Cobb measurements of over 90–100°. In addition, many of them are not very healthy, and repeated surgical interventions necessary with treatments such as growing rods, may not be tolerated. Thus, entertaining a spinal fusion, especially during the juvenile years, may be appropriate. One diagnostic category where this is certainly advantageous is with spinal muscular atrophy. These patients may develop a very severe deformity at a very young age, and they are often not very healthy from a pulmonary standpoint. Thus, it is doubly troubling in that not only are they not healthy enough to tolerate an anterior procedure, but they are also young enough to have a high risk of crankshaft phenomenon occurring, if they undergo a posterior-only arthrodesis. However, this has been our approach and a minimum 5-year postoperative review of these patients has shown reasonable radiographic and clinical results following early intervention for progressive, severe spinal muscular atrophy scoliosis [10].

Another category where spinal fusion has been performed at a very young age is congenital kyphotic deformities of the lumbar spine and those patients with a high-level myelomeningocele. Once a lumbar congenital kyphosis reaches over 100° or so, nothing advantageous is going to happen to that region of the spine, and hence, reconstruction via a kyphectomy and spinal fusion is indicated. Most surgeons would attempt to "grow" the middle and upper thoracic spine with implants such as a Luque-trolley or other growth guided techniques such as Shilla if at all possible, to allow further thoracic growth despite the thoracolumbar and lumbar fusion. It is particularly advantageous to avoid the mid and lower thoracic lordotic deformity that often becomes fixed in response to a progressive lumbar kyphosis below.

Most patients with cerebral palsy who have a scoliosis deformity can be observed, braced, or undergo wheelchair modification during the infantile and juvenile years, in order to avoid spinal fusion until the adolescent time-frame. However, once again, for those with severe deformities, greater than 100–125°, that are relentlessly progressive, continued observation seems inappropriate when so much growth remains. Obviously, if they are healthy enough to undergo multiple surgical procedures, then some type of posterior growing rod construct may be advisable. However, many of these patients are frail and debilitated, and a better option might be a one-time performance of a posterior spinal fusion utilizing intraoperative halo-femoral traction to maximize correction and sitting balance while minimizing complications [3]. Careful discussion with the caregivers is essential for understanding the full ramifications of a spinal fusion at such a young age. However, it has been our experience that these patients with such severe deformities are often best treated in this manner with the caregivers ultimately being appreciative of that fact.

42.2.6 Salvage Procedures

Unfortunately, many young patients are treated either appropriately or inappropriately leading to a progressive deformity requiring revision surgery. Some patients treated with growing rods or actual fusion procedures in the past have severe and progressive deformities that can be worse than the primary deformity. They present a unique set of challenges in that their spine is invariably stiff, their pulmonary status is usually quite limited, and they have often undergone multiple surgical procedures either from an anterior and/or posterior perspective that renders their spinal column very distorted from an anatomical viewpoint. In addition, they have a much higher rate of impending or actual neurological sequel from their severe deformity and repeated surgical interventions. Revision salvage procedures must be well-thought out and thoroughly performed with the goal being optimal spinal alignment and neurological function for the remainder of the patient's life.

One group of disorders that is notorious for having issues like this is severe dysplastic neurofibromatosis. We know that they are very challenging at the outset. Most of these patients, initially treated at a young age will require circumferential fusion. However, even after that, they are at a very high risk of pseudarthrosis and continued progressive deformity (Fig. 42.2a–l) [8]. Prior to revision surgery, we often find halo-gravity traction helpful to maximize gradual correction of their severe deformity, while optimizing pulmonary and nutritional health along the way. Many of these patients have already had anterior multilevel procedures performed, thus repeating anterior work is fraught with difficulty either on the operated or unoperated side. Risk of spinal cord devascularization is also much higher during their revision surgery because of the abovementioned prior procedures [7].

Recently, the use of posterior vertebral column resection procedures has been quite helpful for these severe revision deformities. Obtaining secure pedicle screw fixation above and below the apex of the deformity followed by resection of one, two, or even three vertebrae from an all posterior approach has allowed dramatic radiographic and clinical correction. Ultimately, a spinal fusion over the entire length of the posterior instrumentation has to be performed; however, that is usually the best option when compared with their preoperative condition. These are very technically demanding operations that require not only the surgeon, but the entire surgical team to be adept at very high-level spinal deformity care for successful execution. At our institution, this has revolutionized the care that we have provided to these patients and the results have been quite encouraging. We now have experience in 73 consecutive posterior vertebral column resections for severe pediatric and adult deformity. Of the 46 procedures that have been performed in the pediatric age range, 30 have been performed for salvage of a prior reconstruction. We have obtained on average, 60% correction, the majority performed under one surgical setting, and there have been no spinal cord neurological deficits postoperative. We attribute this to the standard use of both somatosensory and some type of motor-evoked potential monitoring intraoperatively [7]. There have been some root-level deficits in revision of upper lumbar procedures, but the two occurring in the pediatric revision setting were transient. Only one patient has required revision surgery which was for a deep wound infection. None have required revision for implant-related issues and/or pseudarthrosis so far, with over a 5-year follow-up available at present for the initial patients treated in this manner.

Another rare, but nearly universal indication for performing a spinal fusion in a skeletally immature deformity patient is one with impending or actual neurological deficit. In patients with a primary pediatric spinal deformity, this indication will be extremely rare, except in patients with a few types of congenital anomalies; specifically, congenital dislocation of the spine, or type 1 congenital kyphosis – failure of formation. In both of these congenital types of spinal deformities, an angular kyphosis may impinge upon the ventral spinal cord. In CDS, there is also a fair degree of spinal instability, which may lead to frank paraplegia even at a very young age. In addition, post-tuberculous spinal infection can certainly produce a severe angular kyphotic deformity with neurological deficit. Although rare in the North America, this is still somewhat common in more underdeveloped countries. Fortunately, it is rare to see a primary IIS or JIS deformity present with neurological deficit, even with curves that are quite severe in their coronal Cobb measurement.

Besides the few primary types of deformities discussed earlier, it is a bit more common to have patients present with actual or impending neurological deficit in a revision setting. In previously treated patients, a progressive kyphotic or kyphoscoliotic spinal deformity may lead to myelopathy, paraparesis, or in a very rare circumstance, paraplegia. The most common presentation is a patient with posterior multilevel pseudarthrosis, and an angular type of kyphotic or kyphoscoliotic progressive deformity causing ventral spinal cord

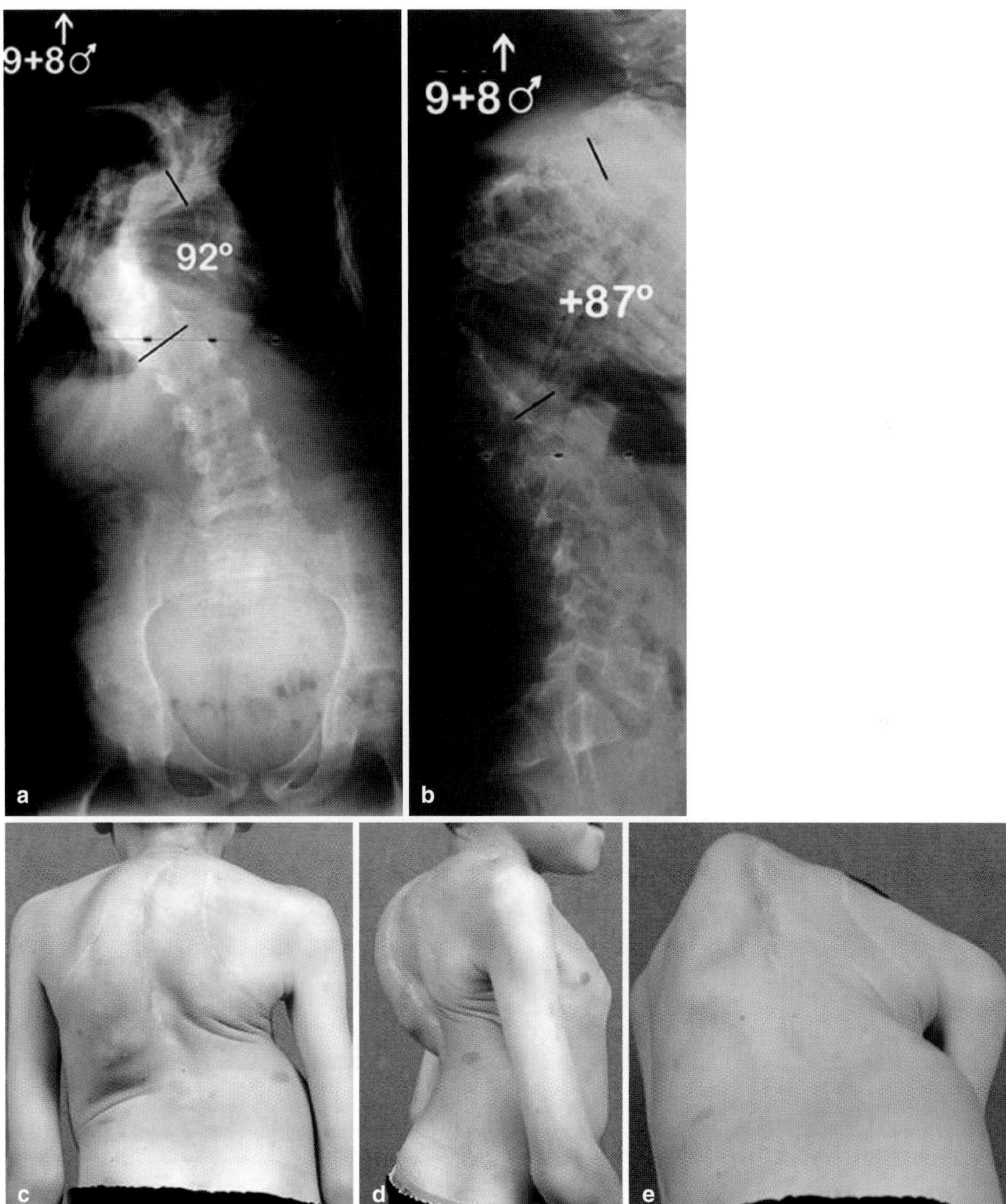

Fig. 42.2 Patient is a 9 + 8-year-old male who was referred to us for treatment of his progressive spinal deformity. He had neurofibromatosis, and had undergone bilateral anterior spinal fusions, as well as three prior posterior spinal fusion attempts, left-sided posterior thoracoplasty, as well as instrumentation removal for prominence following hook pull-off. (**a**, **b**) He presented with a combined 179° kyphoscoliosis. (**c**–**e**) His preoperative clinical photos demonstrated his severe kyphoscoliotic deformity, including bilateral anterior thoracotomy scars, as well as a very severe "rib hump," that was actually his spine since he already has a very aggressive left-sided thoracoplasty performed

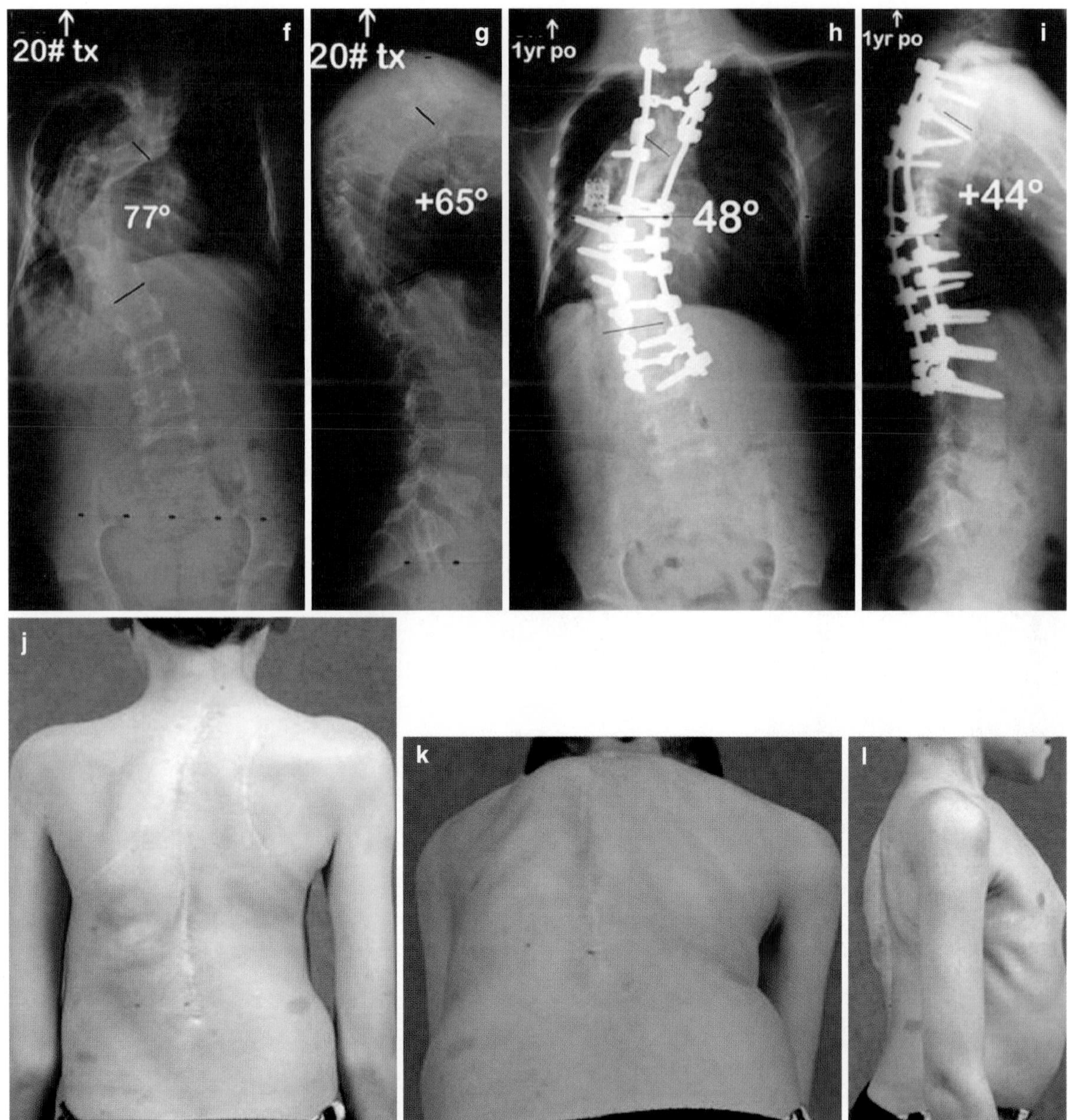

Fig. 42.2 (continued) (**f, g**) He was placed in preoperative halo-gravity traction. With 20 pounds of traction, his scoliosis decreased to 77° and his kyphosis to +65°. (**h, i**) He underwent a posterior three level vertebral column resection and instrumentation and fusion from T1 to L3. This improved his coronal curve to 48° and his sagittal curve to +44° of kyphosis. (**j, l**) His postoperative clinic photos demonstrate the marked improvement in his trunk alignment and also his posterior spine prominence following the posterior vertebrectomy procedure

impingement (Fig. 42.3a–o). Surgical treatment for these patients will necessitate spinal cord decompression and anterior as well as posterior spinal fusion. This can be performed via a formal circumferential approach versus an all posterior approach with a costotransversectomy type of exposure. Even young patients will require fusion over at least the apex of their curve, if not posterior fusion levels required to maintain ultimate coronal and sagittal balance. Potentially, performing an apical fusion with Luque-trolley or Shilla-type pedicle screws at the end of the constructs may be beneficial in an attempt to obtain some growth along the ends of the

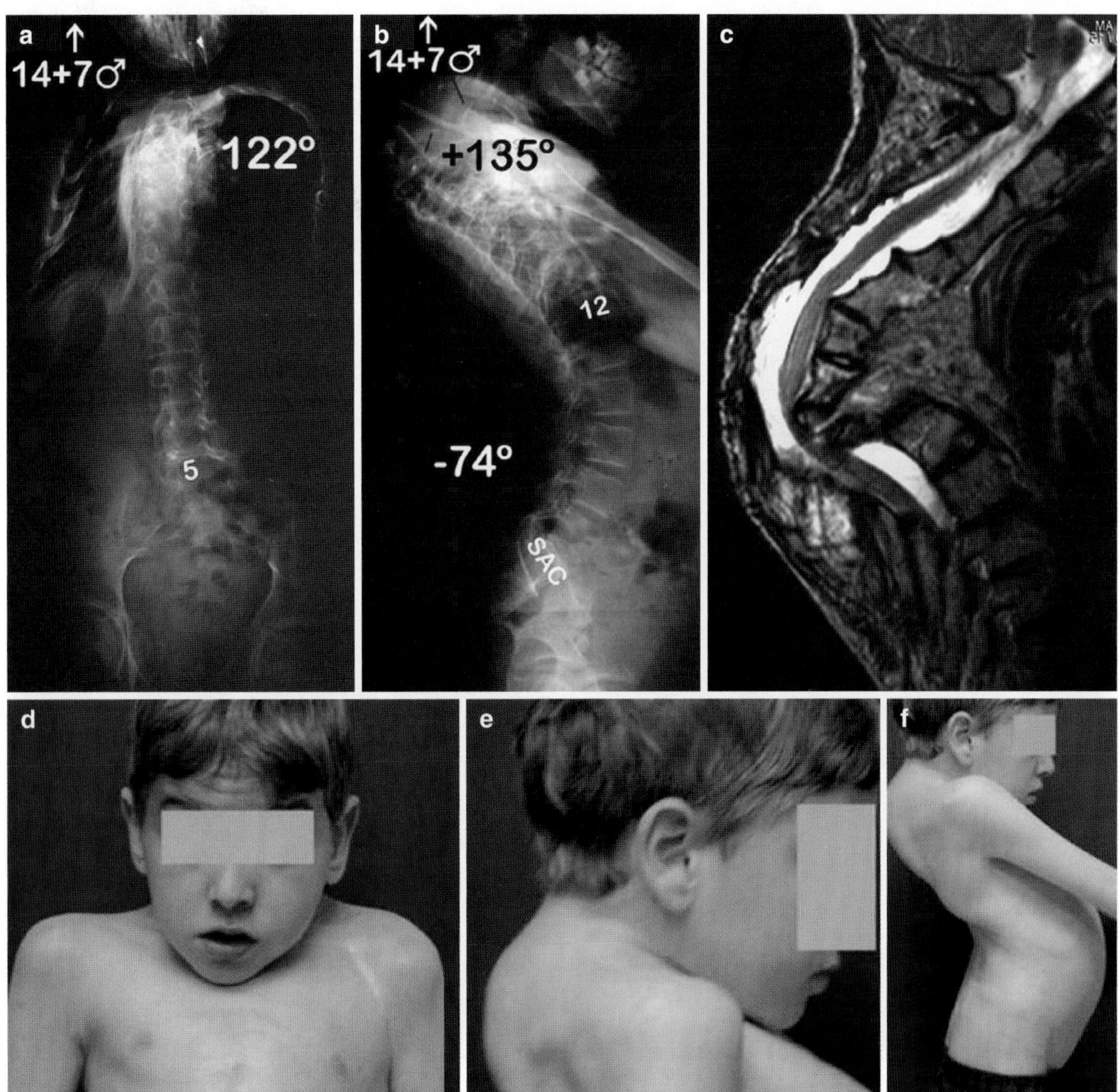

Fig. 42.3 Patient is a 14 + 7-year-old male with neurofibromatosis, who had undergone eight anterior as well as posterior surgical procedures for a severe cervicothoracic kyphosis. (**a, b, c**) He presented with +135° of progressive kyphosis, pseudarthrosis, and myelopathy. His preoperative MRI demonstrated an unresectable neurofibroma anterior to his spine at the cervicothoracic junction, with a dislocation of T4 on T5. (**d, e, f**) His clinical photos demonstrated his fixed cervicothoracic kyphosis and near chin-on-chest deformity and marked hyperlordosis

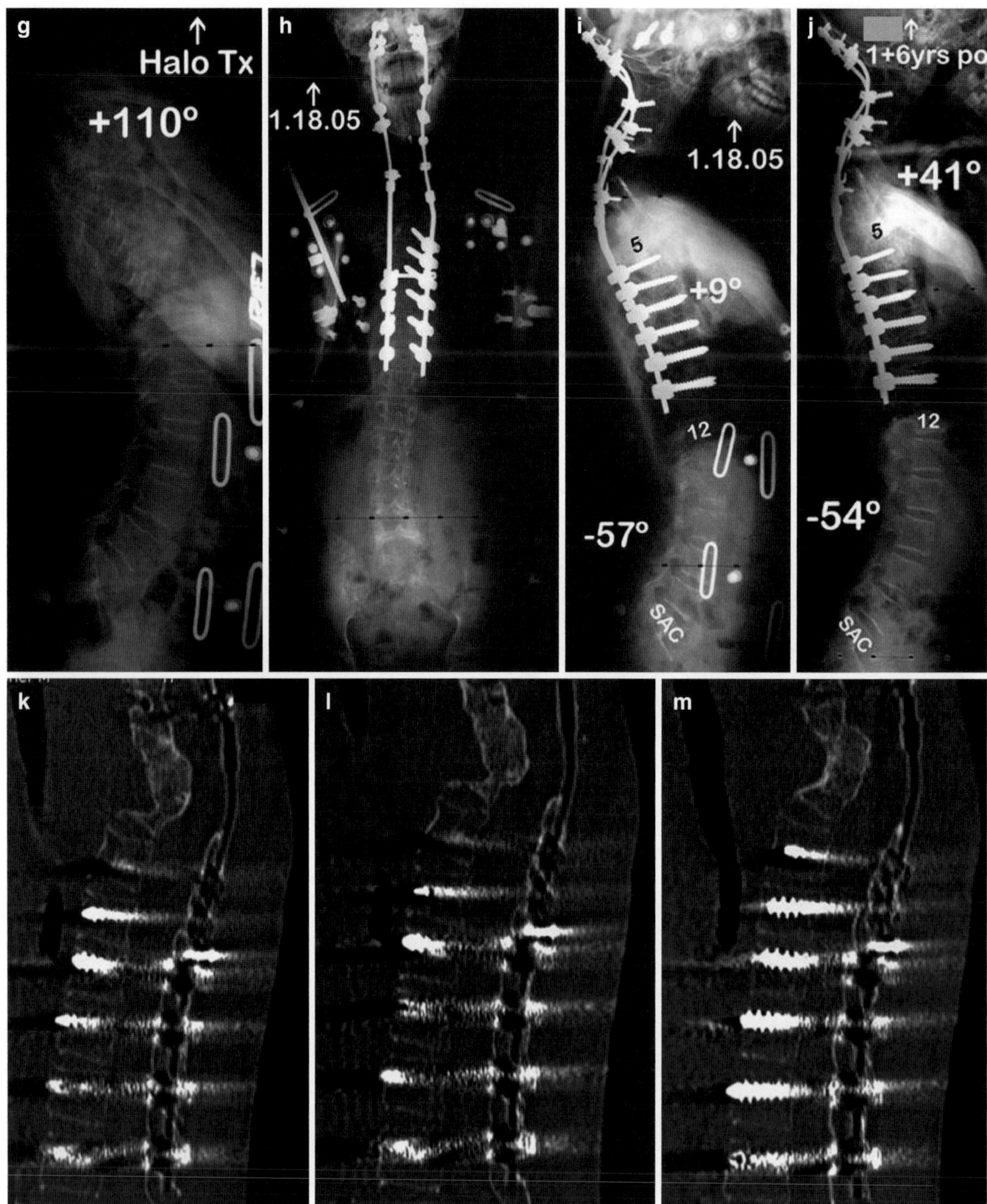

Fig. 42.3 (continued) (**g**) He underwent a period of gentle halo-gravity traction correcting his curve to +110°. (**h, i**) He underwent a posterior T4 and T5 vertebral resection, anterior spinal fusion with BMP-2, and occiput to T11 instrumentation and fusion. He was maintained thereafter for 3 months in a halo vest, and completely resolved his myelopathy. (**j**) At 1 + 6 years postoperative, he has a stable posterior construct, normal neurological exam. (**k, l, m**) A sagittal CT scan showing a solid anterior fusion over his previously decompressed thoracic region between T3 and T6

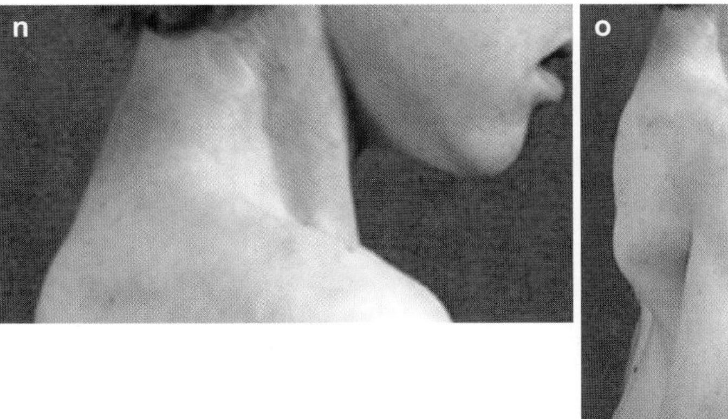

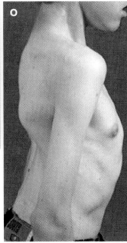

Fig. 42.3 (continued) (**n, o**) Postoperative clinical photos demonstrate his improved clinical alignment

deformity while still securely stabilizing the apex to prevent further neurological deterioration.

42.3 Conclusion

Certainly, there has been much progress made in the last decade in the attempt to avoid or minimize spinal fusion in very young children with progressive spinal deformities. However, as outlined in this chapter, there are certain conditions when performing at least an apical if not longer spinal fusion, which is quite appropriate. Each patient must be individually analyzed and treated. The analysis must include the patient's overlying medical condition, type and progression of deformity, radiographic presentation, and pulmonary function and chest-wall alignment. Treatment will depend on the ability to provide adequate spinal stability, limit progression of the deformity, and maintain optimal chest-wall alignment and function in the long term.

References

1. Ceballos T, Ferrer-Torrelles M, Castillo F et al (1980) Prognosis in infantile idiopathic scoliosis. J Bone Joint Surg Am 62:863–875
2. Dobbs MB, Weinstein SL (1999) Infantile and juvenile scoliosis. Orthop Clin North Am 30:331–341
3. Eberle CF (1988) Failure of fixation after segmental spinal instrumentation without arthrodesis in the management of paralytic scoliosis. J Bone Joint Surg Am 70:696–703
4. Hefti FL, McMaster MJ (1983) The effect of the adolescent growth spurt on early posterior spinal fusion in infantile and juvenile idiopathic scoliosis. J Bone Joint Surg Br 65: 247–254
5. James JI (1954) Idiopathic scoliosis; the prognosis, diagnosis, and operative indications related to curve patterns and the age at onset. J Bone Joint Surg Br 36:36–49
6. Lenke LG, Dobbs MB (2007) Management of juvenile idiopathic scoliosis: the immature spine. J Bone Joint Surg Am 89:55S–63S
7. Lenke LG, O'Leary PT, Bridwell KH et al (2009) Posterior vertebral column resection (VCR) for severe pediatric deformity: Minimum 2-year follow-up of 35 consecutive patients. Spine 34:2213–2221
8. McMaster MJ, James JI (1976) Pseudarthrosis after spinal fusion for scoliosis. J Bone Joint Surg Br 58:305–312
9. McMaster MJ, Macnicol MF (1979) The management of progressive infantile idiopathic scoliosis. J Bone Joint Surg Br 61:36–42
10. Zebala LP, Bridwell KH, Baldus C et al (2008) 5-Year radiographic results of long scoliosis fusion in juvenile spinal muscular atrophy patients: Crankshaft and ultimate correction. In: 43rd Annual Scoliosis Research Society Meeting, Salt Lake City, Utah

43 Outcomes in Children with Early Onset Scoliosis

Michael G. Vitale and James Wright

Key Points

- Traditional radiographic measures inadequately reflect outcomes in the area of early onset scoliosis.
- There is reasonable evidence that early fusion results in negative long-term pulmonary consequences in children with scoliosis.
- Measurement of pulmonary function may require a different set of measures than used in older populations.
- Health-related quality of life (QOL) is also an important endpoint in children with early onset scoliosis.
- We are just beginning to understand the complex relationships between scoliosis, thoracic deformity, lung function, and general health effects in this population, relationships which can be conceptualized using the "framework model of health."
- We have witnessed an expansion in available nonfusion options for patients with early onset scoliosis.
- There are profound obstacles to meaningful research in this area.
- All of these factors contribute to the variability in decision-making in the treatment of these patients.
- Research in this area should be prioritized and incentivized in order to drive innovation, and provide optimal care to these patients.

43.1 Introduction

The term "Orthopaedics" comes from the Greek roots "Ortho" and "Pedics" meaning "straight child." Intuitively, a straight bone seems to imply a good outcome, and radiographic measures have been the historical standard in reports assessing surgical outcomes after orthopaedics surgery. However, in the last 2 decades, there has been a fundamental shift in thinking about how best to measure and describe outcomes. We now look at more broadly defined outcomes including functional status, health-related quality of life (QOL), and cost effectiveness. We utilize more rigorous methods of research design including randomized trials, and we apply more sophisticated means of analysis of data in an attempt to decrease bias and better compare the treatment options.

The last 2 decades have also witnessed an expansion of options in the treatment of the young child with scoliosis and a concomitant increase in attention to important issues in this area. As a result, the treating physician now faces a complex palette of often overlapping and mutually exclusive choices, yet both experience and knowledge base appear insufficient to optimize decision-making.

Should the 18-month-old with infantile idiopathic scoliosis be casted, braced, or observed? Is it better to remove the hemivertebrae and correct the curve or perform a fusion in situ? Is the hemivertebrae better resected from an all posterior approach or from a combined anterior posterior approach? Should the 7-year-old have a growth rod, VEPTR, Shilla procedure, or stapling?

When assigned a position in a debate, we can confidently list our reasons for being so sure that our position is correct, but the reality is that we often lack the appropriate evidence necessary to make optimal decisions for many patients with early onset scoliosis. As a result, even experienced clinicians often disagree strongly about how and even if a particular patient requires treatment.

M. G. Vitale (✉)
MS Children's Hospital of New York, 3959 Broadway, 8 North, New York, NY 10032, USA
e-mail: mgv1@columbia.edu

B. A. Akbarnia et al. (eds.), *The Growing Spine*,
DOI: 10.1007/978-3-540-85207-0_43, © Springer-Verlag Berlin Heidelberg 2011

Variation in decision-making in the area of early onset scoliosis has in fact been documented in a recent survey of members of the Chest Wall and Spinal Deformity Study Group. Vitale et al. [26] demonstrated substantial intraobserver and interobserver variability in decision-making. The 13 surgeons surveyed agreed that *any type* of surgical treatment was indicated in only 8 of 12 hypothetical cases, and there was substantial disagreement regarding details of surgery including bilaterality, instrumentation to the pelvis, and thoracostomy. Among surgeons and cases for which VEPTR was indicated, the same surgeon, when surveyed at two different time points, demonstrated only moderate agreement (kappa = 0.37) with their own previous recommendation (Fig. 43.1). Such variability in opinion, if reflective of actual decision-making, raises concerns about quality of care of patients with early onset scoliosis. Such variability reflects the paucity of definitive evidence in the field and highlights the need for rigorous research including multicenter studies to better define the natural history of early onset scoliosis and rigorously compare various treatment modalities in this heterogeneous and challenging group of patients.

Admittedly, the assessment of outcomes, and the establishment of what constitutes best care for patients with early onset scoliosis, presents a host of unique challenges and rigorous evidence-based studies in this area which are limited [21]. First, patient populations are small and heterogeneous, making it difficult to accrue sufficient numbers of patients and to compare treatments. Second, the pace of evolution of treatment options has been rapid, creating a moving target for patient assessment. Third, treatment of the young child with scoliosis is in-part, an attempt to improve the natural history of disease. However, early onset scoliosis is not a disease, but a symptom of a variety of diagnoses, each with somewhat different comorbidities and natural histories. Fourth, effecting natural history implies following a patient cohort longitudinally over time, and the long periods of follow-up that are necessary represent a major challenge to research in this area. In some situations, treatment does in fact aim to improve short- and medium-term health including aspects of pulmonary function and QOL. Finally, there has been little consensus about how best to measure pulmonary outcomes in this population. In fact, we are just learning how complex the relationships are between early onset scoliosis, treatment, and pulmonary function.

It is clear that many patients with early onset scoliosis have significant issues with a variety of aspects of health-related QOL, but measurement of QOL is fraught with difficulties in this population. Vitale et al. [25] have documented significant perturbations in health-related QOL as measured by the Child Health Questionnaire [18] in older patients who had undergone expansion thoracoplasty in the past. However, generic measures of QOL have been developed and validated primarily in patients >5 years of age limiting the usefulness in this population. Children develop and mature,

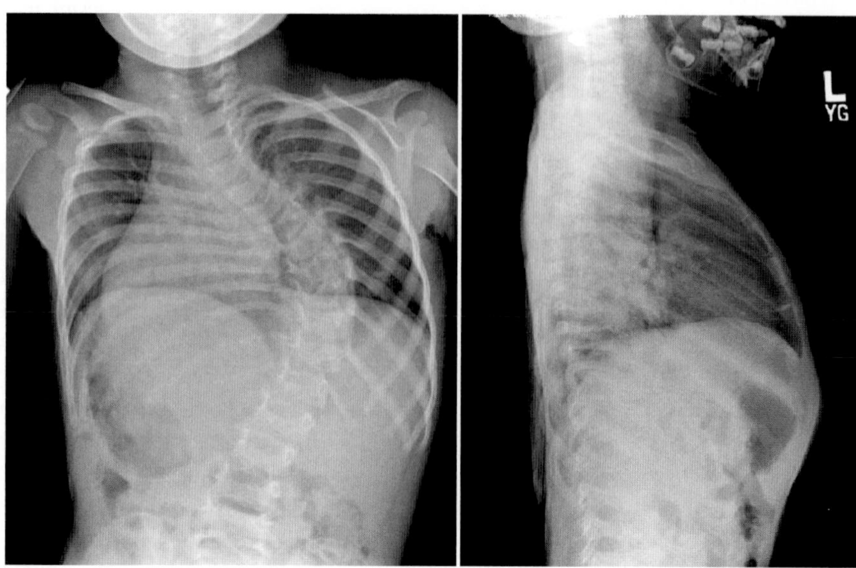

Fig. 43.1 A representative case highlighting difficulty and variability in decision-making in patients with early onset scoliosis. Members of the Chest Wall and Spinal Deformity Study Group exhibited significant inter- and intraobserver variability in treatment recommendations for this child, an 18-month-old Jehovas witness with an undiagnosed mitochondrial disorder and progressive scoliosis

creating a moving target for functional assessment in this population. Finally, health issues in this heterogeneous population can be quite specific, and may not be fully captured with available "off the shelf" measures of health status. Currents efforts by Vitale and collaborators in the Chest Wall and Spinal Deformity Study Group seek to develop and validate a disease-specific measure for children with early onset scoliosis.

Furthermore, new technologies need to be evaluated and approved by the FDA, but the regulatory burdens present significant obstacles. As discussed earlier, it is extremely difficult to amass sufficient populations, and equally challenging is to follow patients in the long term to meet the requirements of post market surveillance imposed by the FDA. Furthermore, while industry plays a role in promoting the necessary research to obtain approval for new technologies in orthopaedics surgery, the small patient populations affected by early onset scoliosis do not draw sufficient interest and may limit available funding.

All of these factors create a "perfect storm," making the design and conduct of high-quality, important clinical evaluative research in this area, a significant challenge.

43.2 Framework for Measurement

The immediate goals of treatment for children with EOS are to minimize physical disability including respiratory symptoms and relieve pain to improve appearance. The long-term aim of treatment is to prevent the onset of new symptoms, minimize future decline in function, and prevent premature death. While several useful frameworks have been proposed to organize outcomes, the International Classification of Functioning [22] has particular relevance to surgery.

The pathway (Fig. 43.2) begins with a disease which in turn leads to an impairment. Impairment is defined as an abnormality of structure of function. Impairments lead to disabilities, defined as the lack of ability to perform an activity in a manner considered normal. Finally, activity restrictions lead to handicap or role limitation which is the inability to fulfill roles, which for children, refer to family friends and school. In the ICF pathway, the disease could be congenital scoliosis leading to spinal, chest wall, and lung deformity. These impairments lead to physical and respiratory disability, limitations in school and play, and possibly, early death. Such a pathway is particularly relevant to the area of early onset scoliosis because our treatments are often directed at reducing spine and chest-wall deformity. If treatments reduce impairments, the hope is that, in turn, we will ameliorate activity restrictions, enhance role function, and prevent early death. However, the pathway is clearly not linear. Furthermore, as discussed earlier, children with EOS often have associated conditions that moderate the pathway, influence the success of treatment, and lead to other impairments with additional consequences. Consider the child with spinal muscular atrophy and early onset scoliosis. Nevertheless, this framework provides a way to categorize measures and draw attention to the important question of what treatment is best at reducing impairments, thereby positively affecting the consequences of disease.

43.3 Available Endpoints and Measures of Outcome

43.3.1 Radiographic Measures

The Cobb angle is a well-accepted primary endpoint in adolescent idiopathic scoliosis. However, Campbell [6–8] has highlighted the complex three-dimensional relationships between early onset scoliosis thoracic

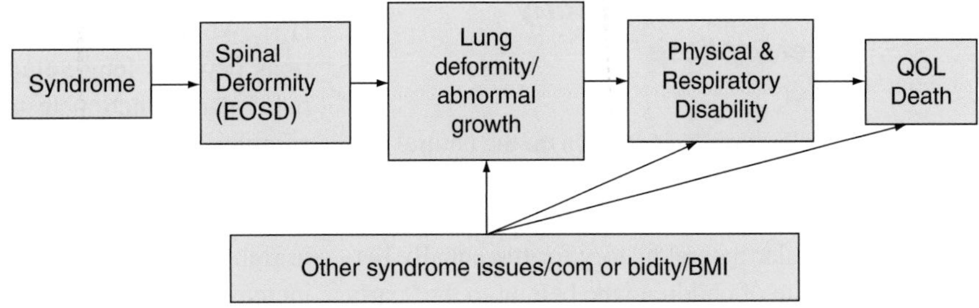

Fig. 43.2 Adapted from the international classification of functioning. Disease leads to impairment, then disability, and then loss of role function

deformity and pulmonary function which are poorly reflected in the unidimensional Cobb measurement. Campbell and others [7, 9] have described a variety of other radiographic measures including the space available for the lung, thoracic height, the spinal penetration index, and the posterior thorax symmetry ratio. Other potential radiographic measures include the interpedicular line ratio, decompensation, shoulder level, and vertebral rotation. Mehta [15] has brought attention to the importance of the position of the ribs in relation to the spine in the idiopathic infantile scoliosis population. A rib vertebral angle difference 20° or more strongly predicted progression in this group. However, even within the diagnostic category of "infantile idiopathic scoliosis," it is not clear that we are examining a single clinical entity. As Fernandes and Weinstein [11] questioned, "Is resolving scoliosis, as opposed to progressive scoliosis, a different entity with a different etiology, or does infantile idiopathic scoliosis have a full spectrum of presentations."

While pulmonary function is of central importance in the early onset scoliosis population, the measurement of pulmonary function in very young children requires special equipment and technique. Furthermore, it is not clear that traditional measures of pulmonary function such as vital capacity and expiratory volumes sufficiently describe the pathology relevant to the children with early onset scoliosis. There are particular concerns with the effect of scoliosis and chest-wall surgery, for example, on chest-wall compliance. Is it better to have a larger thoracic volume even at the expense of more chest-wall stiffness?

Despite the considerable obstacles to meaningful clinical research in this area, research efforts have afforded clinicians some initial understanding of important issues in this area. Following is a brief summary of the available evidence pertinent to the field of early onset scoliosis.

43.3.2 Natural History of Early Onset Scoliosis

Numerous articles have been written on the natural history of early onset scoliosis. However, just as there is no natural history for all children with cerebral palsy, there is no singular natural history for the equally heterogeneous group of children who belong to the "early onset" category. In a much-cited work published in Spine in 1992, Pehrsonn et al. [17] followed patients with infantile onset and juvenile onset to maturity and documented that the age of onset of scoliosis correlated strongly with early demise from cardiopulmonary disease. It is known that scoliosis can lead to pulmonary hypertension and cor pulmonale. This is presumably a result of compression of lung parenchyma, diminution on the size of the thorax, increased stiffness of the chest wall, and increased work of breather caused by the altered mechanics of the pulmonary billows, though we still search for the "right" way to measure these changes before they result in extreme dysfunction. In 1955, Scott and Morgan [20] examined a cohort of patients with significant idiopathic infantile scoliosis and also demonstrated significant cardiopulmonary disability which correlated with the age of curve progression. However, Weinstein's [28] natural history study of AIS demonstrated that cardiopulmonary demise is rare in adolescent idiopathic scoliosis.

43.4 Lung Function

Redding [19] has shown significant alterations in lung function in children with congenital scoliosis, and has hypothesized that scoliosis affects lung function by incursion into the hemithorax, as well as by reducing chest-wall compliance and excursion, producing asymmetry in lung size and function. However, this study of 39 patients with early onset scoliosis did not demonstrate a correlation between Cobb angle and pulmonary measures. On the other hand, another investigation carried out by Vitale et al. [24] showed a positive correlation ($R = -0.5$; $P < 0.005$) with residual thoracic Cobb angle and FEV1 in a cohort of 21 patients with congenital scoliosis who underwent early fusion.

Computerized tomography with three-dimensional reconstructions provides the ability to estimate lung volumes and characterize the intrathoracic deformity [13]. Work by Adams [1] has shown strong correlations between lung volumes as measured by CT and pulmonary function tests. This study highlights the complex nature of spine, thoracic, and lung deformity and discusses the limitations of traditional pulmonary function tests that ignore the significant asymmetries in right versus left lung. However, concerns about the increased risk of malignancy associated with routine and perhaps, repeated CT scans limits its use as a research tool [5]. Magnetic resonance imaging may have similar potential, though investigations in this area are still in their infancy.

43.4.1 *What Do We Know About the Outcomes of Treatment?*

43.4.1.1 Negative Effects of Early Fusion

Several studies have now been published that collectively convincingly demonstrate untoward effects of early fusion in children with scoliosis. Karol et al. [14] examined pulmonary function tests of 28 patients who had undergone a spinal fusion prior to the age of 9 and demonstrated pulmonary function testing with values of 50–60% predicted when compared with norms. Patients at highest risk of restrictive disease were those who had a more extensive thoracic fusion, especially proximal thoracic fusion. Similar results have been reported by other authors including Vitale et al. [24], Goldberg et al. [12], and others. While none of these articles prospectively measured pulmonary function before and after fusion, collectively, this body of work provides substantial evidence that children with early onset scoliosis who have been treated with traditional fusion techniques are at significant risk for considerable problems with pulmonary function. The onus is now on current researchers to demonstrate that new techniques result in an improvement from this dismal picture presented by natural history and early fusion.

43.4.1.2 Outcomes in Patients Treated with "Growing Rods"

In an attempt to avoid fusion at all costs, "growing rods" or more precisely expandable spinal implants have become the standards of care for children with early onset scoliosis. In a multicenter study of 23 patients who underwent dual growing rod constructs for early onset scoliosis, Akbarnia et al. [2] demonstrated significant improvements in Cobb angles and space available for the lung and spinal growth. However, pulmonary and functional outcomes were not assessed. Greater growth and correction seem to be seen in patients who undergo lengthening at interval of less than 6 months. Dual growth rods seem to deliver better radiographic results than single rod constructs [23, 27].

43.4.1.3 VEPTR and Expansion Thoracoplasty in Children with Fused Ribs

As described by Campbell [8], expansion thoracoplasty implies surgical separation of rib fusion and placement of the VEPTR device. Campbell followed a cohort of children with scoliosis and rib fusion who underwent surgery at a mean age of 3.2 years and with mean follow-up of 5.7 years who underwent expansion thoracoplasty [6]. Significant improvements in radiographic measures such as the Cobb angle, space available for the lung, and thoracic spinal height were noted, though pulmonary function at follow-up continued to demonstrate significant perturbations from norms. Vital capacity at follow-up ranged from 44% for those older than 2 years of age at the time of surgery to 58% for those children younger than 2 years of age. In a subset of patients whose lung function was followed longitudinally, there was some improvement in vital capacity, but no significant improvement in percent predicted vital capacity. Of note, 52 complications were encountered in 22 patients through the course of treatment. Motoyoma and collaborators [16] in Pittsburgh showed that PFT during and after expansion thoracoplasty kept up with growth, but did not increase in percent predicted terms.

Emans et al. [10] studied 31 patients with fused ribs and thoracic insufficiency syndrome prospectively. Significant spinal growth and improved lung volumes as measured by CT and pulmonary function tests were noted in this cohort, supporting the role of early nonfusion surgery in this patient cohort.

43.4.1.4 Growth Modulation: Vertebral Stapling and the Shilla Technique

In an effort to improve upon the outcomes of children with scoliosis, clinicians have developed strategies to attempt to modulate or control growth. Betz et al. have pioneered the use of anterior vertebral staples [3, 4]. While this technique has great theoretical appeal and continues to gain popularity, clinical research that is necessary to document that such a technique positively impacts natural history has not been done. McCarthy has developed a novel technique employing an apical fusion with expansion of the rest of the instrumented spine using a specially designed set screw. Again, such innovation is sorely needed, but obstacles to the necessary clinical research documenting success of failure of such new techniques are problematic.

43.4.2 Opportunities for Future Progress

Despite the challenges, there are a number of opportunities to better organize processes that will facilitate clinical research and innovation in this area. A first step would involve some consensus among experts in this area about what should constitute a minimum common set of endpoints. Such a process will require a formal look at available endpoints including broadly defined endpoints, such as QOL. A valid and responsive disease-specific measure of outcome for children with early onset scoliosis would be an important part of this process.

In order to efficiently conduct clinical research in this area, multicenter studies will be critical. Existing today are the Growing Spine Study Group and the Chest Wall and Spinal deformity Study Group, both of which comprise members with significant interest and experience in the area of early onset scoliosis. These groups serve to centralize multicenter efforts in this area, but opportunities to further capitalize on this important infrastructure exist. Such groups should require a minimal common dataset for all studies that are performed by the members. However, many patients with early onset scoliosis are not part of these research efforts, which is a lost opportunity for research and disease understanding. In contrast, the majority of children who receive chemotherapy for childhood cancers are captured as part of a national protocol, which has facilitated meaningful clinical research in this area. Perhaps, use of new investigational techniques and implants on "index" patients with early onset scoliosis should be contingent on contribution of results to a multicenter registry.

Children with early onset scoliosis should be considered as an "orphan population." The small markets and regulatory burdens involved in obtaining approval of new devices in this field hinder innovation. Society must therefore create incentives for innovation in this area. Our national societies and subspecialty organizations can help by funding requests for proposals for research in this area.

These issues have not gone unnoticed by the federal authorities. The Pediatric Medical Device Safety and Improvement Act of 2007 provides several incentives to innovation, including allowing manufacturers to profit from devices approved under the Humanitarian Device Exemption and providing funding through consortia to support innovation in the area of pediatric devices. It remains to be seen if this act will produce the intended effects.

43.5 Conclusion

We are just now entering into a new era in the treatment of early onset scoliosis. The pace of innovation is swift, and a plethora of new options now exist for the treatment of children with scoliosis. The expansion of treatment options has been largely unaccompanied by the appropriate clinical studies necessary to rigorously compare and contrast various treatment options and to optimize decision-making for children with early onset scoliosis, so as to minimize risks and complications and maximize benefit. Treatment in the absence of rigorous evidence may nonetheless be justified based on consensus expert opinion that currently available treatment strategies are likely to provide superior outcomes in contrast to a rather dismal natural history.

In this regard, an analogy can be made to the days of solid organ transplantation. Patients at the beginning of the era of heart transplantation had few viable options, yet techniques of heart transplantation and management post transplantation were rapidly evolving and not well defined. In the course of time, complications decreased dramatically and outcomes improved. Indications became more uniform, based on acquired data of outcomes in various populations.

The same challenge confronts those focused on improving outcomes of children with early onset scoliosis. An improved understanding of patient outcomes in this area is a prerequisite to the timely evolution of care of these children.

References

1. Adam CJ, Cargill SC, Askin GN (2007) Computed tomographic-based volumetric reconstruction of the pulmonary system in scoliosis: trends in lung volume and lung

volume asymmetry with spinal curve severity. J Pediatr Orthop 27(6):677–681
2. Akbarnia BA, Marks D, Boachie Adjei O et al (2005) Dual growing rod technique for the treatment of progressive early-onset scoliosis: a multicenter study. Spine 30(Suppl 17): S46–S57
3. Betz RR, Kim J, D'Andrea LP et al (2003) An innovative technique of vertebral body stapling for the treatment of patients with adolescent idiopathic scoliosis: a feasibility, safety, and utility study. Spine 28(20):S255–S265
4. Betz RR, D'Andrea LP, Mulcahey MJ et al (2005) Vertebral body stapling procedure for the treatment of scoliosis in the growing child. Clin Orthop Relat Res 434:55–60
5. Brenner D, Elliston CD, Hall EJ et al (2001;) Estimated risks of radiation-induced fatal cancer from pediatric CT. AJR Am J Roentgenol 176(2):289–296
6. Campbell RM Jr, Hell-Vocke AK (2003) Growth of the thoracic spine in congenital scoliosis after expansion thoracoplasty. J Bone Joint Surg Am 85-A(3):409–420
7. Campbell RM Jr, Smith MD, Mayes TC et al (2003) The characteristics of thoracic insufficiency syndrome associated with fused ribs and congenital scoliosis. J Bone Joint Surg Am 85-A(3):399–408
8. Campbell RM Jr, Smith MD, Hell-Vocke AK (2004) Expansion thoracoplasty: the surgical technique of opening-wedge thoracostomy. Surgical technique. J Bone Joint Surg Am 86-A(Suppl 1):51–64
9. Campbell RM Jr, Smith MD, Mayes TC et al (2004) The effect of opening wedge thoracostomy on thoracic insufficiency syndrome associated with fused ribs and congenital scoliosis. J Bone Joint Surg Am 86-A(8):1659–1674
10. Emans JB, Caubet JF, Ordonez CL et al (2005) The treatment of spine and chest wall deformities with fused ribs by expansion thoracostomy and insertion of vertical expandable prosthetic titanium rib: growth of thoracic spine and improvement of lung volumes. Spine 30(Suppl 17):S58–S68
11. Fernandes P, Weinstein SL (2007) Natural history of early onset scoliosis. J Bone Joint Surg Am 89(Suppl 1):21–33
12. Goldberg CJ, Gillic I, Connaughton O et al (2003) Respiratory function and cosmesis at maturity in infantile-onset scoliosis. Spine 28(20):2397–2406
13. Hedequist DJ, Emans JB (2003) The correlation of preoperative three-dimensional computed tomography reconstructions with operative findings in congenital scoliosis. Spine 28(22):2531–2534; discussion 1
14. Karol LA, Johnston C, Mladenov K et al (2008) Pulmonary function following early thoracic fusion in non-neuromuscular scoliosis. J Bone Joint Surg Am 90(6):1272–1281
15. Mehta MH (1972) The rib-vertebra angle in the early diagnosis between resolving and progressive infantile scoliosis. J Bone Joint Surg Br 54(2):230–243
16. Motoyama EK, Fine GF, Mutich RL et al (2006) Effects on lung function of multiple expansion thoracoplasty in children with thoracic insufficiency syndrome: a longitudinal study. Spine 31(3):284–290
17. Pehrsson K, Larsson S, Oden A et al (1992) Long-term follow-up of patients with untreated scoliosis. A study of mortality, causes of death, and symptoms. Spine 17(9):1091–1096
18. Raat H, Landgraf JM, Bonsel GJ et al (2002) Reliability and validity of comprehensive health status measures in children: the child health questionnaire in relation to the health utilities index. J Clin Epidemiol 55(1):67–76
19. Redding G, Song K, Inscore S et al (2008) Lung function asymmetry in children with congenital and infantile scoliosis. Spine J 8(4):639–644
20. Scott JC, Morgan TH (1955) The natural history and prognosis of infantile idiopathic scoliosis. J Bone Joint Surg Br 37-B(3):400–413
21. Sponseller PD, Yazici M, Demetracopoulos C et al (2007) Evidence basis for management of spine and chest wall deformities in children. Spine 32(Suppl 19):S81–S90
22. Stucki G, Cieza A, Ewert T et al (2008) ICF-based classification and measurement of functioning. Eur J Phys Rehabil Med 44(3):315–328
23. Thompson GH, Akbarnia BA, Kostial P et al (2005) Comparison of single and dual growing rod techniques followed through definitive surgery: a preliminary study. Spine 30(18):2039–2044
24. Vitale MG, Matsumoto H, Bye MR et al (2008) A retrospective cohort study of pulmonary function, radiographic measures, and quality of life in children with congenital scoliosis: an evaluation of patient outcomes after early spinal fusion. Spine 33(11):1242–1249
25. Vitale MG, Matsumoto H, Bye MR et al (2008) Health-related quality of life in children with thoracic insufficiency syndrome. J Pediatr Orthop 28(2):239–243
26. Vitale MG, Matsumoto H, Bye MR (2010) Variability of expert opinion in treatment of early onset scoliosis. Clinical orthopaedics and related research. In press
27. Wattenbarger JM, Richards BS, Herring JA (2000) A comparison of single-rod instrumentation with double-rod instrumentation in adolescent idiopathic scoliosis. Spine 25(13): 1680–1688
28. Weinstein SL, Dolan LA, Spratt KF et al (2003) Health and function of patients with untreated idiopathic scoliosis: a 50-year natural history study. JAMA 289(5):559–567

44 Current Research in Growth Modulation and Future Outlook

Peter O. Newton and Vidyadhar V. Upasani

Key Points

- Modulation of spinal growth has the potential to eliminate spinal fusions in the treatment of scoliosis in children and adolescents.
- Current research in the field is focusing on anterior and posterior spinal approaches as well as methods to modulate the chest cage growth.
- The goal of spinal growth modulation is to redirect the power of spinal growth to drive scoliosis correction rather than scoliosis progression, while preserving functional spinal mobility.

44.1 Introduction

Surgical instrumentation and fusion is currently the definitive treatment for children with spinal deformities. Although midterm follow-up studies with modern instrumentation systems and techniques have demonstrated satisfactory outcomes in terms of deformity correction, maintenance of correction, and patient satisfaction, it is well accepted that spinal fusions sacrifice spinal flexibility, alter stresses on adjacent unfused segments, and may lead to problems with spinal imbalance in the long term [9, 19, 20, 26, 29, 40]. Concerns with outcomes in the long term have motivated investigators to study more physiologic treatment options that would maximize axial growth and allow spinal motion to maintain intervertebral disc health, while limiting deformity progression. This chapter discusses the rationale behind growth modulation techniques, summarizes current research endeavors in this field, and provides some insights into future developments for fusion-delaying spinal surgery.

44.2 Biologic Growth Modulation

44.2.1 Hemiepiphyseodesis

The use of a unilateral fusion, often termed a hemiepiphyseodesis, as a means of altering spinal growth has been used primarily in congenital scoliosis. The technique has had mixed outcomes, but in some cases, deformity correction has been noted (if the age is less than 5 years, deformity less than 50°). The downside of this approach is the loss of motion associated with the arthrodesis and the relatively low reliability of true growth modulation with the technique. The term is somewhat of a misnomer, suggesting a unilateral closure of the growth plate as performed regularly in the long bone of adolescent patients for genu varum and valgum. In fact, the procedure is a hemiarthrodesis, with the hope that a boney tether will alter spinal growth favorably.

44.2.2 Rib Shortening/Lengthening

The three-dimensional structural deformity in idiopathic scoliosis involves not only the spine but also the ribs, the pelvis, and the thoracic and abdominal viscera. The rib prominence is one of the main sources of patient

P. O. Newton (✉)
University of California San Diego, Rady Children's Hospital and Health Center, 3030 Children's Way, Suite 410, San Diego, CA 92123, USA
e-mail: pnewton@rchsd.org

B. A. Akbarnia et al. (eds.), *The Growing Spine*,
DOI: 10.1007/978-3-540-85207-0_44, © Springer-Verlag Berlin Heidelberg 2011

dissatisfaction, and most approaches to surgical treatment of scoliosis do not address this thoracic deformity directly [46, 49]. Instead, a secondary improvement in rib cage geometry is accomplished by attempting to restore three-dimensional alignment of the spinal column. Although the primary interest in convex-side costoplasty is to treat the cosmetic deformity of the posterior rib hump, clinical investigators have provided evidence for the effect of rib asymmetry in the pathogenesis of idiopathic scoliosis [51]. Experimental studies have shown that scoliosis can be corrected by rib length modulation (shortening or lengthening), taking into account the growth potential of the spine and rib cage [3, 13, 58]. Forces transmitted from the sternum to the vertebral column by the ribs are thought to balance growth of the thoracic spine. Concave-side rib shortening or convex-side rib lengthening have been shown to be helpful in the management of scoliotic deformities by slowing down the rate of deformity progression or by even causing retrogression of the curve, to delay posterior spinal fusion [3, 13, 25].

These procedures, however, have yet to gain wide acceptance, as their biomechanical effects on the spine are not well understood. A 2002 study by Grealou et al. [22] evaluated the biomechanical action of different surgical approaches on the rib cage using a patient-specific finite element model to analyze the resulting geometry and load patterns in the ribs, costovertebral articulation, and vertebrae. They supported the concept of using rib-modifying procedures to induce correction of spinal scoliotic deformity. Carrier et al. [18] performed a similar biomechanical analysis and showed that concave-side rib shortening induced load patterns on vertebral endplates that could act against scoliosis progression, resulting in a decrease in thoracic apical vertebral wedging and a decreased lateral spinal curvature. However, both the rib hump and vertebral axial rotation were found to increase on average by 4° at the curve apex in their models. Future studies need to evaluate the effects of spinal growth modulation from induced loads, in biomechanical and animal models, to more effectively prove the usefulness of rib shortening/lengthening procedures.

44.2.3 Vertebral Neurocentral Synchondrosis Asymmetry

Asymmetrical growth at the neurocentral synchondrosis (Fig. 44.1) has been considered as another possible etiology for the three-dimensional spinal deformity

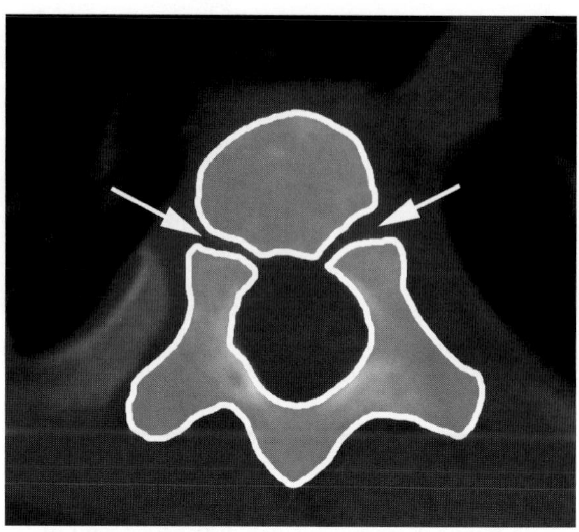

Fig. 44.1 Axial CT image of a 14-month-old spine demonstrating bilateral open neurocentral synchondroses (*white arrows*)

seen in AIS. In theory, an abnormality at the neurocentral junction is thought to produce pedicle length asymmetry, thus leading to vertebral rotation [34]. Vertebral wedging is then thought to result from rotation induced increases in compressive loads on the vertebral growth plates [4]. Once the initial deformity is present, scoliosis is thought to develop due to the propagation of asymmetric loads by the Hueter–Volkmann effect.

Previous anatomic studies of normal and scoliotic vertebrae have found an association between a longer pedicle and vertebral rotation [47, 52, 55]; however, a causative relationship could not be established. A recent 2007 biomechanical simulation with asymmetrical pedicle geometry was not able to produce significant scoliosis, vertebral rotation, or wedging [27], and concluded that asymmetry of pedicle growth rate alone was not sufficient to cause scoliosis. On the other hand, asymmetric epiphysiodesis of the neurocentral synchondrosis (NCS) was performed in a growing porcine model and was able to create a scoliotic deformity with axial vertebral rotation. In addition, the magnitude of the deformity created was found to correlate with the degree of NCS physis closure [59].

44.3 Asymmetric Vertebral Growth

Temporal relationships between scoliosis development and deformity progression, with periods of rapid spinal growth, have encouraged investigators to evaluate etiologic theories of vertebral and spinal growth abnormalities. The spinal deformity in main thoracic idiopathic scoliosis has been associated with relative anterior thoracic spinal overgrowth and a lordotic apical region [44, 50]. Dickson et al. [21] theorized that axial rotation and lateral deviation of the thoracic spine occurred in an attempt to balance asymmetric growth in the sagittal plane. In addition, several morphological studies have identified intravertebral deformities in patients with idiopathic scoliosis [30, 31, 39]. In 2003, Guo et al. [23] proposed that the pathomechanism behind vertebral body asymmetry was disproportionate endochondral and membranous growth. Thus, asymmetric spinal growth and biomechanical imbalance, perpetuated by the Hueter–Volkmann effect, has been postulated as a possible etiology for the progressive deformity observed in idiopathic scoliosis. Ideally, a treatment option would be available that would correct the vertebral growth asymmetry while preserving spinal mobility and long-term function.

44.4 Spinal Growth Modulation Techniques

In the young child, spinal growth modulation provides an important alternative to treat spinal deformity [33]. In a study by Braun et al. [11] a variety of fusionless scoliosis implant strategies were tested in the rat tail model. This study used both rigid and flexible implants to modulate vertebral body growth. The results from their study demonstrated that dynamic loading of the vertebrae provided the greatest growth modulation potential. Aronsson et al. similarly showed that alternating compression and distraction applied to adjacent vertebrae in the calf tail could modulate vertebral growth, suggesting that dynamic motion would be preferred [2].

44.4.1 Anterior Vertebral Staples

Vertebral body stapling was first described in 1951 by Nachlas and Borden [35], using principles learned from growth modulation of the long bones. Vertebral staples were placed across physeal end plates in a canine scoliosis model, resulting in restriction of curve progression and even deformity correction in some cases. There were however several instances of implant failure, thought to be caused by poor staple design and because some of the staples spanned multiple motion segments. In 1954, Smith et al. [48] presented outcomes after vertebral stapling in patients with congenital scoliosis. Their results were disappointing, however, likely because the children had limited growth remaining and because the curves treated were quite severe.

Advancements in staple design have lead to more promising results. Staple hemiepiphysiodesis has been performed by Wall et al. [56] in a porcine model to consistently create spinal deformities in the coronal plane averaging 22.4 ± 2.8°. Braun et al. [8, 9, 12] have tested recently developed nitinol staples in an immature goat scoliosis model, showing them to be safe and efficacious in the treatment of curves less than 70°. Nitinol staples are made out of a shape memory nickel–titanium alloy. The staple prongs are straight when cooled and clamp down into the shape of a "C" when warmed to body temperature [24]. When used in attempts to correct experimentally created scoliosis in an animal model, however, anterior vertebral staples were not able to fully reverse the Hueter–Volkmann effect and only controlled progressive vertebral wedging [11]. In addition, a recent biomechanical study evaluating spinal flexibility after instrumentation with nitinol staples found that staples significantly restricted motion, especially in axial rotation and lateral bending [43].

In 2003, Betz et al. [5] presented the first large clinical case series on anterior vertebral body stapling, reporting on 21 skeletally immature patients with adolescent idiopathic scoliosis. Indications for the procedure were either brace noncompliance or progression of the deformity despite bracing. The authors concluded that the procedure was feasible, safe, and able to stabilize curve progression in the short term. With increasing experience, 87% of the patients who were older than 8 years and had curves less than 50°, had less than 10° curve progression [6]. During this follow-up period, 2 out of 39 patients (5%) required a definitive fusion procedure, one patient's course (3%) was complicated by a diaphragmatic hernia, and five patients (13%) experienced minor complications. The surgical indications for this procedure continue to be refined, and several factors including age (less than 13 years in girls and 15 year in boys), maturity (Risser 0 or 1 and/or 1 year of growth remaining on wrist radiograph), and deformity (coronal curve less than 45° with minimal rotation and flexibility to less than 25°, and sagittal thoracic curves less than 40°) need to be considered. Preliminary clinical results of stapling in patients with idiopathic scoliosis have been encouraging; however, further clinical studies with controls are needed (Fig. 44.2a–d).

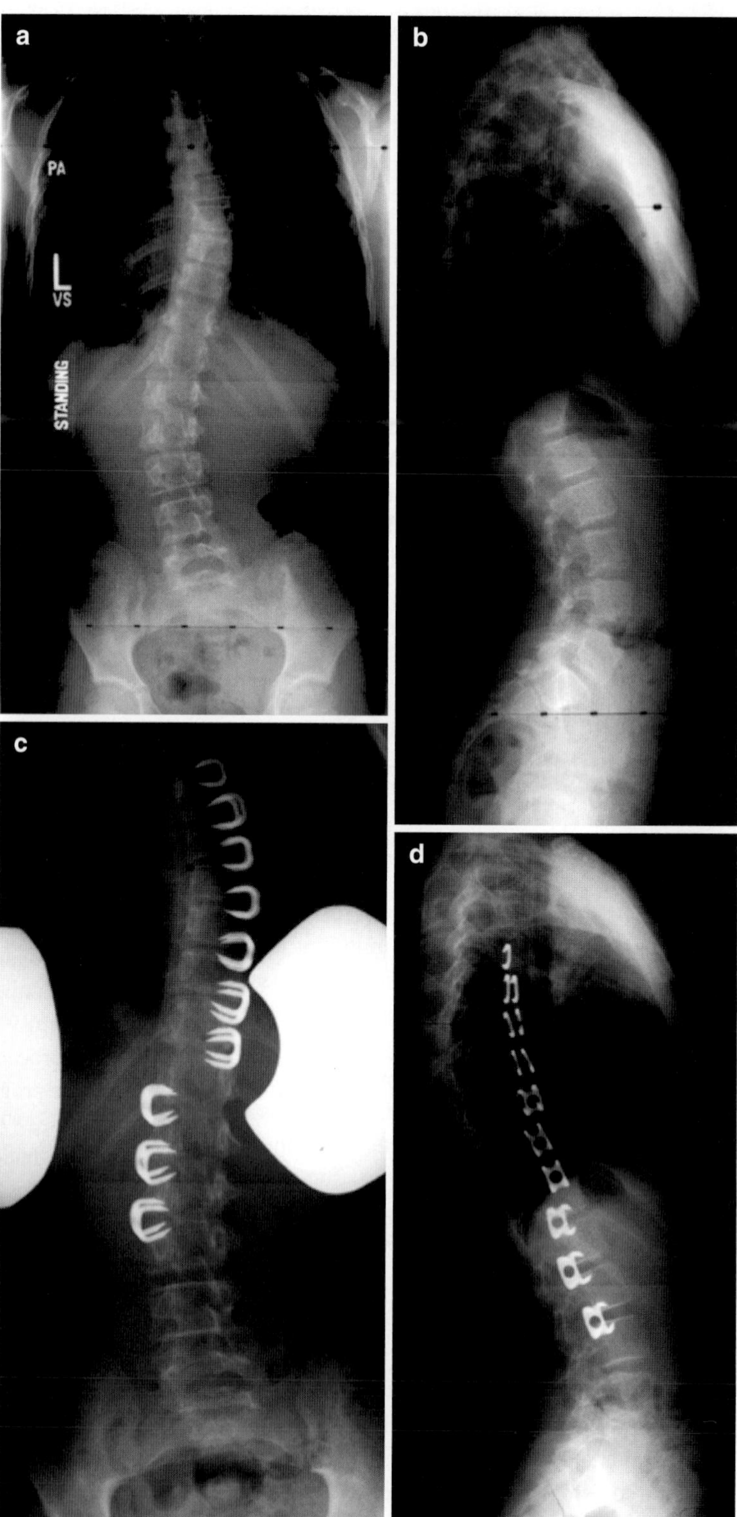

Fig. 44.2 Preoperative posterior–anterior (PA) and lateral radiographs (**a, b**) of a 10-year-old female with juvenile idiopathic scoliosis. Two-year postoperative radiographs after anterior vertebral staples were placed on the convexity of the thoracic and lumbar curves (**c, d**). (Courtesy of Randal Betz, MD)

44.4.2 Anterolateral Spinal Tethering

Anterior vertebral body tethering provides an alternate approach for spinal growth modulation. Similar to vertebral staples, the tether creates a compressive load on the anterior vertebral body and, through the Hueter–Volkmann principal, attempts to correct the asymmetric anterior spinal overgrowth described by Guo et al. [23]. A theoretical advantage over vertebral staples, however, is that anterior tethering may provide a less rigid construct, and thus be less detrimental to long-term intervertebral disc health and spinal motion.

Anterolateral spinal tethering has been tested previously in various animal models. In 2002, Newton et al. [36] evaluated the effects of flexible mechanical tethering of a single motion segment. Eight immature calves were instrumented with anterior vertebral body screws over four consecutive thoracic vertebrae. Two screws were connected by a stainless steel tether and two were left unconnected. After 12 weeks of growth, coronal and sagittal plane deformities were consistently created over the tethered motion segments, compared to control segments. In addition, vertebral body wedging was observed, indicating that physeal growth had decreased on the side of the tether (Fig. 44.3). Biomechanical analyses revealed that the tether restricted lateral bending range of motion. However, this motion was found to return to control levels when the tether was removed. A follow-up study evaluating multilevel growth modulation in the bovine model concluded that given adequate bony fixation, the flexible tether was able to consistently create a biplanar spinal deformity without having a detrimental effect on spinal motion [37].

In 2005, Braun et al. [10] compared the ability of shape memory alloy staples and bone anchor ligament tethers to correct an experimental scoliosis in 24 Spanish Cross-X goats. The flexible ligament tethers were found to improve scoliosis from an average of 73.4–69.9°, while scoliosis actually progressed in the goats treated with staples from an average of 77.3–94.3°. Pull-out testing demonstrated that the bone anchors had improved integration into the vertebral bodies, while the staples were found to loosen. Histologic evidence of a halo of fibrous tissue around the staple tines was also presented and was thought to be responsible for staple loosening.

The next step in the development of the vertebral tether was to evaluate intervertebral disc health after spinal growth modulation. As discussed above, fusionless treatment strategies need to preserve the intervertebral disc if they are to be successful in the long-term. Histologic and biochemical evaluation of intervertebral disc health after spinal growth modulation was reported by Newton et al. [38]. Intervertebral discs from seventeen bovine instrumented with a multilevel flexible steel cable were compared with discs

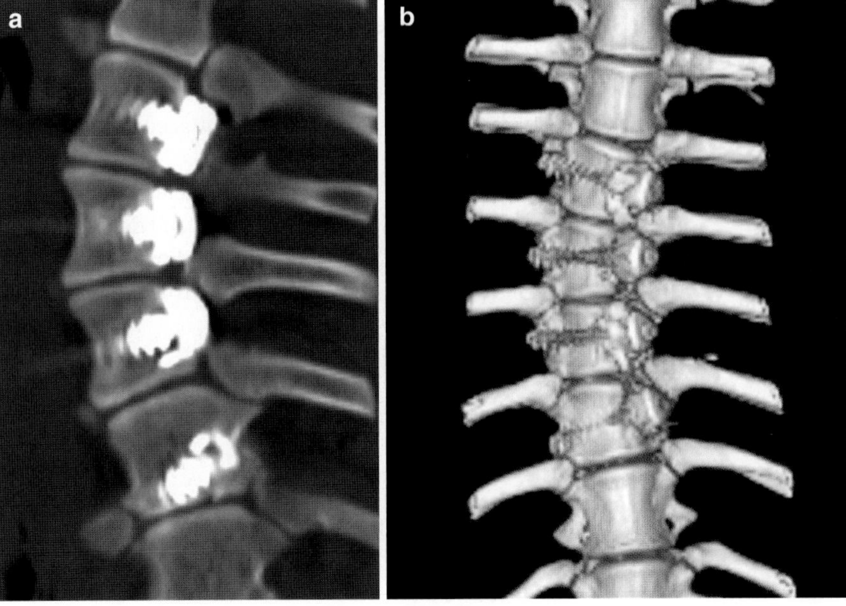

Fig. 44.3 Representative midcoronal 2d CT image (**a**) and 3d CT anterior–posterior image (**b**) of a porcine spine instrumented with an anterolateral spinal tether demonstrate deformity creation and vertebra body wedging after 12 months of spinal growth modulation

from 19 bovine that underwent a control sham surgery (screw-only). A double screw-double tether construct was required in this rapidly growing model to achieve adequate bony fixation. No change in disc water content or gross morphological grading was observed between the two groups; however, decreased disc thickness, increased proteoglycan synthesis, and a change in collagen distribution was present in the tethered discs. Further studies of disc health with noninvasive imaging modalities for the detection of early degeneration and after long-term growth modulation are required.

Clinical application of the anterior vertebral tether has been performed by Lenke (personal communication) in two patients. The curve in the first case reduced from 50° to 25° and was held over a 2-year follow-up period with no complications (Fig. 44.4a–h). The second case was that of an 8-year-old girl with a 30° left thoracic curve, which has corrected to 0° in the coronal plane over a 2-year postoperative follow-up period. Future clinical trials will be required once the effect of anterolateral spinal tethering on intervertebral disc health and the vertebral physis has been thoroughly evaluated.

Although, long-term clinical data with vertebral staples or the tether are not available at this time, anterior spinal growth modulation provides an exciting alternative to controlling progressive scoliosis, while maintaining spinal motion. Its ideal application will likely be in the treatment of preadolescent idiopathic scoliosis with 20–40° curves that have a high likelihood of progression. The staples or the tether would act like an internal brace and limit curve progression, or possibly even improve the deformity during the patient's growth spurt, to delay or eliminate the need for a definitive fusion procedure.

44.5 Posterior Spinal Growth Modulation Techniques

44.5.1 Posterior Spinal Tether

Vertebral tethers have also been used in the posterior spine to modulate spinal growth. In 2006, Lowe et al. [32] evaluated the ability of polyethylene cords to effect sagittal alignment in an immature nonfusion segmental pedicle screw sheep model. At 13 months after surgery, the tethered animals had significantly less kyphosis and vertebral body wedging that the control animals. The authors concluded that the posterior tether may be a potential treatment for adolescents with Scheuermann's disease.

44.5.2 Shape-Memory Metal Instrumentation

A nickel–titanium alloy, similar to that used in nitinol anterior vertebral staples, was used to develop a posterior spinal instrumentation system that would achieve a gradual three-dimensional scoliosis correction [45]. It was theorized that the shape memory metal instrumentation would continue to load the spine postoperatively and take advantage of the spine's viscous properties to obtain further deformity correction over time. Historically, a single-rod construct was used in conjunction with a posterior spinal fusion as an attempt to prevent implant failure associated with motion [57]. It was thought that the additional postoperative correction would occur before arthrodesis formation. The authors' reported induction of a significant scoliosis (average 40°) in all test animals intraoperatively. Postoperatively (6-weeks and 3-months), however, there were no significant changes in deformity magnitude observed, and gross evaluation of the harvested spines (3-months postop) revealed that the instrumentation was nearly overgrown with newly formed bone. Of note, implant corrosion, tissue discoloration, and nickel accumulation were not observed in any of the animals. Additional in vivo animal studies are currently underway to evaluate deformity creation using single- and dual-rod shape memory metal instrumentation without fusion in a porcine model (Newton et al., unpublished document 2008).

44.5.3 Expandable Spinal Instrumentation

Growing rods or expandable spinal implants have been used for decades to control spinal deformity while allowing patient maturation and spinal growth.

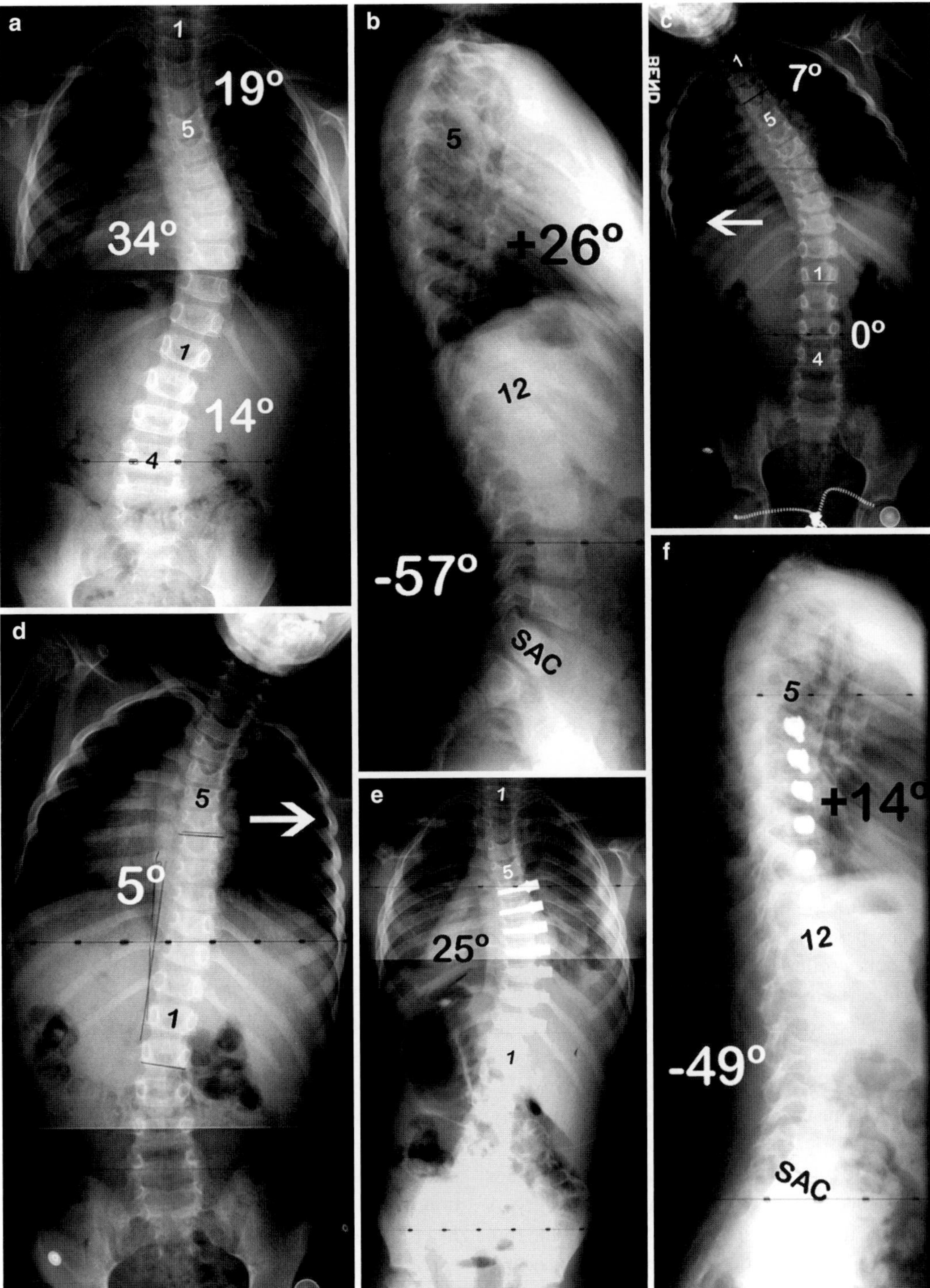

Fig. 44.4 Preoperative posterior–anterior (PA), lateral and side-bending radiographs (**a–d**) of a 8-year 4-month-old boy with juvenile idiopathic scoliosis demonstrate a 34° right thoracic curve with 85% flexibility and a 14° left lumbar curve with 100% flexibility. An anterior spinal tether was placed through a thoracoscopic approach from T6 to T12. Immediate postoperative radiographs (**e, f**) demonstrate a 25° right thoracic curve (26% correction).

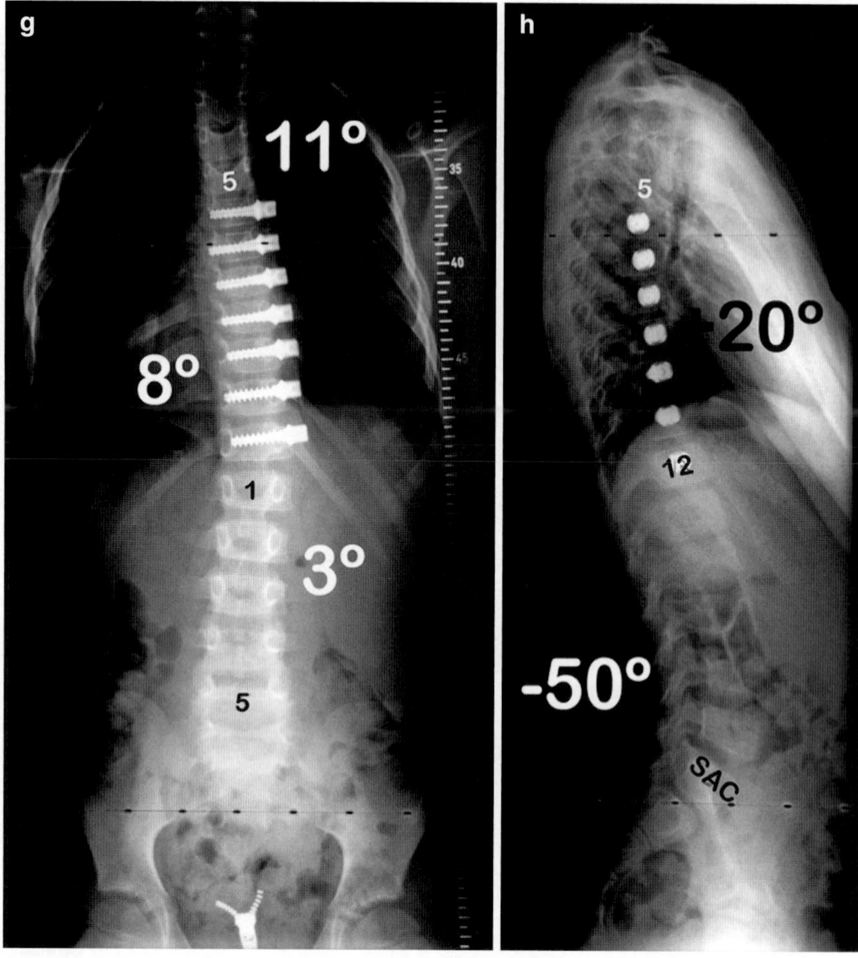

Fig. 44.4 (continued) At 2-year postoperative, radiographs (**g, h**) demonstrate an 8° right thoracic curve (76% correction). (Courtesy of Lawrence Lenke, MD)

Historically, periodic lengthening of a single Harrington rod or Luque trolleys used to support spinal alignment during growth were commonly used [28, 41, 42]. Although these techniques resulted in satisfactory deformity control, complication rates associated with implant failure and spontaneous autofusion were unacceptable, and spinal growth was limited. More recently, Blakemore et al. [7] presented a preliminary report using a submuscular Isola rod with a proximal and/or distal segmental claw for added construct stability. A postoperative orthosis was also used to protect the rod, and a limited apical fusion was performed in nearly 40% of the cases. With an average follow-up of 41 months (range, 11–65 months), the authors reported an improvement in the average coronal deformity from 66 to 47° and a 24% incidence of complications, including: five hook displacements, three rod breakages, and one superficial wound infection (Fig. 44.5a–h).

Periodic lengthening with dual growing rod instrumentation has recently been popularized by Akbarnia et al. [1]. Minimum 2-year follow-up of 23 patients treated with dual growing rods revealed a significant improvement in deformity from 82 ± 20° preoperatively to 38 ± 15° at last follow up. In addition, they reported an overall spinal growth rate (T1–S1) of 1.2 ± 0.7 cm/year. The authors concluded that this technique provided superior stability and maintenance of correction; however, a total of 13 complications were reported in 11 of the 23 patients (48%).

A comparison of single and dual growing rod techniques [53, 54] indicated that both procedures were effective in controlling spinal deformity. Dual growing rods were better able to achieve an initial deformity correction and maintain the correction at 2-years postop; however, the single rod resulted in improved frontal and sagittal plane balance. Future studies with

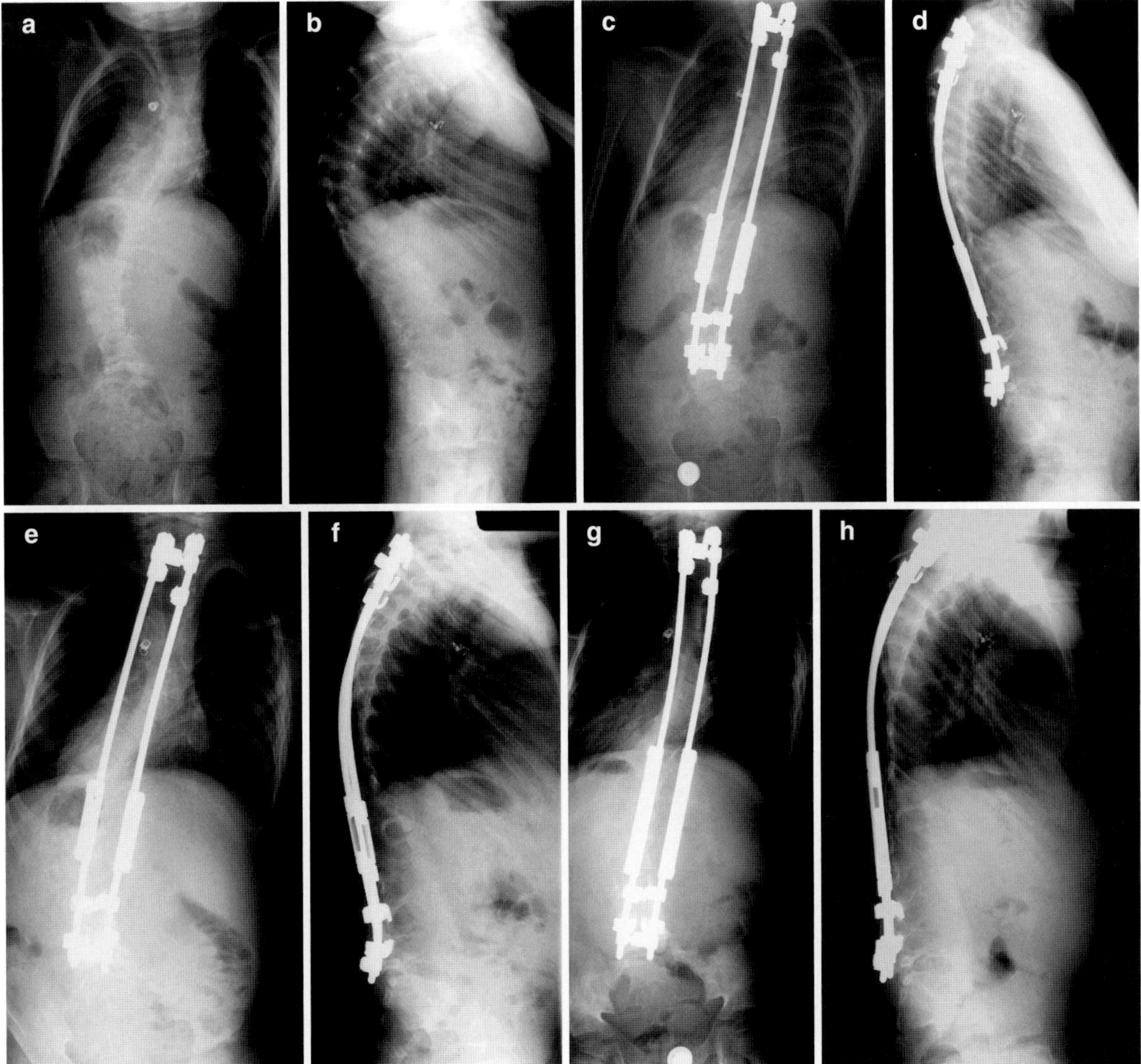

Fig. 44.5 Preoperative posterior–anterior (PA) and lateral radiographs (**a, b**) of a 3-year 5-month-old boy with neuromuscular kyphoscoliosis associated with lateral meningocele syndrome, demonstrate a 71° right thoracic curve with 46% flexibility, a 76° left lumbar curve with 42% flexibility, and a thoracic kyphosis of 88°. Radiographs and spinal MRI were negative for congenital vertebral or intraspinal anomalies. He underwent a posterior spinal fusion at T1-2 and L4-5 with implantation of a dual growing rod construct from T1 to L5. A 1-cm lengthening was performed at 8 months postop (**c, d**) and 14 months postop (**e, f**). At 2-year postoperative, radiographs demonstrate no implant failure, an improved sagittal profile, and maintenance of the coronal plane deformity (**g, h**)

growing rods need to evaluate techniques to further improve construct stability and decrease complications associated with rod breakage and hook displacement. In addition, evaluation of transverse plane deformity correction, intervertebral disc health, facet degeneration, and adjacent segment disease is required to predict long-term outcomes after growing rod treatment.

44.6 Vertical Expandable Prosthetic Titanium Rib

The vertical expandable prosthetic titanium rib (VEPTR) can be used to treat patients with infantile idiopathic or early onset scoliosis associated with a constrictive chest wall deformity [15]. The treatment

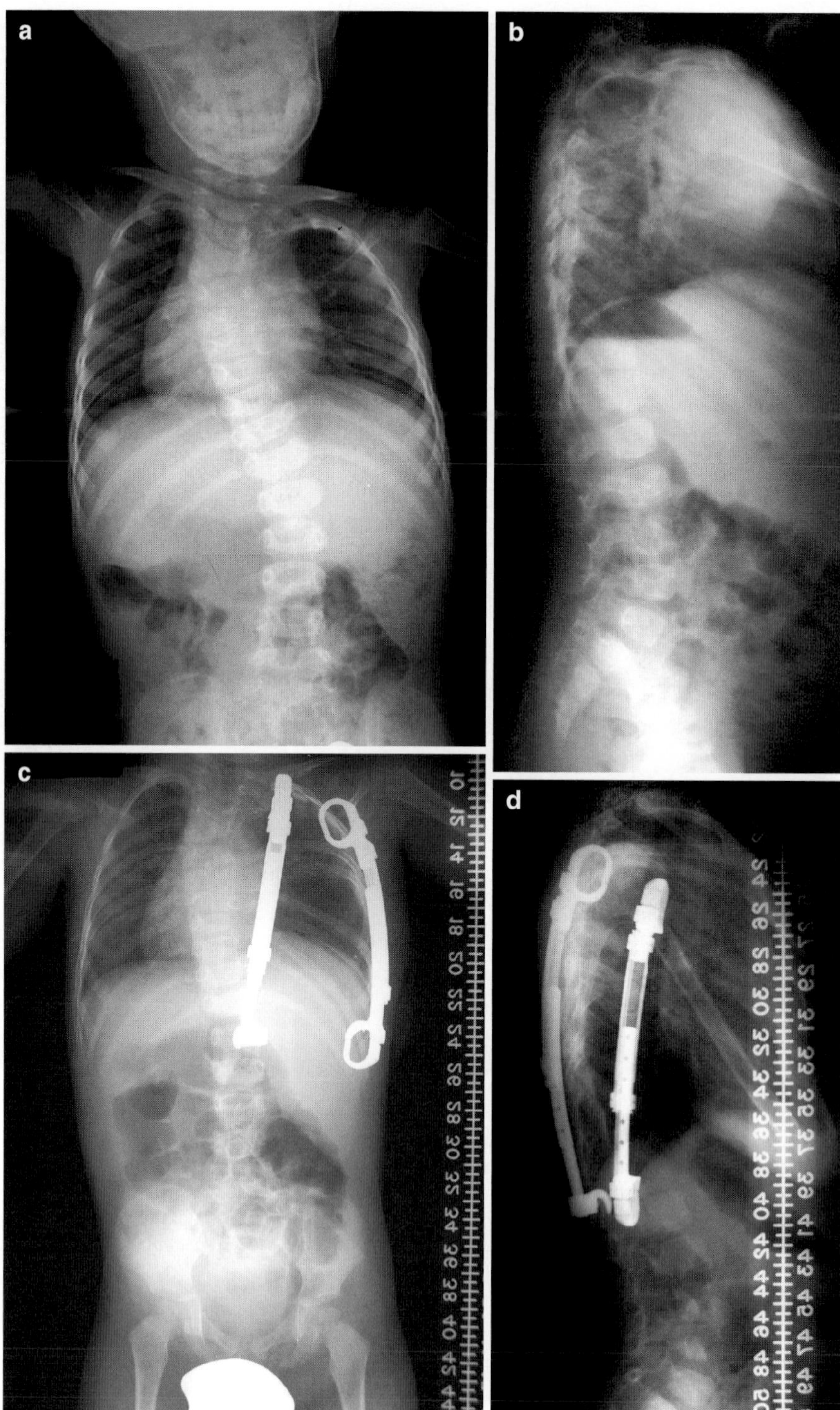

Fig. 44.6 Preoperative posterior–anterior (PA) and lateral radiographs (**a, b**) of a 21-month-old girl demonstrate a 55° rigid left thoracic congenital scoliosis with multiple fused ribs on the right (T1-4, T6-7 and T8-10), a concave bar (T4-7), a convex T8 hemivertebra, and a hemimetameric shift between T4 and T5. Cervical spine radiographs and spine MRI were normal. She underwent an expansion thoracoplasty at T5-6, with a hybrid VEPTR implant placed from T3 to L1 and a rib-to-rib VEPTR implant placed from T3 to T10 (**c, d**).

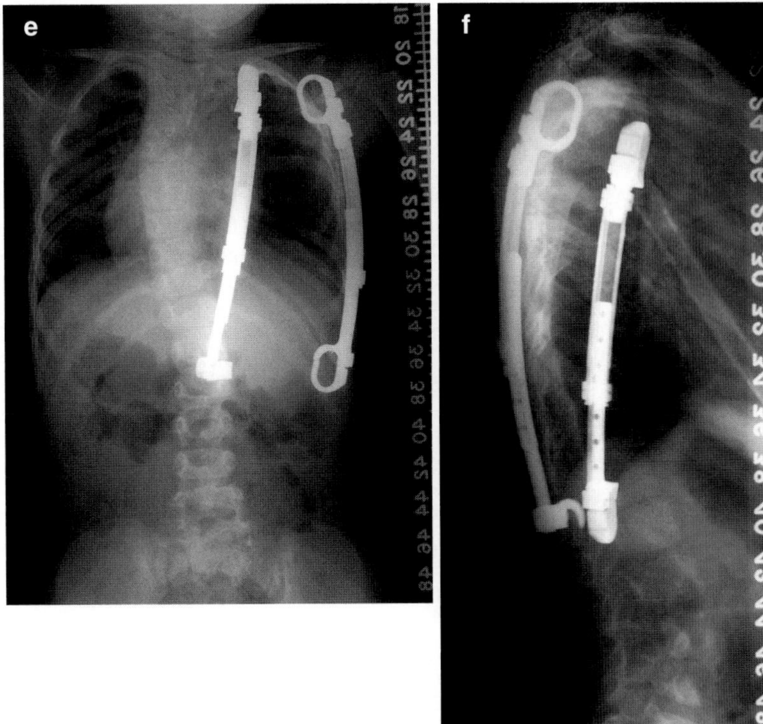

Fig. 44.6 (continued) After three expansions at 6-month intervals, her 18-month postoperative radiographs (**e, f**) demonstrate a well-expanded right thoracic cavity and a 38° left thoracic curve. (Courtesy of Randal Betz, MD)

strategy in these patients is to maximize thoracic volume and symmetry by performing an opening wedge thoracostomy on the concavity of the spinal deformity, either through intercostal muscle lysis or through an osteotomy of fused ribs [14, 16, 17]. The scoliotic spinal deformity is thus corrected indirectly, and the thoracic reconstruction can be stabilized by an additional rib to rib, rib to spine, or rib to pelvis VEPTR construct. Serial lengthenings can be performed every 4–6 months to allow expansion of the constricted hemithorax and delay spinal fusion until skeletal maturity (Fig. 44.6a–d).

Clinical results in patients with congenital scoliosis have been promising. With an average follow up of 5.7 years, Campbell et al. [17] reported an improvement in thoracic spinal deformity in 27 patients from an average of 74° preoperatively to 49° at last follow up. Thoracic spinal growth was noted to be 0.71 cm/year on average and a significant increase in the space available for the lung ratio was observed; however, there were a total of 52 complications reported in 22 patients. The authors concluded that the VEPTR was particularly beneficial in patients with congenital scoliosis and compromised pulmonary function, to treat thoracic insufficiency while controlling spinal deformity and allowing growth of the thoracic spine and rib cage, however, recommended that the technique be performed by a multidisciplinary team after specialized training. Future studies with a greater number of patients are required to better define the indications for this innovative technique and identify the predictors of implant failure.

44.7 Conclusions

Both spinal motion and spinal growth are unfortunately commonly sacrificed in the treatment of young patients with spinal deformity. New treatment solutions to overcome this current limitation are required. While several nonfusion treatment strategies to preserve motion and growth are under investigation, it is likely that more than one solution will be required to account for the numerous complexities of spinal deformity in the growing child. By understanding normal and pathologic spinal growth, it is hoped that solutions to modulate spinal growth can be created to successfully correct spinal deformities in childhood and adolescence without the need for a spinal fusion.

References

1. Akbarnia BA, Marks DS, Boachie-Adjei O et al (2005) Dual growing rod technique for the treatment of progressive early-onset scoliosis: a multi-center study. Spine 30(Suppl 17): S46–S57
2. Aronsson DD, Stokes IA, Rosovsky J et al (1999) Mechanical modulation of calf tail vertebral growth: implications for scoliosis progression. J Spinal Disord 12(2):141–146
3. Barrett DS, MacLean JG, Bettany J et al (1993) Costoplasty in adolescent idiopathic scoliosis. Objective results in 55 patients. J Bone Joint Surg Br 75(6):881–885
4. Beguiristain JL, De Salis J, Oriaifo A et al (1980) Experimental scoliosis by epiphysiodesis in pigs. Int Orthop 3(4):317–321
5. Betz RR, Kim J, D'Andrea LP et al (2003) An innovative technique of vertebral body stapling for the treatment of patients with adolescent idiopathic scoliosis: a feasibility, safety, and utility study. Spine 28(20):S255–S265
6. Betz RR, D'Andrea LP, Mulcahey MJ et al (2005) Vertebral body stapling procedure for the treatment of scoliosis in the growing child. Clin Orthop Relat Res (434):55–60
7. Blakemore LC, Scoles PV, Poe-Kochert C et al (2001) Submuscular Isola rod with or without limited apical fusion in the management of severe spinal deformities in young children: preliminary report. Spine 26(18):2044–2048
8. Braun JT, Ogilvie JW, Akyuz E et al (2003) Experimental scoliosis in an immature goat model: a method that creates idiopathic-type deformity with minimal violation of the spinal elements along the curve. Spine 28(19):2198–2203
9. Braun JT, Ogilvie JW, Akyuz E et al (2004) Fusionless scoliosis correction using a shape memory alloy staple in the anterior thoracic spine of the immature goat. Spine 29(18):1980–1989
10. Braun JT, Akyuz E, Ogilvie JW et al (2005) The efficacy and integrity of shape memory alloy staples and bone anchors with ligament tethers in the fusionless treatment of experimental scoliosis. J Bone Joint Surg Am 87(9):2038–2051
11. Braun JT, Hines JL, Akyuz E et al (2006) Relative versus absolute modulation of growth in the fusionless treatment of experimental scoliosis. Spine 31(16):1776–1782
12. Braun JT, Hoffman M, Akyuz E et al (2006) Mechanical modulation of vertebral growth in the fusionless treatment of progressive scoliosis in an experimental model. Spine 31(12): 1314–1320
13. Broome G, Simpson AH, Catalan J et al (1990) The modified Schollner costoplasty. J Bone Joint Surg Br 72(5):894–900
14. Campbell RM Jr, Hell-Vocke AK (2003) Growth of the thoracic spine in congenital scoliosis after expansion thoracoplasty. J Bone Joint Surg Am 85-A(3):409–420
15. Campbell RM Jr, Smith MD, Mayes TC et al (2003) The characteristics of thoracic insufficiency syndrome associated with fused ribs and congenital scoliosis. J Bone Joint Surg Am 85-A(3):399–408
16. Campbell RM Jr, Smith MD, Hell-Vocke AK (2004) Expansion thoracoplasty: the surgical technique of opening-wedge thoracostomy. Surgical technique. J Bone Joint Surg Am 86-A(Suppl 1):51–64
17. Campbell RM Jr, Smith MD, Mayes TC et al (2004) The effect of opening wedge thoracostomy on thoracic insufficiency syndrome associated with fused ribs and congenital scoliosis. J Bone Joint Surg Am 86-A(8):1659–1674
18. Carrier J, Aubin CE, Villemure I et al (2004) Biomechanical modeling of growth modulation following rib shortening or lengthening in adolescent idiopathic scoliosis. Med Biol Eng Comput 42(4):541–548
19. Cheh G, Bridwell KH, Lenke LG et al (2007) Adjacent segment disease following lumbar/thoracolumbar fusion with pedicle screw instrumentation: a minimum 5-year follow-up. Spine 32(20):2253–2257
20. Danielsson AJ, Cederlund CG, Ekholm S et al (2001) The prevalence of disc aging and back pain after fusion extending into the lower lumbar spine. A matched MR study twenty-five years after surgery for adolescent idiopathic scoliosis. Acta Radiol 42(2):187–197
21. Dickson RA, Lawton JO, Archer IA et al (1984) The pathogenesis of idiopathic scoliosis. Biplanar spinal asymmetry. J Bone Joint Surg Br 66(1):8–15
22. Grealou L, Aubin CE, Labelle H (2002) Rib cage surgery for the treatment of scoliosis: a biomechanical study of correction mechanisms. J Orthop Res 20(5):1121–1128
23. Guo X, Chau WW, Chan YL et al (2003) Relative anterior spinal overgrowth in adolescent idiopathic scoliosis. Results of disproportionate endochondral-membranous bone growth. J Bone Joint Surg Br 85(7):1026–1031
24. Guille JT, D'Andrea LP, Betz RR (2007) Fusionless treatment of scoliosis. Orthop Clin North Am 38(4):541–545
25. Harding IJ, Chopin D, Charosky S et al (2005) Long-term results of Schollner costoplasty in patients with idiopathic scoliosis. Spine 30(14):1627–1631
26. Hilibrand AS, Robbins M (2004) Adjacent segment degeneration and adjacent segment disease: the consequences of spinal fusion? Spine J 4(Suppl 6):190S–194S
27. Huynh AM, Aubin CE, Rajwani T et al (2007) Pedicle growth asymmetry as a cause of adolescent idiopathic scoliosis: a biomechanical study. Eur Spine J 16(4):523–529
28. Klemme WR, Denis F, Winter RB et al (1997) Spinal instrumentation without fusion for progressive scoliosis in young children. J Pediatr Orthop 17(6):734–742
29. Lerner T, Frobin W, Bullmann V et al (2007) Changes in disc height and postero-anterior displacement after fusion in patients with idiopathic scoliosis: a 9-year follow-up study. J Spinal Disord Tech 20(3):195–202
30. Liljenqvist UR, Link TM, Halm HF (2000) Morphometric analysis of thoracic and lumbar vertebrae in idiopathic scoliosis. Spine 25(10):1247–1253
31. Liljenqvist UR, Allkemper T, Hackenberg L et al (2002) Analysis of vertebral morphology in idiopathic scoliosis with use of magnetic resonance imaging and multi-planar reconstruction. J Bone Joint Surg Am 84-A(3):359–368
32. Lowe TG, Wilson L, Chien JT et al (2005) A posterior tether for fusionless modulation of sagittal plane growth in a sheep model. Spine 30(Suppl 17):S69–S74
33. Mente PL, Aronsson DD, Stokes IA et al (1999) Mechanical modulation of growth for the correction of vertebral wedge deformities. J Orthop Res 17(4):518–524
34. Michelsson JE (1965) The development of spinal deformity in experimental scoliosis. Acta Orthop Scand Suppl 81:1–91
35. Nachlas IW, Borden JN (1951) The cure of experimental scoliosis by directed growth control. J Bone Joint Surg Am 33(A:1):24–34
36. Newton PO, Fricka KB, Lee SS et al (2002) Asymmetrical flexible tethering of spine growth in an immature bovine model. Spine 27(7):689–693

37. Newton PO, Faro FD, Farnsworth CL et al (2005) Multilevel spinal growth modulation with an anterolateral flexible tether in an immature bovine model. Spine 30(23):2608–2613
38. Newton PO, Farnsworth CL, Faro FD et al (2008) Spinal growth modulation with an anterolateral flexible tether in an immature bovine model: disc health and motion preservation. Spine 33(7):724–733
39. Parent S, Labelle H, Skalli W et al (2004) Thoracic pedicle morphometry in vertebrae from scoliotic spines. Spine 29(3):239–248
40. Park P, Garton HJ, Gala VC et al (2004) Adjacent segment disease after lumbar or lumbosacral fusion: review of the literature. Spine 29(17):1938–1944
41. Patterson JF, Webb JK, Burwell RG (1990) The operative treatment of progressive early onset scoliosis. A preliminary report. Spine 15(8):809–815
42. Pratt RK, Webb JK, Burwell RG et al (1999) Luque trolley and convex epiphysiodesis in the management of infantile and juvenile idiopathic scoliosis. Spine 24(15):1538–1547
43. Puttlitz CM, Masaru F, Barkley A et al (2007) A biomechanical assessment of thoracic spine stapling. Spine 32(7):766–771
44. Roaf R (1966) The basic anatomy of scoliosis. J Bone Joint Surg Br 48(4):786–792
45. Sanders JO, Sanders AE, More R et al (1993) A preliminary investigation of shape memory alloys in the surgical correction of scoliosis. Spine 18(12):1640–1646
46. Sanders JO, Polly DW Jr, Cats-Baril W et al (2003) Analysis of patient and parent assessment of deformity in idiopathic scoliosis using the Walter Reed Visual Assessment Scale. Spine 28(18):2158–2163
47. Sevastik B, Xiong B, Sevastik J et al (1995) Vertebral rotation and pedicle length asymmetry in the normal adult spine. Eur Spine J 4(2):95–97
48. Smith AD, Von Lackum WH, Wylie R (1954) An operation for stapling vertebral bodies in congenital scoliosis. J Bone Joint Surg Am 36(A:2):342–348
49. Smith PL, Donaldson S, Hedden D et al (2006) Parents' and patients' perceptions of postoperative appearance in adolescent idiopathic scoliosis. Spine 31(20):2367–2374
50. Somerville EW (1952) Rotational lordosis; the development of single curve. J Bone Joint Surg Br 34-B(3):421–427
51. Stokes IA, Laible JP (1990) Three-dimensional osseo-ligamentous model of the thorax representing initiation of scoliosis by asymmetric growth. J Biomech 23(6):589–595
52. Taylor JR (1983) Scoliosis and growth. Patterns of asymmetry in normal vertebral growth. Acta Orthop Scand 54(4):596–602
53. Thompson GH, Akbarnia BA, Kostial P et al (2005) Comparison of single and dual growing rod techniques followed through definitive surgery: a preliminary study. Spine 30(18):2039–2044
54. Thompson GH, Akbarnia BA, Campbell RM Jr (2007) Growing rod techniques in early-onset scoliosis. J Pediatr Orthop 27(3):354–361
55. Vital JM, Beguiristain JL, Algara C et al (1989) The neurocentral vertebral cartilage: anatomy, physiology and physiopathology. Surg Radiol Anat 11(4):323–328
56. Wall EJ, Bylski-Austrow DI, Kolata RJ et al (2005) Endoscopic mechanical spinal hemiepiphysiodesis modifies spine growth. Spine 30(10):1148–1153
57. Wever DJ, Elstrodt JA, Veldhuizen AG et al (2002) Scoliosis correction with shape-memory metal: results of an experimental study. Eur Spine J 11(2):100–106
58. Xiong B, Sevastik JA (1998) A physiological approach to surgical treatment of progressive early idiopathic scoliosis. Eur Spine J 7(6):505–508
59. Zhang H, Sucato DJ (2008) Unilateral pedicle screw epiphysiodesis of the Neurocentral synchondrosis produces idiopathic like scoliosis in an immature animal model. J Bone Joint Surg Am. 90(11):2460–9

Non-Fusion Anterior Stapling

45

Randal R. Betz, Jahangir Asghar, and Amer F. Samdani

Key Points

- Vertebral body stapling is an option for the growing child with progressive scoliosis as an alternative to bracing or for the opportunity to obtain curve correction.
- The technique of staple insertion is one of thoracoscopic insertion in the thoracic spine and the use of minimal access tubes for thoracolumbar or lumbar curves.
- Clinical experience has lead to the following indications and strategies for adjuncts to stapling alone:
  - Age: less than 13 years in girls and less than 15 years in boys
  - Growth remaining: Risser 0 or 1; 1 year of growth by wrist radiograph; Sanders digital stage less than or equal to 4
  - Thoracic and lumbar coronal curve less than 45°; minimal rotation, flexible to less than 20°
  - Thoracic kyphosis less than 40°
  - If a thoracic curve measuring 35–45° does not bend below 20°, consider adding posterior rib to spine hybrid construct at the same time (do posterior first).
  - If on first erect film the curves are not less than 20°, put child in corrective brace until the curve measures less than 20°.

45.1 Introduction

The current standard of care for skeletally immature patients with progressive scoliosis measuring greater than or equal to 25° is a thoracolumbosacral orthosis (TLSO). These braces are used in an attempt to prevent curve progression, but the efficacy is variable [1, 8, 9, 12]. Some children have a problem with the stigmata associated with wearing a brace, especially those who have to wear a brace for many years [6]. Hence, there exist significant issues of compliance with brace wear.

The literature is highly varied on the compliance of brace wear, varying from 20 to 90% [11, 13]. However, objective studies using a manometer or a temperature gauge find that compliance is, at best, around 60% [7]. Also, while brace treatment is noninvasive and preserves growth, motion, and function of the spine, it does not correct an established deformity. While most orthopaedists, families, and patients agree that it is reasonable to wear a scoliosis brace for short periods if it means preventing an operation, a more difficult situation is encountered in the young child who faces the prospect of wearing a brace for more than 4 years with no guarantee of a favorable outcome. It is for these children that fusionless treatment options hold the greatest potential.

Many current growing options have centered on addressing large, progressive curves in the growing child with posterior growing devices. The goals of these treatments are to allow for spinal growth and prevent progression. However, in the vast majority of these patients, the endpoint to the treatment is a fusion of the deformity.

The greatest potential benefit to fusionless scoliosis surgery may be provided in the population that is traditionally braced. In this instance, the endpoint is not only to allow spinal growth but also to wholly prevent

R. R. Betz (✉)
Shriners Hospitals for Children,
3551 North Broad Street, Philadelphia, PA 19140, USA
e-mail: rbetz@shrinenet.org

B. A. Akbarnia et al. (eds.), *The Growing Spine*,
DOI: 10.1007/978-3-540-85207-0_45, © Springer-Verlag Berlin Heidelberg 2011

the need for a definitive spinal fusion and its potential sequelae.

The goal of this procedure is to harness the patient's inherent spinal growth and redirect it to achieve correction, rather than progression, of the curve. The anterior fusionless techniques are theoretically more advantageous than external bracing because they address the deformity directly at the spine and not via the chest wall and ribs and because they eliminate problems with patient noncompliance. Furthermore, minimally invasive thoracoscopic and lumbar techniques to access to the spine are aesthetically less extensive than those for posterior instrumented surgery. Our discussion will outline our experience with the anterior vertebral body stapling technique and outcome.

45.2 Historical Overview

In 2003, our institution published the results of a patient cohort that had undergone anterior vertebral body stapling for adolescent idiopathic scoliosis (AIS) [2]. The significance of the study was rooted in the 87% of curves that were held using the stapling technique. This was contrary to a previous disappointing reports from 1954 on correcting and preventing the progression of scoliosis with anterior fusionless techniques [14]. Convex apical vertebral body (hemiepiphyseal) stapling theoretically affords immediate and possibly reversible cessation of growth of the anterior vertebral physes. Animal studies using a rat tail model confirm its ability to modulate vertebral growth plates with skeletal fixation devices. The concept of using staples for growth modulation of long bones has been repeatedly tested and is fundamentally sound. Staples for epiphysiodesis of long bones in angular deformity have been used for over 50 years. Similarly, the potential benefits in the spine were noted around the same time. In 1951, Nachlas and Borden [10] were initially optimistic about their ability to create and correct lumbar scoliosis in a canine model using a staple that spanned several vertebral levels. Many of the dogs exhibited some correction, and some of the animals exhibited arrest of their curve progression. Some of the staples failed because they spanned three vertebrae. The enthusiasm for this new treatment was lost after the application of their stapling technique in three children with progressive scoliosis yielded poor results. Other investigators have, similarly, been dissatisfied with convex stapling as a means of controlling progressive scoliosis.

In 1954, Smith et al. [14] presented disappointing results for human patients with congenital scoliosis. The scoliosis correction was limited because the children had little remaining growth and the curves were severe, with considerable rotational deformity. Some staples broke or loosened, possibly because of motion through the intervertebral discs. While the concept of stapling the anterior vertebral endplates/physes for growth modulation and curve stabilization seemed sound, the staples designed for epiphyseal stapling about the knee were prone to dislodging in the spine because they were not designed to function across the intervertebral disk and accommodate to the movement in functional spinal unit.

45.3 Basic Science Overview

Recent work has shown the efficacy of anterior growth modulation in animals. Despite the successful use of staples for epiphysiodesis of long bones in angular deformity, staples for growth modulation around the spine were not nearly as successful. The obvious issue was that staples designed for the long bones were prone to dislodge in the spine because they were not designed for movement that occurs in the spine. Furthermore, the morbidity of staple implantation and the subsequent sequelae were unreasonably high.

However, the development of the Nitinol (Nickel Titanium Naval Ordnance Laboratory) staple (Medtronic Sofamor Danek, Memphis, TN) has resolved the first issue. The staple has current 510(k) approval from the Food and Drug Administration (FDA) specifically for use as an anterior spinal staple. The uniqueness of this staple is that it is made out of a shape memory alloy in which the prongs are straight when cooled but clamp down in a "C" shape in the bone for secure fixation when the staple returns to body temperature. Nitinol is a biocompatible shape memory metal alloy of 50% nickel and 50% titanium. The temperature at which the staples will undergo the shape transformation can be controlled by the manufacturing process. Injury to surrounding tissues through the transformation temperature has not been seen in animal or human experience with cervical spinal fusions.

Nitinol has a very low corrosion rate and has been used in orthodontic appliances. Implant studies in animals have shown minimal elevations of nickel in the tissues in contact with the metal; the levels of titanium are comparable to the lowest levels found in tissues of titanium hip prostheses, and titanium is considered a biologically safe implant material. No method of sterilization used in operating rooms has been shown to have any effect on the metal's properties. Although sensitivity to nickel occurs in a very low percentage of the population, it is not anticipated to occur through use of the Nitinol staple. The crystal structure in Nitinol is different than the small amount of nickel crystal structure in stainless steel such that the nickel does not leach out in Nitinol compounds as it can on occasion with stainless steel. The Nitinol staple has been tested in a goat model by Braun et al. [4, 5] and was shown to be safe and have utility for arresting the iatrogenic curves of less than 70° in the goat.

45.4 Clinical Outcomes

In 2003, Betz et al. [2] reported on the use of the Nitinol staple in 21 skeletally immature patients with AIS. Indications for the procedure were either brace noncompliance or the inability of the brace to prevent progression of the curve. They found the procedure to be safe and effective, with the results comparable with that of what would have been expected from bracing. In 2005, the same authors [3] reported on 39 patients and their increased experience with the procedure. Stabilization of the curve was seen in 87% of those patients older than 8 years at the time of stapling who had a curve of 50° or less with at least 1 year of follow up. No curve less than 30° at the time of stapling progressed more than 10° at follow-up.

Most recently, 2 year outcome data consisted of 41 curves (26 thoracic and 15 lumbar). Thirteen patients had both curves stapled. The average age was 9.4 years. Curves decreasing by greater than 10° were considered "improved." Curves within 10° of their preoperative measurement were considered "no change," and those progressing greater than 10° were considered "worse." Success was defined as "improved" or "no change." Thoracic curves measuring less than 35° had a 79% success rate. Curves measuring less than 20° on first erect radiograph had an 86% success rate. In patients with thoracic curves greater than 35°, 6 of 8 progressed past 50°. Seventy-one percent of patients with hypokyphosis showed improvement to a normal sagittal profile. One patient demonstrated worsening of kyphosis associated with coronal progression. Lumbar curves had an overall 87% success rate, with only one patient with a preoperative curve of 40° progressing to 50°. Five patients lost greater than 10° of lordosis, but the final lumbar lordosis remained in the normal range. Complications were minimal with an average blood loss of 214 mL.

On the basis of this review, we have altered our strategy for when to use staples alone and when to use additional strategies, as follows. If the thoracic curve measures 35–45° and does not bend below 20°, consider adding a posterior rib to spine hybrid construct at the same time (do posterior first). If on the first erect film, the curve does not measure below 20°, brace the child until the curve measures below 20°.

45.5 Clinical and Technical Overview

45.5.1 Indications and Contraindications

Patients who have at least 1 year of growth remaining, a scoliosis deformity that would be considered for brace treatment, or may have failed or refused bracing, are good candidates for the stapling procedure. Lenke 1, 3, 5, and 6 scoliosis curves are ideal for treatment with vertebral stapling. Other indications are as follows: Age less than 13 years for girls and less than 15 for boys; Risser 0 or 1, at least 1 year of growth remaining by wrist radiograph, or Sanders digital stage less than or equal to 4; thoracic and lumbar coronal curves less than 45°, with minimal rotation and flexible to less than 20°; and sagittal thoracic curve less than 40°.

Medical contraindications are the same as for any anterior spine or chest procedure and include systemic infection, active respiratory disease such as uncontrolled asthma, or conditions with increased anesthetic risk. Significantly compromised pulmonary function may be a relative contraindication.

We do not perform vertebral stapling for curves over 45° because our early experience has yielded poor results. Kyphosis greater than 40° is also a relative contraindication, because of the potential for the creation of hyperkyphosis with growth.

Surgeons with experience in anterior spine surgery and especially minimally invasive techniques should be able to perform this procedure. It may be helpful to enlist the assistance of an experienced general or thoracic surgeon. Using thoracoscopic and minimally invasive techniques for lumbar curves, scoliotic vertebrae from T3 to L4 can be stapled while limiting the total scar length. Placement of instrumentation at other levels will depend on anatomic variances in the location of the subclavian, azygous, or iliac vessels, and the size of the psoas muscle.

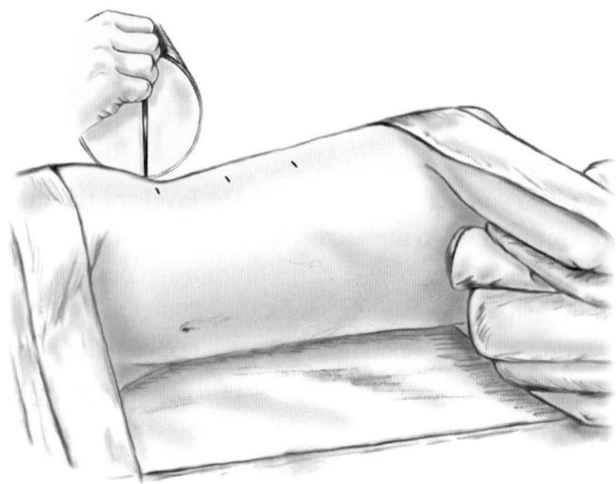

Fig. 45.1 The patient is placed in a lateral decubitus position. Using fluoroscopic imaging, the levels of the spine to be stapled are confirmed

45.5.2 Technical Overview

Under general anesthesia, the patient is placed in the lateral decubitus position with the convex side of the scoliosis curve in the up position. The table is not flexed, and only a small axillary roll is placed. Patient positioning is critical and can be used to maximize correction.

This procedure lends itself to the use of minimally invasive surgical techniques. If video-assisted thoracoscopy is being used for insertion, then one-lung ventilation will be necessary, unless carbon dioxide (CO_2) gas insufflation is available to displace the lung for visualization of the spine and surrounding structures. After positioning the patient, biplanar fluoroscopy is used to determine the exact location for the intercostal portals before the patient is prepped and draped (Figs. 45.1 and 45.2). In the thoracic spine, most incisions will be close to or within the area of the posterior axillary line. Two oblique incisions are usually required for placement of the staple (Fig. 45.3). The incisions are about 2.5–3 cm long following the slope of the ribs. Each incision can then be used to make two to three internal intercostal portals. This allows several levels to be stapled through each skin incision and accommodates the size of the instruments and implants. Both fluoroscopy and direct visualization with the thoracoscope are reliable methods for planning the incision. In the lumbar spine, we currently use tubular retractors and a lateral approach to the spine. The incision length is 2.5–3 cm and, similar to the thoracic spine, is localized based on the image intensifier. Three lumbar levels can be reliably accessed through each incision. It is imperative that nerve root monitoring is performed since the approach is transpsoas.

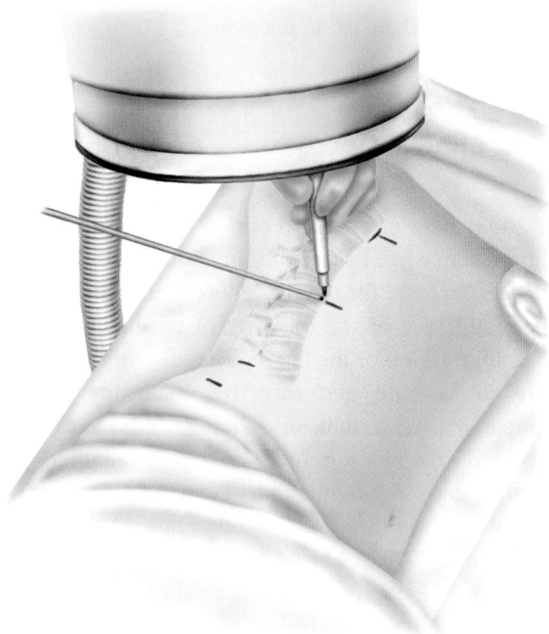

Fig. 45.2 A lateral/medial image is used to again confirm the vertebral levels to be stapled and also to center the portals in the posterolateral line

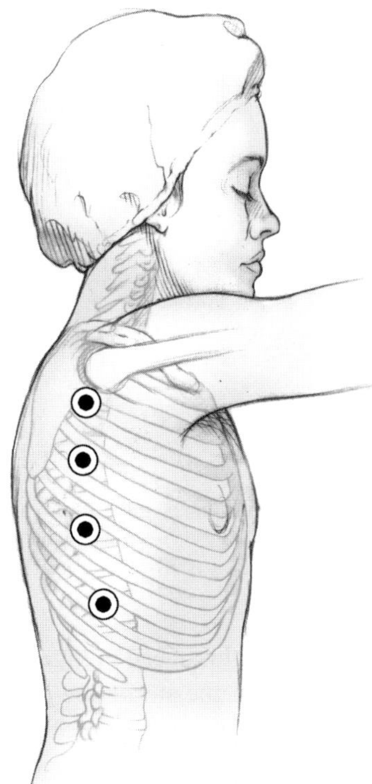

Fig. 45.3 Generally two but up to four portals in the posterolateral line are used, with the thoracoscope being inserted in the anterior axillary line at the apex of the curve

While the patient is in the lateral decubitus position, often the flexible main thoracic curve reduces. To further reduce the curve while placing the staples, lateral pressure to the apical ribs can be applied. The dull staple trial may also be used to push at the apex of the convexity, further reducing the curve before staple impaction (Fig. 45.4). This may be important because preliminary evaluation of data from patients who have already undergone the procedure suggests that patients who had the greatest correction at the time of surgery maintained that correction best.

The insertion device that holds the single two-prong staples is 10 × 14 mm wide. The staples come in many sizes, with the 12-mm four-prong, double staple being the widest, longest object (at 14 × 12 mm) that has to pass between the ribs. Rigid, autoclavable plastic portals (Medtronic Sofamor Danek, Memphis, TN) have been custom made for this specific use. They allow for maintenance of the intercostal portal space, quick removal of the staple trial, and placement of the appropriate sized staple while protecting the muscle and pleura from repeated trauma. Small pediatric Finochietto retractors or nasal speculum distractors can also be used to enlarge the intercostal portals and may be used in place of collapsible or rigid portals. These are ideal in the setting of CO_2 insufflation, since they are collapsible and better preserve intrathoracic pressure to maintain a collapsed lung.

Using fluoroscopy, the appropriate size trial is selected to span the distance across the disk, apophyses, and physes (Fig. 45.4a, b). The desired location in the vertebral body for the tines is as close to the endplates as possible. Once the correct size for the trial is determined, it is tapped into place where the staple will be located. Two single staples (two prongs) or one double staple (four prongs) is placed at each

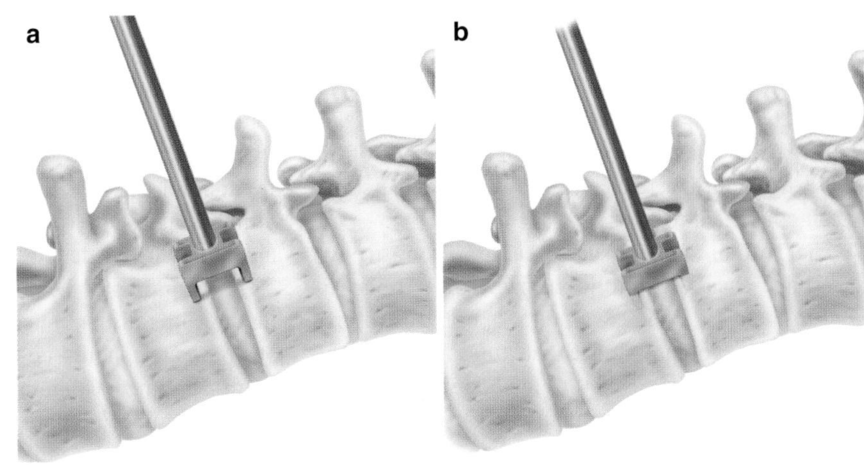

Fig. 45.4 Four-prong trial. (**a**) The staple trial is passed through one of the posterolateral portals and centered over the intervening disc space for staple sizing. The surgeon should place the prongs as close to the end plates as possible. (**b**) Once the position is confirmed through an AP image, starting holes are created. Generally, the posterior holes are created first, just anterior to the rib heads

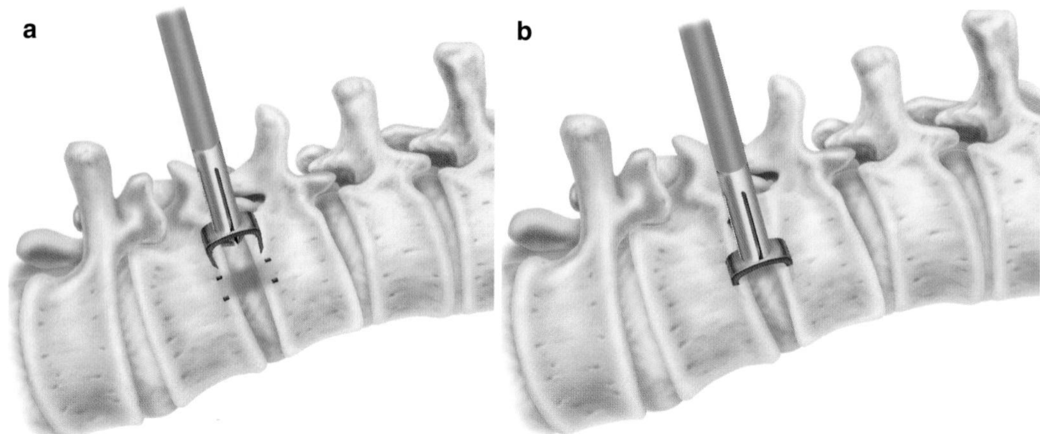

Fig. 45.5 Four-prong staple and inserter. (**a**) The staple is inserted into the pilot holes and the position confirmed with a fluoroscopic image. (**b**) The staple is impacted into the pilot holes

level. In very small children, the most proximal vertebra is often small, and only one single staple can be placed safely. The tines of the trial are used to create the pilot holes for the staple tines. If the tines of the trial come close to the segmental vessels, then the pleura is incised and the vessels are retracted gently while the pilot holes are created and until the staple is seated in place.

The pilot holes will act as a guide for the staple tines to ensure correct placement. The trial is removed and the appropriate sized straightened staple is quickly inserted (Fig. 45.5a, b). The decision to insert a two- or four-prong staple is based on the width of the vertebral body as seen in the operating room. The four-prong staples provide the desired amount of compression with less time required for insertion and fewer instrument passes into the chest. Once the staple is in the desired position, the staple inserter is removed, and if the staple is not flush against the bone, an impactor is used to drive the staple deeper. This must be done quickly before the tines are fully deployed. The dull staple trial can be used to help push at the apex of the convexity to further reduce the curve while the staple is being inserted.

The Nitinol staple's sharp, curved prong design and shape-changing abilities allow for insertion parallel to the cartilaginous vertebral apophyses to provide endplate compression. Staple tines are sharp and are designed to pass easily through bone. The staple's prongs are straightened manually and are then cooled by immersion in a sterile ice-bath. The scrub nurse or technician can perform this ahead of time. The staples must pass quickly from the sterile ice-water bath to the vertebral bodies to prevent staple warming and tine deployment. The tines will remain straight until the staple begins to return to normal body temperature when they deploy to their original curved shape. Complete tine transformation may take a minute. If the staple is completely seated within the vertebral bodies when the prongs deploy, then the staple position is secure.

Staples are placed anterior to the rib heads, and if the patient has severe hypokyphosis or thoracic lordosis, the staples can be placed more anterior on the vertebrae to help produce kyphosis with the patient's growth. If possible, a double and a single staple are placed across the two apical discs such that anterior growth can be further modulated to reduce the hypokyphosis (Fig. 45.6a, b). In the lumbar spine, the staples should be placed as far posteriorly on the vertebral body as possible, at least in the posterior half of the body, to maintain a normal lordosis.

If the staples are being placed thoracoscopically, the addition of CO_2 allows for collapse of the lung without single-lung ventilation. Specialized equipment and portals are needed for this technique. Low-pressure CO_2 also promotes hemostasis in the bleeding bone, but after it is discontinued, brisk bleeding is possible. Gas pressures should be kept low to prevent a lateral shift of the mediastinum, which may cause a drop in blood pressure. Vaseline gauze can be helpful to place over portals to reduce the leakage of CO_2.

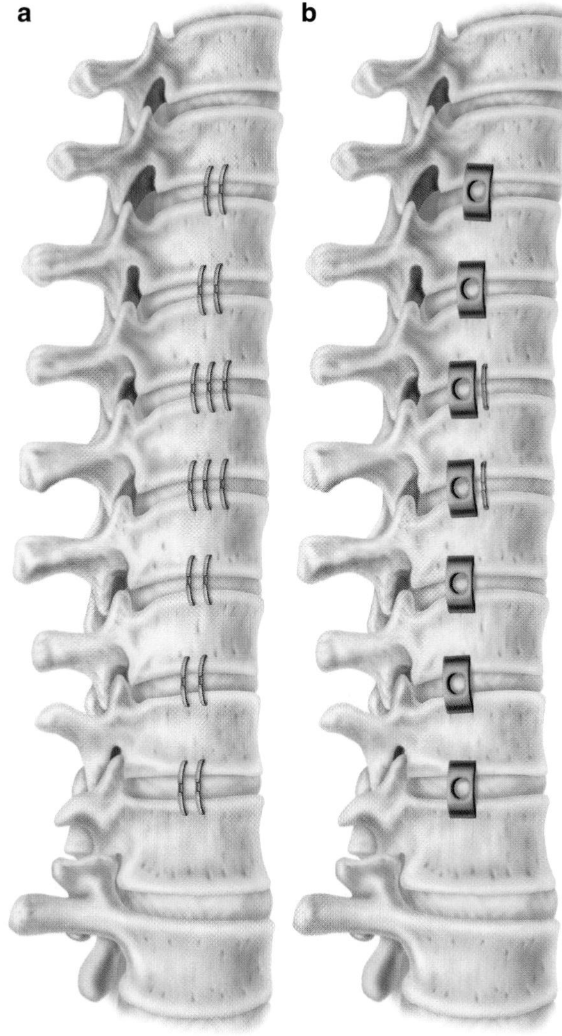

Fig. 45.6 (**a**) Generally, two staples are used at each vertebral segment. This can be in the form of two single staples, which provides the flexibility of adding a third anterior staple if desired. (**b**) To decrease operative time, a double staple is used when appropriate

45.5.3 Postoperative Care

Patients are asked to restrict activities for 4–6 weeks to allow for skin and muscles incised during the surgery to heal. A lumbar corset is used for immobilization for lumbar curves that are stapled. Patients usually return at 3 weeks for a wound check and 6 weeks for initial radiographs. At 6 weeks, any remaining restrictions are lifted, after which the patients are followed every 3 months.

45.5.4 Complications

In our experience, there has been one documented major complication: a rupture of a preexisting, unrecognized congenital diaphragmatic hernia in a 4-year-old child that ruptured at 6 weeks postsurgery and required emergency repair. Other lesser complications include injury to segmental vessels and conversion of the thoracoscopic portal to a mini thoracotomy (1 case), a chylothorax (1 case), development of mild pancreatitis, and clinically significant atelectasis.

Some early patients had prolonged chest tube drainage beyond 4 days. However, in a vast majority of cases, we maintain chest tubes less than 24 h. Three 4-prong staples (early design) fractured at the waist. Pain has been reported by one child, whose preoperative curves were more than 50° when stapled. Her thoracic curve progressed, and she required fusion. The stapled lumbar curve actually corrected. Two distal lumbar segments that were stapled did not require fusion. Two months after fusion, she had pain in the lumbar spine, and a bone scan showed increased uptake at the staple-bone interface. Three weeks after removal of the two distal staples, the patient had no pain. We have, also, had one curve over correct.

45.6 Summary

The recent investigations of convex anterior vertebral body stapling, both in animal models and in juvenile and adolescent scoliosis, offer solid early results with use of improved implants and techniques. The use of a shape memory alloy staple tailored to the size of the vertebral body, the application of several staples per level, the instrumentation of the Cobb levels of all curves, and the employment of minimally invasive thoracoscopic and lumbar approaches, all offer substantial improvements over previous fusionless techniques. Patient selection may also play a role in the current success of these fusionless treatments, with perhaps the ideal candidates for this intervention possessing smaller and more flexible curves. Still, reports on the clinical success of these stapling procedures are based on short term results (Figs. 45.7a–h). Long-term results of the effects on the instrumented motion segments and adjacent spine are not yet available.

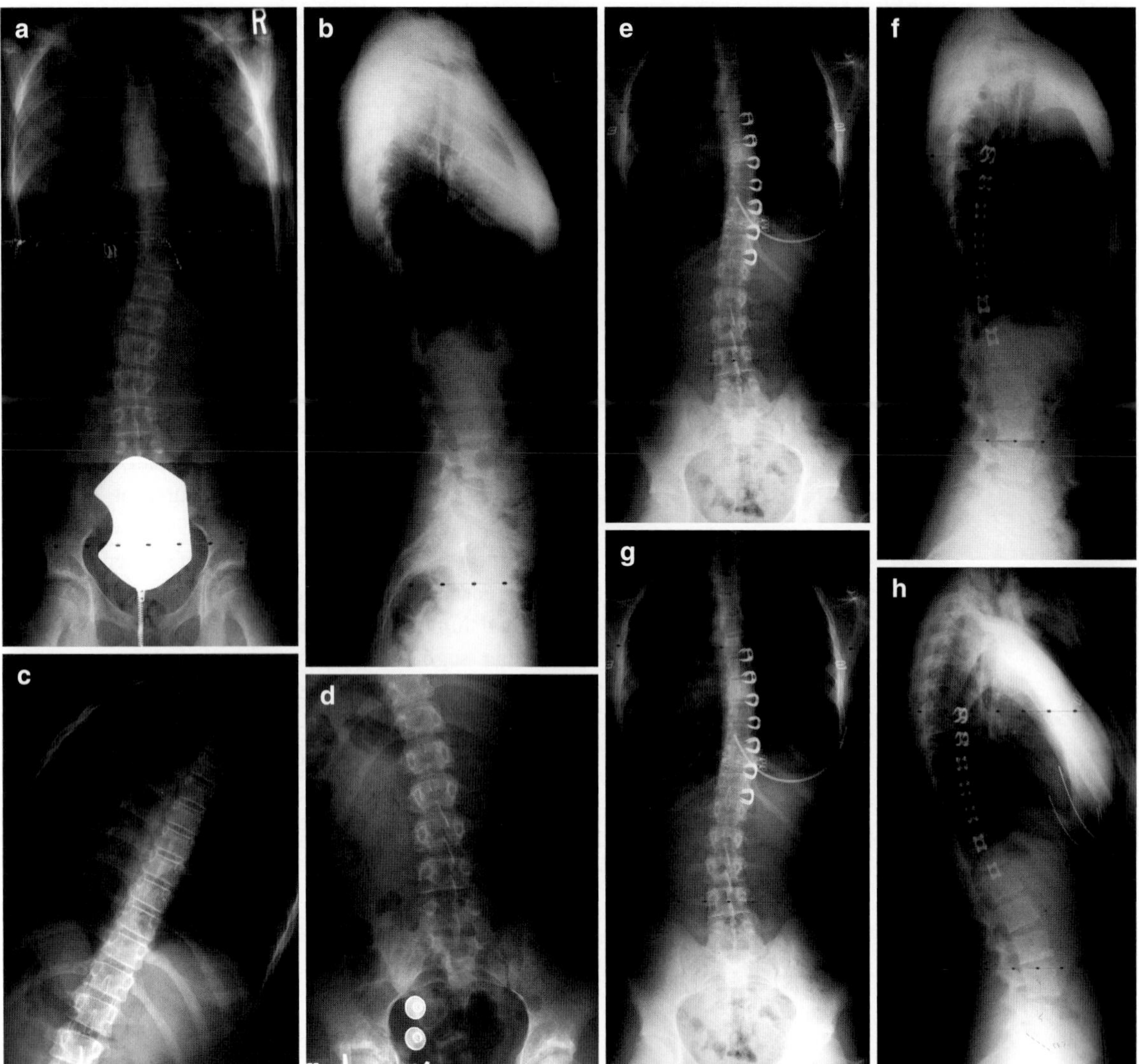

Fig. 45.7 PA (**a**) and lateral (**b**) erect radiograph of a 12-year-old girl demonstrating a 31° right thoracic curve and 15° thoracic kyphosis. Preoperative bend films (**c, d**) demonstrate the flexibility of the curve. Patient underwent a thoracoscopic VBS from T5–T12. Her postoperative radiographs (**e, f**) demonstrated curve correction to 19°. Latest follow-up (**g, h**) at 4.1 years postop demonstrates maintenance of curve correction at 22° and a thoracic kyphosis of 28°

References

1. Allington NJ, Bowen JR (1996) Adolescent idiopathic scoliosis: treatment with the Wilmington brace. A comparison of full-time and part-time use. J Bone Joint Surg Am 78: 1056–1062
2. Betz RR, Kim J, D'Andrea LP et al (2003) An innovative technique of vertebral body stapling for the treatment of patients with adolescent idiopathic scoliosis: a feasibility, safety, and utility study. Spine 28:S255–S265
3. Betz RR, D'Andrea LP, Mulcahey MJ et al (2005) Vertebral body stapling procedure for the treatment of scoliosis in the growing child. Clin Orthop Relat Res 434:55–60
4. Braun JT, Ogilvie JW, Akyuz E et al (2003) Experimental scoliosis in an immature goat model: a method that creates idiopathic-type deformity with minimal violation of the spinal elements along the curve. Spine 28:2198–2203
5. Braun JT, Ogilvie JW, Akyuz E et al (2004) Fusionless scoliosis correction using a shape memory alloy staple in the anterior thoracic spine of the immature goat. Spine 29: 1980–1989

6. Cheung KM, Cheng EY, Chan SC et al (2007) Outcome assessment of bracing in adolescent idiopathic scoliosis by the use of the SRS-22 questionnaire. Internat Orthop 31:507–511
7. Helfenstein A, Lankes M, Ohlert K et al (2006) The objective determination of compliance in treatment of adolescent idiopathic scoliosis with spinal orthoses. Spine 31:339–344
8. Karol LA (2001) Effectiveness of bracing in male patients with idiopathic scoliosis. Spine 26:2001–2005
9. Nachemson AL, Peterson LE (1995) Effectiveness of treatment with a brace in girls who have adolescent idiopathic scoliosis. A prospective, controlled study based on data from the Brace Study of the Scoliosis Research Society. J Bone Joint Surg Am 77:815–822
10. Nachlas IW, Borden JN (1951) The cure of experimental scoliosis by directed growth control. J Bone Joint Surg Am 33:24–34
11. Rahman T, Bowen JR, Takemitsu M et al (2005) The association between brace compliance and outcome for patients with idiopathic scoliosis. J Pediatr Orthop 24:420–422
12. Rowe DE, Bernstein SM, Riddick MF et al (1997) A meta-analysis of the efficacy of non-operative treatments for idiopathic scoliosis. J Bone Joint Surg Am 79:664–674
13. Shaughnessy WJ (2007) Advances in scoliosis brace treatment for adolescent idiopathic scoliosis. Orthop Clin N Am 38:469–475
14. Smith AD, Von Lackum WH, Wylie R (1954) An operation for stapling vertebral bodies in congenital scoliosis. J Bone Joint Surg Am 36:342–348

46 Spinal External Fixation

Koki Uno

Key Points

- Spinal external fixation is a new, novel treatment for severe spinal deformities.
- It uses a two-phase approach – apical release and application of the device and, based on the age and growth potentials, is followed by either a growing rod or a posterior spinal fusion.
- Complications, such as infection and implant failure, are high but manageable.

46.1 Introduction

The treatment of severe scoliosis can be very challenging despite the benefits of modern spinal instrumentation techniques. Rapid correction of these deformities can increase the risk of neurological compromise. Halo-gravity traction is an accepted method of treatment, but the main disadvantages are the need for patient confinement to a bed or a wheel chair and inconsistent speed of correction [3]. Also, using the technique is limited and not very effective, as it supplies traction only in a single direction. Above all, traction force to the deformity is applied by way of the cervical spine, which may cause pain and neurological complications. Halo-pelvic traction allows patient mobility; however, serious complications, such as necrosis of the dens, cranial nerve palsy, and bowel perforation, have been reported. Application of the external fixator to the spine is not new. Magerl [1] reported the use of a skeletal external fixation device, applied to the lower thoracic and lumbar spine for a variety of instability problems. Reyes-Sanchez et al. [2] reported the use of spinal external fixation for the dynamic correction of severe scoliosis using Debastiani's external fixation device. In Japan, Uno et al. [4] reported the experience of Illizarov external fixator correction for severe scoliosis. This chapter describes the indication, operative technique, postoperative management, and complications of this challenging treatment method.

K. Uno
National Hospital Organization, Kobe Medical Center
3-1-1 Nishiochiai Sumaku, 654-0155 Kobe, Japan
e-mail: uno@kobemc.go.jp

46.2 Indications

Indications for the spinal external fixation are primarily idiopathic or syndromic scoliosis of 120° or more. Congenital scoliosis of 80–90° or more may also be candidates. The author recommend spinal external fixator in patients with severe trunk decompensation, those with failed previous spinal fusion surgery and significant progression of deformity, in patients whose trunk shift is not amenable to standard instrumentation techniques, and in patients who have spinal cord pathology, such as tethering. Lastly, children whose pulmonary status places them at the risk of anterior approach may also be considered for spinal external fixation.

46.3 Operative Technique (External Fixator Application)

The surgical protocol has two phases. In the first phase, a posterior release is performed, and the spinal external fixation device is applied. In the second phase, when the

B. A. Akbarnia et al. (eds.), *The Growing Spine*,
DOI: 10.1007/978-3-540-85207-0_46, © Springer-Verlag Berlin Heidelberg 2011

correction has been finished, the external fixation device is removed, and a posterior spinal fusion with segmental spinal instrumentation is performed. The author has developed a rod for connecting pedicle screws and the external fixator. The diameter of the rod is 6 mm with a 15-cm length. It is threaded so that it can provide secure connection between screws and the external fixator.

The pedicle screws can be inserted by an open or minimally invasive method. In the open technique, spinal exposure includes two to three vertebrae above the upper end vertebrae and two to three vertebrae below lower end vertebrae of the curve.

After exposing posterior laminae, pedicle screws are inserted. Usually four pedicle screws are used proximally and four pedicle screws caudally (Fig. 46.1a–c). Posterior release around apex region is performed with separate skin incision, and the incision is closed. Then, the rod is inserted percutaneously and connected to the pedicle screws (see Fig. 46.1a). After skin closure, the rods are connected to the Illizarov carbon ring, which is already cut to adjust to the local anatomic requirements.

Finally, lengthening devices are attached at both sides (see Fig. 46.1b).

46.4 Lengthening Procedure

Postoperatively, the ring is tilted to the concave side. Correction is then performed at the bed side, which is usually 5–10 mm of lengthening on the concave side and 5–10 mm shortening on the convex side per day. This is started on the first or second postoperative day. When the rings are parallel, the amount of correction is usually adequate (see Fig. 46.1c). The patient is brought to the OR again for final fusion. The period for bed side adjustment for correction depends on the severity of the curve. In the authors' experience of 20 cases, the correction period is between 2 and 6 weeks.

46.5 Postoperative Care

During correction, patients usually cannot lie in the supine position. By using cushions or large sponges, they can lie in the supine position for a short period of time. A foam mattress with a hole to accommodate the external fixator to enable supine position of the patient may sometimes be beneficial [1]. Usually, the patient

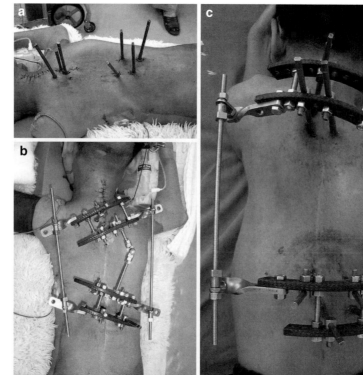

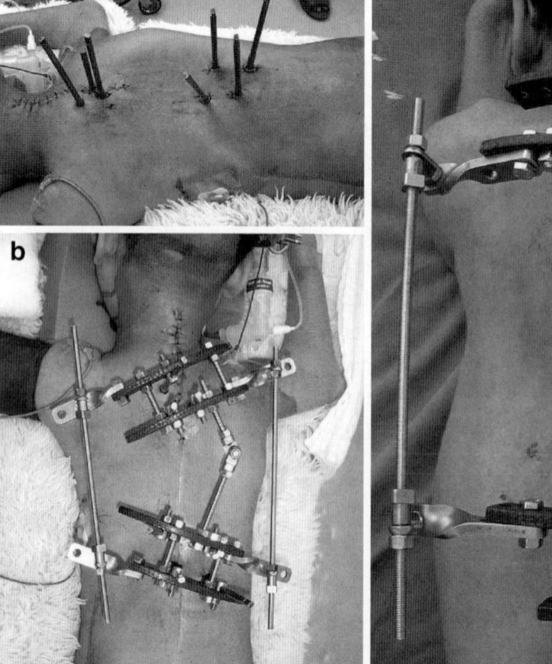

Fig. 46.1 External fixator attachment. (**a**) The rods are connected to the pedicle screws percutaneously. (**b**) Rings and lengthening devices are connected to the rods. (**c**) After correction with the external fixator, rings are parallel

lay in the lateral or prone position. They are mobilized as soon as possible based on comfort. Daily care of the pin sites is, as in other external fixations, mandatory. Sometimes, the patients may complain of pain after daily lengthening, but pain is easily controlled by NSAID.

46.6 Operative Technique (Removal of the External Fixator and Posterior Fusion with Instrumentation)

After endoscopic intubation in the lateral position, the patient is placed in a prone position. When vertebrae in which pedicle screws are inserted for external fixator are not included in final fusion, the operation can be performed with a separate skin incision posteriorly. Otherwise, rings and rods are removed before the posterior spinal fusion. These are usually removed manually together. When the screws are left in the pedicle, they are easily removed percutaneously. After all the rods and screws are removed, prepping and draping are performed, and then, the final posterior spinal fusion and segmental spinal instrumentation is performed.

46.7 Complications

Complications directly related to the external fixator are pain during correction, transient neurological complications, superficial infection, deep infection after final fusion, cerebrospinal fluid fistulae, and implant failure. Most of the complications can be managed nonoperatively. Implant failure, cerebrospinal fluid fistulae, and deep infection require surgical intervention.

46.8 Conclusions

The spinal external fixation correction is still an evolving procedure. However, the author believes it is a safe, well-tolerated method of applying gradual, sustained correction force to maximize postoperative correction, in selected patients without adding the risk of anterior approach in this difficult patient population (Fig. 46.2a–l).

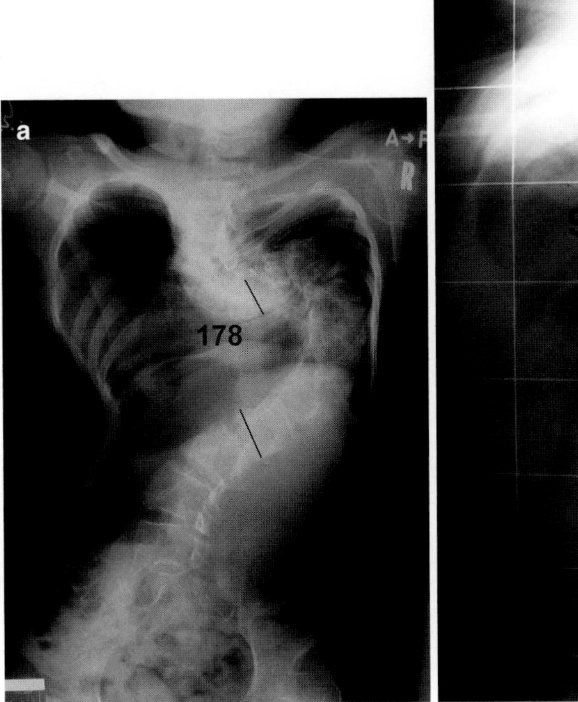

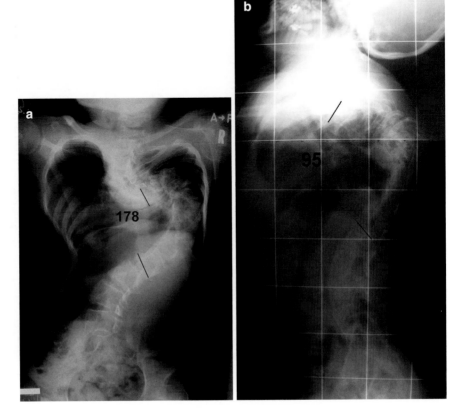

Fig. 46.2 (**a, b**) 13-year-old girl with Larsen syndrome. AP and lateral radiographs showing right thoracic kyphoscoliosis measuring 178° of scoliosis and 95° of kyphosis

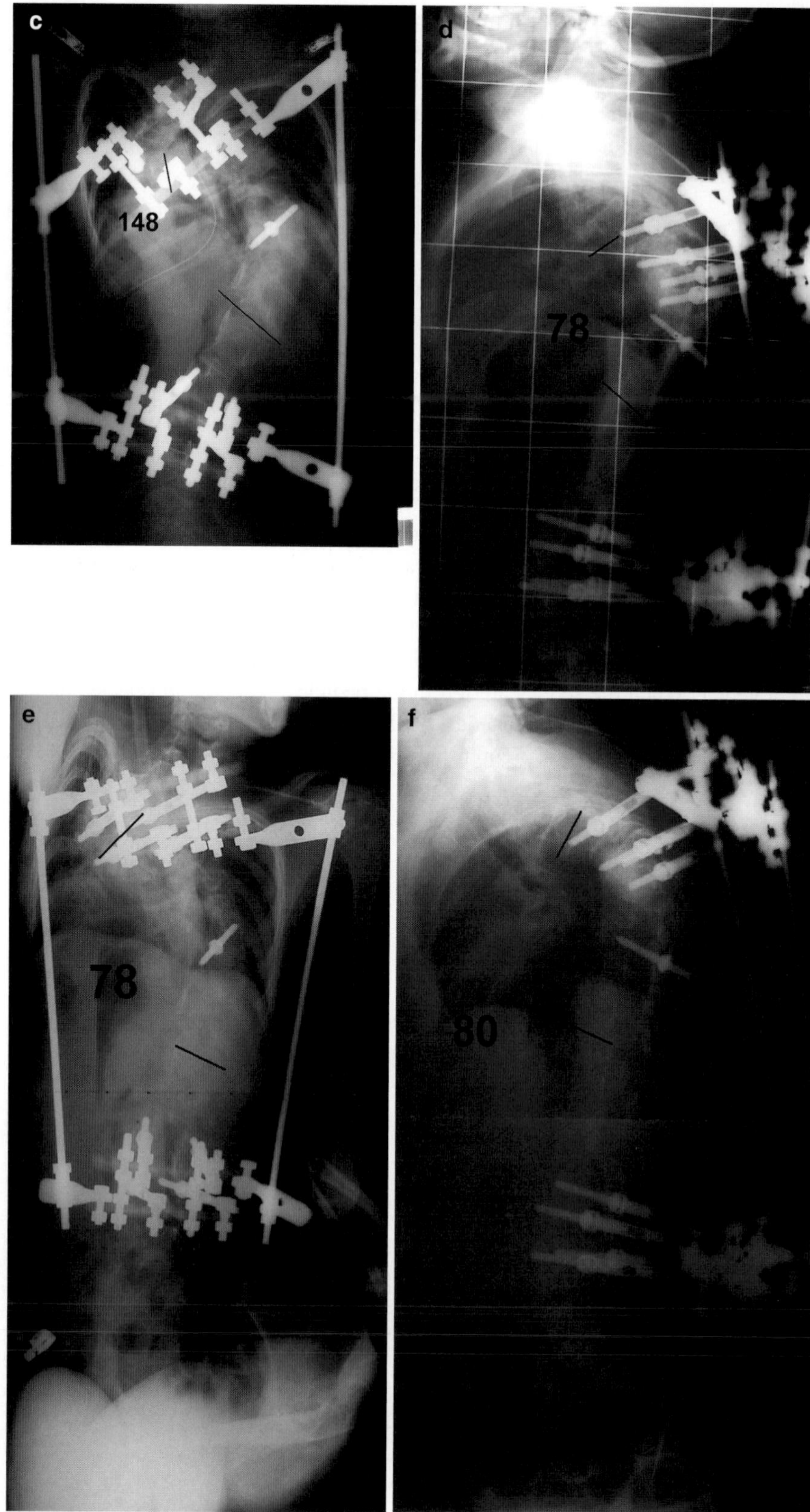

Fig. 46.2 (continued) (**c, d**) Immediately following application of the external fixator. (**e, f**) Maximum correction with the external fixator

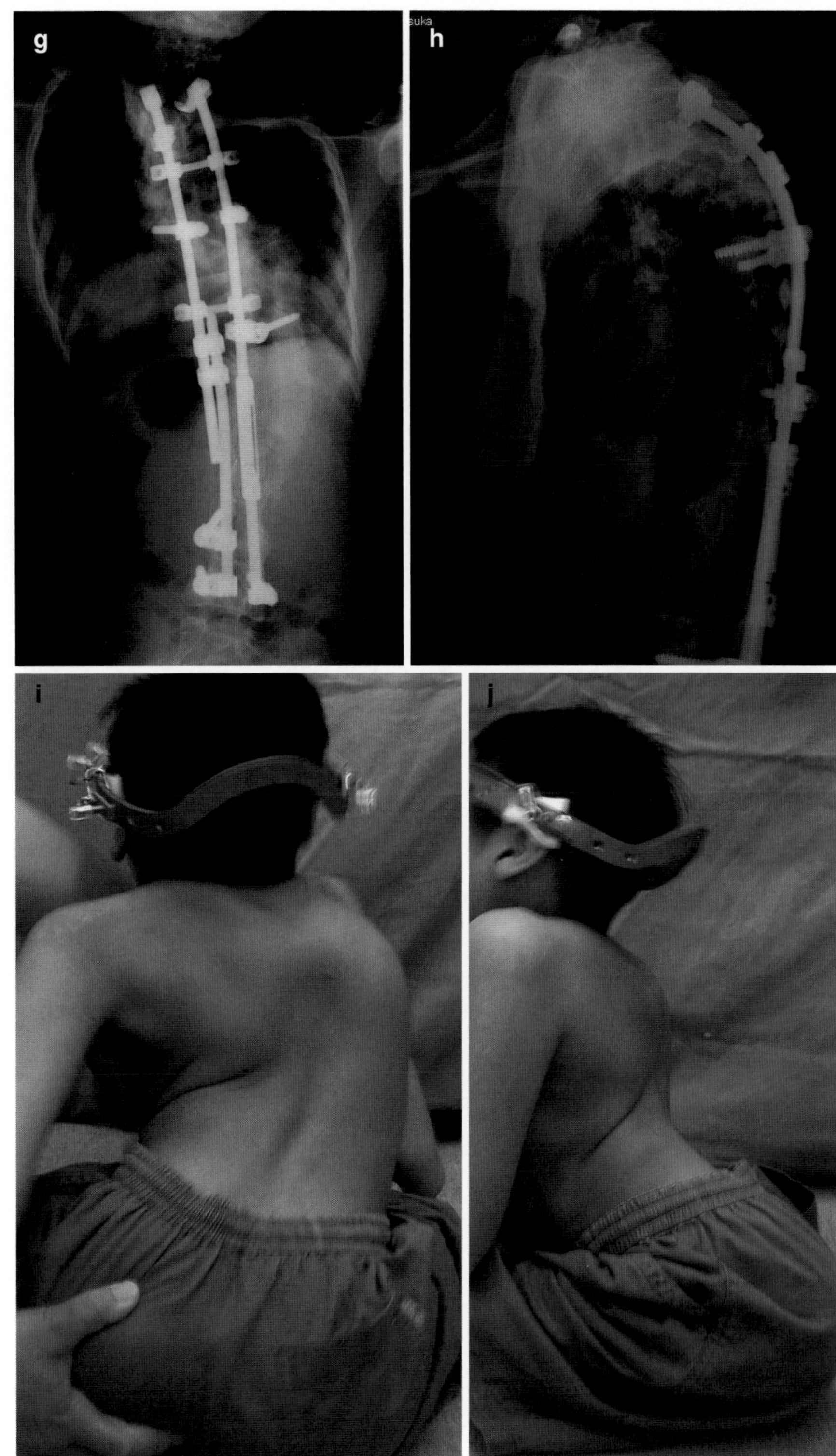

Fig. 46.2 (continued) (**g, h**) Five years follow up after final fusion, the curve was drastically corrected without anterior approach and good trunk balance was obtained. AP and lateral radiographs showing 63° of scoliosis and 60° of kyphosis. (**i, j**) Clinical photo before operation

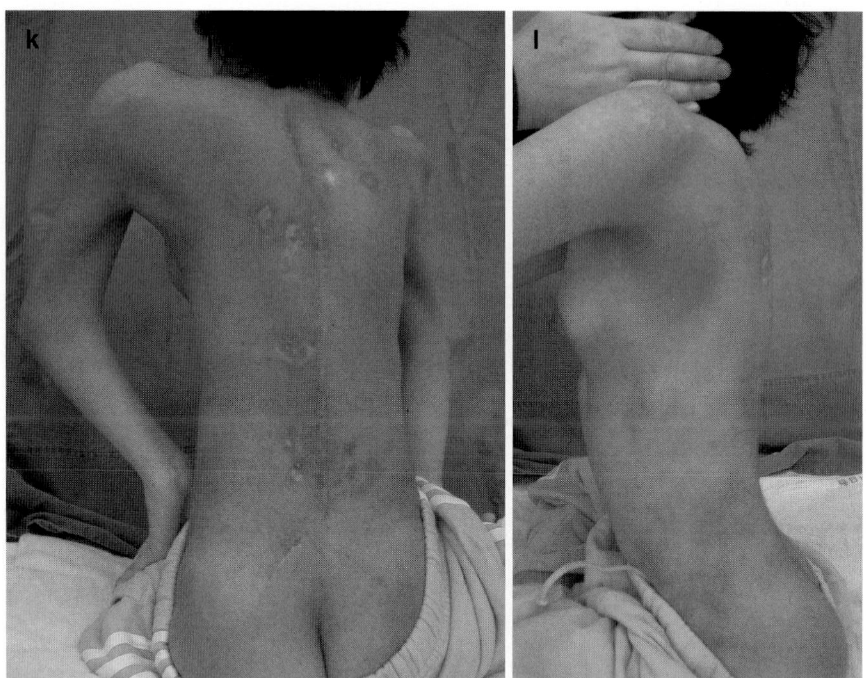

Fig. 46.2 (continued) (**k, l**) Clinical photo after operation

References

1. Magerl FP (1984) Stabilization of the lower thoracic and lumbar spine with external skeletal fixation. Clin Orthop Rel Res 189:125–141
2. Reyes-Sanchez A, Rosales LM, Miramontes V (2005) External fixation for dynamic correction of severe scoliosis. Spine J 5:418–426
3. Sink EL, Karol LA, Sanders J et al (2001) Efficacy of perioperative helo-gravity traction in the treatment of severe scoliosis in children. J Pediatr Orthop 21:519–524
4. Uno K., Kimura T., Tomatsuri M et al (2003) Ilizarov external fixator as a method for severe spinal deformity-Report of a case-. J Japanese Scoliosis Soc 18:118–122

47 Magnetic Powered Extensible Rod for Thorax or Spine

Lotfi Miladi and Jean F. Dubousset

Key Points

- Children who have failure of nonsurgical treatment for progressive scoliosis may require early surgery.
- Standard growing rods that have been used until now require repeated surgeries that increase the risk of complications.
- We present the preliminary results of a new type of growing rod, which is extended by a magnet at home without surgery.
- This technique is safe, easy to use, and has the potential of decreasing the rate of complications, and improving the quality of life of children.
- Longer follow up is necessary to evaluate the real efficacy of this new method.

47.1 Introduction

The use of growing rods may be necessary in early onset scoliosis, deformities associated with abnormalities of the rib cage, and in progressive scoliosis with failure of non-operative treatment regardless of its etiology. Several types of growing rod have been used since introducing of Harrington rod [3, 4, 9, 10, 12]. Growing rods usually require to be elongated every 6 months by repeated surgery, which increases the risk of complications such as infection [1, 2, 5–8, 11, 13]. Jean Dubousset had experienced the same complications in a series of young children who had been operated on with excision of the tumor of lower limbs followed by limb salvage procedures by mechanical growing prosthesis. Then, he asked the medical engineer, Arnaud Soubeiran, to design a prosthesis that is able to be lengthened without the need of multiple surgeries. The first model of this prosthesis was manufactured in 1993. The lengthening was obtained by the expansion of a preloaded spring under the effect of an electromagnetic field. This prosthesis is now used worldwide as limb salvage procedure. His idea was also used to make a spinal rod that can avoid multiple Interventions. The first type of this rod was made in 1997 and used in a small series of children requiring lengthening in outpatient departments. The lengthening was more difficult when the spring was closer to the end of expansion. To solve the problem the same engineer developed a new type of magnetic growing rod in 2004, which may be lengthened at home.

L. Miladi (✉)
Saint Vincent de Paul Hospital, 82 Avenue Denfert Rochereau, 75014 Paris, France
e-mail: l.miladi@svp.aphp.fr

47.2 Technical Specifications

47.2.1 Technique of Lengthening

The lengthening is achieved by a pair of strong neodymium permanent magnets, one is internal (the receiver) and the other external (the controller), to transmit mechanical power to the implanted device. Then, a lever arm is used as a force amplifier and a pair of spring-clutches and screw used to convert the alternating movement of the lever arm into a continuous longitudinal one way movement. The lengthening is controlled through the receiver by a sound feedback, or better with a hap tic feedback. The magnet is rotated 180° alternatively to provide distraction or compression

B. A. Akbarnia et al. (eds.), *The Growing Spine*,
DOI: 10.1007/978-3-540-85207-0_47, © Springer-Verlag Berlin Heidelberg 2011

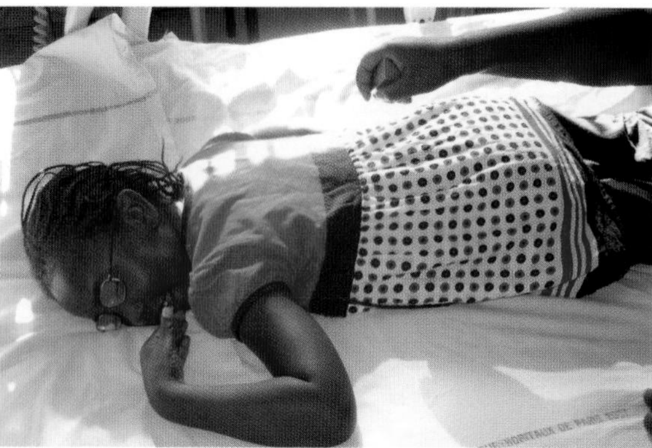

Fig. 47.1 Parent rotating the external magnet

as desired (Fig. 47.1). Therefore, the energy derived from rotation of the external magnet is transmitted through the skin to the mechanical device inserted. The amount of distraction or compression depends on the number and frequency of movements that should be calculated precisely.

47.2.2 Characteristics of the Rod

The rod is made of a resistant Cobalt Chrome alloy. It may have an "I" or "J" form (Fig. 47.2). In the form of "I," the powered part lies between the fixation points of the rod on the spine. This is indicated in the long constructs extended to the entire column, and pelvic fixations in neuromuscular scoliosis. In the form of "J," the powered part is outside the zone instrumented, which allows a harmonious bending of the rod, along its entire length, to better fit the morphology of the trunk of the child, and, especially, it allows a much better correction in the sagittal plane, which is difficult to obtain with other types of growing rod. The diameter of the rod and its reserve of lengthening are chosen by the surgeon, depending on each case, diameters among 3.5, 4.5, and 5.5 mm, and a reserve length from 25 to 60 mm.

47.3 Surgical Instructions

The lengthening device can be fixed to the ribs, vertebras, or both. One or more devices can be used simultaneously in the same patient. The implants are inserted through two small skin incisions at the level of fixation points. The rod is first bent, and then introduced from one incision to the other submuscular.

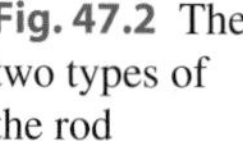

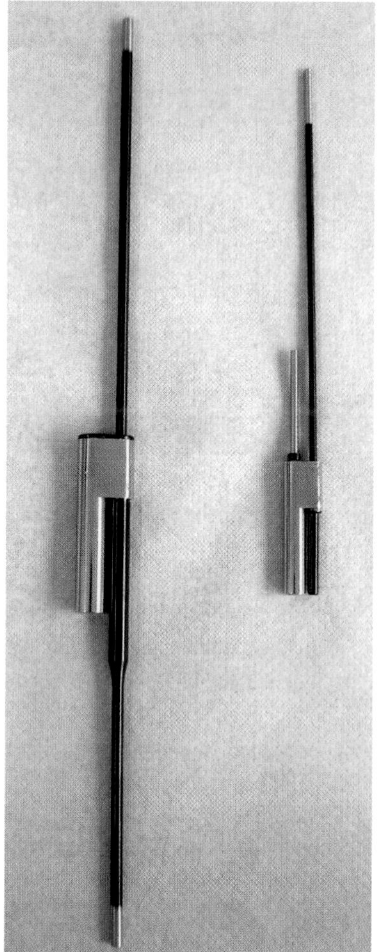

Fig. 47.2 The two types of the rod

47.3.1 Rib Fixation

It is recommended to use a clamp of hooks on two adjacent ribs, without compression, at both ends of the rod, to do a soft distraction, but not to weaken the internal ribs. The preferred diameters of rib fixation rods are 3.5 and 4.5 mm.

47.3.2 Spinal Fixation

At the lower end of the device, it is recommended to use two pedicle screws in two adjacent vertebras or at least a screw in association with a laminar hook on the adjacent vertebras. At the upper end of the device, it is preferred to use pediculo-supra-laminar claw hooks without compression. A soft final distraction is performed on the rod under evoked potential control before closing the skin. The recommended diameter of rod used in spinal fixation is 4.5 or 5.5 mm. If the diameter of 5.5 mm is used, with a solid fixation, the patient may be brace free, but still must avoid doing violent or high risk sports.

47.4 Lengthening Mode

We recommend starting the lengthening 1 month after surgery, at a rate of 20 movements per week, which should lengthen the rod by 1.2 mm/month, and 15 mm/year. The rate can be modified by the surgeon, depending on the case (number of vertebras involved, age of the child, stiffness of the curve, and initial magnitude). The lengthening is done at home by parents or other caregivers of the child, who is dressed lying prone or in sitting position. The external magnet is presented in front of the reservoir of the rod, causing a sensation of push or pull back on the holding hand, depending on the direction of the magnet. The movement of oscillations back and forth next to the reservoir of the rod triggers movements of the magnet, which produce a more or less audible "click," depending on the position of the external magnet. This lengthening is not painful at all; we only need to avoid the presence of metal objects in the immediate vicinity of the magnet, which must also be stored out of reach of children. The only two contraindications to the use of the Phenix rod are a Pacemaker in the vicinity of the patient, and examination by MRI, which is disturbed by the presence of the internal magnet. Radiographs are obtained 3 months after the beginning of the lengthening, then every 6 months.

47.5 Preliminary Results

In this first study, we report the preliminary results of a series of 26 patients who were operated on by a single surgeon, from February 2005 to June 2008. There are 16 girls and ten boys, and the age at the time of operation ranges from 22 months to 13 years and 9 months. Eleven patients had idiopathic scoliosis, seven had congenital scoliosis, and eight had syndromic scoliosis. The average of Cobb angle was 63° preoperatively (from 25 to 130°). An associated anterior convex epiphysiodesis was performed in five cases, because of the big amount of apical rotation. Preparation for surgery by a Stagnara cast was used in three cases, with a halo-pelvic Ilizarov, in one case. Fifteen cases had no postoperative brace. All patients are still being processed; none has yet reached skeletal maturity. The mean postoperative Cobb angle was reduced to 33°, ranging from 4 to 92°. We experienced some complications: dislodgement of a costal hook in one case, transient complete loss of evoked potentials signal perioperatively in one case due to a major correction that required the immediate release, wound infection in two cases, fracture of a 4.5 mm rod in two patients who were brace free, and secondary loss of the correction of scoliosis due to a spontaneous unintentional rotation of the rod in ten cases, of which eight were reoperated on by implanting a new rod which was locked in rotation. The reservoir of the rod was slightly prominent in three cases, which was well tolerated.

Finally, four rods have not grown and have been changed.

47.6 Clinical Cases

47.6.1 Case 1

A 22-month-old boy child with an imbalanced right thoracic curve due to several rib and vertebral malformations (Fig. 47.3a–g). We have done one stage operation by hemivertebrectomy with combined anterior and posterior approach, costal synostosis excision in the concavity of the curve and implantation of two distractors: one with costal fixation and the other with costovertebral fixation (see Fig. 47.3c, d). The radiographic examination performed 8 months (see Fig. 47.3e) and 14 months (see Fig. 47.3f, g) after surgery showed that the rod is lengthened, and the correction is still maintained.

47.6.2 Case 2

A 2-year and 10-month-old girl who had a right thoracic scoliosis with multiple costovertebral malformations (Fig. 47.4a–e). We have performed a

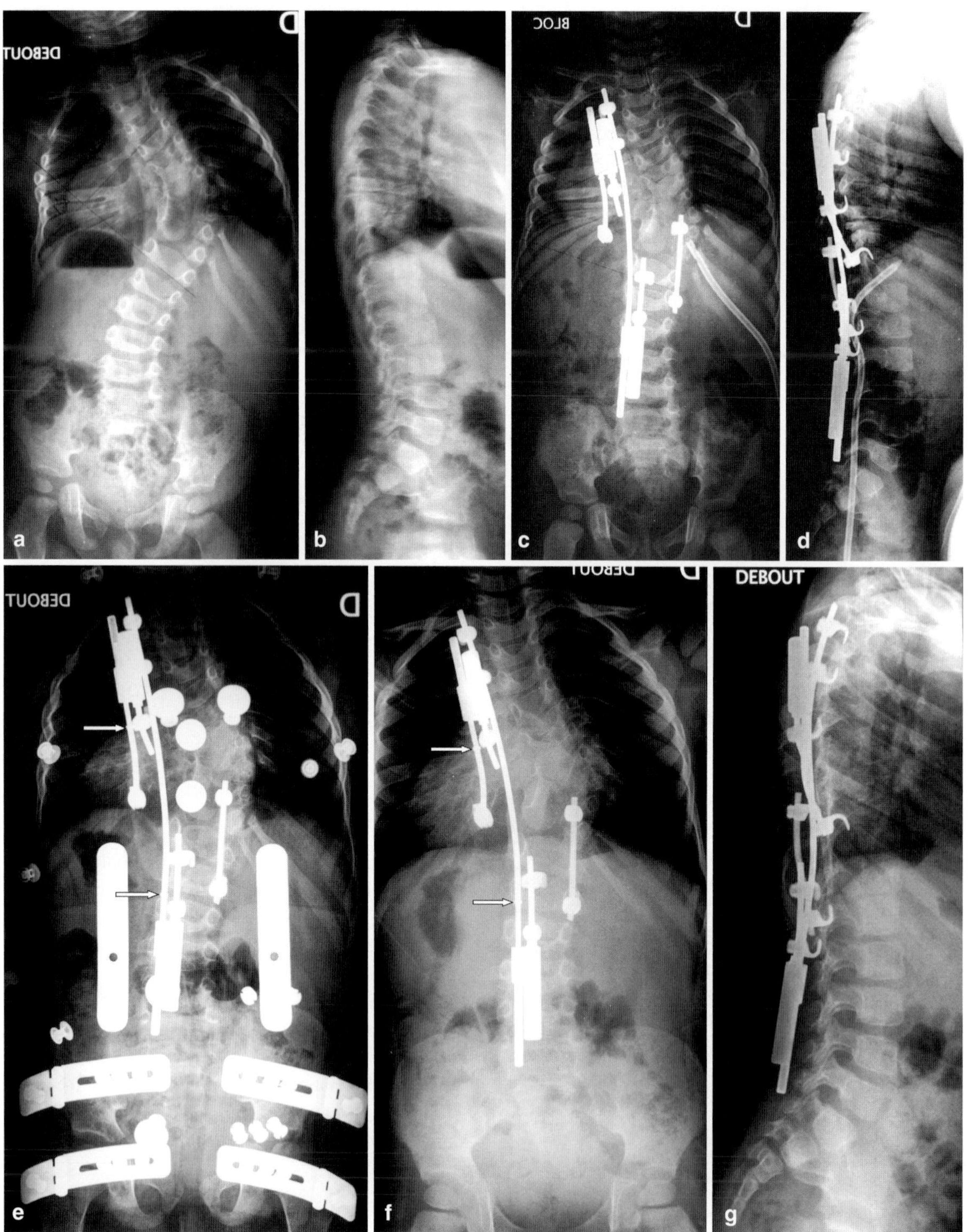

Fig. 47.3 (**a, b**) Posterior–Anterior (PA) and lateral preoperative radiographs. (**c, d**) Posterior–Anterior (PA) and lateral postoperative radiographs. (**e**) 8 months after surgery, with brace. Arrows show the length's increase. (**f, g**) Posterior–Anterior (PA) and lateral radiographs 14 months after surgery

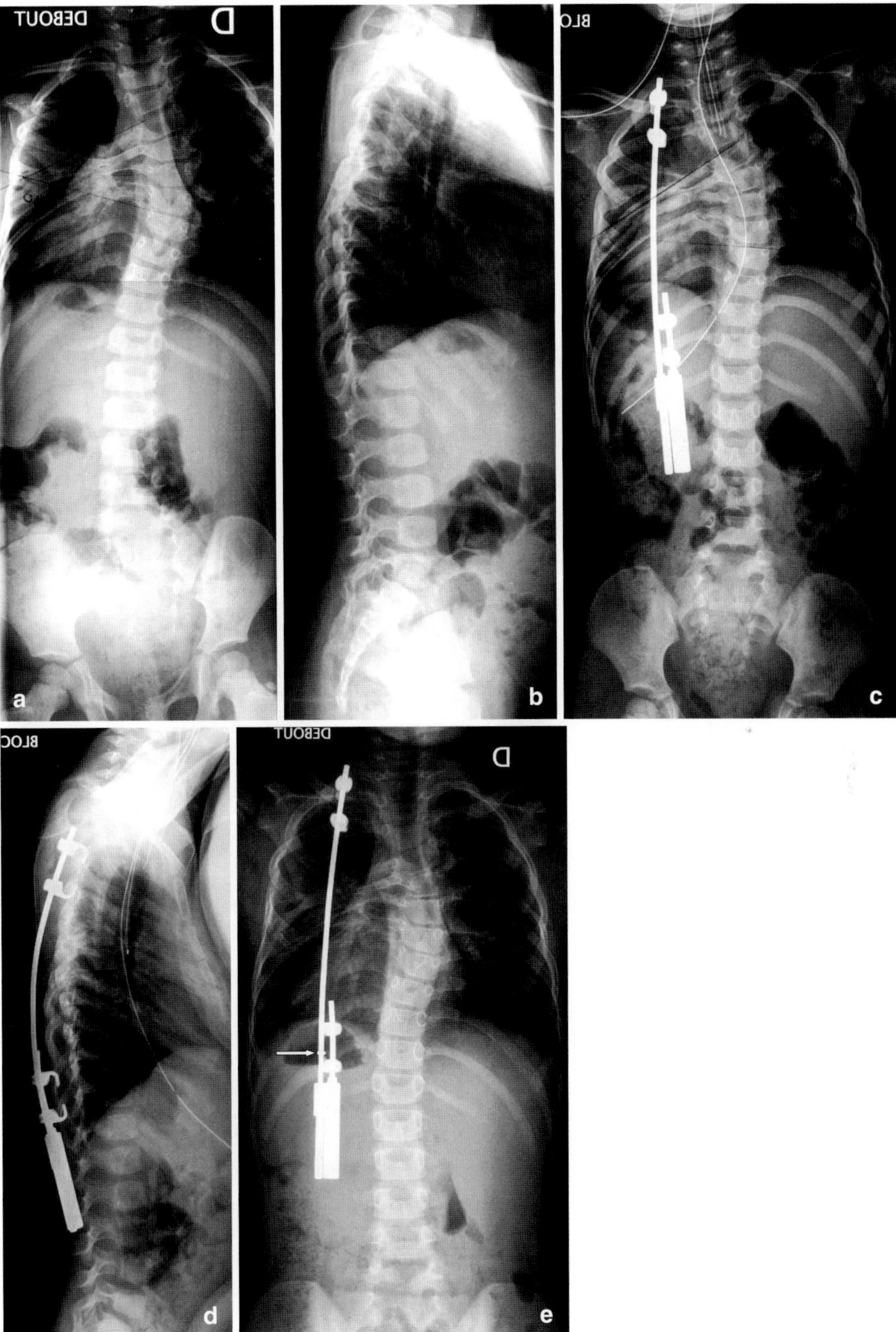

Fig. 47.4 (**a, b**) Posterior-Anterior (PA) and lateral preoperative radiographs. (**c, d**) Posterior-Anterior (PA) and lateral postoperative radiographs. (**e**) 17 months after surgery

rib synostosis excision and put Phenix rod on the ribs (see Fig. 47.4c, d). The roentgenogram performed 17 months after operation shows a decrease of the Cobb angle and decrease of the T1 tilt (see Fig. 47.4e).

47.6.3 Case 3

A 12-year-old girl with neglected advanced juvenile scoliosis and the Cobb angle of 95° (Fig. 47.5a–g). A gradual correction by an elongation cast was

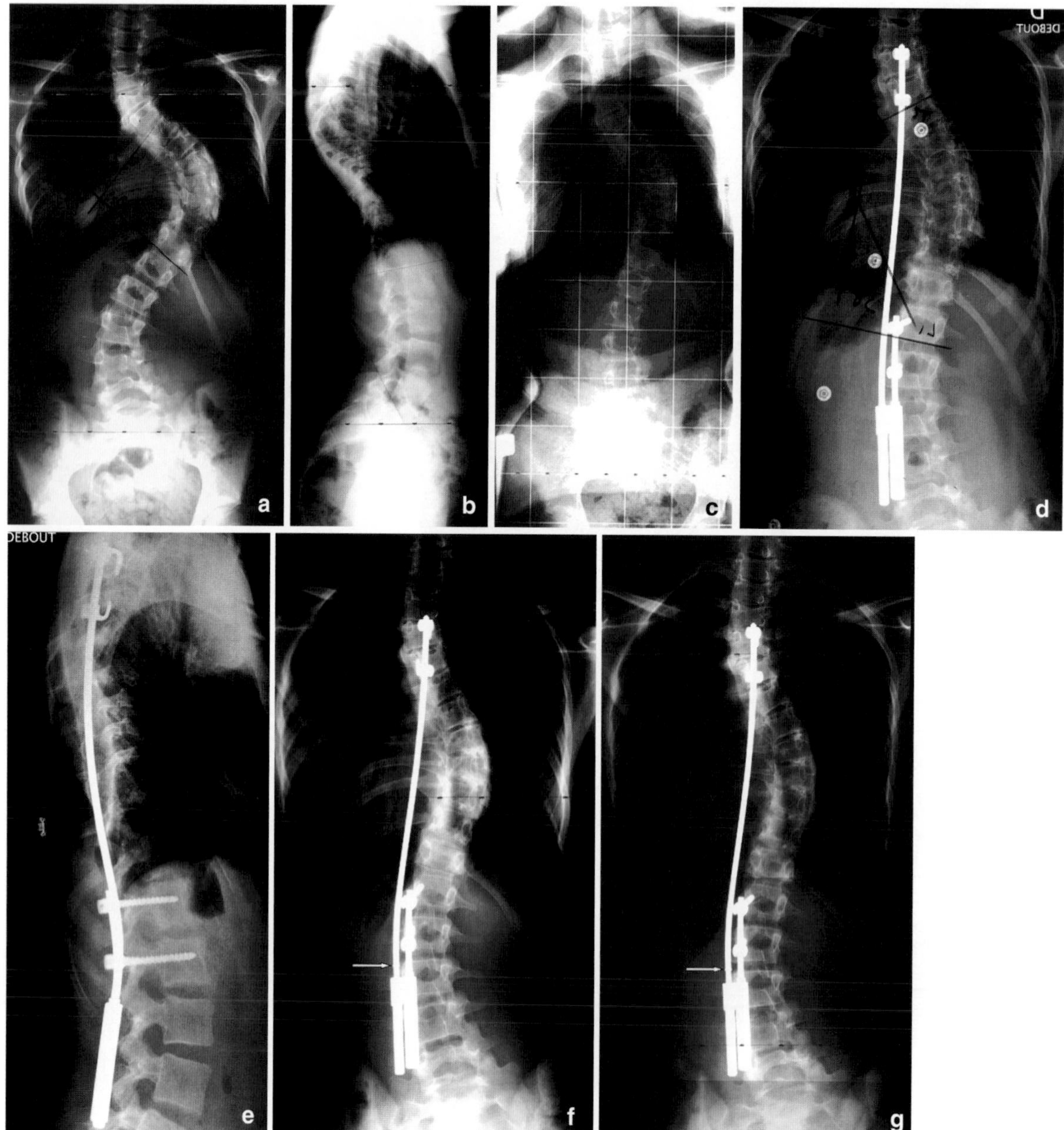

Fig. 47.5 (**a, b**) Posterior–Anterior (PA) and lateral preoperative radiographs. (**c**) Correction obtained by elongation cast. (**d, e**) Posterior–Anterior (PA) and lateral postoperative radiographs. (**f**) 4 months after surgery (**g**) 9 months after surgery

carried out (see Fig. 47.5c) before the surgery, which was followed by anterior convex epiphysiodesis associated with implantation of Phenix rod on the spine (see Fig. 47.5d, e). Postoperative radiograph performed 4 months (see Fig. 47.5f) and 9 months (see Fig. 47.5g) after surgery show rod lengthening and gradual improvement of the deformity.

47.7 Discussion

This is of course a new technique that required a learning curve for its use as well as for its technical refinements. This explains the number of technical complications encountered with finally no damage for the children when surgery was repeated (once) for some patients.

The follow up is of course short, and we cannot present the long-term results of this technique, but the advantages, such as the simplicity of the lengthening, being pain free, no need for anaesthesia, performability of the lengthening by parents at home with control every 6 months as an outpatient, make it an attractive technique for the patients and parents. It is also evident that by using this noninvasive lengthening method and avoiding repeated surgery, infectious complications decrease compared with other techniques. It remains that till now this system has been used only in a distraction mode. One can argue that the effect on apical rotation in the horizontal plane is not directly addressed with the device that presents mainly an anticollapsing mechanical effect to maintain the correction. Will this prevent the crankshaft phenomenon? One may believe that the gentle continuous tension by the magnet rod may do it. Will the presence of the device cause stiffness of the spine at the end of growth? Only the follow up will give us the answer. Would a second rod on the convex side of the curve be useful? This technique opens the way to many discussions and new ideas, thanks to its simplicity for use.

References

1. Akbarnia BA, Marks DS, Boachie-Adjei O et al (2005) Dual growing rod technique for the treatment of progressive early onset scoliosis. A multicenter study. Spine 30:S46–S57
2. Blakemore LC, Scoles PV, Poe-Kochert C et al (2001) Submuscular Isola rod with or without limited apical fusion in the management of severe spinal deformities in young children. Preliminary report. Spine 26:2044–2048
3. Gillespie R, O'Brien J (1981) Harrington instrumentation without fusion. J Bone Joint Surg Br 63:461
4. Harrington P (1962) Treatment of scoliosis: correction and internal fixation by spine instrumentation. J Bone Joint Surg Am 44:591–610
5. Klemme WR, Denis F, Winter RB et al (1997) Spinal instrumentation without fusion for progressive scoliosis in young children. J Pediatr Orthop 17:734–742
6. Luque E, Cardosa A (1997) Segmental spinal instrumentation in growing children. Ortop Trans 1:37
7. Luque ER (1982) Paralytic scoliosis in growing children. Clin Ortop 163:202–209
8. Mineiro J, Weinstein SL (2002) Subcutaneous rodding for progressive spinal curvatures: early results. J Pediatr Orthop 22:290–295
9. Moe JH, Cummine J, Winter RB et al (1979) Harrington instrumentation without fusion combined with the Milwaukee brace for difficult scoliosis problems in young children. Scoliosis Research Society, Cambridge, MA, 1978. Orthop Trans 3:59
10. Moe JH, Kharrat K, Winter RB et al (1984) Harrington instrumentation without fusion plus external orthotic support for the treatment of difficult curvature problems in young children. Clin Ortop 185:35–45
11. Pratt RK, Webb JK, Burwell RG et al (1999) Luque trolley and convex epiphysiodesis in the management of infantile and juvenile idiopathic scoliosis. Spine 24:1538–1547
12. Tello C (1994) Harrington instrumentation without arthrodesis and consecutive distraction program for young children with severe spinal deformities: experience and technical details. Orthop Clin N Am 25:333–351
13. Thompson GH, Akbarnia BA, Kostial P et al (2005) Comparison of single and dual growing rods techniques followed through definitive surgery. A preliminary study. Spine 30:2039–2044

48 Growth Guided Instrumentation: Shilla Procedure

Richard E. McCarthy

Key Points

- The Shilla growing rod system is a growth enabling system designed to direct spinal growth.
- The Shilla device harnesses the growth potential of the spine after correction and fusion of the curve apex.
- Growth continues at the ends of the curve by virtue of Shilla growing screws.

48.1 Introduction

Traditional "Growing Rod" systems are designed to produce a distractive force between the ends of a scoliotic curve and rejuvenate that distractive force on a regular basis. The latter usually requires a return to surgery every 6 months. The goal is to continue this distractive force throughout the period of juvenile and early adolescent growth until a time when sufficient vertebral column growth has been achieved. At that point, the implants are removed and replaced with a permanent rod system and fusion. The patient is sent into adulthood with this system in place.

With regard to idiopathic scoliosis, the Shilla system begins with the ultimate "ideal goal" in mind, namely, sending patients into adulthood with a full length vertebral column in as neutral an alignment as possible, and as mobile as possible, free of implants. The Shilla system is a new and different way of thinking about the treatment of juvenile spinal deformities, which strives to achieve this ideal goal as closely as possible.

The Shilla growing rod system enables growth while directing it into a more normal alignment, harnessing the growth potential of the patient's vertebral bodies. The guiding principles include:

(1) The maximum number of growth centers (34 exist between C7 and S1) should be preserved through the treatment process.
(2) The more unfused segments maintained, the more normal the ultimate mobility.
(3) The deformity is worst at the apex. This is where the maximum corrective forces need to be concentrated and maintained. Therefore, if a growth center has to be sacrificed, it should be at the apex of the deformity.
(4) Bracing or casting compresses the chest wall, compromising pulmonary function while restricting a child's interaction with his/her environment and with others. It also stigmatizes the child as different.
(5) Pedicle screws supply the best, most stable vertebral fixation and can be placed from an extraperiosteal position to maintain growth.

48.2 Historical Perspective

The growth guidance concept grew out of the sliding technique of the Luque Trolley. What was characterized as the "trolley" was an unfused spine instrumented with multiple levels of sublaminar smooth wires place bilaterally and linked to smooth parallel rods placed along the lamina. Some patients with this device continued to grow in spite of the periosteal stripping of the

R. E. McCarthy
University of Arkansas for Medical Sciences, Arkansas Children's Hospital 800 Marshal, Little Rock, AR 72202, USA
e-mail: rmccarthy@uams.com

B. A. Akbarnia et al. (eds.), *The Growing Spine*,
DOI: 10.1007/978-3-540-85207-0_48, © Springer-Verlag Berlin Heidelberg 2011

spine used to place the implants, but the results were inconsistent, and the technique has fallen into disfavor.

The concept was a good one, namely to guide the spine to grow straight. The problem was the anchors causing interlaminar ankylosis and eventually autofusion. The use of an extraperiostally placed pedicle screw allows for continued spinal growth while fixing the vertebral body to a rod and guiding it to grow in a straight manner.

48.3 Experimental Background

Early in its inception, Shilla was implanted into immature goats to address some basic questions. The implants had been tested using an Instron testing machine, and the device itself was shown to be sound. After a million compression cycles, the only instrument defect was metal filings from movement of the rods in the Shilla screws without instrument failures. The in vivo model consisted of 11 immature goats instrumented at approximately 2 months of age with explantation of their spines at 6 months postop. The questions addressed in this model were the following: (1) Could the implant be safely inserted into small pedicles in a manner that would allow for growth? (2) Would bilateral pedicle screws in the thoracic spine produce spinal stenosis? (3) What would be the effects upon the instrumented but unfused facet joints?

The examination at 6 months included gross and radiographic examination of the specimens, manual testing, and microCT studies. The results indicated that the spines grew and the implants slid along the rods as expected. No evidence of spinal stenosis occurred at the apex where the bilateral pedicle screws had been placed; although the facets at the level of the Shilla screws were degenerated, the adjacent levels survived and had preservation of the facet articular cartilage. One goat was paralyzed by the surgery and was sacrificed once this was evident soon after surgery. Autopsy showed one of the thoracic screws significantly encroaching the intrathecal space.

48.4 Method

48.4.1 The Implant Design

The Shilla "growing" screw is a polyaxial screw with a locking plug that fixes to the top of the screw and not the rod. It captures the rod allowing it to slide in a longitudinal direction. The polyaxial head allows the rod a few degrees of side-to-side movement. This movement at the base of the screw head diminishes the stress on the bone/thread interface (Fig. 48.1a, b). The screws placed bilaterally at the apex of the curve are fixed head type to provide maximal correction in all places.

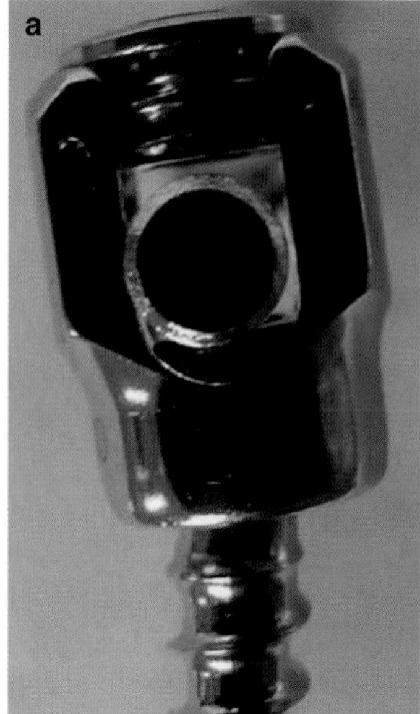

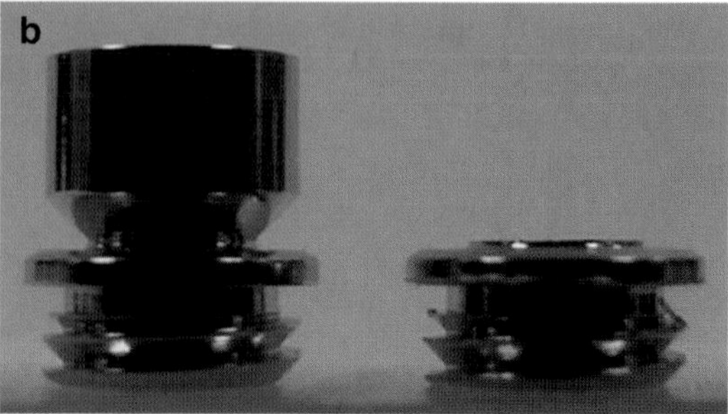

Fig. 48.1 (**a, b**) The Shilla growing screw: A polyaxial pedicle screw with a cap that fixes to the top of the screw and snaps off for a low profile (**b**) and allows for the rod to be captured and able to slide in the screw

The tops of the locking plugs snap off to minimize contour of the implants.

48.4.2 Surgical Technique

48.4.2.1 Preoperative Planning

Preoperative patient planning consists of a careful assessment of the upright coronal and sagittal films coupled with analysis of the flexibility of the curve via supine bend films, fulcrum bend films, or traction films. Determination of the location of the apical vertebral segments is of key importance. Those apical three or four vertebral segments that are least corrected through flexibility testing are the ones that comprise the apical levels for fusion and maximum correction. The goal is to render these segments neutral in all planes. If the surgeon can achieve this through posterior techniques alone, then no anterior release is necessary. For very stiff curves, anterior disc and end plate excision of the interval levels may be necessary before the planned correction. The posterior placed fixation at the apex uses bilateral fixed head pedicle screws. The Shilla growing screws are placed above (cephalad) and below (caudad) the apex to guide the growth of the spine at the ends of the curve and maintain coronal and sagittal correction. These screws are placed through the muscle layer without taking down soft tissues except to cut the fascial planes on each side of the midline. The use of a blueprint based on preoperative planning is helpful for the operating room team (Fig. 48.2).

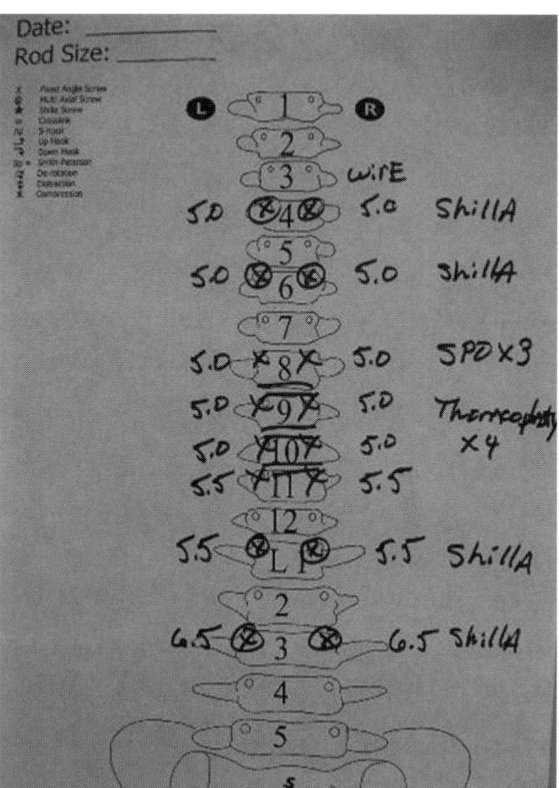

Fig. 48.2 Example of a blueprint planned preoperatively and placed in O.R. where operating room team can refer to it during surgery

A single midline incision has been used to approach the three areas of instrumentation. Before incision of the fascia, radiographs are taken with small needle markers placed in the spinous processes to identify levels. Subperiosteal dissection is isolated to the apical levels only.

The fascia is incised one centimeter off the midline on both sides of the spinous processes from cephalad to caudad merging with the subperiosteal dissection at the apex. With direct visualization and either a free-handed technique or using C-arm fluoroscopy, bilateral pedicle screws are placed throughout the apical levels with fixed head screws. If an apical thoracoplasty is being used to enhance correction of the rib hump or for bone graft harvesting, it can be accomplished from the midline incision through the paraspinal muscle layers, removing the medial 2 cm from the apical deformed ribs.

Ponte osteotomies are performed between the apical segments and will enhance correction in all planes. Apical decortication will be necessary for fusion of these levels.

The Shilla growth guidance screws are placed through the muscular layer without visualization of the bone except radiographically (Fig. 48.3a–f). A cannulated polyaxial screw of sufficient diameter to fill the pedicle is used. The location of the Shilla screws is curve dependent but should extend into the lumbar spine sufficient to control the lordosis and the coronal curve. Avoid stopping the caudal instrumentation at the thoracolumbar junction. The Shilla screws can be placed at bilateral locations or staggered but should be separated apart a sufficient distance on the rod to allow for sliding of the rod easily. The Shilla screws at the top of the construct are subject to pull out forces from kyphosis and are best protected with a sublaminar wire

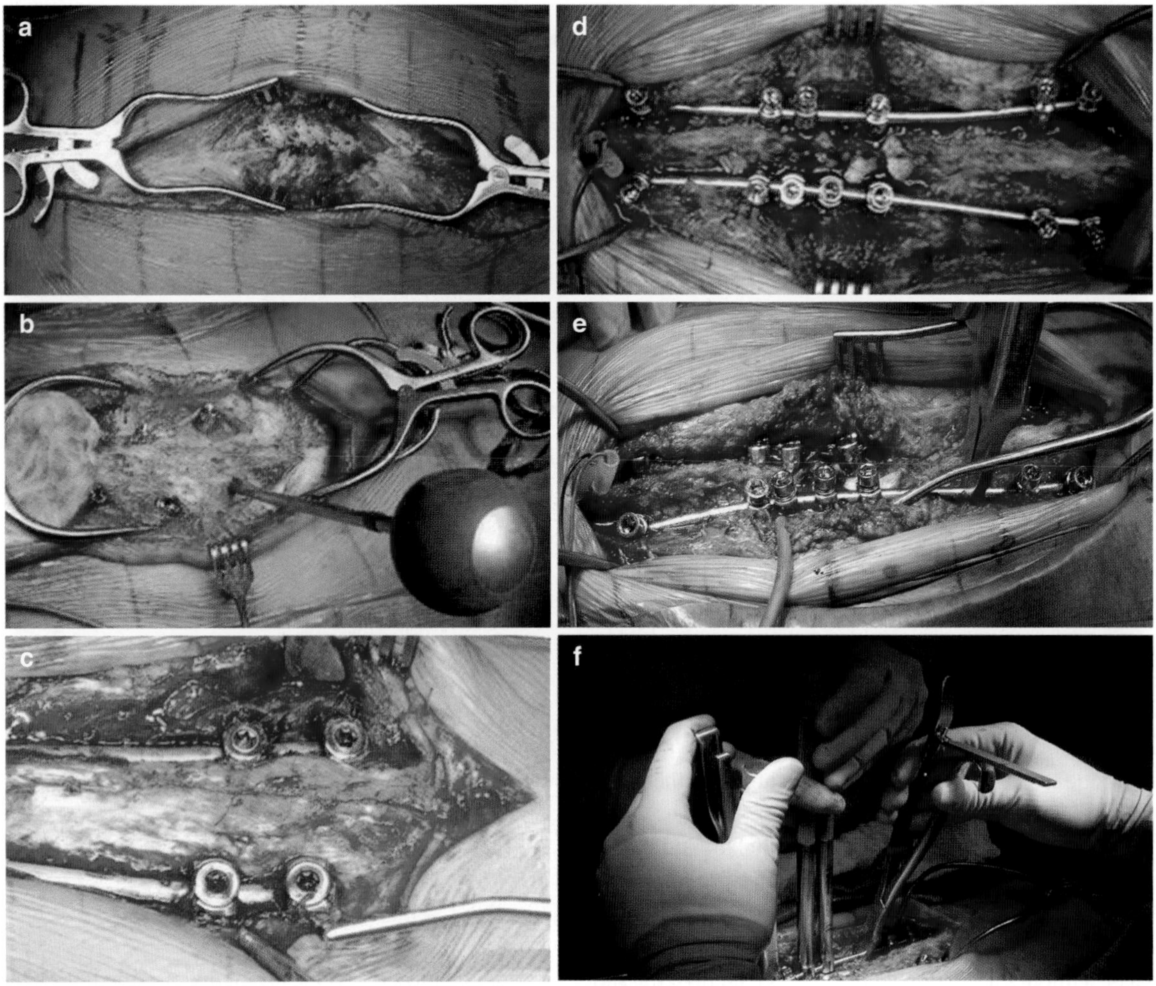

Fig. 48.3 (**a**) A single incision is used, with levels identified using the C-arm, followed by subperiosteal dissection at the apex (cephalad on left, caudad on right). (**b**) Shilla screws are placed through the muscle. (**c**) And with C-arm guidance. (**d**) The rods are placed and rotated into place with normal sagittal contours prebent into the rod. (**e**) Both rods in place. (**f**) Apical derotation with tube derotation

placed one level above the upper screws. The wire can be placed with minimal dissection leaving the inners-pinous ligament intact and removing the ligamentum flavum with a small Kerison ronguer. The double wire can be split after sublaminar passage and passed through the soft tissues to each side without lifting the periosteum. Fiberwire (5 mm) is a good alternative to wire (Fig. 48.4).

The rod diameter is chosen appropriate for the size of the child. The majority of the time a 4.5-mm diameter rod is satisfactory for the apical and lower sections of the rod which transitions to a smaller (3.5) diameter rod in the top section to enhance flexibility and decrease stress on the bone screw interface. The rod is contoured with normal sagittal curves with the rod junction located

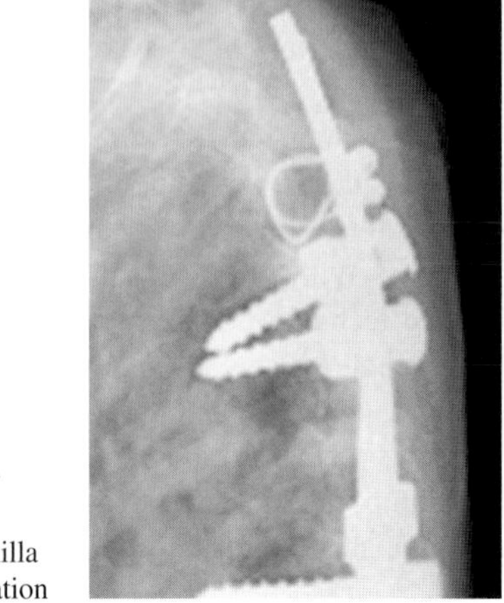

Fig. 48.4 Sublaminar wires can be placed cephalad above the Shilla screws to enhance fixation

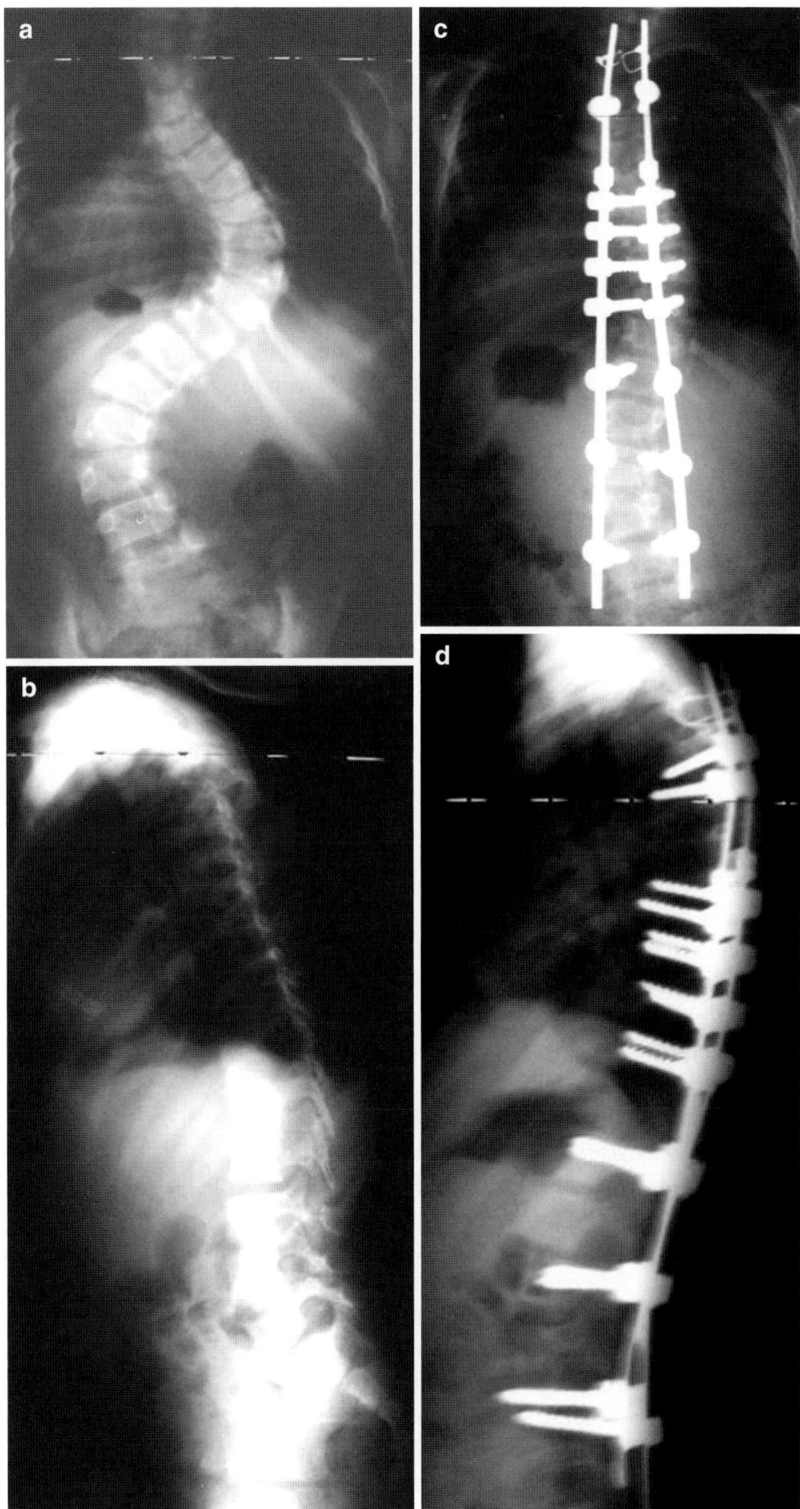

Fig. 48.5 Preoperative (**a, b**) and postoperative (**c, d**) standing AP and lateral radiographs of a 4 year old with Marfan's and scoliosis treated with Shilla procedure

just cephalad to the apical screws. The rod is left one level long at each end for growth (Fig. 48.5a–d).

The apical levels are derotated with tube derotation devices or a vertebral column derotation device, while vice grips hold the rods in place to prevent rod rotation. The fixed head screws lock the rods at the apical screws via the locking set screws that press against the rods, while the Shilla caps capture the rods in the Shilla screws and press onto the polyaxial screw, not the rods. Often a crosslink is used to help control rod rotation. If the child is less than 5 years old, the crosslink should be avoided or a sliding type used to allow for growth in canal diameter. The torque/counter torque device snaps off the caps at a preset torque pressure. Bone graft is placed at the apex only. A small drain is often used.

A bivalved form fitting turtle shell brace for daytime use is recommended for 3 months until the apical fusion is established. Fragile skin may preclude use of the brace. After the initial period of immobilization, a protective brace is not necessary except if excessively vigorous activities are contemplated (Fig. 48.6a–i).

48.5 Clinical Experience

The Shilla has been used in the treatment of curves 40° or greater (range 40–115°; average 77°) where growth is anticipated for at least 4 years or more. Diagnoses for which the Shilla has been used include: infantile and juvenile idiopathic scoliosis, Beale's syndrome, myelomeningocele, Marfan's, spinal muscular atrophy, arthrogryposis, multiple pterygium syndrome, and dwarfism. Ages at the time of surgery have ranged from 23 months to 11 years (average 6½ years). Curve magnitude, potential for worsening deformity and skeletal age have been the key determinants in the decision to operate. Our longest follow up is 5 years and as seen in Fig. 48.6 with a 70% curve improvement at last follow up. She has returned to full activity (see Fig. 48.6).

The Shilla device was implanted in an animal model before widespread use in patients; the results at 6 months showed viable facet joints between the fused apex and the Shilla screws as noted on microCT. Degenerative facet changes were observed in the joints adjacent to the Shilla growing screws. There was no evidence of apical stenosis over the 6 months of implantation (to maturity), and all the specimens reflected growth of the spine.

The first ten patients with greater than 2-year follow-up were reported to reflect similar results with growth in all patients. Five additional procedures occurred beyond the index procedure to treat: one broken rod (4.5 mm), one prominent implant, and one patient who outgrew her rod. Two patients had wound washouts and maintained the implants. These patients when compared with a similar group of patients treated with distraction based growing rods would have had 49 additional procedures beyond their index procedures to accomplish periodic lengthening procedures.

The problems encountered with the Shilla device include bone/screw loosening and prominence of the upper screws. This has necessitated some implant exchanges usually accomplished on an outpatient basis. This issue has been lessened by the use of sublaminar wires or fiberwire (5 mm) placed cephalad to the screws.

Pelvic obliquity when flexible is best treated by placement of Shilla screws at L5 bilaterally, thereby balancing the pelvis. If a larger degree of pelvic obliquity is present especially when stiff, firm fixation must be used on the pelvis with screws at S_1 coupled with iliac crest long screws bilaterally and linked to a cephalad directed rod with an L_4 Shilla screw. This is linked to an uncoupled domino attached to the rod coming inferiorly from the fixed apex. Once this is set up bilaterally, the pelvic obliquity is corrected and able to grow straight through the lower lumbar segments.

48.6 Summary

The Shilla growth guidance system allows for treatment of infantile and juvenile spinal deformities without the need for scheduled lengthenings. The Shilla harnesses the normal growth of the spine and maintains normal sagittal contours. It has the power to correct and maintain correction of pelvic obliquity and is applicable for a multiplicity of disorders causing spinal deformities.

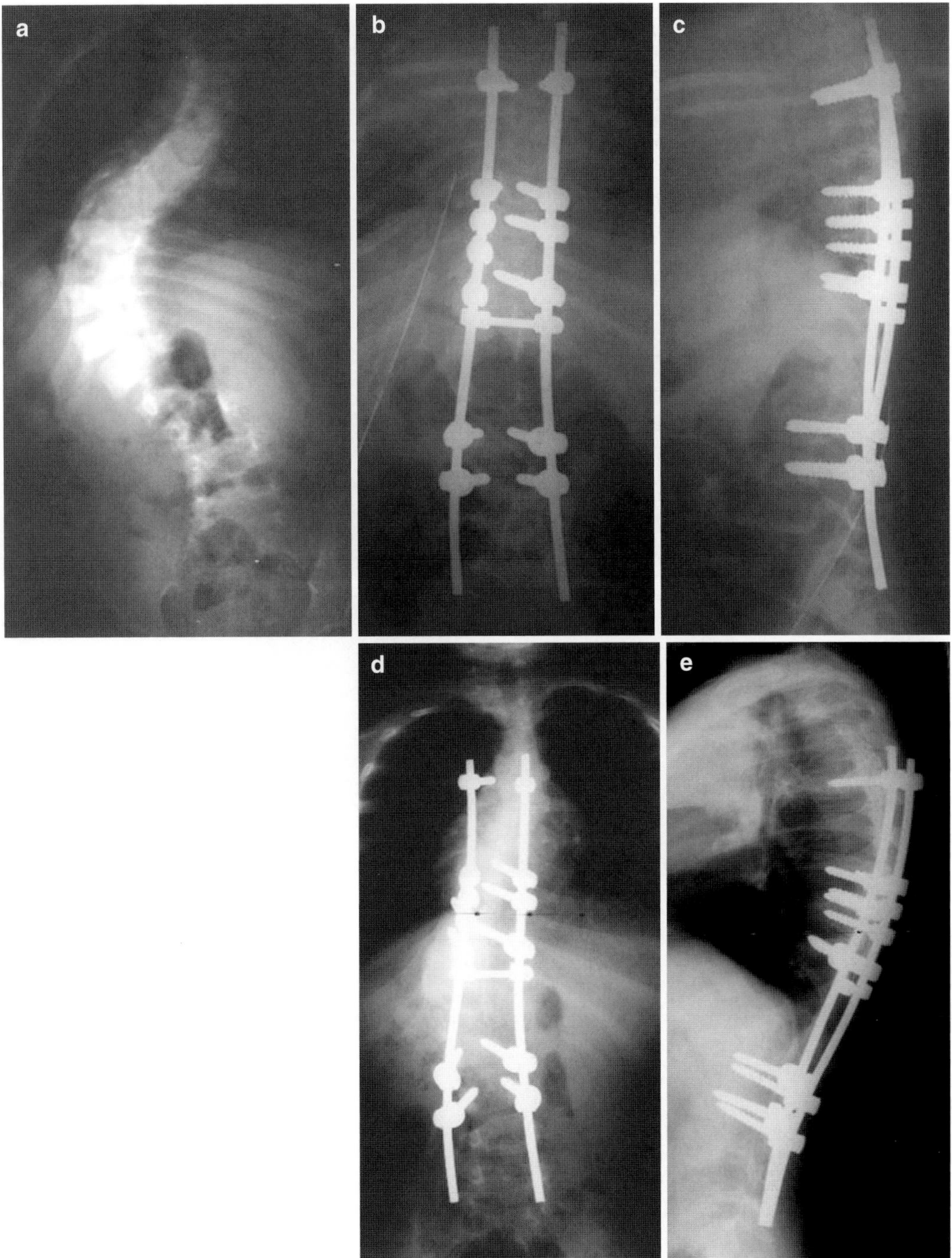

Fig. 48.6 Preoperative (**a**), 6 weeks postoperative (**b, c**), and 5 years postoperative radiographs (**d, e**)

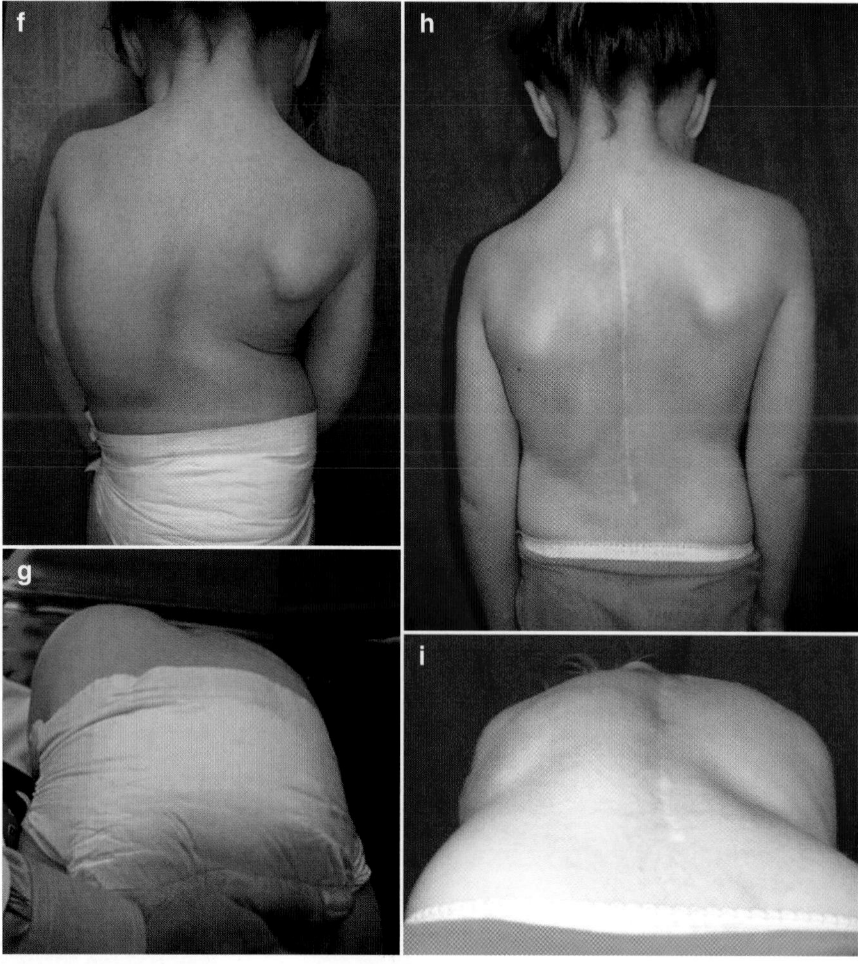

Fig. 48.6 (continued) Clinical photographs preoperatively (**f, g**) and 5 years postoperatively (**h, i**)

Hybrid Distraction-Based Growing Rods

49

David L. Skaggs

Key Points

› Hooks from standard spinal instrumentation systems may be used as rib anchors.
› The use of ribs as anchors for growing rods has the benefit of avoiding dissection and intentional fusion of the upper thoracic spine, which is important for pulmonary development.
› As ribs are mobile, a theoretical benefit of rib anchors is motion preservation, as opposed to spontaneous autofusion observed frequently after extended treatment with rigid standard growing rod constructs.
› Benefits of using standard spinal hooks over specialized rib implants are no special equipment, training, or institutional approval is needed, and multiple ribs at a time may be used for load sharing.
› A thorocotomy, elevation of the scapula, or cutting of tissue between ribs is rarely indicated. Distraction of the concavity of scoliosis leads to expansion of the hemithorax and harmonious separation between ribs.
› Neuromonitoring of the upper extremities is indicated when using ribs as anchor sites.

D. L. Skaggs
Childrens Hospital Los Angeles, University of Southern California School of Medicine, 4650 Sunset Boulevard, #69, Los Angeles, CA 90027, USA
e-mail: dskaggs@chla.usc.edu

49.1 Introduction

Our specialty and patients are indebted to Dr. Robert Campbell (Fig. 49.1) for pioneering treatment of the growing child with thoracic and spinal deformity. He not only first described thoracic insufficiency syndrome [2] but also first described the treatment of this condition with thoracic expansion [1]. A unique feature of his treatment was attachment of distraction-based implants on the ribs.

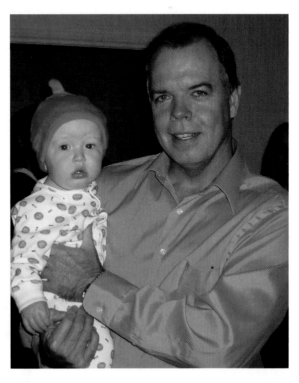

Fig. 49.1 Dr. Robert Campbell holding Clay Skaggs, 2001, Los Angeles (Reproduced with permission of Children's Orthopaedic Center, Los Angeles)

B. A. Akbarnia et al. (eds.), *The Growing Spine*,
DOI: 10.1007/978-3-540-85207-0_49, © Springer-Verlag Berlin Heidelberg 2011

Use of traditional spine hooks on the ribs is considered "off-label" by the Food and Drug Administration of the United States. Whether this is of any significance is questionable, as off-label usage of spine implants in pediatrics is commonplace. The technique of using spine hooks on ribs is becoming common, with at least 6 of 22 orthopaedic surgeons serving as faculty at the first International Congress on Early Scoliosis and Growing Spine (ICEOS) in Madrid, Spain on 2–3 Nov 2007 having used this technique in their practice.

There are many possible benefits for using ribs as anchor sites, the first of which is that the rib attachments may allow for motion preservation. The ribs are attached to the spine via the costotransverse joints (neck of rib to anterior portion of transverse process) and the costovertebral joints (head of rib to vertebral body). The costovertebral joints constitute a series of gliding or arthrodial joints formed by the articulation of the rib head with the facet on the contiguous vertebrae. Ribs 1, 10, 11, and 12 articulate with single vertebral bodies; the remaining ribs attach to two vertebrae [3] (Fig. 49.2a, b). These joints permit a gliding motion. During normal respiration, there is just over 10° of bucket-handle motion of the ribs relative to the spine [11]. In addition, the interface of a hook on the rib is not rigid, and allows for some "slop."

In contrast, traditional growing rods attached to the spine permit little motion of the vertebrae within the construct. As with any diarthrodial joint, prolonged immobilization decreases motion and can lead to spontaneous fusion. It is a common experience upon converting growing rods to a final fusion construct to discover spontaneous fusion of most, if not all, of the vertebrae within the construct. This appears to be a gradual process, and not well documented in the literature. In my experience after about 5 years of traditional growing rods, spontaneous fusion of the vertebrae should be expected. This would be a particular concern when growing rods are placed in young children, i.e., if dual rods are placed in a 2-year-old, the spine may be fused by age 7. In theory, use of the ribs for anchor points will permit motion between vertebrae and prevent or delay spontaneous fusion. This technique is too new to have tested this theory.

Another advantage of using ribs as anchors is to stay out of the spine and preserve a virgin spine for future surgeries. While traditional growing rods aim for a fusion at the top of the construct, methods that attempt nonfusion, such as Luque-Trolley (sublaminar wires and rods without fusion), have been shown to cause fusion in 100% of patients in one series [5]. Fusion in the upper thoracic spine (T1–T3) in young children is particularly harmful to long-term pulmonary function, so avoiding fusion in this region may be an important benefit of this technique [4].

It has been shown that children with thoracic insufficiency are nutritionally depleted, with 79% being below the fifth percentile for weight [9]. Soft tissue coverage of traditional spine implants can be challenging in this population. A further advantage of rib anchors is that they tend to have good soft tissue

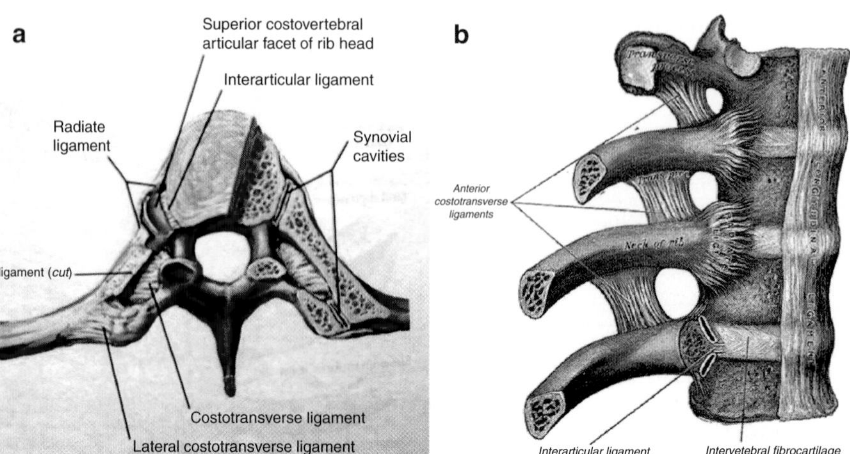

Fig. 49.2 (**a**, **b**) Demonstation of the costotransverse and costovertebral joints

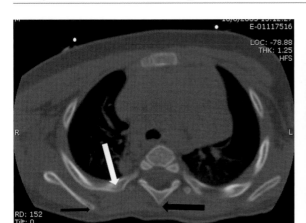

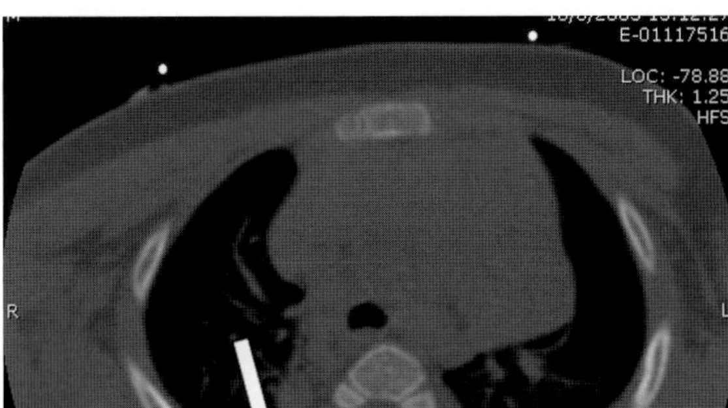

Fig. 49.3 CT of the chest. Note that the attachment point of the rib anchor (*white arrow*) is in a trough with good soft tissue coverage between the spinous process (*thick black arrow*) and scapula (*thin black arrow*). (Reproduced with permission of Children's Orthopaedic Center, Los Angeles)

coverage, as they are located deep to the rhomboids and trapezius, in a valley between the more prominent spine and scapula (Fig. 49.3).

A significant practical advantage of using traditional spine implants on ribs rather than VEPTR is that no special equipment is needed (Table 49.1). Hooks that fit ribs are readily available on all spine implant systems. There are, thus, no special equipment needs, and no special training needed for the surgeon or OR staff. In addition, there is no need for institutional or research approval as traditional spine implant hooks are FDA approved. A particular advantage over the original VEPTR design is that load sharing over multiple ribs is quite simple (Fig. 49.4).

Table 49.1 Possible benefits of spine implants as rib anchors

Motion preservation
No dissection of spine
Good soft tissue coverage
No special equipment, training or institutional approval needed
Load-sharing over multiple ribs
No fusion of the upper thoracic spine, which is important for pulmonary development

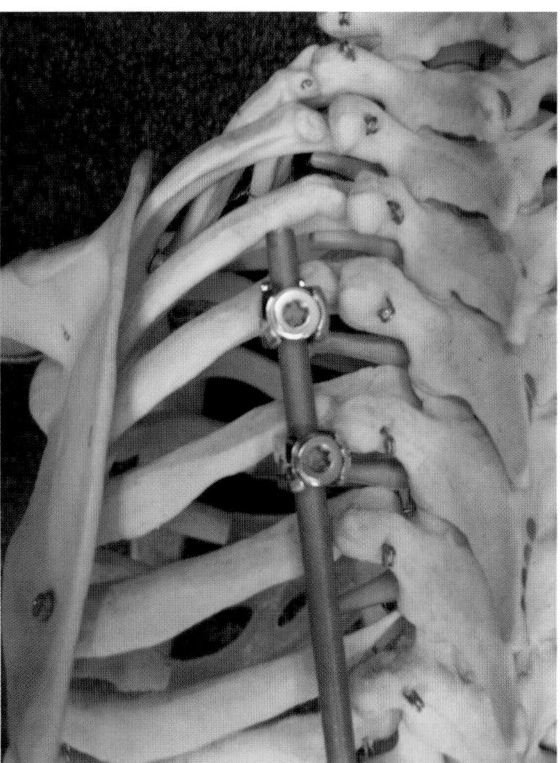

Fig. 49.4 With hooks of standard spine implants, multiple ribs may be engaged to share load over multiple ribs. Note the hooks are immediately adjacent to the transverse process. (Reproduced with permission of Children's Orthopaedic Center, Los Angeles)

49.2 Indications

The indications for use of ribs as anchors in growing systems are evolving. The argument may be made to use rib attachments in children 5 years of age or less, as they would be expected to have growing implants for at least 5 years, and rib attachments may decrease the risk of spontaneous fusion as discussed earlier. Another indication is when there is already a substantial fusion of the mid thoracic spine present (whether from previous surgery or congenital), and one wants to minimize further fusion in the upper thoracic spine. In cases of previous infection of growing implants, the ribs provide an area of new, uninfected tissue as a salvage. Using rib anchors also allow one to avoid sites of previous surgery such as laminectomies.

A strong indication of using ribs as anchors is in cases of significant cervicothoracic scoliosis and head tilt, in which the upper ribs are fused. This is discussed in detail near the end of the chapter.

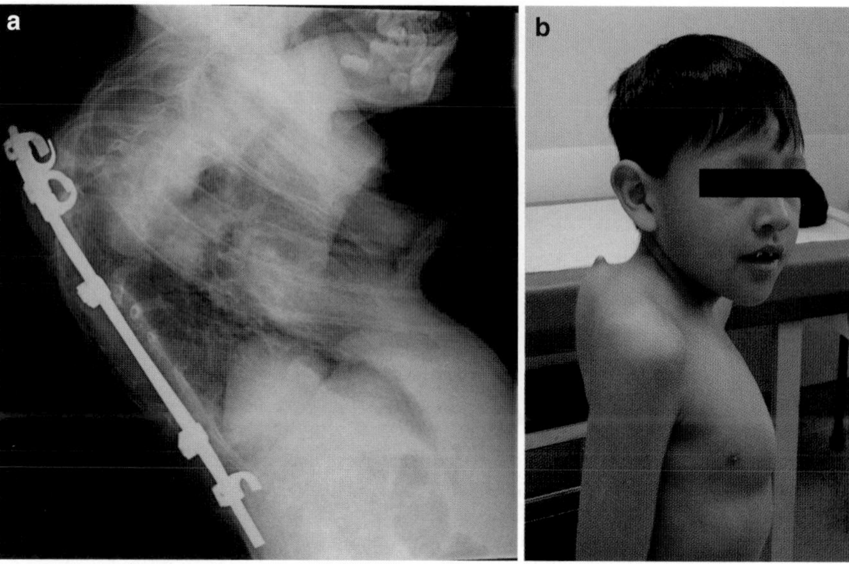

Fig. 49.5 (**a**) Lateral radiograph demonstrating progressive kyphosis despite rib implants. (**b**) Clinical photograph demonstrating rod coming through the patient's skin. (Reproduced with permission of Children's Orthopaedic Center, Los Angeles)

49.3 Contraindications

Rib attachments tend to function poorly in cases of kyphosis as the ribs tend to pull backwards over time as the spine falls forward. In particularly, upper thoracic kyphosis is poorly controlled with rib attachments, and I will use traditional growing rods, bent into kyphosis and attached cephald to the region of kyphosis if possible in this situation (Fig. 49.5 a, b)

49.4 Thorocotomy Generally Unnecessary

It is very uncommon that a formal thorocotomy is used with this technique. It has been shown that a thorocotomy in the treatment of scoliosis leads to a disruption of pulmonary function [6] and is simply not needed to improve spinal and thoracic deformity in the great majority of cases. Soft tissue or osseous release between ribs is rarely needed, except in the truly rare case of multiple rib fusions limiting thoracic expansion. It is natural that ribs are closer together in the concavity of a curve than the convexity, and that is not an indication for tissue destruction between the ribs. When the scoliosis is improved by distraction implants, the spaces between the ribs open up in a harmonious fashion (Fig. 49.6a, b). In contrast, distraction across a formal thoroctomy distracts between the two ribs at the site of the thorocotomy (Fig. 49.7a, b). Any tissue lysis between ribs cannot help but leave scar tissue, which is less mobile and functional than virgin intercostals muscle.

49.5 Surgical Technique

Neurological monitoring should include the upper and lower extremities. The spine is approached through a midline skin incision as it is likely that this incision will be used for the final fusion in the future. Depending on the specifics of the surgery, a long midline incision or separate incisions at the top and bottom of the construct may be made (Fig. 49.8). demonstrates the top incision for the rib attachments is 4 cm in length. The skin is undermined laterally past the transverse processes. The transverse processes are generally palpable as a point of resistance through the muscles. If there is any question, fluoroscopic imaging over a needle placed into bone clarifies the location. A combination of muscle splitting and cautery in a vertical incision should bring one quickly to the ribs with minimal blood loss.

Care should be taken to make certain the dissection is immediately adjacent to the transverse process only. There is a tendency for the hook to slide laterally if soft tissues are dissected laterally. In addition, the implants exert the most control of the spine when they are adjacent to the transverse process, as opposed to a more lateral placement in which the ribs tend to move cephlad in a bucket handle fashion independent of correction of the spine.

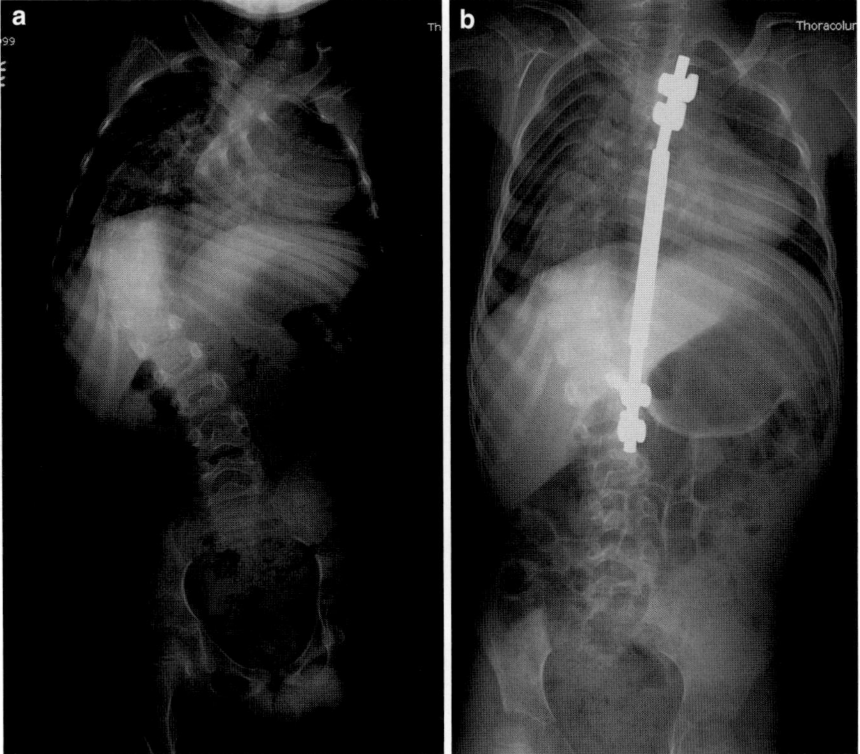

Fig. 49.6 (**a**) A preoperative AP radiograph of 91° scoliosis with ribs on the concave side appearing constricted. (**b**) Evidence of harmonious distraction of the ribs through distraction instrumentation *without* scapula elevation, thorocotmy or any lysis of tissue between ribs. (Reproduced with permission of Children's Orthopaedic Center, Los Angeles)

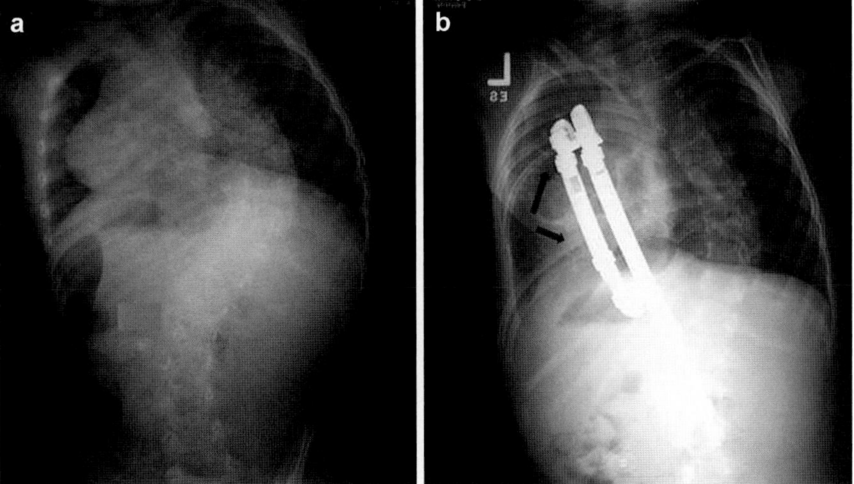

Fig. 49.7 Preoperative (**a**) and postoperative (**b**) radiographs demonstrate large opening of two ribs at a thorocotomy site (between *black arrows*), and compression of rib spaces above the thorocotomy. (Reproduced with permission of Children's Orthopaedic Center, Los Angeles)

Ideally, the periosteum is preserved around the rib to allow the rib to hypertrophy in response to stress. I have found to my surprise that the neurovascular bundle caudad to each rib is really of no consequence in this surgery. To place a hook, a 5-mm transverse incision with a cautery is made just distal to the neurovascular bundle and immediately adjacent but lateral to the transverse process. A freer elevator is then used to dissect soft tissue anterior to the rib, aiming to exploit the plane between the periosteum and the pleura (Fig. 49.9a, b). In reality, this technique has evolved over time to the point where I simply push the hook into position without any preliminary dissection. Usually, a second hook is placed around a second rib as well. Both hooks are up going. There is no need for a down going hook, as distractive forces keep the rib engaged in the hook, and a properly sized hook extends a bit cephlad to the rib (see Fig. 49.9b). I am not aware of any ribs migrating off the top of hooks.

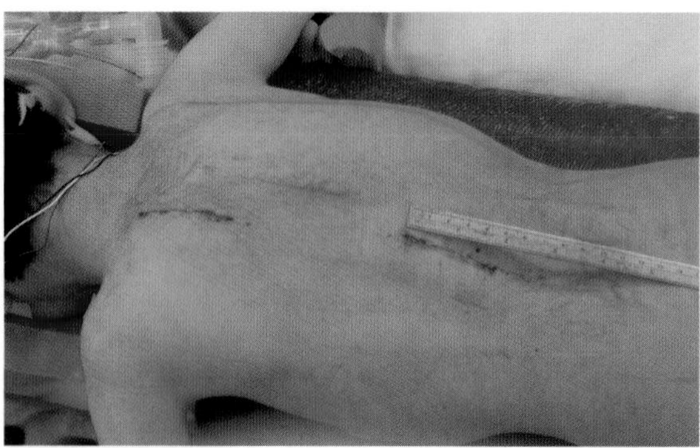

Fig. 49.8 Intra-operative photograph demonstrating a 4- and 5-cm incision for growing rod implants. Same case as Fig. 49.6. (Reproduced with permission of Children's Orthopaedic Center, Los Angeles)

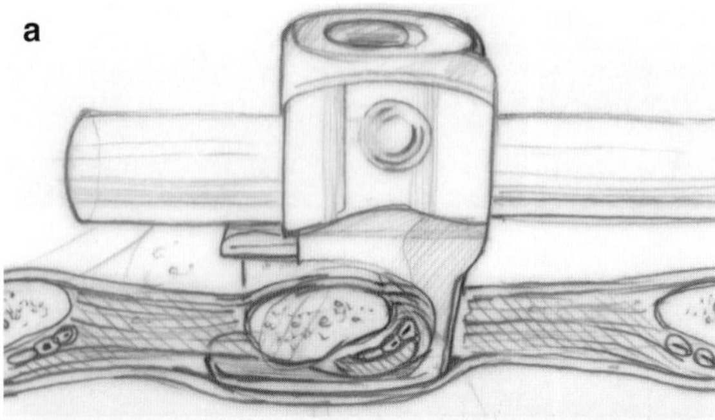

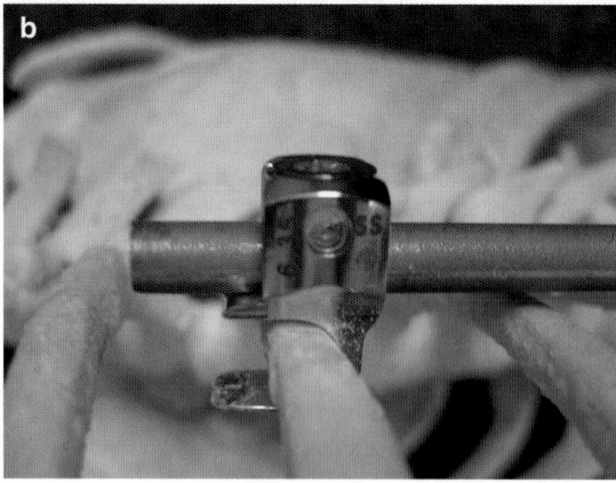

Fig. 49.9 (**a**) Cross-sectional drawing of a lumbar hook engaging a rib. The exact location of the neurovascular bundle within or outside of the hook is not important (From Skaggs et al. [10]). (**b**) Side view of lumbar hook engaging a rib. Note the anterior portion of the hook extends superiorly to the rib, minimizing the possibility of superior migration of the rib away from the hook. The rib is not likely to fall out in a cephlad direction as the hook is distracting the rib. (Reproduced with permission of Children's Orthopaedic Center, Los Angeles)

Attention is then turned to the distal anchor point. Through a midline incision the lamina of the intended vertebrae is subperiosteally dissected. Either one level fixation with a down-going supralaminar hook, or two level fixation with pedicle screws may be used. The theoretical advantage of a one level hook construct is that no fusion is intended, and there is a certain amount of "slop" that may translate to motion and less spontaneous fusion. The disadvantage to using a single hook is that it often migrates posteriorly over time, leading to either a bump that is concerning to the parents, or migration through the lamina and need for revision. A potential pitfall here is to make sure the interspinous ligament is left intact when placing a supralaminar hook or distraction may lead to kyphosis of the distal segment. When using pedicle screws, always place them in at least two segments (unilateral or bilateral) as distal migration over time through pedicle screws could injure nerve roots along the inferior border of the pedicle. The facet joint between the two pedicle screws is destroyed with a narrow rongeur and cortical-cancellous crushed allograft is placed in the joint. The exposed bone is decorticated and bone graft placed *before* the rod is placed to maximize boney contact.

The upper and lower rods may be connected with either a traditional longitudinal growing rod connector or a side-to-side connector with the rods overlapping (Table 49.2, Fig 49.10a, b). If using a side-to-side connector do not rely on only one for the whole system or it may fail over time, perhaps as a result of bending moments in addition to compression forces.

Make a soft tissue tunnel between the two anchor sites with a tonsil clamp, being deep to muscle directly on the ribs. Pull a chest tube through this tunnel and attach an end of the rod into the chest tube, which is then used to safely pass the rod from one anchor to the

Table 49.2 Comparison of side-to-side and end-to-end connectors

Type of connector	Advantage	Disadvantage
Longitudinal connector	Less bulky, only one rod	No sagittal contouring Limited expansion potential
Sid-to-side connector	Sagittal contouring possible More expansion potential	More bulky, two overlapping rods

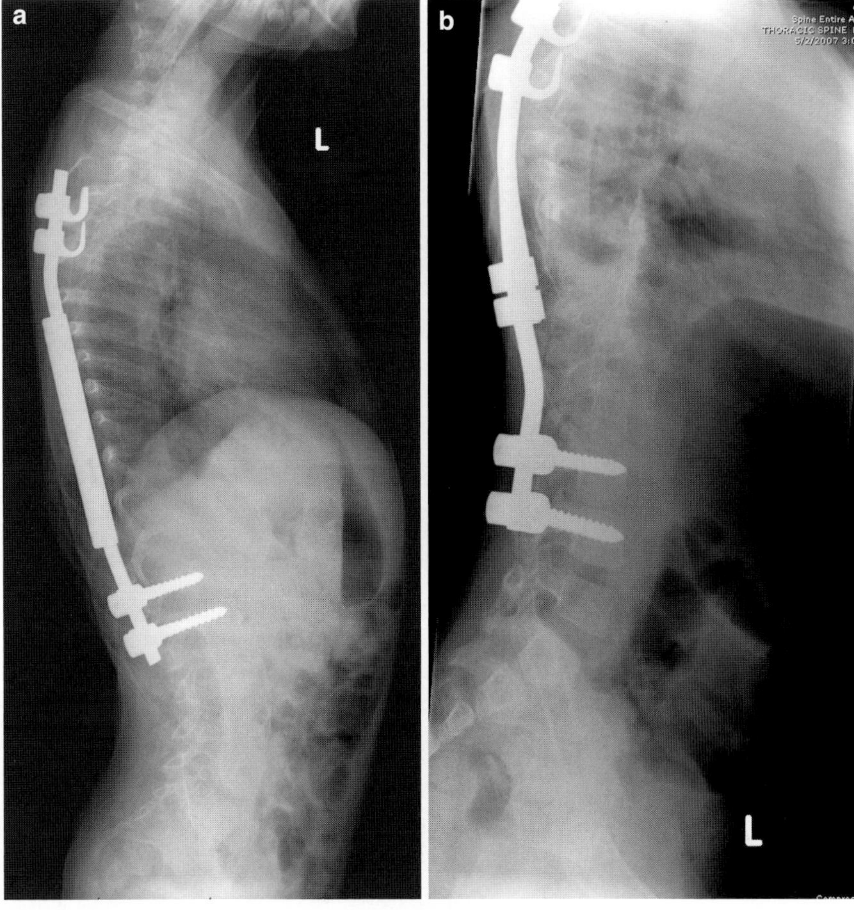

Fig. 49.10 (**a**) Lateral view of a longitudinal growth connector. (**b**) Lateral radiograph demonstrating a side-to-side connector with physiological sagittal contouring of rods. (Reproduced with permission of Children's Orthopaedic Center, Los Angeles)

other in a submuscular fashion. Plan on cutting rods at least 2–3 cm longer than the anchors to permit intraoperative distraction. Once distraction is performed, fill the upper anchor site with warm saline, and ask the anesthesiologist to perform a Valsalva maneuver to look for a pleural leek. If one is present, I place a small hemovac in the chest to function as a chest tube for a few days.

49.5.1 Unilateral or Bilateral Rods

This technique may be used with unilateral rods or bilateral rods. Unilateral rods are minimally invasive but have less anchor points to share load. Both acutely, and more so over time, balancing the curve can become problematic with a single unilateral rod (Fig. 49.11a–c). I rarely use unilateral rods except to span a unilateral bar. In general, bilateral rods seem more stable and less prone to loss of fixation. Bilateral rods also make balancing the spine easier, especially over time, with the ability to preferentially distract one side more than the other. A minor disadvantage of bilateral rods is that more dissection is needed, particularly at the bilateral rib attachments, though this does not affect the spine and is probably of little importance (Fig. 49.12a, b).

49.6 Complications

A unique feature of using ribs as anchor points in distraction-based growing instrumentation is the possibility of neurological injury to the upper extremity. A multicenter prospective study of the VEPTR study group found that neurological injury to the upper

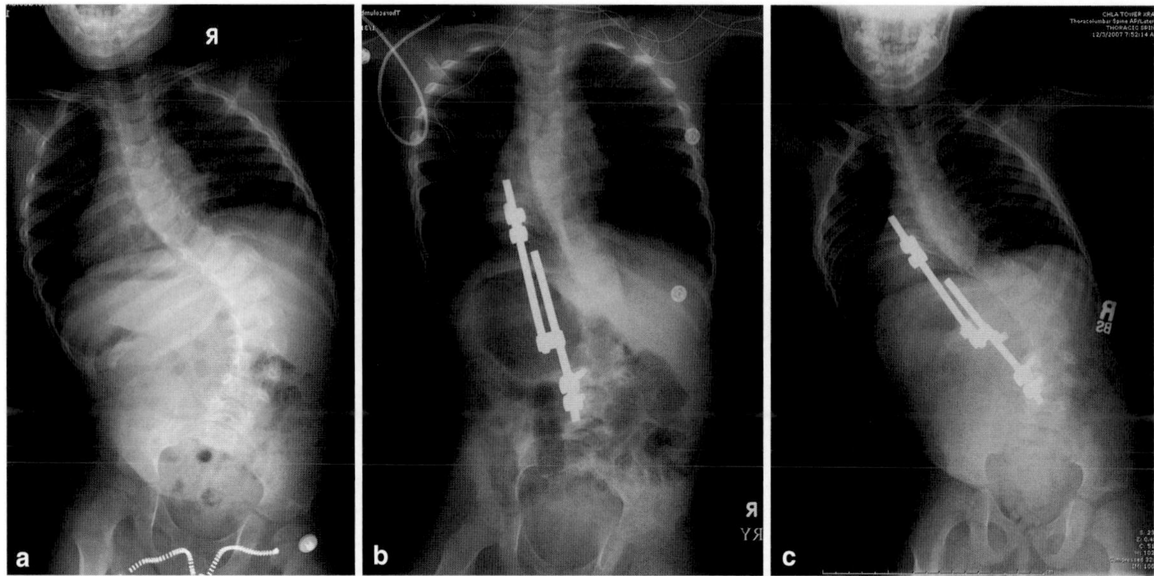

Fig. 49.11 (**a**) Preoperative AP radiograph. (**b**) Postoperative unilateral growing rod. (**c**) Two years later, significant decompensation has occurred. (Reproduced with permission of Children's Orthopaedic Center, Los Angeles)

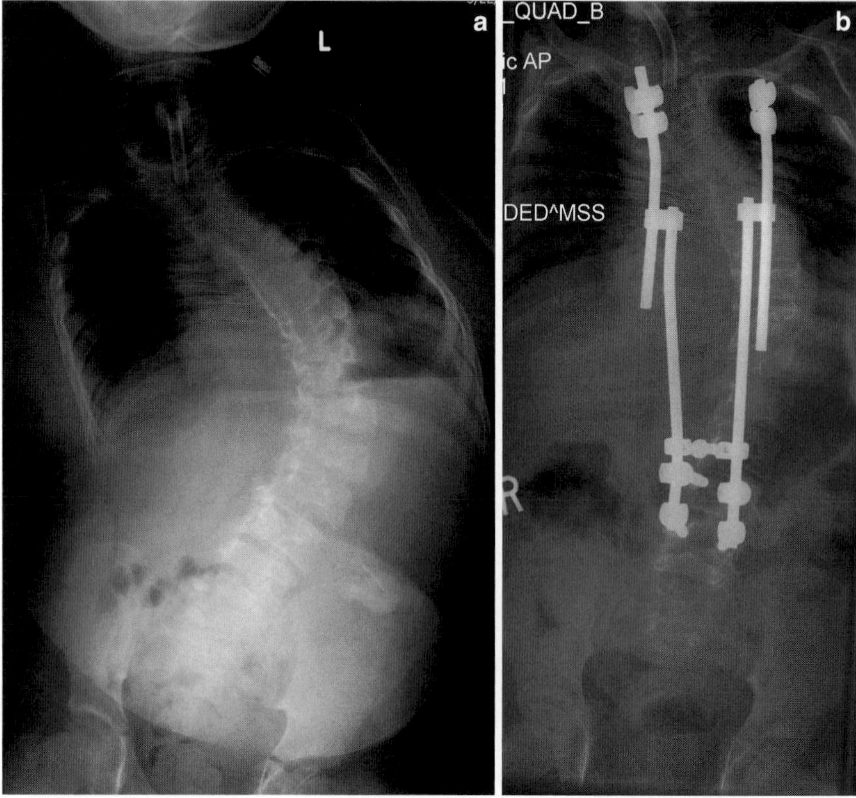

Fig. 49.12 (**a**) AP radiograph demonstrates an 83° curve in this 8 year old with neuromuscular scoliosis and pulmonary problems. (**b**) Postoperative demonstration of bilateral growing rods with hooks as rib anchors. (Reproduced with permission of Children's Orthopaedic Center, Los Angeles)

extremity was six times more frequent than to the lower extremity. The authors conclude the rate of potential neurological injury (neurological injury plus monitoring change) during primary device implantation (2.5%) and device exchange (1.3%) justifies the use of intraoperative neuromonitoring of the upper and lower extremities during primary and exchange VEPTR surgeries [8]. One suspected mechanism for upper extremity injury is direct pressure of the first rib on the brachial plexus (Fig. 49.13). Avoiding placing an anchor on the first rib (unless it is fused to other ribs – see below) is recommended to avoid this complication. Another mechanism of injury, which I have seen on two occasions, is direct impingement of the superior tip of the scapula into the brachial plexus, as the scapula is elevated off the chest wall (Table 49.3). This mechanism is easily avoided as there is no reason to elevate the scapula if a thorocotomy is not being performed, which is the case in the great majority of surgeries.

The hook–rib articulation is mobile, and plowing of the hook through the rib may take place over time. In single unilateral rod constructs with one hook on one rib, this is likely over many years, as has been demonstrated in the case of VEPTR. However, I have never seen a spinal hook plow through a rib when multiple hooks where used or where bilateral rods have been used. If this occurs, it is generally not much of a problem, as the rib grows back, often with more and stronger bone than before, and the same rib can be used again. Often times, there is so much new bone about the rib that a power bur may be needed to cut a slot into the bone mass to allow the hook to be properly seated.

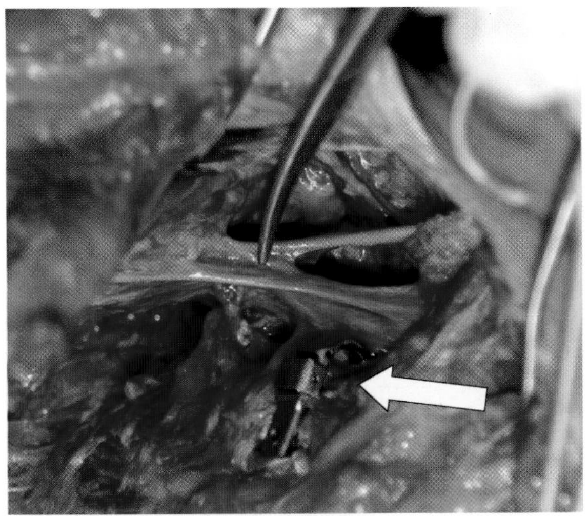

Fig. 49.13 Cadeveric dissection demonstrates the brachial plexus draping over the first rib. White arrow shows a VEPTR cradle on the first rib–rib anchors on the first rib alone should be avoided. (Reproduced with permission of Children's Orthopaedic Center, Los Angeles)

A study at Childrens Hospital of Los Angeles compared 36 children with spinal deformity treated with either dual growing rods, VEPTR, or the hybrid technique described in this chapter with spinal hooks on ribs. The children were a mean of 4 years 10 months at first surgery with a mean of 51 month follow up and a mean of four lengthenings each. The rate of having major complications requiring an unplanned surgery was 230% for growing rods, 237% for VEPTR, and 86% for the hybrid group with spinal hooks on ribs (Table 49.4) [7].

49.7 The Special Case of Cervicothoracic Congenital Scoliosis

Cervicothoracic congenital scoliosis presents a number of unique problems. The head is usually much more tilted than it would be if the same size curve were more caudal, because there are no vertebrae above the curve to create a compensatory curve, and the head tilt is often a very noticeable deformity. In addition, this is an area where spine surgeons do not commonly perform an anterior exposure. The good news is that there are frequently multiple ribs fused at the top, which present a solid fixation point. Although the first rib is generally avoided as a fixation point to prevent migration of the

Table 49.3 Pearls and Pitfalls

Keep the chest wall intact! It is rarely necessary to cut between ribs, do a thorocotomy or elevate the scapula
Keep the dissection and hook as close to the transverse process as possible, or the hook may slid laterally
If using a supralaminar hook for the distal anchor, leave the supraspinous ligament intact, or risk kyphosis of this vertebrae
If in doubt, use a longer construct, especially in younger children, as the curve is likely to add on over time if a short construct is used

Table 49.4 Complications of growing spine surgery

Major complications	Ccx rate (%)	Ccxs/cm growth	Ccxs/year treatment	Ccxs/planned surgeries
Dual growing rods	230	0.20/cm	0.52/yr	0.47/surgery
Spine hook on rib hybrid	86	0.19/cm	0.36/yr	0.29/surgery
VEPTR	237	0.97/cm	0.52/yr	0.44/surgery

cm centimeter; *yr* year; *CCx* complication

rib into the bracial plexus, the fused rib mass is not mobile, and can be used as a fixation point with little risk of brachial plexus injury. Of course, neuromonitoring of the upper extremity is mandatory at the time of the primary surgery if the fused ribs are used. This is the one situation where I will intentionally place the rib hook a distance lateral to the transverse process to take advantage of the moment arm and maximally improve the pathologic tilt of T1 (Fig. 49.14a–e).

In the case of hemivertebrae opposite a unilateral bar, consideration should be given to a instrumented compression and fusion for the hemivertebrae with pedicle screws. This may obtain modest correction acutely, and hopefully prevent future growth anteriorly and posteriorly.

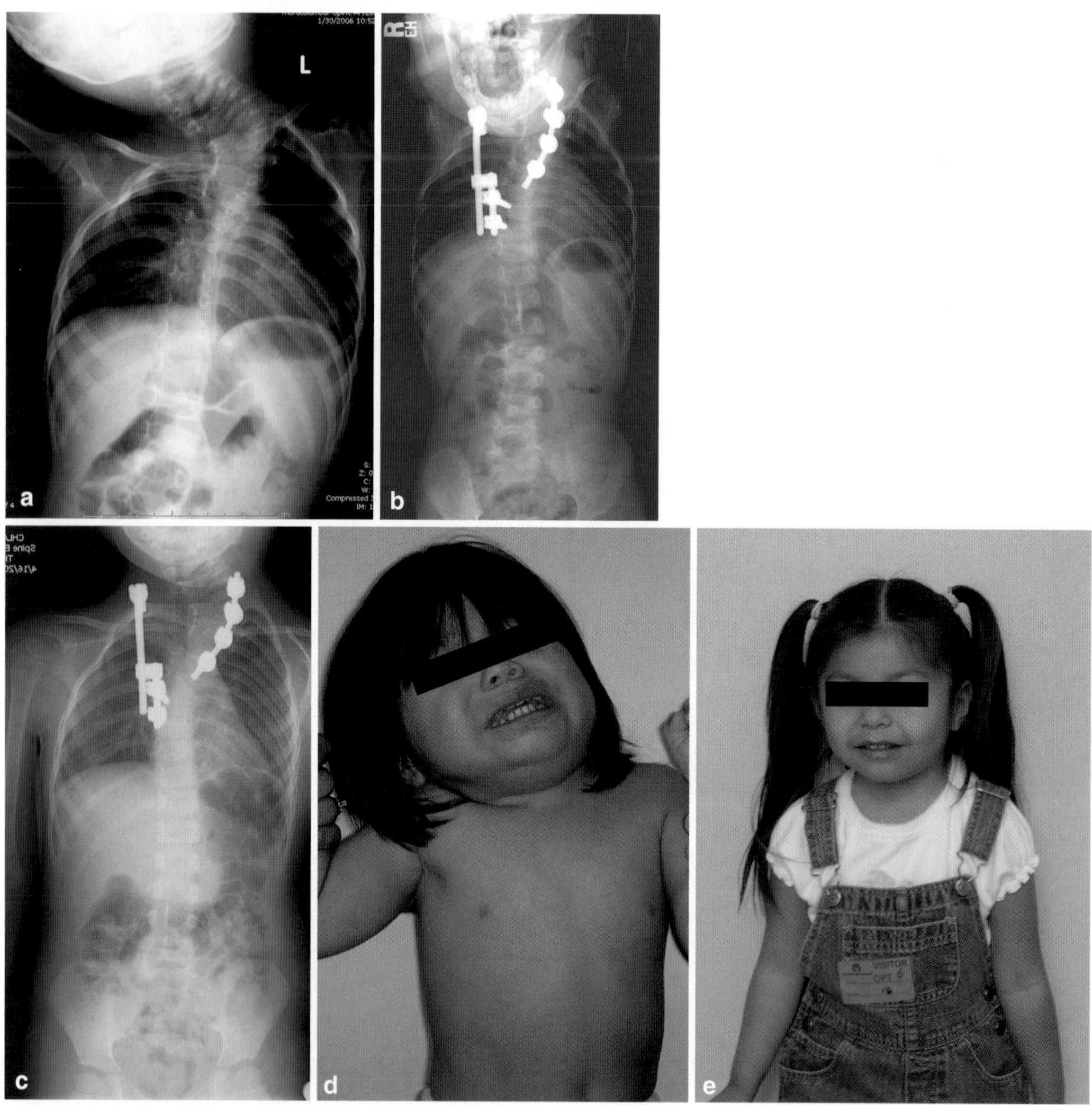

Fig. 49.14 (**a**) Preoperative AP radiograph demonstrates a unilateral bar opposite six pedicles. (**b**) Immediate postoperative AP radiograph. Note improvement in head position. (**c**) AP radiograph 1 year after initial surgery, with one surgical lengthening having been performed in the interim. Not a little migration of the hook on the upper rib, with new rib growing behind it. If this migrates through in the future, the hook could most likely be replaced on the same rib. The head position is significantly improved from preoperative position. (**d**) Preoperative clinical photo. The child's ear almost rested on her shoulder. (**e**) postop clinical photo demonstrating no significant deformity. The child has no pain or complaints. (Reproduced with permission of Children's Orthopaedic Center, Los Angeles)

References

1. Campbell RM Jr, Hell-Vocke AK (2003) Growth of the thoracic spine in congenital scoliosis after expansion thoracoplasty. J Bone Joint Surg Am 85-A(3):409–420
2. Campbell RM Jr, Smith MD, Mayes TC et al (2003) The characteristics of thoracic insufficiency syndrome associated with fused ribs and congenital scoliosis. J Bone Joint Surg Am 85-A(3):399–408
3. Gray H (1918) Anatomy of the human body. Lea & Febiger, Philadelphia
4. Karol L, Johnston C, Mladenov K et al (2008) Pulmonary function following early thoracic fusion in non-neuromuscular scoliosis. J Bone Joint Surg 90:1272–1281
5. Mardjetko SM, Hammerberg KW, Lubicky JP et al (1992) The Luque trolley revisited. Review of nine cases requiring revision. Spine 17(5):582–589
6. Newton PO, Perry A, Bastrom TP et al (2007). Predictors of change in postoperative pulmonary function in adolescent idiopathic scoliosis: a prospective study of 254 patients. Spine 32(17):1875–1882
7. Sankar WN, Acevedo DC, Skaggs DL (2009) Comparison of complications among growing spinal implants In: Pediatric Orthopaedic Society of North America annual meeting, Las Vegas, Nevada, 29 Apr–2 May 2009
8. Skaggs DL, Choi PD, Rice C et al (2006) Efficacy of intraoperative neurological monitoring in VEPTR surgery for early onset spinal deformity. In: 13th International Meeting of Advanced Spinal Techniques (IMAST), Athens, Greece
9. Skaggs DL, Sankar WN, Albrektson J et al (2009) Weight gain following vertical expandable prosthetic titanium ribs surgery in children with thoracic insufficiency syndrome. Spine 34(23):2530–2533
10. Skaggs DL, Buchowski JM, Sponseller P (2008) Temporary distraction rods in the correction of severe scoliosis. In: Tolo VT, Skaggs DL (eds) Masters techniques in orthopaedic surgery: pediatric orthopaedics. Lippincott, Williams & Wilkens, Philadelphia
11. Wilson TA, Rehder K, Krayer S et al (1987) Geometry and respiratory displacement of human ribs. J Appl Physiol 62(5):1872–1877

Basic Science and Future Clinical Perspective

50

James W. Ogilvie

Key Points

- Precise diagnostic and genotype homogeneity of EOS is required.
- Many syndromic EOS may share a common molecular pathway to spinal deformity.
- Translational research may provide the basis for innovative pharmacological treatments in EOS.

Basic science and pharmacology have had a great impact on surgical practice in the preceding decades. The surgical treatment of peptic ulcer disease has been altered as a result of an understanding of the influence of the bacteria *Helicobacter pylorum* and the use of proton-pump inhibitors [10, 21]. A disease that in the past was primarily surgical in nature is now almost exclusively one that is treated medically. Unfortunately, up to this time, such advances have not been common in the treatment of spinal deformity.

Since its wide acceptance in the mid-1980s, the use of magnetic resonance imaging (MRI) has changed the landscape of diagnosis in early onset scoliosis (EOS). Early and routine use of MRI has allowed intraspinal abnormalities to be diagnosed and treated. It has also lessened the number of "idiopathic" cases of EOS, as Chiari malformations, tethered cord, syringomyelia, diastematomyelia, and other difficult to diagnose intraspinal entities were identified. This increasing sophistication in diagnosing the causes of EOS has been paralleled by rapid advances in the field of medical genetics and embryology. New syndromes have been recognized and isolated private mutations identified.

Translational research has brought the prospect of new treatment paradigms that address diseases at the molecular level. As an example, identification of the genetic variation in folic acid metabolism has led to routine dietary folate supplementation during the first trimester of pregnancy [17]. As a result, the incidence of neural tube defects such as anencephaly, encephalocele, and spina bifida has significantly decreased. This multifactorial, e.g., dietary deficiency and genetic predisposition, disorder may be mirrored in other EOS such as infantile idiopathic scoliosis wherein a genetic predisposition and positioning in the cradle or other infant care practices could affect the development of a clinical syndrome.

Research into the molecular basis of Marfan syndrome has led to the prospect of innovative medical treatment options. Marfan knock-out mice can heal their vascular lesions by administration of an antibody to TGF-β [13, 14]. While it is unlikely that such an antibody regimen would find a place in humans, the use of other TGF-β antagonists may herald an era of medical rather than surgical treatment of Marfan syndrome.

As the genetic basis of idiopathic scoliosis is understood, the genes responsible can be sequenced and the mutations identified. Most genetic syndromes that have spinal deformity as a component of their clinical presentation are either chromosomal in origin, i.e., Down syndrome, or single gene disorders, such as achondroplasia and Prader-Willi. Charcot-Marie-Tooth is a neurological disease that is often accompanied by spinal deformity, and 70% of those affected have a

J. W. Ogilvie
Shriners Hospital for Children, 3182 Silver Fork Brighton, Salt Lake City, Utah 84121 USA
e-mail: jwogilvie@msn.com

B. A. Akbarnia et al. (eds.), *The Growing Spine*,
DOI: 10.1007/978-3-540-85207-0_50, © Springer-Verlag Berlin Heidelberg 2011

duplication of one copy of chromosome 17 resulting in an increased production of a peripheral myelin protein. This may contribute to the progressive nature of the disease [12, 15]. Continued research could lead to pharmacological alternative treatment methods.

Muscular dystrophies and atrophies, many of which result in EOS, are the result of complex genetic mutations. Understanding these mutations and the molecular pathogenesis of disease expression offers a promising area for research in pharmacological options of treatment [1, 3–5, 11, 16, 22].

Recent investigations have brought considerable insight into the development of congenital scoliosis [7, 20]. Understanding the molecular basis and sequence of events that leads to failure of vertebral segmentation and formation may ultimately lead to the identification of preventative measures in the first trimester of pregnancy that will lessen the incidence or severity of these congenital malformations.

Juvenile and adolescent idiopathic scoliosis is most likely polygenetic in nature [2]. The markers that are predictive of curve progression in adolescent idiopathic scoliosis are not useful in predicting curve progression in idiopathic EOS. Other recognized polygenetic diseases are primarily neoplastic, including breast cancer, certain types of colon cancer and glioblastoma multiforma [6, 9, 18]. Translational research may give an understanding of the molecular pathway that leads from certain mutations to the development of a curved spine and thus lead to new treatment opportunities. Understanding the pathogenesis of idiopathic scoliosis and other diseases leading to EOS offers the hope that presymptomatic or early medical treatment will lead to better outcomes. This research is multidisciplinary in nature involving molecular biologists, geneticists, biostatisticians, epidemiologists, genotype scientists, and others. Clinical relevance and direction is imperative and this is the role of clinicians. Clinicians are also pivotal in identifying and recruiting cohorts when a particular disease entity is being studied.

In the predictable future, transplantation of hematopoetic stem cells or cord blood will probably be reserved for diseases with an otherwise potentially fatal outcome. EOS secondary to neurological pathology such as cerebral palsy and spinal cord injury may be appropriate areas for emerging research in neurocytokines and ectodermal stem-cell transplants [8]. It is reasonable to anticipate that the use of recombinant proteins and enzymes, now a common practice in lysosomal storage diseases such as Gauchier, Fabry and the mucopolysaccharidoses, may have a place in the treatment of some EOS syndromes.

Bone-marrow transplantation and enzyme replacement therapy in those with Hurler syndrome has allowed survival into adult life. The skeletal dysplasias in general, and spinal deformities specifically, associated with mucopolysaccharidoses remain problematic, however. It is not a simple matter of glycosaminoglycan deposition in bone and soft tissue. There is a complex relationship with glycolipids, esterified cholesterol, and GM2 and GM3 ganglioside deposition that may affect the vasculature and central and peripheral nervous system in addition to tissues of mesodermal origin [19]. More molecular research is needed to explain the metabolic events that produce the crippling and sometimes life threatening complications of thoracolumbar kyphosis and upper cervical stenosis.

Innovative surgical and nonsurgical treatments will continue to have a place in EOS. Evaluating their efficacy is a major challenge and the implementation of well-controlled, multicenter studies can establish the utility of new treatment regimens. This is particularly important in uncommon syndromes such as the mucopolysaccharidoses wherein pooled data from a protocol driven regimen can help in establishing the most effective methods of treatment.

Early onset scoliosis is a wide net that captures many diagnoses. Precise diagnostic identification of these entities may allow a better understanding of the natural history of each cause of EOS, which will in turn permit an accurate assessment of treatment efficacy. Currently, phenotypic heterogeneity of the same disease and genotypic heterogeneity of the same phenotype often make prognostication and outcomes of research in EOS problematic. Continued advances in basic science should present new bench-to-bedside opportunities for more clearly defined diagnostic guidelines and innovative therapeutic options resulting in better outcomes in EOS.

References

1. Alman BA, Raza SN, Biggar WD (2004) Steroid treatment and the development of scoliosis in males with Duchenne muscular dystrophy. J Bone Joint Surg Am 86-A(3): 519–524

2. Braun J NL, Ogilvie J, Ward K (2007) 12 DNA markers with diagnostic and prognostic significance in idiopathic scoliosis. In: Scoliosis Research Society Annual Meeting, Edinburgh
3. Day JW, Ranum LP (2005) Genetics and molecular pathogenesis of the myotonic dystrophies. Curr Neurol Neurosci Rep 5(1):55–59
4. Day JW, Ranum LP (2005) RNA pathogenesis of the myotonic dystrophies. Neuromuscul Disord 15(1):5–16
5. Emery AE (2002) Muscular dystrophy into the new millennium. Neuromuscul Disord 12(4):343–349
6. Irving M, Elmslie F, Berg J (2002) Genetics of breast cancer. Int J Clin Pract 56(9):677–682
7. Kusumi K, Mimoto MS, Covello KL et al (2004) Dll3 pudgy mutation differentially disrupts dynamic expression of somite genes. Genesis 39(2):115–121
8. Kwon BK, Jie L, Lam C et al (2007) Brian-derived neurotrophic factor gene transfer with adeno-associated viral and lentiviral vectors prevents rubrospinal neuronal atrophy and stimulates regeneration-associated gene expression after acute cervial spinal cord injury. Spine 32(11):1164–1173
9. Loader S, Shields C, Rowley PT (2005) Impact of genetic counseling and DNA testing on individuals with colorectal cancer with a positive family history: a population-based study. Genet Test 9(4):313–319
10. Moayyedi P (2007) The health economics of *Helicobacter pylori* infection. Best Pract Res Clin Gastroenterol 21(2): 347–361
11. Mercuri E, Sewry C, Brown SC et al (2002) Congenital muscular dystrophies. Semin Pediatr Neurol 9(2):120–131
12. Meyer zu Horste G, Prukop T et al (2007) Antiprogesterone therapy uncouples axonal loss from demyelination in a transgenic rat model of CMT1A neuropathy. Ann Neurol 61(1):61–72
13. Neptune ER, Frischmeyer P, Arking DE et al (2003) Dysregulation of TGF-beta activation contributes to pahtogenesis in Marfan syndrome. Nat Genet 33(3):407–411
14. Ng CM, Cheng A, Myers LA et al (2004) TGF-beta-dependant pathogenesis or mitral valve prolapse in a mouse model of Marfan syndrome. J Clin Invest 114(11): 1586–1592
15. Niemann A, Berger P, Suter U (2006) Pathomechanisms of mutant proteins in Charcot-Marie-Tooth disease. Neuromolecular Med 8(1–2):217–242
16. Ogino S, Wilson RB (2004) Spinal muscular atrophy: molecular genetics and diagnostics. Expert Rev Mol Diagn 4(1):15–29
17. Pulikkunnel ST, Thomas SV (2005) Neural tude defects: patogenesis and folate metabolism. J. Assoc Physicians India 53:127–135
18. Roversi G, Pfundt R, Moroni RF et al (2006) Identification of novel genomic markers related to progression to glioblastoma through genomic profiling of 25 primary glioma cell lines. Oncogene 25(10):1571–1583
19. Russell C, Hendson G, Jevon G et al (1998) Murine MPS I: insights into the pathogenesis of Hurler syndrome. Clin Genet 53(5):349–361
20. Turnpenny PD, Whittock N, Duncan J et al (2003) Novel mutations in DLL3, a somitogenesis gene encoding a ligand for the Notch signalling pathway, cause a consistent pattern of abnormal vertebral segmentation in spondylocostal dysostosis. J Med Genet 40(5):333–339
21. Vanderhoff BT, Tahboub RM (2002) Proton pump inhibitors: an update. Am Fam Physician 66(2):273–280
22. Yilmaz O, Karaduman A, Topaloglu H (2004) Prednisolone therapy in Duchenne muscular dystrophy prolongs ambulation and prevents scoliosis. Eur J Neurol 11(8):541–544

Index

U

V

W

Printing and Binding: Stürtz GmbH, Würzburg